f

MAGNETIC RESONANCE IMAGING

Second Edition

Volume II

Physical Principles and Instrumentation

C. LEON PARTAIN, M.D., Ph.D.
RONALD R. PRICE, Ph.D.
JAMES A. PATTON, Ph.D.
MADAN V. KULKARNI, M.D.
A. EVERETTE JAMES, JR., Sc.M., J.D., M.D.

Division of Medical Imaging
Department of Radiology and Radiological Sciences
Vanderbilt University Medical Center
Nashville, Tennessee

1988
W.B. SAUNDERS COMPANY
Harcourt Brace Jovanovich, Inc.
Philadelphia   London   Toronto   Montreal   Sydney   Tokyo

W. B. SAUNDERS COMPANY
Harcourt Brace Jovanovich, Inc.

The Curtis Center
Independence Square West
Philadelphia, PA 19106

LIBRARY OF CONGRESS
Library of Congress Cataloging-in-Publication Data

Magnetic resonance imaging (MRI) / [edited by] C. Leon Partain . . .[et al.].
    p. cm.
    Includes indexes.
    Contents: v. 1. Clinical applications—v. 2. Physical principles and instrumentation.
    ISBN 0-7216-1340-3 (set). ISBN 0-7216-2516-9 (v. 1). ISBN 0-7216-2517-7 (v. 2).
    1. Magnetic resonance imaging. I. Partain, C. Leon.
RC78.7.N83M344 1988
616.07'57—dc19   87-26651
                                                   CIP

Listed here is the latest translated edition of this book together with the language of the translation and the publisher.

Japanese (*1st Edition*)—Igaku Shoin/Saunders Ltd., Ichibancho Central Bldg., 22-1 Ichibancho, Chiyoda-Ku, Tokyo 102, Japan

Editor: Lisette Bralow

Developmental Editor: Kathleen McCullough

Designer: W. B. Saunders Staff

Production Manager: Bob Butler

Manuscript Editors: Constance Burton/Susan Thomas

Illustration Coordinator: Brett MacNaughton

Indexer: Alexandra Weir

Magnetic Resonance Imaging (MRI)

Volume I ISBN 0–7216–2516–9
Volume II ISBN 0–7216–2517–7
SET ISBN 0–7216–1340–3

Last digit is the print number: 9   8   7   6   5   4   3   2   1

To
David Blane, Teri Ellyn, and Amy Leigh Partain
Amanda Belle Price
James Allen, Jr., and David Lee Patton
Delores J. Kulkarni
Alton Everette and Pattie Royster James

Contributors

W. J. ADAMS, Ph.D. Software Engineer, Corporate Research and Development Center, General Electric Company, Schenectady, New York
Quantitative NMR Tissue Characterization Using Calculated Images and Automated Image Segmentation

JOSEPH H. ALLEN, M.D. Professor of Radiology and Radiological Sciences, Vanderbilt University Medical Center, Nashville, Tennessee
Tumor Imaging with Gd-DTPA; Pituitary and Parasellar Region

MARY P. ANDERSON, M.S. Office of Radiological Health, National Center for Devices and Radiological Health, United States Food and Drug Administration, Rockville, Maryland
Operational Guidelines: United States

WILLIAM H. ANDERSON, M.S. Research Associate, University of Kansas Medical Center, Kansas City, Kansas
Computer Networks for Medical Image Management

E. R. ANDREW, Ph.D., Sc.D., F.R.S., Graduate Research Professor of Physics and Radiology, University of Florida, Gainesville, Florida
NMR in Medicine: A Historical Review

IAN M. ARMITAGE, Ph.D. Yale University School of Medicine; Yale–New Haven Hospital, New Haven, Connecticut
NMR Evaluation of Tumor Metabolism

TIMOTHY ASHBAUGH, M.S. Graduate student, Vanderbilt University School of Medicine, Nashville, Tennessee
Dynamic Contrast-Enhanced MRI and Mathematical Modeling

T. WHIT ATHEY Lecturer, Electical Engineering Department, University of Maryland, Baltimore, Maryland
Operational Guidelines: United States

LEON AXEL, Ph.D., M.D.   Associate Professor, University of Pennsylvania; Department of Radiology, Hospital of the University of Pennsylvania, Philadelphia, Pennsylvania
Future Directions; MRI of Blood Flow

D. R. BAILES, M.Sc.   Department of Medical Physics, University of Manchester, Manchester, United Kingdom
Artifacts in the Measurement of T1 and T2

D. BALERIAUX, M.D.   Professor of Radiology, Université Libre de Bruxelles; Head of the Neuroradiological Clinic in the Department of Radiology, Erasne Hospital, Brussels, Belgium
Surface Coil Imaging of the Spine

P. T. BEALL, Ph.D.   Department of Biology, Texas Woman's University, Houston, Texas
Distinction of the Normal, Preneoplastic, and Neoplastic States by Water Proton NMR Relaxation Times

M. ROBIN BENDALL, B.Sc. (Tasmania), D.Phil. (Oxford), D.Sc. (Griffith)   Senior Lecturer, Griffith University, Brisbane, Australia
Surface Coil Technology

WILFRIED H. BERGMANN, Ph.D.   Senior Research Associate, Department of Physics and Astronomy, Vanderbilt University, Nashville, Tennessee
Hydrodynamic Blood Flow Analysis with Low Temperature NMR Spin Echo Detection

ALBERT H. BETH, Ph.D.   Assistant Professor of Molecular Physiology and Biophysics, Vanderbilt University School of Medicine, Nashville, Tennessee
Advanced Methods for Spin Density, T1, and T2 Calculations in MRI

FELIX BLOCH, Ph.D. (1905–1983)   Max Stein Professor of Physics, Emeritus, Stanford University, Palo Alto, California. Nobel Prize in Physics (for NMR), 1952
Past, Present, and Future of Nuclear Magnetic Resonance

J. L. BLOEM, M.D.   University Hospital, Department of Diagnostic Radiology, Leiden, The Netherlands
Primary Malignant Bone Tumors

R. G. BLUEMM, M.D.   University of Bochum, Marienhospital Herhe, Herhe, German Federal Republic
Primary Malignant Bone Tumors; Fast, Small Flip-Angle Field Echo Imaging

E. BOSKAMP, Ph.D.   Manager, RF Coil Laboratories, Philips Medical Systems, Best, The Netherlands
Surface Coil Imaging of the Spine

PAUL A. BOTTOMLEY, Ph.D.   Physicist, General Electric Research and Development Center, Schenectady, New York
Frequency Dependence of Tissue Relaxation Times

WILLIAM G. BRADLEY, JR., M.D., Ph.D.   Associate Clinical Professor of Radiology, University of California, San Francisco; Director, MR Imaging Laboratory, Huntington Medical Research Institutes and Huntington Memorial Hospital, Pasadena, California
Inflammatory Disease of the Brain; Intracranial Hemorrhage; Future Directions

THOMAS J. BRADY, M.D.   Associate Professor of Radiology, Harvard Medical School; Associate Radiologist and Assistant in Medicine, Massachusetts General Hopital, Boston, Massachusetts
Iron Ethylene bis (2-Hydroxyphenylglycine) as a Hepatobiliary MRI Contrast Agent; Chemical Shift Imaging

ROBERT C. BRASCH, M.D.   Professor of Radiology and Pediatrics; Director, Contrast Media Laboratory, University of California, San Francisco, California
Free Radical Contrast Agents for MRI

H. G. BRITTAIN, Ph.D.   Research Fellow, The Squibb Institute for Medical Research, New Brunswick, New Jersey
Principles of Contrast-Enhanced MRI

RODNEY A. BROOKS, Ph.D.   Neuroimaging Section, NINCDS, National Institutes of Health, Bethesda, Maryland
Image Reconstruction

MARK S. BROWN, Ph.D.   Research Associate, Yale University School of Medicine, New Haven, Connecticut
Pathophysiological Significance of Relaxation

RODNEY D. BROWN, III, Ph.D.   Research Staff Member, IBM, T. J. Watson Research Center, Yorktown Heights, New York
Relaxometry of Solvent and Tissue Protons: Diamagnetic Contributions; Relaxometry of Solvent and Tissue Protons: Paramagnetic Contributions

GORDON L. BROWNELL, Ph.D.   Professor of Radiological Physics, Harvard Medical School; Professor of Nuclear Engineering, Massachusetts Institute of Technology; Radiological Physics, Massachusetts General Hospital, Boston, Massachusetts
Current and Future Frontiers in Medical Imaging

D. J. BRYANT, Ph.D.   GEC Research, Limited, Wembley, Middlesex, United Kingdom
Artifacts in the Measurement of T1 and T2

LAWRENCE J. BUSSE, Ph.D.   Engineering Staff, General Electric—Aircraft Engines; Adjunct Assistant Professor of Radiology, University of Cincinnati, Cincinnati, Ohio
Gradient Coil Technology

RICHARD B. BUXTON, Ph.D.   Instructor, Department of Radiology, Harvard Medical School; Assistant in Applied Physics, Department of Radiology, Massachusetts General Hospital, Boston, Massachusetts
Chemical Shift Imaging

G. M. BYDDER, M.B., Ch.B., F.R.C.R.   Senior Lecturer, Royal Postgraduate Medical School, Hammersmith Hospital, London, United Kingdom
Tumors of the Central Nervous System; Artifacts in the Measurement of T1 and T2

ROBERT C. CANBY, M.E.E.   Senior Medical Student, University of Texas Southwestern Medical School, Dallas, Texas
Ischemic Heart Disease

GARY R. CAPUTO, M.D.   Resident, Department of Radiology, University of California, San Francisco, California
Magnetic Resonance Imaging of the Heart

FRANK E. CARROLL, JR., M.D.   Associate Professor of Radiology and Radiological Sciences, Vanderbilt University School of Medicine; Director of Diagnostic Radiology, Vanderbilt University Medical Center, Nashville, Tennessee
Lungs

BRITTON CHANCE, Ph.D.   Professor Emeritus, University of Pennsylvania, Philadelphia, Pennsylvania
Phosphorus-31 Spectroscopy and Imaging

JEFFREY A. CLANTON, M.S.   Associate in Radiology, Vanderbilt University School of Medicine; Director, Radio and MRI Pharmacy, Vanderbilt University Hospital, Nashville, Tennessee
Oral Contrast Agents; Dynamic Contrast-Enhanced MRI and Mathematical Modeling

HOWARD T. COFFEY, Ph.D. (Physics)   Sub-Sea Systems, Inc., Escondido, California
Principles of Superconducting Magnets

SHEILA M. COHEN, Ph.D.   Senior Research Fellow, Merck Institute for Therapeutic Research, Merck, Sharp & Dohme Research Laboratories, Rahway, New Jersey
Carbon-13: NMR Spectroscopy

JANET D. COIL, Ph.D.   Philips Medical Systems, Inc., Shelton, Connecticut
Planning and Preparation

THOMAS E. CONTURO, B.A.   Graduate Student and Medical Student (M.D., Ph.D.) Medical Scientist, Training Program of the National Institutes of Health, Vanderbilt University School of Medicine, Nashville, Tennessee
MRI Optimization Strategies; Understanding Basic MR Pulse Sequences; Advanced Methods for Spin Density, T1, and T2 Calculations in MRI

LARRY T. COOK, Ph.D. Associate Professor of Diagnostic Radiology, University of Kansas; University of Kansas Medical Center, Kansas City, Kansas
Breast; Computer Networks for Medical Image Management

GLENDON G. COX, M.D. Associate Professor, University of Kansas; University of Kansas Medical Center (Bell Memorial Hospital), Kansas City, Kansas
Computer Networks for Medical Image Management

F. C. CREZEE, M.D. Academisch Ziekenhuis van de Vrije Universiteit, Department of Radiology, Amsterdam, The Netherlands
Malignant Lesions of the Paranasal Sinuses

LAWRENCE E. CROOKS, Ph.D. Professor of Electrical Engineering, Department of Radiology, University of California, San Francisco, California
Fundamental Limitations

J. CUPPEN, Ph.D. Department of MRI, Philips Medical Systems Division, Best, The Netherlands
Fast, Small Flip-Angle Field Echo Imaging

RAYMOND DAMADIAN, M.D. President, FONAR Corporation, Melville, New York
NMR Scanning

JOHN L. DELAYRE, Ph.D. Department of Radiology, University of Texas Medical School, Houston, Texas
Localization Methods in NMR

J. DEN BOER, Ph.D. Department of MRI, Philips Medical Systems Division, Best, The Netherlands
Fast, Small Flip-Angle Field Echo Imaging

R. G. M. DE SLEGTE, M.D. Academisch Ziekenhuis van de Vrije Universiteit, Department of Radiology, Amsterdam, The Netherlands
Malignant Lesions of the Paranasal Sinuses

TIMOTHY M. DEVINNEY, M.B.A. Assistant Professor, Owen Graduate School of Management, Vanderbilt University, Nashville, Tennessee
Legal Aspects of MRI

L. S. DE VRIES, M.D. Senior Research Fellow, Hammersmith Hospital, Royal Postgraduate Medical School, London, United Kingdom
Tumors of the Central Nervous System

J. DOORNBOS, Ph.D. University Hospital, Department of Diagnostic Radiology, Leiden, The Netherlands
Primary Malignant Bone Tumors; Fast, Small Flip-Angle Field Echo Imaging

LEO F. DROLSHAGEN, III, M.D.   MRI Fellow, Department of Radiology and Radiological Sciences, Vanderbilt University Medical Center, Nashville, Tennessee
Female Pelvis

EDWARD J. DUDEWICZ, Ph.D.   Professor and Chairman, University Statistics Council, Department of Mathematics, Syracuse University, Syracuse, New York
Advanced Statistical Methods for Tissue Characteristics

SAMUEL J. DWYER, III, Ph.D.   Professor of Diagnostic Radiology, University of Kansas Medical Center, Kansas City, Kansas
Breast; Computer Networks for Medical Image Management

WILLIAM C. ECKELMAN, Ph.D.   Vice-President of Research and Development, The Squibb Institute for Medical Research, New Brunswick, New Jersey
Principles of Contrast-Enhanced MRI

WILLIAM A. EDELSTEIN, Ph.D.   Physicist, Corporate Research and Development Center, General Electric Company, Schenectady, New York
Radio Frequency Resonators

KENNETH R. EFFERSON, Ph.D.   President, American Magnetics, Inc., Oak Ridge, Tennessee
Principles of Superconducting Magnets

STEPHEN G. EINSTEIN   Philips Medical Systems, Inc., Shelton, Connecticut
Planning and Preparation

ALAN EISENBERG, M.D.   Resident, Department of Radiology and Radiological Sciences, Vanderbilt University Medical Center, Nashville, Tennessee
MRI Optimization Strategies

JANE E. ERICKSON, M.H.S.   Research Associate, Center for Hospital Finance and Management, Johns Hopkins University, Baltimore, Maryland
The Economics and Regulation of MRI

JON J. ERICKSON, Ph.D.   Associate Professor of Radiology and Radiological Sciences, Vanderbilt University Medical Center, Nashville, Tennessee
Image Production and Display

RICHARD R. ERNST, DR. PROF.   Full Professor, Laboratorium Für Physikalische Chemie, Technische Hochschule, Zürich, Switzerland
A Survey of MRI Techniques

WILLIAM T. EVANOCHKO, Ph.D.   Assistant Professor of Medicine, University of Alabama, Birmingham, Alabama
Ischemic Heart Disease

THEODORE H. M. FALKE, M.D.   Department of Diagnostic Radiology, University Hospital, Leiden, The Netherlands
MRI Optimization Strategies; Adrenal Glands; Blood Flow in MR Imaging; Primary Malignant Bone Tumors; Sonography and MRI

BRIAN D. FELLMETH, M.D., Ph.D.   Resident in Radiology, Vanderbilt University Medical Center, Nashville, Tennessee; Fellow, Vascular Radiology, University of California, San Diego, California
Practical Pediatric MRI

HARVEY V. FINEBERG, M.D., Ph.D.   Dean, Harvard School of Public Health, Cambridge, Massachusetts
Clinical Efficacy: 5000 MRI Cases Between 0.15 and 0.6 Tesla

JAMES J. FISCHER, M.D., Ph.D.   Professor and Chairman, Department of Therapeutic Radiology, Yale University School of Medicine; Chief, Department of Therapeutic Radiology, Yale–New Haven Hospital, New Haven, Connecticut
NMR Evaluation of Tumor Metabolism

MADELEINE R. FISHER, M.D.   Assistant Professor, Department of Radiology, Northwestern University; Medical Director, MRI, Northwestern Memorial Hospital, Chicago, Illinois
Neck; Prostate and Urinary Bladder

ARTHUR C. FLEISCHER, M.D.   Professor of Radiology and Radiological Sciences, Associate Professor of Obstetrics and Gynecology, Vanderbilt University School of Medicine; Director, Ultrasound Section, Department of Radiology and Radiological Sciences, Vanderbilt University Hospital, Nashville, Tennessee
Breast; Sonography and MRI

MARK P. FREEMAN, M.D.   Clinical Assistant Professor, Department of Radiology, Vanderbilt University Medical Center and Baptist Hospital, Nashville, Tennessee
Ischemic Cerebrovascular Disease

G. T. GAUGHAN, Ph.D.   Group Leader, The Squibb Institute for Medical Research, New Brunswick, New Jersey
Principles of Contrast-Enhanced MRI

HARRY K. GENANT, M.D.   Professor of Radiology, Medicine and Orthopaedic Surgery; Chief of Skeletal Radiology, Department of Radiology, University of California, San Francisco, School of Medicine, San Francisco, California
The Spine

G. J. GERRITSEN, M.D.   Academische Ziekenhuis van de Vrije, Universiteit Department of Otolaryngology, Head and Neck Surgery, Amsterdam, The Netherlands
Malignant Lesions of the Paranasal Sinuses

ANTHONY GIAMBALVO, Ph.D.   Vice-President, FONAR Corporation, Melville, New York
NMR Scanning

S. JULIAN GIBBS, D.D.S., Ph.D.   Associate Professor of Radiology and Assistant Professor of Dentistry, Vanderbilt University; Adjunct Professor, University of Tennessee Space Institute; Radiology Service, Vanderbilt University Hospital, Nashville, Tennessee
Bioeffects

EDWARD J. GOLDSTEIN, Ph.D., M.D.   Assistant Professor of Radiology, Hospital of the University of Pennsylvania, Philadelphia, Pennsylvania; Chairman, Department of Radiology, Los Alamitos Medical Center, Los Alamitos, California
Free Radical Contrast Agents for MRI; Hepatobiliary Contrast Agents

J. C. GORE, Ph.D.   Associate Professor of Radiology, Yale University School of Medicine, New Haven, Connecticut
Quantitative NMR Tissue Characterization Using Calculated Images and Automated Image Segmentation; Legal Aspects of MRI; Pathophysiological Significance of Relaxation; NMR Evaluation of Tumor Metabolism

THOMAS P. GRAHAM, JR., M.D.   Professor of Pediatrics, Director of Pediatric Cardiology, Vanderbilt University Medical Center, Nashville, Tennessee
Gated MRI in Congenital Cardiac Malformations

TOM GREESON, J.D., L.L.D.   Professor of Law, Vanderbilt University, Nashville, Tennessee
Legal Aspects of MRI

J. J. HAGAN, Ph.D.   Senior Research Investigator, The Squibb Institute for Medical Research, New Brunswick, New Jersey
Principles of Contrast-Enhanced MRI

A. S. HALL, Ph.D.   GEC Research, Limited, Wembley, Middlesex, United Kingdom
Artifacts in the Measurement of T1 and T2

STEVEN E. HARMS, M.D.   Director of Magnetic Resonance, Department of Medical Imaging, Baylor University Medical Center, Dallas, Texas
Face, Orbit, and Temporomandibular Joint

JOHN H. HARRIS, JR., M.D., D.Sc.   Professor and Chairman, Department of Radiology, University of Texas Medical School; Chairman, Department of Radiology, Hermann Hospital, Houston, Texas
Musculoskeletal System

CECIL E. HAYES, Ph.D.   Senior Physicist, Applied Science Laboratory, GE Medical Systems, Milwaukee, Wisconsin
Radio Frequency Resonators

C. F. HAZLEWOOD, Ph.D.   Professor, Department of Physiology, Baylor College of Medicine, Houston, Texas
Distinction of the Normal, Preneoplastic, and Neoplastic States by Water Proton NMR Relaxation Times

RICHARD M. HELLER, M.D.   Professor of Radiology and Radiological Sciences, Vanderbilt University Medical Center; Chief, Pediatric Radiology, Vanderbilt University Hospital, Nashville, Tennessee
Practical Pediatric MRI

KENNETH S. HENSLEY, M.S.   Research Associate, University of Kansas Medical Center, Kansas City, Kansas
Computer Networks for Medical Image Management

ROBERT J. HERFKENS, M.D.   Associate Professor of Radiology, Director of Magnetic Resonance Imaging Section, Duke University Medical Center, Durham, North Carolina
High Field MRI

CHARLES B. HIGGINS, M.D.   Professor and Vice-Chairman, Department of Radiology, University of California, San Francisco, School of Medicine; Chief, Magnetic Resonance Imaging, University of California, San Francisco, Medical Center, San Francisco, California
Neck; Magnetic Resonance Imaging of the Heart

G. NEIL HOLLAND, M.Phil.   Picker International, Highland Heights, Ohio
Systems Engineering

MYRON HOLSCHER, D.V.M., Ph.D.   Associate Professor of Pathology, Vanderbilt University School of Medicine; Associate Director, Animal Care, Vanderbilt University Medical Center, Nashville, Tennessee
Dynamic Contrast-Enhanced MRI and Mathematical Modeling

HEDVIG HRICAK, M.D.   Professor of Radiology and Urology, University of California, San Francisco; Chief of Uroradiology Section, Department of Urology, University of California, San Francisco, Medical Center, San Francisco, California
Clinical Potential of MRI; Prostate and Urinary Bladder

NOLA M. HYLTON, Ph.D.   Assistant Professor of Physics, Department of Radiology, Radiologic Imaging Laboratory, University of California, San Francisco, California
MRI Parameter Selection Techniques

MASAHIRO IIO, M.D.   Professor and Chairman, Department of Radiology, University of Tokyo, Tokyo, Japan
Current and Future Frontiers in Medical Imaging

JOANNE S. INGWALL, Ph.D. Associate Professor of Physiology and Bio-physics, Department of Medicine, Harvard Medical School; Biochemist, Brigham and Women's Hospital, Boston, Massachusetts
The Physiological Chemistry of Creatine Kinase in the Heart: Phosphorus-31 Magnetization Transfer Studies

A. EVERETTE JAMES, JR., Sc.M., J.D., M.D. Professor and Chairman, De-partment of Radiology and Radiological Sciences, Vanderbilt University School of Medicine; Vanderbilt University Hospital, Nashville, Tennessee
Sonography and MRI; Legal Aspects of MRI; Bioeffects

A. EVERETTE JAMES, III, B.A. Law Student, University of Illinois, Chicago, Illinois
Legal Aspects of MRI

JEANNETTE CROSS JAMES, B.A. Student, The Washington College of Law at the American University, Washington, D.C.
Legal Aspects of MRI

JEROME P. JONES, Ph.D. Diagnostic Physicist, Department of Radiology, Alton Ochsner Medical Foundation, New Orleans, Louisiana
Physics of the MR Image: From the Basic Principles to Image Intensity and Contrast; T1 and T2 Measurement

M. C. KAISER, M.D. Academisch Ziekenhuis van de Vrije Universiteit, De-partment of Radiology, Amsterdam, The Netherlands
Malignant Lesions of the Paranasal Sinuses

ALAN J. KAUFMAN, M.D. Assistant Professor of Radiology and Radiological Sciences, Vanderbilt University Medical Center; Co-Director, Abdominal Im-aging, Vanderbilt University Hospital, Nashville, Tennessee
Gastrointestinal Tract

ROBERT M. KESSLER, M.D. Associate Professor of Radiology, Vanderbilt University School of Medicine; Chief, Neuroradiology, Vanderbilt University Medical Center, Nashville, Tennessee
Ischemic Cerebrovascular Disease

SEYMOUR H. KOENIG, Ph.D. Research Staff Member, IBM, T. J. Watson Research Center, Yorktown Heights, New York; Adjunct Professor of Physics, University of Illinois, Urbana, Illinois
Relaxometry of Solvent and Tissue Protons: Diamagnetic Contributions; Relax-ometry of Solvent and Tissue Protons: Paramagnetic Contributions

W. KOOPS, M.D. Department of Diagnostic Radiology, University Hospital, Rotterdam, The Netherlands
Fast, Small Flip-Angle Field Echo Imaging

KEITH E. KORTMAN, M.D. Assistant Clinical Profesor of Radiology, Uni-versity of California, San Diego; Research Radiologist, Huntington Medical Re-search Institute; Huntington Memorial Hospital, Pasadena; Sharp Memorial Hos-pital, San Diego, California
Inflammatory Disease of the Brain

MADAN V. KULKARNI, M.D. Assistant Professor and Clinical Director, Magnetic Resonance Imaging, Vanderbilt University Medical Center, Nashville, Tennessee
Spinal Cord; Gated MRI in Congenital Cardiac Malformations; Breast; Kidneys and Retroperitoneum; Female Pelvis; Musculoskeletal System; Sonography and MRI Correlation; Pitfalls and Artifacts in Clinical MRI; NMR of ^{23}Na in Biological Systems

RANDALL B. LAUFFER, Ph.D. Assistant Professor, Department of Radiology, Harvard Medical School; Director, NMR Contrast Media Laboratory, Massachusetts General Hospital, Boston, Massachusetts
Iron Ethylene bis (2-Hydroxyphenylglycine) as a Hepatobiliary MRI Contrast Agent

RICHARD L. LAWS, B.S. Research Associate, University of Kansas Medical Center, Kansas City, Kansas
Computer Networks for Medical Image Management

JOHN S. LEIGH, JR., Ph.D. Professor of Biochemistry and Biophysics, University of Pennsylvania, Philadelphia, Pennsylvania
Phosphorus-31 Spectroscopy and Imaging

GEORGE C. LEVY, Ph.D. Professor of Science and Technology, Syracuse University; Adjunct Professor of Radiology, S.U.N.Y. Health Sciences Center at Syracuse; Adjunct Professor of Radiology, State University of New York, Health Sciences Center at Syracuse, New York
Advanced Statistical Methods for Tissue Characteristics

OTHA W. LINTON, M.S.J. Associate Executive Director, American College of Radiology, Chevy Chase, Maryland
The Economics and Regulation of MRI

WILFRIED LOEFFLER, Ph.D. Siemens A.G. Medical Engineering Group, Erlangen, German Federal Republic
Systems Optimization

MARK A. LUTHE, B.A. Diasonics, Inc., San Francisco, California
Chemical Efficacy: 5000 MRI Cases Between 0.15 and 0.6 Tesla; Clinical Efficacy: Analysis of 300 MRI Cases at 1.5 Tesla

JAMES R. MacFALL, Ph.D. General Electric Company, Medical Systems Group, Milwaukee, Wisconsin
Impact of the Choice of Operating Parameters on MR Images

S. MAJUMDAR, Ph.D. Associate Research Scientist, Department of Diagnostic Radiology, Yale University School of Medicine, New Haven, Connecticut
Quantitative NMR Tissue Characterization Using Calculated Images and Automated Image Segmentation

ALEXANDER R. MARGULIS, M.D.   Professor and Chairman, Department of Radiology, University of California, San Francisco, School of Medicine, San Francisco, California
Clinical Potential of MRI

R. MATHUR-DE VRÉ, Ph.D   Research Associate, Institut d'Hygiène et d'Epidémiologie, Brussels, Belgium
Biomedical Implications of Relaxation Times of Tissue Water

A. A. MAUDSLEY, Ph.D.   Associate Professor, University of California, San Francisco; Veterans Administration Medical Center, San Francisco, California
Technical Demands of Multiple Nuclei

MURRAY J. MAZER, M.D.   Associate Professor of Radiology and Radiological Sciences; Chief, Angiography Section, Vanderbilt University Medical Center, Nashville, Tennessee
Gated MRI in Congenital Cardiac Malformations

MICHAEL McCURDY, B.S.E.E.   Student, Master of Science in Electrical Engineering, Vanderbilt University, Nashville, Tennessee
Dynamic Contrast-Enhanced MRI and Mathematical Modeling

ALAN C. McLAUGHLIN, Ph.D.   University of Pennsylvania, Philadelphia, Pennsylvania
Phosphorus-31 Spectroscopy and Imaging

SNEHAL D. MEHTA, M.D.   Assistant Professor, University of Texas Health Science Center; Staff, Hermann Hospital, Houston, Texas
Kidneys and Retroperitoneum; NMR of ^{23}Na in Biological Systems

MARK R. MITCHELL, M.D.   Assistant Professor, Department of Radiology and Radiological Sciences, Vanderbilt University Medical Center, Nashville, Tennessee; Simi Valley Adventist Hospital Staff, Simi Valley, California
MRI Tissue Characterization; MRI Optimization Strategies; Understanding Basic MR Pulse Sequences; Advanced Methods for Spin Density, T1, and T2 Calculations in MRI

E. PAUL NANCE, JR., M.D.   Associate Professor of Radiology; Assistant Professor of Orthopaedics and Rehabilitation; Chief, Section of Bone and Joint Radiology, Vanderbilt University School of Medicine; Department of Radiology, Vanderbilt University Hospital, Nashville, Tennessee
Musculoskeletal System

PONNADA A. NARAYANA, Ph.D.   Assistant Professor, The University of Texas Medical School, Houston, Texas
Kidneys and Retroperitoneum; NMR of ^{23}Na in Biological Systems; Localization Methods in NMR

M. O'DONNELL, Ph.D.   Physicist, Corporate Research and Development Center, General Electric Company, Schenectady, New York
Quantitative NMR Tissue Characterization Using Calculated Images and Automated Image Segmentation

WILLIAM H. OLDENDORF, M.D., D.Sc. Professor of Neurology and of Psychiatry, University of California, Los Angeles, School of Medicine; Senior Medical Investigator, VA Brentwood, Veterans Administration, Los Angeles, California
A Comparison of Resistive, Superconductive, and Permanent Magnets

ARNULF OPPELT, Ph.D. Siemens A.G. Medical Engineering Group, Erlangen, German Federal Republic
Systems Optimization

DOUGLAS A. ORTENDAHL, Ph.D. Associate Profesor of Physics, Department of Radiology and Radiologic Imaging Laboratory, University of California, San Francisco, California
MRI Parameter Selection Techniques

C. LEON PARTAIN, M.D., Ph.D. Professor of Radiology, Radiological Sciences, and Biomedical Engineering, Vanderbilt University School of Medicine; Director, Division of Medical Imaging, Vanderbilt University Hospital, Nashville, Tennessee
Breast; Gastrointestinal Tract; Kidneys and Retroperitoneum; Practical Pediatric MRI; Dynamic Contrast-Enhanced MRI and Mathematical Modeling; Legal Aspects of MRI; Future Directions; NMR Physical Principles; Current and Future Frontiers in Medical Imaging

JAMES A. PATTON, Ph.D. Professor of Radiology and Radiological Sciences, Administrative Officer for Radiology, Vanderbilt University Medical Center, Nashville, Tennessee
Thyroid and Parathyroid Glands; Pitfalls and Artifacts in Clinical MRI; Future Directions; Quality Assurance

J. A. PAYNE, B.Sc. GEC-Research, Limited, Wembley, Middlesex, United Kingdom
Artifacts in the Measurement of T1 and T2

ROBERT A. PHILLIPS, Ph.D. Office of Radiological Health, National Center for Devices and Radiological Health, United States Food and Drug Administration, Rockville, Maryland
Operational Guidelines: United States

DAVID R. PICKENS, Ph.D. Assistant Professor of Radiology and Radiological Sciences, Vanderbilt University Medical Center, Nashville, Tennessee
Blood Flow in MR Imaging; Image Production and Display; Gating: Cardiac and Respiratory; Fast Scanning Methods in MRI

GERALD M. POHOST, M.D. Professor of Medicine, Professor of Radiology, University of Alabama School of Medicine; Director, Division of Cardiovascular Disease; Director, Center for NMR Research and Development, University of Alabama Hospitals, University of Alabama at Birmingham, Alabama
Ischemic Heart Disease

C. F. POPE, M.D. Assistant Professor of Radiology, Yale University School of Medicine, New Haven, Connecticut
Quantitative NMR Tissue Characterization Using Calculated Images and Automated Image Segmentation

ANN C. PRICE, M.D. Associate Professor of Radiology, Medical College of Virginia, Richmond, Virginia
White Matter/Multiple Sclerosis; Tumor Imaging with Gd-DTPA; Pituitary and Parasellar Region

RONALD R. PRICE, Ph.D. Professor of Radiology and Radiological Sciences, Associate Professor of Physics and Astronomy, Vanderbilt University; Director, Division of Radiological Sciences, Vanderbilt University Medical Center, Nashville, Tennessee
Blood Flow in MR Imaging; NMR Physical Principles; Quality Assurance; Fast Scanning Methods in MRI; Advanced Methods for Spin Density, T1, and T2 Calculations in MRI; Current and Future Frontiers in Medical Imaging

JAMIE H. PROST, M.S. General Electric Medical Systems, Waukesha, Wisconsin
Impact of the Choice of Operating Parameters on MR Images

EDWARD M. PURCELL, Ph.D. Professor Emeritus, Department of Physics, Harvard University, Cambridge, Massachusetts. Nobel Prize in Physics (for NMR), 1952
Foreword

S. S. RANADE, M.Sc., Ph.D. Member, Ad Hoc Committee in Biophysics, Bombay University; Research Guide Faculty of Biophysics; Officer-In-Charge, Radiobiology Unit, Cancer Research Institute, Bombay, India
Histopathological Correlation

MRUTYUNJAYA J. RAO, M.S. Digital Equipment Corporation, Marlborogh, Massachusetts
Advanced Statistical Methods for Tissue Characteristics

RUSSELL C. REEVES, M.D. Assistant Professor of Medicine, University of Alabama School of Medicine, University of Alabama Hospitals and Clinics, Birmingham, Alabama
Ischemic Heart Disease

BRADFORD J. RICHMOND, M.D. Radiology Staff, Section of Bone and Joint Radiology, Cleveland Clinic Foundation, Cleveland, Ohio
The Spine

STEPHEN J. RIEDERER, Ph.D. Associate Professor of Radiology and Biomedical Engineering, Duke University Medical Center, Durham, North Carolina
MRI Synthesis

F. DAVID ROLLO, M.D., Ph.D.   Visiting Professor of Radiology and Radiological Sciences, Vanderbilt University School of Medicine, Nashville, Tennessee; Executive Vice-President, Humana, Inc., Louisville, Kentucky
Legal Aspects of MRI

CHARLES E. ROOS, Ph.D.   Professor of Physics, Vanderbilt University, Nashville, Tennessee
Principles of Superconducting Magnets

BRUCE R. ROSEN, M.D., Ph.D.   Lecturer, Harvard/MIT Division of Health Sciences and Technology, Cambridge; Instructor in Radiology, Harvard Medical School; Director of Clinical NMR, Massachusetts General Hospital, Boston, Massachusetts
Chemical Shift Imaging

VAL M. RUNGE, M.D.   Assistant Professor, Tufts University–New England Medical Center Hospitals; Chief of Service, Magnetic Resonance, Department of Radiology, New England Medical Center Hospitals, Boston, Massachusetts
White Matter/Multiple Sclerosis; Tumor Imaging with Gd-DTPA; Pituitary and Parasellar Region; Principles of Contrast-Enhanced MRI; Intravenous Contrast Media

GLYNIS A. SACKS, M.D.   Assistant Professor of Radiology and Radiological Sciences (Ultrasound Section), Vanderbilt University Medical Center, Nashville, Tennessee
Thyroid and Parathyroid Glands

BERNIE J. SAKS, M.D.   Department of Radiology, University of California, San Francisco, School of Medicine, San Francisco, California
Prostate and Urinary Bladder

MARTIN P. SANDLER, M.D., F.C.P. (S.A.)   Associate Professor of Radiology and Medicine; Chief, Nuclear Medicine, Vanderbilt University Medical Center, Nashville, Tennessee
Thyroid and Parathyroid Glands; Gated MRI in Congenital Cardiac Malformations; Adrenal Glands

JOHN F. SCHENCK, M.D., Ph.D.   Adjunct Assistant Professor of Radiology, University of Pennsylvania, Philadelphia; Medical Dental Staff, Ellis Hospital, Schenectady, New York; Technical Staff, Corporate Research and Development Center, General Electric Company, Schenectady, New York
Gradient Coil Technology; Radio Frequency Resonators

MITCH SCHNALL, M.D., Ph.D.   Instructor, Department of Radiology, University of Pennsylvania School of Medicine, Philadelphia, Pennsylvania
Phosphorus-31 Spectroscopy and Imaging

ROGER H. SCHNEIDER, M.Sc.   Director of the Division of Electrical Products, Office of Radiological Health, National Center for Devices and Radiological Health, United States Food and Drug Administration, Rockville, Maryland
Operational Guidelines: United States

C. SEGEBARTH, Ph.D.   Scientific Director of the Department for Magnetic Resonance, Erasme Hospital, Brussels, Belgium
Surface Coil Imaging of the Spine

MAX SHAFF, M.D., F.R.C.R.   Associate Professor, Vanderbilt University Medical Center; Chief, Section of Computed Tomography, Department of Radiology and Radiological Sciences, Vanderbilt University Medical Center, Nashville, Tennessee
Adrenal Glands

TERESA SINNWELL, Ph.D.   Department of Radiology, University of Pennsylvania, Philadelphia, Pennsylvania
Phosphorus-31 Spectroscopy and Imaging

FRANCIS W. SMITH, M.D.   Clinical Senior Lecturer in Medicine, University of Aberdeen; Consultant Radiologist, Specialist in Nuclear Medicine, Aberdeen Royal Infirmary, Aberdeen, Scotland
MRI at Low Field Strength

GREG D. SMITH, M.D.   Resident, Department of Radiology and Radiological Sciences, Vanderbilt University Medical Center, Nashville, Tennessee
MRI Tissue Characterization

HYLTON SMITH, Ph.D., F.I.Biol.   Secretary of International Commission on Radiological Protection, Surrey, United Kingdom
On the Safety of Nuclear Magnetic Resonance Imaging and Spectroscopy Systems

H. D. SOSTMAN, M.D.   Professor of Radiology, Duke University; Attending Radiologist, Duke University Medical Center, Durham, North Carolina
NMR Evaluation of Tumor Metabolism

M. SPERBER, M.D.   Formerly, Academisch Ziekenhuis van de Vrije Universiteit, Department of Radiology, Amsterdam, The Netherlands
Malignant Lesions of the Paranasal Sinuses

DAVID D. STARK, M.D.   Assistant Professor of Radiology, Harvard Medical School; Assistant in Radiology, Massachusetts General Hospital, Boston, Massachusetts
Liver and Spleen

JOHN W. STEIDLEY, Ph.D.   Philips Medical Systems, Inc., Shelton, Connecticut
Planning and Preparation

ALAN A. STEIN, Ph.D., M.B.A.   Diasonics, Inc., San Francisco, California
Clinical Efficacy: Analysis of 300 MRI Cases at 1.5 Tesla; Thin-Slice MRI

EARL P. STEINBERG, M.D., M.P.P. Henry J. Kaiser Foundation Faculty Scholar in General Internal Medicine, Assistant Professor of Medicine and of Health Policy and Management, The Johns Hopkins Medical Institutions; Director, The Johns Hopkins Program for Medical Technology and Practice Assessment, Full-Time Active Staff, The Johns Hopkins Hospital, Baltimore, Maryland
The Economics and Regulation of MRI

R. E. STEINER, M.D., F.R.C.R., F.R.C.P. Emeritus Professor of Diagnostic Radiology, University of London Royal Postgraduate Medical School; NMR Unit, Hammersmith Hospital, London, United Kingdom
Role and Scope of MRI in Diagnostic Medicine

W. HOYT STEPHENS, M.S. Senior Associate in Radiology and Radiological Sciences; Director, Center for Medical Imaging Research, Vanderbilt University Medical Center, Nashville, Tennessee
NMR Physical Principles

BERT TE STRAKE, M.D. Department of Radiology, University Hospital, Groningen, The Netherlands; Consulting Radiologist, MRI, King Faisal Specialist Hospital and Research Centre, Riyadh, Kingdom of Saudi Arabia
Adrenal Glands

A. H. M. TAMINIAU, M.D., Ph.D. Department of Orthopaedic Surgery, University Hospital, Leiden, The Netherlands
Primary Malignant Bone Tumors

ROBERT W. TARR, M.D. Chief Resident in Radiology, Vanderbilt University Medical Center, Nashville, Tennessee
MRI Optimization Strategies; Gastrointestinal Tract; Understanding Basic MR Pulse Sequences

ALBERT TEDESCHI, M.D. Riverview Medical Center; Fellow, Magnetic Resonance Imaging, Vanderbilt University Medical Center, Nashville, Tennessee
Gastrointestinal Tract

ARCH W. TEMPLETON, M.D. Professor and Chairman, Department of Radiology, University of Kansas Medical Center, Kansas City, Kansas
Computer Networks for Medical Image Management

STEPHEN R. THOMAS, Ph.D. Professor of Radiology, University of Cincinnati College of Medicine, Cincinnati, Ohio
Gradient Coil Technology; The Biomedical Applications of Fluorine-19 NMR

JACK TISHLER, M.D. Professor of Radiology, University of Alabama Medical School; University of Alabama Hospitals, Birmingham, Alabama
Gated MRI in Congenital Cardiac Malformations

M. F. TWEEDLE, Ph.D. Director of Research, The Squibb Institute for Medical Research, New Brunswick, New Jersey
Principles of Contrast-Enhanced MRI

B. G. TWEEDY, Ph.D. Chairman, Chemistry Department, Agriculture Division, Ciba-Giegy Company, Greensboro, North Carolina
Dynamic Contrast-Enhanced MRI and Mathematical Modeling

J. VALK, M.D. Professor of Radiology, Academische Ziekenhuis van de Vrije Universiteit, Department of Radiology, Amsterdam, The Netherlands
Malignant Lesions of the Paranasal Sinuses

P. VAN DER MEULEN, M.Sc. Department of MRI, Philips Medical Systems Division, Best, The Netherlands
Fast, Small Flip-Angle Field Echo Imaging

P. VAN DIJK, M.Sc. Department of MRI, Philips Medical Systems Division, Best, The Netherlands
Fast, Small Flip-Angle Field Echo Imaging

A. T. VAN OOSTEROM, M.D. Department of Oncology, University Hospital, Antwerpe, Belgium
Primary Malignant Bone Tumors

ARNOUD P. VAN SETERS, Ph.D. Teacher in Endocrinology, University Medical Center; Staff Member, Department of Endocrinology, University Hospital, Leiden, The Netherlands
Adrenal Glands

W. RICHARD WEBB, M.D. Professor of Radiology, University of California, San Francisco, California
Mediastinum and Hila

P. W. WEDEKING, Ph.D. Research Investigator, The Squibb Institute for Medical Research, New Brunswick, New Jersey
Principles of Contrast-Enhanced MRI

FELIX W. WEHRLI, Ph.D. General Electric Medical Systems, Waukesha, Wisconsin
Impact of the Choice of Operating Parameters on MR Images; Advanced Statistical Methods for Tissue Characteristics

JEFFREY C. WEINREB, M.D. Associate Professor of Radiology, Columbia University College of Physicians and Surgeons; Director of MRI, St. Luke's/Roosevelt Hospital Center, New York, New York
Obstetric Problems

JOSEPH D. WEISSMAN, M.D., Ph.D. Technicare Corporation, Solon, Ohio
Thin-Slice MRI

M. ROBERT WILLCOTT, Ph.D. President, NMR Imaging, Inc., Houston, Texas
NMR Chemical Principles

ALAN C. WINFIELD, M.D.   Professor of Radiology, Vanderbilt University School of Medicine; Director, Abdominal Imaging Section, Vanderbilt University Hospital, Nashville, Tennessee
Breast

GARY L. WISMER, M.D.   Clinical Fellow, Neuroradiology, Massachusetts General Hospital, Boston; Staff Radiologist, Nemours Magnetic Resonance Facility, Jacksonville, Florida
Chemical Shift Imaging

GERALD L. WOLF, Ph.D., M.D.   Professor of Radiology, University of Pittsburgh; President and Medical Director, Pittsburgh NMR Institute, Pittsburgh, Pennsylvania
Free Radical Contrast Agents for MRI; Hepatobiliary Contrast Agents

I. R. YOUNG, Ph.D.   GEC Research, Limited, Wembley, Middlesex, United Kingdom
Artifacts in the Measurement of T1 and T2

EBERHARD ZEITLER, M.D.   Professor at the University of Erlangen—Nürnberg; Head of the Diagnostic Department, Radiological Center, General Hospital, Nuremberg, German Federal Republic
Overview of MRI Clinical Applications in Germany

B. G. ZIEDSES DES PLANTES, JR., M.D.   Stichting Deventer Ziekenhuizen, Deventer, The Netherlands
Malignant Lesions of the Paranasal Sinuses

Foreword

It is nearly 400 years since the practice of medicine and the study of magnetism were combined in the career of Sir William Gilbert, physician to Queen Elizabeth I, president of the Royal College of Physicians, and author of *De Magnete*, one of the great scientific treatises our civilization has produced. Gilbert studied the magnetic field of the Earth, as revealed by the behavior of compasses, and the interaction of small magnets of lodestone (magnetite: Fe_3O_4) or iron. A tireless experimenter and acute observer, Gilbert was an early practitioner of the scientific method. The lore of the lodestone had become encrusted with myths—such as the efficacy of garlic as a demagnetizing agent. Much worse, the essential difference between *electric* attraction (of rubbed amber for bits of straw) and *magnetic* attraction (of a lodestone for pieces of iron) was not recognized. All of this Gilbert straightened out. He showed that magnetically the Earth resembles a giant lodestone sphere. He had an idea of a magnetic field, which he called an *orb of virtue* in the space surrounding a lodestone, and he emphasized the virtue's extraordinary penetrating power. "No hindrance," Gilbert wrote, "is offered by thick boards, or by walls of pottery or marble, or even metals; there is naught so solid as to do away with this force, or check it, save a plate of iron."

Gilbert made other discoveries in what we now call the physics of ferromagnetism. Magnetic effects *not* enhanced by the peculiar properties of iron were far beyond the reach of his experiments, even if he had known what to look for. *De Magnete* was published in 1600. The next significant advance in our understanding of magnetism did not come until 220 years later, with Oersted's discovery that an electric current in a wire can influence a nearby compass needle.

As a physician, Gilbert recorded no notable discoveries. However, Sir William Harvey, whose revolutionary book on the circulation of blood was published in 1628, was an enthusiastic admirer of Gilbert's scientific investigations and may have derived some inspiration from them. Perhaps that should count as Gilbert's most valuable contribution to medical science. In any case, if one indulges in the familiar fantasy of summoning a figure from the past to witness a scientific advance of the present, one would like to tell *both* William Gilbert and William Harvey about the medical uses of magnetism—not omitting observation of the flow of blood, which is described in Chapters 36 and 98 of this book. Dr. Gilbert himself might be more astonished by the total dependence on ferromagnetism of a society that now stores most of its information, whether on tape or disk, in powdered lodestone!

Even physicists of today, accustomed as they have become to rapid growth in the range and power of their instruments, are awed by the resolution of detail that has been achieved in the NMR image. As for those of us who were exploring the physics of NMR 40 years ago, I believe that few could comment on the pictures in this book without using the word *marvelous*. Yet in retrospect one can trace, as Professor Bloch has done in Chapter 1, a path leading, step by logical step, from I. I. Rabi's molecular beam to today's sagittal section. That seems to be the way science, in our century, produces a genuine marvel.

The development of imaging by nuclear magnetic resonance presents a striking contrast to the beginning of roentgenography. When Roentgen discovered x-rays in November 1895, physics could not even explain, let alone predict, the penetrating power of the mysterious radiation. The electron itself was unknown; the structure of atoms would remain a puzzle for the next 20 years. Nevertheless, within weeks of Roentgen's discovery, eager experimenters on both sides of the Atlantic were displaying pictures of bones and medical applications were already being reported. By June 1896 there existed a journal devoted to x-ray shadowgraphs, termed *skiagraphy*.* From discovery to world-wide medical use: less than one year!

The history of nuclear magnetic resonance was quite different. A long sequence of developments, with branches and several turning points, preceded its eventual use in medicine. That an atomic nucleus can have a magnetic moment was deduced around 1925 from certain features in atomic spectra. The magnetic moment of the proton was measured by Otto Stern in 1933 using a beam of hydrogen molecules. Further developments by I. I. Rabi at Columbia, reviewed in the first chapter by Professor Bloch, led to the molecular beam resonance method. In the thirties, nuclear magnetic moments were interesting mainly as clues to nuclear structure. The collective behavior of the nuclear magnets in condensed matter, properly called *nuclear magnetism*, concerned only a few physicists—notably C. J. Gorter in Leiden, and B. Lazarev and L. Schubnikov in Moscow. In 1937 the Russian physicists were able to demonstrate the magnetization of solid hydrogen in a strong field at low temperature, the protonic analogue of electronic paramagnetism. Gorter actually tried a resonance experiment, but without success, in 1942. So matters stood at the end of World War II, when the experiments at Stanford and at Harvard were conceived, and the proton magnetic resonance was observed in ordinary matter.

By 1950, plus or minus a year or two, the basic physics that underlies NMR imaging was for practical purposes completely understood. That includes: the magnetic dipole moments and electric quadrupole moments of relevant nuclei; the relaxation times $T1$ and $T2$ and their dependence on molecular viscosity; the dynamical behavior of spins of all sorts in oscillating fields, both continuous and pulsed; the chemical shifts that were soon to open up an immense field of application in organic chemistry. No physicist working with NMR at that time would have been surprised to see a proton resonance with a mouse, or a human finger, in the coil. Its amplitude, as in the case of any other largely aqueous substance, would have been quite predictable. Yet with all this knowledge ready to apply, the realization of medically useful NMR images lay more than 20 years in the future. What essential ingredients were lacking?

For one thing, sensitivity. In our first proton resonance in 1945, the sample was nearly 1 kilogram of paraffin. Recalling that, as I look at the image in Figure 2–7, I realize that one millionth of our sample, a 1-milligram lump of paraffin, would shine out in that image as a conspicuous anomaly, possibly identifiable through paraffin's exceptionally short $T1$. Of course, that kilogram of paraffin was an absurdly large sample by our later standards. The real advance in sensitivity in the decades after 1950, although difficult to define neatly, was more like 10^3 than 10^6, still a spectacular gain.

---

* Encyclopedia Brit. *23*:845, 1942. "Archives of Skiagraphy" (see O.E.D. for skiagraph).

The key was computer power and the great advance in sophisticated signal-processing techniques that became feasible as computer speed and memory grew by their own powers of ten. Through that period the active frontiers in NMR were expanding from physics to chemistry and biochemistry. Several ingenious and powerful techniques were developed by chemists using NMR to study molecular structure. In addition to increasing sensitivity by one form or another of signal averaging, computer power is, of course, essential for tomographic reconstruction of the NMR image. In short, NMR imaging could hardly have been developed to its present state, no matter how well established its base in physics, without the modern computer.

But something even more essential was lacking in 1950: the *idea* that a useful interior image was in principle obtainable, and was a goal worth pursuing. For that P. C. Lauterbur, P. Mansfield, and R. Damadian deserve enormous credit. Several more ideas that were needed to accelerate developments were forthcoming, when the time was ripe, from other NMR practitioners.

NMR imaging is so powerful, so general, and at the same time so gentle a diagnostic procedure that it is likely to become part of most people's experience. That seems obvious now, even to an antiquated NMR expert like myself who did *not* foresee it. The prospect must be exhilarating for the scientists involved, from physicists to physicians, very well represented by the contributors to this book. It is challenging to me as a teacher of physics, for I feel that some general public understanding of the essential facts is both desirable and attainable.

How fortunate we are that most ordinary matter, as Gilbert observed, is freely penetrated by a magnetic field. To that we owe both the power and the safety of NMR imaging of today. But the layman undergoing this rather mysterious procedure may ask how one can be so confident that magnetic fields are benign. Weren't x-rays considered harmless at first? The concern is understandable. There is a good answer, an answer based solidly on the fundamental physics and chemistry we have learned in this century: *The interaction of a magnetic field with a molecule is so very slight that neither can seriously perturb the other.*

The explanation is simple. It begins with another fact first recognized by Gilbert: Electricity and magnetism are essentially different. We know now that matter, including living tissue of every sort, is at the molecular level an *electrical* structure. Within it electrons are held in atoms, atoms are bound into molecules, and molecules are linked with one another by the forces of attraction and repulsion between *electric charges*. Magnetism is not directly involved. Nothing like a *magnetic charge* has been found in nature. Physicists have searched assiduously, but in vain, for a magnetic monopole, as it would be called. There is not even one such particle among all the electrically charged particles in the human body—some 10^{28} protons and electrons. Magnetic effects in matter arise exclusively from the *motion* of electric charge—an electron orbiting in an atom or spinning around an axis, a proton orbiting or spinning in an atomic nucleus. Magnetism in matter is a by-product, a side effect, so to speak, of the electrical structure of the atom, and as such it is intrinsically feeble.

To emphasize the point with one important example, consider the water molecule

$$H \diagdown \qquad \diagup H .$$
$$O$$

Its "boomerang" shape gives the molecule an electric dipole moment, thereby making liquid water a powerful solvent. That shape represents an equilibrium of *electrical* attractions and repulsions within the molecule, with quantum mechanics governing the motions of all the protons and electrons. The structure is stiff. To bend the molecule straight (H—O—H) by brute force would cost in energy about 50 kcal/mole, roughly five times as much energy as it would take to vaporize the water. Now there is also in this molecule a magnetic interaction, of central importance in NMR, between the two hydrogen nuclei. It is the interaction of each nuclear magnet with the magnetic field of the other. Expressing it in the same units, the energy of this magnetic dipole-dipole interaction is about 10^{-9} kcal/mole, less than one ten-billionth of the energy involved in any major alteration of the molecule's shape. The interaction of one nuclear magnetic dipole with the strong field of an NMR imaging coil can be a few thousand times larger (as in a field of 1 tesla) but is still less than one millionth of the energy exchanged in a typical biochemical reaction. The largest increment of energy associated with the effect of a steady magnetic field on a molecule is the energy required to reverse an electron's spin. In a field of 1 tesla that is 0.003 kcal/mole.

The various oscillating magnetic fields used in NMR imaging, with frequencies up to a few hundred megacycles/second, are generally stronger than, but not different in character from, the alternating magnetic fields in radio waves and around a-c wiring, which imperceptibly pervade our bodies much of the time. As for possible physiological effects of such low-frequency magnetic fields, the ultimate guarantor of safety is the quantum law, $E = h\nu$, which governs the absorption of energy by an individual atom or molecule. If the frequency of alternation ν is lower than 1000 megacycles/second, the quantum energy is less than one-millionth that of a quantum of ultraviolet light. An atom absorbs one quantum at a time. One "x-ray" quantum absorbed by an atom can blow it apart. The disturbance one "radio" quantum can make is so slight that it would be swamped merely by the ever-present thermal agitation of the molecular surroundings.

This assurance that the quantum law gives us is important, for it holds whether the oscillating field is magnetic or electric. As remarked earlier, magnetic interactions with an electrical structure like a molecule are intrinsically weak. No physiological observation I can imagine will tell me whether my hand is penetrated by the Earth's magnetic field (as it has been all my life) or by a steady field ten thousand times stronger. An *oscillating* magnetic field, on the other hand, is necessarily accompanied by an oscillating electric field, induced in accordance with Faraday's law. An oscillating electric field can deposit energy, in the form of heat, in bulk matter and does so readily in a material whose dielectric properties are dominated by the presence of polar molecules, such as water. The result, when it occurs in tissue, is literally nothing but smoothly distributed heat. It is not necessarily negligible, but the precautions called for are the same as in any form of diathermy. I believe that in routine NMR imaging as currently practiced, the amplitudes of alternating electric fields can be kept well below the level at which warming of tissue might be a concern. This question and others related to safety will be thoroughly discussed in Chapters 84 to 86. The point I want to emphasize here is the fundamental difference between the alteration of a specific biochemical structure or process by a low-frequency oscillating field—which appears to me, in view of the quantum law, nearly impossible—and the general warming of a mass of tissue, no more mysterious than if the heat were generated by internal friction.

I write as a physicist, not a biochemist, which is one reason for the qualifying word *nearly* in the preceding sentence. Arguments based on such immutable facts as the electrical nature of matter and the quantum law are compelling, but it would surely be foolish to claim that every potential physiological effect has been thought of and can be categorically ruled out. Nothing can substitute completely for observation over a long period of time of living organisms in a magnetic field. For such empirical testing physics can offer some guidance. Suppose there is some relatively small but definite effect of a magnetic field on a molecular process, unforeseen and awaiting discovery. Imagine, for instance, that the rate of a certain biochemical reaction is changed in the presence of the field. An argument based on a general principle of symmetry in electromagnetism (which I shall not develop here) leads directly to the prediction that the effect of a constant magnetic field upon an electrical structure must be proportional to the *square* of the magnetic field strength, if not to an even higher power. Therefore, a search for new effects should be carried out at the highest possible field strength, in the expectation that a 5-tesla field will be 25 times as effective as a 1-tesla field in evoking a response. Conversely, if a biological system behaves quite normally in a 5-tesla field, confidence that fields of 0.5T or less will not perturb it is greatly strengthened.

My own confident expectation is that clinical experience (accumulating at a rate that may for a while seem exponential) and empirical testing in the 10-tesla range (which ought to be part of a systematic long-term program) will eventually prove beyond question that the extension of William Gilbert's "orb of virtue" into the human body is in the deepest sense benign.

EDWARD M. PURCELL, PH.D.
Gerhardt Gabe University Professor Emeritus
Harvard University

Preface

The continuing developments in MRI techniques and applications following publication of the first edition of Nuclear Magnetic Resonance (NMR) Imaging have been both dramatic and significant. It appears that MRI rapidly is becoming the most comprehensive and efficacious diagnostic imaging modality in medical history. Therefore, we felt the need to initiate a second edition almost immediately after the publication of our first text owing to the rapidity, significance, and number of new developments. It has been a challenge to find a stop frame in the motion picture of innovation in which the current capabilities of MRI techniques will be documented and described most successfully. The refinement of MRI fluoroscopy, MRI angiography, flow measurement, fast scan, cine-mode, and three dimensional imaging, to name a few areas of research and innovation, continues to revolutionize clinical applications of this discipline. Further, the organ substrate metabolism capability of nuclear magnetic resonance spectroscopy (NMRS) is so important an area that it must be given proper emphasis. This text, then, is an effort by the five editors to summarize the collective experience of many leading scientists and clinical investigators in a comprehensive overview of the field of magnetic resonance diagnostic inquiry.

In order to retain the comprehensive nature of the text and to expand the coverage of research to include more from international laboratories, a two-volume set became a necessity. From a first edition of 40 chapters, this second edition has expanded in size and content to 107 chapters. The group of 90 contributors to the 1983 edition, almost all of whom are represented once again, are joined by 80 additional clinicians and investigators. A second reason for a two-volume set is that even the most diligent will not utilize a cover-to-cover analysis in attempting to master this often complex, and sometimes overwhelming, material. Therefore, the two volumes have been organized as a Clinical Volume I and a Basic Sciences Volume II. This is intended to simplify for the reader the location of that information which is deemed most relevant and timely.

Volume I is composed of 11 subdivisions. Following a historical overview and basic sciences introduction, there are sections on clinical imaging experience in various parts of the body, special applications including contrast media, and a concluding section that forecasts and analyzes future expectations. New to this edition are the four chapters on tissue characterization and the five chapters on the use of contrast enhancement in MRI. Six primary subdivisions appear in Volume II, exploring physics and chemistry, relaxation/relaxometry, instrumentation, MRI site planning, NMR spectroscopy, and new areas of research and development. It is evident that many of the exciting advances found in the research section were in their infancy at the time of the first edition. These include relaxation measurement, flow and organ perfusion measurement, medical imaging networks, contrast agents, in vivo NMRS, and thin-section and fast-scan MRI. Many have been or are about to be introduced clinically.

One often has a sense of inadequacy when charged with the responsibility of recognizing the multiple talents involved with such a monumental project as this. We are deeply indebted to our contributors and hope that they will rejoin us when the need arises to update this text in the future. The editors are especially grateful to the Vanderbilt University Medical Center administration for their enthusiastic interest and support, to our colleagues in Radiology and Radiological Sciences, to the Center for Medical Imaging Research, to our residents and students who stimulate our most creative productivity, and to the publication staff at W. B. Saunders. Finally, the responsibility for the reality of any text often rests with the dedicated efforts and editorial skills of a few significant and special people. For this text, our three very special people are Margaret W. Moore and Pamela S. Moore at Vanderbilt and Kathleen McCullough at Saunders, and to them we express our deepest appreciation.

Participation in the evolution of magnetic resonance imaging and the generation of this book represents opportunities that are tremendously exciting and fulfilling for each of us personally and professionally. It is our hope that a portion of that excitement and satisfaction will be transmitted to the reader as he identifies his areas of interest within these volumes.

C. LEON PARTAIN, M.D., PH.D.
A. EVERETTE JAMES, JR., SC.M., J.D., M.D.

Contents for Volume 1

Contents for Volume 2

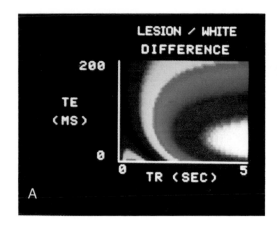

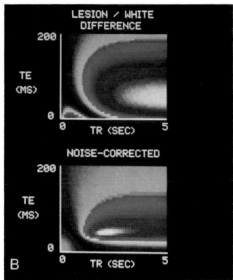

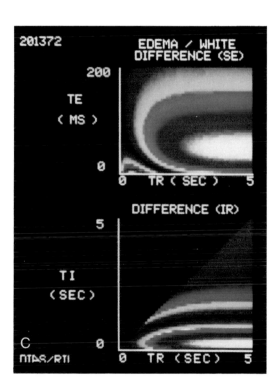

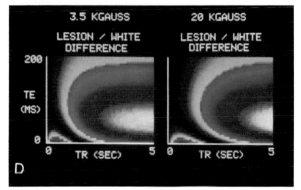

PLATE I

A, ASD map is shown for the patient of Figure 105–5. *B*, ASD and noise-corrected ASD maps for lesion/white contrast for the patient of Figure 105–7. *C*, ASD maps for both spin echo and inversion recovery are shown for the patient of Figure 105–10 for edema versus white matter. The IR map is calculated at TE = 45 ms. *D*, ASD maps are shown for field strengths of 3.5 and 20 kgauss for the patient of Figure 105–14. Equivalent signal difference requires longer TR values at higher field.

XII

PHYSICS AND CHEMISTRY

NMR Physical Principles

RONALD R. PRICE
W. HOYT STEPHENS
C. LEON PARTAIN

A thorough understanding of the physical basis of the nuclear magnetic resonance (NMR) phenomenon and its extension to NMR imaging requires a knowledge of magnetic fields: their origin, their interactions, and their measurements. The purpose of this chapter is to explore basic phenomena associated with magnetic fields and to relate these to the clinical NMR imaging system.

Magnetic fields (identified as B in the figures of this chapter) have their origin as a result of moving charged particles. A magnetic field may be produced easily in the laboratory by connecting a battery to a loop of wire. The current flowing through the wire loop consists of moving charged particles (electrons); the result is a magnetic field whose lines encircle the wire. Magnetic fields are called "vector" fields, since in order to specify a magnetic field at a location in space, one must specify both the magnitude of the magnetic force and the direction in which that force would act on another magnet if it were located at that position. A magnetic field, as opposed to an electric field, is defined in terms of the forces between moving charged particles (current elements). These forces are to be distinguished from electrostatic forces, which are forces resulting from the charge that a particle possesses (e.g., like charges repel, while opposite charges attract) rather than from the motion of those charges. Even though the above explanation is also valid for permanent magnets, it may not be easy to visualize the origin of the moving charges. It is hoped that this will be made clearer in subsequent sections.

MAGNETIC DIPOLES AND MAGNETIC MOMENTS

Almost everyone is familiar with a bar magnet and its behavior in the field of another magnet. Like electrical charges, which have been arbitrarily assigned negative or positive values, magnets have been assigned south-seeking and north-seeking poles. The designation of these poles is based on the orientation that a freely supported magnet assumes when suspended in the earth's magnetic field. As with electrical charges, like poles repel and opposite poles attract. Unlike electrical charges, however, an isolated south pole or north pole (sometimes called a "monopole") does not seem to exist in nature. Thus, the basic element of magnetism is the dipole, and to the best of our knowledge all magnets possess both a south pole and a north pole. An important discovery relative to understanding magnetic fields is that a simple current-carrying loop of wire will produce a field (Fig. 59–1) identical to that of a bar magnet.

The magnetic field intensity ($\overline{B}$) is defined in terms of the magnetic moment ($\overline{M}$) of a small bar magnet or equivalently of a small current-carrying loop. $\overline{M}$ is also a vector quantity; that is, to specify $\overline{M}$ one must specify both its direction and its mag-

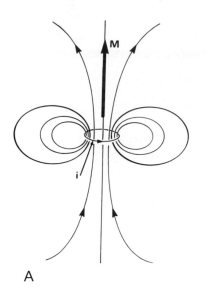

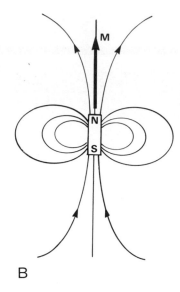

Figure 59–1. Magnetic field lines due to a current loop (*A*) and a small permanent magnet (*B*). At most distances for the loop and the magnetic dipole the magnetic field lines of force are identical. The field lines show lines of equal forces which would be exerted on a small magnet placed at the position. The arrow tips indicate the direction in which the force will be exerted.

A

B

nitude. The direction of $\overline{M}$ is defined as pointed from the south-seeking end to the north-seeking end of a magnet. In the case of a current-carrying loop this direction is conveniently found by the "left-hand" rule. If the fingers of the left hand are wrapped along the coil in the direction of the electron current, then the thumb will point in the direction of M. It should be noted here that error often arises in determining the direction of $\overline{M}$ as a result of confusing conventional current flow with electron flow. In conventional current flow (a convention used by electricians and electrical engineers), the convention is to assume the flow direction to be the direction of an effective positive charge flow. The result is that the conventional current flow direction will be opposite the actual electron flow direction. If the positive current flow convention is used, then the direction of $\overline{M}$ should be determined by using an equivalent application of a "right-hand" rule. In this chapter, we will assume current flow to be in the direction that the electrons are actually flowing.

The magnitude of $\overline{M}$ is most easily defined in terms of the current loop:

$$\overline{M} = NIA \tag{1}$$

where N is the number of turns or loops in the wire, I is the current being carried by the loop, and A is the area of the loop. Thus, $\overline{M}$ can be increased by increasing the number of turns, by increasing the current, or by increasing the diameter of the loops.

As indicated earlier, magnetic fields are defined in terms of forces between current elements. Of interest to us is what happens to a bar magnet or alternatively a small current loop when placed in a field produced by another magnetic source, i.e., an external field. If the external field is uniform, then the field will exert equal and opposite forces on both the south poles and the north poles of either the bar magnet or the current loop. Since this action results in no net force on the magnetic element, the force does not cause it to move linearly along the field direction; rather the effect is to cause a rotation about the center of the magnetic element (Fig. 59–2). A force that tends to rotate rather than translate is called a "torque."

The bar magnet suspended in an external field will thus experience a torque, which will rotate it so that it aligns with the external field lines. The current loop will experience a similar torque and will rotate to align itself so that the plane of the loop is perpendicular to the field lines (Fig. 59–2), or equivalently until its magnetic moment ($\overline{M}$) is aligned parallel to the field lines. The direction of the magnetic field intensity

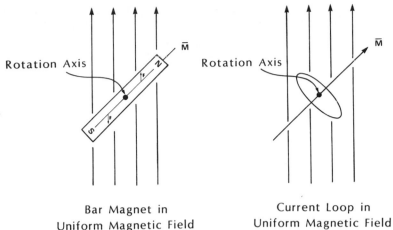

Figure 59–2. When a magnetic element (either a magnetic dipole or a current loop) is placed in a uniform magnetic field, a torque consisting of equal and opposite forces (F) will tend to rotate the element about its center.

Bar Magnet in
Uniform Magnetic Field

Current Loop in
Uniform Magnetic Field

$(\overline{B})$ at a point in space is, therefore, defined as the direction in which the magnetic moment vector $(\overline{M})$ of a small magnet or loop tends to turn when placed at that point in the field. The magnitude of that torque will be directly proportional to the magnitude of the magnetic moment and the field intensity.

MAGNET PROPERTIES OF MATERIALS: PARAMAGNETISM, DIAMAGNETISM, AND FERROMAGNETISM

The previous discussion of magnetic fields assumed the field to be in "free space," that is, without a significant amount of matter around. Air is actually a reasonably good representation of free space in most applications.

When matter is placed in the magnetic field, the matter itself becomes affected by the field and is caused to establish its own magnetic field. In most materials the new field is in the same direction as the external field. In this case, the material is referred to as a *paramagnetic* material. In some materials the new field is in the opposite direction to that of the external field. These materials are called *diamagnetic* materials. Thus the field within a paramagnetic material will be stronger than the external field and the field within a diamagnetic material will be weaker. In most materials these effects are very small and are generally unimportant. However, in a small group of materials called *ferromagnetic* materials these effects can be quite large and of great importance. Ferromagnetic materials can be used with a relatively weak magnetizing force to produce large magnetic fields. For example a current-carrying wire wrapped around a piece of soft iron produces a much larger magnetic field than would be produced by the wire alone without the iron.

All paramagnetic, diamagnetic, and ferromagnetic effects are explained by the motion of individual charges that are associated with atoms and molecules within the material. These moving charges include both electrons and nucleons and as such produce magnetic fields in a manner identical to the current-carrying loop of wire.

The ratio of the magnetization produced within a material to the applied magnetizing force is called the magnetic susceptibility of a material and is usually identified by the Greek letter chi (χ). Table 59–1 is a small list of materials and their magnetic susceptibility. The value of χ is usually small except for ferromagnetic materials and will be positive for paramagnetic materials and negative for diamagnetic materials.

Table 59–1. MAGNETIC SUSCEPTIBILITY OF SELECTED METALS

Magnetic Metal	Susceptibility X (10^{-6} cgs)
Copper	−5.46
Silver	−19.5
Antimony	−99.0
Chromium	+180
Vanadium	+255
Manganese	+529
Cerium	+5160
Nickel, cobalt and iron	ferromagnetic

ANGULAR MOMENTUM

Angular momentum is a quantity that is used to describe rotational motion of a body. Angular momentum is also a vector quantity and thus is specified by both a direction and a magnitude. Angular momentum may be changed by applying a torque to the rotating body. An applied torque may increase or decrease the rotational motion, or it may change the direction of the rotational axis. The direction of the angular momentum vector is determined by the application of a "right-hand" rule (Fig. 59–3). If the fingers of the right hand are wrapped in the direction that an object is rotating, the direction of the angular momentum vector is defined as the direction in which the thumb is pointing.

Two categories of rotational motion are of interest to us. These are orbital and spin angular momenta. Examples of these motions are found in our own solar system with the motions of earth around the sun. Oribital angular momentum is represented by the earth's yearly orbit around the sun, and spin angular momentum is represented by the earth's daily rotation on its own axis. The magnitude of angular momentum is proportional to the mass distribution of the object and the velocity of its rotational motion. The two independent motions of the earth add together (in a relatively complicated way) to yield the earth's total angular momentum. Its orbital angular momentum is proportional to its orbital velocity around the sun (one rotation per year). Its spin angular momentum is proportional to its angular velocity of rotation on its own axis (one rotation per day).

As noted, these angular momenta do not add together in a simple manner; their sum rather depends both on their relative magnitudes and on their relative directions. For example, two objects with equal and oppositely directed angular momenta would

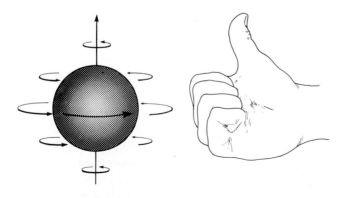

Angular Momentum   "Right-Hand" Rule

Figure 59–3. For a rotational object, the direction of the angular momentum vector can be determined by curving the fingers of the right hand in the direction of the rotation. In this position the direction of the thumb is the direction of the angular momentum vector.

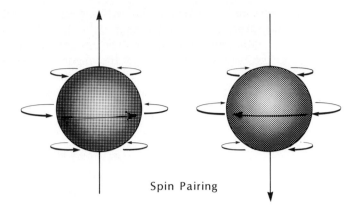

Figure 59–4. In a two-particle system, the preferred (most stable) configuration is when the spinning particles are paired, with their angular momenta vectors pointing in opposite directions, "spin-pairing."

Spin Pairing

result in a total angular momentum of zero, while any other orientation would yield a nonzero value, with the maximum value being obtained when the two are parallel. In nature, particles and structures prefer to exist in their lowest (most stable) energy state. Thus, the lowest energy state of a two particle system would result when the angular momenta were paired in an equal and opposite direction (no net angular momentum). Pairing has been recognized both on the atomic level with paired orbital electrons and on the nuclear level with paired protons and paired neutrons (Fig. 59–4). Since protons and neutrons are not identical particles, protons do not pair with neutrons.

MAGNETIC PROPERTIES OF ELECTRONS AND NUCLEONS

When a single electron orbits about the nucleus, it constitutes an electric current loop and as such possesses a magnetic moment. If the electron is in the smallest possible orbit (K-shell), the value of this magnetic moment is referred to as a Bohr magneton.

In addition to the orbital motion of an electron, the electron is also known to possess an intrinsic rotational motion that is referred to as spin. The spin of all electrons is known to be the same and is equal to a spin quantum number times a fundamental unit of angular momentum called Planck's constant. For electrons the spin quantum number is equal to $\frac{1}{2}$; thus it is generally stated that the spin of an electron is equal to $\frac{1}{2}$. Since intrinsic spin also constitutes a current-carrying loop, the electron also possesses an intrinsic magnetic moment due to its spin in addition to the magnetic moment resulting from its orbital motion. The value of the spin magnetic moment is also equal to 1 Bohr magneton. The Bohr magneton (μ_B) is given by

$$\mu_B = \frac{eh}{4\pi m} \tag{2}$$

where e is the charge of the electron, m is the electron mass, and h is Planck's constant. The value of

$$\mu_B = 9.27 \times 10^{-24} \text{ joules/tesla}, \tag{3}$$

where the joule is a unit of energy and the tesla (10^4 gauss) is a measure of the magnetic field strength.

Like electrons, nucleons (protons and neutrons) are also known to possess an intrinsic spin angular momentum and thus an associated magnetic moment. If we replace the mass of the electron in the equation of the Bohr magneton with the proton mass, we have the nuclear magneton (μ_N). Because of the complex arrangement of nucleons in various nuclei, the magnetic momenta of complex nuclei are not calculated but rather measured for each individual nucleus.

Magnetic moments may be either positive or negative. When the magnetic moment is positive, this implies that the angular momentum (using the right-hand rule) and the magnetic moment are in the same direction. Negative magnetic moments imply that they are in opposite directions. The magnetic moments for the proton (μ_p) and neutron (μ_n) are

$$\mu_p = 1.41 \times 10^{-26} \text{ joules/tesla} \qquad (4)$$

$$\mu_n = -9.66 \times 10^{-27} \text{ joules/tesla} \qquad (5)$$

The fact that the neutron possesses a magnetic moment and that it is also negative presents an interesting aside. Even though the neutron does not have a net charge, the fact that it possesses a magnetic moment leads one to conclude that it must be composed of charges and that they must in some manner be in motion. The fact that the neutron is composed of a relatively complex charge distribution has been confirmed experimentally by bombarding neutrons with high energy electrons.

MAGNETIC PROPERTIES OF THE NUCLEUS

By combining our knowledge of magnetic moments and angular momentum with a knowledge of nuclear structure, we can now begin to understand the origin and nature of nuclear magnetism.

The nucleus of an atom is composed of neutrons and protons. Protons possess one unit of positive charge, which is equal to and opposite the negative charge of the electron. The neutrons and protons bound together form the atomic nucleus. The force that binds the nucleons together is clearly not electrical in nature, since the like charges of the protons would actually tend to push the nucleus apart rather than hold it together. It is now known that there exists a much stronger "nuclear" force that counteracts the repulsive electrical forces and binds the nucleons together to form the nucleus. Even though the protons and neutrons do not actually maintain their original identity after being bound by the nuclear force, for the present, to aid in the development of our nuclear magnetism model, we will assume they do.

As mentioned earlier, protons and, separately, neutrons tend to exist in the nucleus as spin-up/spin-down pairs. Spin pairing cancels out the angular momentum of the pair (equal to zero) and thus will not contribute additional angular momentum to the nucleus. (Being unlike particles, protons and neutrons will not pair.) Thus, one must conclude that it is the angular momentum of the *unpaired* nucleons (either proton or neutron) that adds to the oribital angular momentum and that is thus the primary factor that determines the total angular momentum of the nucleus.

Table 59–2. ANGULAR MOMENTUM OF COMPLEX NUCLEI

Nuclear Configuration	Angular Momentum
1. One unpaired nucleon A-odd	Multiple of 1/2

2. Two or more unpaired
    nucleons
    A-even
    Z-odd
	Multiple of 1

3. No unpaired nucleons
    A-even
    Z-even
	0

The spin of a complex nucleus is more complicated than the electron spin (which is always equal to $\frac{1}{2}$). Nuclear spins may be either zero, a multiple of $\frac{1}{2}$ ($\frac{1}{2}$, $\frac{3}{2}$, $\frac{5}{2}$, etc.), or a whole number, depending upon the unpaired nucleons. Which of these three categories of spins that a nuclide fits into can be determined by its atomic mass A (sum of protons and neutrons) and its atomic number Z (number of protons) (Table 59–2).

INTERACTIONS OF NUCLEAR MAGNETS WITH EXTERNAL MAGNETIC FIELDS

As noted previously, there exist certain "magnetic" nuclei with unpaired nucleons that possess both a magnetic dipole moment and a net spin angular momentum. When a nucleus is placed in an external magnetic field, it is these companion properties of a nucleus that cause the nucleus to execute a unique motion. This motion is a periodic rotational motion of the spin axis of the nucleus about the direction of the external field. This motion is called "precession." The frequency of this precessional motion is called the Larmor frequency. Every nucleus possesses a unique Larmor frequency, and it is this signature that allows us to "tune in" to and measure selected nuclei in MR imaging and NMR spectroscopy.

Precessional motion occurs in symmetric spinning objects when a torque is applied perpendicular to the object's angular momentum. The most familiar example of this is the spinning toy top or a toy gyroscope when it experiences a torque due to the gravitational pull of the earth (Fig. 59–5). When the top tips slightly off center, the pull of gravity tries to rotate the top about its point. The result of this external torque is to push the top into a circular motion about a vertical axis parallel to the direction of gravity. In the case of the top, the friction between the floor and the top will continue to slow the top, the tip will become progressively larger, and the top will eventually fall to the floor.

The toy top analogy can also be used to extend the idea of precession to spinning nuclei if one simply replaces the toy top with the nucleus and the gravitational torque with the torque produced by the external magnetic field (Fig. 59–6). Unlike the toy top the nucleus experiences no frictional forces and thus will not slow down and tip over.

The frequency of the Larmor precession depends upon the strength of the magnetic field (B_0) and the gyromagnetic ratio (γ) of the nucleus. The gyromagnetic ratio is equal to the ratio of the magnitude of the magnetic moment of the nucleus to the magnitude of its spin angular momentum. The equation relating the Larmor frequency (f_L) to the magnetic field is

$$f_L = \frac{\gamma}{2\pi} B_0 \qquad (6)$$

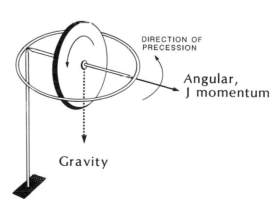

Figure 59–5. The spinning gyroscope with angular momentum, J, is pulled by gravity, producing a torque that tends to rotate the gyroscope about its point. The gyroscope responds by moving in a circle about its point. This motion is called precession.

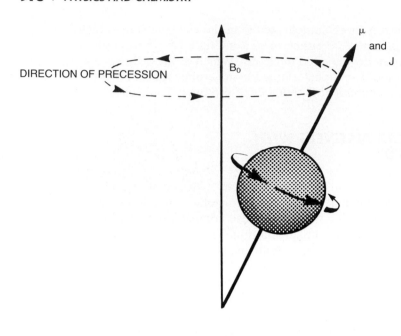

DIRECTION OF PRECESSION

B_0

μ and J

Figure 59–6. A spinning nucleus with angular momentum J and magnetic moment μ under the influence of an external magnetic field B_0 will precess about B_0 at a frequency proportional to B_0.

Some values of the gyromagnetic ratio and the Larmor frequency for some medically important nuclei are shown in Table 59–3.

MAGNETIZATION AND THE MAGNETIZATION VECTOR

In the absence of an external magnetic field the magnetic moments of individual atoms and nuclei within a material will have no preferred direction (Fig. 59–7A). The individual moments will therefore point in random directions with the result being a zero net magnetic moment or zero net magnetization of the material.

If the same material is subjected to an external magnetic field, the individual magnetic moments will tend to align with the applied field. In most materials this alignment is not very strong, and the thermal interactions between atoms will tend to destroy the alignment by randomly bumping individual moments into other directions. From a time-averaged statistical point of view, however, there will exist a net alignment with a small excess fraction of nuclei (on the order of a few per million) finding a preferred direction along the external field. (This is the paramagnetic effect that was described earlier.) If all the magnetic moments of the nuclei making up this excess that is responsible for the net alignment of the material are added together, the resulting sum will be the net magnetization vector ($\overline{M}$) (Fig. 59–7B).

The net magnetization $\overline{M}$ will be a vector, since it will have both magnitude and direction. In addition, since each of the individual nuclei possessed an angular momentum, there will be a total angular momentum associated with the entire sample.

Table 59–3. MAGNETIC PROPERTIES OF MEDICALLY IMPORTANT NUCLEI

Nucleus	Gyromagnetic Ratio 1/Tesla·sec	Larmor Frequency (MHz) for B = 1 Tesla
^1H	26.8×10^7	42.58
^{13}C	6.7×10^7	10.70
^{23}Na	7.1×10^7	11.26
^{31}P	10.8×10^7	17.24

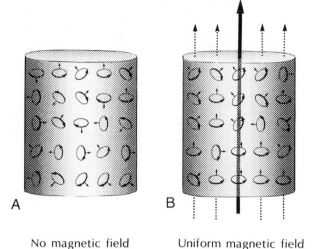

Figure 59–7. *A*, In the absence of an external magnetic field individual nuclei will be randomly oriented. *B*, In the presence of an external uniform field there will be a slight excess of nuclei oriented along the field direction. The result is a net magnetization (*M*) that will have its orientation directly along the uniform field direction.

A   B

No magnetic field   Uniform magnetic field

The importance of the idea of a net magnetization vector is that all of the material in our sample will behave like a single magnet with a net magnetization $\overline{M}$ and an associated total angular momentum. Even though the net magnetization results from an excess of only about 1 nucleus out of a million, when the sample size is on the order of 10^{23} nuclei, we still have a very large number (10^{17}) of nuclei contributing to $\overline{M}$. The advantage is that by measuring $\overline{M}$ we have moved from a microscopic to a macroscopic phenomenon, which can now be measured with macroscopic components in the laboratory.

The summation process leaves the gyromagnetic ratio of $\overline{M}$ identical to the individual nuclei composing it; thus we can tune in the precessional frequency of $\overline{M}$ just as if it were a single nucleus. However, for the precession of $\overline{M}$ to be detected there needs to be a net (unbalanced) torque perpendicular to the angular momentum of $\overline{M}$ which produces a net transverse component of the magnetization. In the equilibrium situation, there will be no net torque on $\overline{M}$ due to the external magnetic field and thus no net transverse magnetization.

The angular momentum vector of individual nuclei will generally not fall along the external field direction, but rather at some angle that will have components both parallel and perpendicular to B_0. The component perpendicular to B_0 is the source of the precessional motion. The perpendicular components of the individual nuclei will be oriented in random directions (having no particular correlation or phase with their neighbors). In this case the perpendicular components will cancel out, since, on the average, for every nucleus pointing in one direction, there will be another nucleus pointing in the opposite direction (Fig. 59–8). For this reason $\overline{M}$ has no perpendicular angular momentum component (M_t) and $\overline{M}$ thus points wholly along B_0.

For $\overline{M}$ to undergo a precessional motion then we must establish a component of the magnetic moment perpendicular to B_0 (M_t). This is accomplished by tipping or displacing $\overline{M}$ away from the B_0 direction by applying an additional magnetic field perpendicular to B_0 (Figure. 59–9). We refer to this perpendicular field as B_1. The simple application of a new static magnetic field, however, would be of little help, since all of the individual nuclei would quickly realign and begin precessing around the new external field direction. The new field direction would be the vector sum of the old B_0 field and the new field B_1. Following realignment, $\overline{M}$ would simply be oriented along the new field direction and would still not be precessing. It has been determined that the best way to produce a precession that can be sustained for a period of time long

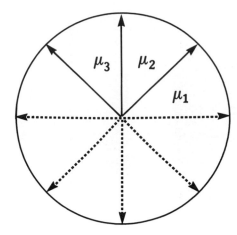

Figure 59–8. View of precessing nuclei from above, looking down upon the B_0 direction. The magnetic moments of individual nuclei (μ_i) will be precessing about B_0 in random order. On average, in this situation, the transverse magnetization will equal zero, since the nuclei will be spread evenly about the axis, thus canceling M_T.

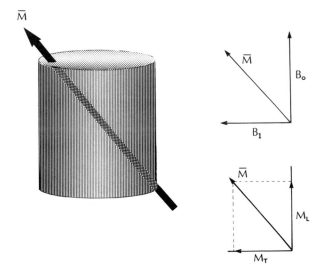

Figure 59–9. A transverse component (M_T) of the magnetization vector $\overline{M}$ can be produced by applying a transverse magnetic field B_1, which will tip $\overline{M}$ away from the B_0 direction. As M_T increases, the longitudinal component (M_L) will decrease. When $\overline{M}$ lies in the transverse plane, $M_T = \overline{M}$ and $M_L = 0$.

enough to make measurements is to use a time-varying magnetic field. This is accomplished by producing short pulses of rf (radiofrequency) waves from a transmitting coil or antenna.

RF (RADIOFREQUENCY) MAGNETIC FIELDS

The perpendicular rf field is produced in a manner similar to the static $\overline{B}$ field. That is, we use a coil of wire (a solenoid) and pass an electric current through it. As we saw earlier, the direction of the field will be perpendicular to the plane of the coil. If we pass the current through the coil in one direction, we have a field produced in the appropriate direction as determined by the right-hand rule. If we reverse the direction of the current flow, we reverse the field direction. If we replace the steady (DC) current flow with an alternating current, the $\overline{B}$ field will oscillate from one direction to the other at the frequency of the applied current.

If the solenoid is placed within the external field magnet in an orientation so that the new solenoid's axis is perpendicular to the axis of the external field magnet, we now have the desired perpendicular oscillating (rf) magnetic field. Typically, the os-

Figure 59–10. When the rf field (B_1) is applied at the resonant frequency, $\overline{M}$ will precess in an ever-increasing circle about the B_0 direction. When $\overline{M}$ reaches the transverse plane, the transverse component M_T will be at its maximum. The pulse that moves $\overline{M}$ from its equilibrium position to the transverse plane is called a 90 degree pulse.

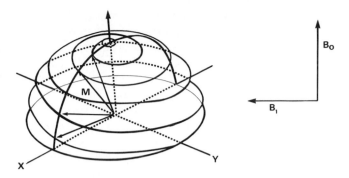

cillating rf field is considerably smaller than the external static field, being only a few gauss relative to the external field, which is typically measured in the kilogauss range.

When the rf-produced $\overline{B}$ field (B_1) is turned on, it appears perpendicular both to $\overline{M}$ and to the angular momentum of $\overline{M}$, with the result being that $\overline{M}$ will try to precess around B_1 with the effect that $\overline{M}$ tips away from its original orientation. When this happens, $\overline{M}$ acquires a component that is perpendicular to B_0, causing it to also try to precess around B_0. With B_1 constantly changing (megahertz or millions of times per second) at an arbitrary frequency, $\overline{M}$ just wobbles about its original orientation. However, if we choose the frequency of the B_1 field to be equal to the Larmor frequency of the B_0 field, we produce a condition called *resonance*. In resonance the effect of the much smaller B_1 field is cumulative, causing the angle of the tip to continue to become larger and larger. From the outside $\overline{M}$ seems to be moving in an ever-increasing spiral as long as the B_1 field is on (Fig. 59–10). The combination of the relative strength of B_1 and how long it is left on determines the degree that $\overline{M}$ is tipped from the B_0 direction.

If the B_1 field is left on long enough to rotate $\overline{M}$ by 90 degrees, we call this a 90 degree or a $\pi/2$ rf pulse. For a rf pulse that results in $\overline{M}$ being rotated 180 degrees (that is, directly opposed to its original direction), we call it either a 180 degree pulse or a π pulse. These two types of pulses are important in most NMR experiments.

THE NMR SIGNAL

When the magnetic field lines-of-force of a magnet pass through a conductor (usually a coil of copper wire), there is a force induced on the free electrons in the conductor that causes the electrons to move. This force is called an electromotive force (emf) and is measured in terms of volts. The moving electrons constitute an electric current that is measured in amperes. This phenomenon is familiar to most of us as the mechanism used by an electrical generator. As with the generator, the current flow is alternating in polarity, flowing first in one direction for a half-cycle and then in the other direction during the following half-cycle and then continuing the same pattern (alternating or AC current). The alternating current is a result of the fact that the magnetic field is dipolar (having both north and south poles). As the north pole field lines cross the conductors the emf is in one direction, and then when the south pole field lines cross the conductors the emf is in the opposite direction.

The magnitude of the induced voltage is directly proportional to the strength of the magnet and to the number of conductors. If the strength of the magnet remains constant and the coil of wire remains constant, then the amplitude of the alternating current will also remain constant.

The frequency at which the current (also the emf) alternates is determined by the rate at which the magnet rotates. The United States standard electrical wall current alternates 60 times per second, that is 60 cycles/second, or 60 hertz.

The NMR signal is produced in a manner very similar to the method described above for producing an alternating current. The rotating magnet used to produce the NMR signal is the precessing net magnetization vector $\overline{M}$ and the conductors are the NMR head, body, or surface coils. In analogy with the AC generator, the magnitude of the NMR signal is directly proportional to the magnitude of $\overline{M}$. The magnitude of $\overline{M}$ is in turn directly proportional to the number of nuclei present (proton density for hydrogen imaging) and the strength of the external field. That is, the tissue magnetization ($\overline{M}$) will be larger at higher field strengths and will thus produce a larger NMR signal. The alternating frequency of the NMR signal will be equal to the precessional frequency of $\overline{M}$.

RELAXATION TIMES AND THE FREE INDUCTION DECAY (FID)

As indicated earlier, in an equilibrium state without the application of a resonant rf pulse, $\overline{M}$ will not be precessing and will be pointed along the B_0 field. Thus in this state, there will be no NMR signal induced into the receiver coils. Following the rf pulse $\overline{M}$ will be tipped from its original direction, producing a transverse component (M_T) of magnetization (see Fig. 59–9). The direction along the B_0 is referred to as the longitudinal direction; the direction perpendicular to B_0 is called the transverse direction. At equilibrium M is all in the longitudinal direction (M_L) and has zero component in the transverse direction ($M_T = 0$).

During a 90 degree rf pulse M_T will begin to increase and M_L will decrease until $\overline{M}$ reaches the transverse plane. At that time M_L equals zero and M_T is equal to $\overline{M}$ (Fig. 59–11, Step 2). In most systems the receiver coils are positioned such that the maximum signal is obtained when M_T is at a maximum. After the 90 degree pulse is turned off, the magnetization will "relax" back to its equilibrium state, during which time M_L will begin to increase and M_T will decrease (Fig. 59–11, Steps 3 and 4) until $M_T = 0$.

Following a 90 degree pulse there will be a maximum signal induced in the receiver coil. However, unlike the AC generator the magnitude of the signal will begin to decrease immediately owing to relaxation until there is no longer a detectable signal. This characteristic signal is called the free induction decay (FID) (Fig. 59–12). The rate at which it decays is related to the magnetic properties of the material (tissue) being studied. Specifically, the FID decay rate is related to how fast the individual nuclei contained in $\overline{M}$ lose their magnetization in the transverse plane. This rate is referred to as the transverse relaxation time, spin-spin relaxation, or simply *T2*. All relaxation phenomena are exponential in time and are therefore specified by the exponential time constant, which is equal to the time it takes the signal to decay to 1/e (37 percent) of its initial value.

For ideal systems and perfectly uniform magnetic fields the rate of the FID signal decay would be equal to the *T2* relaxation rate. Unfortunately, dephasing is accelerated by a non-tissue source of field inhomogeneities caused by imperfect magnets; the result is to cause the FID to decay at a rate faster than the true tissue *T2* (this accelerated rate is called *T2**—*T*-two star). In nonuniform fields, nuclei will experience different field strengths, causing them to precess at different frequencies, resulting in a more rapid loss of coherence than if all were precessing at the same rate.

In the dephasing process due to the nonuniform field some nuclei will precess

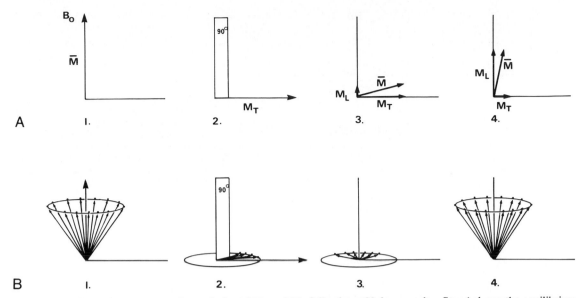

Figure 59–11. A, Steps 1 to 4 show the evolution of M_T and M_L following a 90 degree pulse. Step 1 shows the equilibrium state with $M_T = 0$ and $M_L = \overline{M}$. In Step 2 following the 90 degree pulse, $M_T = \overline{M}$ and $M_L = 0$. Intermediate times (Steps 3 and 4) show the recovery of M_L and the corresponding decrease of M_T. B, Steps 1 to 4 illustrate that $M_T = 0$ before the application of the 90 degree pulse because of the uniform distribution of the individual magnetic moments about B_0. Following the 90 degree pulse (Step 2) the nuclei will be moved to the transverse plane and will also be in phase resulting in a nonzero M_T. As time evolves, M_T will once again begin to diminish as the individual nuclei come out of phase and return to the same equilibrium state (Step 4). The rate of dephasing in the transverse plane is referred to as T_2 relaxation. The rate of magnetization recovery in the longitudinal plane, which is also present but generally occurring at a much slower rate, is referred to as T_1 relaxation.

faster and some slower and will soon fan out in a uniform pattern in the transverse plane (Fig. 59–13).

A measure of true tissue *T2* thus must remove the effects of inhomogeneities in the magnetic field. This is accomplished by the use of the spin-echo technique. When applied properly, the spin-echo technique is a specific set of rf pulses (pulse sequence) that allows the NMR signal to be analyzed to yield true *T2* rather than *T2**.

The spin-echo sequence is initiated by a 90 degree pulse, followed by a delay time (t) and then a 180 degree pulse (Fig. 59–13c, d). The length of the delay determines the extent to which the FID will have decayed. The effect of the 180 degree pulse is to rotate all of the individual nuclei about the transverse axis, placing the nuclei back into the transverse plane but in reverse order. The result is to put the slower precessing

Figure 59–12. Free-induction decay (FID) following a 90 degree pulse. The signal decays at a rate specified by *T2**. The frequency of the oscillation is equal to the Larmor frequency.

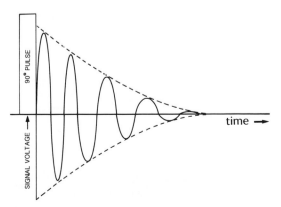

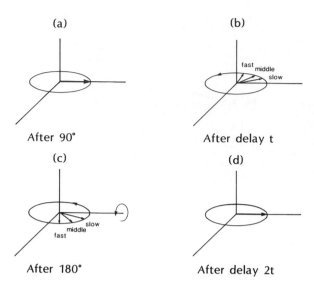

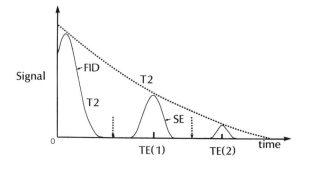

(a)

After 90°

(b)

After delay t

(c)

After 180°

(d)

After delay 2t

Figure 59–13. Magnetization following a 90 degree pulse (*a*). After a delay, *t*, nuclei influenced by different local field strengths will precess at different frequencies (*b*). Following a 180 degree pulse with the proper phase, the individual nuclei will in effect be rotated about the *y* axis, with the result of reversing the order of the individual nuclei (*c*). Nuclei will now rephase at a time equal to 2*t* to give an echo (*d*).

nuclei in front of the faster ones. Since the nuclei are all precessing at a constant (though different) speed, they will all come back into phase at a time after the 180 degree pulse equal to two times the delay time. The rephasing nuclei again regain their transverse magnetization and produce a NMR signal. This signal is called an echo. The shape of the echo is first to increase in intensity up to the time when exact rephasing occurs and then once again to decay with another FID shaped signal as the nuclei once again dephase. The time from the 90 degree pulse to the time of the center of the echo is called the echo time (*TE*). *TE* is equal to two times the delay time (2*t*). An echo signal has been described as back-to-back FIDs.

The spin-echo sequence used to measure true *T2* consists of a single 90 degree pulse followed by a succession of 180 degree pulses, each of which is followed by an echo. Each successive echo amplitude will be smaller, decreasing in an exponential manner. It is this decrease in echo amplitude that is the true *T2* relaxation rate (Fig. 59–14).

The rate of magnetization along the B_0 direction is called the longitudinal, spin-lattice, or simply *T1* relaxation. The *T1* relaxation rate is most often measured using an "inversion recovery" pulse sequence. Again, since $\overline{M}$ is oriented along B_0, there will be no signal produced until we produce a transverse component. Thus, even though we are interested in the rate of change of the magnetization along B_0, we must occasionally use an rf pulse which places the magnetization in the transverse plane just in order to detect the signal. A pulse use for this purpose is called a "measuring" pulse. The inversion-recovery sequence utilizes a series of these measuring pulses.

As the name implies, the inversion-recovery sequence is initiated by a 180 degree

Figure 59–14. Classical spin-echo sequence where the envelopes of the successive echoes are displayed. The peak amplitudes of the echoes are used to determine true *T2*. The decay of the FID is equal to *T2** rather than *T2*.

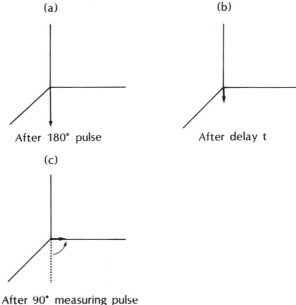

(a) After 180° pulse

(b) After delay t

(c) After 90° measuring pulse

Figure 59–15. Inversion recovery pulse sequence is initiated by an inverting 180 degree pulse (*a*), which leaves the net magnetization oriented in the direction opposite to B_0. After a delay, *t*, often called inversion time (TI), the magnetization will begin to recover to its equilibrium state along B_0 (*b*). In order to measure the remaining longitudinal component, a 90 degree measuring pulse must be applied to move M_L into the transverse plane where a FID will be observed (*c*). The initial amplitude of the FID signal will be proportional to M_L.

pulse, which serves to invert the magnetization vector into the negative B_0 direction (Fig. 59–15). As time elapses the nuclei will begin to reorientate to their equilibrium state, in which there is a slight excess orientation in the positive B_0 direction. At some point during the recovery to the equilibrium state there will be an equal number of nuclei in the inverted and positive B_0 direction. In this case there will be no net magnetization of the sample and thus no signal regardless of measuring pulses.

If after the initial 180 degree inverting pulse one delays a time (*t*) and then applies a 90 degree measuring pulse (Fig. 59–15*c*), the remaining longitudinal magnetization will be rotated into the transverse plane, where an FID will be observed. The magnitude of FID will depend upon the delay time and the longitudinal relaxation rate. If a series of experiments are carried out of the variety:

$$180° - t_N - 90° - \text{delay},$$

where t_N implies N different experiments with N different delay times, a plot of the signal amplitude versus t_N yields an exponential function. The time constant of this exponential function is defined as *T1* (Fig. 59–16).

Figure 59–16. A plot of M_L versus the inversion time (TI) delay for two different tissues with different *T1* relaxation rates. The inversion time that yields the best contrast separation between the two types of tissues can be chosen from plots such as these.

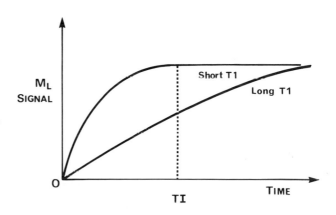

M_L SIGNAL

Short T1

Long T1

O

TI

TIME

THE NMR SPECTRUM

So far we have discussed how a signal is produced in the case of identical nuclei precessing at the Larmor frequency. If other nuclei present in the sample are subject to different field strengths, either because of an external "gradient" used for spatial encoding or because of internal local field variations, the FID will no longer oscillate at a single frequency. It will instead be a sum of many FIDs, all with different frequencies. To unravel this complex signal waveform, a mathematical calculation called a Fourier transform is carried out on the composite signal. The result of this mathematical transformation is the spectrum of frequencies that went into making up the composite "time-domain" signal. The "frequency-domain" representation that results tells us both what frequencies were present (which can be used to tell us where the nuclei are located, since each spatial location will produce its own unique Larmor frequency) and how much of each nucleus was present (reflected by the amplitude of the signal at each frequency).

The ideas presented in this chapter should serve as a basis for understanding the extension of NMR techniques to the study of multinuclear samples (spectroscopy) as well as to NMR imaging. NMR spectroscopy comes about by selecting only the unique Larmor frequency of the nuclei of interest and thus tuning out all the others or alternatively by using "broad-band" pulses to tune in everything and Fourier transforms to sort out which nuclei are present and in what quantities.

As mentioned previously, imaging is achieved by causing nuclei located at different spatial locations to have different resonance frequencies by deliberately producing a nonuniform field. Of particular note, the use of linear gradient fields for this purpose was first used for imaging by Dr. Paul Lauterbur in the early 1970s. It was this early pioneering event that moved NMR out of the chemistry laboratory and into the world of diagnostic imaging.

Suggested Readings

Crooks LE, Kaufman L: Basic Physical Principles. *In* Margulis AR, Higgins CB, Kaufman L, Crooks LE (eds): Clinical Magnetic Resonance Imaging. San Francisco, Radiology Research and Education Foundation, 1983.

Curry TS, Dowdey JE, Murry RC: Nuclear magnetic resonance. *In* Christensen's Introduction to the Physics of Diagnostic Radiology. 3rd Edition. Philadelphia, Lea & Febiger, 1984, pp 461–503.

Goble AT, Baker DK: Elements of Modern Physics. New York, The Ronald Press Company, 1962.

Mansfield P, Morris PG: NMR Imaging in Biomedicine. New York, Academic Press, 1982.

Partain CL, Jones JP: Physics of magnetic resonance. *In* Taveras JM, Ferrucci JT (eds): Radiology: Diagnosis, Imaging, Intervention. Philadelphia, JB Lippincott, 1986.

Partain CL, Patton JA: Magnetic resonance imaging systems. *In* Taveras JM, Ferrucci JT (eds): Radiology: Diagnosis, Imaging, Intervention. Philadelphia, JB Lippincott, 1986.

Segre E: Part II: The Nucleus. *In* Nuclei and Particles. WA Benjamin, Inc., 1964, pp 187–251.

NMR Chemical Principles

M. ROBERT WILLCOTT

The phenomenon of nuclear magnetic resonance (NMR) demonstrated by Purcell, Pound, Bloch, and Hansen in 1946 was immediately important to physicists. Within a decade, chemists discovered that an NMR spectrum, obtained from a small volume of highly homogeneous solution, could help to solve a wide variety of chemical problems. In the late 1950s and 1960s, diverse branches of chemists came to rely on NMR spectroscopy to elucidate molecular structure. Two developments in the early 1970s greatly enhanced the power of NMR spectroscopy for solving complex and intricate chemical and biochemical problems: very homogeneous and intense magnetic fields produced by superconducting solenoids, and the application of Fourier transform techniques for data acquisition and manipulation. These improvements in instrumentation and experimental techniques established high-resolution NMR spectroscopy as a ubiquitous tool for chemical structural analysis. These advances did not, however, make analyses easier; rather they increased the accuracy, scope, and amount of information available. By the end of the 1970s biochemists were able to make meaningful NMR studies of inhomogeneous material, that is, biological tissue, by dividing tissue samples into small regions (voxels) and displaying the results as an image. At present, bulk NMR properties of biological tissue (spin density [SD], $T1$ and $T2$) are determined for voxel arrays; in the future, more subtle NMR properties as determined by high resolution NMR spectra will be obtained for each voxel.

Supplementing NMR imaging with NMR spectroscopy adds a whole new dimension of available information to in vivo biochemistry studies. In addition to noninvasively accessing the biochemistry of human tissue, one can also study biochemical dynamics. NMR spectroscopy provides qualitative differences between normal and diseased tissues, information that is simply unavailable in NMR imaging.

NMR IMAGE

An NMR image is a collection of voxels with varying signal strengths that are displayed on the CRT as pixels with varying shades or colors. A two-dimensional medical image is a digital representation, i.e., a pixel by pixel representation of the NMR signal strength within a plane of voxels (no signal means no picture; lots of signal results in a bright picture). A pixel is a picture element or two-dimensional shape. A voxel is a volume element or three-dimensional shape which has a particular spatial location with reference to the magnet (n units up, n units back, n units left or right). A collection of voxels that produce varying signal strengths makes up the completed three-dimensional NMR image. The difference between adjacent voxels provides the basis for image interpretation. If there were no differences, an image would be a solid color or shade.

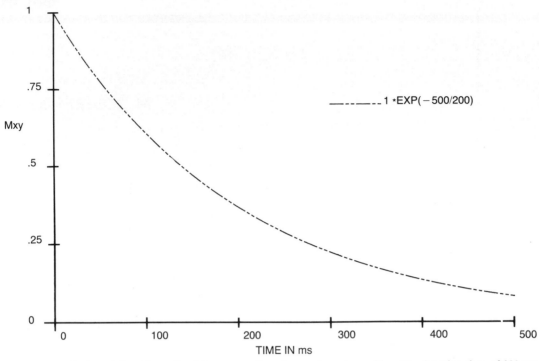

Figure 60–1. A plot of signal intensity, M_{xy}, versus time for a spin system with a *T2* relaxation time of 200 ms.

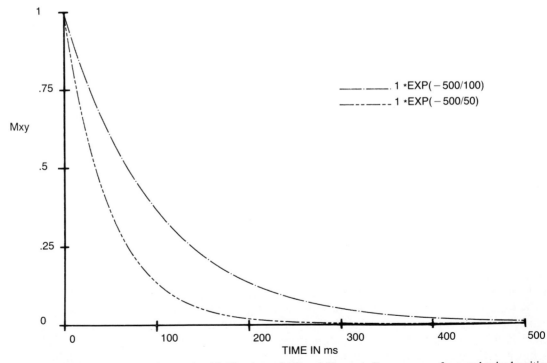

A

Figure 60–2. Differential behavior of 2 voxels with *T2* values of 100 and 50 ms. *A*, Decay curves for equal spin densities. *B*, Decay curves for greater spin density associated with long *T2* value. *C*, Decay curves for lesser spin density associated with long *T2* value.

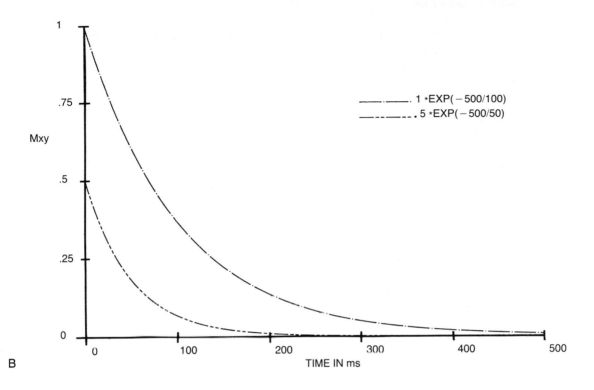

B

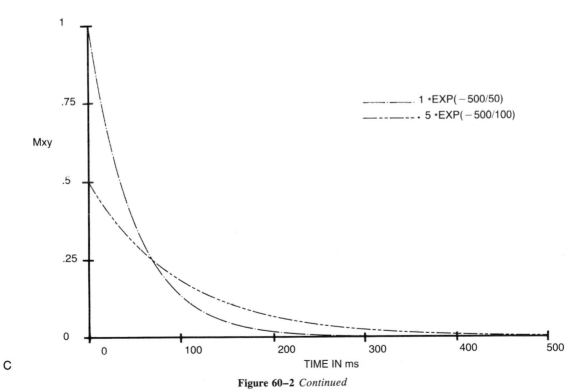

C

Figure 60–2 *Continued*

NMR Parameters

Every voxel can be characterized by a set of NMR parameters: spin density (SD) and time constants, *T1* and *T2*.

Spin density represents the total number of resonating hydrogen nuclei within the sample. SD varies in simple, linear terms, i.e., 1 unit yields a signal; two units double the signal, and so on.

T2 is an intrinsic relaxation time. *T2* does not have an obvious, direct precise relationship with signal intensity, i.e., doubling *T2* does not double image brightness. Indeed, *T2* can cause subtle changes in the NMR image. The curve representing the decay of the signal with time is defined as $M_0 e^{-t/T2}$. The value of the expression can be calculated on most pocket calculators by determining $t/T2$ (where t equals the time after excitation and *T2* equals the relaxation time constant), changing it to the negative, and punching the "exp" key. Figure 60–1 represents this definition.

Even though *T2* is an intrinsic property of the sample, the time (t) after excitation at which the measurement is made does bias the measurement. The biased measurement can best be illustrated by comparing two voxels: voxel *A*, which has a long decay time, $T2_A$, and voxel *B*, which has a short decay time $T2_B$. In the first case, the two voxels have the same SD.

Figures 60–2*A, B,* and *C* show three different cases. Decay curves in the upper trace (*A*) show equal spin densities and *T2* values of 50 and 100 ms. At any time (*t*) shown on the *x* axis, the ratio of the M_{xy} values describes the contrast between the two decay curves. By 500 ms this contrast is maximal, even though the total intensity is quite low.

Analysis of spin density interaction depicted in Figures 60–2*B* and *C* takes two forms. (1) Contrast increases constantly with time (*B*), and (2) contrast reverses with time (*C*). In Figure 60–2*B*, the 100 ms $T2_A$ value curve starts at a spin density (M_{xy}) of 1, while the corresponding spin density for the 50 ms $T2_B$ curve starts at a spin density of 0.5. In the case with the longer *T2* value, the intensity of the voxel is always greater than the intensity of the voxel with the shorter *T2* value. The contrast is again maximal at 500 ms; however, the signal intensity is reduced.

Figure 60–2*C* shows the complexity of this analysis. The curve with the 100 ms $T2_A$ has a spin density of 0.5 while the 50 ms $T2_B$ has a spin density of 1. In this case, the intensities of the two voxels are equal at around 60 ms; therefore, there is no contrast. More important, the contrast reverses from this point, that is, the brighter voxel before the point of equal contrast intensity becomes the darker voxel after passing this point.

Thus generalizations about *T2* behavior must be carefully qualified. Despite the *t* bias, *T2* provides reliable, significant information on which clinical diagnoses can be made. The history of NMR imaging attests to the veracity of the information.

The other relaxation time, *T1*, is also an intrinsic property. *T1* is the time constant associated with the polarization of the nuclei in an NMR observation. Hydrogen nuclei in the *T1* NMR study influence the interpulse delay T_R, such that T_R shows up as *T1* effect. In particular, the recovered magnetization available at the start of each pulse sequence is given by:

$$M_Z = M_0(1 - e^{-TR/T1}) \tag{1}$$

As with *T2*, this expression can be evaluated on a hand-held calculator. It is significant that when T_R is much longer than *T1*, the magnetization available for observation, M_Z, is maximal. For short T_R (compared to *T1*), the signal is minimal.

SD, *T1*, and *T2* characterize all voxels. The contrast in any NMR image is the result of the interaction of these parameters. Chemists and biologists find *T1* and *T2* information to be inadequate, i.e., hard to understand, incomplete, and/or unrelated to problems in their particular disciplines. Instead these scientists use chemical shift as a more accurate and complete picture of molecular structure.

This chapter provides a cursory overview of NMR spectroscopy and the information it adds to each voxel's description without attempting an in-depth explanation of complex theories and applications.

SPECTROSCOPY

NMR spectroscopy of hydrogen provides important medical and chemical information because all hydrogen nuclei do not in fact have the same resonant frequency. A hydrogen atom responds according to its chemical environment, i.e., hydrogen nuclei in H_2O are not identical to hydrogen nuclei in C_6H_6. In general, the effect of one proton on the resonance of another proton or group of equivalent protons depends on the number and kind of intervening chemical bonds and on the stereochemical relationships of interacting groups. An NMR spectrum is a plot (intensity versus frequency) of the chemical shift and the effects of coupling constants.

Chemical Shift

Chemical shifts refer to the differences in absorption-line positions (single or multiple resonance peaks appear at characteristic ''slots'' on the spectrum) for the same kind of nuclei located in different molecular environments. Chemical shifts originate in the diamagnetic and paramagnetic shielding effects produced by the circulation of bonding and nonbonding electrons in the neighborhood of the nuclei. These effects are directly proportional to the magnitude of the applied field H_0. In practice, the magnitude of a chemical shift is always taken with reference to a standard. The customary, external (to the sample) reference standard for protons has been the resonance-line position of water protons, and the internal reference is tetramethylsilane mixed with laboratory samples.

Coupling Constant J

Fine structures appear on many resonance peaks as a result of the small magnetic interactions that occur between the nuclei of neighboring atoms. Coupling constant J represents the distance expressed in hertz (Hz) between the adjacent peaks of a multiplet. For a particular multiplet, the distances between peaks are the same. Unlike chemical shifts, coupling constants are independent of the magnetic field strength. While coupling constants may seem to make a precise spectrum messy, they enable the spectroscopist to interpret variances and to ascertain precisely what is responsible for the complicated absorptions.

HIGH RESOLUTION NMR SPECTROSCOPY

Making high-resolution NMR spectroscopy meaningful to a diverse group of scientists, physicians, and technicians who seek to employ it as an investigative tool in their respective areas requires broad explanations. Traditionally, a nuclear magnetic resonance spectroscopist has been a scientific specialist who produces, measures, and interprets electromagnetic spectra—the frequency range versus the intensity of electromagnetic waves absorbed within the sample being investigated. The author's approach, selected illustrations, and thought patterns are those of an NMR spectroscopist with thirty years of experience in the field, the last ten of which have concentrated on applications within a medical setting.

Before setting out on this task, a back-to-the-future idea for making NMR spectroscopy even more exciting might be the following. Suppose each voxel were very small (less than the dimension of a cell) and we could obtain a high resolution NMR spectrum for all individual voxels of a human organism simultaneously. Then by carefully orchestrating the data, we could understand in detail how the entire human organism functions at the molecular level. Unfortunately, the time for such a wonderful observation is still on the horizon. In the meantime, a thorough knowledge of NMR spectroscopy in 1988 will bring us all closer to realizations of the future.

Anyone intending to become a nuclear magnetic resonance imaging practitioner should spend as much time as possible learning the fundamental concepts. Expectations will be realistic, and results will be meaningful. Collecting NMR data and interpreting NMR images will become easier, more informative, and perhaps more diagnostically rewarding. NMR observations can be made by an investigator who ignores the underlying mathematics that govern the process. However, the investigator who chooses this mode of operation is at peril, and in the long run, doing so would be as effective as hiring a cricket bowler to be the new star pitcher on a professional baseball team. It can indeed be done, but with no real expectation of success.

A few fundamental expressions or concepts serve as building blocks in the construction of a comprehensive foundation for high-resolution NMR spectroscopy, which is a discipline with few short cuts. Each concept has a well-defined mathematical form, and most have equally informative graphic interpretations or representations. We will show the mathematical form in all but one case, and we will explain precisely what can be learned from the solution of these mathematical expressions.

Fourier Transform

Presentation of essential mathematics begins with the range of transformations employed in the modern practice of NMR spectroscopy. The Fourier transform (FT), a mathematical algorithm for relating two functions, is an essential tool for understanding a wide assortment of principles and techniques, which include communications theory, image processing, some thermodynamic properties, FT NMR spectroscopy, NMR imaging, single crystal diffraction processes, and seismic exploration, among others. The first and perhaps most fundamental transformation involved, notwithstanding the expressions that govern nuclear spins, etc., is the Fourier transform integral, known also as the Fourier transform or FT. The continuous FT of a function $f(t)$ is given by the following, where ω = frequency and t = time:

$$F(\omega) = \int_{-\infty}^{\infty} f(t)e^{-i\omega t}\, dt \qquad (2)$$

Because we cannot feed a continuous function into a digital computer, we sample the function at discrete points and use an approximation to the FT known appropriately as the discrete Fourier transform (DFT). In the following equation, N is the total number of data points, v is the sampling frequency, and F_v is the frequency domain spectrum.

$$F_v = \sum_{t=0}^{N-1} f_t e^{-2\pi i v t/N} \qquad (3)$$

Sampled or digitized data is collected using the FT algorithm, which is then transformed using a discrete Fourier transform. FT NMR spectroscopy captures a data set in the time domain, and the Fourier transform converts the data to the frequency domain or a spectrum (Fig. 60–3.) The information in the two data sets is equivalent, but interpreting sampled data is assuredly easier in the frequency domain.

Two very logical questions may arise. Why take the trouble of employing a seemingly complicated transform to make a spectrum? Why not simply collect the data in the frequency domain to begin with and forget the complicated mathematics? For twenty-five years, NMR spectrometers collected data in the frequency domain using continuous wave (cw) radiofrequency (rf) excitation. However, when it was demonstrated that pulsed rf excitation followed by data acquisition using the Fourier transform saves from 10- to 100-fold the time of the first method spectroscopists quickly adopted the method.

The Fourier transform is not limited to converting time and frequency. Any set of data can be Fourier transformed to yield a new set of data, and the inverse Fourier transform may then be performed to regenerate the original data. Some operations, such as convolution, can be performed more efficiently on the transformed data, and the process will alter the properties of the original data in useful ways. As an example, a representation in direct space can be Fourier transformed to give the same data in reciprocal space and then multiplied by some function to enhance the image—the convolution operation. Inverse Fourier transformation then recovers the image in direct space. In this case the recovered image will not be an exact replica of the original image; instead, it is an image in which faulty focusing has been corrected; edges have been enhanced, or other improvements have been effected.

Heisenberg Uncertainty Principle

The Heisenberg uncertainty principle, a property derived from the time-frequency Fourier transform pair, states that increased precision in frequency determination re-

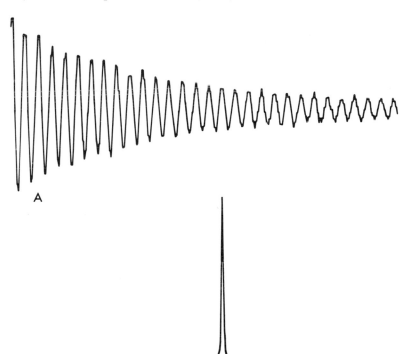

Figure 60–3. Examples of Fourier transformation applied to a simple spin system. *A*, A time domain signal of an exponentially decaying sine wave, or free induction decay. *B*, The frequency domain plot of the Fourier transform of the signal in the trace above.

quires longer observation times. A number of common examples make this principle clear. Even people with a keen ear for music cannot exactly identify a musical note by hearing only a short burst of the tone. However, listening to a tone for several seconds leads to certain identification of the frequency. In FT NMR spectroscopy, the same is true. Gathering data for only 100 ms limits both time and frequency information content. If a time domain NMR signal is observed for only a few ms, the frequency domain definition will be in 100 hertz (Hz) steps. The precision of frequency specification improves considerably when data is acquired for several seconds, i.e., data obtained for several seconds will provide exquisite NMR detail at resolution of 1 Hz or less.

Bloch Equations

The phenomenologic description of magnetic resonance is based on a coupled set of differential equations known as the Bloch equations. Even though the symbols seem complicated, an intense study session with the Bloch equations will provide the reader an excellent insight into the behavior of spins in the imaging experiment.

$$dM_x/dt = \gamma(M_y H_0 + M_z H_1 \sin \omega t) - M_x/T2,$$

$$dM_y/dt = \gamma(M_z H_1 \cos \omega t - M_x H_0) - M_y/T2, \tag{4}$$

$$dM_z/dt = \gamma(M_x H_1 \sin \omega t + M_y H_1 \cos \omega t) - (M_z - M_0)/T1$$

In 1946, Bloch published these equations within a few weeks after his announcement of the discovery of "nuclear induction," which has come to be known as nuclear magnetic resonance. The most remarkable feature of this set of three coupled differential equations is their clarity of exposition. Bloch's description of the NMR phenomenon has withstood the test of time. In addition to providing the background for understanding most NMR experiments conducted since 1946, the Bloch equations are applicable to other areas of physics. Scientists compare the power of these equations to the powerful Maxwell's equations, which relate electric and magnetic fields to electric charges and currents.

Graphical solution of the Bloch equations takes two forms, the laboratory frame of reference, too complex to be of general use, and the commonly utilized rotating frame of reference, shown in Figures 60–4 and 60–5, respectively.

Even though these frames of reference are alien to many, the clarity of the Bloch equations removes their mystery and enables NMR newcomers to understand both NMR and NMR imaging with facility. Describing the motion of the simple carousel commonly found in an amusement park illustrates the laboratory and rotating reference frames. A description of the motion of a given horse on that carousel from a vantage point off the carousel (like a revolving sinusoid of sorts) is relatively complicated and represents a situation analogous to that posed by the laboratory frame of reference.

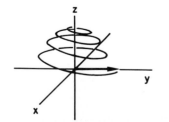
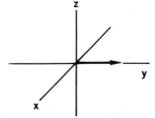

Figure 60–4. Laboratory frame of reference used in NMR discussions.

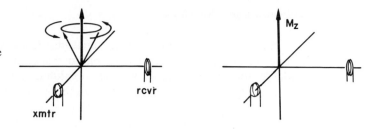

Figure 60–5. Rotating frame of reference used in NMR discussions.

The description of the same horse's motion from a vantage point on the carousel is a linear up and down trajectory. Rotating frame experiments are easier to comprehend and are equivalent to describing nuclear magnetic resonance events in the more complex laboratory frame of reference.

Three terms of the Bloch equations have particular significance: two time constants ($T1$ and $T2$) and a term H_1, the applied external rf field. These three terms effectively permit the observer to move a magnetic vector in space and follow its subsequent observation under multiple conditions. Bulk magnetization behavior is completely specified by solving the Bloch equations illustrated by Figures 60–4 and 60–5.

The laboratory frame of reference in Figure 60–4 is an ensemble of vectors coaligned in the direction of the applied magnetic field, and H_0 represents the net magnetic moment of the sample. These vectors are precessing or rotating about the axis of the H_0 field at the Larmor or resonant frequency of the nuclide under observation. Applying an external rf field, H_1, has the effect of tipping these vectors into the xy plane, where the magnetization can be detected by the receiver coils. The precession does not cease when the ensemble is tipped from the z axis; instead, it continues to precess at the Larmor frequency. The transverse or spin-spin relaxation time constant, $T2$, governs the loss of signal received, while the longitudinal or spin-lattice relaxation time constant, $T1$, governs the re-establishment of equilibrium magnetization.

In the rotating frame of reference, Figure 60–5, the entire coordinate system rotates at the Larmor frequency, which has the effect of "freezing," vectors making their description considerably simpler, as described in the carousel analogy.

Scalar Couplings

Solving the Bloch equations by numerical integration is useful when dealing with only one frequency, like water in a biological system; however, mathematical solutions become cumbersome when a number of different nuclei are considered simultaneously. The NMR description of organic compounds requires that nuclei types be sorted and specified by their chemical shifts. For example, three different regions of rf energy absorption are in the proton or ^{1}H-NMR spectrum of a simple molecule like ethanol, C_2H_6O. In the ethanol molecule, there are two different ^{13}C frequencies and a single ^{17}O signal with individual resonance frequencies which are quite far removed from the proton's signal. Signal intensities in the proton NMR spectrum also reveal the relative numbers of atoms from which they are obtained, in the intensity ratio array $1:2:3$. Incorporating the three frequencies or chemical shifts into the Bloch equations gives a quick prediction of the spectrum's appearance. However, the predicted patterns will be in sharp contrast to the actual spectrum. Scalar couplings (J) between the nuclei in any given molecule are manifested in the spectrum as splittings of the resonance frequencies. These splittings and other complications of NMR spectra constitute additional gauges for structure determination and require a framework for their utilization.

Schroedinger Equation

Employing the Schroedinger equation, easily implemented on digital computers, is now so routine that most investigators are unaware that they are performing formidable matrix operations as they evaluate a high resolution NMR Hamiltonian. McConnell recognized quite early that the solution of the Schroedinger equation:

$$H\psi = E\psi,\tag{5}$$

where the Hamiltonian operator, H, is chosen for high-resolution magnetic resonance, gave an exact prediction of the NMR spectrum for a given set of NMR parameters. The spectrum that is computed from an estimated set of parameters will, however, be similar but not identical to the experimental one shown by the example in Figure 60–6. Both spectra are correct but represent different situations; one is estimated, while the other is observed.

A variety of schemes exist for adjusting the parameters in the calculation so that a better agreement can be reached between experimental and calculated spectra. The spectroscopist certifies the match as good enough when the error is about the level of the experimental uncertainties. At the very least, he will have found a set of NMR parameters, chemical shifts, and coupling constants which used in conjunction with the Schroedinger equation will replicate the experimental spectrum. While there is no logical assurance that these parameters must be correct, they are considered correct.

Mathematical computations that rely on frequencies and intensities of spectral lines to describe the spectrum result in a calculated spectrum that is or is nearly superimposable over the experimentally determined spectrum. Comparison of the calculated spectrum obtained in this manner with the experimentally determined spectrum assumes that all lines are essentially equal in shape and have the same width at half height. Both of these assumptions are likely incorrect because dynamic events at the molecular level can cause substantial deviations from the "equal line shape and half-width" condition. Resolving this problem in a pragmatic match of calculated and experimental spectra is more complex than calculating the simple spectrum.

Density Matrix

The density matrix, a sophisticated and computationally demanding device, elucidates spectral line shapes and dynamic events. In certain selected cases, solution of the density matrix is straightforward. Analytical expressions derived from the density matrix treatment of a two particle, spin $\frac{1}{2}$ system, i.e., ^1H, reduce to a statement of the Bloch equations. Analytical expressions for larger spin systems are much more cumbersome, and finding them is regarded as an intractable problem.

Ernst's analysis of multidimensional nuclear magnetic resonance spectroscopy is the most exciting use of the density matrix. This new technique differs from conventional spectroscopy in that an individual resonance may be defined as a function of two frequencies, $S(F_1, F_2)$. It is possible that there may be cases that can be defined as functions of more than two frequencies, but this discussion is limited to two dimensions. Two-dimensional Fourier transform nuclear magnetic resonance (2DFT NMR) is significant because it correlates the two dimensions, F_1 and F_2, in chemically interesting ways. At a very simple level, the chemical shifts of carbon atoms can be matched with the fine structure caused by directly bonded hydrogen atoms, as shown in Figure 60–7.

The partial two-dimensional spectrum shown in Figure 60–7 seems overwhelming, but taken step by step it becomes quite meaningful. The *x* axis along the bottom of the

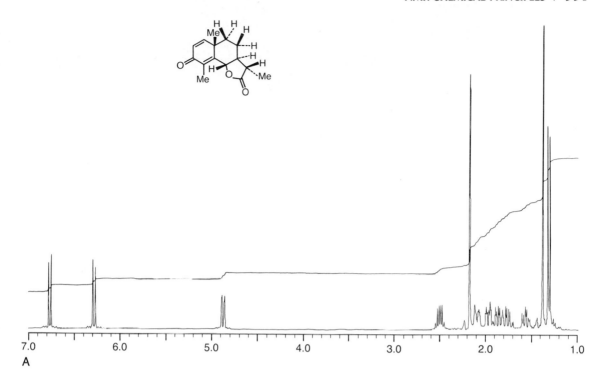

A

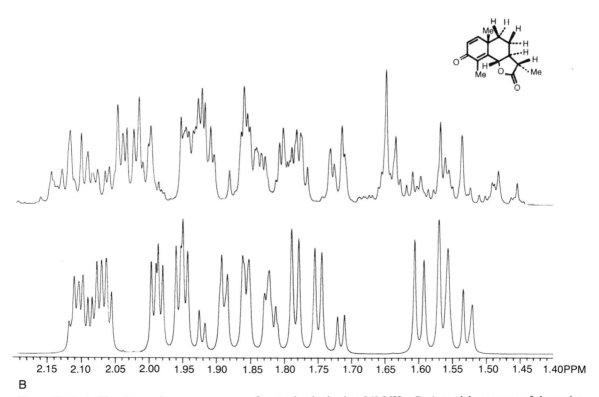

B

Figure 60–6. *A*, The observed proton spectrum of santonin obtained at 360 MHz. *B*, A partial spectrum of the region between 1.4 and 2.2 ppm generated by solution of the Schroedinger equation.

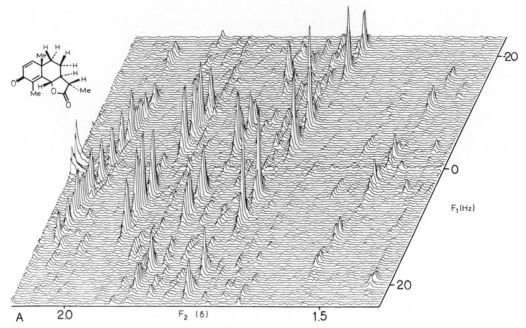

Figure 60–7. *A*, A two-dimensional spectrum displayed as a three-dimensional map of the aliphatic hydrogen atoms in santonin.

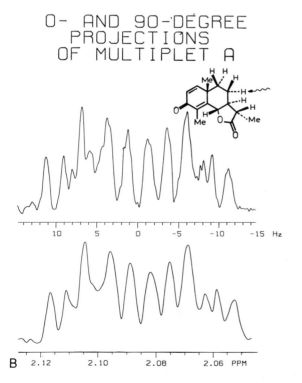

Figure 60–7. *B*, A profile through the signals at 2.2 ppm showing fine structure due to proton interactions.

plot is a chemical shift scale (ppm referred to tetramethylsilane), while the y axis is a J or scalar coupling dimension. The "mountain tops" depict the intensities of interactions between J and chemical shift. The inordinate visual interpretation problem can be reduced by exhibiting profiles (Fig. 60–7B) of all fine structures shown for a given chemical shift. Interpretation is now more straightforward.

Sorting fine structure by chemical shift reveals the functionality of all carbon atoms as methyl, methylene, etc. The spectrum itself can be understood without recourse to the density matrix, but details of experimental conduct require the density matrix. A much more interesting correlation in 2DFT NMR occurs when the directly bonded carbon atoms are correlated by way of their two-quantum transition behavior. Even though the structural meaning of this experiment can be made clear to any scientist in a matter of minutes, no readily understood physical description exists. A full and proper understanding of the origins of the observations must come from the density matrix. Likewise, the same is true for NMR imaging. Technicians can all make images with a turn-key commercial system, but all accomplished NMR imge practitioners will have to revert to the underlying mathematics in order to understand properly the remarkable pictures, to improve image quality, and to increase information content even more.

Two-dimensional NMR can lead to a correlation of the conventional NMR signal with a geometric co-ordinate of the sample or image. A two- or three-dimensional image using NMR spectroscopy will be obtained with an efficient, polished technique, such as a two- or three-dimensional Fourier transform zeugmatogram. Implementing this technique to perform a three-dimensional study at the console of a computer/spectrometer may be several years away. This delay offers the advantage of giving current practitioners time to assimilate and understand appropriate mathematical and physical concepts.

High-Resolution NMR Spectra

As an indication of the practical results expected by demanding NMR spectroscopists, we will now present some of the spectra associated with high-resolution nuclear magnetic resonance spectroscopy. The santonin molecule, used as an illustration earlier in this chapter, illustrates the uses of high-resolution NMR. A spectrum of santonin at 470 MHz emphasizes the sensitivity of a very high field spectrometer operated in the Fourier transform mode. A modern spectrometer can detect very small amounts of material and very small amounts of impurities without bias. The spectrum of the same compound santonin can be studied over a range of frequencies such as 360 MHz and 150 MHz to reveal the detailed appearance of the spectrum in the aliphatic region.

It is possible to see that most hydrogen resonances are all distinct at 470 MHz, i.e., they have different intrinsic chemical shifts. Even so, there are still some overlapping lines, a feature that can easily cause the novice to wonder if NMR spectroscopy is really a useful tool. Computer enhancement (sharpening) of the resonance lines alters the spectrum cosmetically without altering the information content. The sharpest resonances in this spectrum approach 0.05 Hz in width or 1 part in 10^{10} of their resonance frequency. Furthermore, spectroscopists can ascertain frequencies of the individual lines to the same degree of precision.

At 360 MHz, the overlap of some spectral patterns occurs as in Figure 60–8C, but a sharp-eyed observer can still see sufficient detail to understand both the spectrum and the structure of the santonin molecule. When the same study is conducted at 150 MHz (Fig. 60–8B), the overlap of lines, changes in intensity, and overall appearance are sufficient to disguise the spectral and structural information even for an expert.

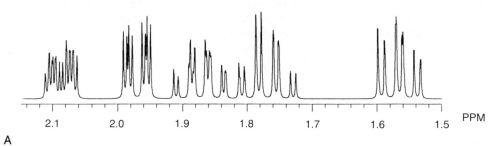

A

Figure 60–8. *A*, Calculated santonin spectrum as it appears at 470 MHz.

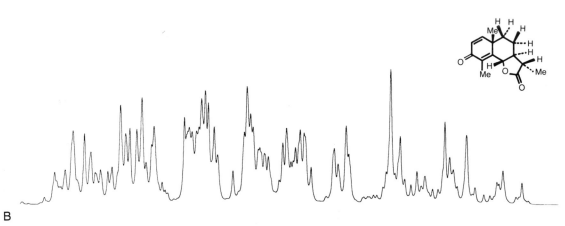

B

Figure 60–8. *B*, Calculated santonin spectrum at 150 MHz.

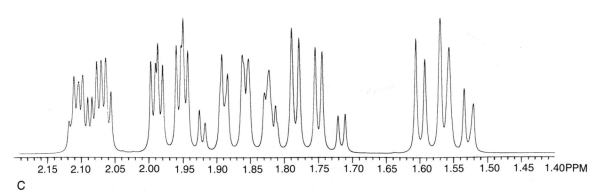

C

Figure 60–8. *C*, Calculated santonin spectrum at 360 MHz.

Hence, the prevalent notion of "high field is better," which originates with spectroscopy, is being extrapolated to NMR imaging.

A water spectrum (not shown) points out two experimental problems. The first problem is that the water resonance is so intense that it completely overwhelms most of the other resonances contained in the spectral window. The second problem is the dynamic range; dilute signals are also displayed in the same spectrum. The basis for the problem is concentration. Water is 110 M with respect to hydrogen, while biologically interesting molecules are micromolar in concentration. One can easily extrapolate this result to water in living systems. The water resonance in the spectra of biological materials dwarfs the materials of the cell structure. Furthermore, the diversity of biological molecules found in living systems will appear at all frequencies as a continuum in which no content distinction can be confirmed.

The chemical shift is a function of a variety of physical causes such as pH, cell structure, tissue type, temperature, or other influences. One expects the spectrum of a simple homogeneous biological sample to be a water line with a chemical shift that is constant to within a few tenths of parts per million (ppm). In a complicated heterogeneous sample, the chemical shift varies from voxel to voxel by more than a part per million, that is, the spectrum actually shifts. This spectral characteristic, the shift, is especially important to imaging because the imaging process sorts geometrical co-ordinates by frequency. If the chemical shift or frequency changes, the image will become blurred. Good experimental design will minimize, but will not eliminate, this bothersome complication of the chemical shift.

In summary, the practice of high-resolution NMR spectroscopy parallels the practice of NMR imaging; each is a well developed technique and discipline. In good cases, we can understand nearly every spectral feature in structural terms. Generally, the more detailed spectrum requires greater effort to interpret but provides a better understanding and an enhanced comprehension of the study subject. The more spectral information we want to decipher in geometrical space, the harder we will have to work. Spectroscopists will continue to concentrate on water, treating its chemical shift as invariant. As time progresses and methods become more sophisticated, NMR spectroscopy will probe deeper and deeper into the precise chemistry of living systems. The future of NMR imaging is bright indeed.

Suggested Reading

The intellectual development of NMR for physics, chemistry, and biochemical and medical applications employs a common thread of NMR theory adapted to specific applications followed by one or more seminal books in the specialty. The author routinely refers to the books on this list. The list includes personal preferences and is by no means comprehensive. Any reader thoroughly interested in medical applications of NMR, both present and potential, will find that these readings form the basis of an interesting professional library.

Abragam A: The Principles of Nuclear Magnetism. New York, Oxford University Press, 1961.
  Simply the best NMR account ever written! WARNING: This is a very rigorous book and not suitable for leisure reading.

Advances in NMR: New York, Academic Press. An annual series from 1965 to present.
  The series, edited by John Waugh, presents reviews of specialized topics in NMR, often prepared by the chief proponent of a technique or viewpoint. The quality is consistently high. Some articles have already become classics of NMR literature. Of special interest is the single volume from this series by Mansfield and Morris, which is listed separately here.

Bax A: Two-Dimensional Nuclear Magnetic Resonance in Liquids. Delft, Holland, Delft University Press, 1982.
  An account of two-dimensional NMR for the specialist. Applications are to chemistry; however, the same two-dimensional techniques are and will be applicable to medical imaging in the future.

Chodorow M, Hofstadter R, Rorschach H, Schawlow A (eds): Felix Bloch and Twentieth-Century Physics. Rice University Studies 66:3, 1980.
  A festschrift for Bloch on his 75th birthday. This volume is not widely known. The authors provide a

unique overall view of Bloch's impact on physics and emphasize the fact that NMR was but one of Bloch's outstanding contributions to science.

Farrar T, Becker E: Pulse and Fourier Transform NMR. New York, Academic Press, 1971.
A concise introduction to the use and understanding of Fourier transform techniques in NMR with frequent reference to organic chemistry.

Mansfield P, Morris P: NMR Imaging in Biomedicine, Supplement 2. Advances in Magnetic Resonance. New York, Academic Press, 1982.
The volume in the Advances in Magnetic Resonance Series which is most pertinent to medical imaging.

Pople J, Schneider W, Bernstein H: High-resolution Nuclear Magnetic Resonance. New York, McGraw-Hill, 1959.
This is a comprehensive account of the experimental device and the intellectual background of NMR in 1959. Applications are shown to illustrate the general utility of NMR in chemistry.

Roberts J: An Introduction to the Analysis of Spin-Spin Splitting in High-Resolution Nuclear Magnetic Resonance Spectra. New York, W. A. Benjamin, Inc., 1962.
A companion volume to Roberts' NMR listed below, this introduction to the quantum mechanical formulation of nuclear spin states and transitions successfully shows how the knowledge and careful use of quantum mechanics lead to greater interest, skill, and understanding of NMR spectra in chemistry.

Roberts J: Nuclear Magnetic Resonance. New York, McGraw-Hill, 1959.
This brief textbook, which demythologizes the role of NMR in chemistry, has enabled many organic chemists to become comfortable with the principles of NMR.

Slichter C: Principles of Magnetic Resonance. Heidelberg, Springer-Verlag, 1978.
This second edition coupled with the first edition leaves little to the imagination of the reader. The broad brush approach to NMR has considered all of the interactions likely to be seen in any NMR measurement, with an emphasis on organized states, liquid crystal, crystal, and solid.

Weuthrich K: NMR in Biological Research: Peptides and Proteins. Amsterdam, North-Holland Publishing Company, 1976.
This comprehensive account of NMR, and its application to peptides and proteins, shows how the technique is becoming suited to the explanation of subtle problems in molecular biology.

61

Physics of the MR Image: From the Basic Principles to Image Intensity and Contrast

JEROME P. JONES

Magnetic resonance imaging (MRI) is probably the most complex of all currently available imaging modalities. In addition to rather formidable physics, there are considerable economic pressures. MR imagers are a multimillion dollar expenditure in a climate of cost containment efforts, so high throughput is needed (to keep costs per patient down) while still providing the desired clinical information. Although MR imaging is very sensitive to some diseases (e.g., multiple sclerosis), it has also been shown that lesions appear most clearly on a few pulse sequences, less clearly on others, and not at all on still others. When no lesions are observed for a patient with suspected pathology, one must choose between (a) no lesions present, (b) lesions present but not detectable by MR, and (c) lesions present and detectable with the proper sequence. If this last possibility is acted upon, one must then find the proper sequence in a reasonable time. Thus, economic, physics, and medical questions must all be considered in order to work out the clinical role of MR imaging.

This chapter will confine itself to physics, tracing the entire imaging process with as little mathematics as possible. The goal is to give the reader sufficient background to deal with the problems that will arise in the clinical service, especially the fundamentals of image contrast and how it can be manipulated.

As a gross overview, MR imaging involves the placement of the subject in a strong and highly uniform magnetic field to align the atomic spins. A radiofrequency (rf) magnetic field is then applied, which rotates the spins of the atoms to be measured (normally hydrogen) away from their equilibrium direction. The signal they emit as they realign (also rf) is measured, and gradient magnetic fields are switched on and off in a prescribed way to determine how much of the (measured) total signal comes from each point in the subject. Thus, each image pixel contains a number proportional to the amount of signal emitted from it at the time of measurement. Its value depends upon the concentration of rotated atoms at that location and upon how quickly the atoms realign; these factors are described by the spin density and two realignment parameters called the *T1* and *T2* relaxation times.

THE STATIC MAGNETIC FIELD

The large magnet is designed to produce a powerful, highly uniform and unidirectional magnetic field within the imaging volume. This magnet's field creates a much weaker field in the subject; the subject's field will point either in the same direction (paramagnetic) or the opposite direction (diamagnetic) as the magnet's field.

The subject's field is the sum of atomic fields throughout the imaging volume. As a general rule, each atom has three intrinsic fields: an electron orbital field, an electron spin field, and a nuclear spin field. The magnitudes of these fields vary from one atomic species to another, and one or more of these fields can be zero. In general, the electron orbital field is diamagnetic, while both spin fields are paramagnetic. The overall properties of the sample depend upon which field predominates, but most substances are diamagnetic.

The magnetism of each atom is permanent, but without the magnetic field, thermal energy and atomic collisions result in random orientation of the atoms and hence no net field from the subject. The magnet's field imposes a slight amount of order upon this chaos; at any instant, an extra one atom per million will be aligned along the magnet's field. Thus the subject's field is far weaker, but disturbing its equilibrium and monitoring its realignment are the fundamental operations of all MR studies.

LARMOR PRECESSION

The basic kinematics of a weak magnetic field out of alignment with a strong one is Larmor precession. The motion is very analogous to that of a spinning top in a gravitational field; in fact, there are so many similarities that a discussion of the top is in order.

If a top is inclined at an angle to the vertical and released, its response will be one of two possibilities. If the top is not spinning, it simply falls over. If the top is spinning, it does not fall over; instead, its axis rotates smoothly around the direction of the earth's gravitational field (the vertical) with its angle to the vertical not changing. The rate of rotation depends upon the mass and shape of the top, its spin rate, and less evident, the strength of the earth's gravitational field.

If a weak magnetic field is somehow inclined at an angle from a strong one and then "released," the situation is virtually the same. The motion of the weak field depends upon whether or not a spin or other angular motion is associated with it. If the atoms making up the weak field have no spin, then the weak field simply aligns itself directly (analogous to the top falling over). If the atoms do have spin, the weak field precesses around the strong field at a steady rate, with the angle between them remaining fixed. The rate of precession depends upon the spin, the mass of the spinning atom, etc., and upon the magnitude of the strong field. All the atomic properties are lumped together into a constant called the gyromagnetic ratio, and the rate of precession, f_L, is given by:

$$f_L = (2\pi)^{-1}\gamma B_0 \text{ revolutions/sec} \tag{1}$$

where f_L is called the Larmor frequency, γ is the gyromagnetic ratio, and B_0 is the magnitude of the strong field. Figure 61–1 shows the geometry for the Larmor precession of the subject's magnetic field $\overline{M}$ about B_0. The tip of $\overline{M}$ traces out a circle parallel to the xy plane, rotating clockwise when viewed from above. The projection of $\overline{M}$ onto B_0, called the longitudinal magnetization, M_L, remains absolutely constant during Larmor precession. The projection of $\overline{M}$ onto the *xy* plane, called the transverse magnetization M_T, remains constant in magnitude but rotates clockwise around the *xy* plane. Both these components figure prominently in MR, as will be shown.

The gyromagnetic ratio is not a fundamental constant that can be calculated from first principles; it is measured empirically. In principle, there is a gyromagnetic ratio for each of the three general atomic fields, provided each field has an associated angular

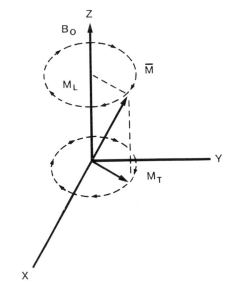

Figure 61–1. The Larmor precession geometry. $\overline{M}$ traces out a circle parallel to the xy plane; its component M_L remains fixed, while the other component M_T traces out a similar circle in the xy plane. The motion is clockwise when viewed from above.

momentum. Both electronic ratios are found to be about 1000 times larger than the nuclear ratio, and all vary somewhat from one particular type of atom to another. So for each type of atom in B_0, there is a single Larmor frequency for each of the electronic and nuclear fields, provided each has a defined gyromagnetic ratio. Thus Larmor precession is potentially a highly selective motion of the atoms, provided one can somehow tip their magnetic fields away from B_0.

SPIN FLIP

This tipping is called the spin flip; it is actually a second Larmor precession perpendicular to the first. However, it is not completely straightforward, as illustrated in Figure 61–2. A third magnetic field B_1 is introduced orthogonal to both B_0 and $\overline{M}$. B_1 is much stronger than $\overline{M}$, much weaker than B_0, and for the moment, stationary. $\overline{M}$ begins a Larmor precession around B_1, which pulls it out into the yz plane away from B_0. But as soon as $\overline{M}$ pulls away from B_0, B_0 starts pulling $\overline{M}$ into a Larmor precession around it. Since B_0 is stronger than B_1, B_0 wins, and $\overline{M}$ rotates toward the xz plane. As it gets closer to this plane, B_1 pulls down on $\overline{M}$ less vigorously and tries to push $\overline{M}$ back to the yz plane more vigorously. When $\overline{M}$ reaches the xz plane, the push of B_1 is entirely parallel to the y axis, and as $\overline{M}$ breaks the xz plane, B_1 begins pushing $\overline{M}$ back up toward B_0 (as well as pushing back against the direction of $\overline{M}$'s motion). By halfway around, B_1 is pushing $\overline{M}$ entirely back toward B_0, and a similar effect follows the rest of the cycle. The net effect is that there has not been a sustained pulling of $\overline{M}$ away from B_0; $\overline{M}$ only wobbled around B_0 a little.

The reason B_1 failed to produce a spin flip was that B_0 pushed $\overline{M}$ toward B_1; as $\overline{M}$ approached B_1, the force between them also changed, leading only to a wobble. From the geometry, a sustained pulling of $\overline{M}$ away from zero can occur only if B_1 is always perpendicular to $\overline{M}$, and a simple way to assure this is to make B_1 rotate in the same direction as $\overline{M}$, and at the rate f_L. This is also indicated in Figure 61–2. With B_1 rotating at this rate, $\overline{M}$ remains perpendicular to it while Larmor precessing around it at the rate:

$$f_{sf} = (2\pi)^{-1}\gamma B_1$$

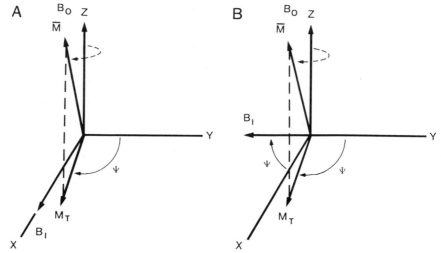

Figure 61–2. The spin flip effect. *A*, B_1 is stationary along the *x* axis. It pulls $\overline{M}$ clockwise away from the *z* axis, but B_0 also pushes $\overline{M}$ toward the *xz* plane. M_T has rotated through the angle ψ, changing the angle between B_1 and $\overline{M}$ (and hence the force on $\overline{M}$). *B*, B_1 has been rotated at the same rate as M_T; this keeps the angle between $\overline{M}$ and B_1 fixed, and hence the force on $\overline{M}$ is the same, pulling $\overline{M}$ away from B_0 even further.

where f_{sf} is the spin flip precession rate. If B_1 does not rotate at the rate f_L, or if it rotates in the opposite direction at any rate, B_1 and $\overline{M}$ will not remain perpendicular, and the result will be a wobble of $\overline{M}$ rather than a sustained spin flip. When B_1 is rotating at the rate f_L, B_1 is said to be in resonance with $\overline{M}$, meaning that the two motions are perfectly timed so that both can occur without interfering with each other.

Since the gyromagnetic ratio differs between electronic fields and nuclear fields, and varies from one type of atom to another, each of these particular fields can be selectively spin flipped while the others only wobble a little. That is, a B_1 rotating at the f_L for hydrogen nuclei will flip them but have little effect upon other nuclei or upon any electronic fields. Thus the choice of the rotation rate of B_1 allows one to study resonance effects in nuclear (called NMR) or electronic (called ESR and EPR) magnetic fields. All MR imaging to date has been NMR because nuclear gyromagnetic ratios give f_L values in the 1 to 100 MHz range (rf), while electronic ratios give f_L values 1000 times greater (microwave range), which have far too many technical problems for imaging. In addition, almost all NMR imaging has been with hydrogen because of its high natural abundance in tissues. Both carbon-12 and oxygen-16 have high natural abundance but they have no spin, and hence no Larmor precession or spin flip. Almost all other nuclei are present in the body in concentrations too small for routine imaging; sodium-23 and phosphorus-31 are of great interest and do have spin, but sodium images have been coarse, and phosphorus has not been imaged.

The last topic for this section is how to generate a magnetic field rotating at the prodigious rate of 1 to 100 million revolutions per second. As with many MR techniques, this is accomplished in a simple but indirect way. One first realizes the mathematical identity that any sinusoidal magnetic field can be thought of as the sum of two rotating fields. Each rotating field has a constant magnitude of one half the sinusoid's amplitude and rotates at a rate equal to the sinusoid's frequency; their only difference is that they rotate in opposite directions. This is illustrated in Figure 61–3, where the reader can test the relationship at various points through the cycle.

This is used with the knowledge that all alternating currents are sinusoidal and produce a sinusoidal magnetic field of the same frequency. By merely sending an al-

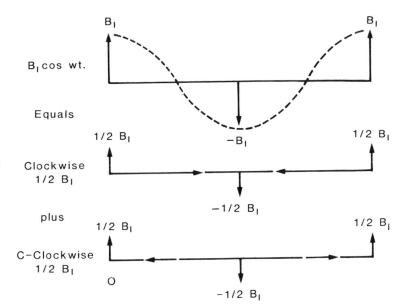

Figure 61–3. An illustration of the decomposition of a sinusoidal wave into two rotating vectors of constant magnitude, equal to half the amplitude of the sinusoid, and rotating in opposite directions.

ternating current through a coil of wire at frequency f_L, a B_1 is produced that varies sinusoidally at that frequency. Half this power rotates clockwise and causes the spin flip, while the other half rotates counterclockwise and only wobbles $\overline{M}$ a little bit (and is essentially wasted). Then if B_1 is turned on for a time t and switched off, $\overline{M}$ will rotate to an angle away from B_0 given by:

$$\theta = (2\pi)^{-1}\gamma(\tfrac{1}{2})(B_1)t \text{ revolutions} \qquad (2)$$

where θ/t equals the spin flip frequency (f_{sf}). If B_1 and t are chosen so that $\theta = \tfrac{1}{4}$ revolution, then B_1 is called a 90 degree pulse. If $\theta = \tfrac{1}{2}$ revolution, then B_1 is called a 180 degree pulse. Flip to any angle is possible, but 90 degrees and 180 degrees are the primary angles used in MR imaging. Other angles can be advantageous in spectroscopy, but their use in imaging has been limited.

It should be noted that reality is not as simple as Equation (2) suggests. Any B_1 pulse contains many frequencies; it is impossible to produce a finite pulse with precisely one frequency. Therefore, the $\tfrac{1}{2}B_1$ must refer to the amplitude of that portion of the pulse having frequency f_L. While this is often used, there are further problems, especially in imaging. They come about because a frequency very near f_L will cause $\overline{M}$ to spin flip, but not as far as Equation (2) predicts, since the resonance is not perfect. Essentially, these frequencies are producing a large-angle but very slow wobble of $\overline{M}$, which does not cancel itself out before B_1 is turned off. The practical result is that Equation (2) is not fully accurate, and 180 degree and 90 degree pulses must be adjusted empirically.

SIGNAL DETECTION

Actual settings for B_1 and t are deduced from the observed signal, which is detected by electromagnetic induction. Figure 61–4 illustrates the idea, which can be set up as a demonstration experiment. A bar magnet (the stronger, the better) is rotated about its short axis, and a detector coil is placed just beyond the end of the magnet (A). As the magnet rotates, the changing field produces a weak current in the coil, which may be displayed on an oscilloscope. The frequency of the alternating current is equal to

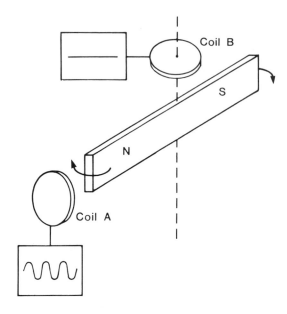

Figure 61–4. A rotating bar magnet with a coil placed at position *A*. The current induced by the coil is the sinusoid displayed below it. A coil in position *B* shows no current, as indicated by the flat line.

the frequency with which the magnet is rotating, and the amplitude of the current is proportional to both the strength of the magnet *and* its rotation frequency. If the coil is moved above the magnet to position B, little or no current is observed because the field of the bar magnet is not sweeping across the coil; it is simply rotating in the plane of the coil. Thus, the largest signal is detected for high rotation rates, strong magnets, and the detector coil (called a pickup coil) oriented perpendicular to the plane of rotation and as near the magnet as possible.

During Larmor precession after a spin flip, the rotation of $\overline{M}$ is similar to this rotating magnet; its component perpendicular to B_0, known as M_T (see Figure 61–1), is exactly like the rotating bar magent. Thus, a pickup coil oriented with its plane parallel to the yz plane will have a weak alternating current produced by the rotation of M_T. MR imagers use fancier coils than this to assure uniform sensitivity throughout the imaging volume, but otherwise, this is their principle of operation. Since the rotation ratte of M_T is f_L, it is even possible to use the same coil for generating the B_1 pulse and detecting the current produced by M_T. Some systems operate in this way, but most use separate transmit/receive rf coils.

To adjust the B_1 pulse to make it a 90 degree pulse, one simply observes that a 90 degree pulse produces the largest M_T possible (equal to $\overline{M}$). Then trial and error adjustment of B_1 and t to give the largest current amplitude in the receive coil gives the 90 degree pulse settings, with some care taken to assure that this is not a 270 degree pulse, or 450 degree pulse, etc. Similarly, a 180 degree B_1 pulse should have approximately twice the amplitude or duration as a 90 degree pulse and produce no current in the receive coil. In practice, the magnitude of B_1 and t are finely adjusted until minimal current is observed in the receive coil. The sharpness of these settings depends upon, among other things, the shape of the B_1 pulse; a sharp, rectangular pulse (called a hard pulse) contains many frequencies and can be difficult to set properly. A more rounded pulse (called a soft pulse) contains fewer frequencies and is more easily set.

The signal number actually stored by the system for image construction is the amplitude of the detected current (or a number proportional to the amplitude). Despite many complications, the end result is that the contents of a pixel are proportional to the amplitude of current produced by the precessing M_T at that point in the imaging volume.

TUNED CIRCUITS

The electronic circuitry used to produce the B_1 pulse and measure the subject's response is tuned circuitry similar to a radio tuner. The tuning is to the frequency f_L because the most intense transmission and greatest receiving sensitivity should be at this frequency. In addition, other frequencies should be transmitted as weakly as possible, with minimal receiving sensitivity.

The principles behind tuned circuits can be illustrated with the simple LRC series circuit of Figure 61–5. It contains an alternating current voltage source, an inductance L, capacitance C, and resistance R, all in series. The resistor is a passive circuit element, but L and C are active in that the impedance they offer depends upon the frequency of the alternating current voltage. More importantly, L and C oppose each other, and at just the right frequency, cancel each other out. This frequency is called the resonant frequency of the circuit and is given by the expression shown. If one then measures the amplitude of alternating current in this circuit as a function of alternating current frequency, the curve of Figure 61–5 results. The current is far larger near the resonant frequency because the cancellation of L and C leaves less impedance (only R) in the circuit. The circuit is said to be tuned to its resonant frequency, and its Q value expresses how sharply peaked this response curve is. Note that both Q and the value of the resonant frequency depend upon L and C.

The ideal, clearly, is to make Q as large as possible and make this circuit resonant at frequency f_L—the Larmor frequency of the subject. The process of assuring that this is so, as well as properly adjusting the 90 degree and 180 degree pulses, is referred to as tuning the rf circuitry.

Two problems arise. The presence of the subject inside the rf coil changes the inductance and capacitance of the circuit by an amount dependent upon the size of the subject, and at higher rf frequencies, B_1 may be attenuated within the subject. The first problem, called loading, is not so difficult to correct. It moves the resonant frequency of the circuit away from its proper value of f_L, so that most of the transmitting power and receiving circuitry are tuned to the wrong frequency. If uncorrected, noisy, displaced, and distorted images will result. Fortunately, a simple frequency check and (less simple) Q check will allow adjustment of variable capacitors and/or inductors to offset the effects of the subject. This correction should be made for each subject, and with most imagers, is a simple step. Attenuation of B_1 is a more difficult problem because there is no adjustment of frequency, power, or duration of B_1 that can correct

Figure 61–5. The frequency response of a series LRC circuit. The current peaks at the resonant frequency; the resonant frequency divided by the full width at half maximum (FWHM) is Q, a measure of the sharpness of the peak. Q can also be related to the values of R, L, and C as shown.

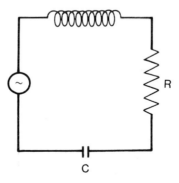

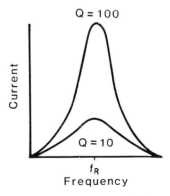

$$f_R = (2\pi)^{-1}(LC)^{-1/2}$$
$$Q = (2\pi R)^{-1}(L/C)^{1/2}$$
$$Q = f_R/\text{FWHM}$$

for attenuation; the spin flip of deep atoms will simply be less than that of atoms at the surface, so one simply adjusts the 90 degree pulse for most signal and the 180 degree pulse for least signal. If there is too much attenuation, accurate spin flips will be impossible, and image degradation will be severe. This is one limitation to high-field imaging of hydrogen and offsets the advantage of higher signal strength in stronger magnetic fields.

RELAXATION

Following a spin flip, $\overline{M}$ does not stay at its flipped position. Atomic collisions, local electric and magnetic fields, and other atomic motions combine to make $\overline{M}$ lose energy and realign with B_0. The realignment process is called relaxation, but it is not a simple realignment, nor is it a spin flip in reverse. It is a completely different process in which atomic magnetic fields exert their influences atom by atom.

During a spin flip, $\overline{M}$ retains a constant magnitude because B_1 is present throughout the imaging volume, making the atoms flip in a more or less coordinated movement. During relaxation, B_1 is absent, so with nothing to coordinate their movement, the atoms realign more chaotically. In fact, $\overline{M}$ seems to lose its identity altogether, making description focus on M_T and M_L.

During relaxation, M_L grows from its spin-flipped value toward an equilibrium value of $\overline{M}$ in a fully relaxed sample. The rate of relaxation is *assumed* to be proportional to the difference between M_L's current value and its equilibrium value at full relaxation. Mathematically, this is the same as observed for a hot body's temperature as it equilibrates with its surroundings, so the growth of M_L is sometimes ascribed to the "cooling" of "hot" spins. The time constant of this relaxation is called *T1*, and the growth of M_L is also referred to as *T1* relaxation. Another common term is spin-lattice relaxation, but the reason for this terminology is irrelevant to MR imaging.

At the same time, M_T decreases to zero as it rotates at the rate f_L around the *xy* plane. In the same way, its rate of decrease is *assumed* to be proportional to the difference between the current magnitude of M_T and its equilibrium value of zero. The time constant of this relaxation is called *T2*, and the decay of M_T can ideally be called *T2* relaxation. Another common term is spin-spin relaxation, but this terminology is also irrelevant to MR imaging. (However, these terms can be helpful in some spectroscopic applications.) For MR imaging, one needs to remember only that *T1* describes the growth of M_L (specifically *T1* is the time for M_L to grow from zero to 63 percent of its equilibrium value), and *T2* describes the decay of M_T (the time for M_T to fall to 37 percent of its initial value).

It should be clear that the coil current during relaxation is due entirely to M_T; M_L makes no contribution. Figure 61–6 shows the coil current following a 90 degree pulse; the oscillations are caused by the rotation of M_T, and their decreasing amplitude is due to the decay of M_T. This particular decay is called a free induction decay (FID), and

Table 61–1. ANGULAR SEPARATION BETWEEN TWO MAGNETIC FIELDS ROTATING AT A DIFFERENCE OF 1 PPM AT 10 MHz

$\Delta\phi = (\Delta w/w)\,(wt)$ (revolutions)	t (milliseconds)
0.1	10
0.2	20
0.3	30
0.4	40
0.5	50

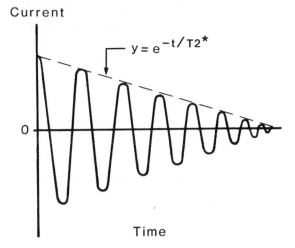

Figure 61–6. An FID. The current peaks decrease as a single exponential, but its time constant is called $T2^*$.

its decreasing amplitude does follow the form of a pure $T2$ decay. However, the time constant is not called $T2$. This complication comes about because $T2$ should be a purely atomic property, while experience shows that the decay of the FID depends upon the specific system being used, even if all else is constant. To denote this property, the decay of the FID is usually called $T2^*$ decay.

The explanation of $T2^*$ decay lies in small variations in the strength of B_0, which will vary from one magnet to another. If B_0 were perfectly uniform, the M_T in each point of the imaging volume would rotate in unison with the others at exactly the same rate (f_L). Thus, each will decay by true $T2$ decay, as will their sum M_T. However, a perfectly uniform B_0 is impossible; in MR imagers, a field with variations not exceeding 40 parts per million is considered highly uniform. This 0.004 percent difference at first seems too small to consider, but it has a strong effect. Table 61–1 shows the angular separation of two M_T's rotating at a 1 ppm difference at 10 MHz. Only 50 ms pass before these two M_T's are opposing one another and cancel each other out. Carrying this over to many M_T's in the imaging volume and the more typical 40 ppm nonuniformity makes it clear that the FID decay is due almost entirely to nonuniformities rather than true $T2$ decay.

Figure 61–7 shows an alternative view of the situation. The pixel M_T's are noted with a lower case letter (m_T); initially all m_T are pointing in the same direction. Since they rotate at slightly different rates, they start spreading apart, with the fastest moving

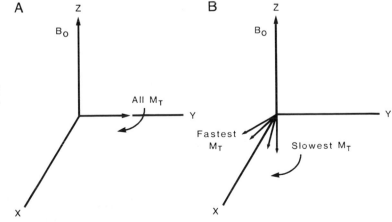

Figure 61–7. The slow spreading of the M_T as they rotate, due to inhomogeneities in B_0.

ahead of the slowest. Note that if the positions of the m_T could be swapped (slowest to the front and fastest to the rear), they would begin moving together at exactly the same rate they spread apart. For an instant they would come together again and then start spreading apart once more. Their sum M_T would actually increase as they came together, reach a peak when they are together, and then decrease once more. At the moment M_T peaks, it will be decreased from its initial value by true *T2* decay during this time, and the effects of nonuniformity will be eliminated.

ECHOES

This swapping is made with a 180 degree pulse; Figure 61–8 illustrates the principle. For clarity, it is assumed that the fastest m_T have not yet lapped the slowest m_T, and the direction of B_1 is through the middle of the pack of m_T's. If the spread of rotation rates of the m_T's is small enough, the 180 degree pulse will rotate them all almost exactly 180 degrees around the direction of B_1. This completes the swap; the coil current then begins growing, reaches a peak when all m_T come back together, and then decreases in another FID. The packet of growth, peak, and decay is called an echo, and another echo can be produced with another 180 degree pulse, and another, and so on, until true *T2* decay reduces all the m_T to zero. A very useful feature of echoes is that if the 180 degree pulses are evenly spaced, each echo peak will occur halfway between successive 180 degree pulses. This simplifies programming of the imager for the echo peak measurement, which will be made at a known time after the 180 degree pulse.

Two complications should be addressed. One is the effect when B_1 is not in the center of the m_T, and the other is why true *T2* decay is not reversed by the same technique. The first can be seen from Figure 61–8 once more; if B_1 were oriented along the $-y$ axis, the fastest m_T would move around B_1 to just short of the $-x$ axis, while the slowest m_T would move to just ahead of (to the right of) the $-x$ axis. This is the desired swap, and an echo will form in the same time as before, and with the same amplitude, though a phase shift will occur (which causes little problem).

The last question is why true *T2* decay does not echo in a similar way as B_0 inhomogeneities. Note that the m_T in this discussion are tacitly assumed to not interact with each other; each nucleus precesses around B_1 independently of the others. This

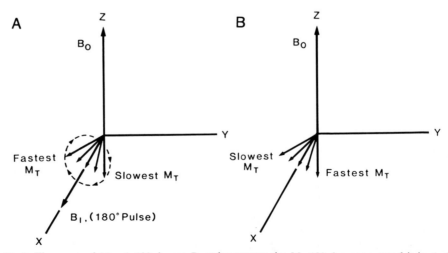

Figure 61–8. The swap of M_T. A 180 degree B_1 pulse rotates the M_T 180 degrees around it in *A*. *B*, B_1 is turned off, and the two M_T are swapped, to begin moving together as they continue to rotate.

means that no energy is exchanged between the m_T, and their spreading can be reversed. True *T2* decay occurs at the atomic level and is due to interactions between the various atomic fields. These fields lose energy as they interact, and this loss cannot be reversed by a 180 degree pulse because the motions of these interacting fields are much more complex than Larmor precession. Therefore, true *T2* decay is due to energy-losing, atom-to-atom interactions and cannot be reversed; magnet nonuniformities are reversible if the fields do not interact.

SPATIAL ENCODING

Since the measured signal is that from the entire imaging volume, some means are necessary to code spatial information into the signal so that the image can be constructed. This begins with Equation (3), which shows that the Larmor frequency is proportional to the magnetic field strength.

$$f_L = (2\pi)^{-1}\gamma B_0 \text{ revolutions/sec} \qquad (3)$$

If it were possible to make B_0 have a slightly different value at each point in the imaging volume, then each point would have a unique value of f_L associated with it. So simply by spin flipping the sample with a broad range of B_1 frequencies and measuring the signal (e.g., the echo) one obtains a current that is the sum of all these frequencies.

Calculating the amplitude of each frequency in a complex signal is possible by the techniques of Fourier analysis. The Fourier transform is the amplitude of each frequency (or the amplitude can be found from it, depending upon exact mathematical definition), so one simply picks a frequency of interest and calculates its contribution to the signal from the Fourier transform equations. In the end, one has a set of Fourier transforms given as a function of frequency; such a data set is sometimes called the spectrum of the signal, but here it represents each image pixel value.

This approach, which requires only one rf sequence and measurement, is not used on any commercial system. The reason is that too much data would have to be handled at once. A full volumetric data set would be $256 \times 256 \times 256$ voxels, each requiring a Fourier transform calculation. Such a vast set would require digitizing the coil current at a faster rate than is now possible, and this scheme would be impossible to upgrade to $512 \times 512 \times 512$ voxels. Finally, the design of the necessary magnetic field would not be trivial because magnetic fields are inherently symmetric. Thus other approaches have been used.

The most commonly used one has been a Fourier transform–based method called the two-dimensional Fourier transform (2DFT) method. It produces tomographic slice images of various possible thicknesses by first limiting the spin flip to only the atoms in the desired slice and then computing the intensity emitted from each pixel in the slice. However, it is not done in a straightforward way.

Slice selection is accomplished by applying a gradient magnetic field at the same time that a B_1 with a narrow range of frequencies is applied. Conceptually, a gradient field is produced using a set of coils as shown in Figure 61–9. The currents in the loops run in opposite directions so that the magnetic field produced by each loop opposes the other. The important property of the total gradient field is that there is some position between the coils where the gradient field is zero (halfway between if each coil carries the same current; otherwise, closer to the coil carrying less current). To the left of this null point, the gradient field points in one direction, while to the right, it points in the opposite direction. Over a range of distances from the null point, the gradient field changes linearly with position, with its slope dependent upon the total current in the two coils. So the strength of the gradient is determined by the total coil current, and

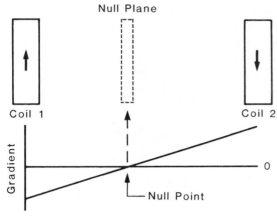

Null Plane

Coil 1

Coil 2

Gradient

0

Null Point

Position between Coils

Figure 61–9. Gradient coils carrying currents in opposite directions (arrows). The fields they produce oppose, creating a plane of no net field somewhere between them.

the null point position is determined by the relative current in each coil; both can be readily controlled.

This gradient is placed in the magnet so that the gradient field is aligned with B_0. Then a very narrow range of frequencies centered around f_L is pulsed (B_1) to produce a spin flip of atoms in a plane centered at the gradient null point. The thickness of the plane will depend upon how narrow the range of frequencies is (high Q circuit) and upon how steep the gradient is; the narrower the frequency range and/or the steeper the gradient, the thinner the slice. Gradients of this type are built into the system for the z direction (direction of B_0) as well as the x and y directions. The z gradient is a pair of loops as described here (called a Maxwell pair), while the x and y gradient coils are more complex (called Golay coils). They produce a gradient field that points in the z direction, but its strength varies linearly with x or y.

With the slice selected, the slice selection gradient is turned off, and other gradients are switched on for the signal read-out. If the gradients could be adjusted so that each pixel in the slice is in a unique magnetic field strength, each would have a unique f_L, and there would be little problem in calculating 256 × 256 or 512 × 512 Fourier transforms for the image. However, no commercial system does this either; they all resort to a tedious data collection scheme that uses both frequency and phase encoding. In the scheme, slice selection is achieved as described above. Then a phase encoding gradient is switched on and back off, followed by a frequency encoding gradient that is left on during signal measurement. The Fourier transform calculation gives a phase-distorted projection of the object, i.e., one distorted line of the image. The sequence is repeated with a different phase encoding, but otherwise all else is the same; the read-out gives the second line of the image. This is continued until all 256 lines are collected; then the phase distortions are removed by an additional Fourier transformation in the phase direction. In general, each line requires about one second to complete, so a typical image takes over four minutes to obtain—a very long time when one considers that anywhere from 10 to 30 images may be required in a typical study.

The role of the frequency encoding gradient should be clear, but the phase encoding is not as clear; in fact, phase itself is often unclear, and what it has to do with imaging is even less clear. Figure 61–10 shows the rotating bar magnet of Figure 61–4 once more, only here the two coils are both located perpendicular to the plane of rotation, but 90 degrees apart (one along the x axis and the other along the y axis). The current observed in each is also shown; it is the same sinusoid with the same amplitude and frequency. Yet the currents are not the same at a given instant of time; the current at the y coil is one-fourth of a cycle ahead of the current at the x coil. This is clearly

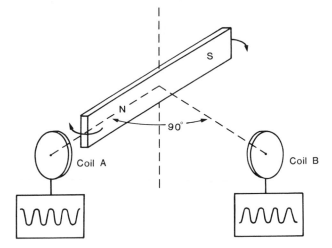

Figure 61–10. Two coils in the transverse plane but located 90 degrees apart. The signals produced have the same amplitude and frequency, but are 90 degrees out of phase.

because the coils are 90 degrees apart, so their physical separation has led to a shift in the currents detected. This shift is called the phase difference, phase shift, or simply the phase; the important point is that the phase shift of the measured current can be related to an angular separation in the xy plane. Note that the same effect would occur if there were only one coil and two noninteracting bar magnets rotating together. If the magnets are separated by 90 degrees as they rotate, the currents produced by them will be 90 degrees out of phase. If the magnets are separated by θ degrees, then their currents will be θ degrees out of phase. Here, the shift in phase of the current gives the angular separation between two magnets rotating at the same rate.

Following a spin flip, all the pixel-by-pixel m_T in the selected slice rotate with the same phase (no phase shift) and at the same rate; they are completely in unison. When the phase encoding gradient is turned on, they begin rotating at different rates depending upon their positions between the phase encoding gradient coils. The line of pixels at the null point is unaffected while lines to either side rotate faster or slower. When the phase encoding gradient is turned back off, all m_T again rotate at the same rate, but they are no longer in unison. There is a constant phase shift from one line to the next due to the difference in rotation rates while the phase encoding gradient was on. The total phase difference between any m_T and the m_T at the null point is proportional to the distance of the m_T from the null point, so one coordinate is coded into the phase of the signal. During read-out, the frequency encoding gradient, orthogonal to the phase encoding gradient, is turned on while the coil current is measured. This gives the position information for each pixel; one coordinate is encoded in the phase, and the other encoded in the frequency. All one needs is the amplitude of each phase and frequency of the coil current, and the image is constructed. Figure 61–11 shows the coordinate encoding for a slice; the y coordinate is determined by the phase (y gradient is the phase encoding gradient) and the x coordinate by the frequency (x gradient is the frequency encoding gradient).

The measured coil current is then the sum of these frequencies and phases. However, Fourier transforms give only the amplitude of each frequency, not the phase. Fourier analysis gives only a single effective phase for each frequency, not the amplitude of each phase at each frequency. More sequences, with different phase encoding in each, must be collected before the image can be constructed. This has been called "sampling the phase distribution,"[3] which is a helpful way to regard it. In essence, the phase encoding gradient is made slightly stronger, and by the same amount, from one sequence to the next. The increment is chosen so that the phase increase at any

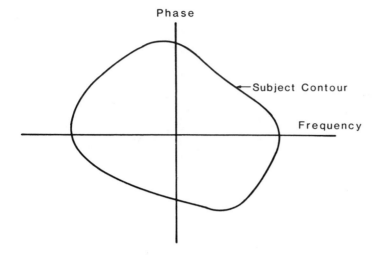

Figure 61–11. Phase encoding is used to determine the *y* coordinate and frequency encoding the *x* coordinate. Note the center corresponds to no phase shift and a frequency f_L because it is at the null point for both gradients.

pixel (other than the null point) from one sequence to the next equals the phase increase from that pixel to the adjacent one on the first sequence. Figure 61–12 may help set this forth more clearly. Pixel *p* has some phase shift relative to the null point on the first sequence; pixel *p* + 1 has a slightly larger phase shift, while pixel *p* − 1 has a slightly smaller one. However, the difference in phase between pixels *p* and *p* − 1 is the same as the difference between pixel *p* + 1 and *p*; i.e., the phase encoding is linear. For the second sequence, the phase encoding gradient is strengthened so that the phase of pixel *p* equals the phase that pixel *p* + 1 had on the first sequence. The third sequence uses a still stronger phase encoding to give pixel *p* the phase that pixel *p* + 2 had on the first sequence, and so on. The Fourier transforms of each sequence measurement are stored line by line in computer memory, so that by the end of the data collection one has an image that is badly phase distorted.

To remove the phase distortion, one notes that each column of data (Fourier transforms as a function of phase for each frequency) describes a complex function of sequence number and phase. Each can be Fourier transformed with respect to sequence number to compute the amplitude of each phase; and when this is done, the phase distortion is removed. The increment of phase encoding must be chosen with some

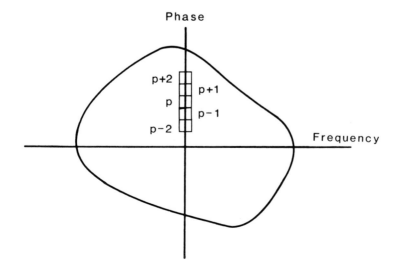

Figure 61–12. The phase encoding of different pixels on the sequences.

care, although this is not the only possible way to "sample the phase distribution." If the increment is too small, the image as constructed in the phase dimension will not cover the range of the imaging volume, while if the increment is too large, the image will be zoomed. Some trial and error adjustment is usually needed to set the increment correctly.

Having to collect repeated sequences causes many problems and is perhaps the weakest feature of MR imaging. First, it simply takes too long, considering the economic and medical pressures. Secondly, the phase encoding produced by the phase and frequency encoding gradients on one sequence must be erased or accounted for on the next sequence to keep the sequences from interfering with each other. This leads to some creative use of gradients; sometimes the read-out gradient is bipolar (i.e., reverses direction) to erase any pulse encoding it might produce, while effects from slice selection and phase encoding gradients are handled in various ways. However, these problems are handled by the vendors in a manner transparent to the user. A third problem is that the signal intensity from each pixel must not be biased from one sequence to the next. It must have the same frequency and same amplitude on each sequence (only the phase varies); this puts some restrictions on the design and use of pulse sequences, but these restrictions are seldom a practical problem.

OTHER ACQUISITION METHODS

The acquisition method just described is called the two-dimensional Fourier transform (2DFT) method and is the basic image construction method. However, the most important methods are probably multislice and multiecho, although three-dimensional methods are of some interest, and projection imaging and gating are also commonly used. Flow imaging is another matter altogether, and discussion of it will be deferred to a later section.

Projection imaging is simply 2DFT without slice selection; it produces a "scout view" of the total thickness of the subject somewhat like a radiograph and can be useful for slice positioning. Otherwise, projection imaging has not proved to be clinically helpful.

The three-dimensional methods are called 3DFT, and they are "simply" an extension of 2DFT to three dimensions. Slice selection is not performed here either; the slice position is phase encoded. So the entire volume is spin flipped, then a phase encoding gradient for the slice position is applied, followed by an orthogonal phase encoding gradient, which is followed by the frequency encoding (read-out gradient). On the next sequence, the first phase encoding gradient is incremented while the second is kept fixed and so on, until the first row of all slices has been obtained. Then the second row of all slices is obtained, then the third, etc., until the data collection is completed. Fourier transformations from slice to slice and along the columns of each slice are required to remove the phase distortions, and care must be taken not to confuse one phase encoding with the other. Two types of 3DFT collections can be made. In isotropic 3DFT, the increments in the two phase encodings are the same, which gives the same resolution in these two dimensions. The reconstructed voxels are then cubes and can be reformatted for any view desired. In anisotropic 3DFT, the slice selection gradient is incremented in larger steps, giving voxels that are thicker than their breadth. While the reconstructed slices have good resolution (and are thick slices), reconstruction of other views suffers markedly from loss of spatial resolution. Neither 3DFT method is in common use because of the time required. If TR is the time per pulse sequence, then the total acquisition time for any sequence is

$$\tau = \text{(number of phase encoding steps)(number of averages)}(TR).$$

For a *TR* of 1 sec with two averages, this is 512 sec ($8\frac{1}{2}$ min) for a 256 × 256 2DFT (256 phase encoding steps × 256 frequencies) and the impressive total of 16,384 sec (273 min or 4.55 hr) for a 256 × 256 × 32 slice 3DFT. Actual 3DFT times are typically 30 to 45 min, however, because *TR*s of 0.25 sec and less are used whenever possible. In addition, interpolation may be used to further reduce the acquisition time. But despite these efforts, 3DFT acquisitions often are just too time consuming to be practical.

This brings one to multislice (MS) acquisition. This is basically a 2DFT, except the next slice is begun while waiting for the first to recover. As many as eight to sixteen slices can be collected in about the time needed to collect a single 2DFT image. Figure 61–13 illustrates all rf excitation, gradient firing, and read-out occurs early in the sequence, so most of the *TR* time is spent waiting for enough *T1* recovery to start the next sequence. MS uses this time to start sequences at other slice positions, one after the other, until the first *TR* period is over. Then the second round is begun, giving the second line of each slice, and the third round gives the third line of each slice, etc., until all slices are completed. Each column of each slice must be Fourier transformed to remove the phase distortion, but no other calculations are needed.

The total acquisition time is slightly more than the time for a single 2DFT with the same *TR*, depending upon how many slices are collected. One limitation of MS is that it is usually better to leave a gap between slices because slice width is not precisely defined; it depends upon the rf band width, degree of tuning, and other factors that blur the slice edges. If the MS collection is made with contiguous slices, some atoms near the boundary between slices might be spin flipped with each other, distorting both images. A relatively small gap is sufficient to assure that this crosstalk will not occur, but this gives an option for the choice of gap size. One can survey a large volume with contiguous slices using two MS acquisitions and a slice gap equal to the slice width, or one can save time using one MS acquisition using slices with a minimal gap (e.g., 2 mm), on the gamble that an abnormality in only the gap will not be overlooked. However this option is handled, MS is a great time saver for examining large volumes, taking roughly the same time of a single 2DFT.

Multiecho (ME) imaging is another great time saver, though it is used for comparing the *T2* relaxation rates of different structures in the image. It takes the same length of time as a simple 2DFT, but the 180 degree pulse is repeated several times to produce several echoes. Figure 61–14 illustrates the process. The slice selection is generated as usual, followed by the phase encoding. An echo is produced and read out, then

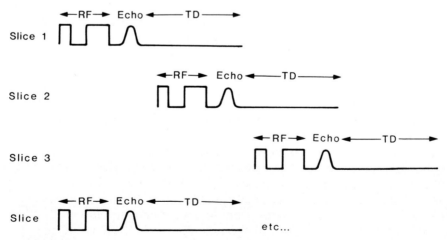

Figure 61–13. SA multislice collection, here showing all *F* for three slices. The additional slices are begun while slice 1 recovers; as many as can have their echo measured before TD on slice 1 elapses can be collected. The actual rf sequence does not matter, so MS is usable for all pulse sequence types.

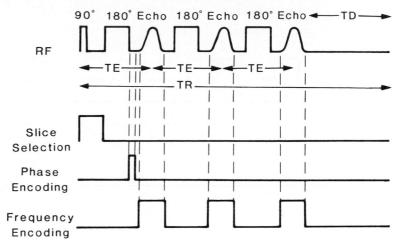

Figure 61–14. A multiecho collection. Each 180 degree pulse produces an echo that is measured. A single slice selection pulse is used, and in this example, a single phase encoding gradient. The frequency encoding gradient (readout gradient) is applied for each echo; any phase encoding that it introduces is erased, however (not shown).

another produced and read out, etc., giving the first row of several successive images. The next sequence gives the second row of these images, and so on, until all are acquired. 2DFT is used to remove the phase distortion from each image, but no further processing is required. The images are all at the same slice location, but they show pixel-by-pixel T2 decay. A structure with a short T2 will darken quickly, while a structure with longer T2 will darken less quickly. This can be helpful in identifying unknown masses, for example. Comparing the T2 decay of the mass with the T2 decay of a known structure will show whether or not the mass has characteristics similar to that of any known structures.

MS and ME can be combined, and this combination sequence is probably the most efficient for routine screening examinations. It allows a survey of the entire imaging volume with several echoes at each slice, all in the same time as for an ordinary 2DFT image. However, the number of usable echoes is sometimes reduced to only two or three because of various hardware restrictions (e.g., memory available, eddy currents produced). Even so, this is still acceptable for a screening, and more detailed examinations can be confined to suspicious areas as indicated.

SIGNAL INTENSITY

The measured signal intensity (more properly, the amplitude of the coil current) is not particularly dependent upon the type of imaging performed (2DFT vs. MS/ME). It is most dependent upon the type of rf pulse sequence used and the time between rf pulses. Numerous sequences have been used in spectroscopy, but imagers have largely been confined to two: spin echo (SE) and inversion recovery (IR); both are diagrammed in Figure 61–15. Of the two, SE is most commonly used because IR sequences usually take longer. However, IR has some important contrast advantages over SE and should not be neglected.

The goal of the next few sections is to compare the contrasts these sequences can produce; this first requires a knowledge of how the signal intensity depends upon the interpulse times, $T1$, and $T2$ for each sequence. Since SE is simpler, it will be considered in detail to illustrate a technique for finding the signal intensity of any sequence.

The SE sequence may be written as $(90° - TE/2 - 180° - TE/2 - \text{measure} - TD)_n$, and the technique will be to determine M_L and M_T at each event in the sequence. This is done in Table 61–2; initially $\overline{M}$ is aligned with B_0, so $M_L = M$ and $M_T = 0$. Following the 90 degree pulse, $M_L = 0$ and $M_T = M$, with both $T1$ and $T2$ relaxation beginning

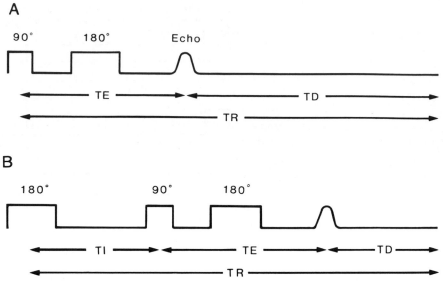

Figure 16–15. Radio-frequency pulses and timing parameters for spin echo (*A*) and inversion recovery (*B*) pulse sequences (this nomenclature follows ACR recommendations). The sketches are not to scale; typically TE is much less than any of the other times, and TR is measured from the center of the first pulse to the center of the first pulse on the next sequence.

and allowed to continue (as an FID) for a time $TE/2$. The relaxation equations are the following (where M equals the magnitude of $\overline{\mathrm{M}}$):[4]

$$M_L(t) = M(1 - e^{-t/T1}) + M_L(0)e^{-t/T1} \tag{4}$$

$$M_T(t) = M_T(0)e^{-t/T2} \quad \text{(true } T2 \text{ decay)} \tag{5a}$$

$$M_T(t) = M_T(0)e^{-t/T2*} \quad \text{(FID decay)} \tag{5b}$$

where $M_L(0)$ is the value of M_L immediately following an rf pulse, t is any time after the pulse, and similarly for M_T. Using Equations 4 and 5b gives the values of M_L and M_T when $t = TE/2$, and the 180 degree pulse serves only to invert M_L, with no effect upon M_T. The time of measurement is at the echo peak, and M_T has the magnitude shown. Since M_T is proportional to the current amplitude, the signal intensity expression can be written as

$$I_1 = kMe^{-TE/T2}$$

where I_1 is the intensity measured on the first sequence and k is a proportionality constant that depends upon the coil. By the end of the sequence, M_T has decayed to the value shown by $T2*$ relaxation, and M_L has grown by $T1$ relaxation.

Since this sequence will be applied repeatedly for imaging (256 times for a 256 ×

Table 61–2. THE FIRST SPIN–ECHO SEQUENCE

Event	M_L	M_T
Start	M	0
90°	0	M
TE/2	$M(1 - e^{-TE/2T1})$	$Me^{-TE/2T2*}$
180°	$-M(1 - e^{-TE/2T1})$	$Me^{-TE/2T2*}$
TE/2	$M(1 - 2e^{-TE/2T1} + e^{-TE/T1})$	$Me^{-TE/T2}$ ⟵ measure
End	$M(1 - 2e^{-(TR - TE/2)/T1} + e^{-TR/T1})$	$Me^{-TE/T2}e^{-TD/T2*}$

256 image), it must produce the same signal amplitude on each sequence; otherwise an intensity gradient will run through the image. This, in turn, requires that both M_L and M_T have the same values at the end of the sequence as at the start. Table 61–2 shows this is little problem for M_T; if TD, the delay time (see Fig. 61-5), is long enough, $T2^*$ decay will make M_T practically zero by the end of the sequence. Most imagers require a TD of at least 50 ms, which is not a restriction, since typical TD values are 500 ms or more.

This is a problem for M_L. The same value will result if TR, the repetition time (see Fig. 61-15), is enough larger than $T1$, but $T1$ values are typicaly 200 to 1000 ms, requiring TR values as long as 3 s. This is simply not practical, and M_L ends the sequence at a value smaller than that with which it started. However, note that M_L is fully relaxed at the start of the first sequence, but only partially relaxed at the end. Since this partial relaxation was recovery from the 90 degree and 180 degree pulses, it will likely give the same partial relaxation on succeeding sequences. Table 61–3 shows that this is true; it follows the second sequence, and M_L does end with the same partially relaxed value with which it started. So if the first sequence is ignored, M_T has the same magnitude on all other sequences, and the signal intensity can be written as

$$I_{SE} = kM(1 + e^{-TR/T1} - 2e^{-(TR-TE/2)/T1})e^{-TE/T2} \tag{6}$$

A similar analysis for the inversion-recovery sequence $(180° - TI - 90° - TE/2 - 180° - TE/2 -$ measure $- TD)_n$ is an exercise in algebra, which gives

$$I_{IR} = kM(1 + 2e^{-(TR-TE/2)/T1} - e^{-TR/T1} - 2e^{-TI/T1})e^{-TE/T2} \tag{7}$$

Both Equation 6 and Equation 7 show the same $T2$ dependence, which is controlled by the choice of TE. Both also show the same M dependence, which cannot be controlled. TR exerts the primary control over $T1$ dependence in Equation 6, although TE does have a small effect, while TI exerts the primary control in Equation 7. In practice, TR is much greater than TE, so both equations can be reduced to

$$I_{SE} - kM(1 - e^{-TR/T1})e^{-TE/T2} \tag{8}$$

$$I_{IR} - kM(1 - 2e^{-TI/T1} + e^{-TR/T1})e^{-TE/T2} \tag{9}$$

For a spin echo image, I is increased if TE is made smaller or TR is made larger. In a given image, a structure will be brighter if it has a larger M, a shorter $T1$, or a longer $T2$. Thus, M and $T2$ have the same direction of effect upon I, while $T1$ opposes them. For an inversion-recovery image, the quantity in parentheses can be either positive or negative. If it is positive, then the dependence upon M, TE, and $T2$ is the same as a spin echo image. In addition, a longer TI, longer TR, or shorter $T1$ produce a larger signal. If the quantity in parentheses is negative, everything reverses. Increasing M and $T2$ decreases I (makes it more negative); decreasing TE decreases I; and longer TI, longer TR, or shorter $T1$ produces a more negative signal. The negative signal does present some problems; it is detected as a 180 degree phase shift (it means that M_L was pointing down rather than up when the 90 degree pulse was applied). Some com-

Table 61–3. THE SECOND SPIN–ECHO SEQUENCE

Event	M_L	M_T	
Start	$M(1 - 2e^{-TR - TE/2)/T1} + e^{-TR/T1})$	≈ 0	
90°	0	$M(1 - 2e^{-(TR - TE/2)/T1} + e^{-TR/T1})$	
TE/2	$M(1 - e^{-TE/2T1})$	$M(1 - 2e^{-(TR - TE/2)/T1} + e^{-TR/T1})e^{-TE/2T2^*}$	
180°	$-M(1 - e^{-TE/2T1})$	$M(1 - 2e^{-(TR - TE/2)/T1} + e^{-TR/T1})e^{-TE/2T2^*}$	
TE/2	$M(1 - 2e^{-TE/2T1} + e^{-TE/T1})$	$M(1 - 2e^{-(TR - TE/2)/T1} + e^{-TR/T1})e^{-TE/T2}$	$\longleftarrow$ measure
End	$M(1 - 2e^{-TR - TE/2)/T1} + e^{-TR/T1})$	$M(1 - 2e^{-(TR - TE/2)/T1} + e^{-TR/T1})e^{-TE/T2} e^{-TD/T2^*}$	

mercial imagers never account for this and always use signal magnitudes. This makes I_{IR} always positive, so that $T1$ always opposes the effects of M and $T2$. Other systems can account for this phase shift, but the correction is sometimes complicated and inaccurate. In principle, $T1$ and TR can be chosen so that M, $T1$, and $T2$ all affect I in the same way, but the procedure is tricky and of very unclear clinical utility.

CONTRAST

Equations 6 and 7 are valid pixel by pixel throughout the image, and signal differences are due to differences in either M, $T1$, or $T2$. Since M is proportional to the number of affected spins in each pixel, it is often called the spin density (or proton density when hydrogen is imaged, since a hydrogen nucleus is a proton). Pixel-by-pixel signal differences are called contrast, and an observed contrast is always due to the sum of spin density, $T1$, and $T2$ differences. However, the sum is a weighted sum:

$$\text{Contrast} = W_M(\Delta M/M) + W_{T1}(\Delta T1/T1) + W_{T2}(\Delta T2/T2) \tag{10}$$

where each W is the weighting factor and the terms in parentheses are the percent differences in M, $T1$, and $T2$ between two given pixels. The values of the W's depend upon the type of pulse sequence and the value of the timing parameters (TE, TR, TI) as compared to $T1$ and $T2$. Analytical expressions for the W's can be derived and analyzed, but the reader will be spared this and simply given the results. For a spin-echo image,

$$W_M = I_{SE} = kM(1 - e^{-TR/T1})e^{-TE/T2} \tag{11}$$

$$W_{T1} = -kM(TR/T1)e^{-TR/T1}e^{-TE/T2} \tag{12}$$

$$W_{T2} = (TE/T2)I_{SE} = kM(1 - e^{-TR/T1})(TE/T2)e^{-TE/T2} \tag{13}$$

Inspection of these equations shows that W_M is largest when TR is large and TE is small, and that both W_{T1} and W_{T2} are virtually zero under these conditions. Such an image is said to be spin density weighted because the contrast is due entirely to spin density differences. $T1$ and $T2$ have no effect. Continuing with W_{T1}, its magnitude is maximum when $TR = T1$ and TE is small. W_{T2} is virtually zero under these conditions as well, but W_M is larger than W_{T1}, as Table 61–4 shows. Structures in an image whose $T1$ is equal to TR and and whose $T2$ is much longer than TE are said to be $T1$ weighted. Note that the *image* is *not* $T1$ weighted; different structures will have different $T1$ values and hence different degrees of $T1$ weighting (the image is said to contain $T1$ weighting). Note also that even with maximum $T1$ weighting, spin density differences carry almost twice as much weight as $T1$ differences. Even so, $T1$ effects are evident in such images; the reason is that spin density differences are themselves small (a few percent) while $T1$ differences are large (up to a factor of 2 or 3).

The last inspection is of W_{T2}; it is maximum when TR is large and $TE = T2$; under these conditions, W_{T1} is virtually zero and W_M is equal to W_{T2}. Note also that as TE further increases, W_{T2} exceeds W_M. However, W_M is rapidly falling to zero, so W_{T2} itself is decreasing as TE increases. Interestingly, the maximum difference between

Table 61–4. WEIGHTING SUMMARY FOR SPIN–ECHO IMAGES

Weighting	Conditions		Contrast
Spin density	$TR \gg T1$	$TE \ll T2$	$kM\,(\Delta M/M)$
$T1$	$TR = T1$	$TE \ll T2$	$0.63\,kM(\Delta M/M) - 0.37\,kM(\Delta T1/T1)$
$T2$	$TR \gg T1$	$TE = T2$	$0.37\,kM(\Delta M/M) + 0.37\,kM(\Delta T2/T2)$

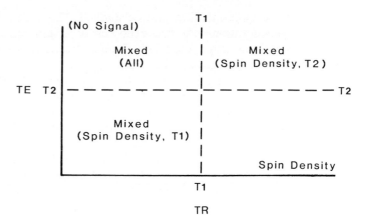

Figure 61–16. Regimes of weightings on the TE-TR plane. The regimes are divided by the *T1* and *T2* values of the structure of interest. Only the lower right quadrant gives regimes where only one parameter dominates the weighting; all other areas have mixed weightings.

these weights occurs for $TE = 2T2$, so *T2* contrast accounts for more of whatever contrast is observed at this longer *TE* value (but the total contrast is greater when $TE = T2$). Table 61–4 is a summary of these weighting conditions, and Figure 61–16 indicates regimes of different weightings in the *TE–TR* plane.

Inversion recovery follows a similar pattern. The weights are:

$$W_{\mathrm{M}} = I_{\mathrm{IR}} \tag{14}$$

$$W_{\mathrm{T1}} = kM[(TR/T1)e^{-TR/T1} - 2(TI/T1)e^{-TI/T1}]e^{-TE/T2} \tag{15}$$

$$W_{\mathrm{T2}} = (TE/T2)I_{\mathrm{IR}} \tag{16}$$

and Table 61–5 summarizes the various weightings. Spin density and *T2* weighting are very similar to spin echo; it is the *T1* weighting that is striking. At maximum, the *T1* weight is almost three times as much as the spin density weight. In fact, a slightly smaller *TI* ($TI = T1$ 1n2) will make $W_{\mathrm{M}} = 0$, keep $W_{T2} = 0$, and have W_T nonzero, giving total *T1* weighting. However, the signal will be zero from such structures, and they may be hard to distinguish from air or bone filled ($M = 0$) structures.

PROTOCOLS

The simplest way to design protocols is to find out what everybody else does and do the same. This is a good way to start, but as more experience is gained, changes in some or all protocols will be desired. Protocol development comes down to two considerations: (1) cover the volume to be imaged as fast as possible, or (2) choose pulse sequences giving good contrast.

The first consideration almost always leads to a multislice or MS/ME techique. This requires that a view be chosen (transverse, sagittal, or coronal), and in some cases

Table 61–5. WEIGHTING SUMMARY FOR INVERSION–RECOVERY IMAGES

Weighting	Conditions			Contrast
Spin density	$TI \gg T1$	TD–any value	$TE \ll T2$	$kM(\Delta M/M)$
	$TI \ll T1$	$TD \gg T1$	$TE \ll T2$	$-kM(\Delta M/M)^{*}$
T1	$TI = T1$	$TD \gg T1$	$TE \ll T2$	$0.26\ kM(\Delta M/M) - 0.74\ kM(\Delta T1/T1)$
T2				
	$TI \gg T1$	TD–any value	$TE = T2$	$0.37\ kM(\Delta M/M) + 0.37\ kM(\Delta T2/T2)$
	$TI \ll T1$	$TD \gg T1$	$TE = T2$	$-0.37\ kM(\Delta M/M) - 0.37\ kM(\Delta T2/T2)^{*}$

more than one view may be desired. The multiecho addition is recommended on both considerations; the first echo can be a spin density weighted image, and the last a *T2* weighted image, especially if several echoes are usable. Further, no added acquisition time is required for the other echoes.

Spin echo is the sequence used in most MS/ME implementations. The choices to make are of *TR, TE,* and the number of echoes. TR should exceed at least 2.5 times the longest *T1* of interest in the image (*TR* ≫ *T1* is required for both spin density and *T2* weighted images) and will probably be at least 2 s. The number of echoes should be at least two and the first *TE* chosen as small as possible. Since *T2* values of normal tissues will rarely exceed 100 ms, the *TE* value should at least reach 100 ms for the last echo. So in a period of 20 minutes, one will obtain a high-resolution screening evaluation based upon spin density weighted images and *T2* weighted images at each slice position. Such a set of images should be very sensitive to the presence of lesions, especially those with a *T2* difference, but may not be as specific as desired.

Specificity may be improved with *T1* weighting for which an inversion recovery image at the plane of interest is targeted either to the *T1* value of the organ around the lesion or the *T1* of the lesion itself (which is more likely to be unknown). A MS acquisition can be used if desired, but an ME collection will introduce *T2* weighting, which will offset some of the *T1* weighting. If the image is too "contrasted," a spin-echo *T1* weighted image may be preferred, owing to its lower contrast. Thus, an important first step for any NMR imaging facility is to examine various sequence combinations so that weightings can be targeted to contrast abnormalities as efficiently as possible.

OTHER TOPICS

There are several other topics that have some relation to MR physics and/or are in development at this time. These are gating, flow, contrast agents, gradient echoes, and surface coil development. Both gating and flow are used to collect special information. This is somewhat true with contrast agents and surface coils, but one major role of these areas as well as of gradient echoes is to help speed up data acquisition.

Thoracic imaging is of poor quality owing to cardiac and respiratory movement during acquisition; the 2DFT reconstruction fails if the object being imaged moves. Both cardiac gating and respiratory gating have been used to help reduce the effects of these movements. For a single gating (e.g., cardiac gating), the idea is to start each pulse sequence in phase with a gate trigger (e.g., R-wave detector). As long as the gate frequency remains fixed (a steady heart rate), this works fine. *TR* can be set equal to the gate interval (either manually or by software) and either 2DFT, MS, ME, or 3DFT imaging performed. Note that both MS and ME image sets have a time delay from one image to the next, so each image in either an MS or ME set will show the heart at a later point in the cardiac cycle (a typical delay is 45 to 100 ms). Neither simple 2DFT, projection imaging, nor 3DFT has this problem, but they may take longer to obtain the same information.

The gating is fine so long as the gate interval remains constant, but irregularities in the gate interval are a problem. If *TR* is allowed to change with gate interval variations, the *T1* weighting will change from one sequence to the next, at least with spin-echo images (note that inversion-recovery images are not as sensitive to *TR* changes: *TI* controls their *T1* weighting, so inversion recovery may be a better sequence). If *TR* is kept fixed, the sequences will be out of phase with the gate cycles, and the data cannot be collected until the pulse sequences and gate cycles are somehow in phase once more. So the choice is either extremely long acquisition times or image artifacts (varying $T1$ contrast or out of phase images); both are bad choices. If both respiratory and cardiac gating are used simultaneously, the problem is compounded, but either a respirator or coaching of a cooperative patient can help minimize variations in respiration time.

Cardiac variations are not as easily minimized. Most systems simply let TR follow the R-R interval time, but a very short cardiac cycle followed by a very long one will give markedly different signal levels. Despite these timing problems, good quality images of cardiac patients have been reported.[5]

Flow can reasonably be divided into two types: tissue perfusion and flow through major arteries (or CSF flow). Tissue perfusion may be assessable through M, $T1$, or $T2$ changes; at least, infarcted and ischemic tissues show differences in signal intensity from normal tissue, although other factors related to the tissue's response may be responsible for the differences. This area remains to be investigated at this time.

Flow through major arteries is also under investigation, and the best approaches have yet to be determined. The basic principle is that flow perpendicular to the imaging plane moves spin-flipped atoms out of that plane by the time of measurement, replacing them with unflipped or partially flipped atoms. The question is how to extract this information and relate it to flow, especially pulsatile flow.

Flow in the imaging plane is not measured and leads to artifacts, since both the phase and frequency encoding are distorted by the flow. Flow perpendicular to the imaging plane gives a signal change that depends upon how the gradients are switched on and off and may or may not lead to artifacts. For example, if the slice selection gradient is left on long enough for the flipped spins to flow completely out of the slice, the spins will increase or decrease their precession rate (and signal frequency) according to how far they flow and the steepness of the gradient. When the slice selection gradient is turned off, the flow will be phase encoded, and care must be taken not to confuse this phase encoding with that introduced for 2DFT image construction. If this can be done, then the flow distribution is phase encoded, and the flow can be measured if some way can be found to decode the phase information. If the 180 degree pulse producing the echo is nonselective (i.e., no gradients on when the pulse is fired), the flowing spins will contribute to the measured signal. If the 180 degree pulse is selective (slice selection gradient on), the flowing spins will not contribute to the measured signal. This latter choice has been used for qualitative assessment of blood flow;[5] the decrease of signal, as compared with stationary blood, depends upon what fraction of the flipped spins flow out of the slice, creating flow voids. However, there is a compensating effect at low flow velocities. If the flow is so slow that not all spin-flipped blood leaves the slice during TR, the next sequence will encounter a mix of partially relaxed blood from the previous sequence and fully relaxed blood that has flowed into the slice since then. The fully relaxed blood will give a stronger signal than the partially relaxed blood, producing an enhancement as compared with stationary blood. Techniques that take any or all these effects into account have been proposed for flow measurements, but so far all are experimental and require further evaluation for clinical use.

Paramagnetic contrast agents are now under clinical trial and may prove to be important in several ways. Selective uptake by a diseased tissue or part of a diseased tissue may provide additional information not otherwise available, and selective uptake by an organ system can simplify its visualization and allow a functional evaluation similar to radiotracer evaluations. Paramagnetic contrast agents are pharmaceuticals with a paramagnetic ion label; this ion has an unusually strong intrinsic magnetic field, which speeds the normal relaxation rates. Thus, an accumulation of contrast agent will shorten both the $T1$ and $T2$ values of the structure they accumulate in, and the amount they shorten it will depend upon the chemical form of the paramagnetic ion, the type of ion (e.g., Gd vs. Cr vs. Fe), and its concentration. The change in $T1$ and $T2$ so induced is quite strong, and the volume of concentration is usually very contrasted from the surrounding areas (brighter if the shorter *T1* predominates, darker if the shorter *T2* predominates). Contrast agents may make it possible to find abnormalities much faster (almost any pulse sequence will show the contrast, so optimized sequences are less important), evaluate how organ systems handle certain agents (similar to an IVP or nuclear medicine study), or even monitor the levels of certain therapeutic drugs (e.g., chemotherapy) to assure maximum benefit. However, there are also some potential problems. Cost, possible toxicity, and metabolic breakdown of the pharmaceuticals may limit their usefulness. Interestingly, radiographic contrast agents also provide some MR contrast, though the effect is simply a different *T1* and *T2* from surrounding tissues rather than a paramagnetic effect. Thus, there are many, many possibilities, making this an active area in the literature.[6,7]

Gradient echo sequences can be used to speed up imaging by giving reasonable signal levels at very short TR values (≤ 0.1 s). These sequences use a tip angle less than 90 degrees to preserve a nonzero M_L, and form the echo by read-out gradient reversal instead of a 180 degree pulse. This avoids inversion of M_L and greatly reduces rf absorption levels. However, there are some problems. Gradient-induced echoes are more sensitive than ordinary spin echoes to field inhomogeneities, patient motion, etc., and thus are more prone to artifacts. In addition, they have *T2** rather than *T2* dependence, and a contrast behavior more complicated than ordinary SE or IR. These sequences will no doubt have a clinical role, especially for reducing study time, but this role is not yet clear. Perhaps the best way to reduce study time would be to eliminate phase encoding altogether and find a way to frequency encode a slice so that the image could be constructed from one *TR* per slice instead of 256 *TR*'s per slice. If calculated fast enough, nearly "real-time" MR images would be possible.

The last topic of this section will be surface coils, which are receive-only coils whose geometry can be optimized for a particular application. Recall with the rotating magnet of Figure 61–4 that the closer the coil to the magnet, the stronger the signal. Surface coils simply implement this principle and are designed to fit closely to an organ of particular interest. There are now surface coils for the spine, thyroid, eye, breast, and other body sections. The coils provide greater signal to noise for the organs they are intended to image and in most cases better resolution, since the gradients are made stronger than usual to magnify the relatively small field of view of the coil. The drawbacks of these coils are their small field of view and curvilinear distortions in the images. In addition, they must be aligned properly to avoid induction currents from the switching gradients, and they can be amazingly difficult to tune. In a typical design, copper tubing is bent to the desired shape and variable capacitor networks added for tuning. The tuning is approximated before patient use, but since it is an entire circuit which must be tuned, final tuning must be made with the patient in place in the magnet.

CONCLUSION

This chapter has been an attempt to describe the physics of magnetic resonance in some detail, but with a minimum of mathematics. This leads to more verbiage, but it is hoped that the material presented will help fill the gaps in knowledge and alleviate the frustration many nonphysicists endure when physicists explain how MR imaging works.

Though detailed, the coverage has not been exhaustive. Chemical shift and other spectroscopic topics have received little mention. This is partly because many excellent discussions already exist[1,8] and partly because chemical shift work requires uniformities better than 1 ppm—beyond the uniformity of present imagers. Very high fields are also required, although there has been a pseudochemical shift technique reported using a commercial system.[9] This may prove to be the best way to separate two populations of chemicals (Dixon separated fat from water), but its extension to more than two populations is very uncertain. Similarly, flow has received only a superfluous treatment, since more work remains to determine how to best assess it with MR imaging.

ACKNOWLEDGMENTS

The author wishes to express his thanks to Juanita Shipman for her tireless typing, to Marion Stafford for editorial expertise, to Barbara Siede for the art work, and to Dr. C. L. Partain for his encouragement in conceiving and completing this chapter.

References

1. Mitchell MR, Conturo TE, Gruber TJ, Jones JP: Two computer models for selection of optimal magnetic resonance imaging (MRI) pulse sequence timing. Invest Radiol *19*:350–360, 1984.
2. Brown TR, Vgurbil K: Nuclear magnetic resonance. *In* Rousseau DL (ed): Structural and Resonance Techniques in Biological Research. Orlando, Florida, Academic Press, 1984, pp 1–88.
3. Hinshaw WS, Lent AH: An introduction to NMR imaging: From the Bloch equation to the imaging equation. Proc IEEE *71*:338–350, 1983.
4. Jones JP, Partain CL, Mitchell MR, et al: Principles of magnetic resonance. *In* Kressel HY (ed): Magnetic Resonance Annual 1985. New York, Raven Press, 1985, pp 71–111.
5. Soulen RL, Higgins CB: Magnetic resonance imaging of the cardiovascular system. *In* Kressel HY (ed): Magnetic Resonance Annual 1985. New York, Raven Press, 1985, pp 27–43.
6. Wolf GL, Burnett KR, Goldstein EJ, Joseph PM: Contrast agents for magnetic resonance imaging. *In* Kressel HY (ed): Magnetic Resonance Annual 1985. New York, Raven Press, 1985, pp 231–266.
7. Runge VM, Clanton JA, Lukehart CM, et al: Paramagnetic agents for contrast enhanced NMR imaging: A review. Am J Roentgenol *141*:1209–1215, 1983.
8. Gadian DG: Nuclear Magnetic Resonance and Its Application to Living Systems. Oxford, Clarendon Press, 1982.
9. Dixon WT: Simple proton spectroscopic imaging. Radiology *153*:189–194, 1984.

62

Fundamental Limitations

LAWRENCE E. CROOKS

In this chapter I attempt to define some of the limits placed on magnetic resonance imaging (MRI) both by the physics of the resonance and by practical considerations. Proclaiming a limit beyond which things cannot go is a risky business. There is always a clever person who sees a different or better approach to pursue. There is also the rare case in which a limit is surpassed by accident. The power of magnetic resonance derives from the many different ways that any problem can be solved. One can thus attack every limit from many different directions. In the area of practical applications, limits change daily as technology advances and are thus almost a matter of personal preference. There are also imaging approaches that are not appropriate for studying humans or animals but address fundamental limits. With these thoughts in mind I will discuss several types of limits: theoretical limits that are far from present practice; theoretical limits that are close to present practice; and practical limits as they currently exist.

IMAGE SPATIAL RESOLUTION

Of fundamental interest are image spatial resolution and contrast (including signal-to-noise). As imagers have developed, image quality has improved by increases of these two parameters. Human imagers presently provide voxels of $0.5 \times 0.5 \times 2.5$ mm, and small animal imagers are close to providing voxels 5 times smaller in all dimensions. This gives a spatial resolution of 100 micrometers, 10 times the size of an *Escherichia coli* organism or red blood cell. Will we be able to image an *E. coli?* Probably, if it is held still enough and is in a small sample. It is not enough just to keep it from swimming through the sample while it is being imaged. One of the limits to resolution in liquid samples is the random thermal motion of the imaged molecules, in most cases the water in tissue. The water in tissues is moving about randomly at a rate of about 2.5×10^{-5} cm^2/sec. This means that a water molecule can move the length of an *E. coli* in 40 ms. If one is trying to image the water and it moves out of a voxel during the time required to record the resonance, the resulting image will be blurred. There is also a more subtle effect, due to random motion, than the water moving out of view. The random position of the water in the imaging field gradient randomly changes the phase of the resonance of each molecule. The randomized phases will have a progressively increasing destructive interference, and the total signal will decay in a way very similar to *T2*. This effectively shortened *T2* limits the time over which the resonance is observable in any given gradient. The reduced observation time limits the resolution that can be achieved. Mansfield[1] has calculated that for a typical tissue with a gradient of 100 G/cm the resolution can be 6 micrometers. This is just at the size of an *E. coli* using a gradient

100 times stronger than usually used for human imaging. With gradient switching such a value would exceed United States Food and Drug Administration guidelines for human exposure. Since it is unlikely that such a switched gradient can be achieved at the human size, such imaging will be done on small samples surrounded by small gradient coils to provide the strong gradients.

Diffusion is reduced by lowering sample temperature. In water samples freezing moves one into solid state MR, which has a different set of limits as discussed below. For cryogenic liquids freezing occurs at lower temperatures and diffusion could be less of a problem. Liquid He^3 is attractive for this reason and for its low noise environment at 4° K.

Another influence with high resolution and strong gradients is variation of magnetic susceptibility within the sample. The magnetic field in a heterogeneous sample can vary because different molecules magnetize by different amounts. Consider the water next to a lipid layer in a cell wall. The magnetic field in the water is one value while the field in the lipids is another value. The difference is only a few parts per million, but the field gradient near the lipid surface is very strong. If this gradient is of about the same strength as the imaging gradient, the apparent positions of lipid or the water change. Also all the water that is enclosed in the cell wall can be at a different field strength than the water outside, giving it an apparent position shift. Thus the magnetic heterogeneity of the structures being imaged distort the image, just as a magnetic implant distorts a human MR image. Here the frequent opportunity of taking an MRI problem and turning it to advantage arises. From two images with different dependences on the magnetic susceptibility, a susceptibility image can be derived. Such an image might tell us something useful.

The above high resolution and microscopy discussion has assumed there is enough signal from the small voxels to overcome noise and produce a reasonable image. Since predicting absolute signal-to-noise (S/N) from first principles[2-4] is complex, I will make some scaling arguments which should be within two orders of magnitude of the actual result. A brain imaged at 15 MHz in a 30 cm diameter coil provides a S/N of more than 30:1 for $1 \times 1 \times 10$ mm voxels in 17 minutes. Reducing the dimensions of the voxel by a factor F reduces its volume and thus its magnetization by F^3. Reducing the coil's dimensions by F increases its sensitivity to the magnetization by F. The coil's inductance also decreases. When F is 100, the resolved voxel is $10 \times 10 \times 100$ micrometers and the rf coil is 3 mm in diameter. The magnetization is a million times smaller while the coil is 100 times more sensitive. Including the inductance change gives a net loss of 1000 in S/N, resulting in a value of 0.03. Hoult has also shown[3] that as size is reduced the tissue conductivity noise rapidly drops. At these sizes the conductivity is not a problem, and increasing the magnetic field improves S/N as field to the 3/2 power. A field increase of a factor of 30, to 500 MHz, gives a 160 times S/N improvement. The resulting value of 4.8 could be enhanced by further reduction of the coil size. Considering the uncertainty in the above scaling, the result is hopeful that at high field there is sufficient S/N to perform microscopy. In addition to the small rf coil the gradient coils will also have to be designed to provide the very strong gradients over the small sample dimensions.

When the sample to be imaged is solid, the diffusion limits are tremendously reduced compared with the liquid case. Mansfield[1] has calculated that diffusion in solids would allow 2 to 5 Angstrom resolution, the size of a single atom. The problem with solids is that since they are rigid, like atoms are strongly coupled and $T2$ is very short. Special pulse sequences[5] can overcome this strong coupling and would allow resolution of about 4 micrometers with a 100 G/cm gradient[1] and the S/N described above. Using these pulse sequences to achieve atomic resolution requires a gradient of 5 million G/cm. Even if such a gradient can be produced, the signal from individual atoms will be incredibly small compared with noise. Cryogenic cooling seems to be the only hope for noise reduction in this case.

IMAGING TIME

Imaging times of a few minutes yield clinical images in most imaging systems. This is with voxel volumes of 5 mm^3 giving S/N of 30 in the brain. Two years ago this performance would have required four times the scan time. Imager S/N improvement has contributed to this speed increase. Given further S/N improvements it is clear that trading S/N for speed will require different imaging "modes" than are now used. The fastest imaging mode is the Echo Planar technique of Mansfield.[6,7] It reduces imaging time to about 100 ms.

The typical two minute Fourier imaging scan measures 256 spin echoes each 0.5 s apart. Each of these echoes is a different image projection. When taken together they resolve an object into 256 lines, each line with 256 points. These echoes each last about 18 ms. Echo planar imaging collects all the echoes in one fast burst. Each echo is shortened to last only 1 ms and a train of 128 of them are collected in 128 ms. These 128 echoes are reconstructed into an image of 128 lines, each with 128 points. Some resolution has been sacrificed. Why not take more echoes with more points to improve resolution? Because all the echoes must be collected before the resonance has decayed due to $T2$ relaxation, $T2$ being less than 100 msec for many tissues sets a maximum time duration for echo planar imaging. Shortening the time required for each echo is possible by increasing the signal bandwidth per pixel. The associated increased noise reduces S/N. Now the practical limitations begin to appear. To have a 1 ms duration echo with 128 sampled points giving 2 mm spatial resolution requires a field gradient of 1 gauss/cm. To collect the train of echoes in close to 100 ms requires that the gradient be switched on and off in 100 μs. So far this rapid switching of strong gradients is limited to small gradient coils, big enough for children only. To appreciate the problem of going faster, consider reducing the echo duration to 0.5 ms with no resolution change. The gradient must double to shorten the time. This requires twice the coil current, and since this new current level must still be achieved in 100 μs, the power supply voltage must also double. This means that the supply power increases by a factor of four. This rapid increase in power (and cost) provides the technological challenge of echo planar imaging. In addition to practical limits of the gradients there is another implication: exposure to rapidly changing magnetic fields (the gradients) with their associated induced voltages. The 1 gauss/cm field gradient switched in 100 μs gives a 10 tesla/s field change at 10 cm from the center of the gradient. This begins to impinge on exposure guidelines. Fast imaging is possible; its limits are the achievable gradients, exposure limits for the gradients, and the available S/N.

At the other extreme is the question of what is the longest possible imaging time. For human studies this is usually the time over which a person can hold still in the imager. For well-motivated subjects this is close to one hour. When inanimate objects are the subject, we move into the realm of the *Guinness Book of World Records*. Spectroscopic studies of low sensitivity nuclei are run (accumulating many signals to improve S/N) over a weekend. Longer runs will require that the computer word size that accumulates the signal be large, but this limit is easy to surmount. Next are considerations such as filling a cryogenic magnet without disturbing the experiment, reliability of the system electronics, frequency of electric utility failures (about 2 per year at our laboratory), time between natural disasters (the next BIG earthquake is due during the next 50 years here in California). Before going too far in this direction you need to ask: Is there any question that MR can answer that I am willing to wait 20 years for and for which I can get funding?

SIGNAL-TO-NOISE PERFORMANCE

As mentioned above, image S/N is a prime factor in image quality. The signal of interest in MR imaging is the difference in intensity of a pathology compared with its surrounding tissue, the image contrast. Noise degrades the ability to distinguish such a difference. Improving S/N thus improves an imager's ability to demonstrate tissue differences. Imaging time, resolution, and S/N can usually be traded back and forth. Increased S/N cannot always be converted into faster imaging. In typical Fourier imaging the *TR* value limits speed but has to be on the order of seconds to provide high sensitivity to pathologies in the brain.[8] As shown above for echo planar imaging, S/N exceeds the needs of present imaging speeds, because speed is limited by gradient performance.

When considering the S/N that is available from other nuclei, scaling the performance of hydrogen is useful. The sensitivity, relative to hydrogen, of all nuclei are well known constants. Of the stable nuclei, hydrogen is the strongest signal producer. For S/N comparison the most effective approach is to consider the case in which all nuclei resonate at the same frequency. The comparison is then independent of the frequency dependencies of the receiver coil and electronics on complex variables such as tissue conductivity. The cost of this direct comparison advantage is that the magnetic field to reach the chosen frequency can be many times larger than the hydrogen field value (^{31}P requires 2.47 times the field strength). This approach also allows one to retain all the benefits of optimizing the electronics at your operating frequency.

The sensitivity constants are stated per nucleus. To use these constants the natural abundance must be factored in along with the atomic mass to have a result in mass units (useful for looking up the elemental composition of tissues). Carbon-13 has a sensitivity of 25 percent of hydrogen, a relative abundance of 1.1 percent, and a mass of 13, giving a sensitivity of 0.00021 for a gram of carbon compared with a gram of hydrogen. Once such numbers are computed they can be weighted by elemental composition of the tissues to provide in vivo sensitivities. Collections of such comparisons are available.[9,10] These give close to the best case results for sensitivity. The MR signal is proportional to the sensitivity, and the receiver noise will be the same in all cases, since we are considering constant frequency, so this gives the best case S/N. The signal can also be reduced by other mechanisms. In the case of phosphorus five sixths of it is bound into rigid lattices, has a short *T2*, and is not observable in vivo, further reducing S/N. Not all the other nuclei have simple spin quantum mechanics. Sodium has four possible spin alignments compared with two for hydrogen. The result for sodium is much faster relaxation times. The resulting short *T1* is an advantage in that more signals can be collected from sodium in a given time. The extra signals improve S/N. The reduced *T2* makes the signal decay faster and reduces S/N. The impact is that while relaxation time considerations modify S/N, the extent is usually small. Nuclei that have many chemically shifted lines will distribute the signal among the lines. This reduces the S/N for any line according to its relative population. Destructive interference between lines will reduce the S/N of an image that combines the lines in an incoherent way.

To image these other nuclei the lower S/N must be accommodated by larger voxels, longer imaging time, or poorer contrast. The sensitivity of all other nuclei in tissues is less than about one thousandth that of hydrogen. With this as a factor, what performance can be achieved? The performance of hydrogen imaging is a moving target with ever improving S/N. The earlier mentioned value of S/N = 30 for 1 × 1 × 10 mm resolution can be achieved for 10 × 10 × 100 mm resolution in the same time with a nucleus that gives 1000 times less signal. A cube 1 cm on a side would have a S/N of 3 in this case. Increased imaging time improves the situation slowly. Four times the imaging time would improve the S/N to 6 for the 1 cm cube. That images are possible with the signal available from sodium has been demonstrated.[11-13] Higher sensitivity to pathology available from such other nuclei may offset part of the S/N loss.[11] The S/N that can be achieved with spectroscopy of other nuclei can also be calculated when the tissue volume contributing to the signal is known. The signal will be distributed among all the peaks in the spectrum.

Spatial resolution continues to improve in MR images. The prospects for microscopic resolution in small samples are good. Even smaller resolution is theoretically achievable in solids. Echo planar imaging is providing 100 ms imaging times, and further reductions are possible. As S/N in systems improve, all nuclei benefit. The sensitivity of direct observation of other nuclei wil! always be more than 1000 times less than protons. Larger resolved volumes for these nuclei provide more S/N in reasonable imaging times. Their clinical utility is being actively pursued.

References

1. Mansfield P, Grannell PK: "Diffraction" and microscopy in solids and liquids by NMR. Physical Review B *12*:3618–3634, 1975.
2. Hoult DI, Richards RE: The signal-to-noise ratio of the nuclear magnetic resonance experiment. J Magn Reson *24*:71, 1976.
3. Hoult DI, Lauterbur PC: The sensitivity of the zeugmatographic experiment involving human subjects. J Magn Reson *34*:425–433, 1979.
4. Hoult DI: Field, contrast, and sensitivity in imaging. *In* James TL, Margulis AR (eds): Biomedical Magnetic Resonance. San Francisco, Radiology Research and Education Foundation, 1984, pp 35–45.
5. Waugh JS, Huber LM, Haeberlen U: Applications to high resolution NMR in solids. Phys Rev Lett *20*:180, 1968.
6. Mansfield P, Pykett IL: Biological and medical imaging by NMR. J Magn Reson *29*:355–373, 1978.
7. Mansfield P: Real-time echo-planar imaging by NMR. Br Med Bull *40*:187–190, 1984.
8. Brant-Zawadzki M, Norman D, Newton TH, Kelly WM, Kjos B, Mills CM, Dillon W, Sobel D, Crooks LE: Magnetic resonance of the brain: The optimal screening technique. Radiology *152*:71–77, 1984.
9. Crooks LE, Hoenninger JC, Arakawa M, Kaufman L, McRee R, Watts J, Singer JR: Tomography of hydrogen with NMR and the potential for imaging other body constituents. SPIE *206*:120, 1979.
10. Kramer DM: Imaging of elements other than hydrogen. *In* Kaufman L, Crooks LE, Margulis AR (eds): Nuclear Magnetic Resonance Imaging in Medicine. New York, Igaku-Shoin, Inc., pp 184–203.
11. Hilal SK, Maudsley AA, Simon HE, et al: In vivo NMR imaging of tissue sodium in the intact cat before and after cerebral stroke. AJNR *4*:245–249, 1983.
12. Perman WH, Hayes CE, Glover G, et al: The physics of in-vivo human sodium NMR imaging (abstract). Presented at the Meeting of the Society of Magnetic Resonance in Medicine, New York, August 1984.
13. Feinberg DA, Crooks LE, Kaufman L, Brant-Zawadzki M, Posin JP, Arakawa, Watts JC, Hoenninger J: Magnetic resonance imaging performance: A comparison of sodium and hydrogen. Radiology *156*:133–138, 1985.

XIII

RELAXATION/ RELAXOMETRY

63

Relaxometry of Solvent and Tissue Protons: Diamagnetic Contributions

SEYMOUR H. KOENIG
RODNEY D. BROWN, III

Understanding magnetic relaxation of protons of diamagnetic tissue at the molecular level requires not only extensive data over a substantial range of values of magnetic field and temperature, but also the development of a model that describes the microscopic dynamical behavior of tissue water. The initial step is to discover whether tissue must be regarded as liquid or solid, to first order, since the theoretical description of relaxation of water protons is quite different in the two cases. In particular, the longitudinal and transverse relaxation rates $1/T1$ and $1/T2$ are closely related in liquids, whereas in solids predominant contributions to $1/T2$ can exist that have no correspondence in $1/T1$. We discuss data on the magnetic field dependence of $1/T1$ (NMRD, nuclear magnetic relaxation dispersion, profile) for a range of diamagnetic proteins, cell suspensions, and tissue—the latter both normal and abnormal—that indicate that tissue behaves as a liquid as regards the relaxation of the protons of tissue water. Thus, the water molecules of tissue are quite mobile, rapidly sampling the intra- and extracellular environment of tissue, and the relaxation rates of their protons arise from the explorations made by these water molecules averaged over a relaxation time. The justification for this view, and aspects of its limitations, are considered below, as are means by which the relaxation rates could become altered by disease. Understanding the latter is the goal, since the ultimate utility of NMR imaging (MRI) will depend on its ability to distinguish normal from abnormal tissues.

BACKGROUND

Contrast in MRI is influenced by many physical and chemical parameters of tissue. Among the most important, for proton imaging, are the longitudinal and transverse magnetic relaxation rates $1/T1$ and $1/T2$ of tissue protons. A major reason, of course, is that the density of protons—to which the image signal from any point in space is directly proportional—varies very little among tissues, certainly far less than do the characteristic relaxation rates. Much has been learned about these relaxation rates in vivo in the relatively short period that high resolution images have been available, and much more can, and will, be learned. However, such knowledge is limited to the specific magnetic field strength used and the physiological conditions of temperature, pH, etc. at which image data are collected. In addition, accuracy is limited by the fact that experimental protocols for obtaining optimal image quality in a given time are not necessarily optimal for deriving values of the relaxation parameters themselves.

Ultimately, the utility of NMR imaging will relate to its ability to detect disease, to distinguish abnormal from normal conditions; resolution and perfection of the images will be of lesser importance. Advances in diagnostics, and prognostics as well, will certainly require a more fundamental understanding of the determinants of nuclear relaxation rates than we now have, ultimately at the molecular level, in order to relate observed changes in proton relaxation rates to changes in the state of tissue, both retrospectively and predictively. To achieve such basic understanding requires measurements in regimes beyond the limited range of thermodynamic parameters, particularly field and temperature, proscribed by imaging instrumentation. What is necessary, though far from sufficient, is to study relaxation behavior in vitro both in tissue samples and in solutions and suspensions of its molecular components, using instrumentation specialized for this function. We have, in the past,[1] referred to such instruments as "relaxometers" and research in this area as "relaxometry." In the present chapter, we discuss relaxometry of diamagnetic tissue in its many aspects. The emphasis will be on the $1/T1$ NMRD profiles (the dependence of $1/T1$ over almost four decades of field) of a variety of in vitro samples of diamagnetic protein solutions, cell suspensions, and tissue, the latter both normal and abnormal.

TISSUE: SOLID OR LIQUID?

It is straightforward to define $1/T1$ and $1/T2$, and $1/T1_\rho$, a quantity only recently introduced into the MRI literature,[2] in terms of the dynamics of the macroscopic magnetization of an ensemble of proton spins—e.g., the water protons of a piece of liver—in a fashion that is, in essence, a prescription for measuring these rates. In mathematical terms, these are the Bloch equations;[3] they are purely phenomenological and make no reference to mechanisms of relaxation. In words, a prescription follows:

Place an ensemble of proton spins in a static magnetic field B_0 of, say, 1 tesla, pointing in the z direction, and wait a few seconds—until the spin system reaches thermal equilibrium. At this point, the orientations of the spins are no longer completely random (though almost so); rather, there is a bias such that the z components of the spins tend to be parallel rather than antiparallel to B_0, while the x and y components remain randomly distributed. The bias is minuscule, producing an equilibrium magnetization of the proton ensemble, M_0, equivalent to about 1 spin in 10^6 pointing along B_0. M_0 is a macroscopic classical vector quantity that is parallel to the vector B_0. $1/T1$ and $1/T2$ describe the rates of response of the components of M_0 to a sudden change of B_0. Now that M_0 has been established in B_0, change B_0 rapidly, in direction if not also in magnitude, to a new value B_0', and watch the magnetization "relax" to its new equilibrium value M_0'. The magnetization component parallel to B_0' (the "longitudinal" component) and that perpendicular to B_0' (the "transverse" component) will both approach their new equilibrium values exponentially (in most cases), generally with *different* rate constants. The longitudinal component of magnetization will either decay or grow to M_0' with a longitudinal relaxation rate $1/T1$, and the transverse component of magnetization will decay to zero with a transverse relaxation rate $1/T2$.

The rates $1/T1$ and $1/T2$ are in general functions of B_0'. It is often the case that a transverse radio frequency field B_1 is present, rotating in resonance with the precessing magnetization M_0. A sufficiently large value of B_1 can reduce the value of $1/T2$. Under such circumstances the transverse relaxation rate with respect to the direction of B_1 (in the rotating frame) is called $1/T1_\rho$, for "relaxation in the rotating frame." It becomes equal to $1/T2$ when B_1 is negligibly small. Its value is very sensitive to B_1, at a given value of B_0, whenever $1/T1$ is sensitive to B_0 at comparably low fields. As will be seen from the figures that follow, this is the case for most soft tissue, so that $1/T1_\rho$ may have application potential in MRI.

The foregoing defines the phenomenology of relaxation in terms of measurable quantities, $1/T1$, $1/T2$, and $1/T1_\rho$, the parameters that characterize the time dependences of the longitudinal and transverse components of the magnetization of any proton ensemble. Relating these rates, which describe the dynamics of a macroscopic parameter, to the microscopic dynamics of the individual, quantum mechanical spins is the realm of relaxation theory and is best left for other discussions, except for noting that there are fundamental differences between relaxation in solids and liquids. The latter is far simpler to describe, since (in most instances) $1/T1$, $1/T2$, and $1/T1_\rho$ are but different aspects of the same interaction or set of interactions. In solids, by contrast, the major contribution to $1/T2$ often has no influence on $1/T1$. Their values can be widely disparate; $T1$ can be weeks and $T2$ milliseconds. Not so for liquids, for which (generally) the two rates are equal for $B_0 \to 0$, and may differ 10- to 100-fold, but rarely by more, at fields of several tesla. What then of tissue? Is it to be regarded as liquid or solid, to first order?

We have been investigating the relaxometry of protein solutions, both diamagnetic[4-8] and paramagnetic,[9-12] for many years, extending the capability, accuracy, and efficacy of our specialized instrumentation[1,11] as needed to relate the data to theory, and elaborating the theory[13,14] as required by the systems investigated. In particular, we have developed a relaxometer that can measure $1/T1$ of water protons in solutions of protein, or samples of tissue, over the field range 0.01 to 60 MHz (proton Larmor frequency) and the temperature range -10 to 40°C. The data, generally the NMRD profiles of $1/T1$ at a fixed temperature, are accumulated under program control, over any preset sequence of field values. The absolute reproducibility of $1/T1$ is typically 1 percent for sample volumes ~ 0.5 ml when $1/T1$ is in the range 0.3 to 30 s^{-1}; rates within a factor of three of these limits can be measured with reduced accuracy. It is possible to measure $1/T2$ profiles as well, but it is technically more difficult at present.

Our experience to date has been that, to first order, the NMRD profiles of tissue resemble those of homogeneous, isotropic (liquid) protein solutions.[10,15-17] This was noted a decade ago for blood,[10] admittedly a very specialized tissue but one that contains no more water than, for example, liver. These data indicate that the hydrodynamic behavior of hemoglobin in erythrocytes is the same as that of a homogeneous hemoglobin solution at the same concentration, and that the water molecules exchange rapidly between the intra- and extracellular regions of the sample. Modeling erythrocytes as sacs of hemoglobin, pervious to water, is realistic for describing these NMRD profiles.

More recent data indicate that this approach is reasonable for suspensions of more complex cells, and for more complex tissues as well.[16,17] Thus, in a time interval comparable to a relaxation time, it would appear that a typical water molecule explores the intra- and extracellular environment of tissue over a region several cell diameters in extent; its relaxation behavior derives from an average of its interactions within this region. Undoubtedly this is a simplification and, for some specialized tissues, may be an oversimplification, or may even be inapplicable.[18] Nonetheless, this view has served us well in correlating a wide range of observations, and it is the experimental facts that have brought us to this view, which we would like to reiterate in this chapter in addition to noting results that suggest limitations to this view. First, however, a digression on relaxation and "motional narrowing."

THE DETERMINANTS OF 1/T1 AND 1/T2 IN LIQUIDS

Intuitively there is no great conceptual leap to be made in relating the phenomenological macroscopic relaxation parameters of the Bloch[3] equations to some microscopic mechanism that causes the spins of individual protons to reorient. Here, however, one must be careful; after all, spins in a magnetic field are continually reorienting owing to their Larmor precession. The kind of reorientation that relaxes the magnetization differs from this steady secular motion in a fundamental way; it requires a reorientation that randomizes, in some statistical sense, the orientation of the several components of the spins of the protons. More particularly, this reorientation must arise through interactions that contain the chaos that characterizes the randomness of all movement associated with thermal motion and thermal equilibrium. For diamagnetic solutions, including tissue, these interactions are relatively few and rather weak. Moreover, the random, thermal motion of the water is so very rapid that the actual interaction is almost averaged out; the appropriate theory becomes a theory of "motional narrowing," in which the interaction is reduced to an effective interaction that can be regarded as a small uncertainty in the energy of the spins. The concomitant uncertainty in time, from the uncertainty principle, is the lifetime of a spin in a given state, and thereby the lifetime and relaxation time of the magnetization.

As an example of the foregoing, consider proton relaxation in pure water, in the spirit of the classic work of Bloembergen et al.[19] almost four decades ago. The coupling of a given proton to the thermal motion, i.e., the reservoir of thermal energy, is through the time-varying magnetic field produced by the magnetic moments of its neighboring protons, which is in fact dominated by the intramolecular partner of the given proton. Were the water molecules stationary, this field would have a time dependence that reflects only the Larmor precession frequency of the protons in the field B_0, and a magnitude and direction that depend on the orientation of the water molecule with respect to B_0. The mean amplitude value of this local field is about 5 gauss (5×10^{-4} tesla), corresponding to an interaction energy $\sim 10^5$ rad s^{-1}. However, relaxation occurs only because the waters are not stationary but reorient on a time scale in the range of 10^{-11} to 10^{-12} s^{-1}; this modulates the proton–proton interaction at $\sim 10^6$ times the interaction frequency, reducing it 10^6-fold to an effective interaction $\sim 10^{-1}$ rad s^{-1}, corresponding to an uncertainty in time of about 10 s. The observed values of $T1$ and $T2$ of 4 seconds near 25°C are in remarkable agreement with this rough estimate. This is the essence of motional narrowing, but it is something more, since $T2$ as well as $T1$ in a liquid derive from the same, motionally narrowed, interaction.[19]

Implicit in the foregoing, and also in the Bloch[3] equation that defines $T1$, is that a change in the z component of the magnetization, that parallel to B_0, represents a change in energy, the Zeeman energy of the proton ensemble in B_0. Thus longitudinal relaxation is indeed to be equated with energy relaxation; accordingly, $T1$ is often termed the "spin-lattice relaxation" to convey the idea that energy is exchanged between the spin system and the "lattice," the latter suggesting the solid state, but here referring to the bulk of the liquid (less its protons) as the reservoir of thermal energy. In a liquid, however, $T2$ also derives from exchange of energy alone, a point not readily apparent, or at least not generally stressed, in the usual derivations of $T2$. That is, spin-lattice interactions produce $1/T1$, $1/T2$, and $1/T1_\rho$ in a liquid. (However, these three rates vary differently with field so that their values are usually different.) It is mainly in solids that interactions among the proton spins themselves, "spin-spin" interactions, without a lattice component, dominate $T2$, making $T2 \ll T1$ even for $B_0 \to 0$. This is an extremely important point,[20] particularly if tissue can be regarded as liquid, and is a strong argument for using the terms "longitudinal" and "transverse," terms that *describe* relaxation rather than *attribute* its causes. (It is a bit ironic that, in the example given, spin-lattice relaxation proceeds through the intermediary of the spin-spin interaction of neighboring protons and thus of the proton ensemble. It need not be confusing, however. In other systems, e.g., solutions of paramagnetic ions, interactions of protons with other protons make a minor contribution to energy relaxation; interactions with the ions dominate, and the mutual interactions of protons can usually be ignored for both $1/T1$ and $1/T2$.)

HEMOGLOBIN AND ERYTHROCYTES

Figure 63–1 shows the observed NMRD profile of carbonmonoxyhemoglobin[10] (which is diamagnetic) at 6°C, a profile typical in form to those of other globular proteins: a field-independent contribution D; and a dispersive contribution, of magnitude A at low fields, that inflects at field ν_c, and approaches zero at high fields.[5] The buffer (water) background for the longitudinal relaxation rate $(1/T1_w)$ is also shown. The buffer background for the transverse relaxation rate $(1/T2_w)$ is the same as $1/T1_w$ except near neural pH,[21] where interactions with ^{17}O in natural abundance can more than double the values of $1/T2_w$. The solid curve through the data derives from a least squares fit to a heuristic equation with four adjustable parameters:[5] A, D, ν_c, and a variable that adjusts the slope of the curve at ν_c. The dashed curve is the *prediction*[16] for $1/T2$ (using no additional parameters), which, judged from the few data available, holds quite well for protein solutions.

There are few data in the literature giving $1/T2$ at more than one field for homogeneous protein solutions, and even fewer for tissue. (It is difficult to measure the NMRD profile of $1/T2$). Nonetheless, some generalizations can be made that have an impact on the idea of tissue as liquid. Figure 63–2 shows data from the literature:[22] the $1/T1$ NMRD profile of serum albumin; values of $1/T2$ at a few values of field, and our heuristic fit and consequent prediction for the $1/T2$ profile. The agreement is excellent. The essence of the prediction is that the D term (Fig. 63–1), which does not disperse in the range shown, contributes identically to both $1/T1$ and $1/T2$, whereas the A term, which disperses to 0 for $1/T1$, goes to 0.3 of A at high field for $1/T2$. The latter is a very general result that arises from the condition that liquids are isotropic; the result depends on geometry and not on the details of the relaxation processes. It has been long established that ν_c is inversely proportional to the rotational reorientation time of the protein molecules (it varies appropriately with molecular weight and shape, solvent viscosity, temperature, and protein–protein interactions); that A is proportional to the ratio of protein concentration to ν_c; and that the dispersive contribution to the NMRD profile reflects the rotational Brownian motion of the protein molecules.[4] The D term

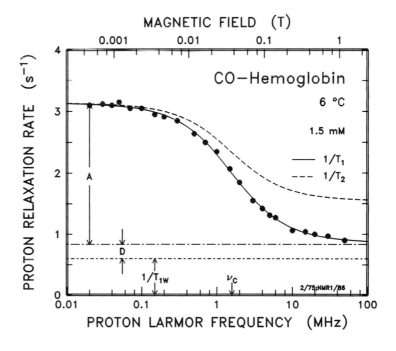

Figure 63–1. $1/T1$ NMRD profile of a 1.5 mM solution of carbonmonoxyhemoglobin (which is diamagnetic) at 6°C, pH 6.25. The solid curve through the data points (●) derives from a least squares comparison of the data with a heuristic theory with four adjustable parameters: A, the low field magnitude of a contribution that disperses to zero at high fields, and inflects at field ν_c; a field-independent contribution D that adds to the buffer background $1/T1_w$; and a parameter (not shown) that adjusts the slope of the curve at ν_c. The upper dashed curve is the prediction for $1/T2$. (Data after reference 10.)

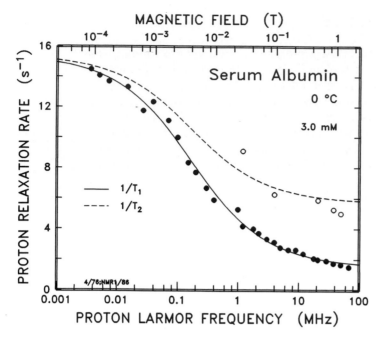

Figure 63–2. $1/T1$ NMRD profile of a 3.0 mM solution of bovine serum albumin at 6°C (●), and more limited data for $1/T2$ (○). The curves associated with the data points derive as in Figure 63–1. (Data after reference 22.)

arises from collisions of the water molecules with the surface of the protein molecules; these collisions are uniformly short-lived ($\sim 10^{-9}$ to 10^{-10} s), too short to sense the rotational motion of the protein. D is in fact the only contribution attributable to the traditional "hydration shell" of the macromolecules. From extensive analysis of a large amount of data, there is little question that the time spent by a typical water molecule in this region is the time for it to approach, collide, and escape from the surface; this time is short on the scale of protein reorientation times but relatively long on the scale of the reorientation time of a water molecule in water.[5–7,16]

Figure 63–3 shows the NMRD profile of a suspension of erythrocytes,[10] for which about 1/3 the volume is occupied by cells, compared with the profile of a homogeneous

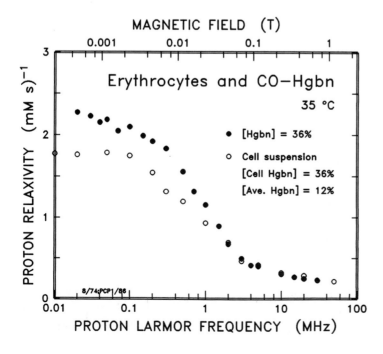

Figure 63–3. Comparison of the $1/T1$ NMRD profiles of a suspension of red blood cells (erythrocytes) and a solution of human hemoglobin at 35°C, with the concentration of the hemoglobin adjusted to equal the intracellular hemoglobin concentration of the suspension. The data are expressed as relaxivity, the incremental rate over the buffer background, per mM of total protein present. Carbonmonoxyhemoglobin was used in each case to prevent oxidation of the iron to Fe^{3+}, and thus avoid an artifactual paramagnetic contribution to the observed rates. (After reference 10.)

solution of hemoglobin, under the same buffer conditions, with the concentration of protein throughout the solution adjusted to equal the intracellular hemoglobin concentration of the cells in suspension. The data are plotted as relaxivity, the contribution to $1/T1$ per mM of protein in the sample, independent of the protein spatial distribution. (The measured rates, of course, are about threefold different.) The close agreement of these two curves shows that the relaxation of water protons in the presence of hemoglobin is independent of the spatial distribution of the protein molecules; clearly, solvent water molecules explore the intra- and extracellular space of the suspension uninhibited by the presence of the cell membrane, at 35°C. (There is a small, but detectable, influence at 6°C.) From Figure 63–3, the phenomenology shows that for a simple tissue, composed of one cell type containing essentially a single type of protein, the liquid model works well.

RAT LIVER CELLS

Figure 63–4 shows the NMRD profiles of rat liver, an organ with a single predominant cell type (hepatocyte), and two suspensions of liver cells.[16] The cells were obtained by enzymatic treatment of the supporting tissue matrix, separated by centrifugation, and kept alive in an appropriate growth medium. For the initial NMRD run, the cells were allowed to settle under gravity and the supernatant was then siphoned off. For the subsequent run, the same sample was compacted two- to three-fold by centrifugation and the supernatant again removed.

The macromolecular content of liver cells is more varied than for erythrocytes, and the shape of the NMRD profiles in the figure reflects this. It is not difficult to simulate these profiles by superimposing NMRD profiles for proteins of various sizes, appropriately weighted. However, the profile for hepatocyte suspensions has not, as yet, been shown to derive directly from the NMRD profile of solutions of the cellular constituents, as is the case for erythrocytes (Fig. 63–3).

The solid curves through the data, Figure 63–4, result from the same heuristic fit used for the other figures; the curves have no other significance for the present dis-

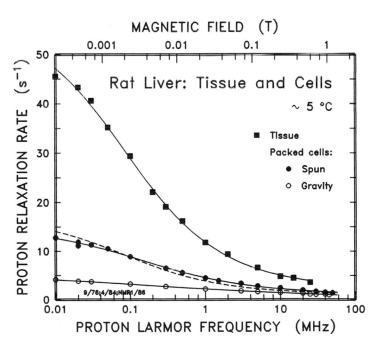

Figure 63–4. $1/T1$ NMRD profiles for rat liver tissue at 6°C (■), and a suspension of rat hepatocytes at two cell concentrations, at 5°C (●, ○). The solid lines through the data derive as in Figure 63–1, while the dashed curve is that of liver tissue scaled by the factor 0.29, after correction for a field independent water background rate of 0.6 s^{-1}. (Cell data after reference 16.)

cussion. The dashed curve, Figure 63–4, was scaled from the curve through the tissue data by a factor of 0.25 and includes a small correction for the water background contribution. It is reasonable, from these results, to regard the sample of centrifuge-packed cells as "diluted liver tissue"; it has previously been shown that, in effect, the cells packed under gravity can be regarded as a further dilution.[16] Thus for liver, water has rapid access to the intra- and extracellular regions of assemblages of cells, in this case hepatocytes, whether organized in tissue or suspended in water. Moreover, the behavior is analogous to erythrocytes in blood, the major difference ostensibly arising from the more complex cellular composition of hepatocytes. We infer from the foregoing that the essence of relaxometry of liver is that liver can be regarded as a liquid as appropriately as can blood. Thus, the morphology of tissue is not a guide to its relaxation properties, suggesting that changes in gross tissue morphology due to disease may not be easily detectable by MRI. On the other hand, changes in tissue histology, such as in the type or quantity of tissue constituents, amount of intra- or extracellular water, or lipid content should be detectable by MRI.

SPECIFICITY OF NMRD PROFILES (NORMAL TISSUE)

Longitudinal Relaxation

The NMRD profile of rat liver (Fig. 63–4) is similar in form to most other tissues, as seen in the data for rabbit tissues[16] in Figure 63–5. These results are very much like corresponding data for other species, including rat, dog, and human:[1,15] the rates for liver are highest and for spleen lowest; muscle and kidney are similar; and the profile for fat has a notably different form. We have not as yet attempted to correlate the magnitudes of profiles with the cellular constituent of the different tissue types, except to note that the data for adipose tissue generally contain contributions from both water and aliphatic protons and that the signal is observably composite (all the tissue protons are included in our signals, and the magnetization decay for adipose tissue can be resolved into the sum of two relaxation rates within experimental error).

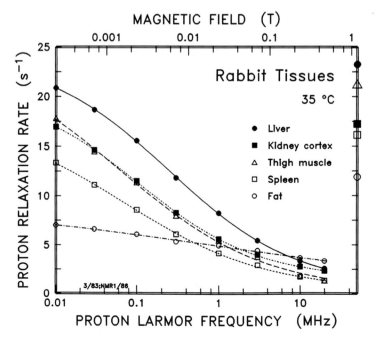

Figure 63–5. $1/T1$ NMRD profiles of various rabbit tissues at 35°C. The curves through the profiles derive as in Figure 63–1. Also shown, on the right hand scale, are values for $1/T2$, from Table 12 of reference 21, at unspecified field values. (The $1/T1$ data after reference 16.)

Figure 63–6 shows the NMRD profiles of white and gray matter from dog brain. The animal was a relatively large mongrel dog so that the dissection could be done with relative ease. The difference between the profiles for white and gray matter in Figure 63–6 is relatively insensitive to field strength, but perhaps decreases somewhat at higher fields. The effect on $1/T1$ is almost a factor of two at the high fields now popular for imaging, though the "intrinsic" effect is not as great: the larger relative difference at high fields arises mainly as a chance concomitant of the insensitivity to field of the NMRD contribution of whatever is responsible for the difference between the behavior of white and gray matter. This difference resembles the profile of fat tissue (Fig. 63–5), and it is tempting to invoke a contribution from myelin lipid of the axons of white matter to explain this difference. However, the situation appears to be rather complex, and it is not at all clear (as yet) to what extent these lipid protons contribute to the signal intensity[23] or influence the observed rates by cross relaxation.[8]

Transverse Relaxation

There is a great quantity of diverse data reported for $1/T1$ and $1/T2$ of a range of tissue types, generally at one value of B_0 (frequently not stated) and often under unspecified conditions of temperature, sample handling, etc. Bottomley et al.[24] have recently assembled, collated, and displayed these many disparate results and we will draw heavily on that effort, as summarized in their Table 12, in what follows.

There are but few reports of NMRD profiles of both $1/T1$ and $1/T2$ for the same sample of tissue; one of these is replotted in Figure 63–7, which shows data for frog muscle[25] at 25°C. The solid curve through the $1/T1$ profile derives from the heuristic fit used in the preceding figures. The prediction for the $1/T2$ NMRD profile, assuming the validity of using the same procedure[16] as for Figures 63–1 and 63–2, substantially underestimates the actual values of $1/T2$, though its relative insensitivity to B_0 at higher fields, common to most tissues, is predicted.

Predicting $1/T2$ NMRD profiles requires knowledge of A, a parameter that can be obtained with reasonable certainty only when the $1/T1$ NMRD profile has a clearly

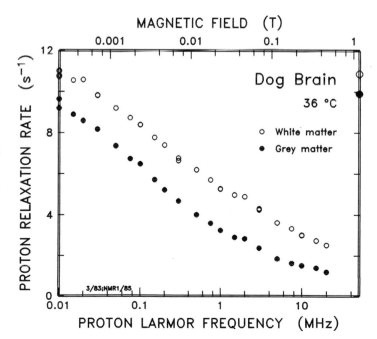

Figure 63–6. $1/T1$ NMRD profiles of white and grey matter from a dog brain at 36°C. Also shown, on the right hand scale, are values for $1/T2$, from Table 12 of reference 24, at unspecified field values.

defined inflection, as in Figures 63–1 to 63–3. For most tissues (other than blood; see Figure 63–5 and particularly Figure 63–7) the data do not show a clear enough inflection to permit extrapolation of the $1/T1$ profile to zero field to obtain A (even assuming that no unforeseen dispersive contributions appear below 0.01 MHz). This makes the prediction of the magnitude of the $1/T2$ NMRD profile quite uncertain, but the predicted functional form should be realistic. (Early data[26] on $1/T1_\rho$ of tissue indicate that $1/T1$ of several tissue types continues to increase substantially below 0.01 MHz, but the quantitative implications of these findings on the present discussion have not yet been considered in detail.)

An example of the relation of $1/T1$ profiles to the high field values of $1/T2$ is shown in Figure 63–5, where values for $1/T2$ from Table 12 in Bottomley et al.[24] are indicated on the right-hand scale. Despite the species differences, the ordering of the $1/T2$ data mimics that of the low field $1/T1$ measurements. Indeed, it appears to be an empirical rule, of general applicability to diamagnetic tissue, that the high field values of $1/T2$ roughly equal those for $1/T1$ at 0.01 MHz. (For homogeneous protein solutions, the ratio, as indicated earlier, is $\lesssim 0.3$.)

Another example of the relation of the $1/T1$ NMRD profile to the high field values of $1/T2$ is indicated in Figure 63–6, where data for $1/T2$ are again indicated on the right-hand scale. If the difference between the two profiles is attributed to an incremental contribution from white matter (as yet of undetermined origin), as this contribution has little dispersion, the *difference* in the respective values of $1/T2$ should be about that between the $1/T1$ profiles. The absolute values of $1/T2$, from the empirical rule, should be near the 0.01 MHz values of $1/T1$. Both these points are seen to be true.

The data presented so far indicate that tissue can be regarded (certainly as a useful approximation) as an isotropic liquid, with each tissue water molecule relatively free to explore its intra- and extracellular local environment. When this holds, both $1/T1$ and $1/T2$ NMRD profiles derive from the same molecular interactions, and knowledge of one, plus insight into mechanisms, should allow prediction of the other. In particular, knowledge of $1/T1$ NMRD profiles (the easier to measure) should allow prediction of $1/T2$ profiles, as is the case for homogeneous protein solutions. This appears to be

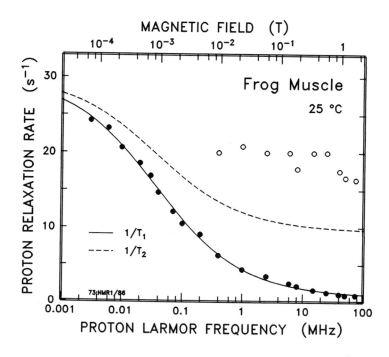

Figure 63–7. $1/T1$ (●) and $1/T2$ (○) NMRD profiles of frog muscle tissue (*R. escutenta*) at 25°C. The solid and dashed curves derive as in Figure 63–1. (Data after reference 25.)

possible for tissue as well, noting, however, that we cannot as yet obtain the proper low field limit of the dispersive A term. The convenient empirical relation, that A is about 3.3 times $1/Tl$ at 0.01 MHz, circumvents this problem for the present.

NMRD PROFILES OF ABNORMAL TISSUE

Differences in relaxation rates of abnormal (meaning, here, tumorous) and normal tissue can arise from numerous sources. Two main classes should be distinguished, however: tumors that are transformations of the major cell type of a given tissue, such as hepatomas, and those that arise either from transformation of a local minority cell type or from metastases. An example of the latter class, Figure 63–8, has been discussed before:[27] an invasive carcinoma of the breast by a tumor of ductal origin. The dramatic distinction between the two dispersion profiles corresponds to the difference (Fig. 63–5) between the forms of the profiles of fat tissue and most others. This is an extreme example of how contrast between normal and abnormal tissue can arise in NMR images: the source of the contrast derives from displacement of one type of cell by another with (in this case) a dramatically different dispersion profile.

An example of the first class, though admittedly somewhat artificial, is shown in Figure 63–9, in which the NMRD profile of rat liver is contrasted with those of thigh-implanted tumors derived from two lines of transformed hepatocytes, one slow growing, the other rapid growing. The results are consistent with an often-expressed (but incorrect) view that tumors always have lower relaxation rates than the corresponding normal tissue. It will take further investigation to clarify these changes, but it must be stressed that extensive edema can be a large component of any observed change in rates.

To the extent that edema occurs in association with tumor, it will, of course, influence NMR images. The problem, however, is to detect the abnormality that underlies the edema and verify its nature with reasonable certainty. Experiments that indicate this possibility are shown in Figure 63–10, in which the NMRD profiles of

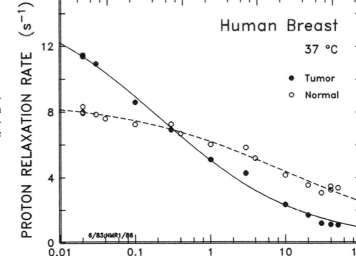

Figure 63–8. $1/Tl$ NMRD profiles of a resected ductal carcinoma of the human breast (●) and nearby uninvolved "normal" tissue (○), at 37°C. (After reference 27.)

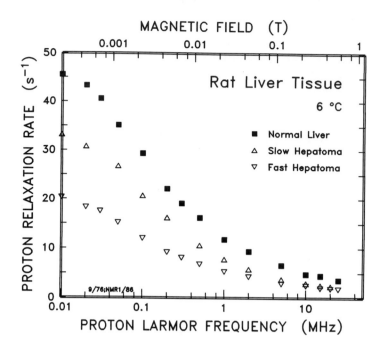

Figure 63–9. 1/*T1* NMRD profiles of normal rat liver (■) and two hepatomas grown in the thigh, one slow growing (▲), the other fast growing (▼), at 6°C.

surgically resected tumors are contrasted with the profiles of uninvolved neighboring tissue. The *sign* of the distinction is different in the two cases, an observation made previously[27] for adenocarcinomas of the transverse colon from two different patients. Though in neither case do we have a baseline to indicate whether the profiles of the uninvolved tissue are shifted systematically from those of normal tissue in healthy individuals, it is clear that one cannot yet generalize regarding the changes in relaxation rates that are induced by neoplastic transformation.

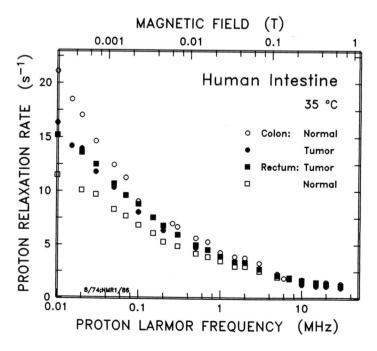

Figure 63–10. 1/*T1* NMRD profiles of two resected adenocarcinomas, of the colon (●) and rectum (■) and of nearby uninvolved "normal" tissue (○, □), at 35°C.

SUMMARY

We have found that a liquid model of tissue is extremely useful as a guide for research into the relaxometry of diamagnetic tissue. Not only is its use rationalized, and justified, by the data presented here, but a large body of data on tissue with substantial contributions from paramagnetic ions also lend support to this approach.[1,17,18,27] There are problems, of course, or at least complications, and it will be the subject of future research to elaborate and refine the foregoing ideas to incorporate them into a more global view. Among these, the question of cross relaxation between separate, but interacting, ensembles of protons will have to be addressed,[8] as indeed will cross relaxation between protons and other nuclei.[15,28,29,30] Thus, transfer of magnetization between, for example, protein protons and water protons in tissue remains to be investigated; this is known to influence the NMRD profiles of homogeneous protein solutions.[8] Additionally, relaxation between water protons and aliphatic protons in adipose tissue must be examined; cross relaxation effects are certain to arise here and possibly in brain tissue as well.

The investigation of cross relaxation, particularly magnetization transfer among different proton ensembles, is not only important for a fundamental understanding of relaxation at the molecular level, but for a practical reason as well. It may be possible, by a proper choice of pulse sequence, to use the transfer of magnetization to advantage by enhancing contrast in some critical circumstances (a potentiality that remains to be explored).

As studies of relaxation of diamagnetic tissue progress, complications relating to the specific structure of tissue are certain to arise. Organs in which the compartmentalization of water is part of their role, as in the ascending tubules of the kidney medulla, will manifest relaxation behavior that is composite: more than one exponential will be required to characterize changes in both the longitudinal and transverse components of the proton magnetization.[18,31] It has been pointed out that such composite behavior is difficult to resolve, even when the two rates differ by a factor of three, unless the noise is very low and the accuracy of the data is very high. Nonetheless, with advances in technology, and continued motivation, many of these problems will be addressed successfully, to the advantage of fundamental science on the one hand, and clinical medicine and patient care on the other.

ACKNOWLEDGMENTS

The rat liver data, Figure 63–4 and all the data and Figure 63–9, were obtained in collaboration with Drs. R. Nunnally and D. Hollis; the brain data, Figure 63–6, with Dr. D. Adams; the breast data, Figure 63–8, with Dr. Y. Wang; and the colon data, Figure 63–10, with Drs. T. R. Lindstrom and C. F. Brewer.

References

1. Koenig SH, Brown III RD: Relaxometry of tissue. *In* Gupta RK (ed): NMR Spectroscopy of Cells and Organisms. Boca Raton, CRC Press, 1987, pp 75–114.
2. Sepponen RE, Pohjonen JA, Sipponen JT, Tanttu JI: A method for $T1_\rho$ imaging. J Comput Asst Tomogr 9:1007–1011, 1985.
3. Bloch F: Nuclear induction. Phys Rev 70:460–474, 1946.
4. Koenig SH, Schillinger WE: Nuclear magnetic relaxation dispersion in protein solutions. I. Apotransferrin. J Biol Chem 244:3283–3289, 1969.
5. Hallenga K, Koenig SH: Protein rotational relaxation as studied by solvent ^1H and ^2H magnetic relaxation. Biochemistry, 15:4255–4264, 1976.
6. Koenig, SH, Hallenga K, Shporer M: Protein-water interaction studied by solvent ^1H, ^2H, and ^{17}O magnetic relaxation. Proc Nat Acad Sci USA 72:2667–2671, 1975.

7. Koenig SH: The dynamics of water-protein interactions: Results from measurements of nuclear magnetic relaxation dispersion. *In* Water in Polymers. ACS Symposium Series *127*:157–176, 1980.

8. Koenig SH, Bryant RG, Hallenga K, Jacob GS: Magnetic cross-relaxation among protons in protein solutions. Biochemistry *17*:4348–4358, 1978.

9. Koenig SH, Schillinger WE: Nuclear magnetic relaxation dispersion in protein solutions. II. Transferrin. J Biol Chem *244*:6520–6526, 1969.

10. Lindstrom TR, Koenig SH: Magnetic-field-dependent water proton spin-lattice relaxation rates of hemoglobin solutions and whole blood. J Magn Reson *15*:344–353, 1974.

11. Brown III RD, Brewer CF, Koenig SH: Conformation states of concanavalin A: Kinetics of transitions induced by interaction with Mn^{2+} and Ca^{2+} ions. Biochemistry *16*:3883–3896, 1977.

12. Koenig SH, Brown III RD, Lindstrom TR: Interactions of solvent with the heme region of methemoglobin and fluoro-methemoglobin. *In* Ho C (ed): Hemoglobin and Oxygen Binding. New York, Elsevier Biomedical, 1982, pp 377–385.

13. Koenig SH: A novel derivation of the Solomon-Bloembergen-Morgan equations: Application to solvent relaxation by Mn^{2+}-protein complexes. J Magn Reson *31*:1–10, 1978.

14. Koenig SH: A classical description of relaxation of interacting pairs of unlike spins: Extension to $T1_\rho$, $T2$, $T1_{\rho\text{off}}$, including contact interactions. J Magn Reson *47*:441–453, 1982.

15. Koenig SH, Brown III RD, Adams D, Emerson D, Harrison CG: Magnetic field dependence of $1/T1$ of protons in tissue. Invest Radiol *19*:76–81, 1984.

16. Koenig SH, Brown III RD: The importance of the motion of water for magnetic resonance imaging. Invest Radiol *20*:297–305, 1985.

17. Koenig SH, Brown III RD, Goldstein E, Wolf GL: Magnetic field dependence of tissue proton relaxation rates with added Mn^{2+}: Rabbit liver and kidney. Magn Reson Med *2*:159–168, 1985.

18. Koenig SH, Spiller M, Brown III RD, Wolf GL: Magnetic field dependence (NMRD profile) of $1/T1$ of rabbit kidney medulla and urine after injection of Gd-DTPA. Invest Radiol *21*:697–704, 1986.

19. Bloembergen N, Purcell EM, Pound RV: Relaxation effects in nuclear magnetic resonance absorption. Phys Rev *73*:679–712, 1948.

20. Slichter CP: Principles of Magnetic Resonance. 2nd ed. Berlin, Springer-Verlag, Berlin, 1978. (An intermediate level discussion)

21. Meiboom S: Nuclear magnetic resonance study of proton transfer in water. J Chem Phys *34*:375–388, 1961.

22. Grösch L, Noack F: NMR relaxation investigation of water mobility in aqueous bovine serum albumin solutions. Biochim Biophys Acta *453*:218–232, 1976..

23. Wehrli FW, MacFall JR, Glover GH, Grigsby N, Haughton V, Johanson J: The dependence of nuclear magnetic resonance (NMR) image contrast on intrinsic and pulse sequence timing parameters. Magn Reson Imag *2*:3–16, 1984.

24. Bottomley, PA, Foster TH, Argersinger RE, Pfeifer LM: A review of normal tissue hydrogen NMR relaxation times and relaxation mechanisms from 1-100 MHz: Dependence on tissue type, NMR frequency, temperature, species, excision, and age. Med Phys *11*:425–448, 1984.

25. Held G, Noack F, Pollak V, Meltons B: Protonenspinrelaxation und Wasserbeweglichkeit in Muskelgewebe. Z Naturforsch *28c*:59–62, 1978.

26. Knipsel RR, Thompson RT, Pintar MM: Dispersion of proton spin-lattice relaxation in tissue. J Magn Reson *14*:44–51, 1974.

27. Koenig SH, Brown III RD: Determinants of proton relaxation rates in tissue. Magn Reson Med *1*:437–449, 1984.

28. Winter F, Kimmich R: NMR field-cycling relaxation spectroscopy of bovine serum albumin, muscle tissue, *Micrococcus luteus*, and yeast. $^{14}N^1H$ quadrupole dips. Biochim Biophys Acta *719*:292–298, 1982.

29. Koenig SH: Theory of relaxation of mobile water protons induced by protein NH moieties, with application to rat heart muscle and calf lens homogenates. Biophysical J (in press).

30. Beaulieu CF, Clark JI, Brown III RD, Spiller M, Koenig SH: Magnetic field dependence of $1/T1$ in calf lens cytoplasm in vitro: solvent-protein cross relaxation. Sixth Annual Meeting, Society of Magnetic Resonance in Medicine, New York, 1987 (Abstract).

31. Barroilhet LE, Moran PR: NMR relaxation behavior in living and ischemically damaged tissue. Med Phys *3*:410–414, 1976.

64

Relaxometry of Solvent and Tissue Protons: Paramagnetic Contributions

SEYMOUR H. KOENIG
RODNEY D. BROWN, III

Bloch,[1,2] for the first observation of proton magnetic resonance in a liquid, added ferric nitrate to a sample of water to shorten the relaxation time of the protons. The concern was that $T1$, the longitudinal relaxation time, might be too long, which would prevent recovery of the magnetization of the proton ensemble between successive attempts to observe a signal, thereby precluding the observation of NMR in liquids altogether. Since that time, over four decades ago, the influence of solute paramagnetic ions on the relaxation rates of solvent protons has been the subject of continuous research, initially for studying the chemistry of small solute paramagnetic chelate complexes and, later, for investigating the structure and function of paramagnetic macromolecular complexes, mainly metalloproteins. There is a long, well-documented history of the study of water solutions of paramagnetic ions, recently reviewed,[3,4] from which it is apparent that most of the solution results are relevant to the relaxation behavior of water protons in tissue containing paramagnetic ions.[5-7]

Those aspects of relaxation-enhancement by paramagnetic ions that are relevant to MRI may be classified in a number of ways. A particularly convenient division is between endogenous and exogenous agents. The first group would include iron in its various states of oxidation and oxygenation in hemoglobin, transferrin, ferritin, hemosiderin, and perhaps smaller complexes as well; O_2 in blood and lungs; free radicals, conceivably; and other paramagnetics that could accumulate as a result of trauma or disease, for example, Cu^{2+} in Wilson's disease. The second group would include small chelate complexes such as Gd-DTPA and analogous structures; macromolecular derivatives of these chelates, hopefully with site specificity;[8] and both paramagnetic and ferromagnetic particulates with desirable macroscopic magnetic properties.

We will group all the above under the rubric of "contrast-enhancing agents" (or simply, contrast agents), though the endogenous paramagnetic ions are not really agents, and some of the particulates actually obliterate parts of the image, an effect that may be useful in its own way. Having done that, it is convenient to distinguish between agents that alter $1/T2$ predominantly at typical imaging fields, with little influence on $1/T1$, and all others. The issue is as follows. The contribution of any agent to the relaxation *rates* (not times) generally adds to the background values (the relaxation rates of the nonparamagnetic tissue) and, for paramagnetic complexes that act as independent centers, the incremental contributions to $1/T1$ and $1/T2$ are usually comparable and related. At typical imaging fields, generally $1/T2 \gg 1/T1$ for tissue, so that the *fractional* changes in rates are far less for the transverse than the longitudinal relaxation rates. By contrast, localized assemblages of paramagnetic complexes (e.g., deoxyhemoglobin in erythrocytes;[9] perhaps Fe^{3+} ions in the core of ferritin;[10] and particles of iron oxide) produce inhomogeneities in the magnetic field in their vicinity. The effect is to alter the Larmor precession frequency of nearby protons. The accumulated precessional phase shifts[11] produce a contribution to $1/T2$, called "secular," that has no equivalent for $1/T1$.

The utility of any contrast agent will ultimately relate to the balance between relaxivity and toxicity, relaxivity being defined as the change in relaxation rate per unit concentration of ion. Intuitively, the relaxivity of a particular paramagnetic agent should depend on how closely tissue water molecules can approach the complexed paramagnetic ion and probe its magnetic aspects. But this view is often inadequate. For example, water molecules complex directly to the iron of Fe^{3+} hemoglobin (methemoglobin), but the lifetime of this complex is so long (about 10^{-4} s) that the effect of the interaction is markedly reduced.[12] In this case, the relaxivity contribution from "inner sphere" complexation is small, comparable to the integrated "outer sphere" effects that arise as water molecules diffuse in the vicinity of, but not too close to, the paramagnetic ions and sense the fields that they generate.

Toxicity tends to go as the inverse of relaxivity. Those paramagnetic complexes that are tight and long-lived, as a consequence, often exclude water from their inner coordination sphere. An example, and an exception that at the same time illustrates the point, is Gd-DTPA. DTPA (diethylenetriaminepentaacetic acid) is an octadentate chelate that forms extremely stable complexes with many metal ions. Gd-DTPA not only remains essentially undissociated in vivo but does not even interact with the cellular components of tissue.[7] Its relaxivity, one-fourth that of the hydrated Gd^{3+} ion,[13] is, nonetheless, relatively large because lanthanides are large ions, with room for nine inner-coordinated ligands. The relation of relaxivity to toxicity, as in this example, is going to depend on subtleties of ligand physical chemistry and how this influences the exchange rate of ligands from the inner coordination sphere of the ion. Moreover, the ligand environment determines the paramagnetic properties of the ions, in particular, the relaxation rates of the electronic paramagnetic moments of these ions. This, in turn, affects the correlation time of the ion-proton interaction[4] (a quantity that will not be emphasized here, except to note that it has a strong influence on paramagnetic relaxivities).

The theory of relaxation by paramagnetic centers is rather well developed and complete.[4] However, because of the many chemical parameters that describe a given paramagnetic complex, it is still difficult to choose values for the variables that enter into the theory in a particular case. To date, the theory has not been too useful for prediction of relaxation by paramagnetic centers; the emphasis in this chapter, therefore, is on the phenomenology. As in the earlier chapter in this volume on the relaxometry of diamagnetic tissue, the information presented will be the magnetic field dependence of the longitudinal relaxation rates (NMRD profiles) for a wide range of samples, all in vitro and mostly solutions rather than tissue. Most studies of relaxation by paramagnetic ions have been carried out for solutions. However, the limited NMRD data on tissue containing paramagnetic agents indicate that their relaxivity in tissue is closely related to their solution behavior, so that the data considered here have a direct and immediate bearing on the principles that underly contrast enhancement in MRI.

RELAXOMETRY OF Fe^{3+} AND Fe^{2+} IONS

Iron is certainly the most ubiquitous endogenous paramagnetic ion. The high spin Fe^{3+} oxidation state, with its relatively long electronic relaxation time,[3,4] makes the greater contribution to proton relaxation.[10,12] However, the relaxivity of Fe^{3+} complexes is quite complicated,[14] owing in part to the nature of the aqueous chemistry of Fe^{3+}, in part to the relatively slow rates of ligand exchange, and in part to the tendency of the ground electronic state of Fe^{3+} ions to split into levels[15,16] in a manner that makes prediction of relaxation effects from first principles difficult.[17,18]

The clinical relevance of Fe^{3+} ions is multifaceted. Management of hematomas could in principle be aided by imaging the ions that oxidize to Fe^{3+} as hemoglobin in the hematomas breaks down. The increased production of the iron-storage proteins ferritin and hemosiderin, made in response to excess iron, can be monitored by NMR imaging.[19] Such excess iron can result from transfusion treatment of patients who lack a gene for proper hemoglobin production, and death can ensue when the storage mechanisms are ultimately overwhelmed. As another example, transferrin is a circulating protein that transports iron, as Fe^{3+}, from the gut to the bone marrow for incorporation into hemoglobin. Normally the two binding sites per molecule are about 30 percent saturated with Fe^{3+}, an occupancy that can increase under abnormal conditions. A question that arises is whether changes in the iron loading of transferrin are detectable by MRI. Finally, certain strongly associated chelates of Fe^{3+} ions are taken up differentially by the liver and have potential therefore as hepatobiliary contrast agents.[20] An examination of the NMRD profiles of solutions of Fe^{3+} complexes, relevant to all the above, with discussions of the salient features of the relaxation profiles, follows.

Fe^{3+} Aquoions

Fe^{3+} ions are insoluble in water above pH 3 and therefore must be complexed either to protein or small chelates to be useful under physiological conditions different from those found in the stomach. This point is made explicit in the NMRD profiles[14] of Figure 64–1. There are multiple equilibria among the several hydrolyzed forms of the aquoion, so that the exact pH dependence of the relaxivities at intermediate pH values depends on the Fe^{3+} concentration. Nevertheless, Figure 64–1 is more than

Figure 64–1. Longitudinal NMRD profiles of solvent protons in a 0.68 mM solution of $Fe_2(SO_4)_3$, for several values of pH, at 25°C. The sample was initially at pH 1.25 (●), and the pH was raised by addition of concentrated KOH. The data have been corrected for the effects of dilution, which was at most 7 percent. The solid curve through the upper set of data points results from a least squares comparison of the data with the usual theory of relaxation by dipolar interactions within a complex, with rapid ligand-solvent exchange. Outer sphere contributions (about 5 percent, cf. Fig. 64–2) were ignored in the fit. (Data after reference 14.)

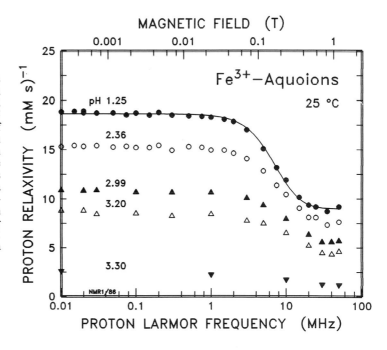

adequate to illustrate the point that Fe^{3+} aquoions do not relax water protons in the physiological pH range.

The NMRD profiles of Figure 64–1 arise from the Fe^{3+}-proton magnetic dipolar interaction. The single dispersion, i.e., the inflection of the NMRD profile centered near 10 MHz, results from the condition $\omega_S\tau_c = 1$, where ω_S is the Larmor precession frequency of the paramagnetic moments of the Fe^{3+} ions. (The correlation time τ_c is dominated by the rotational reorientation of the aquoion[4] due to thermal motion; from the inflection points of the curves (Fig. 64–1), one obtains $\tau_c \sim 2.5 \times 10^{-11}$ s.) The relaxivity is mainly due to proton exchange between the bulk solvent and the inner sphere of the Fe^{3+} ions, presumably acid-catalyzed exchange of protons rather than exchange of water molecules, since the latter are known to exchange very slowly for Fe^{3+} aquoions. The contribution from solvent molecules diffusing in the outer sphere environment of the aquoions is about 5 percent of the total (see below).

Small Chelate Complexes of Fe^{3+} Ions

Fe^{3+} ions can be maintained in solution at physiological pH by complexation with small chelates, either by using a large excess of a chelate that forms a weak complex or by stoichiometric combination with a chelate that forms a tight complex.[14] Citrate is an example of the former. It is the dominant anion of certain dietary supplements meant to correct iron deficiency and as such has been tried on human volunteers as a contrast agent for the gut.[21] Examples of tight complexes are DTPA (diethylenetria-minepentaacetic acid)[13] and EHPG (ethylene bis-(2-hydroxyphenylglycine)),[20] which occupy the entire inner Fe^{3+} coordination sphere; and EDTA (ethylenediaminetetra-acetic acid), which tends to force Fe^{3+}, which is normally 6-coordinate, into a 7-coordinate configuration.[22] The NMRD profiles of these chelates are shown in Figure 64–2 near physiological conditions of pH and temperature.

The excess relaxivity of the EDTA complex compared with the other three is evident, though the difference is not as great as one-sixth the inner sphere values (Fig. 64–1), as 7-coordination might imply, nor equal to that of the isoelectronic Mn^{2+}-EDTA

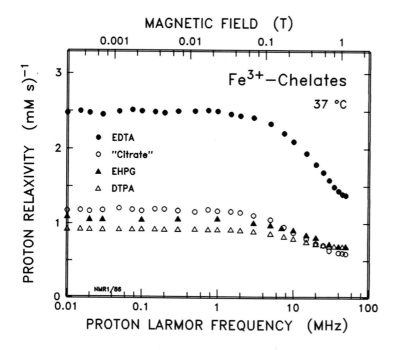

Figure 64–2. NMRD profiles of solutions of several chelate complexes of Fe^{3+}, near pH 7, at 37°C. EDTA (ethylenedi-aminetetraacetic acid) (●) is hexaden-tate, but the iron becomes (partially) 7-coordinate in this complex; "citrate" (○) here is the dietary supplement Geritol, in which a large excess of ammonium ci-trate maintains Fe^{3+} in solution, even near pH 7; EHPG (ethylene bis-(2-hy-droxyphenylglycine)) (▲) is a hexaden-tate ligand taken up preferentially by liver; and DTPA (diethylenetriaminepen-taacetic acid) (△) is an octadentate li-gand. The near equivalence of the lower three profiles suggests that outer sphere relaxation dominates the relaxivity in all three cases. (Data, in part, after refer-ence 14.)

complex, which has a value of 5 $(mM \ s)^{-1}$ at low fields, at 37°C. However, a quantitative analysis to ascertain the source of the excess relaxivity would require knowing whether the 7-coordinate bond length is that of the aquoion, or is somewhat longer, and whether or not there is a mixture of coordination configurations in solution.

The relaxivity profiles of the other three complexes (Fig. 64–2) are ostensibly due to outer sphere effects, for which the several published theories[23–26] have been recently reconsidered.[27] Of note in Figure 64–2 is that the high field extreme of these profiles does not disperse to the expected 0.3 of the low field limit, a technical point indicating that the correlation time for the interaction is a function of magnetic field.[4] To handle this theoretically requires the recent generalization[27] of the results of Freed.[25] However, application of the theory to the rather featureless data for outer sphere relaxation (Fig. 64–2) is premature, since we find that a wide range of values for the several parameters of the theory fit the data equally well, and there is as yet no realistic way of deciding on their relative validities.

The major point to note is that Fe^{3+} can be made soluble near physiological pH by small chelates but at a cost of roughly a 5- to 10-fold reduction in relaxivity from the aquoion values (Fig. 64–1), which makes them quite low. The situation is only somewhat improved by complexation with protein, if at all.

Fe^{3+}-Transferrin

Transferrin, a circulating serum protein of 84 kDa required for transport of iron, has two iron-binding sites per protein molecule, both very similar though not identical, that are essentially noninteracting. The concentration of transferrin in the blood is ~0.04 mM, and the transferrin molecules are about one-third saturated with Fe^{3+} under normal conditions.[28] Although crystallographic data are not yet available at high resolution, many physical and biochemical investigations have led to the consensus that the Fe^{3+} ions are 6-coordinate, with four protein-donated ligands, and with OH^- and HCO_3^- contributed by solvent. HCO_3^- is required for tight binding of Fe^{3+} and, in vivo, is always present unless specific mechanisms exist to remove it.[28]

Figure 64–3 shows the NMRD profiles of Fe^{3+}-saturated and apotransferrin,[29,30] at 37°C. It is now generally agreed that the paramagnetic contribution to the relaxivity results from rapid exchange of a second sphere, hydrogen bonded water molecule, with one proton about 3 Å from an Fe^{3+} ion. (Exchange of a hydroxyl proton near physiological pH is not sufficiently rapid to contribute observably to relaxation without resort to an unusual mechanism of exchange.[31]) This type of second sphere exchange, originally postulated for fluoromethemoglobin,[12] and dubbed[30] the "fluoromet mechanism," also appears to account for relaxation in solutions of cupric and vanadyl transferrin derivatives[32] and protein-bound nitroxide radicals.[27]

The functional form of the paramagnetic contribution of the Fe^{3+} ions (Fig. 64–3) is complex.[12,14] What is germane for questions of MRI, however, is the relatively low magnitude of the paramagnetic relaxivity, in the range 3 to 4 $(mM \ s)^{-1}$ at all fields. Given the low concentration of transferrin in the circulation, saturation under iron overload conditions would contribute a rate increase of about 0.1 s^{-1} to $1/T1$ at all fields (and comparably to $1/T2$), which is at the edge of observability.

Fe^{3+}-Hemoglobin

The paramagnetic relaxivity of the Fe^{3+} ions of methemoglobin is even smaller than that of Fe^{3+}-transferrin; the greater potential utility of hemoglobin in MRI comes

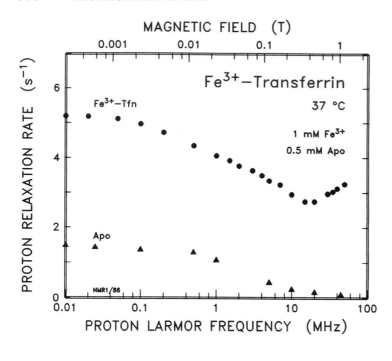

Figure 64–3. NMRD profiles of an 0.5 mM solution of human transferrin saturated with Fe^{3+} (●), near pH 7, at 37°C, and that of the apo (demetallized) protein (▲). (Data after references 29 and 30.)

about because of the greater concentration of hemoglobin relative to transferrin. Figure 64–4 shows the NMRD profiles of Fe^{3+}-hemoglobin and a diamagnetic control, carbonmonoxyhemoglobin, at 35°C. For ease of comparison with MRI data, the hemoglobin concentration in the sample was that of normal blood. The paramagnetic relaxivity (per Fe^{3+}) is very low, comparable to the outer sphere contribution of small chelates of Fe^{3+} ions. It has previously been shown[12] that about half the methemoglobin relaxivity is outer sphere, with the remainder due to slow exchange of the inner coordinated water molecules of the heme groups. Displacing these waters by fluoride

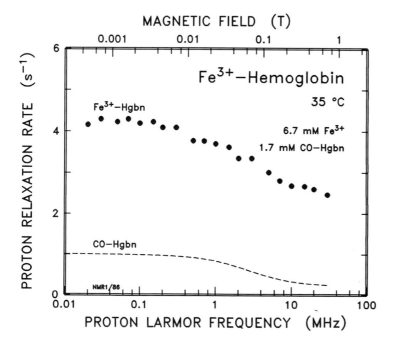

Figure 64–4. NMRD profiles of a 1.7 mM solution of carbonmonoxyhemoglobin (dashed curve), which is diamagnetic, near pH 7, at 35°C, and a similar solution of methemoglobin (●). The latter includes the diamagnetic background of the lower curve as well as the paramagnetic contribution of the four Fe^{3+} ions per protein molecule. (Data after reference 12.)

gives a 10-fold enhancement of the relaxivity, in vitro, due to the fluoromet mechanism mentioned above.[30]

Oxidation of hemoglobin iron to Fe^{3+}, at physiological concentrations, will certainly produce a detectable change in a *T1* weighted image provided that rapid access of water to the heme pocket is maintained. The incremental contribution to $1/T2$ will be similar, but the fractional effect in an in vivo imaging situation will be much smaller, as discussed above.

Ferritin

Ferritin, an iron storage protein of 447 kDa, has a spherical protein shell of about 130 Å outer diameter and 70 Å inner diameter, that is assembled from 24 nearly identical subunits. Channels of both threefold and fourfold symmetry lead to an inner core that, in the native state, may contain as many as 3000 Fe^{3+} ions in a solid-state crystalline array of an unusual ferric oxyhydroxide that is ostensibly paramagnetic at physiological pH.[33,34] Figure 64–5 shows the NMRD profiles for solutions of horse spleen apoferritin, ferritin with one Fe^{3+} per subunit, and ferritin with rather fully loaded core.[10] The 24:1 data were obtained by titration of iron into apoferritin, with subsequent oxidation of the complexed iron to Fe^{3+}, whereas the 900:1 sample was natural ferritin. As might be expected, loading the core makes little contribution to the $1/T1$ relaxivity profile; the 30 Å thick protein shell isolates the solution from the core very effectively. The theory of outer sphere relaxation is in agreement with this and also predicts that the contribution to $1/T2$ should be comparably small.[23,24]

The surprise is that MRI of patients with iron overload disease shows dark livers and spleens,[19] indicative of a very short *T2* caused by the presence of iron-induced ferritin formation, but at concentrations such that little if any effect would be expected on the basis of theory coupled with the data of Figure 64–5; rather, the $1/T2$ profiles should be much like the $1/T1$ profiles, as appears to be the case for the 24:1 sample. For the 900:1 sample, $1/T2$ is anomalously large, with a rate of 5 s^{-1} at 20 MHz in vitro. No mechanism has as yet been proposed that accounts for this anomaly.

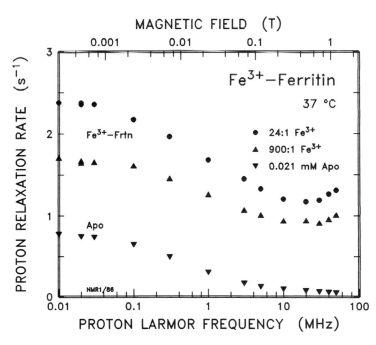

Figure 64–5. NMRD profiles of a 21 μM solution of apo (demetallized) horse spleen ferritin (▼), near pH 7, at 37°C, and similar solutions with the ferritin containing respectively 24 (●) and about 900 (▲) Fe^{3+} ions per protein molecule. (Data after reference 10.)

Summary of Fe^{3+} Relaxometry

The role of ferric iron for contrast enhancement in MRI is now mainly as an endogenous agent. The limitation is that Fe^{3+} complexes generally have low relaxivities, due in the main to the extensive chelation needed to maintain Fe^{3+} in solution and to slow exchange of coordinated water molecules. Two endogenous complexes appear useful as present; methemoglobin and ferritin (including hemosiderin, which appears to be the product of the partial degradation of ferritin[35]). For methemoglobin, the low relaxivity can be offset by the large concentrations of paramagnetic protein that can occur in disease or trauma. The major influence will be on $1/T1$. Ferritin, on the other hand, appears to have a large secular relaxivity[10,19] that, by definition, contributes to $1/T2$, and not to $1/T1$; although the reasons are not clear, the presence of excess ferritin is associated with very high transverse relaxation rates.

A theoretical description of the NMRD profiles of Fe^{3+} complexes is still rather difficult in general, in part due to the varied (and unpredictable) biochemistry involved and in part to the anisotropy of the ligand fields of the Fe^{3+} ions that complicates computational aspects of the theory.

Fe^{2+} Ions

The relaxivity of Fe^{2+} ions is very low, 50-fold less than that of Fe^{3+} ions under comparable conditions,[10] and its contribution to $1/T1$ and $1/T2$ of solvent protons is rarely considered. For example, the heme centers of hemoglobin are paramagnetic in the deoxygenated state, but the oxy to deoxy transition has never been detected by relaxivity techniques applied to hemoglobin solutions.[12] On the other hand, effects have been reported for blood,[9] demonstrably related to the confinement of the paramagnetic species within erythrocytes, which arise because the magnetic susceptibility of the sample varies spatially on a cellular scale. What is observed is an increase of $1/T2$ of the water protons of blood upon deoxygenation, with no change in $1/T1$. The magnitude of the effect increases with the square of the static magnetic field.

Several authors have considered the theory of secular relaxation in a form applicable to samples with inhomogeneous magnetic properties,[36,37] including blood and highly structured diamagnetic tissues such as muscle.[38] There are as yet but few data to compare with this theory, in part because the effects are small except at high fields (since they vary quadratically with the field), so that it is premature to say how well understood this area is. Two points, quite unrelated, should nonetheless be noted. (1) The magnitude of the effects will depend on whether in blood, for example, water exchanges rapidly between the intra- and extracellular environments or only senses the extracellular magnetic field inhomogeneities. (2) The theory is equally applicable to the effects of particulate ferromagnetic contrast agents. There is little question, given the structure of tissue and the increasingly high fields being used in MRI and in in vivo spectroscopy, as well as the fact that these secular effects alter $1/T2$ predominantly, that research in this area will grow rapidly in interest and in relevance to MRI.

RELAXOMETRY OF Mn^{2+}

Manganese is probably the most studied paramagnetic relaxation agent. In the early years of applications of NMR to solution chemistry, it was discovered that the longitudinal and transverse relaxivities of Mn^{2+} in aqueous solution were markedly different,[39] which led to the realization that the Mn^{2+}-proton interaction in the aquoion had a relaxivity contribution in addition to the usual magnetic dipolar interaction,[40] called the scalar or hyperfine interaction. This offered the possibility of using this interaction to prove the nature of ligand orbitals. Though the technical details are not too relevant to MRI, the scalar term does alter the NMRD profile in a useful way,[4] as will be seen. Subsequently, when interest developed in applying relaxometry to studies of macromolecular systems, the fact that Mn^{2+} could substitute for Mg^{2+} in many weak macromolecular complexes made possible studies of the kinases,[41] including their interactions with substrate and ATP, as well as studies of various nucleic acids.[42-44] Mn^{2+} also has the following desirable properties: it is soluble at physiological pH; it has an EPR spectrum that is readily observable, and identifiable, in solutions of the aquoion and some protein complexes; and it can often substitute for diamagnetic ions in many metalloproteins without altering substantially the biological properties of the native proteins. Much of our understanding of the mechanisms of solvent proton relaxation has come from studies of Mn^{2+} complexes,[45,46] and it is appropriate to consider some of these results here. Nonetheless, the utility of Mn^{2+} as a contrast agent in MRI has been limited to date, in large part because its complexes tend to dissociate in vivo,[6] and free Mn^{2+} is toxic.

NMRD Profiles of Mn^{2+} Complexes

Figure 64–6 shows the NMRD profiles of solutions of three complexes of Mn^{2+}: the hexa-aquoion; Mn^{2+} complexed tightly with excess EDTA; and Mn^{2+}-concanavalin A, a well-studied lectin[46] that contains Mn^{2+} in the native state. These data illustrate how the form of the NMRD profiles for a single type of paramagnetic ion varies with its chemical environment. The reasons for the differences in the profiles are understood quantitatively,[4] and will not be considered here except to note one salient feature of the profile for the protein-bound Mn^{2+} ion not contained in the profiles of the smaller complexes: the peak in the NMRD profile at the higher fields.[45,46] It arises when two conditions are met: the paramagnetic ion must be complexed with a macromolecular entity sufficiently large that the rotational thermal motion of the complex no longer

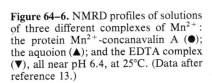

Figure 64–6. NMRD profiles of solutions of three different complexes of Mn^{2+}: the protein Mn^{2+}-concanavalin A (●); the aquoion (▲); and the EDTA complex (▼), all near pH 6.4, at 25°C. (Data after reference 13.)

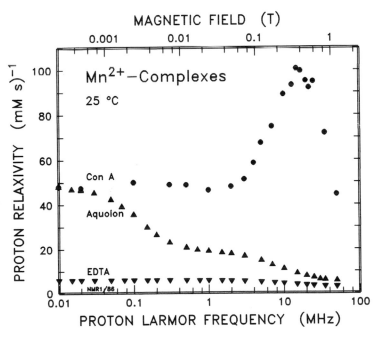

influences the relaxation process (something greater than about 20 kDa) and the relaxation parameters of the paramagnetic moment of the ion itself must be a function of magnetic field. These conditions, which maximize the relaxivity in the MRI range, are satisfied routinely with Mn^{2+} and, as will be seen, with Gd^{3+}, which is a reason for further investigation of both these paramagnetic cations.

Outer Sphere Relaxation of Chelated Mn²⁺

The relaxivity of certain chelate complexes of Mn^{2+} is due only to outer sphere interactions. NOTA, a triazacyclononane with three acetate groups coordinated to the nitrogens, is a highly symmetric hexadentate molecule that forms a relatively rigid chelate complex with Mn^{2+}, which remains 6-coordinate. DOTA, the analogous four-nitrogen molecule, is octadentate. Solutions of complexes of these chelates with Mn^{2+}, as well as Mn-DTPA, have nearly identical NMRD profiles,[13,47] as seen in Figure 64–7. The relaxivities are about half those of Mn-EDTA, indicating that it, like ferric-EDTA, is 7-coordinate.[48]

The solid curve through the profile for Mn-DTPA (Fig. 64–7) results from a least squares comparison of the data with a theory of outer sphere relaxation. Not surprisingly, the theoretical fit is not unique; the solid curve is a representation of two sets of values for the parameters of the theory, both of which give the identical fit over the field range illustrated. At present we have no reason to prefer one set of values over the other, nor are we certain that there are not other equally good sets of values for the parameters. The major point, however, is that the agreement of data and theory establishes the utility of the theory and provides a baseline for the magnitude of outer sphere effects. As will be seen, this becomes particularly important for understanding the relaxivity of analogous chelated complexes of Gd^{3+}.

Mn²⁺ in Tissue

Mn^{2+} is an exogenous contrast agent (though there is some evidence that it can accumulate in the liver of rabbits and contribute observably to the liver relaxation rate

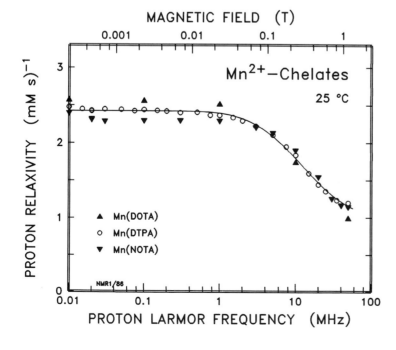

Figure 64–7. NMRD profiles of solutions of several chelate complexes of Mn^{2+}, near pH 6.5, at 25°C. NOTA (a polycyclic triazacyclononane) (▼), is hexadentate, whereas DTPA (○) and DOTA (a polycyclic tetraazacyclododecane) (▲) are both octadentate. The near equivalence of the three profiles suggests that outer sphere relaxation dominates the relaxivity in all three cases. The solid curve through the Mn-DTPA data points results from a least squares comparison of the data with the theory of outer sphere relaxation. (Data, in part, after reference 47.)

when the rabbit's food intake is restricted to certain prepared chows,[6] so that it can be endogenous in this sense). The experience to date with externally introduced Mn^{2+}, given either by intravenous injection or by mouth, chelated or as the chloride, is that it accumulates predominantly and uniformly in the liver, separated from chelate (if any) and complexed with some macromolecular structure.[4,5] This is illustrated in Figure 64–8, in which the NMRD profiles of (excised) livers of normal rabbits before and after intravenous injection of a weak chelate complex of Mn^{2+} are compared. The injections were 12 and 36 µMoles per kg body weight of Mn^{2+}-propanoldiaminetetraacetic acid (PDTA); the animals were sacrificed 15 min after injection. The mean concentration of Mn in the livers, indicated in Figure 64–8, was measured by ICP (inductively coupled plasma) analysis.

The lowest set of data, a control, is a profile of the liver of an uninjected rabbit. Runs on numerous controls show little individual variation other than the slight rise in the 10 to 20 MHz region. This rise, attributable to Mn^{2+} in the food, has been ignored in fitting the solid curve through these data, a curve used later to correct the profiles of the Mn-containing livers for the diamagnetic background. There are three points to note: the concentration of Mn found in the liver is proportional to the total amount injected in the limited range shown;[49] there is a marked enhancement of the relaxation rates; and this enhancement is not linear in Mn concentration for the examples used here. In fact, we know from earlier work[4] that there is indeed a saturation in the relaxation rates with Mn-PDTA dosage and from more recent work[49] that this saturation arises from chemical saturation of the liver with Mn at about 0.5 to 0.7 mM Mn. In fact, when this saturation regime is approached, the relaxation data become nonexponential and the entire situation more complex. Accordingly, we consider only the data for the lower Mn-PDTA dosage, replotted in Figure 64–9 as the paramagnetic contribution to the liver NMRD profile per mM of Mn.

The data in Figure 64–9 have a clear peak, indicative of solvent-accessible Mn^{2+} bound to macromolecules. The relaxivities are high, at least 10-fold greater than the outer sphere relaxivities of small Mn^{2+}-chelate complexes. Based in part on the fact that administration of aqueous Mn^{2+} gives the same results, we argue that the data of Figure 64–9 represent macromolecular-bound Mn^{2+} ions freed from chelate.[6] It is not

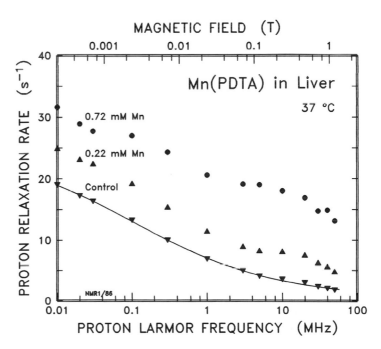

Figure 64–8. NMRD profiles of normal rabbit liver (▼), and livers from two rabbits injected with different total amounts of Mn-PDTA (propanoldiaminetetraacetic acid), at 37°C. The rabbits were sacrificed 15 min after injection. The Mn contents of the livers were subsequently determined to be 0.72 mM (●) and 0.22 mM (▲) for the two samples. (Data after reference 6.)

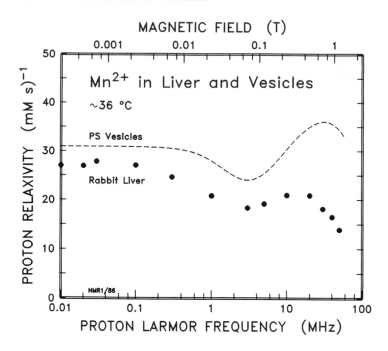

Figure 64-9. The paramagnetic contribution of Mn^{2+} to the NMRD profile of the liver of Figure 64-8 containing 0.22 mM Mn (●), near 36°C, indicated in relaxivity units. The dashed curve is the profile of a solution of Mn^{2+} bound to phosphatidyl-serine vesicles. (Kurland and Koenig, unpublished.)

yet clear where these ions are bound. Addition of Mn^{2+} ions to a suspension of liver cells, removed enzymatically from their tissue substrate, gives very similar NMRD profiles immediately after Mn^{2+} addition,[5] suggesting that the Mn^{2+} may be bound to the exterior of the cells and associated with the cell membranes. On the other hand, in vivo data indicate that Mn^{2+} accumulates in the bile, which can only occur if these ions pass through the hepatocytes. Although this is not of present concern, it should be noted that physiological questions of this sort can be addressed by NMRD measurements, perhaps more readily than by any other technique.

The dashed curve, Figure 64-9, is the dispersion profile of Mn^{2+} ions added to a solution of phosphatidyl-serine vesicles,[50] the intent being to compare the liver data with a system that mimics cell membranes. Although the exact form and amplitude of the vesicle profiles are sensitive to the ionic strength and cationic content of the solution, nonetheless, the qualitative similarity of the two profiles in Figure 64-9 suggests a generalized interaction of Mn^{2+} ions in liver with the exterior polar groups of the cell membranes.

Remarks on Mn^{2+} Relaxometry

The finding[6] that several chelates of Mn^{2+} dissociate in the liver is a good reason to look elsewhere for paramagnetic contrast agents useful for clinical MRI. Current interest centers around chelates of Gd^{3+}, which tends to be 9-coordinate, so that chelation by even an octadentate ligand would leave an inner sphere site for solvent exchange. Because of the toxicity of Mn^{2+}, its utility as a contrast agent will be restricted, for the present, to animal experiments of the type indicated here, centered around liver function and chemistry, bile production, and gall bladder activity. The unique relaxometry properties of Mn^{2+}, as summarized in Figure 64-6, make it rather clear that such interest will continue. However, Mn^{2+} complexes have the highest relaxivities ever reported,[4] and advances in chelate chemistry may make it possible to take advantage of this property in the clinical environment.

RELAXOMETRY OF Gd³⁺

Trivalent gadolinium has a half-filled f-shell and, accordingly, has a relatively long electronic relaxation time (though generally not as long as Mn^{2+}), which is favorable for high relaxivity.[4] The ion is large and highly charged so that the coordination number tends to be high, typically nine, as compared with six for Mn^{2+}. Hexadentate chelates exist that form very strong complexes with Gd^{3+}, leaving three coordinated waters in rapid exchange in aqueous solution. Gd-DTPA, a complex with an octadentate chelate with one coordinated water, is used extensively at present for clinical MRI. It is small, highly stable, and very soluble under physiological conditions and excreted in the urine within several hours after intravenous introduction.[7] Its toxicity is low, as is its relaxivity in aqueous solution,[14] though the latter is greater than the comparable Mn^{2+} and Fe^{3+} complexes because of both a higher spin (7/2 vs 5/2) and a larger inner sphere coordination capacity.

Applications of Gd-DTPA to date[51] have been to the circulatory system, e.g., to look for breaks in the blood-brain barrier. The relatively low and comparable values of $1/T1$ and $1/T2$ of blood, and body fluids in general, favor independently acting paramagnetic ions as contrast agents, since they generally make comparable contributions to the *changes* in $1/T1$ and $1/T2$. Until recently, little was known about the interaction of Gd-DTPA with blood protein and cells and with tissue. Data are beginning to become available that indicate that this chelate remains intact in vivo, interacting minimally with tissue, and is excreted intact.[7] These results, along with related background information, follow.

NMRD Profiles of Gd³⁺ Complexes

Figure 64–10 shows the NMRD profiles[13] of solutions of four complexes of Gd^{3+}: the aquoion,[52] Gd-EDTA; Gd-DTPA; and Gd^{3+}-concanavalin A. In many ways the behavior of Gd^{3+} is much like that of Mn^{2+}, particularly when allowance is made for

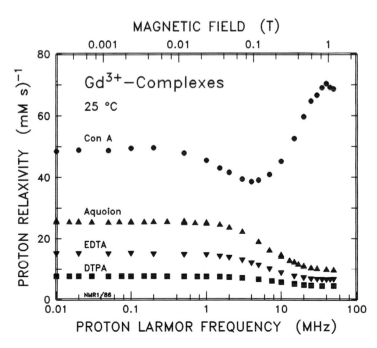

Figure 64–10. NMRD profiles of solutions of four different complexes of Gd^{3+}: The protein concanavalin A, with the native Mn^{2+} replaced by Zn^{2+} and the Gd^{3+} bound nonspecifically (●); the aquoion (▲); the EDTA complex (▼); and the DTPA complex (■), all near pH 6.4, at 25°C. (Data after reference 13.)

their different coordination numbers. The main distinction between the results in Figures 64–6 and 64–10 is in the profiles of the aquoions: Gd^{3+}, because its deep-lying f-shell is not part of the ligand environment as is the d-shell of Mn^{2+}, has no detectable hyperfine contribution. As a result, the profiles of chelates of Gd^{3+} and that of the Gd^{3+} aquoion are very similar in form, making it difficult in general to tell from the NMRD profile whether Gd^{3+} in a sample exists as the aquoion or complexed in a small chelate; the total Gd^{3+} content must be obtained from other measurements and the paramagnetic contribution to the relaxation rates then calculated from the known relaxivities. This is quite unlike the situation for Mn^{2+}, for which the magnitude of the observed hyperfine contribution is a quantitative measure of the concentration of Mn^{2+} aquoions.[45,46]

Small Chelate Complexes of Gd^{3+}

The relaxivity of small chelate complexes of Gd^{3+} is turning out to be rather intriguing; the results to date suggest that the meaning of outer sphere relaxation must be re-examined and, in particular, that attention must be given to the possibility of hydrogen bonding of water molecules in the second coordination environment of the chelated Gd^{3+} ions, with resident lifetimes sufficiently long to influence the relaxivity.[27,31,53] A hint of this phenomenon comes from a comparison of the NMRD profiles of Gd-EDTA and the aquoions (Fig. 64–10). EDTA, being hexadentate, should remove two-thirds of the waters coordinated in the aquoions. Since the inflection frequencies for the two profiles are about the same, the low field relaxivity of Gd-EDTA might be expected to be about 8 $(mM\ s)^{-1}$; the observed value is twofold greater, a significant effect. The paradox is more apparent in Figure 64–11.

In Figure 64–11 the NMRD profiles of Gd-DOTA and Gd-NOTA, octa- and hexadentate chelates, respectively,[47] are compared. Over the entire field range, Gd-DOTA, which ostensibly has one-third the number of coordinated waters of Gd-NOTA, nonetheless has the higher relaxivity. Moreover, the relaxivities of both are greater than those of Gd-DTPA, also octadentate. Though the variation in profiles among these

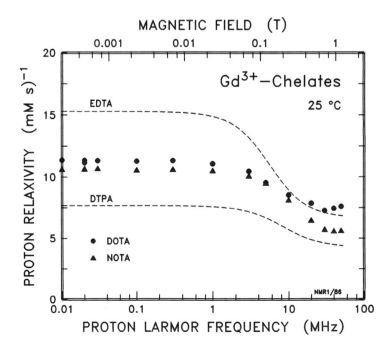

Figure 64–11. NMRD profiles of Gd-DOTA (●) and Gd-NOTA (▲), near pH 6.4, at 25°C. The relaxivity of the former, with ostensibly one-third the number of coordinated water molecules of the latter, is nevertheless greater at all fields. The dashed curves indicate the profiles of Gd-EDTA and Gd-DTPA, for ease of comparison. (Data after reference 47.)

several chelate complexes can be ascribed, in part, to differences in correlation times (good EPR data are needed[4]), it does appear that some of the chelate complexes have an excess relaxivity beyond that which can be accounted for by the sum of the inner coordination and the traditional outer sphere contributions.

This excess relaxivity may be another example of the fluoromet mechanism, a point worth expanding, since it is appearing in an increasing number of different situations. For example, displacement of the Fe^{3+} coordinated water in methemoglobin by F^- increases the paramagnetic part of the relaxivity (Fig. 64–4) about 10-fold. This was attributed to hydrogen bonded, second-sphere waters, for which the protons coordinated to the F^- ions are not much farther from the paramagnetic ions than the protons of coordinated first-sphere water molecules would be. The labile hydrogen bond permits rapid exchange and an enhanced relaxivity. This fluoromet mechanism has been invoked to account for the relaxivity profiles of Fe^{3+}-transferrin[30] (Fig. 64–3) as well as those of Cu^{2+}- and VO^{2+}-transferrin.[32] More recently, it was suggested as the main determinant of the relaxivity of protein-bound nitroxide radicals.[27] The values for the lifetime of the hydrogen-bonded complex in all these cases would appear to be no shorter than about 10 ns. The question is whether water molecules hydrogen bonded to those carboxylate oxygens coordinated directly to chelated Gd^{3+} ions, for example, can have sufficiently long residence times so that their contributions must be considered separately from the usual diffusional outer sphere contributions. This is an open question, at present, and an extremely important one for NMR imaging, in which the optimal balance between toxicity and relaxivity invariably is sought. Another question is: Why is this effect not observed in analogous complexes of Mn^{2+} and Fe^{3+}?

Unchelated Gd^{3+} in Tissue

There are as yet no data for Gd^{3+} comparable to those of Figure 64–8 for Mn^{2+}, i.e., no instance in which the presence of protein-immobilized Gd^{3+} in tissue is evident from a high field peak in the NMRD profile. One problem is that it is difficult to get Gd^{3+} into tissue. Chelated Gd^{3+} introduced intravenously is concentrated in the kidney medulla and excreted in the urine, unlike chelated Mn^{2+}, which accumulates predominantly in the liver (until the liver is saturated), dissociates, and passes to the bile. Also, Gd^{3+} injected into the blood as the aquoion "disappears"; i.e., it becomes relatively "relaxation silent," and does this despite the fact that serum albumin is known to bind, though weakly, to and enhance the relaxivity of Gd^{3+} in water and buffer solutions.[54] The reason, only recently clarified,[55] is that Gd^{3+} interacts with the normal levels of bicarbonate (and inorganic phosphate) in blood and precipitates. Thus, to take advantage of the high relaxivities of macromolecular complexes of Gd^{3+} for in-vivo tissue studies will require an approach different from those tried to date, one that will yield macromolecular complexes with low dissociation constants.

Chelated Gd^{3+} in Tissue

Since Gd^{3+} is widely used in human clinical medicine as the Gd-DTPA complex,[51] it is not surprising that the majority of the investigations of the relaxivity of Gd^{3+} complexes in vivo have also involved this particular complex. The chelate is removed from the circulation by the renal (kidney) cortex and accumulates in the renal medulla, where it is concentrated by active countercurrent processes for ultimate excretion in the urine. Results for rabbit urine[7] are shown in Figure 64–12. Here, the observed profiles are compared with those expected for water solutions of Gd-DTPA equal in

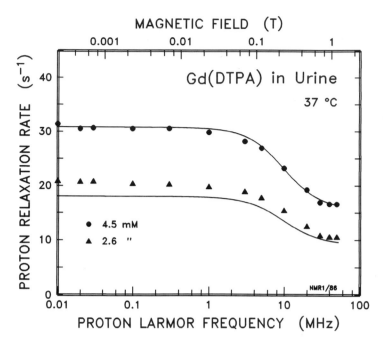

Figure 64–12. NMRD profiles of two samples of rabbit urine, at 37°C, found to contain, respectively, 4.5 mM (●) and 2.6 mM (▲) total Gd. The dashed curves associated with the data points are the profiles expected for solutions of the same respective concentrations of Gd-DTPA in water, at physiological pH and 37°C. (Data after reference 7.)

concentration to the measured total Gd content of the samples. The agreement is extremely good, indicating, within the experimental uncertainty, that Gd^{3+} remains chelated in its passage through the rabbit. Complementary results can be obtained by radioactive tracer techniques, for example, but these only determine total Gd; few techniques other than NMRD can so readily demonstrate the chemical state of the contrast agent.

Demonstration of the chemical state of Gd in the medulla itself is more difficult, owing in part to the function-related structure of this organ. Since its function is to concentrate solute ions for excretion, it must have compartments between which the rate of water exchange can be controlled. If, in addition, the distribution of Gd-DTPA becomes spatially nonuniform, with differential access by the tissue water, then the time dependence of the magnetization data that leads to each data point of an NMRD profile becomes subtly multiexponential.

An attempt to resolve each point of an NMRD profile of tissue into two contributing relaxation rates has only recently been successful.[7] There are several intrinsic difficulties: the data set that is to be resolved into two exponentials can generally be described quite adequately by a single exponential with an uncertainty of less than ±3 percent. For reasonable values of the signal-to-noise ratio, it is almost a mathematical truism that two exponentials can often be simulated by one;[3] accordingly, a large data set must be accumulated with rather high accuracy. An example is shown in Figure 64–13, in which 108 points were collected along the magnetization decay curve of a sample of excised renal medulla containing Gd-DTPA, for a single field. (For the profiles in the previous figures, 23 points were taken for each point on the profiles, and the fit to a single exponential was invariably better than ±1 percent.) The results are interesting in their own right in that it will be necessary to include the anatomy and physiology of the renal medulla in a very specific way in order to model the relaxation data. However, further study is required to prove that the Gd in the medulla is present as Gd-DTPA; an additional approach is necessary, one in which the tissue structure is partially disrupted to allow tissue water uniform access to the exogenous Gd.

Figure 64–14 shows data for three samples of rabbit renal medullas with differing

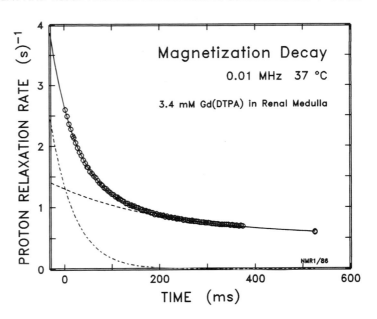

Figure 64–13. An example of the time dependence of the proton magnetization of a sample of rabbit renal medulla containing about 3.4 mM Gd-DTPA from which a single typical point of an NMRD profile is computed, here 0.01 MHz, at 37°C. Because of the high load of Gd in this sample, the data were measurably nonexponential. A fit of a single exponential to the magnetization decay gives a rate of 12.1 s^{-1} with a standard deviation of 3.6 percent, whereas a fit of two exponentials gives rates of 20.1 s^{-1} and 4.2 s^{-1} with an uncertainty of 0.76 percent. The relative amplitudes of the two fits are about 3:1, obtained by extrapolating the data back to −30 ms (which is a reasonable procedure for the instrument settings used). 108 points were taken along the decay curve, including eight at the long time extreme.

measured concentrations of Gd. Two samples were aged (for 11 weeks) at 5°C to permit a certain amount of enzymatic degradation and, perhaps, extensive diffusion of water and contrast agent. A control, with no Gd, was treated similarly. A third sample, fresh, was cut into millimeter-size pieces and subjected to repeated cycles of freezing and thawing. The profiles of all four samples were measured in the usual way to obtain the single-exponential NMRD profiles. In every case, the data were well described by a single exponential, within the experimental uncertainty. The profile of the aged control was indistinguishable from that of fresh tissue, and that for the lowest dosage was also little changed. However, the amplitudes of the profile of the intermediate dosage sample increased by 50 percent and that of the most heavily dosed sample by 100 percent from the respective single exponential profiles of the same samples when fresh and intact.

The profiles (Fig. 64–14) compare well with the profiles expected from water solutions of Gd-DTPA at concentrations of Gd equal to those found in the tissue samples, as shown by the smooth curves. (The curves are adjusted to take account of the 20 wt. percent solids content of the tissue, which makes the Gd concentration in tissue water greater than its measured mean value.) The comparison of the curves with the data for the aged samples is excellent, this being the strongest evidence to date that not only is Gd present in the renal medulla as Gd-DTPA but the microviscosity sensed by Gd-DTPA in tissue water is essentially that of neat water at the same temperature. The agreement is quite reasonable for the freeze/thaw sample and would probably be improved by further disruption of the tissue structure. In all, the main point—that, when all the Gd^{3+} can be accessed by tissue water, the data are single exponential and the paramagnetic contribution to the NMRD profile is precisely that expected for Gd-DTPA—would appear proven.

Chelated Gd^{3+} in Blood and Plasma

As remarked above, the main clinical applications of chelated Gd^{3+} have been to the circulatory system. But in order to estimate the anticipated changes in contrast it is necessary to know the relaxivity of the chelate in blood and this depends on the physical-chemical interactions of the chelate molecules with the components of blood.

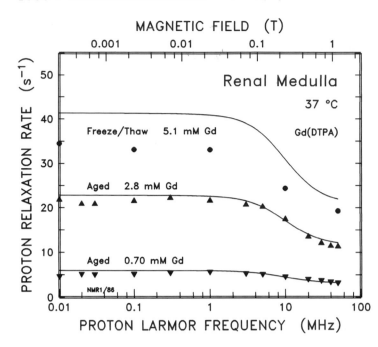

Figure 64–14. Paramagnetic contribution to the NMRD profiles of three samples of rabbit renal medulla, at 37°C, found to contain respectively 5.1 mM (●), 2.8 mM (▲), and 0.70 mM (▼) total Gd. The data are for samples in which the tissue structure has been partially degraded, either by several cycles of freezing and thawing or by autocatalysis due to long-term (11 weeks) storage at 5°C. The magnitude of the upper profile increased about 100 percent, the center one about 50 percent, and the lower one hardly at all as a result of these procedures. After this treatment, all the data could be well represented by single exponentials. The curves associated with the data points are the profiles expected for solutions of the same respective concentrations of Gd-DTPA in water, at physiological pH and 37°C, but including a correction for the volume occupied by the solid content of tissue (about 20 wt. percent). (Data after reference 7.)

The NMRD profiles of Gd-DTPA in blood have only recently been reported,[56] from which a basic understanding of the relaxivity of the complex can be obtained. Representative results for a sample of rabbit blood, and plasma derived from it, are shown in Figures 64–15*A* and *B*. From these data, one can conclude that Gd-DTPA remains extracellular; that it binds neither to blood protein nor to erythrocyte membranes; and that its rotational mobility is the same as it is in water solution. Figure 64–15*A* shows the NMRD profiles of blood and plasma before intravenous injection with chelate, as controls, and after injection with 600 μMoles/kg of Gd-DTPA. The measured concen-

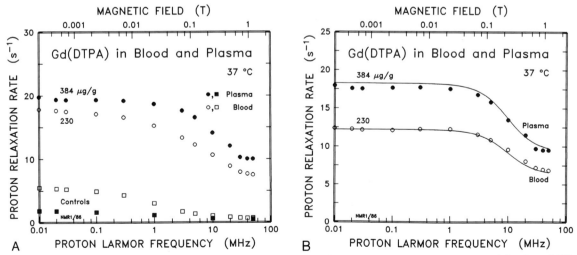

Figure 64–15. *A*, NMRD profiles of blood drawn from a rabbit before (□) and after (○) intravenous injection of 600 μMoles/kg of body weight of Gd(DTPA), and the plasma obtained from the same samples, (■) and (●), respectively, at 37°C. The total Gd content of the samples, obtained from ICP (inductively coupled plasma) analysis, is indicated in each case. (Data after reference 56.) *B*, The paramagnetic contribution to the NMRD profiles of blood (○) and plasma (●) for the data of *A*. The curves through the data points are the NMRD profiles of water solutions of Gd-DTPA with the same concentrations of Gd as were found in the blood and plasma samples (with a correction for the partial volume effects of the protein in the blood and plasma).

trations of total Gd in the samples are indicated. The first point to note is that the plasma has the higher Gd concentration. This means that as the red cells settle they leave the chelate behind, thereby increasing its concentration in the plasma. A quantitative analysis of these results, assuming a normal hematocrit for the sample, shows that no Gd is removed by the red cells; i.e., the chelate neither enters the cells nor binds to their exteriors.

Figure 64–15*B* shows the data of the Gd-containing blood and plasma corrected for their respective diamagnetic backgrounds. The curves through the corrected data are the *predictions* for the NMRD profiles assuming that all the Gd is present as Gd-DTPA and that the profile of the chelate in plasma is identical to that in water. (To obtain these curves, corrections must be made for the volume occupied by the protein in the samples, a correction that is 7 percent for the sample of plasma and 21 percent for the blood.) The conclusions, from the results of Figures 64–15*A* and *B*, are unequivocal; no interaction of Gd-DTPA, either physical or chemical, with the components of blood is observed.

Summary

As with the results for diamagnetic tissue discussed in an earlier chapter, the major conclusion is that results for homogeneous solutions of paramagnetic complexes—for which there is an extensive and sophisticated literature—can, to first order, be carried over to the study of these complexes in tissue. At this level, the structure of tissue can be regarded as morphological, something that constrains tissue water without restraining its microscopic mobility. At a finer level, the details of the structure of specific tissues will influence the relaxivity of complexes of paramagnetic ions in a manner that relates to tissue function. The goal, of course, is to use the observed changes in relaxation rates, and the associated changes in MRI contrast, to detect tissue dysfunction associated with disease.

References

1. Bloch F: Nuclear induction. Phys Rev *70*:460–474, 1946.
2. Bloch F, Hansen WW, Packard M: The nuclear induction experiment, Phys Rev *70*:474–485, 1946.
3. Koenig SH, Brown III RD: Determinants of proton relaxation in tissue, Magn Reson Med *1*:437–449, 1984.
4. Koenig SH, Brown III RD: Relaxation of solvent protons by paramagnetic ions and its dependence on magnetic field and chemical environment. Magn Reson Med *1*:478–495, 1984.
5. Koenig SH, Brown III RD: The importance of the motion of water for magnetic resonance imaging. Invest Radiol *20*:297–305, 1985.
6. Koenig SH, Brown III RD, Goldstein E, Burnett KR, Wolf GL: Magnetic field dependence of tissue proton relaxation rates with added Mn^{2+}: Rabbit liver and kidney. Magn Reson Med *2*:159–168, 1985.
7. Koenig SH, Spiller M, Brown III RD, Wolf GL: Magnetic field dependence (NMRD profile) of 1/*T1* of rabbit kidney medulla and urine after intravenous injection of Gd(DTPA). Invest Radiol *21*:697–704, 1986.
8. Lauffer RB, Brady TJ, Brown III RD, Baglin C, Koenig SH: Ternary complexes of protein, chelates, and metal-ions. Magn Reson Med *2*:541–548, 1986.
9. Thulborn KR, Waterton JC, Matthews PM, Radda GK: Oxygenation dependence of the transverse relaxation time of water protons in whole blood at high field. Biochim Biophys Acta *714*:265–270, 1982.
10. Koenig SH, Brown III RD, Gibson JF, Ward RJ, Peters TJ: Relaxometry of ferritin solutions and the influence of the Fe^{3+} core ions. Magn Reson Med (in press).
11. Cf. Slichter CP: Principles of Magnetic Resonance. 2nd ed. Berlin, Springer-Verlag, 1978, (An intermediate level discussion).
12. Koenig SH, Brown III RD, Lindstrom TR: Interactions of solvent with the heme region of methemoglobin and fluoro-methemoglobin. *In* Ho C (ed): Hemoglobin and Oxygen Binding. New York, Elsevier Biomedical, 1982, pp 377–385.
13. Koenig SH, Baglin C, Brown III RD, Brewer CF: Magnetic field dependence of solvent proton relaxation induced by Gd^{3+} and Mn^{2+} complexes. Magn Reson Med *1*:496–501, 1984.

14. Koenig SH, Baglin CM, Brown III RD: Magnetic field dependence of solvent proton relaxation in aqueous solutions of Fe^{3+} complexes. Magn Reson Med 2:283–288, 1985.

15. Dowsing RD, Gibson JF: Electron spin resonance of high-spin d^5 systems. J Chem Phys 50:294–303, 1969.

16. Aasa R: Powder line shapes in the electron paramagnetic resonance spectra of high-spin ferric complexes. J Chem Phys 52:3919–3930, 1970.

17. Koenig SH: A novel derivation of the Solomon-Bloembergen-Morgan equations: application to solvent relaxation by Mn^{2+}-protein complexes. J Magn Reson 31:1–10, 1978.

18. Koenig SH: A classical description of relaxation of interacting pairs of unlike spins: extension to $T1_\rho$, $T2$, $T1_{poff}$, including contact interactions. J Magn Reson 47:441–453, 1982.

19. Brasch RC, Wesbey GE, Gooding CA, Koerper MA: Magnetic resonance imaging of transfusional hemosiderosis complicating thalassemia major. Radiology 150:767–771, 1984.

20. Lauffer RB, Greif WL, Stark DD, Vincent AC, Saini S, Weeden VJ, Brady TJ: Iron-EHPG as an hepatobiliary MR contrast agent: initial imaging and biodistribution studies. J Comput Asst Tomogr 9:431–438, 1985.

21. Wesbey GE, Brasch RC, Engelstad BL, Moss AA, Crooks LE, Brito AC: Nuclear magnetic resonance contrast enhancement study of the gastrointestinal tract of rats and a human volunteer using nontoxic oral iron solutions. Radiology 149:175–180, 1983.

22. Bloch J, Navon G: An NMR study of iron (III) EDTA in aqueous solution. J Inorg Nucl Chem 42:693–699, 1980.

23. Pfeifer H: Der Translationsanteil der Protonenrelaxation in wäßrigen Lösungen paramagnetischer Ionen. Ann Physik (Leipzig) 8:1–8, 1961.

24. Pfeifer H: Protonenrelaxation und Hydration in wäßrigen Lösungen des Manganions. Z Naturforschg A 17:279–287, 1962.

25. Freed JH: Dynamic effects of pair correlation functions on spin relaxation by translational diffusion in liquids. II. Finite jumps and independent $T1$ processes. J Chem Phys 68:4034–4037, 1978.

26. Albrand JP, Taieb MC, Fries PH, Belorizky E: NMR study of spectral densities over a large frequency range for intermolecular relaxation in liquids: pair correlation effects. J Chem Phys 78:5809–5815, 1983.

27. Bennett HF, Brown III RD, Koenig SH, Swartz HM: Effects of nitroxides on the magnetic field and temperature dependence of $1/T1$ of solvent water protons. Magn Reson Med 4:93–111, 1987.

28. Aisen P, Listowsky I: Iron transport and storage proteins. Ann Rev Biochem 49:357–393, 1980.

29. Koenig SH, Schillinger WE: Nuclear magnetic resonance relaxation dispersion in protein solutions II: transferrin. J Biol Chem 244:6520–6526, 1969.

30. Koenig SH, Brown III RD: Coordinated solvent molecules in metalloenzymes and proteins studied using NMRD. In Bertini I, Drago RS, Luchinat, C (eds): The Coordination Chemistry of Metalloenzymes. Dordrecht, Reidel, 1983, pp 19–33.

31. Koenig SH, Brown III RD, Bertini I, Luchinat C: Water exchange at the active site of carbonic anhydrase; a synthesis of the OH^- and H_2O models. Biophys J 41:179–187, 1983.

32. Bertini I, Briganti F, Koenig SH, Luchinat C: Magnetic relaxation of solvent protons by Cu^{2+}- and VO^{2+}-substituted transferrin: Theoretical analysis and biochemical implications. Biochemistry 24:6287–6290, 1985.

33. Clegg CA, Fitton JE, Harrison PM, Treffry A: Ferritin: molecular structure and iron-storage mechanisms. Prog Biophys Molec Biol 36:53–86, 1980.

34. Rosenberg LP, Chasteen ND: Initial iron binding to horse spleen apoferritin. In Saltman P, Henenaur J (eds): The Biochemistry and Physiology of Iron. New York, Elsevier Biomedical, 1982, pp 405–407.

35. Weir MP, Gibson JF, Peters TJ: Haemosiderin and tissue damage. Cell Biochem Funct 2:186–194, 1984.

36. Robertson B: Spin-echo decay of spins diffusing in a bounded region. Phys Rev 151:273–277, 1966.

37. Luz Z, Meiboom S: Nuclear magnetic resonance study of the protolysis of trimethylammonium ion in aqueous solution—order of the reaction with respect to solvent. J Chem Phys 39:366–370, 1963.

38. Packer KJ: The effects of diffusion through locally inhomogeneous magnetic fields on transverse nuclear spin relaxation in heterogeneous systems. Proton transverse relaxation in striated muscle. J Magn Reson 9:438–443, 1973.

39. Laukien G, Schlüter J: Impulstechnische Messungen der Spin-Gitter- und der Spin-Spin-Relaxationszeiten von Protonen in wäßrigen Lösungen paramagnetischer Ionen. Z Physik 146:113–126, 1956.

40. Bloembergen N: Proton relaxation times in paramagnetic solutions. J Chem Phys 27:572–573, 1957.

41. Cohn M: Magnetic resonance studies of enzyme-substrate complexes with paramagnetic probes as illustrated by creatine kinase. Quart Rev Biophys 3:61–89, 1970.

42. Peacocke AR, Richards RE, Sheard B: Proton magnetic relaxation in solutions of E. coli ribosomal RNA containing Mn^{2+} ions. Mol Phys 16:177–189, 1969.

43. Danchin A, Gueron M: Proton magnetic relaxation study of the manganese-transfer-RNA complex. J Chem Phys 53:3599–3609, 1970.

44. Eisinger J, Shulman RG, Szymanski BM: Transition metal binding in DNA solutions. J Chem Phys 36:1721–1729, 1962.

45. Koenig SH, Brown RD, Studebaker J: On the interpretation of solvent proton magnetic relaxation data with particular applications to the structure of the active site of Mn-carboxypeptidase A. Cold Spring Harbor Symp Quant Biol 36:551–559, 1971.

46. Cf. Brewer CF, Brown III RD, Koenig SH: Metal ion binding and conformational transitions in concanavalin A: A structure-function study. J Biomol Struct Dynam 1:961–997, 1983.

47. Geraldes CFGC, Sherry AD, Brown III RD, Koenig SH: NMRD investigation of Mn^{2+} and Gd^{3+} NOTA complexes, and comparison with the analogous EDTA complexes. Mag Reson Med 3:242–250, 1986.

48. Oakes J, Smith EG: Structure of Mn-EDTA^{2-} complex in aqueous solution by relaxation nuclear magnetic resonance. J Chem Soc Faraday Trans 2, 77:299–308, 1981.
49. Spiller M (unpublished).
50. Koenig SH, Brown III RD, Kurland R, Ohki S: Relaxivity and binding of Mn^{2+} ions in solutions of phosphatidyl serine vesicles. Magn Reson Med (submitted).
51. Cf. Wolf GL (ed): Contrast enhancement in biomedical NMR: A symposium. Physiol Chem Phys 16:1984.
52. Koenig SH, Epstein M: Ambiguities in the interpretation of proton magnetic relaxation data in water solutions of Gd^{3+} ions. J Chem Phys 63:2279–2284, 1975.
53. Desreux JF, Koenig SH (unpublished).
54. Reuben J: Gadolinium (III) as a paramagnetic probe for proton relaxation studies of biological molecules. Binding to bovine serum albumin. Biochemistry 10:2834–2838, 1971.
55. O'Hara PB, Koenig SH: ESR and magnetic relaxation studies of Gd (III) complexes with human transferrin. Biochemistry 25:1445–1450, 1986.
56. Koenig SH, Spiller M, Brown III RD, Wolf GL: Relaxation of water protons in the intra- and extracellular regions of blood containing Gd(DTPA). Magn Reson Med 3:791–795, 1986.

Additional References

1. Koenig SH, Brown III RD: Relaxometry of paramagnetic ions in tissue. *In* H. Sigel (ed): Metal Ions in Biological Systems. Vol 21. New York, Marcel Dekker, 1986, pp 229–270.
2. Lyon RC, Faustino PJ, Cohen JS, Katz A, Mornex F, Colcher D, Baglin C, Koenig SH, Hambright P: Tissue distribution and stability of metalloporphyrin MRI contrast agents. Magn Reson Med 4:24–33, 1987.
3. Koenig SH, Brown III RD, Spiller M: The anomalous relaxivity of Mn^{3+}(TPPS$_4$). Magn Reson Med 4:252–260, 1987.
4. Gillis P, Koenig SH: Transverse relaxation of solvent protons induced by magnetized spheres: applications to ferritin, erythrocytes, and magnetite. Magn Reson Med 5:323–345, 1987.
5. Bennett H, Swartz HM, Brown III RD, Koenig SH: Modifications of relaxation of lipid protons by paramagnetic materials: feasibility and clinical potential. Invest Radiol 22:502–507, 1987.
6. Koenig SH, Spiller M, Brown III RD, Wolf GL: Investigation of the biochemical state of paramagnetic ions *in vivo* using the magnetic field dependence of 1/$T1$ of tissue protons (NMRD profile): applications to contrast agents for magnetic resonance imaging. Nucl Med Biol, Int J Radiat Appl Instrum Part B (1987, in press).

65

Pathophysiological Significance of Relaxation

JOHN C. GORE
MARK S. BROWN

Nuclear magnetic resonance (NMR) images have high intrinsic contrast primarily because tissues possess different relaxation properties. Anatomic cross sections are heterogeneous distributions of relaxation times so that sequences that produce signals sensitive to $T1$ or $T2$ are able to differentiate subtle tissue differences and thereby delineate regions of abnormal relaxation characteristics. Thus the fundamental significance of relaxation lies in the fact that pathological conditions often produce alterations in those factors that account for the observed relaxation behavior of tissues. A better understanding of those factors would assist in the interpretation of NMR images and possibly lead to more specific tissue descriptions for more accurate tissue classification. At this time it should be emphasized that the detailed interactions governing relaxation in heterogeneous tissues are either not well understood or are quantified with only poor precision. There do not exist any accurate quantitative models that explain why, for example, gray and white matter differ in the manner and to the extent observed.

A more precise understanding of tissue relaxation may evolve at various levels. First, we need to understand the phenomenological significance of each tissue component at the macromolecular level, in particular the contributions to relaxation that arise from different types of protein, lipid, or polysaccharide. Second, we need to appreciate the significance, if any, of the manner in which such contributions are affected by the macroscopic organization of tissue constituents at the cellular or organelle level. In particular, we may question whether tissue is merely an aqueous suspension of macromolecules, or whether compartmental effects, or structural organization and integrity, are also important. Third, at a more fundamental level, we are interested in the individual molecular interactions that determine the efficacy as relaxation agents of tissue molecules, although this level of understanding may impact little on the practical interpretation of bulk relaxation properties, except perhaps when any individual process is affected by physiological changes such as pH or ionic content.

There exists a large and growing literature reporting studies of the molecular interactions that determine the relaxation of individual resonances in macromolecules, but there has hitherto been much less interest in the bulk relaxation effects of macromolecules in water. Proton relaxation times in aqueous media largely reflect the manner in which water molecules tumble and diffuse by Brownian motion and represent bulk averages of the detailed history of many interactions with other water molecules or macromolecular surfaces in the medium. In the presence of long chain or large globular molecules (including proteins and polysaccharides) the relaxation times should be dramatically affected by the size of the average molecule (since this affects the correlation time for the motion of the macromolecule) and by the nature of the surface of the macromolecule (in particular, the area, the electrostatic charge density, and the nature of any labile protons). Various types of NMR and other physical measurements have been used to support the conclusion that the following processes may be important:

(a) Water in the close vicinity of macromolecules ("hydration layers") may show different motional characteristics, because of hydrogen or other bonding to the surface, from "bulk" water, thereby decreasing its relaxation times. Water may be translating or rotating anisotropically, or even bound irrotationally, while evidence has also been adduced that supports the existence of a long-range hydrodynamic or "slosh" effect whereby the tumbling effect of the macromolecule itself is felt over many water molecule diameters.[1]

(b) Water exchanges through the different phases in a heterogeneous system; and this exchange, if fast, causes an averaging effect of the influence of each environment. The exchange time is itself an important parameter affecting the overall rate.

(c) Water protons and water molecules may exchange chemically with acidic protons on the outer surface of macromolecules.

(d) Water protons may exchange nuclear magnetization with macromolecular protons, and such cross relaxation effects may provide an efficient means for depositing magnetization from the bulk water into the macromolecular manifold, in which it may then dissipate by spin diffusion.[2]

It is not well understood what the relative importance of each of these processes is, nor which of them is altered in pathological states. It is clear, however, from measurements of the proton and deuterium relaxation in deuterated tissues that the mean correlation time for water molecules is substantially longer in tissue compared to water alone, while the intramolecular dipole-dipole coupling that dominates pure water relaxation is of much reduced significance in tissue,[3] which is consistent with cross relaxation being the dominant process. Direct evidence for cross relaxation effects has been provided by high resolution studies of protons in model systems and lipid preparations (including bile) in which transient Overhauser effects are measurable in, for example, methylene resonances, when the solvent water peak is selectively inverted, demonstrating a magnetic exchange between the two components.

With regard to composition, it is clear that *T1* and *T2* are dependent on the percentage composition of water and protein. Experimental measurements of relaxation time and water content have led to arguments that alterations in water content alone can account for most of the variations in relaxation seen. A simple two compartment fast exchange model is often invoked when considering the data. Such a model predicts that the relaxation rate is expected to be inversely proportional to the fractional water content. However, at moderate imaging fields, tissue longitudinal relaxation rates usually fall in the range of 1 to 3 s^{-1}. A change in water content of 1 percent will correspond to a 1 percent change at most in the protein content. A 10 percent change in the tissue relaxation time, viz., 0.1 to 0.3, would require that the tissue protein produce a relaxation rate change of 0.1 to 0.3 per percentage change. The relaxation rates per unit concentration of several proteins are presented in Table 65–1. For the above argument to be true (and 10 percent changes in *T1* for 1 percent changes in water content are not atypical[4]) requires the identification of proteins significantly more effective at relaxing water than those reported in Table 65–1. Indeed, it is the quantitative discrepancy between observed protein behavior and that needed to explain the results obtained in tissues that undermines the validity of this simple approach.

The precise dependence of *T1* on water content has been contradicted in several previous reports. There seems to be a quantitative difference in the correlation between *T1* and water content when comparing large changes in water content between different tissues or tissues subjected to partial dehydration (when 1/*T1* and 1/water content are strongly correlated) with the normal variations, usually smaller, that occur within the

Table 65–1. RELAXATION RATE CHANGES, ΔR, PER UNIT CONCENTRATION OF PROTEIN $(s^{-1} \% ^{-1})$ AT 20 MHz*

Material	Molecular Weight	ΔR_1
Bacitracin	1,400	.017
Lysozyme	14,300	.043
Carbonic anhydrase	30,000	.025
β-Lactoglobulin	37,100	.056
Hemoglobin	64,500	.106
Serum albumin	68,500	.033
Hexokinase	102,000	.046
γ-Globulin	153,000	.036
Urease	483,000	.248

* At 37°C, pH = 7.2, in 0.1M MOPS buffer.

same tissue type or as a result of some insult. In our studies of a large series of mice tissues, in which the mice were matched for age, sex, and nutritional status and in which the tissues were excised fresh and measured under identical conditions, the variation in water content of each tissue was less than ±1 percent about the mean values, while the standard deviation of *T1* was approximately 5 percent. However, no significant correlations were found between the fluctuations about the mean water content and the mean *T1*, although in heart and liver the water content was correlated with *T2* (Table 65–2). From such studies it may be concluded that significant alterations in relaxation can occur without changes in the water content.

It is often conjectured that relaxation in cells can be derived from "an appropriately weighted superposition of the relaxation rates of homogeneous solutions of the cellular constituents."[5] Furthermore, spin-spin relaxation rates are supposedly dominated by the Brownian motion of cell globular protein and are "thus influenced predominantly by the distribution of molecular weights of intracellular protein." This view is not, however, convincingly supported by a close examination of experimental results. For example, Figure 65–1 shows the histograms of protein molecular weights present in homogenates of rat brain, liver, and kidney. These plots were obtained from quantitative microdensitometer tracings of high resolution SDS gels in which the protein distribution was dispersed by electrophoresis.

Table 65–2. RELAXATION TIMES OF NORMAL ADULT FEMALE CF1 MICE

(a) Normal Variation of Relaxation Times and Water Content

	Liver			Heart		
	T1	T2	% Water	T1	T2	% Water
Mean	321	35.7	69.90	593	45.6	76.56
Standard Deviation	20	2.6	.74	32	6.6	.68

(b) Regression of Water Content vs. Relaxation Times

	Liver (N = 34)		Heart (N = 26)	
	Correlation Coefficient	P Value	Correlation Coefficient	P Value
$1/T1$ vs. $1/\%H_2O$	.106	N.S.	.051	N.S.
$1/T2$ vs. $1/\%H_2O$	.504	.003	.422	.04

	Spleen (N = 10)		Kidney (N = 10)	
$1/T1$ vs. $1/\%H_2O$	.042	N.S.	.392	N.S.
$1/T2$ vs. $1/\%H_2O$	.118	N.S.	.222	N.S.

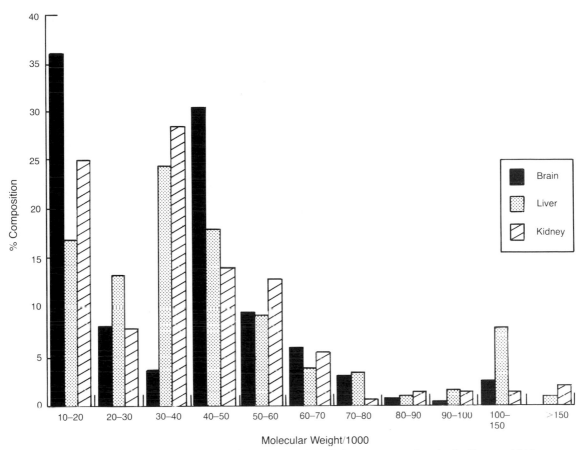

Figure 65–1. Histograms of protein molecular weights present in homogenates of rat brain, liver, and kidney.

The mean molecular weights of rat brain, kidney, and liver are 38, 40, and 45 kd, respectively, and clearly there are differences in the shapes of these histograms. Unfortunately, these distributions do not permit a straightforward calculation of the overall relaxation rate at the frequencies used in clinical imaging. The reason lies in our lack of adequate data, at these higher fields, on the relationship between relaxation rate and protein type. For example, Koenig and Brown[5] have argued that $1/T1$ at high fields depends strongly on the total surface area of the protein molecules, while $1/T2$ is directly related to τ_c, the time for protein molecules to reorient, which is directly proportional to the molecular weight for spherical proteins. However, the results depicted in Table 61–1 show that no obvious relationship exists between molecular weight and the relaxation rate changes per unit concentration of protein, ΔR, when this is measured at 20 MHz, 37°C, and pH = 7.2. Indeed, Table 65–1 confirms two important facts. First, there is no significant correlation between ΔR and molecular weight for the nine proteins considered in the molecular weight range of 0 to 150,000. Second, in all cases, the value of ΔR is substantially too low to account for tissue relaxation. It is this quantitative discrepancy that leads to the conclusion that, as yet, we do not have an adequate model of tissue relaxation.

The relaxation data do not support the idea that tissue is a simple mixture of proteins acting independently so that the overall relaxation rate is merely the sum of the individual constituents. This result is also confirmed by visual inspection of the NMRD profiles of Koenig and Brown.[5] For example, they show that at 1 MHz the relaxation rates of 5 percent solutions of various proteins with molecular weights of

Table 65–3. PROTEIN (PERCENT) COMPOSITION OF VARIOUS RAT TISSUES

Tissue	Percent Protein	Percent Total Lipid
Brain	11.8%	7.5%
Heart	8.8	2.4
Kidney	15.2	3.1
Liver	19.6	3.7
Muscle	4.7	1.3
Spleen	11.4	1.8

14,000 to 160,000 lie in the range 0.5 to 1.5 s^{-1}, where pure water has a rate of approximately 0.4. At the same frequency, rabbit tissues show rates of 5 to 8 s^{-1}. Table 65–3 records the total protein contents measured by the method of Lowry for freshly excised rat tissues. Combining these measurements with our knowledge of the distribution of molecular weights in the sample and our measured relaxation rate constants for representative proteins leads to the conclusion that superimposing the contribution of single, simple proteins would underestimate the tissue relaxation rates by at least a factor of 2 and more probably an order of magnitude for both *T1* and *T2*.

There are some other obvious factors not yet discussed that can modulate tissue relaxation. We have ourselves previously reported that glycogen is a weakly effective agent for modifying tissue relaxation.[6] There are diurnal and other temporal variations that will have some influence. Metal ions are a possible source of major discrepancy, particularly for the liver, where they are usually more abundant, while other simple ions can be effective in altering molecular associations and may have some effect on relaxation. But none of these factors would appear to provide a reason for the quantitative discrepancy described above. If brain is composed of 12 percent protein of mean molecular weight 38,000, and the relaxation times are *T1* = 600 ms, *T2* = 70 ms, then the mean protein relaxation rates required to achieve this are 0.14 $s^{-1} \%^{-1}$ (for *T1*) and 1.2 $s^{-1} \%^{-1}$ (for *T2*), respectively, rather higher than the protein rates measured by us or reported by Koenig and Brown.

The preceding comments do not help clarify what the pathophysiological factors are that may alter tissue relaxation times. It is our opinion that a myriad of small independent factors may each contribute to the overall relaxation process in tissue. However, the influence of several such factors can be evaluated independently by careful measurements on tissues and model systems. A better understanding of the contributing processes at the molecular level would aid the interpretation of relaxation changes in pathological conditions.

References

1. Hallenga K, Koenig SH: Protein rotational relaxation as studied by ^{1}H and ^{2}H magnetic relaxation. Biochemistry *15*:4255–4263, 1976.
2. Kalk A, Berendsen JC: Proton magnetic relaxation and spin diffusion in proteins. J Magn Reson *24*:343–366, 1976.
3. Brown MS, Armitage IM, Gore JC: Proton relaxation times derived from deuterium relaxation in solution. Submitted to J Magn Reson.
4. Morris PG: Nuclear Magnetic Resonance Imaging in Medicine and Biology. Oxford, Oxford University Press, 1986, p 262.
5. Koenig SH, Brown RD: Relaxometry of tissue. *In* CRC Handbook on NMR in Cells. Boca Raton, CRC Press, 1986.
6. Gore JC, Brown MS, Mizumoto CT, Armitage IM: Influence of glycogen on water proton relaxation times. Magn Reson Med 3:436–466, 1986.

66

Frequency Dependence of Tissue Relaxation Times

PAUL A. BOTTOMLEY

Longitudinal (*T1*) and transverse (*T2*) nuclear magnetic resonance (NMR) relaxation times play a pivotal role in the understanding of molecular level organization of biological systems in general and in NMR imaging in particular. Differences among proton (¹H) NMR relaxation times of normal and pathological tissue are key to NMR image contrast and the discrimination of disease, a fact responsible for their widespread use as diagnostic parameters in clinical NMR imaging. They directly affect the selection of imaging pulse sequence timing parameters and consequently the total image scan times and patient throughput, and even influence the choice of magnetic field strength used for NMR imaging because of their significant variation with NMR frequency.

Since the early ¹H relaxation time studies on animal and human tissue by Odeblad et al. in the late 1950s,[50,67–71] the observation of elevated *T1*'s in cancer by Damadian in 1971,[17] and the more general *T1* variations in pathologies reported by Eggleston et al. in 1975,[27] the literature has burgeoned with hundreds of investigations of relaxation time behavior in biological tissue. We recently undertook a review and compilation of the published ¹H relaxation time data from animal tissues as a function of tissue type, NMR frequency, species, temperature, time after excision, in-vitro versus in-vivo measurement, and age.[7] Our goal was to determine just what the ¹H NMR relaxation times of tissue are under the physical and physiological conditions operating in a clinical NMR imaging instrument. Since whole body ¹H NMR imaging systems currently operate within the frequency range about 1 to 85 MHz,[6] with even higher frequencies imminent, data extending over the frequency range of 1 to 100 MHz were examined.

The frequency dispersions of the relaxation time data also provide valuable insight into the physical mechanisms responsible for NMR relaxation in tissue as well as the state of water therein. The traditional theoretical description invokes dipole-dipole interactions between protons and a fast exchange two state (FETS) model for tissue water to explain the observed relaxation dispersions. In the FETS model, water in biological tissue undergoes rapid exchange between an essentially free phase and a phase that is bound or adsorbed on macromolecule surfaces.

This chapter presents the normal tissue *T1* and *T2* ¹H relaxation data compiled from the literature and reviews the theoretical models used to explain the relaxation dispersions. Simple, empirically determined expressions describing the dispersions are also examined. These enable rapid computation of *T1* and *T2* at any desired frequency in the range of 1 to 100 MHz.

RELAXATION DATA

Frequency Dependence

Normal tissue relaxation time data were obtained from a subset of about 150 papers published up to the end of 1983 and tabulated elsewhere.[7] The papers were located using a computer literature survey or by cross-referencing personal files of papers collected since 1975. Even so, not all of the useful data published during this period was discovered and much more was deliberately omitted. The latter included data from dehydrated, homogenized, soaked, preserved, embalmed, fetal, or immature tissue; data obtained from tissue in vitro more than 12 hours after excision; data obtained from diseased animals; and data derived from experiments performed at unspecified NMR frequencies or field strengths.

T1 relaxation was typically characterized by a single-component exponential on a time scale >2 ms except in several reports of in-vivo and in-vitro measurements of mouse liver,[3] in-vivo newt tails,[77] in-vitro rat muscle,[13] and in-vitro human breast tissue,[63,57,8] where dual, relatively long (>50 ms) *T1* components of comparable magnitude were measured. Dual *T1* components with one short component (≤10 ms) constituting ≤8 percent of the magnetization have also been reported in mouse kidney, muscle, and spleen when long (~150 μs) inversion pulses were employed in the inversion-recovery *T1* experiment.[2]

The *T1* frequency dispersions of normal liver, skeletal and heart muscle, kidney, spleen, brain, adipose, breast, and lung tissue are plotted in Figures 66–1 to 66–8. Each data point represents an average of up to 101 individual measurements with a typical number of around 10 measurements.[7] The mean cited standard deviation for each relaxation data point expressed as a percentage of the *T1* and *T2* values is about (10 ±

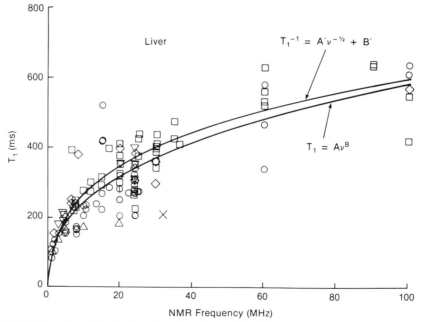

Figure 66–1. *T1* dispersion data for liver fitted to $T1 = A\nu^B$ with $A = .000534$, $B = .3799$ and standard deviation from the curve of 22 percent using a method of least squares. A least squares fit to the Escanye et al. expression $T1^{-1} = A'\nu^{-1/2} + B'$ gave the same standard deviation and a best fit with $A' = 9807$, $B' = .689$. These parameters are the same as determined previously with less data.[28] The mean cited standard deviation for each point expressed as a percentage of the *T1* value is about (9 ± 5) percent. Different symbols denote different species: X = chicken; △ = dog; ◇ = human; □ = mouse; ▽ = rabbit; ○ = rat.

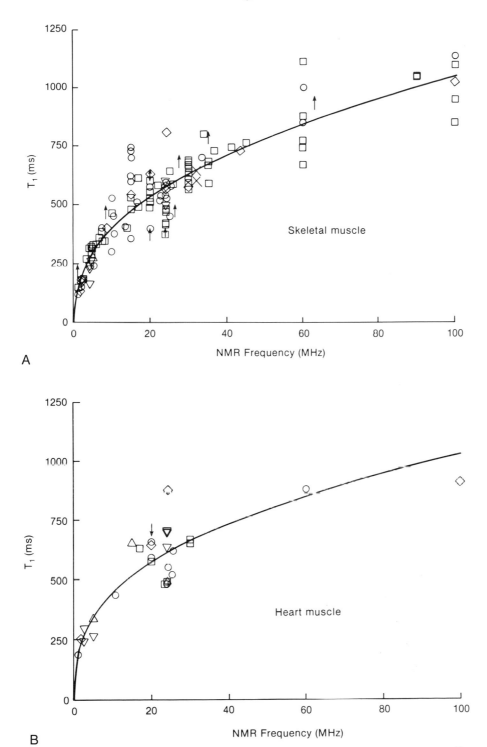

Figure 66–2. *T1* dispersion data for skeletal muscle (*A*) and heart muscle (*B*) fitted to $T1 = A\nu^B$. Fitting parameters are listed in Table 66–1. The mean cited standard deviation for each point expressed as a percentage of the *T1* value is about (5 ±3) percent. Different symbols denote different species: X = chicken; △ = dog; ↑ = frog; ◇ = human; □ = mouse; ↓ = pig; ▽ = rabbit; ○ = rat.

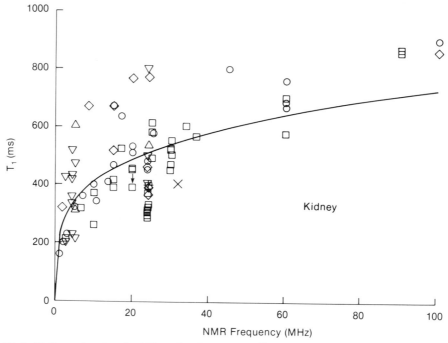

Figure 66–3. *T1* dispersion data for kidney fitted to $T1 = A\nu^B$ with parameters listed in Table 66–1. Cortex and medulla are undifferentiated. The mean cited standard deviation for each point expressed as a percentage of the *T1* value is about (6 ±5) percent. Different symbols denote different species: X = chicken; △ = dog; ◇ = human; ↓ = pig; ▽ = rabbit; ○ = rat.

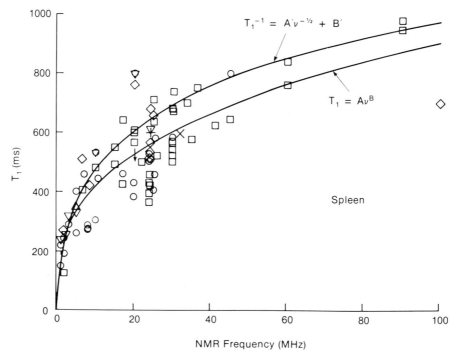

Figure 66–4. *T1* dispersion data for spleen fitted to $T1 = A\nu^B$ with Table 66–1 fitting parameters (standard deviation = 19 percent). A best fit to Escanye et al.'s equation, $T1^{-1}\ A'\nu^{-1/2} + B'$ with $A' = 5036$, and $B' = .520$, gave a 21 percent standard deviation.[28] The mean cited standard deviation for each point expressed as a percentage of the j*T1* value is about (8 ±5) percent. Different symbols denote different species: X = jchicken; △ = dog; + = hamster; ◇ = human; □ = mouse; ↓ = pig; ▽ = rabbit; ○ = rat.

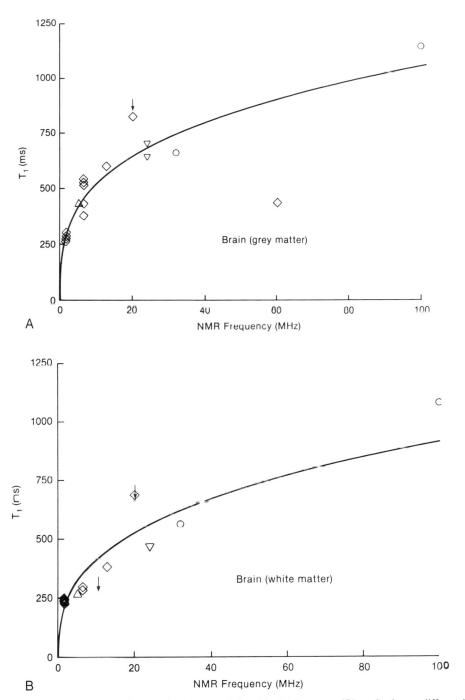

Figure 66–5. *T1* dispersion data for grey brain matter (*A*), white brain matter (*B*), and other undifferentiated brain tissue (*C*), fitted to $T1 = Av^B$ with Table 66–1 fitting parameters. The mean cited standard deviation for each point expressed as a percentage of the *T1* value is about (7 ±4) percent. Different symbols denote different species: △ = dog; ★ = gerbil; ◇ = human; □ = mouse; ↓ = pig; ▽ = rabbit; ○ = rat.

10) percent for all tissues. Different symbols denote different species and include human, rat, mouse, chicken, cow, pig, dog, gerbil, hamster, rabbit, frog, and newt contributions. No differentiation is made here between data recorded in-vitro and in-vivo data obtained by NMR imaging techniques (see sections Other Variables, and Errors). Skeletal and heart muscle (Fig. 66–2), and gray and white brain matter (Fig.

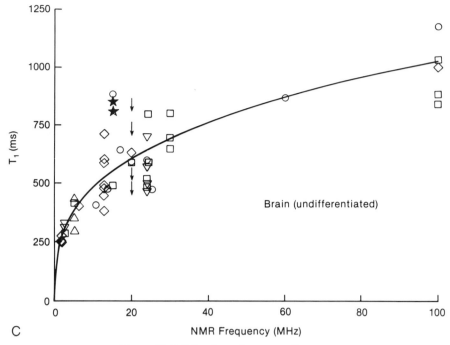

C

Figure 66–5 *C* See legend on preceding page

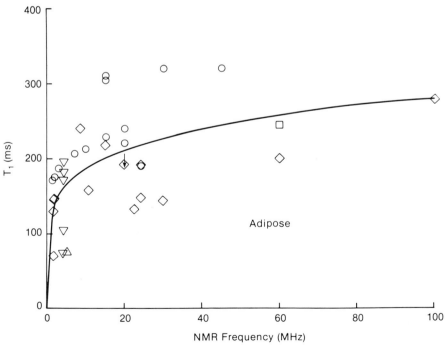

Figure 66–6. *T1* dispersion data for adipose tissue fitted to *T1* = *Av*^B with Table 66–1 fitting parameters. The mean cited standard deviation for each point expressed as a percentage of the *T1* value is about (12 ±6) percent. Different symbols denote different species: △ = dog; ◇ = human; □ = mouse; ↓ = pig; ▽ = rabbit; ○ = rat.

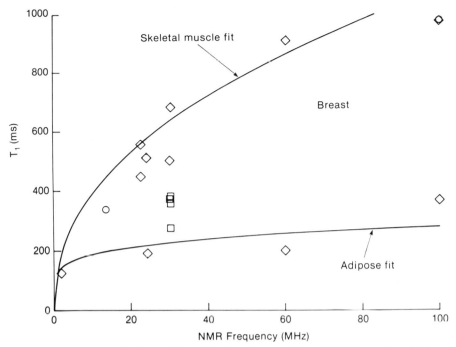

Figure 66–7. *T1* dispersion data for breast tissue. The best fit curves from skeletal muscle and adipose tissue are superimposed for comparison. The mean cited standard deviation for each point expressed as a percentage of the *T1* value is about (12 ± 13) percent. Different symbols denote different species: ◇ = human; □ = mouse; ○ = rat.

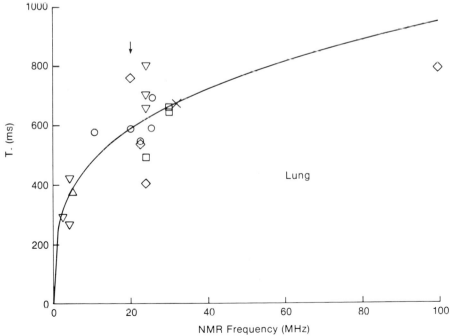

Figure 66–8. *T1* dispersion data for lung tissue fitted to $T1 = A\nu^B$ with Table 66–1 fitting parameters. The mean cited standard deviation for each point expressed as a percentage of the *T1* value is about (10 ± 10) percent. Different symbols denote different species: X = chicken; △ = dog; ◇ = human; □ = mouse; ↓ = pig; ▽ = rabbit; ○ = rat.

66–5) have different *T1*'s and are therefore differentiated where possible. Similarly, kidney cortex and medulla have significantly different *T1*'s, but because few authors make such a distinction, segregation of the kidney plot was impractical. Thus Figure 66–3 should be regarded cautiously, as an organ average only. Note that for a given tissue type, there are no significant systematic differences in the *T1* data due to differences in species (Figs. 66–1 to 66–8).

Curves of the form

$$T1 = A\nu^B \tag{1}$$

where A and B are constants, and ν is the NMR frequency, are fitted to the liver, muscle, kidney, spleen, brain, adipose, and lung *T1* dispersions using the method of minimizing the sum of the squares of the fractional differences of *T1* data from the curves. Conventional fitting routines that minimize the sum of the squares of the absolute differences between the curve and the data preferentially weight the less numerous high frequency points, generating curves that appear better fitted but that have slightly higher fractional errors. The applicability of the curve fitting algorithm to individual *T1* dispersion data is demonstrated in Figure 66–9 with measurements from the muscle and liver data sets published by Escanye et al.[28] and Koenig et al.[56]

Fits of the dispersion data to other standard functions were also sought. Power series expansions, and the dipolar expression for *T1* with a single correlation time (see Spin Lattice Relaxation), diverged or were less successful at fitting data at extreme frequencies. However, an expression for the frequency dispersion due to Escanye et al.[28],

$$T1^{-1} = A'\nu^{-1/2} + B' \tag{2}$$

(A', B', constants) yielded quite comparable results. Best fits to the Escanye et al. expression are plotted in Figures 66–1 and 66–4 for comparison.

Values of the fitting coefficients and the percentage standard deviations (assuming random distributions) of *T1* values from the curves for each tissue are tabulated in Table 66–1. The curves are not weighted with the number of samples averaged for each

Table 66–1. MEAN ¹H TISSUE *T1* AND *T2* RELAXATION TIMES

Tissue	*T1*[a]			*T2*[b]	
	A	*B*	*SD (%)*	*T2 (ms)*	*SD (ms)*
Muscle					
Skeletal	.000455	.4203	18	47	13
Heart	.00130	.3618	16	57	16
Liver	.000534	.3799	22	43	14
Kidney[c]	.00745	.2488	27	58	24
Spleen	.00200	.3321	19	62	27
Adipose	.0113	.1743	28	84	36
Brain					
Gray matter	.00362	.3082	17	101	13
White matter	.00152	.3477	17	92	22
Unspecified	.00232	.3307	19	76	21
Lung	.00407	.2958	19	79	29
Marrow[d]				59	24
Breast[e]				49	16

[a] $T1 = A\nu^B \pm SD\%$, where ν = ¹H NMR frequency in Hz; SD = standard deviation expressed as a percentage of *T1*; *T1* in sec.
[b] Assumes *T2* is independent of frequency. Multicomponent data are omitted from the computations. *T2* is in ms. SD = standard deviation in ms.
[c] Averages medulla and cortex.
[d] Insufficient data for a *T1* fit.
[e] Use skeletal muscle and/or adipose *T1* fits.

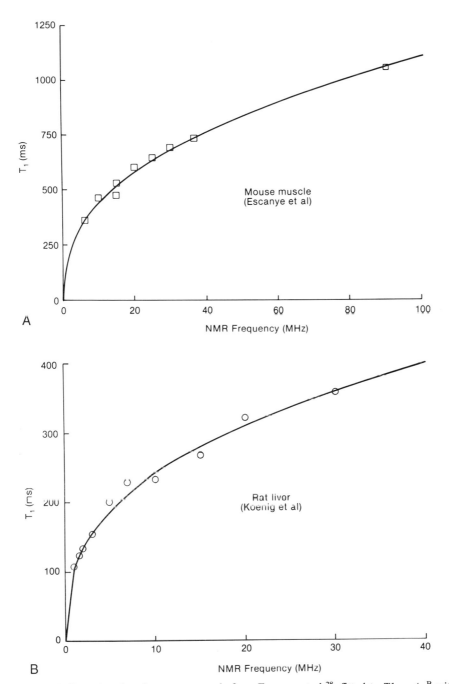

Figure 66–9. *A, T1* dispersion data for mouse muscle from Escanye et al.[28], fitted to $T1 = A\nu^B$ with $A = .000645$, $B = .4044$, and standard deviation 3.7 percent. The Escanye et al. fit, $T1^{-1} = A'\nu^{-1/2} + B'$ with $A = 6225$, $B = .300$ yielded the same standard deviation. *B, T1* dispersion data for rat liver from Koenig et al.[56] fitted to $T1 = A\nu^B$ with $A = .000741$, $B = .3592$, and standard deviation 3.9 percent. The latter data were derived from relaxation rate curves and probably contain reading errors.

point because the scatter in *T1* values measured at the same frequency often greatly exceeds the cited standard deviations. The concentration of disagreeable data around 15 MHz and 20 MHz attests to this. Thus curves computed from weighted data were essentially congruent with the unweighted curves and showed comparable standard deviations. For breast tissue (Fig. 66–7), where the scatter exceeds 100 percent, curves from muscle and adipose plots (Figs. 66–2*A* and 66–6) are superimposed on the data, suggesting tissue heterogeneity is the main cause. Breast tissue is apparently a mixture of fibrous and fatty components.

Figure 66–10 illustrates the *T2* dispersion for liver. *T2* data scatter is significantly greater than that for *T1* and obscures any frequency dependence. Many researchers reported multiple (≤5) *T2* components that constituted between 6 and 76 percent of the observed tissue NMR signal intensity.[7,12,22,42,74] Only the single *T2* component values are used in Figure 66–10 and in computing the average *T2* values listed in Table 66–1. The latter calculations assume that *T2* is independent of NMR frequency.

Other Variables

The vast majority of plotted relaxation data were measured either at room temperature (~23° C) or at physiological temperatures (~37° C). The effect of temperature on *T1* over this temperature range is evident from Fung and colleagues' study of mouse muscle and liver *T1*'s from 0.01 to 100 MHz.[36–38] Increases in *T1* of approximately 20 percent, 30 percent, and 40 percent between 17° C and 37° C at 7.5 MHz, 35 MHz, and 60 MHz, respectively, were reported. *T1* varied linearly with the reciprocal of the absolute temperature (1/T). Also, Lewa and Majewska[58] presented data from rat and cow liver, muscle, heart, spleen, and lung tissue at 16 MHz indicating that *T1* increases by about 10 percent between room and physiological temperatures. As for tissue *T2*'s, Finch and Homer[32] found no change in frog muscle between 4° C and 25° C at 23 MHz, within experimental error. Belton et al.[5] reported a slight decrease in the major frog muscle *T2* component with increasing temperature from 0° C to 25° C.

In-vitro relaxation time data were recorded within 12 hours following excision or

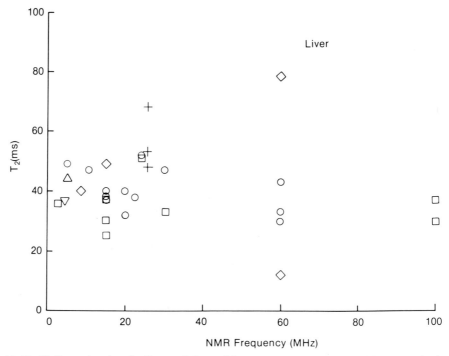

Figure 66–10. *T2* dispersion data for liver omitting multicomponent measurements. The mean cited standard deviation for each point expressed as a percentage of the *T2* value is about (10 ± 10) percent. Different symbols denote different species: △ = dog; + = hamster; ◇ = human; ▽ = rabbit; ○ = rat.

death. The dependence of tissue relaxation on time after excision is another potential source of variation among in-vitro data. However, no appreciable changes in the *T1* and *T2* of human and animal tissues up to 24 hr after excision were observed by Frey et al.,[33] Hollis et al.,[48] and Pearson et al.[73] Thickman et al.[86] reported no changes in rat liver and spleen *T1*'s up to 6 hr post excision, but decreases in *T1* of up to 18 percent ensued after 24 hr. No changes in the corresponding *T2*'s occurred up to 48 hr post excision. Changes in *T1* of less than 10 percent in human and animal liver, spleen, kidney, and brain up to 14 hr post excision[13,16,17] and a 10 percent decrease in breast *T2* over a 24 hr period[79] have been reported elsewhere.

Also, negligible or less than 10 percent variations in *T1* occur when animal and human tissues are refrigerated at 4 to 5° C for periods of up to a week post excision according to Frey et al.,[33] Damadian et al.,[18] Parish et al.,[72] and Koenig et al.,[56] although larger variations have been reported by Beall[4] and Small et al.[79] No differences have been observed between autopsy and surgically removed tissue within experimental error.[39,72] Moreover, a comparison of in-vitro relaxation time measurements with in-vivo data measured by ^{1}H NMR imaging showed no significant systematic differences that could not be attributed to variations in temperature.[7]

Dramatic elevations in relaxation times of up to 2.7 times normal adult values have been reported in neonatal tissue,[9,43,52–54,59,64,80] persisting a few weeks in animals to at least several months after birth in humans. This is the reason for omitting fetal and immature tissue data from the plots. Also, minor fluctuations in *T1* of about 12 percent with circadian rhythm have been observed by De Certaines et al.[21] in rat liver excised as a function of time. *T1* peaked at midday and was lowest at dawn. No corresponding fluctuation in *T2* was measured.

Error

Other factors potentially responsible for the large scatter among *T1* and *T2* tissue dispersion data are inherent tissue heterogeneity, sample handling techniques, the NMR measurement methods, and the existence of multiple *T2* components as well as presently unidentified sources. Tissue heterogeneity is unlikely to influence scatter significantly because of the large number of samples typically represented by each data point and the relatively small standard deviations quoted for individual *T1* points.[7] Sample handling is a key issue for in-vitro studies, addressed in depth by Beall,[4] but the plotted data have been screened to exclude measurements from abused tissue (see Frequency Dependence).

The techniques used for measuring *T1* in vitro were the multiple point inversion recovery, partial saturation, or saturation recovery methods, or the less accurate single point null method. The few investigators who employed the null technique almost invariably verified their experimental accuracy by comparing their results with measurements obtained by other methods. In-vitro *T2* measurements were performed mainly by the standard Carr-Purcell or Carr-Purcell-Meiboom-Gill methods. Therefore, one cannot objectively discriminate against in-vitro *T1* or *T2* data on the basis of measurement technique.

However, more dubious practices abound in the measurement of relaxation times in vivo using NMR imaging techniques. To expedite patient scan times, *T1* and *T2* measurements are typically performed using only two points on the nuclear magnetization relaxation curves for each image picture element.[10,11,19,20,24,40,45–47,49,60,61,65,66, 75,80–84,87] The standard expressions employed for computing *T1* from inversion or saturation recovery with two samples of the transient magnetization presume precise 90 degree or 180 degree radio frequency (rf) NMR pulses at each and every picture element in the image plane.[25] This is extremely difficult to achieve in conventional NMR transmitter coil designs. The effect of imprecise rf pulses due to rf field homogeneity is to render the derived T1 values dependent upon the time after initial excitation at which they are measured. For example, Gore et al.[40] reported dramatic T1 variations of up to 60 percent as a result of increasing the relaxation recovery time, t, from 0.2 s to 0.4 s! A prudent approach to accurate T1 measurement in the presence of inhomogeneous rf fields in NMR imaging may be to use a three-parameter fit to the signal intensity $S = P + Q \exp(-t/T1)$, where P, Q, and T1 are fitting constants.[31] Obviously, more than two data points would be required.

The situation is worse for in-vivo T2 studies, since multiple components are widely identified in vitro. Hence, Gore et al.[40] tabulated variations in T2 of up to 350 percent, comparing values computed from spin echoes occurring at 32 ms and 64 ms after the initial 90 degree rf pulse. Worse still, the pulsed gradient spin echo imaging experiment employed in T2 imaging studies is a facsimile of the standard Stejskal and Tanner pulsed gradient diffusion measurement technique.[85] Since bulk tissue diffusion coefficients are significant fractions of pure water values,[41,42] attenuation of computed T2's by diffusion effects is quite predictable. Diffusion and ignorance of multiple components may thus substantially account for the sad state of the T2 data.

MECHANISMS AND MODELS

Spin-Lattice Relaxation

T1 characterizes the time taken for the longitudinal nuclear magnetization to return to equilibrium. The time dependence of the longitudinal magnetization, as described by the Bloch equations in a frame of reference rotating about the longitudinal axis at the resonance frequency ν, is proportional to only transverse magnetic field components.[1] This is due to the presence of a vector cross product of the nuclear magnetization and the magnetic field in the Bloch equations. T1 relaxation is induced only by fluctuations in the transverse field that are static in the rotating frame of reference. For protons in biological tissue, the major source of magnetic field fluctuations is the thermal motion of neighboring dipoles. In a nonrotating, laboratory frame of reference, thermal fluctuations at the resonance frequency (2ν) and at twice that frequency (2ν) satisfy the criteria for T1 relaxation. The 2ν effect arises because a motion at 2ν may reverse the sense of rotation of a nuclear spin, thereby enabling relaxation via the counter-rotating component of magnetic field fluctuations that occur at frequency ν.

The intensity of fluctuations in the transverse field at the resonance frequency and at 2ν are measured by the spectral density functions, $J(\nu)$ and $J(2\nu)$. Their intensities and the strength of the interaction jointly determine the value of T1. Since protons exhibit the strongest naturally occurring nuclear magnetic moments and are ubiquitous in biological tissue, proton dipole-dipole interactions dominate normal tissue ^{1}H relaxation. In general, these interactions can involve both intramolecular and intermolecular protons on both macromolecules and water molecules.

The monotonic increase in T1 with frequency from 1 to 100 MHz evident in Figures 66–1 to 66–9 reflects a corresponding reduction in $J(\nu)$ and the intensity of high-frequency thermal motion of the tissue protons. The frequency dependence of T1 derives from the general expression for T1 relaxation via magnetic dipole-dipole interactions:

$$\frac{1}{T1} = \frac{9}{8} \gamma^4 \bar{h}^2 [J^1(\nu) + J^2(2\nu)] \tag{3}$$

where $\gamma = 2.675 \times 10^8 \ s^{-1}T^{-1}$ is the proton gyromagnetic ratio, $\bar{h} = 1.055 \times 10^{-34}$

J·s is Planck's constant divided by 2π, and $J^1(\nu)$ and $J^2(2\nu)$ are the spectral density functions for the various motions evaluated at the resonance frequency and at twice that frequency.[1]

Intramolecular processes involve mainly rotational motion with spectral density functions

$$J^1(\nu) = \frac{J^2(\nu)}{4} = \sum_{i,j} \frac{4C_{ij}}{15r_j^6} \left[\frac{\tau_{ij}}{1 + 4\pi^2\nu^2\tau_{ij}^2} \right] \quad (4)$$

where r_j is an intramolecular (H–H) distance between nuclear dipoles, C_{ij} are weighting coefficients independent of frequency, and the τ_{ij} are correlation times for the ith characteristic mode of motion of the jth intramolecular dipole pair.[1,32,38,54,88] The correlation times represent average periods between atomic collisions of the nuclei in various states of motion. Intermolecular $T1$ interactions involving rotational or translational motion have spectral density functions with the same frequency dependence as Equation (4), but with r_j an intermolecular dipole distance between the jth intermolecular dipole pair. For intramolecular interactions, Equation (4) can be simplified by ignoring the macromolecular hydrogen, whereupon the j-summation can be omitted and r_j set as the average separation between hydrogens in water molecules.

Many established models describing the behavior of water in biological tissue invoke two components of water undergoing rapid exchange relative to the NMR observation time. These consist of a large free water compartment and a bound water compartment hydrogen-bonded to macromolecules and proteins to form hydration layers.[15,22,23,28,29,32,34,35,42,51,53,55,76] The observation of a nonfreezing water component in many tissues, often directly identified with the bound phase, is key evidence for this fast exchange two state (FETS) model.[62] A hypothesis, due to Ling, in which all intracellular water exists in an ordered, polarized state has also been invoked.[17,37,42]

The relaxation rate in the FETS model is a weighted average of the two states:

$$\frac{1}{T1} \sim \frac{b}{T1_b} + \frac{1-b}{T1_f + \tau_e} \quad (5)$$

where $T1_b$ is the $T1$ of the bound fraction ($b \ll 1$) of water, $T1_f$ is the $T1$ of the free water fraction, and τ_e is the residence time of water in the bound compartment.[32,42] $T1_f$ is approximately equal to the $T1$ of tap water (~ 2 s) and constitutes ~ 75 to 99 percent of the total observed water ($b \sim .01$ to .25). Free water undergoes rapid translational and rotational diffusion, that is, $4\pi^2\nu^2\tau_f^2 \ll 1$ for $\nu \leq 100$ MHz with a free water correlation time $\tau_f \sim 1$ ps. Thus $T1_f$ is essentially independent of frequency. The frequency dependence of the measured $T1$ is therefore determined by $T1_b$.

That this is so for biological tissue is evidenced by $T1$ experiments performed by Fung at 5 MHz, 30 MHz, and 100 MHz in which b is varied by soaking tissue samples in solutions of different osmolarity.[35,78] The extrapolated intercept from Equation (5) is identified as $\sim 1/T1_f$ provided that $\tau_e \ll T1_f$, and corresponds to $T1_f \sim 1.7$ s independent of frequency.[35] Also Escanye et al.[28] determined $T1_f \sim 1.8[^{+1.3}_{-.5}]$ s independent of frequency from 6.7 MHz to 90 MHz as a tissue average over normal and cancerous muscle, spleen, liver, and kidney. This results from equating Equation (5) with their dispersion Equation (2), whereupon $B' = \sim (1 - b)/T1_f$.

The simplest model characterizes the rate $1/T1_b$ by isotropic rotational motion and a single correlation time, implying, from Equations (3–5), $T1 \propto \nu^2$. Such behavior was fitted by Knispel et al.[55] to $T1$ data measured over 17 to 45 MHz, but this model clearly does not satisfactorily cope with the extended 1 to 100 MHz range investigated here.[28] Thus multiple or continuously distributed correlation times are required. A dual correlation time model involving intramolecular interactions with anisotropic reorientation of bound water fitted Escanye et al.'s data[28] but required excessive free water fractions in the range $.98 \leq 1 - b < 1$. Here, one correlation time would correspond to rapid motion about an axis perpendicular to the H–H direction; and the other, to slow reorientation of this axis under the influence of macromolecular motion.[88]

While correlation times associated with intramolecular interactions are dominated by rotation, intermolecular interactions usually involve mainly translational motion. However, rotation and translation of water molecules in free water are strongly coupled, suggesting that the same correlation times might be used to characterize both motions. This, and the similarity between the spectral density functions describing intermolecular and intramolecular interactions, offers some justification for floating C_{ij} and r_j to intermolecular/intramolecular averages and computing $T1_b$ from Equations (3–5) with a single summation over the i correlation times.[32] Finch and Homer fitted such a model to frog muscle dispersion data to within experimental accuracy (5 percent). However nine fitting parameters, including five discrete correlation times for the bound compartment and a single correlation time for the free compartment, were needed to fit only 19 data points.[32] The resultant weighting coefficients (C_i) are plotted against correlation time in Figure 66–10.

These results may seem consistent with the existence of several hydration layers bonded to macromolecules with increasing mobility in outer layers and suggest a distribution of residence times (τ_e) rather than the single value assumed. The estimates of $(1 - b)$ and τ_e, however, again appear somewhat excessive at .97 and 0.8 ms, respectively.

Models incorporating distributed correlation times for the molecular motion of the bound water fraction were preferred by Held et al.,[44] Fung and McGaughy,[38] Fung et al.,[37] and Escanye et al.[28] All attempted a log-Gaussian distribution function of intramolecular correlation times for rotation

$$g(\tau) = \frac{\alpha}{\tau\sqrt{\pi}} \exp\left[-\left[\alpha \ln \left(\frac{\tau}{\tau_0} \right) \right]^2 \right] \tag{6}$$

(α, τ_0 empirically determined constants), not dissimilar from the discrete distribution of Figure 66–10, to provide a good fit to muscle frequency dispersion data recorded between 3 KHz and 75 MHz. This requires replacement of the Equation (4) summation, $\sum C_{ij}$, by the integral $\int g(\tau) \, d\tau$, which is then evaluated numerically.[38] Both intramolecular and intermolecular contributions are again incorporated implicitly by empirically fitting the parameters.

Escanye et al.[28] also proposed a model involving distributed correlation times to explain their fit to Equation (2). In this model, $T1$ relaxation is dominated by intermolecular interactions that consist entirely of translational diffusion of bound tissue water treated as spheres. The spectral density functions for isotropic, uniform translational diffusion are

$$J^1(\nu) = \frac{J^2(\nu)}{4} = \frac{M}{dD} \int_0^\infty [J_{3/2}(u)]^2 \frac{u \, du}{u^4 + 4\pi^2\nu^2\tau_d^2} \tag{7}$$

where M is the ^{1}H spin density; $J_{3/2}(u)$ is a Bessel function of order 3/2, $u = rd$, where r is the distance variable between diffusing molecules and d is the distance of closest approach; D is the diffusion coefficient and $\tau_d = d^2/2D$ is the diffusion jump time.[1,28] Assuming $d = 5$ Å and a 50 ns jump time, the model[28] yields a bound water diffusion coefficient of 2.5×10^{-8} cm^{-2}·s^{-1} that is about 400 times less than Hazlewood et al.'s bulk muscle tissue measurements.[41,42] However, the latter must be considered as free/bound fraction averages.

The empirical expression for the $T1$ dispersions, $T1 = A\nu^B$, bears close resemblance to the Escanye et al.[28] expression, Equation (2). Unfortunately numerical evaluation of Equations (3) and (7) using similar values of τ_d, d, and D in the isotropic diffusion model yields curves nonlinear in $\log(T1)$ versus $\log(\nu)$ over 1 to 100 MHz, contrary to the requirements of both Equations (1) and (2), as shown in Figure 66–11. Therefore either a distribution of diffusional correlation times is necessary, or intramolecular or intermolecular rotational contributions cannot be totally neglected.

An alternative approach to fitting tissue $T1$ dispersions has been adopted by Koenig et al.[56] who used the heuristic Cole-Cole expression

$$\frac{1}{T1} = \frac{1}{T1_f} + G + \frac{H[1 + (\nu/\nu_c)^{\beta/2} \cos(\pi\beta/4)]}{1 + 2(\nu/\nu_c)^{\beta/2} \cos(\pi\beta/4) + (\nu/\nu_c)^{\beta}} \tag{8}$$

where $T1_f$, G, H, ν_c, and β are five empirically determined parameters. This expression has been used extensively to fit tissue electrical permittivity dispersions. It has the advantage that dispersions exhibiting multiple inflections can be accommodated, as is the case for $T1$ when the frequency range is extended down to the KHz region. Its disadvantage is its complexity for computing $T1$ in the more restricted NMR imaging range of 1 to 100 MHz, in comparison to Equations (1) or (2).

Indeed all of the semiempirical multiparameter models are susceptible to the criticism that given enough variables, success is virtually guaranteed, particularly since the experimental dispersions are apparently continuous, slow-varying, and monotonic. In this context the empirical relationship, $T1 = A\nu^B$, holds the nontrivial advantage of providing as good or better average fit to the tabulated data than the Escanye group's equation (Figs. 66–1 and 66–4) and an excellent if not superior fit to the individual tissue dispersions of Escanye et al. and Koenig et al. (Fig. 66–9) with minimal fitting coefficients compared to Equations (3) to (8), even though its physical significance, if any, is yet to be determined. Ultimately, close scrutiny of predicted variables will be necessary to determine the physical validity of all of the various models.

Estimates of the relative importance of intermolecular and intramolecular interactions to bound water relaxation are also open to ambiguous interpretation. A priori, the r_j^{-6} dependence of the dipole-dipole interaction (Eq. 4) strongly favors dominance

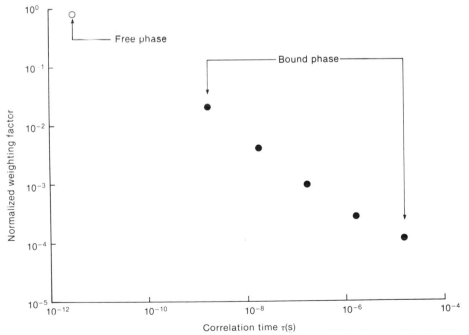

Figure 66–11. Discrete distribution of six correlation times and their weighting factors fitted by Finch and Homer[32] to frog muscle $T1$ and $T1_\rho$ dispersions using Equations (3) and (4) and omitting the j^- summation.

by intramolecular processes. However, both intermolecular and intramolecular models can be fitted to the *T1* dispersions with essentially equivalent ease or difficulty because both contain terms quadratic in frequency (compare Eqs. 4 and 7).

To elucidate the relative importance of the intermolecular and intramolecular mechanisms, Civan and Shporer[14] and Fung[36] observed the ^{1}H *T1*'s of muscle and brain tissue bathed in various concentrations of deuterated water (^{2}H$_2$O) in Krebs solution for an hour. Since the gyromagnetic ratio of ^{2}H is 0.15 that of ^{1}H, the substitution of ^{2}H$_2$O for ^{1}H$_2$O in bulk water reduces the strength of intermolecular H$_2$O–H$_2$O dipolar interactions for ^{1}H. It also reduces the intramolecular H–H dipolar interaction, since ^{1}H$_2$O and ^{2}H$_2$O undergo rampant chemical exchange to ^{1}HO^{2}H. Thus bulk water *T1* rapidly increases as the ratio [^{2}H$_2$O/^{1}H$_2$O] increases. In tissue, the increase is much less: about 20 percent extrapolating to complete substitution compared with a factor of 24 for bulk water. Rustgi et al.[76] extended these measurements over the frequency range 15 to 60 MHz for muscle tissue, recording essentially the same observation.

This somewhat surprising and significant result is interpreted as evidence that tissue ^{1}H relaxation is dominated by intermolecular interactions between macromolecules and water molecules in the first hydration layer. This is the only remaining relaxation mechanism that is transparent to the ^{2}H$_2$O substitution.[36] The small 20 percent change observed is possibly attributable to chemical exchange between macromolecules and water deuterons. The implication is that tissue *T1* relaxation entirely hinges on the interaction between macromolecules and a single adsorbed layer or less of water. The relaxation mechanism may be either translational or rotational and likely involves the stronger H–H interactions. To explain the dispersion data, a distribution of correlation times in the neighborhood of 10 to 100 ns is necessary. If the interaction responsible for relaxation is principally translational diffusion of water molecules at the macromolecule surface, as in the Escanye et al.[28] version of the FETS model, then the residence time τ_e that a water molecule remains in the bound phase cannot be much longer than the translational diffusion jump time of $\tau_d \sim 50$ ns. Indeed, if translational diffusion is dominant and the hydration water consists of only a single layer or less of water molecules, then it would be difficult to argue that τ_d and τ_e are not identical.

Finally a further intricacy concerning relaxation at the macromolecule/hydration water interface should be noted. Cross relaxation is a relaxation mechanism involving the transfer of magnetization between two different nuclear spin species via mutual spin flips. Recently this mechanism has been invoked to describe the intermolecular interaction between protons on the hydration water and protons on macromolecules at the interface.[2,26,30] Edzes and Samulski's[26] theoretical description introduces several new variables or fitting parameters, including the rate of exchange of spin-energy across the interface, and the hypothetical *T1*'s of the macromolecule and hydration protons calculated in the absence of cross relaxation. Experimental evidence for the mechanism is provided by the observation of multicomponent *T1*'s in biological tissue when long (>100 μs) inversion pulses are used in the inversion-recovery *T1* experiment.[2,26,30] Such pulses have restricted bandwidths and therefore selectively invert only the water proton components which exhibit longer *T2* values than the macromolecule components.[26] However, the cross relaxation term is dipolar and has the same frequency dependence as Equations (4) and (7).[26] Therefore, consideration of this mechanism adds little insight to the explanation of the tissue *T1* frequency dispersions.

Spin-Spin Relaxation

The Bloch equations describing transverse relaxation in the rotating frame of reference contain magnetic field components in both transverse and longitudinal directions. Fluctuations in the magnetic field that are static in the rotating frame induce $T2$ relaxation. Thus, like $T1$, $T2$ processes can arise from fluctuations in the transverse field in the laboratory frame of reference which occur at the resonance frequency and at 2ν. But unlike $T1$, $T2$ processes can also involve variations in the longitudinal field. Since a static magnetic field in the longitudinal direction in the rotating frame of reference transforms to a static magnetic field in the laboratory frame of reference, $T2$ relaxation processes also include a static field or zero frequency contribution in the laboratory frame.

The expression for the $T2$ dispersion corresponding to Equation (3) is thus

$$\frac{1}{T2} = \frac{3}{4}\gamma^4\bar{h}^2 \left[\frac{3}{8} J^0(0) + \frac{15}{4} J^1(\nu) + \frac{3}{8} J^2(2\nu) \right] \qquad (9)$$

where $J^0(0)$ is the static component of the spectral density function[1] and includes here effects due to microscopic and molecular level field heterogeneity in biological tissue. Thus $T2$ is independent of frequency if the last two terms in Equation (9) are small compared to the first, static contribution. Furthermore, since $J^1(\nu)$ and $J^2(2\nu)$ terms appear in both Equations (9) and (3), the presence of the static term in Equation (9) also ensures the frequency independence of $T2$ if $T2$ is much less than $T1$. This is true of virtually all of the nonfluid tissues, except perhaps for the longest of $T2$ components in those studies reporting multiple $T2$ components,[12,22,42,74] and for adipose whose $T1$ dispersion is essentially constant above 10 MHz anyway (Fig. 66–6). The dispersions of long $T2$ components presumably follow those of the corresponding $T1$'s. Like $T1$, $T2$ can also be equated to a sum of contributions from free and bound components in an expression analogous to Equation (5). The static intramolecular spectral density function due to rotation is $J^0(0) = 6J^1(0)$ as defined in Equation (4), and the static intermolecular spectral density function due to isotropic translational diffusion is $J^0(0) = 2N/15dD = 2\pi N\eta/5kT$ where η is the viscosity and k, Boltzmann's constant.[1]

Evidence for multicomponent relaxation times is more compelling for $T2$ than for $T1$. The sparse multicomponent $T1$ data reported are largely explicable by sample or chemical heterogeneity or by cross relaxation, as noted earlier. For example, in adipose tissues, ^1H chemical shift spectroscopy reveals two principal components associated with H_2O and $-CH_2-$ (macromolecular) hydrogens[6] with different $T1$ and $T2$ relaxation times thus far neglected in the above analyses. Breast or other tissues with large fatty components, tissues with high blood content, or tissues with other heterogeneity such as gray and white brain matter or kidney cortex and medulla can easily yield multicomponent relaxation values. Multicomponent $T2$'s that are not attributable to macroscopic/microscopic heterogeneity are difficult to explain at a molecular level. Given the similarity of mechanisms responsible for $T1$ and $T2$ relaxation, a key question is whether multicomponent $T2$'s can coexist with single-valued $T1$'s.

Hazlewood, Chang, and colleagues interpreted the multicomponent $T2$ data as evidence against the fast exchange model.[12,42] However, slow exchange would require residence times τ_e of the order $T2$ ($\sim$10 ms), which could be expected to generate observable multicomponent $T1$ data. Diegel and Pintar responded that the different behavior of $T1$ and $T2$ is explicable via the static $T2$ spectral density term,[22] $J^0(0)$. They observed dual component tissue $T1_\rho$'s (effectively, the $T1$ at extremely low frequency) from $\sim$0 to 60 KHz equivalent to the dual component $T2$ values. The two components were principally attributed to intercellular (150 ms) and intracellular (53 ms) water, because intercellular water could be expected to contain a much smaller fraction of hydrated water.

The fact that both the $T1_\rho$ and $T2$ values are shorter than corresponding $T1$'s can be accounted for by a $\sim$10 μs correlation time associated with the residence time τ_e for exchange diffusion of water molecules between the free phase and the hydration layer.[22,55] This 10 μs correlation time arises directly from the $T1_\rho$ dispersion studies.[22,55] The 10 μs exchange diffusion correlation time is too slow to directly affect $T1$ relaxation between 1 and 100 MHz, but since $\tau_e \ll T1$, it strongly averages the different $T1$ values in the various compartments, leaving the observed $T1$ more or less single-valued in the >1 ms range. $T1_\rho$ measurements in normal and deuterated muscle, spleen, and kidney by Rustgi et al.[76] confirm the importance of exchange diffusion as a relaxation process at extremely low NMR frequencies. The exchange diffusion can directly affect tissue water $T2$'s by exposing water molecules to local static field inhomogeneities at the exchange interface: Fung and McGaughy[38] note microscopic field inhomogeneity as a likely explanation of why $T2 < T1$ in tissue.

This aspect of the FETS model is incompatible with the Escanye et al.[28] view of $T1$ dispersions dominated by translational diffusion because Escanye et al. require $\tau_e \sim \tau_d$, and 10 μs ≠ 50 ns. It is, however, compatible with the intramolecular/intermolecular rotational model of $T1$, or the model involving cross relaxation at the interface, or even a modified Escanye et al. scenario in which $T1$ dispersion is dominated by rotational diffusion rather than translational diffusion at the hydration layer. In the latter case, rotational diffusion would be characterized by the same diffusion jump time τ_d. The free water correlation time is still ~1 ps, much faster than both the exchange diffusion correlation time $\tau_e \sim 10$ μs and either the rotational diffusion time $\tau_d \sim 50$ ns or the distribution of correlation times τ in the range of 10 to 100 ns responsible for $T1$ relaxation.

Some additional information on multicomponent $T2$'s is provided by Peemoeller et al.,[74] who analyzed the relative contributions of water and macromolecular hydrogens to each $T2$ component in mouse muscle by comparison with tissue soaked in an osmotically balanced ^2H_2O solution for four hours. They ascribe a 143 ms and a 24 μs $T2$ component to macromolecules, a 40 ms component to water alone, and a 5 ms component to both water (70 percent) and macromolecules (30 percent). This is a more explicit allocation of $T2$ components than the Diegel and Pintar intercellular/intracellular assignment,[22] and is consistent with the aforementioned observation of discrete H_2O and $-CH_2-$ peaks in some tissue ^1H NMR spectra.[6] Aside from chemical exchange, macromolecular components cannot be expected to participate in fast exchange.

CONCLUSIONS

Tissue Relaxation Data

The principal determinants of $T1$ relaxation in normal biological tissue in the range of 1 to 100 MHz are NMR frequency (ν) and tissue type. All of the tissue $T1$ dispersions studied obey the simple relationship $T1 = A\nu^B$, where A and B are parameters dependent on tissue type and $B \sim 1/3$. This expression gives an equivalent or better fit to $T1$ data than previously used expressions and models and is simple enough to enable rapid computation of $T1$ values at any desired frequency between 1 and 100 MHz. The standard deviations of $T1$ from the fitted curves are about 20 percent, reflecting mainly systematic errors not readily identifiable with species, temperature, in-vivo versus in-vitro status, time after excision, or age differences. Fetal and immature tissue excluded from this analysis exhibit dramatically elevated $T1$ values. Most data are recorded at room temperature or physiological temperature, but there is a dearth of the latter measurements above 20 MHz. Evidence that the temperature dependence of $T1$ increases significantly at higher frequencies could therefore result in our mean curves underestimating the high frequency physiological temperature data (Fig. 66–12).

Virtually all researchers report single-component $T1$ values. However, breast tis-

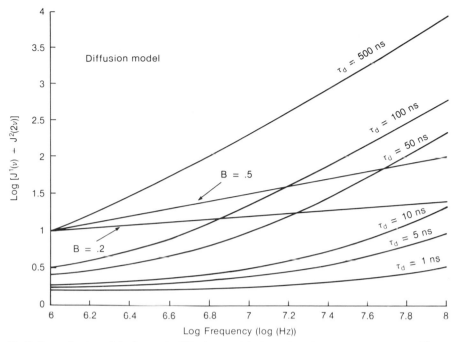

Figure 66–12. Investigation of the isotropic diffusion model of *T1* relaxation in the bound phase.[28] The curves were obtained by numerical integration of Equation (7) as a function of frequency from 1 to 100 MHz with different diffusion correlation times τ_d. Since $1/T1 \propto J^1 (\nu) + J^2 (2\nu)$, the model satisfies the empirical equations (1) and (2) when a τ_d is found for which the curves are linear. Straight lines with gradients of .2 and .5 depict the actual range of *B* values observed (Table 66–1).

sue *T1* dispersions can be resolved into two components comprising adipose and fibrous tissue that have essentially equivalent dispersions to those of skeletal muscle and adipose. Dual components can arise from macroscopic tissue heterogeneity or from the discrete chemical species H_2O and $-CH_2-$ on macromolecules when these are sufficiently mobile to be detectable on the time scale of the NMR experiment.

The principal determinant of *T2* relaxation in normal biological tissue in the range of 1 to 100 MHz is tissue type. No substantial dependence on NMR frequency, temperature, in-vivo versus in-vitro status, time after excision, or age can be differentiated within systematic errors of about 30 percent. Therefore average *T2* values are tabulated as constants for each tissue. Substantial evidence for multiple *T2* components exists. In muscle, the major component ($T2 \sim 40$ ms), constituting about 75 percent of the signal, derives from tissue water. There exist very long ($T2 \sim 140$ ms) and very short ($T2 \sim 20$ μs) *T2* components from macromolecules contributing about 7 percent and 11 percent each, and a short *T2* component ($T2 \sim 5$ ms) of about 7 percent derived from both water and macromolecules. Multicomponent *T2*'s and diffusion in the presence of imaging gradients are deleterious factors affecting in-vivo *T2* measurements which must be dealt with.

It is imperative that guidelines be established for the measurement of tissue proton NMR relaxation in vivo if *T1* and *T2* are to be useful as reproducible diagnostic parameters independent of a particular imaging system.

Best-Guess FETS Model

The observed tissue *T1* and *T2* relaxation data and their frequency dispersions can be substantially accounted for by the FETS model with free and bound phases of water undergoing rapid exchange. There is disagreement concerning the detailed mechanisms responsible for relaxation; however, the following scenario, which is consistent with the reviewed data and which incorporates elements from the models of Fung et al., Diegel and Pintar, and the results of the deuterated water exchange experiments of Fung, Rustgi et al., Civan and Shporer, and Peemoeller et al., is tentatively offered. This model is illustrated in Figure 66–13.

Water in the free phase undergoes rapid, probably correlated, rotational and translational motion with a correlation time of order 1 ps. This is too fast to directly affect relaxation between 1 and 100 MHz so the $T1$ of the free phase is long ($T1_f \sim 1.7$ s), like ordinary water, and independent of frequency. In muscle, the bound phase constitutes about 10 percent of the total tissue water content and consists of a single hydration layer or less, adsorbed on the surface of macromolecules. The intramolecular rotational correlation time of these water molecules is probably still about 1 ps, but faster relaxation of water hydrogen is facilitated by intermolecular interactions involving mainly macromolecular hydrogen. The latter mechanism requires a log-Gaussian or similar distribution of correlation times for motion, probably rotational or involving cross relaxation, of order 10 to 100 ns to cause $T1$ relaxation in the NMR frequency range 1 to 100 MHz. This faster intermolecular relaxation process is primarily

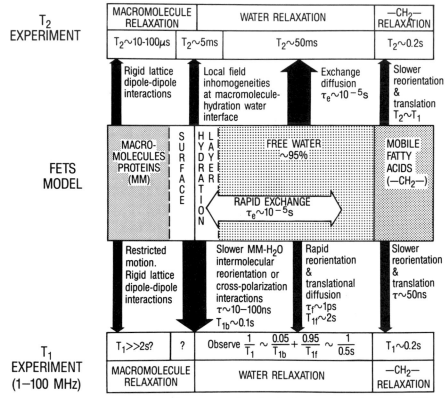

Figure 66–13. The best-guess FETS model for proton relaxation in tissue. Three chemically different proton species are identified horizontally: macromolecular protons excluding mobile fatty acids, water protons, and mobile fatty acid protons, denoted —CH₂—. These exist in up to five phases, depicted at center. Dipole-dipole interactions within each phase give rise to $T1$ and $T2$ relaxation times indicated by solid arrows. The dominant relaxation mechanisms in each phase and their corresponding times, τ, are noted next to the arrows. Widest arrows denote the largest $T2$ component, and the principal $T1$ relaxation mechanisms. Thus the $T2$ experiment (*top*) yields four $T2$ components including two water components, whereas the $T1$ experiment (*bottom*) yields just one water component, a fatty acid component, and one or two macromolecule components.

responsible for the observed dependence of $T1$ on frequency from 1 to 100 MHz and tissue type.

The bound water undergoes exchange diffusion with the free component with a slower correlation time of about 10 μs, which may be identified as the residence time in the bound state. This exchange diffusion correlation time is too long to facilitate $T1$ relaxation directly in the 1 to 100 MHz range but could provide an important relaxation mechanism for $T1_\rho$ and $T2$. Nevertheless, it is sufficiently short to prohibit resolution of the free and bound water $T1$'s on the time scale of the $T1$ experiment. Thus the observed water $T1$ relaxation rate ($1/T1$) is essentially equal to the sum of the free and bound water relaxation rates.

Unlike $T1$, $T2$ largely measures the low frequency and static components of molecular motion and can therefore discriminate free and bound water and macromolecule proton phases. The bound water and the corresponding macromolecular adsorption surface must share the same low frequency/static motional environment and can therefore be assigned the joint short $T2$ component of about 5 ms in muscle.[74] The major free water component exhibits a unique, significantly longer $T2$ value (~40 ms in muscle)[74] reflecting its greater mobility. However the free water component $T2$ value is much less than the free water $T1$ values (~25 ms) owing to an exchange diffusion relaxation mechanism. Thus the free water component $T2$ relaxation rate ($1/T2$) is equal to the sum of the rate due to exchange diffusion at the exchange interface and the much slower rate in the true liquid water phase. The exchange diffusion rate decreases with decreasing temperature, causing the free water $T2$ component to increase slightly. Since this is the majority component, and $T2$ varies with tissue type, the exchange diffusion correlation time is likely tissue dependent. A physical candidate for the exchange diffusion $T2$ relaxation mechanism is local static field gradients between the exchange interface and the free phase due to the presence of the macromolecules.

The remaining two macromolecular $T2$ components have no water counterparts. The extremely short component of around 20 μs in muscle[74] probably corresponds to rigid membrane or protein structures not normally observable in the NMR experiment, and the very long 140 ms component to highly mobile hydrogen on fatty acids, with essentially no hydration layer. The dominant role of low frequency relaxation mechanisms for all $T2$ components except the very long component ensures $T2$ dispersions independent of the NMR frequency. The 140 ms fatty acid $T2$ component[74] may be associated with the comparable valued $T1$ observed in adipose tissue, in which case its frequency dispersion will be similar. This component also probably corresponds to the $-CH_2-$ resonance observed in the ^1H chemical shift spectra of most tissues.

Further effort is necessary to evaluate the full range of fitting parameters for the model peculiar to each tissue.

ACKNOWLEDGMENTS

I thank T. H. Foster, R. E. Argersinger, L. M. Pfeifer, and W. A. Edelstein for their contributions to reference 7, on which this chapter is based. I also thank C. J. Hardy for useful discussions and R. W. Redington for technical support.

References

1. Abragam A: The Principles of Nuclear Magnetism. Oxford, Oxford University Press, 1978, pp 291–303.
2. Bakker CJG, Vriend J: Multi-exponential water proton spin-lattice relaxation in biological tissues and its implications for quantitative NMR imaging. Phys Med Biol 29:509–518, 1984.
3. Barroilhet LE, Moran PR: Nuclear magnetic resonance (NMR) relaxation spectroscopy in tissues. Med Phys 2:191–194, 1975.
4. Beall PT: Practical methods for biological NMR sample handling. Magn Reson Imag 1:165–181, 1982.

5. Belton PS, Jackson RR, Packer KJ: Pulsed NMR studies of water in striated muscle. I. Transverse nuclear spin relaxation times and freezing effects. Biochim Biophys Acta *286*:16–25, 1972.
6. Bottomley PA, Hart HR Jr, Edelstein WA, Schenck JF, Smith LS, Leue WM, Mueller OM, Redington RW: Anatomy and metabolism of the normal human brain studied by magnetic resonance at 1.5 tesla. Radiology *150*:441–446, 1984.
7. Bottomley PA, Foster TH, Argersinger RE, Pfeifer LM: A review of normal tissue hydrogen NMR relaxation times and relaxation mechanisms from 1–100 MHz: Dependence on tissue type, NMR frequency, temperature, species, excision, and age. Med Phys *11*:425–448, 1984.
8. Bovee W, Huisman P, Smidt J: Brief communication: Tumor detection and nuclear magnetic resonance. JNCI *52*:595–597, 1974.
9. Buonanno FS, Pykett IL, Brady TJ, Vielma J, Burt CT, Goldman MR, Hinshaw WS, Pohost GM, Kistler JP: Proton NMR imaging in experimental ischemic infarction. Stroke *14*:178–184, 1983.
10. Bydder GM, Steiner RE, Young IR, Hall AS, Thomas DJ, Marshall J, Pallis CA, Legg NJ: Clinical NMR imaging of the brain: 140 cases. AJR *139*:215–236, 1982.
11. Chandra R, Pizzarello DJ, Keegan AF, Chase NE: A study of proton relaxation time (*T1*) in rat tissues at various times after intracardiac manganese injection. Proc. 2nd Annual Meeting of the Society of Magnetic Resonance in Medicine. August, 16–19, 1983, pp 90–91.
12. Chang DC, Hazlewood CF: Comments on PMR studies of tissue water. J Magn Reson *18*:550–554, 1975.
13. Chang DC, Hazlewood CF, Woessner DE: The spin-lattice relaxation times of water associated with early post mortem changes in skeletal muscle. Biochim Biophys Acta *437*:253–258, 1976.
14. Civan MM, Shporer M: Pulsed nuclear magnetic resonance study of 17O, 2D, 1H of water in frog striated muscle. Biophys J *15*:299–306, 1975.
15. Coles BA: Dual-frequency proton spin relaxation measurements on tissues from normal and tumor-bearing mice. JNCI *57*:389–393, 1976.
16. Cottam GL, Vasek A, Lusted D: Water proton relaxation rates in various tissues. Res Comm Chem Pathol Pharmacol *4*:495–502, 1972.
17. Damadian R: Tumor detection by nuclear magnetic resonance. Science *171*:1151–1153, 1971.
18. Damadian R, Zaner K, Hor D, DiMaio T: Human tumors detected by nuclear magnetic resonance. Proc Natl Acad Sci USA *71*:1471–1473, 1974.
19. Davis PL, Kaufman L, Crooks LE, Margulis AR: NMR characteristics of normal and abnormal rat tissues. *In* Kaufman L, Crooks LE, Margulis AR (eds): Nuclear Magnetic Resonance Imaging in Medicine. New York, Igaku-Shoin, 1981, pp 71–100.
20. Davis PL, Sheldon P, Kaufman L, Crooks L, Margulis AR, Miller T, Watts J, Arakawa M, Hoenninger J: Nuclear magnetic resonance imaging of mammary adenocarcinomas in the rat. Cancer *51*:433–439, 1983.
21. de Certaines JD, Moulinoux JP, Benoist L, Bernard A, Rivet P: Proton nuclear magnetic resonance of regenerating rat liver after partial hepatectomy. Life Sciences *31*:505–508, 1982.
22. Diegel JG, Pintar MM: Origin of the nonexponentiality of the water proton spin relaxations in tissues. Biophys J *15*:855–860, 1975.
23. Diegel JG, Pintar MM: Brief communication: A possible improvement in the resolution of proton spin relaxation for the study of cancer at low frequency. JNCI *55*:725–726, 1975.
24. Doyle FH, Pennock JM, Banks LM, McDonnell MJ, Bydder GM, Steiner RE, Young IR, Clarke GJ, Pasmore T, Gilderdale DJ: Nuclear magnetic resonance imaging of the liver: Initial experience. AJR *138*:193–200, 1981.
25. Edelstein WA, Bottomley PA, Hart HR, Smith LS: Signal noise and contrast in nuclear magnetic resonance (NMR) imaging. J Comp Assist Tomogr *7*:391–401, 1983.
26. Edzes HT, Samulski ET: The measurement of cross-relaxation effects in the proton NMR spin-lattice relaxation of water in biological systems: hydrated collagen and muscle. J Magn Reson *31*:207–229, 1978.
27. Eggleston JC, Saryan LA, Hollis DP: Nuclear magnetic resonance investigations of human neoplastic and abnormal nonneoplastic tissues. Cancer Res *35*:1326–1332, 1975.
28. Escanye JM, Canet D, Robert J: Frequency dependence of water proton longitudinal nuclear magnetic relaxation times in mouse tissues at 20 degrees C. Biochim Biophys Acta *721*:305–311, 1982.
29. Escanye JM, Canet D, Robert J, Brondeau J: NMR proton longitudinal relaxation times in tissues of the tumour-bearing C3H mouse studied as a function of frequency. Cancer Detect Prev *4*:261–265, 1981.
30. Escayne JM, Canet D, Robert J: Nuclear magnetic relaxation studies of water in frozen biological tissues. Cross-relaxation effects between protein and bound water protons. J Magn Res *58*:118–131, 1984.
31. Evelhoch JL, Ackerman JJH: NMR *T1* measurements in inhomogeneous *B1* with surface coils. J Magn Reson *53*:52–64, 1983.
32. Finch ED, Homer LD: Proton nuclear magnetic resonance relaxation measurements in frog muscle. Biophys J *14*:907–921, 1974.
33. Frey HE, Knispel RR, Kruuv J, Sharp AR, Thompson RT, Pintar MM: Brief communication: Proton spin-lattice relaxation studies of nonmalignant tissues of tumorous mice. JNCI *49*:903–906, 1972.
34. Fullerton GD, Potter JL, Dornbluth NC: NMR relaxation of protons in tissues and other macromolecular water solutions. Magn Reson Imag *1*:209–228, 1982.
35. Fung BM: Correlation of relaxation time with water content in muscle and brain tissues. Biochim Biophys Acta *497*:317–322, 1977.
36. Fung BM: Proton and deuteron relaxation of muscle water over wide ranges of resonance frequencies. Biophys J *18*:235–239, 1977.

37. Fung BM, Durham DL, Wassil DA: The state of water in biological systems as studied by proton and deuterium relaxation. Biochim Biophys Acta *399*:191–202, 1975.
38. Fung BM, McGaughy TW: The state of water in muscle as studied by pulsed NMR. Biochim Biophys Acta *343*:663–673, 1974.
39. Goldsmith M, Koutcher J, Damadian R: NMR in cancer. XI. Application of the NMR malignancy index to human gastrointestinal tumors. Cancer *41*:183–191, 1978.
40. Gore JC, Doyle FH, Pennock JM: Relaxation rate enhancement observed in vivo by NMR imaging. *In* Partain CL, James AE, Rollo FD, Price RR (eds): Nuclear Magnetic Resonance Imaging, Philadelphia, W. B. Saunders Co., 1983, pp 94–106.
41. Hazlewood CF, Chang DC, Medina D, Cleveland G, Nichols BL: Distinction between the preneoplastic and neoplastic state of murine mammary glands. Proc Natl Acad Sci USA *69*:1478–1480, 1972.
42. Hazlewood CF, Chang DC, Woessner DE, Nichols BL: Nuclear magnetic resonance transverse relaxation times of water protons in skeletal muscle. Biophys J *14*:583–605, 1974.
43. Hazlewood CF, Nichols BL, Chang DC, Brown B: On the state of water in developing muscle: A study of the major phase of ordered water in skeletal muscle and its relationship to sodium concentration. Johns Hopkins Med J *128*:117–131, 1971.
44. Held G, Noack F, Pollack V, Melton B: Proton spin relaxation and mobility of water in muscle tissue. Z Naturforsch *28c*:59–62, 1973.
45. Heller M, Moon KL, Helms H, Schild H, Chafetz NI, Rodrigo J, Jergesen HE, Genant HK: NMR imaging of femoral head necrosis. Proceedings of the 2nd Annual Meeting of the Society of Magnetic Resonance in Medicine, August 16–19, 1983, pp 152–153.
46. Higgins CB, Herfkens R, Lipton MJ, Sievers R, Sheldon P, Kaufman L, Crooks LE: Nuclear magnetic resonance imaging of acute myocardial infarction in dogs: Alterations in magnetic relaxation times. Am J Cardiol *52*:184–188, 1983.
47. Higgins CB, Stark D, Lanzer P, Botvinick EH, Lipton MJ, Schiller N, Herfkens RJ, Crooks L, Kaufman L. NMR imaging of the heart: Normal and pathologic findings. Proceedings of the 2nd Annual Meeting of the Society of Magnetic Resonance in Medicine, August 16–19, 1983, pp 154.
48. Hollis DP, Economou JS, Parks LC, Eggleston JC, Saryan LA, Czeisler JL: Nuclear magnetic resonance studies of several experimental and human malignant tumors. Cancer Res *33*:2156–2160, 1973.
49. Hricak H, Williams RD, Moon KL Jr, Moss AA, Alpers C, Crooks LE, Kaufman L: Nuclear magnetic resonance imaging of the kidney: Renal masses. Radiology *147*:765–772, 1983.
50. Huggert A, Odeblad E: Proton magnetic resonance studies of some tissues and fluids of the eye. Acta Radiol *51*:385–392, 1958.
51. Inch MR, McCredie JA, Knispel RR, Thompson RT, Pintar MM: Water content and proton spin relaxation time for neoplastic and non-neoplastic tissues from mice and humans. JNCI *52*:353–356, 1974.
52. Kasturi SR, Ranade SS, Shah SS: Tissue hydration of malignant and uninvolved human tissues and its relevance to proton spin-lattice relaxation mechanism. Proc Indian Acad Sci *84B*:60–74, 1976.
53. Kiricuta IC Jr, Simplaceanu V: Tissue water content and nuclear magnetic resonance in normal and tumor tissues. Cancer Res *35*:1164–1167, 1975.
54. Kiricuta IC, Simplaceanu V, Demco D: N.M.R. study on tumor tissue water. *In* Allen PS, Andrew ER, Bates CA (eds): Proceedings of the 18th Ampere Congress, Nottingham. Vol. 1. Amsterdam, North-Holland, 1975, pp 287–288.
55. Knispel RR, Thompson RT, Pintar MM: Dispersion of proton spin-lattice relaxation in tissues. J Magn Reson *14*:44–51, 1974.
56. Koenig SH, Brown RD III, Adams D, Emerson D, Harrison CG: Magnetic field dependence of $1/T1$ of protons in tissue. IBM Research Report RC 10116 (#44807). Yorktown Heights, New York, IBM, Thomas J. Watson Research Center, 1983.
57. Koutcher JA, Goldsmith M, Damadian R: NMR in cancer. X. A malignancy index to discriminate normal and cancerous tissue. Cancer *41*:174–182, 1978.
58. Lewa J, Majewska Z: Temperature relationships of proton spin-lattice relaxation time *T1* in biological tissues. Bull du Cancer *67*:525–530, 1980.
59. Lewa CJ, Zbytniewski Z: Magnetic transverse relaxation time of the protons in transplantable melanotic and amelanotic melanoma and in some inner organs of golden hamster *Mesocricetus auratus,* Waterhouse. Bull du Cancer *63*:69–72, 1976.
60. Mallard J, Hutchison JMS, Edelstein W, Ling R, Foster M: Imaging by nuclear magnetic resonance and its bio-medical implications. J Biomed Eng *1*:153–158, 1979.
61. Mano I, Levy RM, Crooks LE, Hosobuchi Y: Proton nuclear magnetic resonance imaging of acute experimental cerebral ischemia. Invest Radiol *17*:345–351, 1983.
62. Mansfield P, Morris PG: NMR Imaging in Biomedicine. New York, Academic Press, 1982, pp 10–32.
63. Medina D, Hazlewood CF, Cleveland GG, Chang DC, Spjut HJ, Moyers R: Nuclear magnetic resonance studies on human breast dysplasias and neoplasms. JNCI *54*:813–818, 1975.
64. Misra LK, Narayana PA, Beall PT, Amtey SR, Hazlewood CF: Developmental changes in *T1* relaxation times of muscle water protons in muscular dystrophy. Proceedings of the 2nd Annual Meeting of the Society for Magnetic Resonance in Medicine, August, 16–19, 1983, pp 236–237.
65. Moon KL, Genant HK, Helms CA, Chafetz NI, Crooks LE, Kaufman L: Musculoskeletal applications of nuclear magnetic resonance. Radiology *147*:161–171, 1983.
66. Moon KL, Mosley M, Young G, Hricak H: NMR relaxation characteristics of fasting and non-fasting bile in canines. Proceedings of the 2nd Annual Meeting of the Society for Magnetic Resonance in Medicine, August 16–19, 1983, pp 245–246.

67. Odeblad E: Studies on vaginal contents and cells with proton magnetic resonance. Ann NY Acad Sci *82*:189–206, 1959.
68. Odeblad E, Bahr BN, Lindstrom G: Proton magnetic resonance of human red blood cells in heavy-water exchange experiments. Arch Biochem Biophys *63*:221–225, 1956.
69. Odeblad E, Bryhn U: Proton magnetic resonance of human cervical mucus during the menstrual cycle. Acta Radiol *47*:315–320, 1957.
70. Odeblad E, Linstrom G: Some preliminary observations on the proton magnetic resonance in biologic samples. Acta Radiol *43*:469–476, 1955.
71. Odeblad E, Westin B: Proton magnetic resonance of human milk. Acta Radiol *49*:389–392, 1958.
72. Parrish RG, Kurland RJ, Janese WW, Bakay L: Proton relaxation rates of water in brain and brain tumors. Science *183*:438–439, 1974.
73. Pearson RT, Duff ID, Derbyshire W, Blanshard JMV: An NMR investigation of rigor in porcine muscle. Biochim Biophys Acta *362*:188–200, 1974.
74. Peemoeller H, Pintar MM, Kydon DW: Nuclear magnetic resonance analysis of water in natural and deuterated mouse muscle above and below freezing. Biophys J *29*:427–435, 1980.
75. Rupp N, Reiser M, Stetter E: The diagnostic value of morphology and relaxation times in NMR-imaging of the body. Eur J Radiol *3*:68–76, 1983.
76. Rustgi SN, Peemoeller H, Thompson RT, Kydon DW, Pintar MM: A study of molecular dynamics and freezing phase transition in tissues by proton spin relaxation. Biophys J *22*:439–452, 1978.
77. Sandhu HS, Friedmann GB: Proton spin-lattice relaxation time study in tissues of the adult newt *Taricha granulosa* (Amphibia: Urodele). Med Phys *5*:514–517, 1978.
78. Saryan LA, Hollis DP, Economou JS, Eggleston JC: Brief communication: Nuclear magnetic resonance studies of cancer. IV. correlation of water content with tissue relaxation times. JNCI *52*:599–602, 1974.
79. Small WC, McSweeney MB, Goldstein JH, Sewell CW, Powell RW: Handling of in vitro human breast tissue samples: Protocol requirements for accurate NMR relaxation measurements. Biochem Biophys Res Comm *112*:991–999, 1983.
80. Smith FW: The value of NMR imaging in pediatric practice: A preliminary report. Pediatr Radiol *13*:141–147, 1983.
81. Smith FW, Mallard JR, Reid A, Hutchison JMS: Nuclear magnetic resonance tomographic imaging in liver disease. Lancet *i*:963–966, 1981.
82. Smith FW, Reid A, Hutchison JMS, Mallard JR, Path FRC: Nuclear magnetic resonance imaging of the pancreas. Radiology *142*:677–680, 1982.
83. Smith FW, Reid A, Mallard JR, Hutchison MS, Power DA, Catto GRD: Nuclear magnetic resonance tomographic imaging in renal disease. Diagn Imag *51*:209–213, 1982.
84. Stark DD, Bass NM, Moss AA, Bacon BR, McKerrow JH, Cann CE, Brito A, Goldberg HI: Nuclear magnetic resonance imaging of experimentally induced liver disease. Radiology *148*:743–751, 1983.
85. Stejskal EO, Tanner JE: Spin diffusion measurements: Spin echoes in the presence of a time dependent field gradient. J Chem Phys *42*:288, 1965.
86. Thickman DI, Kundel HL, Wolf G: Nuclear magnetic resonance characteristics of fresh and fixed tissue: The effect of elapsed time, Radiology *148*:183–185, 1983.
87. Wesby G, Goldberg HI, Mayo J, Moon K, Stark D, Moss A: In-vivo proton NMR imaging characterization of the normal human liver and spleen. Proceedings of the 2nd Annual Meeting of the Society for Magnetic Resonance in Medicine, August, 16–19, 1983, pp 373–374.
88. Woessner DE: Spin relaxation processes in a two-proton system undergoing anisotropic reorientation. J Chem Phys *36*:1–4, 1962.

67

Biomedical Implications of Relaxation Times of Tissue Water

R. MATHUR-DE VRÉ

In recent years extensive clinical trials of nuclear magnetic resonance (NMR) imaging and rapid progress in instrumentation have revealed a very vast potential for the medical applications of magnetic resonance (MR); at the same time they have revealed a number of deep-rooted problems in obtaining consistent results and in interpreting the data in general. The complexity of MR applications in medical diagnosis and biomedical research stems from the fact that NMR parameters depend on a number of intricately related inherent biological factors and extrinsic physical conditions as well as on instrumental parameters. This chapter analyzes the biophysical aspects of relaxation times of tissue water that are important for assessing their biomedical implications.

BIOPHYSICAL ASPECTS OF MR APPLICATIONS IN MEDICINE

Biophysical concepts provide the essential link between physical parameters characterizing the imaging and spectroscopic results and the various pathophysiological processes. Therefore, an understanding of the biophysical basis of relaxation times of water protons is essential for (i) effectively evaluating the clinical applications of NMR and (ii) providing insight into many practical problems associated with tissue discrimination.

A full understanding of the biophysical basis of the relaxation behavior of water in biological systems requires a knowledge of (1) the state of water in biological systems and the factors that affect it; (2) the physical basis of relaxation times and the time scale of various relaxation processes; (3) the impact of modified water structure on relaxation mechanisms, underlining a link between (1) and (2); (4) different biological and physical factors that affect $T1$ and $T2;$ and finally, (5) the implications of the multiparameter dependence of relaxation times.

The State of Water in Biological Systems

Most biological systems comprise 70 to 90 percent water distributed as intracellular (ICW) and extracellular water (ECW). In general, the total water content as well as the fraction of extracellular water for the newborn is higher than for adults. The decrease in the water content of skeletal muscle with maturation has been attributed to an increase in cellular macromolecules at the expense of tissue water.[1]

The special characteristics of intracellular water that influence the relaxation times of water protons are largely due to specific interactions of H_2O molecules with various charged and polar groups of biological macromolecules. These interactions result in a dynamically oriented structure of water near the surface of macromolecules (hydration water) and constitute an integral part of macromolecular structure. It has been indicated that "order" extends over 1 to 3 molecular dimensions.[2,3] Hydration water plays a crucial role in maintaining the structural and conformational integrity of all biostructures and represents a substantial part of intracellular water. The behavior of water near hydrophobic groups and microtubule[4] organization can also influence the mobility of intracellular water. Most biological processes are closely associated with the structural organization of water at the whole organ, cellular, and subcellular levels.

The state of water near the surface of biological macromolecules comprises (a) a primary hydration layer, or internal water, found inside the macromolecular structure (e.g., associated with charged groups); (b) a secondary hydration layer; and (c) unperturbed water. In fact, bound water refers only to the primary or internal water, whereas the more general term "hydration water" implies both the primary and the secondary hydration layers. The degree of hydration is related to the availability of the surface of biopolymers to H_2O molecules in the medium.

From the preceding discussion it follows that a fraction of biological water exhibits properties different from free water. In general, the dynamic structure within the hydration layer depends on the local structure and configuration of macromolecules. Some characteristic properties of hydration water that are important from the point of view of NMR measurements are the following:

1. Restricted motion involving translation and rotation of water molecules; e.g., τ_c, the average time between molecule collisions (correlation time), varies between 10^{-6} and 10^{-9} s in the hydration layer and has a value of $\sim 10^{-12}$ s for free water.

2. Partial orientation of H_2O molecules with respect to macromolecular chains.

3. Multiple motional frequencies and distribution of τ_c.

4. Anisotropic diffusion and enhanced proton transfer along the hydration layer.

5. Anisotropic rotational and decoupling of translational and rotational motions of H_2O molecules due to macromolecular-water interactions.

6. Differential interaction potential along the charged macromolecular chains.

These characteristics of water, which are influenced by macromolecules, can be affected by many diseases, natural processes, and radiation and chemical therapy.

Tissue Heterogeneity

The behavior of water in biological tissues is characterized by a heterogeneity in space and time that is the basis for MR imaging detection of many disorders and abnormal states of tissues localized in different organs.

Tissue Heterogeneity in Space

Biological water represents a very heterogeneous system at both the microscopic and the macroscopic levels. Individual soft tissues have a unique protein water composition, giving rise to local differences in the state of water at the microscopic level. The inhomogeneous distribution of water content and different metabolic processes further contribute to macroscopic heterogeneity. Space heterogeneity manifests as either localized or systemic effects.

Tissue Heterogeneity in Time

In living systems the continuous evolution of many natural processes, such as metabolic activity, biosynthesis, cell degradation and cell proliferation, maturation of tissues (resulting in age dependence of relaxation times), different phases of cell cycle, and different doubling times for cell population, contributes to tissue heterogeneity in time. The progressive development of pathological conditions and lesions as well as inflammatory processes produces variations in the state of water in the affected regions.

The development of heterogeneity in space and time during natural processes (such as biorhythm, growth, and aging), nutrition, intoxication, stress and strain, and finally the evolution of some pathological conditions result in systemic effects on $T1$ and $T2$.

The Physical Basis of Relaxation Times T1 and T2

NMR relaxation is induced by interactions of nuclei with small fluctuating fields arising from the dynamic structure of neighboring atoms and groups and the surrounding lattice. In the domain of medical applications of NMR, the relaxation times $T1$ and $T2$ are of fundamental importance for two reasons. In all pulsed NMR techniques (spectroscopic as well as imaging), relaxation times impose severe constraints on instrumental parameters, and the relaxation times of tissues are sensitive to the dynamic structure and amount of water in biological systems, thereby making them valuable index parameters for studying the state of tissues. The fundamental role of relaxation phenomena in studying the molecular motion (dynamic state of water) is directly related to the low frequency range characteristic of this technique. The two relaxation times are similar from the mechanistic point of view but differ in their physical significance.

The $T1$ and $T2$ values of water are shortened in the presence of a very low concentration (mM) of paramagnetic materials (discussed elsewhere in this book). Two types of paramagnetic effects on $T1$ and $T2$ of tissue water are significant for biomedical applications: (1) the effects arising from differences in metal ion concentrations intrinsically present in normal and pathological tissues, and (2) the selective relaxation enhancement induced in certain cases by exogenous substances given to living systems and by the presence of paramagnetic O_2 in blood. This is used to enhance the image contrast for differentiating certain pathological features more clearly.

Impact of the Modified Structure of Water on Relaxation Times

The dynamic, heterogeneous, and partially oriented structure of water near the surface of biological macromolecules results in local time-dependent fluctuating magnetic fields. The impact of these field fluctuations on the relaxation mechanisms causes $T1$ and $T2$ to encode details about intrinsic molecular states and the dynamic structure of tissue water and renders them very useful index parameters for discriminating among tissue types.

The effects of special properties of hydration water molecules on $T1$ and $T2$ are averaged over all other compartments in the system by means of exchange, diffusion, and proton transfer. Many details about the intrinsic state of tissue water at the microscopic and molecular levels can be interpolated from in-vitro measurements of $T1$ and $T2$ under different experimental conditions (e.g., by varying temperature, frequency, hydration) and by using appropriate methods of data analysis.

The observed $T1$ rate is given by the following relation:

$$(1/T1)_{ob} = (1/T1)_f X_f + \sum_i (1/T1)_b X_b \tag{1}$$

where $(1/T1)_f$ and $(1/T1)_b$ are the relaxation rates of free and different fractions of bound water, respectively, and X_f and X_b are their corresponding fractions.

The *T1* relaxation is essentially dependent on the fast components of molecular motion (such as rotational motion of H_2O molecules) and is related to total water content and its distribution in different compartments. As a result, *T1* depends on the biological processes involving a change in the total amount of water and its distribution. The correlation time (τ_c) of water molecules influences the rate of fluctuations of local magnetic fields and thereby affects *T1*. The variations in *T2* times are largely due to low frequency components of molecular motion such as those arising from molecular diffusion and exchange, which are modified near the surface of macromolecules. *T2* is a sensitive monitor of water binding as well as of the structure and conformation of hydrated biopolymers. The measurements of *T1* and *T2* provide invaluable complementary information about the molecular state and the dynamic structure of tissue water.

Factors Affecting the Relaxation Times

Various factors that influence *T1* and *T2* are illustrated in Figure 67–1.

THE INHERENT BIOLOGICAL FACTORS

The relaxation times of tissue water are influenced by a delicate balance of the following three factors, collectively termed "water balance": (i) the total water content, (ii) macroscopic and microscopic distribution of water in different sites, and (iii) macromolecular-water interactions. Different tissue types have a characteristic water balance, and disease conditions can alter the state of water in cells and tissues by varying one or all of the aspects mentioned above.

The state of water balance in cells and tissues is perturbed readily but nonselectively by many essential biological processes. This gives rise to a very high sensitivity of NMR for discriminating soft tissues and detecting abnormal states (lesions, tumors) that are associated with a change in the state of water. However, similar effects induced

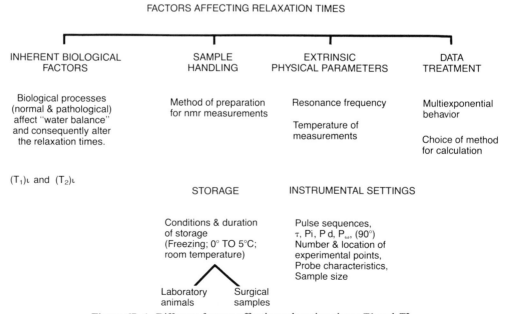

FACTORS AFFECTING RELAXATION TIMES

INHERENT BIOLOGICAL FACTORS	SAMPLE HANDLING	EXTRINSIC PHYSICAL PARAMETERS	DATA TREATMENT
Biological processes (normal & pathological) affect "water balance" and consequently alter the relaxation times.	Method of preparation for nmr measurements	Resonance frequency Temperature of measurements	Multiexponential behavior Choice of method for calculation
$(T_1)\iota$ and $(T_2)\iota$	STORAGE	INSTRUMENTAL SETTINGS	
	Conditions & duration of storage (Freezing; 0° TO 5°C; room temperature)	Pulse sequences, τ, Pi, P d, P_ω, (90°) Number & location of experimental points, Probe characteristics, Sample size	
	Laboratory animals Surgical samples		

Figure 67–1. Different factors affecting relaxation times *T1* and *T2*.

by a number of natural, pathological, and physiological processes on the state of water result in a lack of specificity for unequivocal identification of abnormal states by means of *T1* and *T2* values of tissue water.

The biological processes involving a change in the physiological pH and ionic fluctuations can result in variations in *T1* and *T2* values. The relaxation times of cell water were shown to depend on different phases of cell cycle for synchronized cells and on cell growth.[5] Furthermore, the fast growing tissues (regenerating liver, tumors, fetus) generally exhibit longer relaxation times.

The *T1* and *T2* values of biological tissues from in-vivo and in-vitro studies have been compiled extensively by several authors.[6-8] The following general conclusions are drawn from an analysis of these results.

Normal Tissues. The *T1* and *T2* values for each tissue type fall within a distinct range. Furthermore, the frequency dependence of *T1* of the same organ tissue from different species are also very similar.[9] This similarity is invaluable for extrapolating results from experiments on animals to human cases and for tissue identification. The well-defined range of relaxation times of normal organ tissue from different species could be associated with unique macromolecular-water relationships and similarities in intracellular (nuclear) water embodying the functional role of water in each organ. Nevertheless, the significant spread of values over a distinct range for each tissue type can be attributed to the fact that the water balance of normal tissues is sensitive to the combined effects of (i) biological processes (age and maturation, rate of cell growth, metabolism, phases of cell cycle) and (ii) environmental conditions (food and water regimen, intake of exogenous products such as certain drugs and alcoholic beverages, ambient temperatures, climatic conditions, stress and strain, physical rest).

Pathological Tissues. In many cases of cancer tissues, relaxation times are enhanced and scattered over a very wide range. Several other disease states, such as hepatitis, liver infarction, and some forms of cirrhosis, are associated as well with prolonged *T1* values. The pathological conditions accompanied by increased tissue fluids, such as pneumonia and inflammation, also give longer relaxation times. The values from normal and pathological tissues overlap in many cases, however; and the variations in *T1* and *T2* values for the same tissue from different healthy individuals of a species may be more important than the differences between normal and pathological tissues.

Two important questions have received significant attention.

1. What is the biophysical basis of differences in relaxation times between normal and pathological tissues, particularly between normal and cancerous cells and tumors?

2. What are the causes of the very broad range of *T1* and *T2* values for tumors?

It is generally considered that the increase in *T1* and *T2* values for water protons in certain pathological tissues with respect to the normal state is due to the following:

1. An increase in the total water content.

2. An increase in the ratio of free to bound water.

3. A change in the dynamic structure of water near macromolecules, the structure of intracellular water, and ion concentration (Na^+, K^+, Ca^{2+}).

4. A change in the concentration of paramagnetic ions in certain cases.

A concerted effect of factors (1) to (3) contributes to the relaxation mechanism rather than the discrete action of each individual term. A change in the ratio of different water fractions affects *T1* and *T2* because the relaxation rates are determined by weighted average over different water compartments. The variations in total water content can entail important changes in the free/bound water fraction and macromolecular-water interactions. A loss of structure in cellular water may be accompanied by a simultaneous increase in free water, causing elevated *T1* values. It is likely that changes in the amount of bound water of tumors are associated with changes in macromolecular structure. Diseases in which there is an excessive accumulation of iron and copper in the liver generally give shorter *T1* values. Some forms of cirrhosis are associated with copper buildup in the liver, and in this case the *T1* values decrease.[10] It is becoming increasingly apparent that relaxation times are not only a function of the total water content but that other factors specific to each tissue type also exert a marked influence.

In MR imaging, large variations in *T1* are often observed for tissues exhibiting small changes in water content. This fact can be attributed to large values of relaxation rates $(1/T1)_h$ characteristic of hydration water and important changes in the relative fractions of bound/free and intra- /extracellular water. Changes in the water content have very little effect on *T2* values.

Intrinsic heterogeneity and extrinsic heterogeneity are responsible for very broad range of *T1* and *T2* values for different types of tumors. Intrinsic heterogeneity refers to the fact that tumors contain different amounts of cancer cells and differ in their development stage and growth rate. The specificity of *T1* and *T2* values for categories of tumors and for different stages of tumor development would cause significant variations in their inherent values. Extrinsic heterogeneity refers to the fact that surgically removed samples often contain a considerable amount of fat and adjacent unaffected tissues, introducing experimental uncertainties into the accurate measurements of *T1* and *T2* for an inhomogeneous mass of tissues.

EXTRINSIC PHYSICAL CONDITIONS

Two sets of experimental parameters influence the measurements of relaxation times: (i) those arising from nonideality of experimental and instrumental conditions (sample handling, sample size, pulse characteristics, radio frequency (rf) coil design, etc.) and (ii) those related to inherent structure of cell/tissue water by basic biophysical relationship (temperature of measurements, resonance frequency). Various factors are shown in Figure 67-1.

Sample Handling

Sample handling and storage conditions influence the in-vitro NMR measurements because all biological tissues undergo progressive degeneration following instantaneous changes induced by death and excision of tissues. In view of the limitations imposed by working conditions and priorities for patient care in the case of surgical samples, attention should be paid to certain inevitable differences in handling processes for laboratory animals and surgical samples.

Temperature Dependence The choice and control of temperature at which measurements are performed are very important considerations for tissue discrimination in vitro. The temperature dependence of *T1* and *T2* of biological tissues arises from two important effects: (i) degeneration of tissues in vitro at high temperatures and (ii) thermal control of relaxation mechanisms such as τ_c, rotational motion, diffusion, proton transfer, and exchange. An important dilemma arises in the choice of optimum conditions for measurements in vitro. Owing to sample degeneration at high temperatures, the relative comparison of small variations in *T1* and *T2* for different tissue types in vitro (or the same tissue undergoing evolution) is more meaningful at low temperatures (e.g., 0° to 10° C), whereas the values at about 37° C are required for comparison with results from in-vivo studies of magnetic resonance imaging.

Instrumental Parameters The observed relaxation times of tissue water (in vivo and in vitro) and the image patterns depend upon two types of instrumental conditions: (i) the instrumental characteristics such as field strength and rf coil design, and (ii) variable instrumental settings (data acquisition conditions) such as pulse timings, pulse sequences, 90 degree pulse length, and number of data points and their location (in the case of multiexponential behavior). Important differences in the characteristics of equipment in different laboratories and variations in the performance of a machine require frequent calibration with suitable standard materials and test objects.

Instrumental Characteristics. The relaxation times of macromolecular solutions and of tissue water depend on the resonance frequency.[6] Generally, $T1$ of tissue water is more sensitive than $T2$. Frequency dependence of relaxation times arises from the relaxation rates of water molecules in the primary hydration layer of macromolecules.

The earlier detailed studies of the $T1$–frequency relationship were very useful for revealing the heterogeneous nature of tissue water and for proposing different models describing the state of water. However, in the domain of medical applications and biomedical research, the frequency dependence of $T1$ causes serious experimental problems. The $T1$ changes are more significant in the low frequency range (1 to 40 MHz), which coincides with the most sensitive range for biomedical applications of NMR. In most cases $T1$ discrimination is improved at low frequencies, and the in-vivo whole body imaging studies are usually performed in the range of 1.7 to 20 MHz. The choice of a suitable frequency for optimum contrast between relaxation times of normal and pathological tissues depends on the frequency-dependent behavior of (a) relaxation rates of each type of tissue and (b) the S/N ratio, which is a very important consideration for imaging of patients.

The sample size (sample height) relative to the rf coil also influences the $T1$ and $T2$ values measured in vitro by spectroscopic techniques; this depends on the inhomogeneity of the rf field over the sample volume and is related to probe characteristics.

Variable Instrumental Settings. The optimum conditions of pulse settings need to be determined in each case to obtain reproducible and consistent results in vitro, and to seek the best combination of signal-to-noise (S/N) ratio, contrast and spatial resolution for a given exposure time, and other conditions in imaging in vivo.

Data Analysis and Nonexponential Behavior

The calculation of significant values of relaxation times of water in biological systems is confronted with two major problems. In most cases the magnetization curves are multiexponential, but for simplicity the data is treated so as to calculate single average values; and the calculation of the average $T1$ and $T2$ values depends on the method of data analysis,[11,12] such as linear regression, nonlinear (e.g., exponential) regression, and successive iterations.

The nonexponentiality of the magnetization decay/growth curves arises from (i) local tissue heterogeneity and (ii) nonaveraging of the local field fluctuations and diffusion barrier. Furthermore, nonexponential behavior imposes a careful control of pulse parameters for discriminating tissues with largely different relaxation times.

Implications of the Multiparameter Dependence of Relaxation Times

Two important and unique features of the NMR technique in relation to its medical application are the possibility of using three distinct but interrelated variables (proton density I, $T1$ and $T2$) and the multiparameter dependence of relaxation times. The signal intensity is directly related to the proton density and the total water content in tissues, but it is also affected by certain relaxation processes; whereas $T1$ and $T2$ reflect the dynamic structure of water, $T1$ is also influenced by the total water content. The diffusion constant (related to spin spin relaxation time) is also a useful discriminating parameter important for biomedical applications of NMR.

The relaxation times of tissue water used for identification of biological tissues in vitro and in vivo depend on a number of inherent biological conditions, biophysical factors, and extrinsic instrumental parameters. Therefore great care is needed in interpreting the biomedical implications of $T1$ and $T2$.

The multiparameter relation of NMR terms makes this technique very versatile. Certain features are detected more easily either by *T1* or *T2* or proton density images. However, this flexibility often introduces ambiguity in the interpretation of results and gives rise to many practical problems requiring optimization, standardization, and control of instrumental and physical conditions for measurements. Nevertheless, magnetic resonance can provide detailed pathophysiological information generally nonaccessible by other techniques applicable to living systems. The experimental protocols suitable for in-vitro measurements have been proposed recently.[13,14]

Proton density changes are small within most soft tissues, but important differences are revealed among bones, tissues, and fluids. Therefore proton density images can provide useful details about anatomical features of certain organs. However, in many cases, relaxation times are more useful imaging parameters for high tissue contrast and for discriminating normal from pathological tissues. Individually *T1* and *T2* lack specificity for unequivocal identification of the abnormal state; nevertheless, some methods combining *T1*, *T2*, and proton density information could give much improved specificity.

RELEVANCE OF IN-VITRO MEASUREMENTS TO IN-VIVO STUDIES

In-vitro measurements have relevance to in-vivo studies in two ways: (i) in facilitating basic biophysical studies for understanding the origin of NMR properties in relation to tissue structure and establishing correlations between pathological conditions and NMR parameters and (ii) in allowing determination of the effects of instrumental factors on in-vivo measurements and tissue heterogeneities that are exclusive features of NMR imaging. Important differences mark the NMR studies of biological tissues in vitro and in vivo.

Experimental Conditions

Instrumental characteristics and variable parameters are significantly different for imaging and spectroscopic methods. For example, imaging employs field gradients and long 90 degree pulses (~ms), low resonance frequency, and a limited number of acquisitions. On the other hand, in-vitro measurements by spectroscopic techniques are performed by using a uniform magnetic field and much shorter 90 degree pulses (~μs) and a large number of τ values. Most of the available relaxation time values have been measured at much higher frequencies[6] than those employed for imaging. The most suitable approach is to determine the in-vitro data with imaging equipment. A knowledge of the predetermined range of relaxation times in vitro and full scale M_t vs. τ curves for different types of tissues can be very helpful in correctly setting the pulse parameters for selective discrimination of tissues exhibiting largely different *T1* and *T2* values.

The difference in temperature during measurements of tissues in vitro and in vivo (~37° C) is a serious setback for direct comparison of results.

Differences in Basic Structure and Properties of Water

In any living system, each tissue type is characterized by a unique dynamic structure of water, and water balance is controlled by specific metabolic and other continuously evolving biological processes in each organ tissue. On the other hand, in the case of inanimate biological tissues in vitro the characteristic water balance is perturbed by nonspecific degeneration processes, and they are discriminated by the state and degree of hydration and macromolecular-water interactions. The NMR parameters from in-vivo studies are likely to be more tissue specific, but in practice in-vitro measurements provide more reliable values of *T1* and *T2* under controlled and preselected physical and instrumental conditions. Furthermore, at low fields employed for whole body imaging the signals from water and fat protons are not resolved, whereas in many cases the in-vitro *T1* and *T2* values are determined for the water protons signal.

In general, the relaxation times of an organ tissue from live animals are higher than for the corresponding excised tissues.[15] In spite of this difference between relaxation times of tissues in different biological states, similar trends in variations in *T1* and *T2* values in response to biological effects have been observed in each case. It is likely that the hydration characteristics of cellular biopolymers in live and inanimate tissues remain closely similar, but the amount and distribution of water content differ, resulting in important differences in the dynamic structure of water in these two states. Alterations in the lymphatic system and blood supply of tissues (normal/tumors, live/inanimate) are some of the possible causes of differences in the dynamic state of water in various tissues.

Technological progress in recent years has provided the means for obtaining high quality images and for varying the tissue contrast by carefully controlling the instrumental conditions. However, the biomedical significance of imaging and spectroscopic results are not fully recognized owing to insufficient knowledge of the underlying biophysical aspects. There is an increasing need to optimize and standardize the experimental parameters in order to obtain consistent and meaningful results for experimental studies and clinical applications of magnetic resonance.

An important biomedical aspect of NMR is that the technique is very sensitive for detecting abnormal conditions and pathological states associated with a change in the state of water, but it is nonspecific for the identification of different cases. The impact of a number of extrinsic physical conditions, variable instrumental parameters, and data analysis methods on the observed values of relaxation times must be clearly defined in order to underline the biomedical significance of *T1* and *T2*. The observed values of *T1* and *T2* are not an intrinsic property but exhibit a representative range for a given type of tissue.

ACKNOWLEDGMENTS

The author is grateful to Prof. J. Reisse (University of Brussels) and Dr. C. Segebarth (Erasme Hospital) for reading the manuscript and giving many critical comments. I also wish to acknowledge the help and encouragement of Dr. P. Lejeune.

References

1. Hazlewood CF: A role for interfacial water in the exclusion of intracellular sodium. Colloque Internationaux du C.N.R.S. N246, "L'eau et les systèmes biologiques." 289–296, 1975.
2. Derbyshire W: Dynamics of water in cellular systems. *In* Franks F, Mathias S (eds): Biophysics of Water. New York, John Wiley & Sons, 1983, pp 249–253.
3. Berendsen HJC: Specific interactions of water with biopolymers. *In* Franks F (ed): Water. A Comprehensive Treatise. Vol. 5. New York, Plenum Press, 1975, pp 293–439.
4. Beall PT, Brinkley BR, Chang DC, Hazlewood CF: Microtubule complexes correlated with growth rate and water proton relaxation times in human breast cancer cells. Cancer Res 42:4124–4130, 1982.
5. Beall PT, Hazlewood CF, Rao PN: NMR pattern of intracellular water as a function of HeLa cell cycle. Science *192*:904–907, 1976.
6. Bottomley PA, Foster TH, Argersinger RE, Pfeifer LM: A review of normal tissue hydrogen NMR

relaxation times and relaxation mechanisms from 1-100 MHz: Dependence of tissue type, NMR frequency, temperature, species, excision and age. Medical Physics *4*:425–445, 1984.

7. Mathur-De Vré R: Biomedical implications of the relaxation behaviour of water related to NMR imaging. Br J Radiol *57*:955–976, 1984.

8. Hazlewood CF: A view of the significance of the physical properties of cell-associated water. *In* Clegg J, Drost-Hansen W (eds): Cell Associated Water. New York, Academic Press, 1979, pp 165–259.

9. Koenig SH, Brown RD, Adams D, Emerson D, Harrison CG: Magnetic field dependence of 1/*T1* of protons in tissue. Invest Radiol *19*:76–81, 1984.

10. Doyle FH, Pennock JM, Banks LM, McDonnell MJ, Bydder GM, Steiner RE, Young IR, Clarke GJ, Pasmore T, Gilderdale DJ: Nuclear magnetic resonance imaging of the liver: Initial experience. AJR *138*:193–200, 1982.

11. Riesse J, Wilputte L, Zimmerman D: *T1* measurements and calibration in relation with the so-called *T1* images. *In* Orr JS, Podo F (eds): Proceedings of EEC Workshop on Identification and Characterization of Biological Tissues by NMR. Rome, May 18–20, 1983. Annali dell'Istituto Superiore di Sanità *19*:51–56, 1983.

12. Wehrli FW: Systematic errors in spin-lattice relaxation and nuclear overhauser experiments. Varian Application Note No. NMR-77-2, September, 1977.

13. Beall PT, Amtey SR, Kasturi SR: NMR Data Handbook for Biomedical Applications. New York, Pergamon Press, 1984.

14. Workshop on: Standardization of methodologies for in-vitro studies by NMR, December 11–12, 1984, Brussels (Organiser: R. Mathur-De Vré). EEC Concerted Research Project: Identification and Characterization of Biological Tissues by NMR, II. A protocol for in-vivo proton relaxation studies. Magn Reson *6*:2, 1988.

15. Gore GC, Doyle FH, Pennock JM: Relaxation rate enhancement observed in-vivo by NMR imaging. *In* Partain CL, James AE, Rollo FD, Price RR (eds): Nuclear Magnetic Resonance Imaging. Philadelphia, W. B. Saunders Co., 1983, pp 94–106.

68

Histopathological Correlation

S. S. RANADE

Since 1974, over 1500 samples have been studied using pulsed nuclear magnetic resonance (NMR). These studies were performed on biological tissue samples composed of normal and cancerous tissues from experimental animals or human cancer patients. Subsequent to 1978, the emphasis of these investigations has been on ascertaining the cause underlying the relaxation time (*T1* values). Histopathological study of uninvolved regions of esophageal cancer have demonstrated that areas intermediate between normal and neoplastic tissues, which show a mixed cell population, demonstrated *T1* values intermediate between normal and tumor tissue. This observation[40] was confirmed in uninvolved regions of colon and rectum and has been investigated in uninvolved regions of other body sites.

Studies were also carried out on isolated nuclei. Pellets of cell nuclei isolated from normal and tumor tissues showed that *T1* values of nuclei were higher than *T1* values of tissue of origin. Further, the tumor nuclei showed the highest of the *T1* values. Comparison of *T1* values of nuclear fractions from livers of tumor-bearing animals (Swiss mice) showed higher *T1* values than liver nuclear fractions. A hierarchy of increasing *T1* values was evident in the following order: nuclear fractions from normal liver to liver from tumor-bearing animals to the active tumors themselves.

For the past few years studies have been geared to malignant lymphoma and esophagus. In malignant lymphomas the *T1* values obtained in Hodgkin's lymphomas are lower than those obtained in non-Hodgkin's lymphomas. This has been ascribed to the difference in the proportion of normal and malignant cells. While the Hodgkin's lymphomas have a smaller proportion of malignant cells, the non-Hodgkin's lymphomas are characterized by predominantly malignant cell populations.

A further relationship became apparent in *T1* of non-Hodgkin's lymphomas. The diffuse non-Hodgkin's lymphomas, which have a poor prognosis, were found to show low *T1* values compared with nodular non-Hodgkin's lymphoma, which showed relatively higher *T1* values and better prognosis. These results implicate cell type as an influential factor in relaxation time.

A series of histological features that characterize the regions in normal to tumor zones have been taken into account in an effort to ascertain their influence on the relaxation time of the areas, especially in gastrointestinal regions. The studies presented here were carried out on esophageal regions; areas with dysplasia have been found to singularly influence the relaxation time of the zones where they are encountered.

PULSED NMR AND HISTOPATHOLOGICAL STUDIES ON HUMAN SUBJECTS

Biopsy samples of the involved and uninvolved regions of human tissues were selected from surgically resected material in connection with different types of cancers.

These include carcinoma of the esophagus, colon, rectum, and other regions. The control samples in the present studies have been taken from areas that appeared normal on gross examination and were away from the tumor and have been designated as "uninvolved" in all these studies. In the NMR technique the sample biopsies, about 1 cm in diameter, are placed in a glass test tube (12 mm diameter), which is placed in the probe coil located in the center of the magnet. The magnetic field is fitted to the resonant radio frequency (rf) of the element in the sample one wishes to detect. We were interested in the protons of biological tissue water. The rf signal is applied as a pulse to the sample, and the signal is re-emitted by the atoms of the sample as a signal with its own amplitude and a characteristic frequency. The re-emitted signal is monitored on an oscilloscope screen. The signal falls off exponentially on a logarithmic scale, and the rate at which it falls to zero can be expressed as a rate of decay constant. One of these rate constants is called the spin-lattice relaxation time (*T1*) because of the fact that energy applied as rf is taken up by spins of the atomic nucleus under investigation and then dissipated to the surroundings, i.e., the lattice. The exchange of energy between the spin and the lattice is characterized by the spin-lattice relaxation time studies and is conventionally referred to as *T1* values. In the present studies *T1* measurements were made on a home-made pulsed NMR spectrometer. All *T1* measurements were made at 25.3 MHz, and the details have been published in an earlier paper.[11]

In the present work, the progressive saturation recovery method was employed. A boxcar signal averager (Model 162, Princeton Applied Research Corporation, USA) was used for processing the signal. The *T1* values were obtained by doing the least squares fit of the data. The error in *T1* measurements is about 7 percent based on reproducibility, taking into account the temperature variation and instrument instability, while in single measurements the error is always less than 5 percent. The free induction decay signal monitored in this investigation was entirely due to the water protons alone on account of the long recovery time of the receiver and the positioning of the boxcar gate. The spin-lattice relaxation times have been obtained by fitting the data to a single relaxation function. In each case the correlation coefficient is 99.9 percent or better.

Histopathology of Uninvolved Regions of Esophagus, Colon, and Rectum

The data on *T1* values obtained on cancers from various sites have been presented in the form of a *T1* histogram in Figure 68–1. It becomes apparent that the mean *T1* values of uninvolved and involved regions are distinct. They are, however, more distinct in the case of individual sample pairs, and overlap of *T1* values was not observed. In this respect the data are in accord with those of other workers.[28] However, the distinction between the involved and uninvolved regions was greater in other studies, e.g., Damadian,[12] as the controls came from noncancer patients. On the basis of *T1* and water content data it was concluded that the increase of *T1* value is not just a monotonic function of water content, but a factor intrinsic to malignant cells or tissues.[38,22,54] The histological studies were conceived at this stage when it became apparent that the *T1* values of uninvolved regions appeared to fall into two subgroups: one group in which the *T1* values were less than the mean *T1* value and another group in which the *T1* values were near the mean *T1* value or higher. This group tended to upset the basis of *T1* values and made it essential to look for any clues of this extreme variability of *T1* values. Hence histopathological studies were carried out on the very samples that were

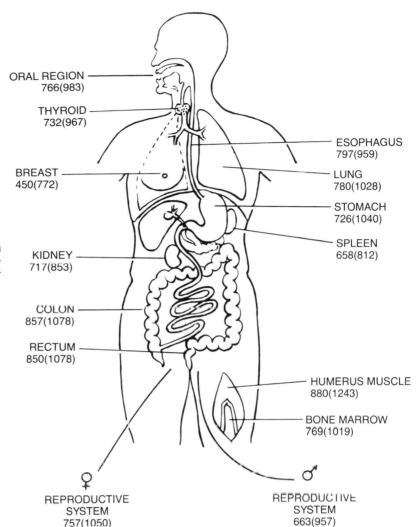

Figure 68–1. *T1* map of human body at 25 MHz. Proton spin-lattice relaxation times of specific organs/tissues.

ORAL REGION
766(983)

THYROID
732(967)

BREAST
450(772)

KIDNEY
717(853)

COLON
857(1078)

RECTUM
850(1078)

ESOPHAGUS
797(959)

LUNG
780(1028)

STOMACH
726(1040)

SPLEEN
658(812)

HUMERUS MUSCLE
880(1243)

BONE MARROW
769(1019)

♀
REPRODUCTIVE
SYSTEM
757(1050)

♂
REPRODUCTIVE
SYSTEM
663(957)

studied by NMR. The special nature of the material used as 'controls' viz., the uninvolved regions, was a second reason for histological investigation. The uninvolved regions were selected from surgically resected material, which on "gross examination" appeared normal. In this respect the selection of control samples was distinct from the selection used by other investigators, who took control material from noncancer subjects.

In Table 68–1 most of the samples were squamous cell carcinoma in esophagus and adenocarcinomas and colloid carcinomas located in the colon and rectum. The uninvolved regions in some cases show a normal histopathological appearance and the *T1* value is relatively close to mean *T1* or lower. The rest of the group shows *T1* values higher than the mean *T1* values of esophagus, colon, and rectum. On the other hand, cases marked as H$^+$ showed the presence of malignant cell groups or clusters, and these samples were registering elevated *T1* values, as seen in Table 68–1, in the uninvolved areas of esophagus, colon, and rectum. It is therefore contended that elevation of *T1* values in the grossly uninvolved H$^+$ cases can be attributed to the presence of malignant cells. Such a conclusion lends support to the observation that malignant cells and tissues display elevated relaxation times.[41,43]

Table 68–1. PROTON SPIN LATTICE RELAXATION TIMES AND HISTOPATHOLOGY OF THE
INVOLVED AND UNINVOLVED REGIONS OF ESOPHAGUS, COLON, AND RECTUM

Sample Number	Diagnosis	*T1* (ms)		Histological Appearance
		Involved Region	*Uninvolved Region*	
Esophagus				
1	Squamous cell carcinoma (no grading)	831	815	H$^+$
2	Squamous cell carcinoma (grade II)	922	804	N
3	Squamous cell carcinoma (grade III)	1213	952	H$^+$
4	Squamous cell carcinoma (grade III)	1122	1018	H$^+$
5	Squamous cell carcinoma (grade III)	1024	984	H$^+$
6	Squamous cell carcinoma (grade II)	1080	568	N
7	Squamous cell carcinoma (grade II)	868	669	N
8	Adenocarcinoma with mucin formation	1122	1042	H$^+$
Colon				
9	Granulocytic sarcoma	1064	1067	H MAC
10	Adenocarcinoma with areas of colloid formation	959	974	H MAC
Rectum				
11	Adenocarcinoma (grade II)	980	644	N
12	Adenocarcinoma (grade II)	1346	1303	H$^+$
13	Adenocarcinoma (grade II)	886	826	H$^+$
14	Adenocarcinoma (grade II)	703	563	N
15	Adenocarcinoma (grade II)	1303	1235	H$^+$
16	Colloid carcinoma	1018	822	H$^+$
17	Colloid carcinoma	1324	979	H MAC
18	Colloid carcinoma	1467	965	MAC

MAC, malignancy associated changes (dysplasia).
H$^+$, presence of malignant cells in the uninvolved region which appeared normal on gross examination.

Histopathological Studies on Miscellaneous Regions

Table 68–2 summarizes the results of studies from other human body sites. The involved and uninvolved sample pairs were first studied for *T1* values. The involved regions had higher values, which is consistent with the theme of NMR relaxation measurements in cancer. The uninvolved regions in Table 68–2 show higher *T1* values than normal (Fig. 68–2) as well as mean *T1* values of respective group (Tables 68–1 and 68–2). Further, the histopathological study of cases 1, 2, 3, 4, 5, 6, 7, 11, and 12, which are taken from different anatomical locations, showed the presence of malignant cells in the uninvolved regions. As such these cases are designated as having the H$^+$ condition. The regions are oral, respiratory, gastric, reproductive, and kidney as well as

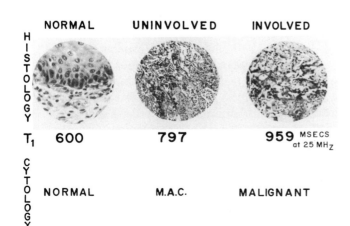

Figure 68–2. Mean *T1* values of normal uninvolved and involved region in human subjects at 25 MHz. Normal at ×240, H & E staining; uninvolved region ×240 H & E staining; regions showing clusters of malignant cells, involved region ×240.

Table 68–2. PROTON SPIN LATTICE RELAXATION TIMES AND HISTOPATHOLOGY OF THE INVOLVED AND UNINVOLVED MISCELLANEOUS REGIONS

Sample Number	Site	Diagnosis	Histological Findings	*T1* (ms) Uninvolved	*T1* (ms) Involved
1	Neck	Uninvolved region	H$^+$	950	1148
		Adenocarcinoma (grade III)	—		
2	Lung	Uninvolved region	H$^+$	843	1174
		Metastasis sarcoma lower lobe	—		
3	Lung	Uninvolved region	H$^+$	783	942
		Epidermoid carcinoma (grade III)	—		
4	Thyroid	Uninvolved region	H$^+$	732	967
		Giant cell carcinoma	—		
5	Kidney	Uninvolved region	H$^+$	773	853
		Renal cell carcinoma	—		
6	Uterus	Uninvolved region	H$^+$	842	1013
7	Stomach	Uninvolved region	H$^+$	766	1201
		Adenocarcinoma (grade III)	—		
8	Stomach	Uninvolved region	MAC	1030	1178
		Adenocarcinoma	—		
9	Cervix	Uninvolved region	MAC	922	1198
		Adenocarcinoma	—		
10	Cervix	Uninvolved region	MAC	981	1267
		Adenocarcinoma	—		
11	Fibula	Uninvolved region	H$^+$	984	1086
		Primary osteosarcoma	—		
12	Humerus	Uninvolved region	H$^+$	882	1159
		Ewing's tumor	—		

MAC, malignancy associated changes (dysplasia).
H$^+$, presence of malignant cells in the uninvolved region which appeared normal on gross examination.

muscle. Despite their diverse origins, the samples show higher *T1* values as well as H$^+$ condition. In keeping with the findings in the esophagus, colon, and rectum, the high *T1* values here too could be attributed to the presence of malignant cells. Case numbers 8, 9, and 10 in Table 68–2 showed areas with malignancy-associated changes—dysplasia. The various elements of dysplasia are abnormal, thus introducing a new factor that could be responsible for the increase of free water content as compared with normal cells and tissues. These areas are encountered in the transition zone between the normal tissue and the tumor.

It may be stated that the presence of groups of malignant cells seems to be the main factor in the observed elevation of *T1* in H$^+$ cases. An increase in the free water content in tissues, due to loss of structure in the cellular organization, is also considered a factor in the increase of *T1* in the malignant state, although there has been no demonstration of any structure.[8,19] The investigations by Fung (1974) have shown that the quantity of nonfreezable bound water is less in tumor than in normal tissues[15a]. Goldsmith et al.[16] observed that normal uninvolved and cancerous areas showed a higher malignancy index than normal tissue, the malignancy index being defined as the sum of *T1* and *T2*. Certaines et al.[10] studied a mixed population of normal and tumor cells with different proportions of tumor cells. The *T1* was found to be increased according to the percentage of tumor cells. These observations also support the conclusions drawn from the present studies, which are illustrated in Figure 68–2.

NMR in Cancer—Some Biochemical Studies

In attempting to explore the basis of elevated relaxation times, concomitant NMR studies and biochemical studies have been done. Hollis et al.[20] had observed that serum protein contents of tissues were lowered in malignant states. Estimated levels of the protein contents of normal and malignant tissues by themselves did not correlate with elevation of *T1* values. In our experience both high and low protein contents are encountered in tumors.[40] In the case of lipids these are seen to be lowered in malignant tumors. The data are shown in Table 68–3 along with the *T1* times of the samples and the mean *T1* of several regions. These studies were extended to the study of proteins and lipoproteins by gel electrophoresis of the tissue homogenates. In a recent observation it has been found that agarose slide gel electrophoresis patterns of protein and lipoproteins of normal and malignant tissues show differences of enormous relevance to NMR studies (Ranade and Javeri, unpublished data).

The agarose slide gel electrophoresis patterns of pairs of involved (I) and uninvolved (U) regions for stomach, esophagus, and colon are seen in Figure 68–3. They have *T1* values of 885 (I) and 765 (U) ms for stomach, 965 (I) and 810 (U) ms for esophagus, 560 (I) and 500 (U) ms for colon. These pulsed NMR studies were done at 20 MHz.

Figure 68–3 shows gel electrophoretic patterns for pairs of uninvolved (U) and involved (I) areas of the stomach, esophagus, and colon. The slides at both extremes of the figure show protein and lipoprotein bands from human serum.

The samples of uninvolved stomach (Fig. 68–3) (U, slide 1) show the presence of

Table 68–3. PROTON SPIN LATTICE RELAXATION TIMES FOR PROTEIN, LIPID, AND WATER CONTENTS OF INVOLVED AND UNINVOLVED HUMAN TISSUES

Sample Number	Organ	Diagnosis	T1 (ms)	Protein Content (%)	Lipid Content (%)	Water Content (%)
1	Tongue	Epidermoid carcinoma recurrent	959	8.49	1.60	82.7
		Uninvolved region	892	12.39	4.59	79.2
2	Mouth	Epidermoid carcinoma of floor of mouth	1004	6.42	0.90	80.7
		Uninvolved region	676	5.26	1.79	—
3	Esophagus	Epidermoid carcinoma (grade II)	922	11.26	0.28	82.5
		Uninvolved region	804	7.49	0.78	83.2
4	Stomach	Colloid carcinoma (infiltrating)	1133	9.0	0.65	85
		Uninvolved region	855	11.65	0.89	83.2
5	Stomach	Adenocarcinoma (grade I)	891	12.25	1.47	80.1
		Uninvolved region	864	15.34	4.31	78.7
6	Stomach	Adenocarcinoma (grade II)	1122	5.81	0.91	81.1
		Uninvolved region	1047	7.65	2.43	83.0
7	Stomach	Adenocarcinoma (grade I)	1033	8.66	0.74	82.6
		Uninvolved region	757	9.41	3.80	79.3
8	Stomach	Adenocarcinoma (grade II)	713	8.96	1.15	73.9
		Uninvolved region	697	5.71	2.13	82.1
9	Lung	Epidermoid carcinoma	750	4.61	4.53	79.2
		Uninvolved region	708	17.72	5.54	77.2
10	Retroalveolar area	Carcinoma of retroalveolar area (grade I)	763	6.70	1.29	80.6
		Uninvolved region	423	4.55	3.3	43.6
11	Breast	Infiltration duct carcinoma (grade I)	330	1.06	20.2	96.25
		Uninvolved region	329	1.45	40.3	68.80
12	Neck node	Metastasis epidermoid carcinoma (grade II)	773	5.14	2.50	77.5
		Uninvolved node	715	10.17	3.66	70.4
13	Penis	Squamous carcinoma (grade II)	1018	3.84	0.65	83.3
		Uninvolved region	988	4.35	0.83	82.1

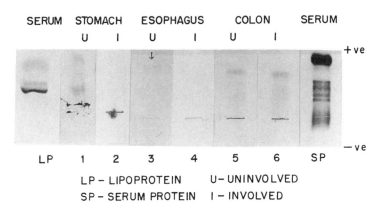

Figure 68–3. Agarose gel slide electrophoretic patterns of sucrose homogenates of the uninvolved and involved gastrointestinal regions. Note absence of lipoprotein band in carcinoma of esophagus.

lipoprotein bands. These bands are missing in the tumor (I slide 2). The tumor was diagnosed as poorly differentiated adenocarcinoma of the fundus of the stomach. Further, a protein band seen in the uninvolved esophagus (U, slide 3) is absent in the involved region (I, slide 4) diagnosed to be a moderately differentiated squamous carcinoma. Slides (U, 5) and (I, 6) show the presence of protein bands in both uninvolved and involved colon. On histopathological examination the latter turned out to be a benign tumor (a fibroid polyp of the colon). The percentage lipid content of the involved region of the gastrointestinal tract is lower than that of the uninvolved region, as seen from Table 68–3. The variation in the percent protein content of the same tissues does not, however, show any correlation with the $T1$ differences.[40]

The $T1$ values and the percent lipid contents of the gastrointestinal tract (Table 68–3) are suggestive of a reduction of lipid content in malignancy, with a concomitant increase in proton spin-lattice relaxation times. The percent protein values of a relatively larger number of samples from the gastrointestinal tract as well as from other regions do not show any correlation with $T1$ variation.[40] Against this background the results of the electrophoretic studies are significant, as they display distinct differences in the profiles of lipoproteins and protein patterns between normal and malignant sample pairs (Fig. 68–3). The difference is evident in the loss of lipoprotein and protein bands from the malignant tissue. This observation has been repeated in the electrophoretic patterns of subsequent samples studied. That the absence of these bands is specific to malignant tissues is confirmed by the electrophoretic patterns showing the presence of the band in a benign tumor as well as in the uninvolved region of the colon (Fig. 68–3).

These studies provide a preliminary yet specific instance of a biochemical difference in malignant and nonmalignant tissue correlating with $T1$ differences and merit consideration for their relevance to NMR studies.

On the basis of the preceding observations and the electrophoretic patterns in normal and malignant tissues shown in Figure 68–3, substantiated with $T1$ data on tissues and isolated nuclei as well as histological studies, it is proposed that macromolecular components play a role in the ordering of cell structure and that a loss of these macromolecules is associated with the loss of structure and the consequent enhancement of free water content, leading to the increased $T1$ values in malignancy. The observed decrease in the lipid content of tumors and the loss of lipoprotein bands in gastrointestinal tract tumors provide experimental evidence in support of this proposal.

Recent studies reveal clear evidence of loss of the membrane lipid vinculin in malignancy. A change in the linking protein spectrin, which attaches microfilaments to membrane, is also observed in malignancy.[33] Although these studies were not done in the context of NMR, they provide independent support for the correctness of the viewpoint developed in the present case correlating biochemical parameters with *T1* differences.

Beall et al.[5] have shown that the serum *T1* pattern is altered in disease states. They found a correlation between increased *T1* values and a lower protein content of the serum and vice versa. Further, gamma globulin, which influences vicinal water, reduces *T1* values.

PULSED MR STUDIES ON NUCLEAR FRACTIONS

Samples for pulsed MR studies on nuclear fractions were obtained from different strains of 6- to 8-week-old mice of either sex.

The tumor mouse fibrosarcoma (MFS) was transplanted into Swiss mice. The tumor was induced by subcutaneously injecting a chemical carcinogen, 6,12 dimethylbenzol-(1,2b,5,4–6')-dithionaphthene (2 mg in 0.2 ml tricaprylin) into the mice. The tumor was maintained in the same host by serial transplantation by injecting 10^6 tumor cells into the hind leg of each animal. For experiments, tumors were used 15 days after transplantation. The other tumor adenocarcinoma was a spontaneous mammary tumor of another mouse strain—ICRC. Animals were sacrificed by cervical dislocation. Tissues were excised, blotted dry, and used for NMR experiments.

The nuclear fractions were prepared by using the procedure of Smuckler et al.[61] This consists of homogenization of tissues and centrifugation in a defined sucrose solution. The nuclear preparations were monitored by acridine orange fluorescence microscopy for homogeneity of nuclei and by electron microscopy for intactness of nuclear structure. The water content of all the tissues and nuclear fractions was determined by lyophilization until constant weights were attained.

The data on *T1* values of various tissues and nuclear fractions are interesting. It has been noted that the *T1* values of nuclei are increased compared with those of tissues of origin. This observation is confirmed in tissues of normal and tumor-bearing animals as well as in tumors in Swiss and ICRC mice (Tables 68–4, 68–5, and 68–6 and Fig. 68–4). An important point emerges from the comparison of nuclear fractions of livers from normal and tumor-bearing mice. The mean *T1* values of nuclear fraction (NF) of normal mouse liver is 693 ms, while the NF of liver from tumor-bearing animals is 804 ms. The latter cannot be attributed to malignant cell invasion, since no abnormal elements of involvement by tumor are seen histologically. The increased *T1* of nuclear fraction of tumor-bearing animal-like tissues can be attributed to a systemic effect. The nuclear fractions of kidney and spleen tissues show mean *T1* values of 873 and 1044 ms, respectively. Here again the increase in *T1* in nuclear fractions is confirmed as in the case of liver NF's. The *T1* values of ICRC mouse are relatively close, but their nuclear fractions show distinct and higher *T1* values. In the MFS and adenocarcinoma tumors the nuclear fractions show *T1* values of 1132 and 1072 ms, respectively. These are the highest *T1* values encountered in these studies.

Other investigations that provide further evidence for present observations come from the work from Adamski et al.[1,2] They studied both the *T1* and the *T2* values of nuclear fractions isolated from human uterine muscle, myometrium, its neoplastic tissue, and a benign tumor. The data are reproduced from the work of Adamski and his colleagues in Table 68–7. They observed that the nuclear fractions have higher *T1* and *T2* values than the tissues of origin. It was further observed that the two relaxation times have a long relaxing component, $T1_A$ and $T2_A$, and a short relaxing component, $T1_B$ and $T2_B$. These are seen in Table 68–7. They found that in tissues and nuclear fractions the values of the longer component are different while the values from the

Table 68–4. PROTON SPIN LATTICE RELAXATION TIMES (*T1*) AND PERCENTAGE WATER CONTENT OF NUCLEAR FRACTIONS FROM TISSUES OF NORMAL AND MFS TUMOR–BEARING SWISS MICE

Sample Type	Tissues*		Nuclear Fractions		Significance†	
	T1 (ms)	*Water Content (%)*	*T1 (ms)*	*Water Content (%)*	*T1 (ms)*	*Water Content (%)*
Liver (normal)	426 ± 12 (26)‡	70.8 ± 0.25	692 ± 20 (37)	75.1 ± 0.65	P < .01	P < .001
Liver (tumor)	615 ± 17 (24)	72.5 ± 0.42	804 ± 37 (36)	79.5 ± 0.85	P < .001	P < .001
Spleen (normal)	712 ± 26 (14)	77.5 ± 1.2	1044 ± 59 (11)	79.0 ± 1.6	P < .001	P < .001
Spleen (tumor)	782 ± 19 (15)	77.4 ± 0.9	—	—	—	—
Kidney (normal)	581 ± 25 (16)	75.2 ± 1.3	873 ± 52 (10)	81.9 ± 0.85	P < .001	P < .001
Kidney (tumor)	669 ± 24 (12)	75.4 ± 1.1	—	—	—	—
Mouse fibrosarcoma tumor (MFS)	944 ± 26	79.1 ± 0.71	1132 ± 45	80.9 ± 0.5	P < .001	P > .05

* *T1* values and water content shown are the mean values and the standard errors of the mean.
† *P* values denote the probability of the significance of the difference in the mean values of tissues and their nuclear fractions calculated by using Student's *t* test.
‡ Number of samples is shown in parentheses.

shorter component are the same for malignant and benign tumors, although they are different from those of normal tissues. It was also found that the elevation of *T1* values is independent of water content.

The relationship between *T1* and water content is one of the factors that has been frequently discussed in relation to the correlation between tissue hydration changes and water proton *T1* value. Many investigators have attributed elevated relaxation times

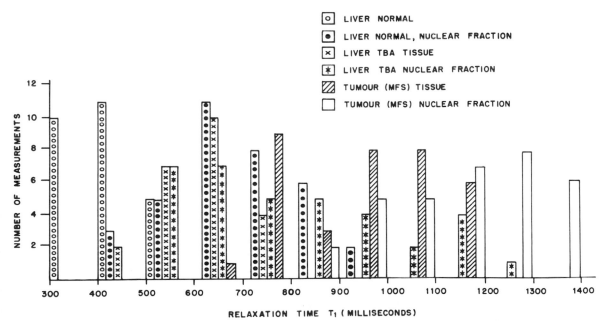

Figure 68–4. Histogram showing water proton spin-lattice relaxation times in tissues and nuclear fractions at 25 MHz (Swiss mice).

Table 68–5. PROTON SPIN–LATTICE RELAXATION TIMES (*T1*) AND PERCENTAGE WATER CONTENT OF NUCLEAR FRACTIONS FROM LIVER TISSUES AND MFS TUMOR–BEARING SWISS MICE

Sample Number	Liver (Normal)		Liver (Tumor Bearing)	
	T1 (ms)	Water Content (%)	*T1* (ms)	Water Content (%)
1	838	80.5	1054	87.9
2	839	77.8	795	85.3
3	738	73.4	901	85.2
4	736	77.1	815	83.1
5	801	76.7	970	80.5
6	678	75.0	971	80.4
7	812	76.0	834	77.6
8	858	76.2	934	78.6
9	975	76.5	1048	80.0
10	906	78.6	594	76.6
11	578	72.9	559	84.0
12	828	77.1	558	81.6
13	693	73.8	798	87.3
14	654	75.9	826	87.2
15	713	73.3	614	82.0
16	656	78.8	593	81.4
17	608	77.1	553	75.0
18	650	77.0	578	74.5
19	636	88.2	576	79.4
20	636	88.2	576	79.4
21	528	81.8	689	70.4
22	630	72.7	703	75.2
23	793	65.2	626	69.5
24	739	75.9	634	78.1
25	668	71.2	644	75.0
26	753	74.6	624	71.4
27	661	72.2	708	77.1
28	692	72.5	757	75.6
29	563	70.6	862	86.6
30	752	71.0	834	85.3
31	746	72.0	657	70.5
32	572	73.9	1178	81.4
33	557	73.4	1197	83.7
34	663	74.5	1276	81.0
35	487	71.0	1145	81.9
36	485	72.5	1119	79.0
37	478	72.0	—	—
Mean ± SEM	692 ± 20 (37)	75.1 ± 0.65 (37)	804 ± 36 (36)	79.5 ± 0.85 (36)

Table 68–6. PROTON *T1* AND PERCENTAGE WATER CONTENT OF TISSUES AND THEIR NUCLEAR REACTIONS IN NORMAL AND ADENOCARCINOMA TUMOR–BEARING ICRC MICE

Sample Number	Sample Type	Tissue*		Nuclear Fractions		Significance†	
		T1 (ms)	Water Content (%)	*T1* (ms)	Water Content (%)	*T1* (ms)	Water Content (%)
1	Liver (normal)	375 ± 29	68.8 ± 2.4	549 ± 25	75.8 ± 1.4	P < .01	P > .05
2	Liver (tumor bearing)	366 ± 17 (3)‡	70.8 ± 0.75	690 ± 60 (5)	76.4 ± 0.48	P < .02	P < .01
3	Adenocarcinoma	653 ± 18	79.0 ± 0.5	1072 ± 42	85.4 ± 1.0	P < .001	P < .01

* *T1* values and water content shown are the mean values and the standard error of the mean.
† *P* values denote the probability of the significance of the difference in the mean values of tissues and their nuclear fractions calculated by using Student's *t* test.
‡ Number of samples is shown in parentheses.

Table 68–7. VALUES OF RELAXATION TIMES (*T1* AND *T2*) AND STANDARD DEVIATIONS (SD) OF HUMAN TISSUES AND NUCLEAR FRACTIONS*

Sample	Tissue				Nuclear Fraction			
	T1A (S)	*T1B* (S)	*T2A* (ms)	*T2B* (ms)	*T1A* (S)	*T2B* (S)	*T1A* (ms)	*T2B* (ms)
Sarcoma	1.99	0.11	116.0	21.0	2.39	0.22	140.0	35.0
	1.80	0.24	108.9	25.0	2.21	0.40	132.0	27.0
Myometrium	1.04	0.44	62.3	22.0	1.56	0.49	120.0	26.0
	1.38	0.11	70.0	24.0	1.35	0.49	117.0	27.0
	0.95	0.18	80.0	37.0	1.64	0.36	116.0	49.0
	1.12	0.44	83.0	28.0	1.65	0.57	97.3	30.0
	1.30	0.57	52.8	30.0	1.64	0.75	70.0	40.0
	1.00	0.25	67.6	35.6	1.50	0.40	122.0	40.0
	1.00	0.27	75.0	30.0	0.40	0.40	119.0	26.0
Mean	1.11	0.32	70.1	29.5	1.56	0.49	108.7	34.0
SD	0.17	0.16	10.4	5.5	0.09	0.13	18.5	8.6
Leiomyoma	0.82	0.11	59.2	30.0	1.15	0.25	60.0	28.0
	0.95	0.23	36.0	11.0	1.04	0.43	50.0	12.1
	1.04	0.11	40.0	11.1	1.26	0.20	47.0	18.4
	0.90	0.20	40.0	12.3	0.90	0.22	50.0	29.9
	1.05	0.30	44.0	12.0	1.15	0.32	48.0	25.1
	0.92	0.20	37.4	10.2	1.02	0.02	102.0	20.0
	1.20	0.18	59.2	24.0	1.13	0.32	75.4	25.6
	1.05	0.18	44.0	22.0	1.20	0.25	49.0	22.4
	1.09	0.31	42.0	15.0	1.35	0.31	41.0	19.9
	1.10	0.13	51.0	12.1	1.28	0.28	71.0	16.0
	0.90	0.13	41.0	16.0	1.00	0.15	46.0	14.0
	1.20	0.17	38.0	15.0	1.49	0.40	40.5	28.1
	0.90	0.17	43.0	10.0	1.10	0.20	42.0	10.0
Mean	1.01	0.19	45.8	15.4	1.17	0.27	55.5	20.7
SD	0.12	0.06	8.2	6.2	0.16	0.08	17.7	6.5

* Adamski J, Bucko J, Pislewski N: Acta Physica Polonica A *63*:287–296,1983.

for malignant tissues or cell lines to increased water content of the tissues. Nevertheless other investigators have shown that there is no linear relationship between hydration changes and *T1* values. Beall et al.[6] have found no correlation between water content and *T1* values of human breast cancer cell lines. Instead, a correlation has been observed by them showing the interaction of water with macromolecular network in influencing water proton *T1*. The water content estimated in the nuclear fractions from different tissues is seen in Tables 68–4, 68–5, and 68–6. It can be noticed that nuclear fractions from tissues of tumor-bearing animals have a statistically significant higher water content than that of corresponding normal tissues.

However, in a continuation of this work by Shah et al.,[55,56] an examination of *T1* times and water content shows the absence of a direct relationship between the two parameters for the following:

1. Normal liver nuclear fractions and tissues.

2. Nuclear fractions from tissues of normal and tumor-bearing animals (Swiss and ICRC mice).

3. MFS tumor and its nuclear fractions.

These data therefore establish that the differences observed between the nuclear fractions of tissues of normal and tumor-bearing animals show elevated *T1* values, which cannot be attributed solely to water content but must be related to factors intrinsic to the nuclear compartment.

Some recent pulsed NMR studies have been carried out on nuclei isolated from human spleen and rat liver and subjected to treatments such as $MnCl_2$ bathing, removal

Table 68–8. TRACE METAL LEVELS IN NUCLEAR FRACTIONS OF HUMAN SPLEEN AND RAT LIVER BEFORE AND AFTER TREATMENT

Samples	Treatment	Metal (μg/Gm Dry Weight)			T1 (ms at 90 MHz)
		Iron	*Copper*	*Manganese*	
Normal human spleen tissues	Nil	651	5.3	3.2	510
Normal spleen NF	Nil	719.8	34.2	3.6	570
Normal spleen NF	Nil	602.2	33.9	5.6	390
Normal spleen NF	Nil	1035.8	10.6	3.5	470
Normal spleen NF	RBC lysis	483.5	60.4	2.1	1050
Normal spleen NF	1% Triton	101.1	26.0	4.3	910
Normal rat liver NF	Nil	567.9	69.9	6.6	560
Normal rat liver NF	*MnCl$_2$ $\frac{1}{2}$ hr	536.3	61.9	6.5	440
Normal rat liver NF	RBC lysis	420.6	88.8	18.7	1150
Normal rat liver NF	0.25% Triton	211.4	—	11.5	560

* 0.15 mM.

of red blood cells, and storage at the low temperature of 2° C. They revealed that the specificity of *T1* values in isolated nuclei was retained and was distinct from tissue *T1* value. This effect was also seen in the response of *T1* and *T2* values of nuclei subjected to altered paramagnetic concentrations of metal ions (loss or gain) and to a lesser extent in detergent-treated nuclear membrane. The reproducibility of *T1* and *T2* at 90 MHz and *T1* at 20 MHz following cold storage provides a clear case for specificity of NMR parameters in tissues in relation to cell nuclei (Ranade and Adamski, unpublished data, Table 68–8).

The role of paramagnetic metal ions in tissues and nuclear fractions has also been studied.[42] Modak et al.[31] studied water proton relaxation times (*T1*) of nuclear fractions of liver and spleen of normal and tumor-bearing animals. At 90 MHz *T1* values for nuclear fractions of tumor-bearing animals were found to be less than those for normal nuclear fractions, contrary to observations at the cellular level,[31] which could be ascribed to DNA–metal ion interaction.

CORRELATION OF MR PARAMETERS AND TISSUE CONSTITUENTS

Histopathological investigations make it evident that *T1* variations can be explored in relation to tissue architecture. This section includes the results on work done to ascertain the role of tissue constituents and their effect on *T1* value.

In these studies surgically resected specimens of carcinoma of lower esophagus were taken. The selection of tissue samples for this study was made on the basis of gross examination of the resected specimens. Samples were taken from the tumor carcinomas and were designated as zones III and IV. Besides these, areas were selected from either side of the tumor (adjoining the tumor) that appeared normal on gross examination, and areas were also selected from the esophageal resection margin, designated as zones I and II, and from the stomach margin included in the resected specimen, designated as zones V and VI (Fig. 68–5).

The samples measured about 1 cu cm. They were stored in sealed vials at 4° C until the *T1* measurements were taken.

Proton spin-lattice relaxation times have been measured on the IJS-2-75 water and oil content pulsed NMR analyser at 32 MHz at the Agriculture and Biology Division, Bhabha Atomic Research Centre, Bombay. The samples were transferred to NMR

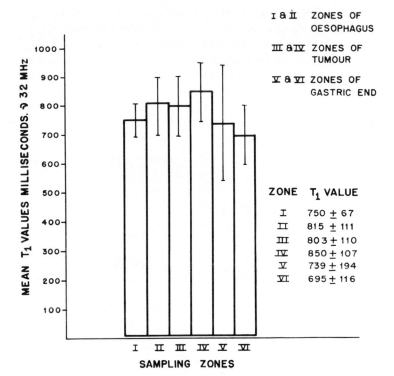

I & II ZONES OF OESOPHAGUS

III & IV ZONES OF TUMOUR

V & VI ZONES OF GASTRIC END

ZONE	T_1 VALUE
I	750 ± 67
II	815 ± 111
III	803 ± 110
IV	850 ± 107
V	739 ± 194
VI	695 ± 116

Figure 68–5. Histogram showing mean *T1* values of zones I to VI in transition from normal to neoplastic areas from esophagus to stomach.

sample tubes 12 mm in diameter and placed in a water bath at 32 to 33° C to bring them to the temperature within the probe coil. The *T1* was then determined using the 90° – τ – 90° pulsed sequence. With this method the magnetization relaxes exponentially according to the relation:

$$M_z(\tau) = M_0(1 \quad e^{-\tau/T1}) \tag{1}$$

where $M_z(\tau)$ is the magnetization measured as a function of τ, which is the duration between the two 90 degree pulses. M_0 is the equilibrium magnetization, and *T1* is the proton spin lattice relaxation time. The slope of the semi-log plot $1-M_2(\tau)/M_0$ versus τ is $1/T1$, from which the *T1* can be calculated.

After the *T1* measurements, the tissues were fixed in 10 percent formalin and processed for histological studies by clearing and embedding the material in paraffin. The paraffin blocks were sectioned on a rotary microtome at 6 μ thickness. The sections were taken on albuminized glass slides and stained with hematoxylin and eosin.

T1 measurements are seen in the histogram (Fig. 68–5) depicting the mean *T1* values, along with standard deviations, of zones I to VI. Zone IV is characterized by the highest *T1* values for the tumor region. Table 68–9 gives *T1* values for zones II and III. These are uninvolved esophagus and the tumor, respectively. The tumors represent a wide variety of types, as seen from the diagnoses provided.

The mean *T1* values of zone III (*T1* = 803 ms) represent a tumor zone close to zone II (*T1* = 815 ms), which represents a zone of uninvolved region of esophagus, and analogous to zone V of stomach (*T1* = 739 ms). Esophageal zones I and VI (*T1* = 695 ms) of gastric end represent uninvolved regions and show lower *T1* values of all the zones.

Measurements of proton spin-lattice relaxation times of cellular water protons of normal and malignant esophageal tissues from zone III and zone IV showed the highest *T1* values, characterizing malignant conditions. Apart from this, the present studies focus attention on transition zones I, II, V, and VI, which appear normal on gross examination. The microscopic observations further reveal that zones I and II showed dysplasia. The cells of these areas are classified as neither normal nor malignant. They showed features in between the two and are considered to represent distinct cell types. It was also observed that dysplastic areas of zones I and II showed higher $T1$ values than the normal samples from noncancer subjects, which were on the order of 600 ms. Further, almost similar $T1$ values were seen in zones II and III (mean $T1$ for zone II is 815 ms and for zone III is 803 ms). This is a striking feature, as zone II represents

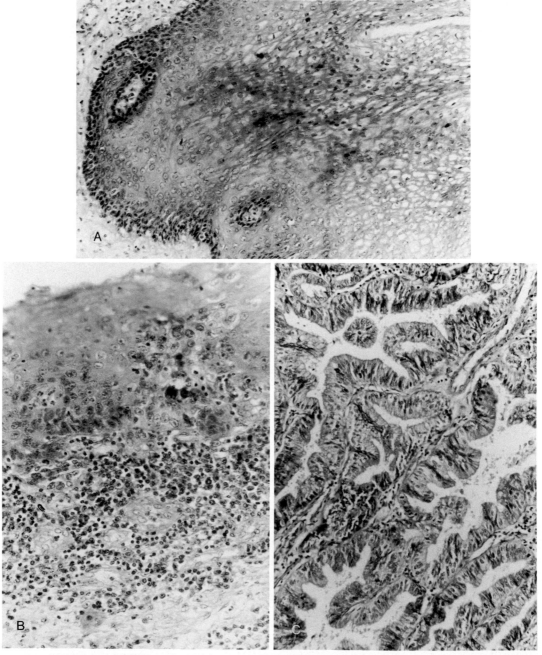

Figure 68–6. *A*, Microphotograph of esophagus showing normal mucosa (×150 H & E staining). *B*, Microphotograph of esophagus showing dysplasia (×240 H & E staining). *C*, Microphotograph of esophagus showing adenocarcinoma (×150).

dysplasia and zone III represents tumor proper. Likewise, comparison of mean *T1* values of zone IV (mean *T1* is 850 ms) and zone V (mean *T1* is 739 ms) shows relatively greater mean *T1* differences. It is also to be noted that zone IV is a tumor zone, while zone V is uninvolved gastric end. The histopathology of zone V shows some degree of metaplasia and hyperplasia but not the predominance of dysplasia at the gastric end, quite unlike the esophageal end (Fig. 68–6A, B, C).

In view of these observations it becomes evident that zone II, where areas of dysplasia are predominantly manifested, are responsible for elevation of *T1* values of these regions. Consequently, one is led to the conclusion that next to the presence of tumor cells (see Fig. 68–2), areas with dysplastic cell type also contribute to the elevation of *T1* values. It can be further seen that there is greater *T1* variation between zones IV and V, which correlates with the histological heterogeneity of these regions. Compared to equivalent zone II, the *T1* variation in zone V could be attributed to the findings of areas with metaplasia. Thus in monitoring zones I to VI, the *T1* variation can be sequentially correlated with histological characteristics.

Zone II represents the outstanding features of these studies—dysplasia. This was repeatedly seen in histopathological studies in 13 samples also studied by NMR. A separate evaluation was carried out by histopathology on similar zones. This independent study of 32 cases also revealed dysplasia in most of the cases, providing support for the contention that *T1* elevation could be attributed to dysplasia.[8]

The correlation linking the NMR parameter with histopathology may be somewhat empirical, but it has been well substantiated from observations enumerated above.[48] The implications of these studies for MR imaging are discussed in the last section of this chapter, Role of Cell Type in the Elevation of Spin Lattice Relaxation Time.

PULSED NMR STUDIES ON MALIGNANT LYMPHOMAS

Pulsed NMR studies of malignant lymphoma were undertaken with a view to ascertain the *T1* variation within the group. These studies were also done to find out if the morphological criteria, which have been emphasized in the classification of this complex class of tumors, show any correlation at all with the *T1* variation encountered in this group.

For this work surgically resected specimens of Hodgkin's and non-Hodgkin's lymphoma were obtained. Normal lymph nodes, which were used as controls, came from autopsy cases of noncancer subjects. The samples were taken in NMR sample tubes. The proton spin-lattice relaxation times were determined on IJS-2-75 water and oil content pulsed NMR analyser at 32 MHz. The method of determination of *T1* values has been described in an earlier section.

Proton spin-lattice relaxation times of lymph nodes of Hodgkin's and non-Hodgkin's lymphomas are seen in Table 68–10. It can be seen that the non-Hodgkin's lymphomas show a range of 851 to 1084 ms with a mean *T1* value of 982 ms. The Hodgkin's lymphomas show a range of 650 to 771 ms with a mean *T1* value of 715 ms. These data indicate that the two main subgroups of malignant lymphomas can be distinguished on the basis of distinct mean *T1* values. Further, within the non-Hodgkin's lymphomas the diffuse and nodular groups show *T1* values of 1012 ms and 796 ms, respectively (Fig. 68–7A and B).

The distinction between *T1* values seen in Hodgkin's and non-Hodgkin's lymphomas is significant. In attempting to see if this could be associated with any morphological feature it became apparent that the relatively lower *T1* values in Hodgkin's lymphoma could be attributed to different proportions of malignant cells. Hodgkin's lymphoma shows a smaller number of malignant cells, among a dominant normal cell population,

Table 68–9. PROTON SPIN–LATTICE RELAXATION TIMES OF ZONES OF ESOPHAGUS FROM TUMOR AND UNINVOLVED REGIONS AT 32 MHz

Sample Number	Zone III		Zone II	
	T1	*Diagnosis*	*T1*	*Diagnosis*
1	1048	Poorly differentiated epidermal carcinoma	1046	Uninvolved esophagus
2	558	Adenocarcinoma (grade II)	556	Uninvolved esophagus
3	820	Poorly differentiated adenocarcinoma	899	Uninvolved esophagus
4	799	Squamous carcinoma	811	Uninvolved region
5	857	Moderately differentiated epidermoid carcinoma	873	Uninvolved esophagus
6	662	Moderately differentiated epidermoid carcinoma	706	Uninvolved esophagus
7	769	Poorly differentiated adenocarcinoma	756	Uninvolved esophagus
8	632	Poorly differentiated adenocarcinoma	728	Uninvolved esophagus
9	896	Epidermoid carcinoma	517	Uninvolved esophagus
10	691	Poorly differentiated adenocarcinoma	—	—
11	993	Poorly differentiated epidermoid carcinoma	—	—
12	558	Adenocarcinoma (grade II)	556	Uninvolved esophagus
13	602	Epidermoid carcinoma (grade II)	648	Uninvolved esophagus
14	593	Epidermoid carcinoma (grade II)	676	Uninvolved esophagus
15	800	Adeno papillary carcinoma	830	Uninvolved esophagus
16	738	Poorly differentiated adenocarcinoma	892	Uninvolved esophagus
17	750	Moderately differentiated squamous carcinoma	830	—

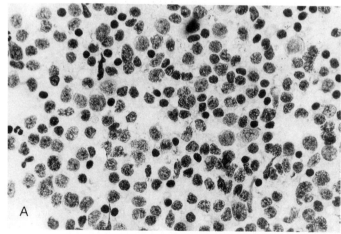
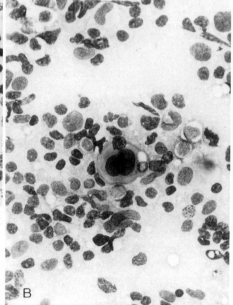

Figure 68–7. *A*, Microphotograph of non-Hodgkin's lymphoma (×400). *B*, Microphotograph of Hodgkin's lymphoma showing Reed-Sternberg cells (×400).

while non-Hodgkin's lymphoma show a predominantly malignant cell population. The correlation of lower $T1$ with normal cell type and higher $T1$ with malignant cell type is well justified in this case and substantiated by the earlier findings in histopathology and nuclear fractions.

Yet another distinction has become apparent within the non-Hodgkin's lymphomas (Table 68–10). The nodular non-Hodgkin's lymphomas are known to have a better prognosis as compared with the diffuse type of non-Hodgkin's lymphoma. It is notable that higher $T1$ values within the non-Hodgkin's lymphoma group are seen in the diffuse type, while the nodular type has relatively lower $T1$ values. This indicates the possibility of relating favorable and unfavorable prognoses of disease to low and high $T1$ values, respectively.[63] Such a conclusion would be of value in subgrouping the malignant lymphomas. In fact, the recent trend in re-emphasizing the value of morphological parameters to classification of lymphomas lends support to the rationale of classification and characterization of malignant lymphomas on the basis of $T1$ values and their relation in turn to the prognostic value. It is pertinent to quote Lennert, whose classification of malignant lymphomas is well known.

Coordinated studies of histopathological and multiparameter data have taught us the significance of morphological findings and established the distinctness of cytological criteria of individual cell types. From our experience reliance on immunological or cytochemical data without correlation with morphological evaluation is generally unreliable.[26]

In earlier studies on $T1$ times of leukemic cells isolated from blood and bone marrow of patients with acute myeloid leukemia, chronic myeloid leukemia and acute lymphoblastic leukemia, it was observed that high $T1$ values were encountered in cells with active stages of disease as well as in recurrence while in cases of patients receiving chemotherapy in remission and normal subjects relatively low $T1$ values were observed. These studies were carried out on isolated cell pellets,[34,56] supporting $T1$ variation as reflecting cell type.

In the case of malignant lymphomas it is known that computerized tomography has limitations in demonstrating lymph node pathology. Pulsed NMR studies of malignant lymphomas are suggestive of a distinction, however, within the lymphoma group, on the basis of $T1$ of cell type and prognosis. We would like to see this speculation substantiated when NMR imaging of lymphomas is accomplished.

As a further step, NMR studies on metastatic lymph nodes were undertaken. It was found that the $T1$ values of metastatic lymph nodes were higher compared with normal lymph nodes. The $T1$ values were in the range of 500 to 780 ms as compared with the range of 200 to 300 ms observed in normal lymph nodes. The mean $T1$ values showed statistical differences at the 1 percent level. Storage of lymph nodes at $2°$ C did not affect the distinction betwen normal and metastatic lymph nodes. Agarose slide gel electrophoresis of these cases further showed two protein bands each in tissue homogenates of Hodgkin's lymphoma, non-Hodgkin's lymphoma, and the metastatic lymph nodes as compared with one protein band obtained in normal lymph nodes. These preliminary studies at 20 MHz of lymph nodes in malignant lymphoma show, however, that a distinction within the subclass of non-Hodgkin's lymphoma was not possible on the basis of $T1$ values alone.[70]

The levels of paramagnetic trace metals and physiologically important cations have been studied in these very samples and have been reported.[45,46,47,64]

ROLE OF CELL TYPE IN THE ELEVATION OF SPIN LATTICE RELAXATION TIME

The account of the histopathology of uninvolved regions has shown effectively that while normal and malignant tissues are characterized by low and high $T1$ values, the intermediate areas with mixed cell populations display intermediate *T1* values. The observations made on regions of gastrointestinal tissue have been confirmed in the uninvolved regions of other body sites (Table 68–2). The observation points to the significance of the role of cell type in influencing the *T1* values of the tissues. In this context it is to be noted that Koutcher et al.[24] have recommended the use of a malignancy index, the sum of *T1* and *T2* values, as being more discriminatory of the normal and the malignant states. The present studies have consistently shown *T1* to be discriminatory. Overlaps of values were rarely observed. The reason for this has to be seen in the choice of the sample. The samples were selected from the resected specimens of the same subject. This point is also relevant in the context of NMR imaging where in-vivo *T1* and *T2* values of normal and pathological states and cancer are determined on the same subject and are found to be discriminatory.[32] The choice of the samples thus merits special mention. The studies also indicate that cell type is a possible basis of *T1* variation.

Detailed histopathological studies of zones I to VI of the involved region of esophagus showed that the occurrence of areas with dysplasia seems to be predominantly responsible for the elevation of *T1* values. This is corroborated by the observed close mean *T1* values of the regions with zone II dysplasia as compared with those of zone III. On the other hand, zone V of gastric end, which does not show dysplasia, is more heterogeneous in terms of constituent elements and shows a larger spread of mean *T1* values, which are lower than the proximal tumor zone IV. It is therefore reasonable to propose that *T1* elevation be attributed to occurrence of dysplasia.

Dysplasia is a precancerous condition well known to pathologists, and as seen in zone II, areas with dysplasia have shown an increase in relaxation time in the detailed histological study of esophagus. The nuclear changes leading to malignancy are manifest, viz. high N/C ratio, hyperchromatism of the nucleus, and increased mitotic activity. It can be argued that dysplastic changes are bound to reflect increased relaxation times compared with normal and cellular areas.

Pulsed MR studies of cell nuclei isolated from normal and malignant tissues of experimental animals have shown that the *T1* values of pellets of malignant nuclei are higher than for nuclei of normal tissues.[31,41,43] Confirmation of the observation that isolated nuclei register specific and higher *T1* values than tissue of origin has been

Table 68–10. PROTON SPIN–LATTICE RELAXATION TIMES IN LYMPH NODES OF HODGKIN'S AND NON–HODGKIN'S LYMPHOMA (AT 32 MHz)

Histopathological Diagnosis	*T1* (ms)
Non-Hodgkin's Lymphomas	
Diffuse lymphocytic	1029
Diffuse lymphocytic	1129
Diffuse poorly differentiated lymphocytic	1080
Diffuse poorly differentiated lymphocytic	1084
Diffuse poorly differentiated lymphocytic	1038
Diffuse histiocytic	1010
Diffuse histiocytic	1027
Nodular poorly differentiated lymphocytic	868
Nodular poorly differentiated lymphocytic	851
Nodular poorly differentiated lymphocytic	861
Nodular mixed histiocytic/lymphocytic	906
Nodular mixed histiocytic/lymphocytic	911
Hodgkin's lymphomas	
Mixed cellularity	661
Mixed cellularity	650
Mixed cellularity	775
Mixed cellularity	771

gathered by Adamski et al.[1] in their studies on nuclear fractions isolated from carcinomas of endometrium and its normal human tissue. This line of investigation represents an area in which to follow the contribution of the subcellular fractions to the overall tissue relaxation phenomenon. Studies on the relaxation behavior of ^{17}O from H_2O in rat lymphocyte pellets has indicated the presence of two fractions, one slowly relaxing fraction ascribed to the nucleus, having a relaxation time of 5.1 ms, and a fast relaxation component with $T1$ of 3.1 ms.[61]

Beall et al.[4] have observed changes of $T1$ with chromatin condensation during various phases of the cell cycle. The difference observed in the normal and malignant cell nuclei could well be attributed to the variation in the chromatin and consequently altered water content. The nuclear fraction makes a pronounced contribution to the cellular $T1$ values. In view of these observations, the arguments favoring the role of nuclear cytology and $T1$ are further substantiated.

In nuclear magnetic resonance imaging, it has been observed that $T1$ values surrounding the tumor being imaged are elevated. This has the effect of making the tumor larger and hence detectable.[3] It is conceivable that these are regions comprised of areas with H^+ in our studies or with zone I or II of esophagus, making the tumor area larger and detectable. With NMR imaging becoming a reality it has become necessary to seek anatomic correlation of the sample with the NMR image. Smith et al.[59] have been able to demonstrate esophageal carcinoma by NMR imaging, making the gastrointestinal tract neoplasms amenable to detection by NMR. Ross et al.[52] were able to identify and differentiate human breast neoplasms from other pathological states by in-vivo $T1$ and $T2$ values. NMR imaging of various anatomic locations has been accomplished.[67,68] These developments validate the importance of correlative studies to the field of NMR imaging. The relevance of the present studies to NMR imaging appears to suggest a promising area of investigation.

A unique cytological feature encountered in the study of the uninvolved regions in addition to the H^+ areas is the presence of malignancy-associated changes (MAC) per the criteria of Nieburgs.[35] These changes are seen in the nuclear chromatin and probably arise as a result of mitotic arrest and are observed in areas in the proximity of tumor in normal cells experiencing mitosis. MAC have been described by Nieburgs[35] and Rilke.[51] This cell type deviates from the normal type and can be considered cytologically intermediate between normal and malignant cell types (Fig. 68–8). With this model and demonstration of increased free water content in malignant cells it can be

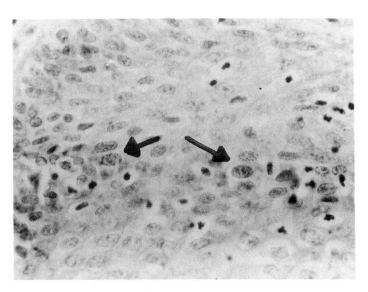

Figure 68–8. Microphotograph of malignancy-associated changes (MAC) in involved regions of human esophagus. Note: MAC seen in nuclear chromatin marked by arrows in plurifocal isolated cells.

proposed that MAC cells would display higher *T1* values than normal cells. Consequently from normal to MAC to malignant cell type a gradient increase in *T1* values can be expected. The increase in the *T1* value would be contributed to by MAC cell type. Such a possibility has been enhanced by identification of MAC in the present specimens.

The studies presented in this chapter and the conclusions reached are, we feel, relevant to NMR imaging, where differences in the *T1* and *T2* values and corresponding information presenting gray scale or color coding is increasingly proving to be of great value in diagnosis of pathological states, especially cancer. It is hoped that the work presented in this chapter contributes to the understanding of the causes of *T1* variation in terms of biological architecture.

ACKNOWLEDGMENTS

The pulsed MR data presented here have been a result of collaboration for a number of years with R. Vijayaraghavan, Ph.D.; S. R. Kasturi, Ph.D.; R. S. Phadke, Ph.D., and R. S. Chaughule, Ph.D. of Tata Institute of Fundamental Research, Bombay; and later with B. B. Singh, Ph.D.; and V. T. Shrinivasan, Ph.D. of Biology and Agriculture Division, Bhabha Atomic Research Centre, Bombay. The sample selection and histopathological studies were done in collaboration with G. V. Talwalkar, M.D., of Pathology Department, Tata Memorial Hospital. The graduate students Mrs. Smita Shah, Mrs. Shubhada Bharade, Miss G. K., Sujata, Miss Jetashri Javeri, Mr. R. P. Mahajan, Miss P. Trivedi, Miss A. Padval, and Mr. B. B. Patil were associated with this work in various phases and have rendered valuable assistance in bringing out this chapter; and thanks are due to R. S. Rajpal, M.S., for useful discussions. Franko Rilke, M.D., and C. Clementi, M.D., of Instituto Nazionale Per Lo Studio E La Cura Dei Tumori, Milano, Italy, identified the MAC in our slides, for which the author is indebted. Thanks are due to Professor N. Pislewski of the Institute of Molecular Physics, Polish Academy of Science, Poznan, Poland, for permission to reproduce Table 68–7 and to Dr. J. Adamski, Clinical Radiospectroscopy Laboratory of Poznan, Poland, for helpful discussion.

References

1. Adamski J, Olzewski KJ, Bucko J, Pislewski N: NMR relaxation times of purified cell nuclei of non-malignant tumors and human uterus muscle. Studia Biophysica *92*:45–49, 1982.
2. Adamski J, Bucko J, Pislewski N: Pulsed NMR studies on human tissues and their nuclear fractions. Acta Physiol Pol *63*:287–296, 1983.
3. Andrew ER, Worthington BS: Nuclear magnetic resonance imaging. *In* Newton TH (ed): Radiology of the Skull and Brain. Technical Aspects of Computed Tomography. Vol. 5. St. Louis, C. V. Mosby, 1981, pp 4389–4405.
4. Beall PT, Medina D, Chang DC, Seitz PK, Hazlewood CF: Systemic effect of benign and malignant mammary tumors on the spin-lattice relaxation time *T1* of water protons in mouse serum. JNCI *59*:1431, 1977.
5. Beall PT, Medina D, Hazlewood CF: The "systemic effect" of elevated tissue and serum relaxation times for water in animals and humans with cancers in NMR in medicine. *In* Diehl P, Fluck E, Kosfeld R (eds): NMR. Basic Principles and Progress. Vol. 19. Heidelberg, Springer Verlag, 1981, pp 39–57.
6. Beall PT, Brinkley BR, Chang DC, Hazlewood CF: Microtubule complexes correlated with growth rate and water proton relaxation times in human breast cancer cells. Cancer Res *42*:4215, 1982.
7. Beall PT, Hazlewood CF, Rutzky LP: NMR relaxation times of water protons in human colon cancer cell lines and clones. Cancer Biochem Biophys *6*:7, 1982.
8. Bharade SH: Significance of histopathology to pulsed nuclear magnetic resonance studies on esophageal cancer. M.Sc. Thesis, Bombay University, 1984.
9. Bovee W, Huisman P, Smidt J: Tumor detection and nuclear magnetic resonance. JNCI *52*:595, 1974.
10. Certaines J de, Gallier J, Lencine G, Bellosi A: Apart de la resonance magnetic nuclear et diagnostic en carcinologie. Quest Med *32*:671–674, 1979.
11. Chaughule RS, Kasturi, SR, Vijayaraghavan R, Ranade SS: Normal and malignant tissues—an investigation by pulsed nuclear magnetic resonance. Indian J Biochem Biophys *11*:256–258, 1974.
12. Damadian R: Tumor detection by nuclear magnetic resonance. Science *17*:1151, 1971.
13. Dodd HJF: Electron spin resonance study of changes during the development of a mouse myeloid leukemia: Paramagnetic metal ions. Br J Cancer *32*:108, 1975.
14. Frey HW, Kniespel RR, Kruuv J: Proton spin-lattice relaxation studies on non-malignant tissues of tumors in mice. JNCI *49*:903, 1972.

15. Floyd RA, Yoshida T, Leigh JS Jr: Changes of tissue water proton relaxation rates during early phases of chemical carcinogenesis. Proc Natl Acad Sci USA 72:56–58, 1975.

15a. Fung, BM: Correlation of relaxation time with water content in muscle and brain tissue. Biochem. Biophys. Acta. 497:317–322, 1977.

16. Goldsmith M, Koutcher J, Damadian R: NMR in cancer XI. Application of NMR malignancy index to human gastrointestinal tumors. Cancer 41:183, 1978.

17. Hazlewood CF, Cleveland G, Medina D: Relationship between hydration and proton nuclear magnetic resonance relaxation times in tissues of tumor bearing and non-tumor bearing mice: Implications for cancer detection. JNCI 52:1849, 1974.

18. Hazlewood CF: A view of the significance and understanding of the physical properties of cell-associated water. In Drost-Hansen W, Clegg JS (eds): Cell-associated Water. New York, Academic Press, 1979.

19. Hazlewood CF, Nichols BL, Chamberlain NF: Evidence for the existence of a minimum of two phases of ordered water in skeletal muscle. Nature (Lond) 222:747–750, 1969.

20. Hollis DR, Economou JS, Parks LC, Eggleston JC, Saryan LA, Czeisler JL: Nuclear magnetic resonance studies of several experimental and human malignant tumors. Cancer Res 33:2156, 1973.

21. Inch WR, McCredie JA, Knispel RR, Thompson RT, Pintar MM: Water content and proton spin-lattice relaxation times for neoplastic and non-neoplastic tissues from mice and humans. JNCI 52:353, 1974.

22. Kasturi SR, Ranade SS, Shah S: Tissue hydration of malignant and uninvolved tissues and its relevance to proton spin-lattice relaxation mechanism. Proc Ind Acad Sci 84B:60, 1976.

23. Kiricuta IC, Simplaceaneau V, Block RE: Factors affecting proton magnetic resonance line widths of water in several rat tissues. FEBS Lett 34:109, 1973.

24. Koutcher JA, Goldsmith M, Damadian R: NMR in cancer X. A malignancy index to discriminate normal and cancerous tissues. Cancer 41:174, 1978.

25. Lauterbur PC: NMR zeumatographic imaging in medicine. J Med Syst 6:591–597, 1982.

26. Lennert K, Collins RD, Lukes RKJ: Concordance of the Kiel and Lukes-Collins classification of non-Hodgkin's lymphoma. Histopathology 7:549–559, 1983.

27. Ling GN, Tucker M: NMR relaxation and water contents in normal mouse and rat tissues and in cancer cells. JNCI 64:1199, 1980.

28. Mathur-De Vré R: The NMR studies of water in biological systems. Prog Biophys Mol Biol 35:103–134, 1979.

29. Mathur-De Vré R: Review article: Biomedical implications of the relaxation behaviour of water related to NMR imaging. Br J Radiol 57:683, 955–976, 1984.

30. Michael LH, Seitz P, McMillan-Wood J, Chang DC, Hazlewood CF, Entamn ML: Mitochondrial water in myocardial ischemia: Investigations with nuclear magnetic resonance. Science 208:1267, 1980.

31. Modak SG, Chaudhary CA, Kasturi SR, Phadke RS, Shah S, Ranade SS: Factors influencing the water proton relaxation in nuclear fractions from tissues of normal and tumor-bearing animals. Physiol Chem Phys 14:41, 1982.

32. Moon KL, Davis PL, Crooks LE, Sheldon PE, Miller TE, Brito AF, Watts JE: NMR imaging of fibrosarcoma tumor implanted in rat. Radiology 148:177–181, 1983.

33. Morrow JS: Spectrins: Mediators of cytoskeletal function. Perspectives in dermatopathology. Am J Dermatopathol 6:573–581, 1984

34. Nadkarni JJ, Nadkarni JS, Advani SH, Ranade SS, Kasturi SR, Chaughule RS: Nuclear magnetic resonance compared with membrane specific immunofluorescence activity. Indian J Cancer 13:76–80, 1976.

35. Nieburgs HE: Recent progress in the interpretation of malignancy associated changes (MAC). Acta Cytol 12:445–453, 1968.

36. Partain CL, James AE, Rollo FD, Price RR (eds): Nuclear Magnetic Resonance Imaging. Philadelphia, W. B. Saunders Co., 1983.

37. Ranade SS, Chaughule RS, Kasturi SR, Nadkarni JS, Talwalkar GV, Korgaonkar KS, Vijayaraghavan R: Pulsed nuclear magnetic resonance studies on human malignant tissues and cells in vitro. Indian J Biochem Biophys 12:229–232, 1975.

38. Ranade SS, Shah S, Korgaonkar KS, Kasturi SR, Chaughule RS, Vijayaraghavan R: Absence of correlation between spin-lattice relaxation times and water content in human tumor tissue. Physiol Chem Phys 8:131–135, 1976.

39. Ranade SS, Shah S, Advani SH, Kasturi SR: Pulsed nuclear magnetic resonance studies of human bone marrow. Physiol Chem Phys 9:297–299, 1977.

40. Ranade SS, Shah S, Talwalkar GV: Histopathological evidence in support of the association of elevated proton spin-lattice relaxation times with the malignant state. Tumori 65:157–162, 1979.

41. Ranade SS, Shah S, Phadke RS, Kasturi SR: Pulsed nuclear magnetic resonance studies on nuclear fractions of normal and malignant tissues. Physiol Chem Phys 11:471–474, 1979.

42. Ranade SS, Shah S, Pallavi H: Transition metals in an experimental tumor system. Experientia 35:460, 1979.

43. Ranade SS, Shah S, Talwalkar GV, Kasturi SR: Significance of histopathologic studies in pulsed NMR studies on cancer. In Partain CL, James AE, Price RR, Rollo FD (eds): Nuclear Magnetic Resonance Imaging. Philadelphia, W. B. Saunders Co., 1983.

44. Ranade SS, Shah S, Phadke RS, Kasturi SR: Pulsed nuclear magnetic resonance studies of water proton in subcellular fractions. Indian J Biochem Biophys 20:180–182, 1983.

45. Ranade SS, Panday VK: Transition metals in human cancer. I. Oesophagus and Bone-marrow. Sci Total Environ 29:177–181, 1983.

46. Ranade SS, Panday VK: Transition metals in human cancer. II. Sci Total Environ *40*:245–257, 1984.
47. Ranade SS, Panday VK: Major metals in human cancer: Calcium, magnesium, sodium and potassium. Sci Total Environ *41*:79–89, 1985.
48. Ranade SS, Bharade SH, Talwalkar GV, Sujata GK, Shrinivasan VT, Singh BB: Significance of histopathology in pulsed NMR studies on cancer. Magn Reson Med *2*:128–135, 1985.
49. Ranade SS, Adamski J, Olszewski KJ: Specificity of the *T1* and *T2* values in the nuclear fractions from human spleen and rat liver and their stability to storage in cold. Unpublished manuscript.
50. Ranade SS, Talwalkar GV, Padwal AJ, Trivedi PN: Pulsed NMR studies in malignant lymphoma: *T1* values of metastatic lymph node. Unpublished manuscript.
51. Rilke F, Clemente C, Pilotti S: Morfologia nuclear nelle biopsie retalli negative e false negative. Tumori *61*:199–209, 1975.
52. Ross RJ, Thompson JS, Kim K, Bailey R: Nuclear magnetic resonance imaging and evaluation of human breast tissue: Preliminary clinical trials. Radiology *143*:195–205, 1982.
53. Saryan LA, Hollis DP, Economou JS, Eggleston JC: Nuclear magnetic resonance studies on cancer. IV. Correlation of water content with tissue relaxation times. JNCI *52*:599, 1974.
54. Shah S: Pulsed NMR studies on cancer. M.Sc. Thesis, Bombay University, 1977.
55. Shah S, Ranade SS, Kasturi SR, Phadke RS, Advani SH: Distinction between normal and leukemic bone marrow by water proton nuclear magnetic resonance relaxation times. Magn Reson Imag *1*:23, 1982.
56. Shah S, Ranade SS, Phadke RS, Kasturi SR: Significance of water proton spin-lattice relaxation times in normal and malignant tissues and their subcellular fractions. I and II. Magn Reson Imag *1*:91–104; 155–164, 1982.
57. Shah S: Significance of water proton spin-lattice relaxation times in subcellular fractions and their elemental profiles to pulsed NMR studies on cancer. Ph.D. Thesis, Bombay University, 1983.
58. Sirsat MV, Doctor VM: Mucosal patterns in carcinoma of the oesophagus. Ind J Cancer *2*:131–134, 1965.
59. Smith W, Huchinson JM, Mallard JR, Johnson G, Redpath TW, Selbei RD, Reid A, Smith CC: Oesophageal carcinoma demonstrated by whole body NMR imaging. Br Med J *262*:510–512, 1981.
60. Smuckler EA, Koplitz M, Smuckler DE: Isolation of animal cell nuclei in subcellular components. Preparation and fractionation. *In* Birnie GD, Rickwood D (eds):Centrifugal Separations in Molecular and Cell Biology. London, Butterworth and Co., 1976, pp 1–58.
61. Spohrer M, Civan MM: Pulsed nuclear magnetic resonance study of ^{17}O from H_2 ^{17}O in rat lymphocytes. Biophys J *16*:606–610, 1976.
62. Sujata GK: Pulsed NMR studies of malignant lymphomas. Ph.D. Thesis, University of Bombay, 1984.
63. Sujata GK, Shrinivasan VT, Ranade SS, Singh BB, Talwalkar GV: Proton spin-lattice relaxation times in lymphnodes afflicted with lymphoma. Indian J Exp Biol *22*:407–409, 1984.
64. Sujata GK, Nair M, Ranade SS: Iron, zinc, copper, manganese and magnesium in malignant lymphoma. Sci Total Environ *42*:237–243, 1985.
65. Wagh UV, Kasturi SR, Chaughule RS, Shah S, Ranade SS: Studies on proton spin-lattice relaxation times (*T1*) in experimental cell cultures. Physiol Chem Phys *9*:167, 1977.
66. Worthington BS: Clinical prospects of NMR. Clin Radiol *34*:3–12, 1983.
67. Abstracts of the 69th Annual Meeting of the Radiological Society of North America, Chicago, Nov. 1983. Radiology *149*, 1983.
68. Abstracts of the 2nd Annual Meeting of the Society of Magnetic Resonance in Medicine, June 1984. Magn Reson Med *1, 2*, 1984.
69. Ranade, SS: Cell type and proton relaxation. Invest Radiol 22:346–347, 1987.

XIV

INSTRUMENTATION

A Comparison of Resistive, Superconductive, and Permanent Magnets

WILLIAM H. OLDENDORF

Fundamental to all magnetic resonance (MR) devices is the need for an intense magnetic field that does not vary with time and that has very nearly the same field strength (is of high uniformity) throughout the anatomical region to be examined. Although technically this is the B_0 (B-zero) field, for clarity, it will be called here the main field, to distinguish it from all of the other much weaker fields that are intermittently superimposed on it in the scanning or measurement process.

A magnetic field is always a result of moving electrical charges. In most clinical MR devices the main field is generated by either superconductive magnets or electromagnets. Helical coils of conductor encircle the region of the body to be examined. They are precisely shaped, and the electron current passing through them is constant.

It is also possible to generate the required movement of charge without generating streams of charges in conductors. A few elements and certain alloys and ceramic substances have an electronic structure such that their atoms align with an applied magnetic field and remain in alignment (ferromagnetism) after the external field is removed, making the entire solid a magnet more or less permanently. When so magnetized, a field is maintained that requires no continued applied voltage and generates no heat.

ELECTROMAGNETS

When an electron current passes along a wire, a concentric magnetic field is created that diminishes in strength at points progressively distant from the wire. When five amperes of current pass along a straight wire, the magnetic field strength 1 cm from the wire is defined as 1 gauss. One ampere passing through each of five such parallel wires generates the same field strength (Fig. 69–1). Because some fields in common use are so strong that the number of gauss becomes cumbersome to use, a larger unit, the tesla (equals 10,000 gauss), has come into common usage. It commonly is abbreviated "T" (e.g., a 15 kilogauss field strength would become 1.5 tesla).

In a clinical scanner the conductor is either a wire or foil of conductor (usually an aluminum foil) or a superconductive (zero resistance) wire. Although aluminum is a good conductor of electrons, it does offer measurable resistance, and such magnets are called resistive. The type of magnet conductor used to make the main field is often used to classify the entire MR apparatus. It is either a "resistive" or a "superconductive" or a "permanent magnet" scanner. Until recently, it was thought that the method of creating the main field was of paramount importance in establishing the

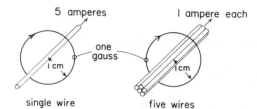

Figure 69–1. A straight wire carrying 5 amperes generates a concentric magnetic field about it. One centimeter from the conductor the field strength is arbitrarily defined as 1 gauss. On the left, 5 amperes are passing through a single conductor; on the right 1 ampere is passing through five insulated conductors. The magnetic field strength at 1 centimeter is still 1 gauss.

quality of a scanner. With experience it has become clear that there is much more to a scanner than the main field and that gradient and antenna coil design, excitation and reception coils, computer software, and scanning strategies are all as important as the magnitude of the main field. This does not diminish the importance of the main field quality, but to classify (and thus judge) the entire scanner on the basis of the main field's strength and the means of generating it is unjustifiable.

RESISTIVE MAGNETS

Most commercial main fields have a strength of 1000 to 5000 gauss, and the two main manufacturers of resistive magnets use a few thousand spirally wound layers of aluminum foil strips (about 15 cm wide) as the conductors, limiting field strength to about 1500 gauss. This limitation is due to the heat dissipated in the aluminum by the very large currents required. The electrical resistance of a typical clinical MR magnet is about 1 ohm. The current needed to make a 1500 gauss field is 200 to 250 amperes. Power dissipation, in watts, is current squared × resistance in ohms. Thus, such a coil generates about 50,000 watts (50 kW) dissipated as heat in the coil. Since the field strength is proportional to current, and power dissipation rises with the square of current, to raise the field strength to 3000 gauss would dissipate 200 kW. The required high-grade power supply is simply impractical, since it is prohibitively expensive and the necessary raw power is not ordinarily available.

Heat from the aluminum foil is dissipated by passing deionized cooling water past one or both edges of each coil assembly to an external heat-exchanger. Fifty kW of heat is approximately the heat produced by a passenger automobile engine and the heat exchanger is equivalent to the automobile's radiator. Fifty kW is manageable, but 200 kW would become a major engineering feat. Surprisingly, high quality, stable, and reliable power supplies are now available that will provide 50 kW at a reasonable cost.

If it were practical to substitute copper foil for the aluminum foil conductor, heat production would fall to about 30 kW. Although prohibitively expensive, substituting silver would drop the power requirement by about another 6 percent over copper. Aluminum is less than one third as dense as copper but has 58 percent of its conductance. A trade-off has been made in favor of aluminum based on cost and weight.

If an infinitely fine wire conductor is spirally wound around a nonmagnetic sphere starting at one point on the sphere and leaving precisely opposite the origin, the cavity of the sphere will have a perfectly uniform field (Fig. 69–2A and B). Such a magnet, however, would leave no access for the patient. Providing holes at the end for patient access allows the field to bulge out, destroying the required internal uniformity. The four coil arrangement approximates this sphere, but the end coils are made smaller to create a slightly higher field near these apertures, thus tending to repel the bulging field back inside, compensating for the defect produced by the access holes.

If two circular coils with the same radius, R, are arranged on a common axis and parallel to each other and separated by R, an arrangement called a Helmholtz pair

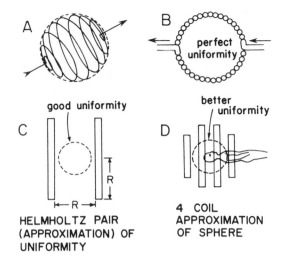

Figure 69–2. The most uniform and strongest field, using the least length of conductor, is made by spirally wrapping a conductor around an imaginary sphere, the current going in from the left into *A* and ultimately emerging opposite its point of entry. *B* shows this spirally wound coil in a cross section, cut through the entry and exit conductors. Within such a spherically wound coil the field is perfectly uniform. *C* shows that if two circular coils are arranged parallel to each other and are separated by a distance equal to their radius, such a "Helmholz pair" forms the largest field of good uniformity possible with two coils. *D* shows the usual arrangement in resistive MR scanners. In addition to the two central coils that approximate the positioning of the Helmholz pair, there is a smaller pair of end coils. The overall configuration of these four coils approximates the surface of the sphere. The end coils are slightly smaller, however, to contain the field, which would otherwise bulge out.

results (Fig. 69–2*C*), and this provides the maximum-sized volume of uniformity in the center of two coils.

The configuration of clinical resistive magnets typically is an extension of the Helmholtz pair. Four coils are arranged relative to each other as shown in Figure 69–2*D*.

Field uniformity is worse with resistive magnets than with superconductive magnets for several reasons. In an attempt to use minimal lengths of conductor (to reduce heat generation), the coils are made small relative to the patient. In general, the larger the magnet relative to the patient, the greater will be the volume of acceptable uniformity. The four independent coil units in the usual resistive systems are difficult to position exactly parallel and undistorted in the presence of the magnetomotive forces to which they are subjected when their fields are on. The electronic current supply is very stable but, inevitably, imperfectly regulated.

Despite its limited field strength, resistive main coils have some attractive features. Their manufacturing cost is low compared with superconductive coils. Their electrical power cost is only 6 to 10 dollars per hour while operating. They can be easily turned on and off when not in use.

Near the center of such a solenoid (a spirally wound coil), 1 meter in diameter, the relationship between field strength, current, and number of turns can be approximated by:

$$\text{Field strength (in gauss)} = \frac{\text{total number of turns} \times \text{amperes}}{200}$$

To produce a 1500 gauss field requires that approximately 200 amperes be passed through 1500 turns of conductor.

FIELD UNIFORMITY

Chemical analytic spectrometers often have fields that differ, within the region examined, by less than one part per billion (10^{-9}) over a 5 millimeter diameter volume. This extreme uniformity is unnecessary in clinical imagers, where the most stringent requirements now foreseen are 1 part per 10 million in tissue volumes perhaps 10 cm in diameter.

If chemical shift spectroscopy is the objective, better than 1 part in 10 million is

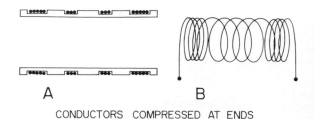

A   B

CONDUCTORS COMPRESSED AT ENDS

Figure 69–3. If the length of coil is of no concern, a simple spirally wound solenoid coil will not create a uniform field near its center unless the coil is very long relative to its width. This can be corrected for short solenoids by making the windings at the end more closely spaced than in the middle, as shown in *B*. *A* shows, in longitudinal section, the general arrangement of superconducting wires wrapped on a precision machined cylinder, usually of aluminum. Although the coils are all wrapped on one cylinder, because there are more turns at the ends, one approaches the four coil approximation of a sphere shown in Figure 69–2*D*. However, considerably greater lengths of conductor are needed to wrap this on a simple cylinder as in *A*. Since this configuration is used only with superconducting magnets, where the length of wire is immaterial, it is a practical way to get the greatest mechanical rigidity for stable positioning of the coil wires. This is particularly so at high field strengths where there is a great magnetostrictive force tending to pull all of these coils toward a common center. This is more rigidly and precisely supported by a single piece of machined aluminum.

necessary. Depending upon spatial resolution requirements and the reconstruction method used, 1 part in 10,000 may be adequate for clinical hydrogen imaging. There is little reason to aim at clinical spatial resolution better than about 0.5 mm, since there is approximately this much movement even in the most cooperative patient due to ballistocardiographic and respiratory effects.

When discussing uniformity, the size of the field must be stated. As this volume gets smaller, any given magnet shows greater uniformity. Although the uniformity for a 50 cm field might be only 1 part in 100,000, and thus unacceptable for spectroscopy, a surface (topical) coil might examine only a 6 to 10 cm region of the total field, and within this smaller volume the uniformity could be quite acceptable for spectroscopy.

No magnet is perfectly shaped, nor are its coils perfectly spaced, nor will its surroundings be entirely nonmagnetic, owing to structural steel and other factors. To allow fine tuning for maximal uniformity (shimming), several movable ferrous rods are placed outside the coils. Threaded adjustments of coil positions are often also provided in resistive systems. Variable electromagnetic coils can also be used for shimming.

In resistive magnets of certain designs, the four coils must be positioned with great precision relative to the others. This is made more difficult by the magnetostrictive forces that result from coil interactions trying to pull the coils toward their common center. Positioning and magnetostriction problems would be helped if the coils could be wrapped about a precision-machined aluminum cylinder with appropriately spaced grooves for the coils on its outer surface. An effect comparable to the hypothetically wrapped sphere could be created by placing more turns of conductor at the ends of a cylinder than near its center (Fig. 69–3). This would use much more resistive coil length and so generate more heat than the sphere approximation. If heat generation were nonexistent, as much conductor as necessary could be used. This is the case with superconductive magnets where the conductor resistance is zero so no heat is generated.

SUPERCONDUCTIVE MAGNETS

Most metals show an electrical resistance that is roughly proportional to their absolute (Kelvin) temperature. Cooling causes their resistance to drop. The resistance of the tungsten filament in an incandescent lamp at room temperature is only about one tenth that when it is lighted.

Progressively cooling a conductor while measuring its resistance shows a nearly linear drop as absolute zero is approached. With many metals, at their individual critical temperatures near absolute zero, the resistance falls to zero (Fig. 69–4), their conductivities become infinite, and they are said to be superconductive. It is difficult to

Figure 69–4. This figure shows the tendency of most metals to show a resistance approximately proportional to absolute temperature. But at some point in the cooling curve, many metals suddenly become superconductors and have no resistance. The boiling point of helium is about 4° above absolute zero (4.2°K). Therefore, helium is the only practical working fluid that can be used to cool a niobium-titanium alloy wire into its superconducting range. Although superconductivity as high as 23°K has been recorded with certain niobium alloys, the niobium-titanium wires in general use are cooled to 4°K. The superconducting magnets decay very slowly, losing perhaps 1 percent per year of their field, mainly because of the junctions between the pieces of superconducting wire. These junctions, which have a very small resistance, are necessary because of the several kilometers' total length of wire used.

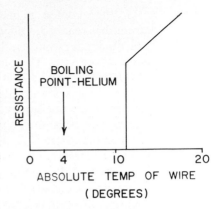

accept the notion that the resistance of a conductor is, literally, zero. The temperature at which this happens is variable. Ordinary lead (Pb) becomes superconductive below 7.4° K. The most practical means of maintaining something that cold is to immerse it in liquid helium, which boils at 4.2° K. It clearly would be desirable to use a conductor that had a critical temperature as high as possible. Certain niobium-titanium alloys have critical temperatures above 20° K. The niobium-titanium alloys used for clinical magnets typically are superconductive at 10 to 15° K. It might be thought that a zero resistance conductor could carry an infinitely large current, but there is a limit for any given conductor at a given temperature and field strength above which it becomes resistive, causing resistive heating.

A superconductive magnet is constructed on a precision-machined cylinder, usually of aluminum. On its outer surface are grooves for the cables of niobium-titanium conductor. The conductors are clustered in groups of four or six, with more conductors near the ends of the cylinder. The cylinder and its coils are then suspended in liquid helium. The helium container is suspended in a vacuum chamber, which, in turn, is surrounded by liquid nitrogen (70° K), and this in turn is surrounded by an evacuated chamber. This rather elaborate assembly (Fig. 69–5) is understandably expensive and requires a very knowledgeable group to make a reliable product. Two commercial companies make essentially all of the clinical superconductive magnets at present.

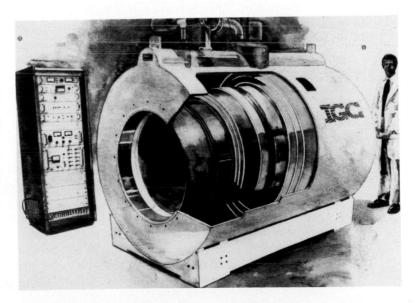

Figure 69–5. The complex internal structure of a modern superconducting magnet is shown in this cutaway view. In addition to the superconductors, there are gradient coils and excitation and data acquisition coils plus the multilayer insulation compartments required to minimize helium boil-off. (Courtesy of Intermagnetics General Corporation, Voorheesville, New York.)

When cooled at installation, the current is started, and when the desired field strength is reached, a superconductive switch is closed and no further power is required. For practical purposes, the current runs indefinitely and only a few gauss drop in field occurs each year. This slow drop is largely due to the junctions between tandem pieces of conductor. Since it is impractical to draw out a single piece of niobium-titanium-copper wire several kilometers long, lesser lengths must be joined together. These junctions are not superconductive and contribute a very small resistance so that, in reality, the coils do not have zero resistance. The field declines so slowly from week to week that there is no practical effect in the short term. No small "ripple" is evident, as is inevitable in resistive power supplies.

Superconductive magnets are permanent magnets in the sense that they maintain field without outside power. Other than replenishing their liquid gases and maintaining vacuum, they should require no maintenance for several years.

The design of these large, delicate devices has greatly improved in the past several years. Typically, the loss of helium is only about 250 ml/hour. This is about one fifth the loss in the early models, some five years ago, and is due largely to improvements in suspension of the various internal supports between chambers, offering a poorer heat conductivity path from the outside room. Preventing the helium from boiling off is a formidable problem and can be best appreciated by thinking of the outside room as an oven some 300° C hotter than the helium.

Superconductivity is a delicate phenomenon and can disappear seemingly without reason. The magnet is said to "quench," and the field drops to zero. Fear has been expressed in the past lest a quench occur with a patient in position. Quenches are most likely to happen while technicians are working on the systems, and a patient is unlikely to be inside during these times. With the advanced design of modern superconductive magnets, several factors make it unlikely that a quench will be dangerous to a patient in the magnet or a person nearby the magnet.

For a variety of reasons, such as mechanical movement of a conductor rubbing against an adjacent conductor (generating a small but significant amount of frictional heat), a section of the conductor can "go resistive." This has been solved by surrounding the niobium-titanium with a substantial layer of copper, which, although it cannot be made superconductive, at 10° K has only about 2 percent of its resistance at room temperature. This acts as a shunt for the small region of resistive niobium-titanium until the niobium-titanium again cools into its superconductive range. In a sense, the copper cladding serves as a bandage and "heals" any small regions of niobium-titanium that are driven out of their superconductive temperature range.

After a total quench, depending on its cause, down time could be several hours to several weeks. The cause must be determined, and this usually is some defect in the liquid helium containment. After the cause has been corrected, the entire helium content of the magnet will likely have to be replaced and, after cooling, the build-up of field cannot be instantaneous, typically being built up over several hours.

Quenching of superconductive magnets might be thought of as the MR equivalent of the x-ray tube failure in computerized tomography, an expensive source of unreliability. Quenching is much rarer than x-ray tube failure, but each event is costly.

Liquid nitrogen is universally available, but liquid helium is not. Its cost is correspondingly variable. It is present in underground gas deposits because of alpha decay of long-lived radioactive substances such as thorium and its daughters. Because it is a noble, monatomic gas and has an atomic mass of only 4, it is highly diffusible and so can be isolated commercially from natural gas either by simple diffusion through a membrane or by liquefaction. Since helium cannot burn, it is a useless component if it remains with the gas. Although easily produced by anyone having a substantial supply of natural gas, there has not been widespread recovery of helium (and particularly its liquefaction) because of the lack of a market. The 1987 liquid helium price in the United States is about five dollars per liter.

If helium loss is a serious economic problem, it is possible (and commercially available) to maintain superconductivity by an entirely closed, multiple stage refrigeration system. Such a refrigerant system could be at some distance from the scanner and would consume 5 to 20 kW.

Superconductive magnets can be quite large relative to the patient. Currently there is interest in coil diameters in the vicinity of 2 meters. Coupled with their inherently constant current, these large, mechanically stable magnets offer high field strengths and great uniformity of field. It is entirely practical to make a 2 to 4 tesla clinical magnet and, indeed, some of the currently installed scanners have a magnet capable of 2 tesla. Whether or not such strong fields will find any wide clinical use is today highly controversial. Most of the currently available superconductive systems use fields of about 0.35 to 0.6 tesla, considerably below their rated maximum. This seems to be adequate for high resolution clinical hydrogen imaging. Very good images are now available from a 0.15 tesla (see legend of Fig. 69–6) and even a 0.09 tesla resistive scanner. One such resistive scanner, with a field of only 200 gauss, is now being marketed (Fig. 69–7). It produces clinically useful images, and the entire question of field strength must be reconsidered. Each company seems to promote the notion that the field strength of its particular scanner is ideal.

The longitudinal field created by most electromagnets results in the positioning of the patient in a deep tunnel in which he or she feels isolated. Access to the patient for conversation, instructions, and life-support systems is limited. This is quite different from the very shallow gantry opening of a CT scanner, where the patient is very accessible and has no sense of confinement and where the machine is essentially noiseless. The large bore diameter of modern superconductive magnets (Fig. 69–6) considerably lessens the feeling of confinement.

When considering the strength of these main fields, the spread of the field (fringe

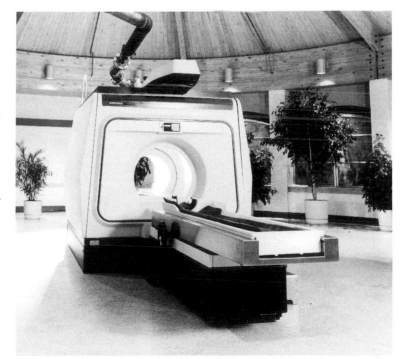

Figure 69–6. A state-of-the-art superconducting gantry installed in a large, circular, nonferromagnetic structure dedicated to this scanner. A vent for cooling gases is shown emerging from the top of the gantry. The same company makes a similar-appearing (but smaller) gantry, which makes excellent pictures even though it has a field strength of only 0.15 tesla, requires much less space and costs about half that of its larger brother shown here. The large bore diameter possible with superconducting magnets makes patients more accessible and lessens their sense of isolation and claustrophobia. (Courtesy of Technicaire Corp., Solon, Ohio.)

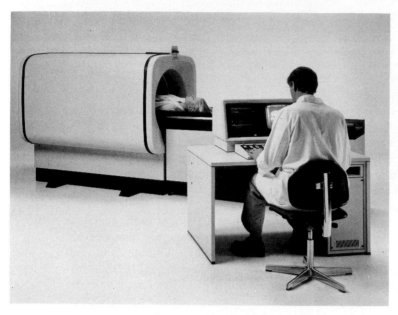

Figure 69-7. This clinical scanner uses a resistive copper solenoid to create a 200 gauss field (0.02 tesla). Actually, this particular machine is operating at 197 gauss, corresponding to a hydrogen frequency of about 800 kHz. The power supply for this magnet provides 3 KW, and the scanner produces 4 slices in 5 minutes. The spatial resolution appears to be 2 to 3 mm but the *T1* or *T2* enhanced images appear to show greater lesion contrast than higher field scanners. The stated installed cost in mid 1985, with electrical shielding and one independent viewing console, is less than $400,000. From initial clinical experience, it appears to be very useful despite its lower spatial resolution. (Courtesy of Instrumentarium Corp., Helsinki, Finland.)

field) must be taken into account (Fig. 69–8). When we state that there is a 1 tesla field in the magnet, we are defining the number of magnetic lines per unit cross section inside the coils. These same lines must have a return path around the exterior of the magnet. This external field spreads out to include all of the surrounding space, but fortunately (in the first 5 to 10 meters) the field strength falls off approximately with the inverse cube of distance rather than by inverse square, as one might intuitively believe. This means that the field strength falls by eight rather than four each time the distance from the magnet is doubled. If it actually fell off with inverse square, it would probably be impractical to consider placing one in a hospital because the space requirement would be prohibitive. Federal regulations require that all space having more than a 5 gauss field strength have controlled public access. High field magnets require correspondingly more controlled space. At any particular distance from the magnet the field strength is proportional to the magnet's strength. This spread of the field is an inherent disadvantage of either type of electromagnet.

As the field converges at both ends of the magnet, large gradients exist and these suck in ferromagnetic materials brought into these regions. This could include wrenches, oxygen tanks, and so on. This is called the missile effect and is a greater problem with stronger magnets (Fig. 69–8).

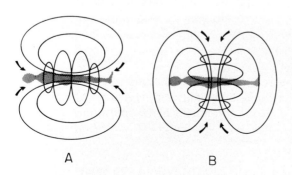

A   B

Figure 69-8. The four-coil arrangement used with resistive systems can either have the field passing longitudinally through the patient, which is the usual configuration as shown in *A*, or have the field pass at right angles to the patient, with the patient positioned between the two center coils (*B*). This latter arrangement has two major advantages. Having the field transverse allows a simple solenoid antenna to be wrapped around the patient, which is considerably more efficient than the saddle coils usually used for this purpose. Another advantage is that the missile effect, which is greatest in the strong gradient regions designated by the arrows, is moved into inaccessible positions above the gantry and near the floor, where they can be covered and are thus less likely to attract any ferromagnetic objects.

It would be desirable, in view of the preceding, to have very little external field and to have a shallow gantry opening with better access to the patient. Among other factors, these are advantages of permanent magnets.

PERMANENT MAGNETS

Many electromagnetic devices that require a strong, constant, and inexpensive field use a permanent magnet to generate this field. Such devices are loudspeakers, galvanometer movements, and small electric motors (Fig. 69–9).

A loudspeaker creates a very strong field (approaching 1 tesla) in a narrow gap in which a circular coil is suspended. This coil is attached to a movable, shallow cone of paper or plastic. Currents passed through the voice coil interact with the constant field, moving the cone to make sound. There are general similarities between a loudspeaker and an MR scanner, since both have a constant field in which a coil is suspended and interactions between the two produce a useful result. Although the main field of loud-speakers was, prior to the end of World War II, generated by resistive electromagnets, the postwar availability of alnico (developed by the Japanese before the War) made much stronger and more permanent fields possible, and resistive magnets were abandoned. Today, no one would consider making a loudspeaker with an electromagnetic source of main field. Although the field strength in a loudspeaker is about as strong as in an MR scanner, its dimensional volume and uniformity are very much less.

MR scanners are elaborations of chemical spectral MR analyzers in which a strong, uniform main field has a small volume of high uniformity in which a 5 to 10 mm specimen is positioned. The original MR scanners were made by inserting the gradient, excitation and data recovery coils into the region normally occupied by a test tube containing the substance to be analyzed. The fundamental differences between the main field require-

Figure 69–9. Several magnetic devices in which a coil is placed in a strong magnetic field and interacts with this field, carrying out some useful function, are shown. *A*, The voice coil of a loudspeaker attached to the loudspeaker cone, with the coil is in a narrow gap in the magnetic path, is shown. In this case, a resistive coil is used to generate the magnetic field. *B*, After World War II, when alnico permanent magnets became available, they were substituted for the earlier resistive source of magnetic field, and essentially all loudspeakers use a permanent magnet as the source of the main magnetic field because it is inexpensive, simple, and permanent. *C* shows a galvanometer movement in which, again, a coil is suspended on a spring-loaded support, which is itself on a bearing and has a pointer attached to it. As current is passed through this coil, interaction of the current and the field in the small gap causes the galvanometer movement to rotate to the right, indicating the amount of current flowing. *D* shows the general arrangement of a simple "H" frame permanent magnet NMR gantry in which the patient is placed between the permanent magnet pole faces.

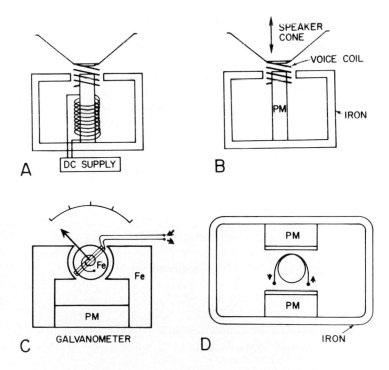

ments of a clinical MR scanner and a chemical analyzer are that the field strength and uniformity requirements are lower and the specimen much larger in the clinical scanner.

Chemical shift spectral analyzers are manufactured by several companies, and each offers a range of quality. At the lower end of each line usually are permanent magnet devices. They have the disadvantage relative to the top of the line, that their field strength is limited to less than about 1.2 tesla because they have iron in their magnetic circuit and iron saturates above this field strength (Fig. 69–10). Electromagnets with air (which is not saturable) as their entire magnetic path medium can generate a very strong field. The extreme uniformity offered by air-path electromagnets, particularly the superconductive magnets, cannot be achieved by permanent magnets.

Although several exotic MR permanent magnet designs have been suggested, most efforts have used a simple "H" configuration (Fig. 69–11) as used in chemical analyzers. An elliptical or rectangular iron frame has within it a pair of permanent magnets forcing magnetic flux through a gap in which the patient is placed. The field is inherently transverse to the long axis of the patient, unlike most MR electromagnets in which the field parallels this axis. If sufficient iron is included in the return path, most of the field will be confined and will not spread into the room. Because there is little external field, much less room area is needed.

Magnetic field lines repel each other much as do electrical charges. If not confined, they tend to bulge out of any gap in the iron magnetic path. In chemical analyzers, the pole faces are machined very flat and moved very close to each other relative to their diameter (a small gap to width ratio). The field bulge at the edges of the gap is minimal and does not much affect the uniformity at its center, where the small test tube is to be placed. The edge bulge effect on the center field uniformity can be lessened by building an electrical conductor around the pole face edges, thus building up the field, or by raising the edge by a layer of ferromagnetic foil. The slight increase in field strength at the pole edge pushes the more central field toward the pole face center. The percentage of the pole face diameter used is about 1 percent. If such a magnet were simply scaled up to include a volume large enough for human scanning, the weight of magnet, and particularly the iron return path, would be impractically great.

To be of a practical size and weight, it is necessary to use a much larger fraction of the pole face diameter and to increase the gap to width ratio considerably by pulling the pole faces apart. This results in a considerably greater bulge at the edge of the field and destroys the uniformity at the center. To enlarge the central volume of uniformity, the pole faces must deviate considerably from flat. The shape of these pole faces has not yet been optimized, but obtaining an acceptably large volume of uniformity probably will require some combination of pole face shaping supplemented by a final shimming by electromagnetic means but probably requiring little electrical power.

Several types of permanet magnet materials can be used. These include alnico, ceramic, and rare-earth magnets. The latter are probably too expensive to consider.

MAGNETIZATION

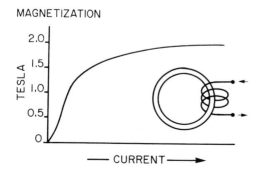

Figure 69–10. In an iron doughnut with a coil wrapped around it, the iron becomes magnetized more strongly as the current through the coil increases. Although fairly linear up to about 1 tesla, the iron becomes saturated at about 2 tesla and cannot become further magnetized. This limits the flux density that can be achieved in the iron return paths of a permanent magnet.

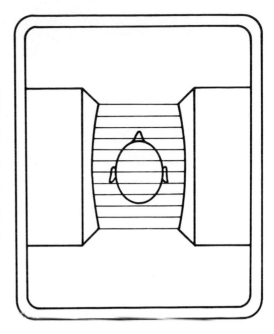

Figure 69–11. A very schematic arrangement in which permanent magnets on either side of the patient's head create a magnetic field in the patient's head and the magnetic lines are returned through the external rectangular iron return paths. The shaping of the pole faces is problematic, and although it is easy to obtain 0.1 to 0.3 tesla magnetic field strength, it is very difficult to shape the pole faces mechanically to produce a useful volume of magnetic flux of high uniformity. If this problem is overcome, permanent magnets have the great advantages of low initial cost, high stability, no power requirement, and no liquid gas requirement. Since the field is contained within the iron frame, there is essentially no fringe field, allowing it to be placed in a relatively small space. One commercial permanent magnetic scanner is shown in Figure 69–12.

Because of their low cost and long life, ceramics are attractive. Although some of the exotic magnetic materials, such as samarium-cobalt, generate a strong field per unit weight, the savings in weight are much less than expected because the iron in the return path must still be provided and therein lies most of the total magnet weight. The field strength in this return path should be kept below about 1 tesla because higher flux densities cause the field to leave the iron into the surrounding air. Above 2 tesla (at which strength the iron is saturated and cannot carry any more flux) all further attempts at increasing the field in the iron path push the flux into the surrounding space, thus negating one of the major advantages of permanent magnets, their limited fringe field. If the magnetic material itself weighed nothing, the total system weight would be reduced by only $\frac{1}{4}$ to $\frac{1}{3}$. It is probably impractical to make a field strength greater than about 0.3 tesla using permanent magnets unless weight is no consideration.

It appears practical to generate the main field of an MR scanner using permanent magnets as the source. One such unit is commercially available with a field strength of 0.3 tesla (Fig. 69–12). Although very heavy (90,000 kg) it makes excellent images and requires very little power. Its design is proprietary, but it probably generates the field by permanent magnets with supplementary field adjustment (shimming) done electrically. Its initial cost is about the same as superconductive scanners but has no maintenance cost and can be installed in a relatively small (but well-supported) space because of its low fringe field. Importantly, this magnet proves that there are no insurmountable obstacles presented by the proximity (and thus interaction) of the gradient and other coils with the nearby ferromagnetic pole faces. Hopefully, the success of this pioneering magnet will encourage further development of permanent magnets.

Among the major advantages of a permanent magnet should be ease of manufacture, weight under about 3000 to 5000 kg, long life without appreciable field strength loss, low cost, and low external field.

How strong should the main field be? This has been a highly controversial area, having been the center of heated discussion since 1983, when commercialization of scanners began in earnest. Because all of the practical limitations on field strength become worse as the field increases, the ideal field is the least that will "do the job." Since the jobs that MR will be asked to do have not been defined as yet, it is impossible

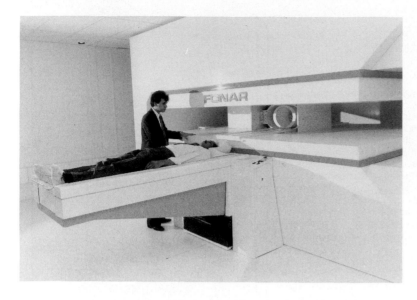

Figure 69–12. A commercially available permanent magnet (0.3 tesla) that makes excellent images. It has large pole faces and a correspondingly massive field return path. This pioneering magnet is heavy (90,000 kg) but proves the feasibility of the permanent magnet for clinical scanning. Having a trivial fringe field, it requires essentially no site preparation other than assuring adequate structural support. (Courtesy of Fonar Corp., Milbrook, New York.)

to suggest an overall ideal field strength. Even so, it is useful to list the two advantages and some of the many disadvantages accrued as the field strength rises (Table 69–1).

ADVANTAGES

The emitted signal strength rises because a larger population of nuclei are available to be driven into their high-energy state. Getting back the most signal is particularly important when examining rare and inefficiently resonant nuclei, such as ^{13}C, ^{23}Na, and ^{31}P.

Table 69–1. ADVANTAGES AND DISADVANTAGES OF RESISTIVE, SUPERCONDUCTIVE, AND PERMANENT MAGNETS

	Advantages	Disadvantages
Resistive magnets	Inexpensive Readily available Can be turned off No liquid gases No vacuum Reliable	Ltd uniformity (10^{-5}) Ltd strength 0.2 tesla max Cooling required Power consumption ± 50 kW Quality power supply Fringe field Poor patient access
Superconductive magnets	High fields possible (greater than 2 tesla) High uniformity better than 1 part/million	High cost Liquid gases required Gas boil off $10–20,000/yr Can quench (rare) Quench costly: time & money Fringe field Poor patient access
Permanent magnets	Can be inexpensive No power consumption No major power supply Weak fringe field No gases Cannot quench No heat generated Good patient access Transverse field	Ltd strength <0.3 tesla Ltd uniformity 10^{-5} max

Stronger fields are important when hydrogen or phosphorus chemical shift spectroscopy (which has a large future) is considered. Not only is the signal from any particular peak stronger, but the peaks are more separated. Chemical shifts of spectral peaks are expressed in parts per million of the resonant frequency. Since the resonant frequency of any particular nucleus is proportional to field strength, the absolute frequency separation of spectral peaks is proportional to field strength; the peaks are moved farther apart at higher fields, simplifying their electronic separation.

DISADVANTAGES

Cost rises with field strength. It is probably impractical to create a resistive magnet stronger than about 0.2 tesla. Permanent magnets probably are limited to about 0.3 tesla. This becomes a crucial field strength threshold because above this level, one must resort to the much more expensive superconductive magnets. It is paradoxical that two of the major manufacturers are selling superconductive scanners that could operate at much higher field strengths but choose to run them at only 0.35 tesla, not far beyond that achievable at much less cost by a resistive or permanent magnet. Superconductive magnets now being routinely delivered are designed to make a 2 tesla field but can be run at any lower field strength desired.

The amount of building space that must be dedicated to the magnet rises because of the fringe field created by electromagnets. The acceptable 5 gauss field line is pushed farther away, and site preparation costs rise. This fringe field can be very annoying in that it will distort TV and computer screen images at considerable distances. Many video cameras cannot be used within 5 to 10 meters of the magnet.

Elongated ferromagnetic materials in the body (such as some vascular clips) experience a torque tending to orient them parallel to the field. This could be a problem in some patients, and the torque would be proportional to field strength. Fortunately, most metallic prosthetic materials implanted surgically are not significantly ferromagnetic.

Effects on cardiac pacemakers can be expected to be greater at high fields. Pacemaker effects are a problem with which we must eventually contend if widespread use of NMR is to be implemented.

Stronger gradient and especially excitation fields are needed at higher field strengths to fully capitalize on the greater signal strength capability, causing more tissue heating.

The strong currents present intermittently in the various gradient coils cause them to act like the voice coil in a loudspeaker and their on-off activity results in a click or thump heard by the patient. With multislice excitation this becomes a very loud and, to some patients, disturbing noise. This gradient coil noise increases with the square of the field strength (assuming a proportionate gradient strength) and undoubtedly contributes to the claustrophobic response of a small percentage of patients.

The energy stored in the field (which must be dissipated during a quench) rises with the square of field strength. Any ill effects of a quench on patients or the apparatus itself increase accordingly. The missile effect, sucking ferromagnetic materials such as wrenches and gas tanks into the ends of the magnet, is greater at high fields.

The resonant frequency of hydrogen rises proportionately with field strength (42 MHz at 1 tesla), causing selective phase shifts and differential absorption by different tissues. This has not been the problem it was feared to be for hydrogen imaging, since very high quality images have been produced at 64 MHz (1.5 tesla).

In conclusion, one should not judge a scanner solely on the means of generating its main field, field strength, or uniformity. There is growing evidence that excellent hydrogen images can be made with field strengths in the range of 0.15 to 0.3 tesla (and very useful images at 0.02 tesla), a range that can be met with relatively inexpensive resistive or permanent magnets. Such small permanent magnets, with their negligible fringe fields, could be placed in a space no greater than required for a CT scanner, thereby creating a large market that will bring the capabilities of NMR imaging to areas that could not justify a much more costly system; costly in original purchase price, site preparation, and maintenance.

ACKNOWLEDGMENTS

The author would like to thank Eddy A. Gosschalk, Leon D. Braun, Richard E. Stelter, Dr. Slade L. Carr, William H. Oldendorf, Jr., and Nancy H. Rose for their help in preparation of the manuscript and editorial assistance.

Suggested Reading

1. Becker JJ: Permanent magnets. Sci Am *223*:92, 1970.
2. Montgomery DB: Solenoid Magnet Design: The Magnetic and Mechanical Aspects of Resistive and Superconducting Systems. New York, Wiley-Interscience, 1969.
3. Kinzler JE, Tanenbaum M: Superconducting magnets. Sci Am *206*:60, 1962.
4. Hulon JK, Matthias BT: High field, high current superconductors. Science *290*:881, 1980.
5. Hulon JK, Kunzler JE, Matthias BT: The road to superconducting materials. Physics Today 34, 1981.

70

Principles of Superconducting Magnets

CHARLES E. ROOS
HOWARD T. COFFEY
KENNETH R. EFFERSON

The images of body organs obtained by whole body nuclear magnetic resonance (NMR) techniques and the potential they offer in medical diagnosis are well documented in Chapters 10 to 45. Some of these images have been obtained using conventional resistive magnets, and others have been obtained using superconducting magnets in the NMR system. The choice between these two types of magnets will be determined to some extent by the magnetic field at which the system is to operate. At high fields, the choice will be in favor of superconducting magnet systems. Currently, some whole body NMR experiments are also being performed with water cooled copper magnets. However, the versatile superconducting magnet systems seem to have already won the contest, since all the major MRI manufacturers are now producing them as rapidly as possible. In fact it has been reported[1] that as many as 600 superconducting imaging system magnets have been manufactured worldwide up to the present time.

As noted earlier, clinical NMR studies of living tissue are most often concerned with the chemistry of hydrogen, carbon, and phosphorus. The electrical conductivity of body tissue and saline fluids limits the penetration of the radio frequency (rf) field into the body and thus limits the useful frequencies of the rf used to excite the NMR. Since the magnetic field and the rf field are directly related, this in turn limits the external magnetic field. For hydrogen studies, high quality images can be obtained in fields of less than 5000 gauss. There are still arguments on both sides as to whether or not much is to be gained in hydrogen imaging parameters by using higher fields. Chemical NMR spectroscopy on the other hand requires fields of 20,000 gauss or higher.

The most outstanding characteristic of superconducting magnets, and the characteristic that makes them most desirable in NMR imaging, is the absence of electrical resistivity in the superconducting state. To operate a superconducting magnet, it must be in a liquid helium environment at $4.2°$ K ($-453.6°$ F). At this temperature, the conductor loses its electrical resistance and conducts current without a power loss.

This highly desirable feature provides several benefits. One of these is the negligible power required for operating the magnet. Another is the extreme stability of the magnet when operated in what is called the persistent mode. This stability permits images to be made with greater resolution. After the magnet is energized, the terminals of the magnet may be electrically shorted using a superconductor to provide a continuous path that is without resistance. Consequently, with no dissipation available, the magnetic field is maintained constant over extended periods of time. This is a somewhat idealized description in that some resistance does occur in joints between conductors and within the conductor itself and can lead to a slight decay of the magnetic field over long periods. Nevertheless, stabilities of 1 part in 10^6 to 1 part in 10^7 per hour can be expected with these systems. Images can be made without adjustments to the magnetic field, and, indeed, the power supply can be turned off and the current leads to the magnet may be removed. With the current leads removed the only power necessary is that required for refrigeration. This refrigeration removes heat conducted into the system from the room and the trivial amount of heat generated in the joints of the magnet. A cryostat typical of the type required for whole body NMR imaging might evaporate about 0.5 liter per hour at a cost of $1.50 to $2.50 per hour, depending on the location in the United States and what sort of terms can be obtained from the liquid helium supplier. These prices may be higher in other countries where liquid helium is less readily available.

Many factors must be considered in designing a superconducting magnet to assure its proper performance. Some of these factors are (1) the magnetic field strength, bore size, and the stored energy in the system, (2) the magnetic field shape or homogeneity of the field, (3) the design of the superconducting wire to be used, (4) the mechanical design as related to the magnetic forces the differential cool down stresses, and (5) the problems associated with the quench (sudden loss of superconductivity) of a magnet.

It is not necessary to address all these topics in detail, but a brief review of some of the more important aspects might assist the practitioner in the selection of a magnet system. First we review a few fundamental concepts.

SUPERCONDUCTIVITY

Superconductivity is a phenomenon occurring in certain metals and alloys and characterized by the absence of electrical resistivity. This phenomenon is currently restricted to very low temperatures, although some active research indicates that higher temperature superconductors may someday become available.

Superconductors are divided into two types depending on their characteristic behavior in the presence of a magnetic field. Type I superconductors are usually pure metals, whereas Type II superconductors are comprised of intermetallic compounds. Only the latter are of interest in magnets; both, however, have one common feature: below a critical temperature, T_c, their resistance vanishes. T_c is as high as 23° K in some materials. In technically useful superconductors, however, T_c is in the range of 9 to 18° K (Fig. 70–1).

Current Density

The maximum current density sustainable by the conductor increases with reduced temperature. Similarly, as the magnetic field, $\overline{B}$, increases, the sustainable current

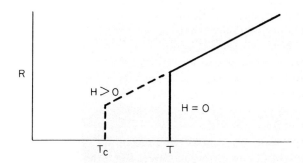

Figure 70–1. Relationship between resistance (R) and temperature (T) for Type II superconductors. T_c is a critical temperature at which R goes to zero.

density decreases. Consequently, the current density (j) magnetic field, and critical temperature are interdependent, j_c being a function of $\overline{B}$ and T, and B_c being a function of j and T. By increasing any of these parameters to a sufficiently high value, super-conductivity can be destroyed and the conductor will revert to the normally conducting state (Fig. 70–2).

Conductor Considerations

One of the most crucial factors in determining the performance of the final magnet is the design of the conductor. This design affects the ultimate field achieved by the magnet, the rate at which the magnet can be energized, and the drift rate in the persistent mode of operation. Several phenomena observed in magnets are caused by the conductor itself.

One of the earliest phenomena observed in superconducting magnets wound of single filament conductors is flux jumping. This arises from current induced in the conductor by the presence of transverse field generated by the magnet.

If the superconductor is placed transverse to the magnetic field, currents are set up in the conductor that shield the bulk of the conductor from the external magnetic field. These circulating currents extend along a length of the conductor, flowing in one direction on one side of the conductor and returning on the other to complete the circuit (Fig. 70–3).

Because the shielding currents are finite, increasing magnetic fields cannot be shielded by the surface currents and the field penetrates deeper into the conductor, exciting new shielding currents as it does. This process generates heat, which must somehow find its way through a very poor thermal conductor to the surface. When the field has penetrated deep enough so that the temperature rise in the superconductor is high enough where superconducting currents can no longer be supported, then an instability occurs wherein the magnetic field penetrates rapidly into the center of the conductor, heating it up to the point where it is no longer superconducting. This is the basic process called a flux jump. Since the conductor carries the basic magnet current in addition to the shielding current, the shielding currents add to the basic magnet current on one side of the conductor and subtract on the other side. This complicating factor can cause flux jumps at fields and currents that are quite low in comparison with expected values, and the conductor is driven into the resistive state. In this state, heat is dissipated in the small normal zone, and the attendant increase in temperature causes the normal zone to expand and propagate both along the length of the conductor and transverse to it. This results in the magnet being discharged as the energy in the magnet

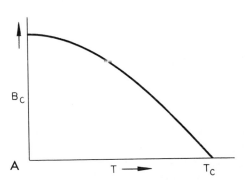
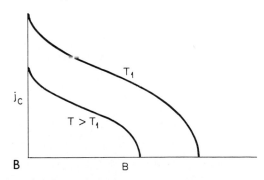

Figure 70–2. *A*, Inverse relationship between magnetic induction (B) and temperature (T). *B*, Similar inverse relationship between current density (j_c) and magnetic induction (B).

is dissipated in the resistive portion of the conductor, a process referred to as a "magnet quench."

It was found that this problem could be partly circumvented by embedding the superconductor in a copper matrix to form a composite conductor. The copper then provides a temporary path for the magnet current while the superconductor sustains a flux jump as well as providing additional heat capacity to reduce the temperature rise. If the resistance of the copper is low enough, it is possible for the temperature of the conductor to remain below the critical temperature and superconductivity will resume after the currents in the superconductor have decayed (Fig. 70–4).

Addition of the copper is effective, but flux jumping is always to be expected in single core copper-clad wire. This type of magnet, obviously, is dissipative, and the heat generated during a flux jump must be conducted to the helium bath. Thus, the magnetic field must be changed slowly to allow time for the heat to be conducted to and dissipated in the liquid helium. Also, the diamagnetic currents in the superconductor contribute to the field generated by the magnet and can reduce its homogeneity.

If, instead of one superconducting filament, many fine filaments of superconductor are used (Fig. 70–5), the screening currents around the individual superconductor filament penetrates easily to the center of the fine filaments. The heat produced during this process is easily transmitted to the cooled copper surfaces because of the short distances involved. Also, flux jumping can be avoided. Wires that have superconducting filaments small enough to eliminate flux jumping are called intrinsically stable conductors. Although this has the desired effect of avoiding flux jumps, if the conductors are parallel in the highly conductive normal matrix, circulating currents can again be formed. In this case, the circulating current is between two or more filaments in parallel with the current crossing over through the normally conductive matrix. The filaments in which the diamagnetic current and the gross transport current add together will reach their critical current much more rapidly than is expected and will cause the magnet to quench. To work at all, the rate at which the magnet is charged must be very slow in order to keep the diamagnetic currents at a low value (Fig. 70–6).

This problem has been largely circumvented in modern conductors by twisting the filaments in the conductor (Fig. 70–7). This causes the voltages due to flux changes from the external magnetic field to alternate in direction through adjacent loops and thus cancel out the long distance diamagnetic currents. This reduction in diamagnetism or hysteresis has two desirable effects. First, it reduces the amount of energy dissipation in the magnet and permits it to be charged more rapidly, and second, the reduced diamagnetism results in a better homogeneity and the current in the magnet is more linearly related to the magnetic field. Conductors of this type are used in producing MRI magnets as well as most other magnet types.

MAGNETS

Magnets, like the conductors with which they are wound, have unique phenomena that can occur in them. One of these is the training effect caused by wire motion.

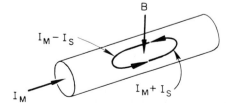

Figure 70–3. Single filament conductor in magnetic field B, with induced currents I_M and I_s.

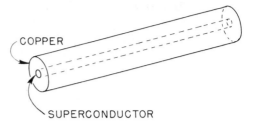

Figure 70–4. Composite conductor formed by embedding superconductor in a copper matrix.

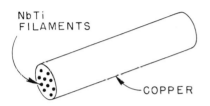

Figure 70–5. Multiple superconducting filaments in a copper matrix.

Figure 70–6. Production of diamagnetism by parallel superconductors tends to limit charging rate.

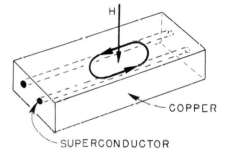

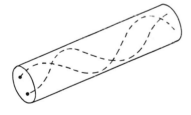

Figure 70–7. Twisting superconducting filaments reduces the diamagnetism effect.

Figure 70–8. Training effect caused by wire motion.

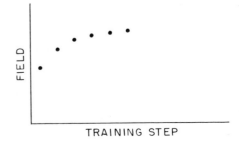

Training

The heat capacities of the materials in a superconducting magnet at 4° K are several orders of magnitude lower than the heat capacities of the same materials at room temperature. Thus, only a small amount of heat dissipated inside the magnet can raise the temperature of the conductor above its critical temperature (Fig. 70–8).

One source of heating is wire motion caused by the Lorentz force on the conductor in the magnet, i.e., the force on the wire caused by the interaction between the current and the magnetic field. Imperceptible motions of the wire can result in frictional heating sufficient to drive the conductor normal at fields well below the anticipated maximum field of the magnet. Upon re-energizing the magnet, it is frequently observed that it will "train" to successively higher fields before quenching. The wire might eventually reach a stable position, allowing the magnet to achieve the design field. In some cases, the wires will remain in their shifted positions and the magnet will perform well. In other cases, however, retraining is required after the magnet is warmed to room temperature and recooled. To avoid this training effect, it is necessary that the conductors be bonded securely in place to prevent the wire from moving. Various epoxies are used for this process. Bonding the conductor in the magnet entails a substantial risk, in that the conductor cannot economically be recovered and reused after it has been secured in place.

Since thermal conductivities are very low at these temperatures, any material used to bond the conductor also limits the thermal conductivity of the magnet. Consequently, the effects of wire motion are amplified, in that the heat generated is less effectively dissipated to the liquid helium. The conductors in most laboratory sized magnets are bonded in epoxy. The technique involves wet winding using a filled high thermal conductivity epoxy that is too viscous for vacuum impregnation.[5] Since each turn of the windings is visible as the magnet is being wound, voids in the epoxy can be avoided. Also, the relatively high thermal conductivity of this epoxy causes the heat generated during a quench to be better distributed throughout the coil, thereby reducing the thermal stresses caused by the quench.

Premature quenching can also occur if the large forces between coil sections result in the motion of one coil with respect to another. This is most likely to occur in magnets having coils that are wound in opposition. Such coils are used in Mossbauer magnets and magnets for nuclear demagnetization, where a low field region is required close to the high field region.

An alternative to bonded windings is to wind the magnet in such a manner that liquid helium permeates the windings. In this case, the liquid helium, which does have a high heat capacity at these temperatures, absorbs the heat generated when the windings move. The conductor used in this type of construction incorporates a much larger amount of copper to limit the electrical resistance and consequently the temperature increase when the superconductor is driven normal. The operating current density in this type of "cryostable" magnet is much lower than in the magnets described earlier. This kind of magnet is generally considered to be a "safe" magnet because it will not self-destruct during a quench by overheating or producing high voltage arcs. In fact, typical practice is to add so much copper to the wire that the copper is able to carry the entire magnet current while maintaining the superconductor at a low enough temperature to insure that it cannot possibly go normal. However, this type of construction is unsuitable for MRI magnets because its bulk and because its ventilated structure makes it difficult to keep the wires from moving due to the magnetic forces and thus ruining the homogeneity.

Quenching

Any superconducting magnet can be quenched by increasing the current and field indiscriminately. A quench in a well-encapsulated magnet typically starts at the location of the highest field in the magnet. One of the effects already discussed causes a small resistive region to occur in the wire. Joule heating (I^2R) then starts in the magnet. The normal zone continues to spread as the current and magnetic field drops rapidly. In high current density magnets like those used in MRI magnets, almost all of the energy contained in the magnetic field is initially dissipated in heating the windings. On a slower time scale the heat contained in the windings is conducted to the helium bath. The rapid discharge of cold helium gas from the quench of a 1.0 tesla, two mega-joule MRI magnet can be quite spectacular.

If the resistance across the terminals of the magnet due to the power supply is low, the magnet can be viewed as an inductor decaying into a time varying resistance $R(t)$. The resistive voltage, $iR(t)$, is counteracted by an inductive voltage, Ldi/dt. Unlike the few volts used in charging the magnet, the voltages encountered during a quench discharge can be measured in kilovolts. Initially, the iR voltage is confined to the layers of windings near the point where the quench originated and internal arcing can occur between layers if sufficient insulation has not been provided.

The voltage and temperature during a quench can be decreased by increasing the ratio of copper to superconductor in the magnet wire. However, this has the undesirable effect of reducing the current density in the magnet and results in a larger magnet to generate the same field. Other important techniques include (1) using conducting bob-bins such as aluminum to slow down the quench and absorb some of the energy and (2) breaking the magnet windings into many sections each of which can be paralleled (shunted) with a resistor to limit the voltage and, hopefully, distribute the quench over a larger portion of the magnet windings via mutual inductance coupling between sec-tions. This limits both the voltage and temperature in the windings. Suppliers of MRI magnets usually work out all these details with their first prototype. The customer then gets a production model that can withstand an accidental quench.

Persistent Mode Operation

After it has been energized, a superconducting magnet can be operated in the persistent mode by short-circuiting the magnet with a superconductor. This is accom-plished by connecting a section of superconducting wire across the terminals of the magnet. This section of superconductor can be heated to drive it into the resistive state so a voltage can be established across the terminals and the magnet can be charged or discharged.

To achieve persistent mode operation, the magnet current is held at a constant value, the heater is turned off, and the switch is permitted to cool into the supercon-ducting state. The power supply can then be turned off and the magnet current will circulate through the magnet and the persistent switch. The decay of the magnet field is given by $H = H_0 e^{-t/T}$ where T is the usual L/R time constant. The small residual resistance in the magnet arises from resistance in the joints or from the flux motion discussed earlier. The problem of flux motion only gets bad when the superconducting wire is carrying close to its maximum current at a given magnetic field. Thus this problem is easily solved by adding more superconductor to the wire than is necessary to achieve the maximum operating field. The problem of low joint resistances is more difficult. Since the typical MRI magnet will use well in excess of twenty miles of wire, it is not practical to wind the magnet with one piece of material. Thus, the magnet will have several joints. As far as is known to the authors, all MRI magnets use multi-filamentary material. A popular material for magnets producing 5000 gauss contains 24 filaments of superconductor. To make a joint, the copper has to be removed from the ends of the wires with nitric acid and the 48 filaments joined into a zero resistance blob. The MRI magnet manufacturers all have their own techniques for doing this, and they have to do it very well, because the failure of only one joint can give a resistance of about 10^{-8} ohms and a drift rate in the magnetic field of the order of 100 ppm per hour when the expected value is as low as 0.1 ppm per hour.

MAGNET DESIGN AND CONSTRUCTION

One of the problems in designing a magnet is to achieve the high homogeneity required for imaging. Since the magnetic field normally peaks at the center of a magnet and falls off rapidly towards the ends, the homogeneous magnet must somehow prevent the field from falling off too fast near the center.

For illustration, consider the following simple solenoid, which is about the minimum size required for whole body NMR purposes. A magnet having an inside winding diameter of 44 inches should permit a room temperature bore (about 85 cm) large enough for various gradient coils, an rf coil, and the patient. Homogeneous magnets are wound with an even number of layers to eliminate the magnetic field due to unpaired current leads coming from the two ends of the magnet, as would happen if an odd number of layers were used. For demonstration, we will choose the minimum case of a two layer homogeneous magnet. We start with a four layer simple solenoid where we have chosen the right length in advance. If we choose a length of 80.758 inches, use four layers with 8205 turns of 1 mm diameter conductor, and a current of 113 amperes we get a simple solenoid that generates 5000 gauss, has an inductance of 32 henries, and a stored energy of about 210,000 joules.

The homogeneity of this simple solenoid is inadequate for NMR imaging, but techniques for improving the homogeneity are available. The magnetic field only 2 inches from the center of the magnet along the axis is 0.07 percent lower than at the center of the magnet, and at a distance of 8 inches along the axis it is lower by approximately 1.1 percent than the central field. In the magnet described, it was presumed that the 8205 turns of conductor were wound on a magnet in four layers. Suppose we now remove the outer two layers from the magnet over a length of 61.812 inches. The magnetic field homogeneity is improved quite radically. We now find that at a distance 2 inches on axis from the center of the magnet, the field has improved in homogeneity from 0.07 to essentially no deviation from the central field, and at 8 inches it has improved from 1.1 to 0.001 percent. Since we have removed some of the turns in the top layers of the magnet, the current must be increased to generate the prescribed 5000 gauss magnetic field. In particular, the current is increased by about 113 to 211 amperes. The inductance is reduced to 12 henries, and the system has approximately 270 kilo-joules of stored energy. The increased energy in the magnet is due to the fact that the magnetic field at the ends of the solenoid had to be increased in order to flatten out the center field. Since all the energy is actually stored in the magnetic field, the higher field over the volume at the ends of the coil accounts for most of the increase.

This example should not be considered a serious magnet design, but it does illustrate one way to obtain NMR homogeneity in superconducting magnets. This particular approach is known as the sixth order homogeneous design. The term "sixth order solution'' means that if the magnetic field is expressed as a polynomial expansion in even orders of the axial distance, z, from the center of the magnet, then the first term in the expansion would be z^6 because the second and fourth orders were canceled out by appropriate choice of the magnet length and the length of the gap in the windings. Other designs, such as eighth order coil systems, can be formulated with three, four, or more symmetrically placed coil sections to yield shorter magnets and give magnetic fields with better homogeneity than the sixth order type. A comparable eighth order magnet comprised of three coils is given in Table 70–1, and the fields of each of these magnets are given in Table 70–2. Since eighth order solutions can be obtained with five, six, or even higher numbers of appropriately chosen symmetrically placed coil sections, the manufacturer is thus free to choose whatever solution is appropriate to his manufacturing technique. The authors assume that all MRI magnet manufacturers are using some sort of eighth order magnet system.

No matter which mathematical solution is chosen, winding errors will reduce the homogeneity. For example, in the sixth order magnet example, the theoretical homogeneity on axis is better than 1 part in 10^6 or 0.0001 percent at distances up to 5 inches from the center of the magnet. If only one turn is omitted from the center of the coil, and we subtract the field generated by this single turn from the field originally calculated for the complete coil, we find that the homogeneity at ± 6 inches is reduced by more than a factor of 10, and the deviation from the central field is approximately 4×10^{-5} of the central field. Obviously, omitting a complete turn is an unlikely occurrence, but incorrectly spacing the conductors will have a fractional effect of what

Table 70–1. MAGNET DESIGN PARAMETERS

	Simple Solenoid	6th Order Magnet	8th Order Magnet		
			Coil 1	*Coil 2*	*Coil 3*
Winding ID	44.000 in	44.000 in	44.000 in	46.000 in	46.000 in
Winding OD	44.315 in	44.315 in	44.157 in	48.362 in	48.362 in
Winding length	80.760 in	80.760 in	42.475 in	1.811 in	1.811 in
Winding center	0 in	0 in	0 in	30.242 in	30.242 in
Layers	4	4	2	46	46
Notch					
Layers		2			
Length		61.812 in			
Turns	8205	3140	2158	1380	1380
Current	113.37	211.28	206.81	206.81	206.81

Table 70–2. AXIAL MAGNETIC FIELDS OF MAGNETS

Axial Position (inches)	Magnetic Field (gauss)		
	Simple Solenoid	*6th Order Magnet*	*8th Order Magnet*
0	5000.000	5000.000	5000.000
1	4999.185	5000.000	5000.000
2	4996.734	5000.000	5000.000
3	4992.634	5000.000	5000.000
4	4986.862	4999.999	5000.001
5	4979.385	4999.997	5000.000
6	4970.160	4999.989	5000.000
7	4959.137	4999.972	4999.997
8	4946.252	4999.937	4999.990
9	4931.433	4999.869	4999.970
10	4914.596	4999.748	4999.926

has been shown here. For example, had this one conductor been misplaced by 0.010 inch, or one fifth of the wire diameter, the resulting homogeneity would still have been reduced to 1 part in 10^5. The object here is to illustrate that designing a magnet of the required homogeneity is not nearly as difficult as constructing it with the required tolerances. In fact, the sensitivity is so great that, in general, one cannot wind the magnet with the required tolerances and the art lies not in winding with precision but in shimming the coil, subsequent to its construction, in such a fashion that the original design homogeneity can be recovered.

It was mentioned that a decay rate of the magnetic field of 1 part in 10^7 per hour is not unreasonable. Let us now determine the resistance that the coil must have in order to achieve this low decay rate. At 1 part in 10^7 per hour and with an inductance of 12 henries, the resistance of the entire magnet must be less than 3×10^{-10} ohm. If we assume that we are able to obtain pieces of superconductor of sufficient length that only eight joints are required, each of these joints would be required to have a resistance of less than 4×10^{-11} ohm. Although such resistances can be achieved, doing so is not a trivial matter, as noted earlier.

BIOLOGIC EFFECTS

There is very limited reliable data on the biologic effects of magnetic fields, and it is not known whether magnetic fields are harmless to all patients. Brechna[2] pointed out that the USSR limits exposure of its citizens to high magnetic fields. There is no clear evidence that magnetic fields are harmful, but St. Lorant[3] noted that some individuals may be more susceptible than the general population, as in the case with "harmless" drugs such as aspirin.

The United States Department of Health and Human Services, Food and Drug Administration, has issued Guidelines for Evaluating Electromagnetic Risk for Trials of Clinical NMR Systems.[4] These guidelines were made available ". . . to assist sponsors and IRB's [International Review Boards] in determining when a study involving a nuclear magnetic resonance (NMR) system might be regarded as significant risk to the subject with respect to exposure to static, changing, or radiofrequency (rf) magnetic fields." Studies exposing patients to field levels above the following guidelines must be individually evaluated with respect to the significance of the risk entailed:

1. Static (DC) magnetic fields ($\overline{B}$). Whole or partial body exposures of 2 tesla (20 kilogauss).

2. Time-varying magnetic fields ($d\overline{B}/dt$). Whole or partial body exposures of 3 tesla/second (30 kilogauss/second).

3. Radiofrequency electromagnetic fields. Exposure to rf fields that results in a specific absorption rate (SAR) that exceeds 0.4 W/kg as averaged over the whole body or 2 W/kg as averaged over any 1 gram of tissue.

If a significant risk exists, a formal application for an Investigational Device Exemption must be made to the Food and Drug Administration.

These effects are discussed more fully in Chapters 83 to 86.

MAGNET COST FACTORS

The specifications for the superconducting magnet are very critical. The cost of the system can increase quite rapidly with size and demands for high field intensity and homogeneity. If these parameters are overspecified, the magnet system will have an excessive cost, while the system can be inadequate if the magnet is underdesigned or the specifications are not met (see also Chapter 69).

The cost and complexity of a superconducting magnet increases rapidly with the energy stored in the magnetic field, the bore size, the magnetic field magnitude, and the homogeneity requested. Some of the difficulties due to the size of the magnet are related to the large stresses caused by the interaction of the current carrying wires with the magnetic field. A useful analogy is to compare the problem of keeping a magnetic field in a volume to that of storing a gas at high pressure. The magnetic pressure increases with the square of the magnetic field. The stress on the walls of a pressure vessel depend on the ratio of the inside to the outside diameter of the vessel. It is very easy to make a small container for high pressure, but large pressure vessels require a very thick wall to keep the stresses at reasonable levels. A 70,000 gauss, niobium titanium solenoid with a 2 cm bore is trivial, since the magnetic stress forces are easily held by the windings. In the 15,000 gauss 2 m bore solenoid built for Cornell, the magnetic forces must be carried by external aluminum windings. The system required extensive engineering design studies and very careful manufacturing techniques. This 2 m × 3 m magnet is shown in Figure 70–9. The most likely effect to be encountered due to stresses is erratic operation. The pressure can make the operation of the magnet unstable due to wire motion as already discussed. The easiest way to reduce the stresses is to reduce the magnetic field intensity or the size of the superconducting magnet or both.

In specifying the diameter of the homogeneous region, it is well to remember that this is proportional to the inside diameter of the magnet. The diameter over which the homogeneity can be readily corrected is about 30 percent of the bore of the solenoid. Thus, one can practically obtain a homogeneity of about 1 part in 10^5 in a 30 cm sphere at the center of a 1 m bore magnet. Even then, additional shim coils may be needed

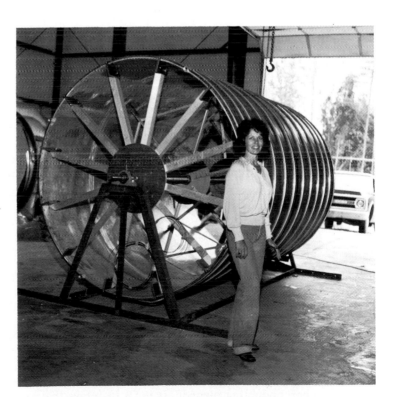

Figure 70–9. A 2 × 3 meter superconducting magnet under construction.

to correct for magnet imperfections as well as for magnetic field variations that occur naturally in the building. The use of special room temperature shimming techniques by Diasonics allows magnets with inhomogeneities of 100 to 200 ppm to be corrected to the lower values. Since trimming with this technique is cheaper and easier than producing a very high homogeneity magnet, the net result is the same high quality field with a cheaper system price.

Whole body NMR imaging systems, designed for hydrogen resonance at magnetic fields below 4000 gauss, can readily be produced in 1 m bore magnets without problems of stress or coil protection. Increasing the magnetic field to 20,000 gauss for phosphorus resonance increases the stress and the stored energy by 25 times, thus requiring much more stringent engineering design techniques to ensure that training does not occur and that the magnet remains undamaged in case of an accidental quench. The 20,000 gauss system also requires much more superconducting material than the 4000 gauss system.

The result of these factors is that the 1 m bore 20,000 gauss whole body NMR magnet is about twice as expensive as the 4000 gauss magnet. A low field MRI magnet, dewar, power supply system can be purchased for about a quarter of a million dollars at this time.

The cost of the gradient coils, RF coils and NMR electronics is a separate expense.

MAGNET AND SYSTEM SPECIFICATIONS

Manufacturers who have completed the larger superconducting systems are usually willing to review specifications and point out features that cause excessive cost. It is also useful to consult with magnet experts, as those who have experience with large magnets will not bid on proposals with strict penalties and specifications that are beyond the state of the art.

The system specifications will usually include the following:
1. Field homogeneity within a certain specified volume.
2. Dimensions of the accessible room temperature region.
3. The maximum field in the homogeneous region.
4. The field decay rate in the persistent mode.
5. The magnet charging time.
6. The dewar helium capacity and the boil-off rate.

The type and dimensions of the superconductor are usually not specified, since each magnet manufacturer will select the superconductor to meet the other specifications. Currently, United States companies producing MRI superconducting magnets are American Magnetics, Inc. (a subsidiary of Diasonics Inc.), G.A. Technology Inc., Intermagnetics General Corporation, and Oxford Airco Inc. (a branch of the English company Oxford Industries). Oxford Airco has been the largest producer of such systems. Various companies throughout other parts of the world are establishing themselves in the MRI magnet manufacturing business.

CRYOSTAT AND ACCESSORIES

In addition to the magnet itself, an operational system must contain a cryostat for maintaining the magnet at liquid helium temperatures and instruments and controls for monitoring and operating the system.

The cryostat is a vessel providing a constant low temperature environment for the superconducting magnet. It must maintain the magnet at liquid helium temperatures for prolonged periods in an economical fashion. This requires that the vessel be well insulated and that the mechanical supports for the magnet have very low thermal conductivities. Insulation is provided by a vacuum space between surfaces at different temperatures to eliminate conductive heat transfer, and multiple layers of metal-coated plastic film to reduce radiant heat transfer. Stainless steel or glass-fiber reinforced epoxy tubes, rods, or belts are generally used for force transmission between components at different temperatures, since their thermal conductivities are quite low.

Although a cryostat can be constructed in which liquid helium (4.2° K) alone is used as a cryogen, more frequently liquid nitrogen (77° K) is used to intercept the major portion of the heat transmitted into the cryostat from the room. The reason for the extra expense of the liquid nitrogen reservoir is that on a per liter basis liquid nitrogen costs less than 10 percent as much as liquid helium but absorbs 60 times as much heat upon evaporation. It is also much easier to liquefy and handle than liquid helium.

Another method of reducing the liquid helium losses is to use a refrigerator in place of the liquid nitrogen. Refrigerator heads are available that can be installed directly on the cryostat and provide cold stations at two temperatures, usually 77° K and 20° K. These "cold heads" employ reciprocating parts in the regenerator, but the main compressor may be located remotely. If the vibration and magnetic interference from the cold head is acceptable for the type of imaging desired, such a refrigerator will allow the system to be used for weeks or months without replenishing the liquid helium. A drawing of a cryostat of this type, employing liquid nitrogen reservoirs as back-up refrigerants in case of a power failure, is shown in Figure 70–10. A photo of an American Magnetics 0.35 tesla magnet using this type refrigeration scheme is shown in Figure

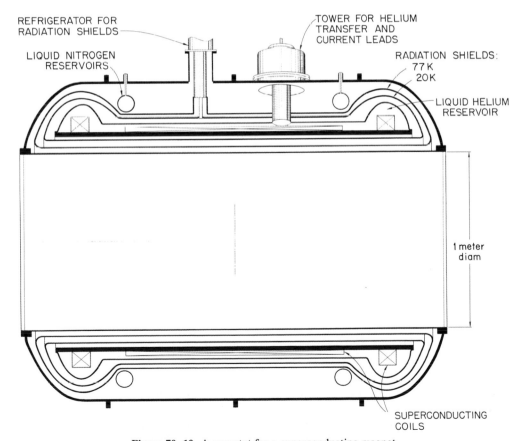

Figure 70–10. A cryostat for a superconducting magnet.

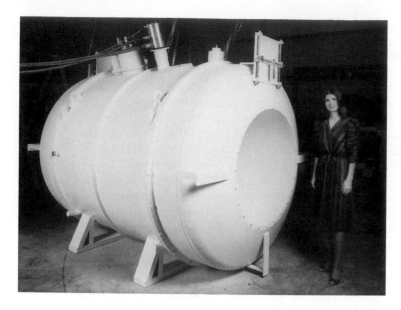

Figure 70–11. A 1.0 meter bore MRI magnet with refrigerator.

70–11. This particular unit has been used by Diasonics for about two years. The refrigerator is run continuously, and no liquid nitrogen is required. Liquid helium losses are less than 200 ml/hr. A range of losses is now covered by the latest AMI magnet system. The system is designed to have a helium loss rate of about 1/liter/hr with no liquid nitrogen cooling. The addition of liquid nitrogen halves this loss. A closed cycle refrigerator can be added so that no liquid helium is lost at all.

The cryostat also serves as a mounting platform for various gradient coils appropriate to the NMR imaging scheme being used. The bore tube is expected to be nonconducting to reduce field distortions caused by eddy currents induced during field gradient pulses. Fiber-reinforced epoxy tubes are ideal for this purpose, since in addition to being nonconducting, they are also nonmagnetic.

After the gradient coils are installed, adequate room must be allowed for the patient to rest comfortably inside the bore tube. This constraint, combined with variation in patient size, governs the size of the cryostat and ultimately the size of the magnet.

The introduction of current into the cryostat with minimal heat input is a crucial factor in the economics of operating the system. The heat generated in the leads can be extracted to a great extent by cooling them with the exiting helium gas. Persistent switches are always supplied with the magnet to produce magnetic field stability and to allow the current leads to be reduced to zero current and possibly removed altogether to reduce liquid helium loses.

INSTRUMENTATION

High-quality instrumentation is not only necessary but can also make operation of the magnet system very simple. A superconducting filament type liquid helium level sensor gives an instantaneous and reliable readout of the level of the liquid helium in the dewar. It is a great assistance in transferring and a must for avoiding operation of the magnet with too little helium.

A current meter is used to determine the magnetic field being generated in the dewar while the magnet is being energized. Once the correct current is attained the magnetic field is monitored by the NMR signal of the imaging system.

A temperature sensor is highly recommended for monitoring the cool-down of the magnet from room temperature. It is true that this need not be done often but when it is necessary a temperature sensor is desirable. The price of the instrument can easily be recovered in the savings of helium if a problem is detected during a transfer.

Most manufacturers furnish a console that contains the power supply, helium level detectors, and so on as a turnkey system that allows complete control of the magnet system.

ACKNOWLEDGMENTS

Portions of this chapter are taken from Cofey HT: Selection Guide: Superconducting Magnets, Magnet Systems, Cryogenic Accessories. American Magnetics, Inc., 1981.

References

1. Larbalestier D, Fisk G, Montgomery B, Hawksworth D: High-field superconductivity, Physics Today *39*, March 1986, p. 24.
2. Brechna H: Limitation of exposure to high magnetic fields, Fifth International Conference on Magnet Technology, Rome 1975, pp 351–366.
3. St. Lorant SJ: Bioeffects of magnetic fields, Sixth International Conference on Magnet Technology, Bratislava 1975, pp 337–345.
4. Villfort JC: Guidelines for Evaluating Electromagnetic Exposure Risk for Trials of Clinical NMR Systems. U.S. Department of Health and Human Resources, Bureau of Radiological Health, 1982.
5. Personal communication, American Magnetics, Inc., Oak Ridge, TN, 1987.

71

Gradient Coil Technology

STEPHEN R. THOMAS
LAWRENCE J. BUSSE
JOHN F. SCHENCK

The gradient coils used for nuclear magnetic resonance (NMR) imaging establish relatively weak spatially varying magnetic fields, which when superimposed on the homogeneous static main field, perform a number of important functions, including (a) encoding of the spatial-frequency information required for planar (two-dimensional) and volumetric (three-dimensional) NMR imaging techniques;[1-4] (b) determination of the plane definition and slice thickness parameters through utilization of two-dimensional, selective irradiation techniques; and (c) production of gradient echoes in specialized pulse protocols (e.g., those involving fast scanning methods).[5] Generally, the three orthogonal gradients provided are linear so that the frequency spectrum corresponds directly to a specific spatial position in a straightforward manner through the Larmor equation

$$\omega_i = \gamma B_i$$

where, as defined elsewhere in this text, ω_i is the resonance frequency associated with the field strength B_i and γ is the gyromagnetic constant for the nuclei of interest. Figure 71–1 provides a schematic representation of the spatial encoding properties of gradient magnetic fields. Examples of the gradient field control during selective radio frequency (rf) excitation, three-dimensional Fourier transform techniques and gradient echo pulse sequences are shown in Figure 71–2. The design of the gradient coils and the associated electronic driving circuits will depend on various aspects of the imaging system, including (a) the main magnet geometry (patient access axial or transverse with respect to the static field); (b) the type of investigation and pulse protocol sequences employed (rapid switching requirements versus driven equilibrium pulse sequences and oscillating gradient slice selection[6]); and, (c) the intrinsic inhomogeneity of the main magnetic field.

The lower limit of the gradient magnitude required is determined by the criterion that the gradient field must be stronger than the main magnetic field inhomogeneity in order to ensure that the spatial-frequency encoding established will not be dominated by the uncontrolled nature of these intrinsic nonuniformities. This consideration has more significance for some pulse protocol sequences and image reconstruction schemes than others; for example, as shown in Figure 71–3, two-dimensional Fourier transform (2DFT) techniques are more forgiving of inhomogeneities in the imaging plane than are projection reconstruction methods. For the former, the nonuniformities are manifest only as geometric distortions within the final image without an accompanying broadening of the effective system response function, as is the case with projection reconstruction.[7,8] For projection reconstruction, the effect of this broadening (which would degrade spatial resolution) should be limited to less than one pixel dimension within

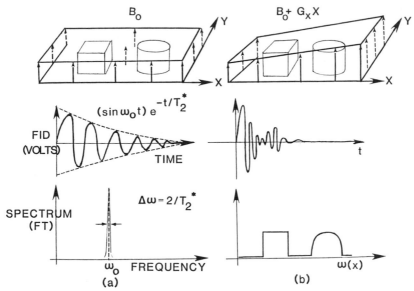

Figure 71–1. A schematic representation of the spatial encoding function of gradient magnetic fields.[2] Under a uniform magnetic field, B_0, the NMR received signal (free induction decay, FID) may be represented as a damped sine wave characterized by the effective spin-spin relaxation time $T2$ (a). The Fourier transform (FT) of this FID provides a single line spectrum centered around the resonance frequency ω_0 (shown with a slightly expanded frequency axis scale to emphasize the line shape). There is no differentiation of the spatial distribution of the signal-producing objects within the region of uniform field. A change in the z component of B is superimposed upon the main magnetic field, here shown as a linear gradient in the x direction, G_x (b). The FID is now a more complicated function as a consequence of the multiple resonance frequencies present. The resultant spectrum, which is spatially encoded through the one-to-one correspondence of frequency to x position, represents a projection of the object space onto the x axis.

the product image. This requires that the following relationship be satisfied:

$$G_m > \Delta B_i(N/D) = (\Delta\omega_i/\gamma)\,(N/D)$$

where G_m is the minimum applied gradient strength, ΔB_i or $(\Delta\omega_i/\gamma)$ represents the maximum intrinsic magnetic field deviation from the central nominal value over the imaging plane field of view (FOV), N is the number of pixels across the image, and D is the diameter of the FOV.[7,8] Therefore, if the homogeneity specification for a 0.15 tesla system were 50 parts per million (ppm) over a 40 cm diameter volume (representing the FOV), the minimum gradient required for a 128 $\times$ 128 back projection technique would be:

$$G_m \geq (50 \times 10^{-6})\,(0.15\text{ T})\,(128/0.4\text{ m}) = 2.4\text{ mT/m} = 0.24\text{ gauss/cm} \qquad (1)$$

Typical values of the gradient field strengths used in various clinical imaging systems range from 0.01 to 1.0 gauss/cm. The higher value mentioned represents a change in field of only 40 gauss across a 40 cm FOV and illustrates the weak nature of these gradient fields relative to the static magnetic field, which may range from 1000 gauss (0.1 tesla) to 20,000 gauss (2 tesla).

In practice, the gradient coils themselves may also be used in an offset current mode to provide additional shimming correction for first-order magnetic field inhomogeneities and thus improve the effective uniformity characteristics over and above the specified intrinsic value. This function is of particular value for those systems that do not have an independent shim coil set.

Another effect, as discussed by Edelstein et al.,[7] relating the minimum gradient strength necessary to the intrinsic inhomogeneity, which has significance for both projection reconstruction and Fourier transform techniques, involves maximizing the sig-

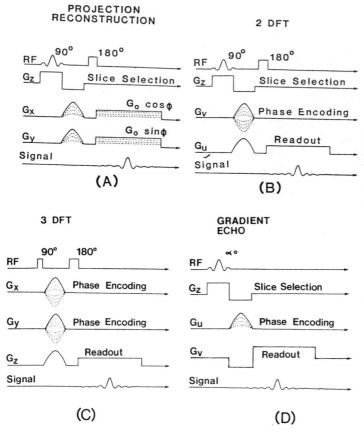

Figure 71–2. Pulse sequences illustrating the relationship between the gradient wave forms and the rf excitation commonly used for imaging techniques. *A*, Projection reconstruction. *B*, Planar two-dimensional Fourier transform (2DFT). *C*, Volumetric three-dimensional Fourier transform (3DFT). *D*, Gradient echo with flip angles less than 90 degrees. In all cases except *C*, the slice selection is provided by selective excitation. The time-to-echo, TE (from the center of the 90 degree pulse to the center of the signal echo), is typically 30 milliseconds for *T1* weighted imaging. The text refers to the phase encoding gradient as G_v and the readout gradient as G_u. (Modified in part from reference 7.)

nal from each voxel. This requires that $T2^*$ for each voxel be much larger than the signal sampling time. This statement is equivalent to the condition that $\Delta B_m \gg \Delta B_s$, where ΔB_m represents the magnetic field change in the imaging plane due to the applied gradient, and ΔB_s is the static field inhomogeneity across one pixel. Continuing with the 0.15 tesla system example given above, the maximum intrinsic gradient for an inhomogeneity specification of 50 ppm across 40 cm would be approximately 0.02 mT/ m. Thus, within a slice thickness of 1 cm, the change in magnetic field, ΔB_s, would be approximately 0.2 μT; and, for a pixel dimension of 3 mm (~40 cm/128 pixels) under the constraint that $\Delta B_m \sim 10 \times \Delta B_s$, the minimum gradient strength required would be approximately 0.7 mT/m (0.07 gauss/cm).

In practice, the magnitude of the gradient employed will be limited by signal-to-noise and bandwidth considerations. It is generally undesirable to utilize gradients any larger than necessary because the frequency bandwidth required for imaging is proportional to the gradient strength. A larger bandwidth introduces more noise and increases the complexity of tuning and matching narrow band, high Q rf coils.[7]

Effect of Field Inhomogeneities

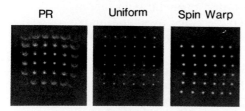

Figure 71–3. An example of the effect of magnetic field inhomogeneities on the reconstructed image. The center panel shows the image of a point array under conditions of uniform field. The introduction of field inhomogeneities produces blurring of the point spread function as well as geometric distortion for projection reconstruction (PR) while introducing geometric distortion only in the direction of the readout gradient for 2DFT (spin warp).[7]

GENERAL MATHEMATICAL DESCRIPTION OF GRADIENT FIELDS

Under conditions of a small gradient magnetic field strength ΔB relative to a large static field B_0 defining the z axis of the spin system, the gradient vector G may be described with three independent orthogonal components $G_x = \partial B_z/\partial x$, $G_y = \partial B_z/\partial y$ and $G_z = \partial B_z/\partial z$ (see the Appendix to this chapter).[9] A linear combination of these components will allow a gradient vector to be established in any arbitrary direction according to the requirements of the image plane orientation. This ability to select a plane electronically and acquire data in any read-out direction without necessitating the mechanical hardware constraints of a moving gantry represents one of the positive aspects of the NMR imaging technique.

The linear gradient fields will be established by the magnetic field produced by current carrying conductors arranged in a geometrical configuration appropriate for the desired gradient orientation. The integrated magnetic field $\bar{B}(r)$ at a point $r-r_\ell$ from a wire displaced r_ℓ from the origin, which carries a current, I, is given by the Biot-Savart law (see Fig. 71–4):

$$\bar{B}(r) = \frac{\mu_0 I}{4\pi} \int_\ell \frac{(\bar{r} - \bar{r}_\ell)}{|\bar{r} - \bar{r}_\ell|^3} \times \overline{d\ell} \tag{2}$$

where μ_0 is the magnetic permeability of free space and $d\ell$ is an element of the wire. The components of $\bar{B}$, such as $B_z(x, y, z)$ etc., may be obtained by expansion of the vector product. The challenge of designing linear gradient coils is then that of determining a spatial distribution for the associated conductors (wires) that will allow the desired gradient pattern to be established in an efficient manner throughout the imaging volume.

Independent coil windings to produce controlled gradient fields have been used historically with NMR spectrometers to (1) correct for the static field inhomogeneities in an attempt to produce as uniform a field as possible over the sample volume as required for high resolution studies and (2) provide the relatively strong gradient fields required for diffusion investigations. Representative papers dealing with these applications are given in references 10 to 17. Although the functional use of the gradient

Vector Representation Associated with the Calculation of $\vec{B}(r)$

using the Biot–Savart Law

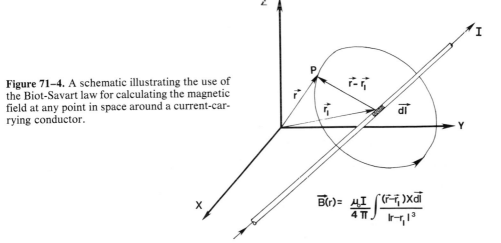

Figure 71–4. A schematic illustrating the use of the Biot-Savart law for calculating the magnetic field at any point in space around a current-carrying conductor.

fields in NMR imaging is unique in relationship to the "classical" purposes listed above, MRI gradient coil design has as its origin these original concepts. In addition, while not the topic of this paper, shim coil configurations utilizing the same theoretical basis are usually employed in MRI systems to provide correction for main magnetic field inhomogeneities.[18]

As outlined in the Appendix to this chapter, because $B_z(x, y, z)$ satisfied Laplace's equation at all points within the image volume of interest (namely $\nabla^2 B_z = 0$), it may be expanded in terms of power functions of r, associated Legendre polynomials, and appropriate constants. The constants will be determined by the shape of the coils and the strength of the currents in them.[19,20] For gradient coil designs under consideration for NMR imaging, the current-carrying conductors will be located most often on a cylinder surrounding the imaging region. This constraint allows simplification of the mathematical expressions. In most cases of concern, the surface current density, $\lambda_\phi(\phi_o, z_o)$ can be expressed as the product of two functions, one depending only on ϕ_o (the azmuthal angle) and one depending only on Z_o (the normalized axial position: $Z_o = z_o/r_o$ where r_o is the cylinder radius and z_o is the axial coordinate position) such that:

$$\lambda_\phi(\phi_o, z_o) = cf_\phi(\phi_o)\sigma_\phi(Z_o) \qquad (3)$$

where c is a constant of proportionality, $f_\phi(\phi_o)$ expresses the angular variation of the surface current density, and $\sigma_\phi(Z_o)$ expresses the variation along the cylindrical axis (z direction). The task of the coil designer is to determine the shape functions $f_\phi(\phi_o)$ and $\sigma_\phi(Z_o)$ that will emphasize the coefficients of the fields desirable for the intended application and that will eliminate or minimize the coefficients of the undesirable contaminating terms. Note that although some z directed current density (λ_z) is present, it will make no contribution to B_z.

AXIAL Z GRADIENT COILS

In general, a linear z gradient in a defined region may be established by cylindrically symmetric coils wound on the surface of a cylinder (with the axis of the cylinder oriented along the z direction of the magnetic field) under the constraint that the current density is antisymmetric. In this case, the surface current density that is in the ϕ direction is given by the simplified expression $\lambda_\phi = c\sigma_\phi(Z_o)$ with the antisymmetry condition that $\sigma_\phi(-Z_o) = -\sigma_\phi(Z_o)$.

The most common design configuration for the z gradient coils in those systems where access is oriented such that the patient axis is parallel to the direction of the main magnetic field involves a Maxwell coil pair. These consist of two flat circular wire coils, each of radius r_o, oriented parallel and coaxial to each other with a separation of $\sqrt{3}r_o$ (Fig. 71–5A). Each carries a current of equal magnitude but opposite in direction, as shown in the schematic of Figure 71–6. This configuration is designed to remove the third order contaminant term in the expansion. An ideal Maxwell coil would have a filament (coil width) of zero diameter with each coil represented by a delta function at $z_o = \pm (\sqrt{3}/2)r_o$. Therefore, the normalized shape function for this idealized coil would be

$$\sigma_\phi(Z_o) = 0.78 \, [\delta(Z_o - \sqrt{3}/2) - \delta(Z_o + \sqrt{3}/2)] \qquad (4)$$

In practice, real coils will have a definite width. For the example in which the width of each coil is 0.2 r_o, the shape function is given as:

$$\sigma_\phi(Z_o) = \begin{cases} 3.945 & \text{for } 0.7751 < Z_o < 0.9751 \\ 0 & \text{otherwise} \\ -3.945 & \text{for } -0.9751 < Z_o < -0.7751 \end{cases} \qquad (5)$$

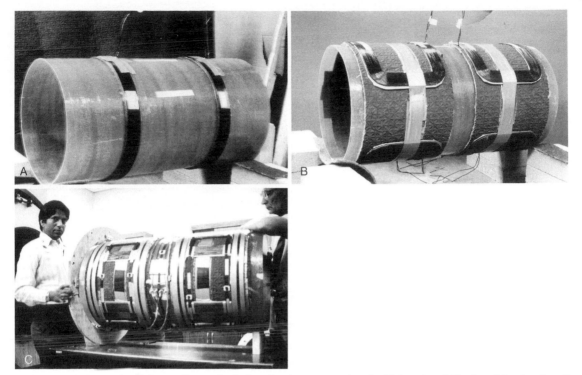

Figure 71–5. Photographs of the gradient coils designed and constructed at the University of Cincinnati for the six-coil, 0.15 tesla whole-body imaging system.[22] The inner radius of the fiber glass former supporting the coils is approximately 25 cm (10 in). Padding has been placed between the coils and the former to reduce the acoustic noise generated through vibration of the coils under pulsed conditions in the magnetic field. *A, z* Gradient coils: Maxwell pair. *B, y* Gradient coils: saddle configuration. The *x*-coils of similar design would be mounted at 90 degrees relative to the *y*-coil set. *C,* The fully assembled gradient coil set.

Photographs of the z gradient coils designed and constructed at the University of Cincinnati for a 6-coil, 0.15 T resistive whole body imaging system[22] are shown in Figure 71–5*A*. A plot of the experimental results obtained when evaluating the z gradient field obtained is shown in Figure 71–7*A*.

The Maxwell pair configuration as discussed above cancels the third order term in the expansion so that the initial term contributing to the nonlinearity is fifth order

Figure 71–6. A schematic representation of the Maxwell coil pair (*z*-coil segment indicated) and the *y*-saddle coil set (one segment indicated) used to establish the z gradient and y gradient, respectively. (*a*) The *x*-saddle coil set is not shown; however, it would be composed of four units identical to the *y*-coils but oriented at 90 degrees with respect to them. The direction of the current in each coil is indicated by the arrows. A first quadrant gradient plot in the $z = 0$ imaging plane of the gradient field generated by the *y*-saddle coils. (*b*) The curves, as interpolated from a computer iteration of the Biot-Savart law, would be symmetrical about the *x* and *y* axes and represent intensity contour plots of the *z* component of the magnetic field produced by the *y*-coils. Each line shown represents a different value of the gradient magnitude in arbitrary nits from 1 toll. (Modified from reference 21.)

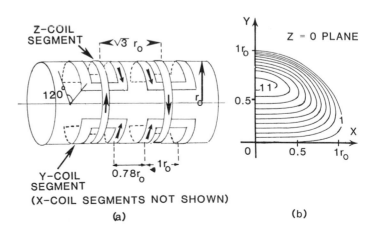

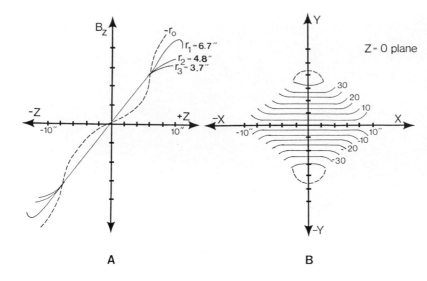

Figure 71–7. Experimental gradient field plots for the coil sets designed and constructed at the University of Cincinnati. *A*, Gradient field produced by the *z* gradient coil set. *B*, Gradient field produced by the *y* gradient coil set ($z = 0$ plane). The curves are labeled with arbitrary relative numbers proportional to the strength of the magnetic field provided by the gradient coils.

(A_5). To provide a greater degree of linearity, it is necessary to cancel these higher order terms. This may be accomplished through the use of additional coil loops. Various two Maxwell pair coil designs have been described by Saint-Jalmes et al.,[23] which increase the overall efficiency by allowing equivalent field linearity with smaller coils utilizing less electrical power (Fig. 71–8). This advantage is even more significant when considering switched power operation. The linearity was demonstrated to be maintained within approximately 0.2 to 0.6 percent over a 0.4 m diameter sphere in the central region as compared to the 5 percent linearity deviation characteristics obtained with a single pair of the same size. To produce this same degree of linearity for the specified gradient strength, a single Maxwell pair would require a larger diameter with dc and switched power consumption 5 times and 15 times greater, respectively.

An analysis of polygonal gradient coils has been performed by Blicharski and Sobol.[16,17] Geometrical considerations are shown in Figure 71–9 along with a schematical representation of the triangular (D3h group) and rectangular (D4h group) symmetries. For the same values of current and radius, the triangular coils produce the highest gradient field strength (2.81 times stronger than that produced by the outer scribed circular coils[16]); however, in practice this advantage may be lost owing to

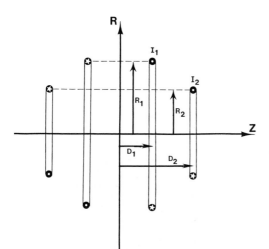

Figure 71–8. A *z* gradient coil design utilizing a 2 Maxwell coil pair configuration. This system increases the overall efficiency by providing the equivalent gradient field linearity as for a single pair while allowing use of smaller coils, which are more power efficient.[23]

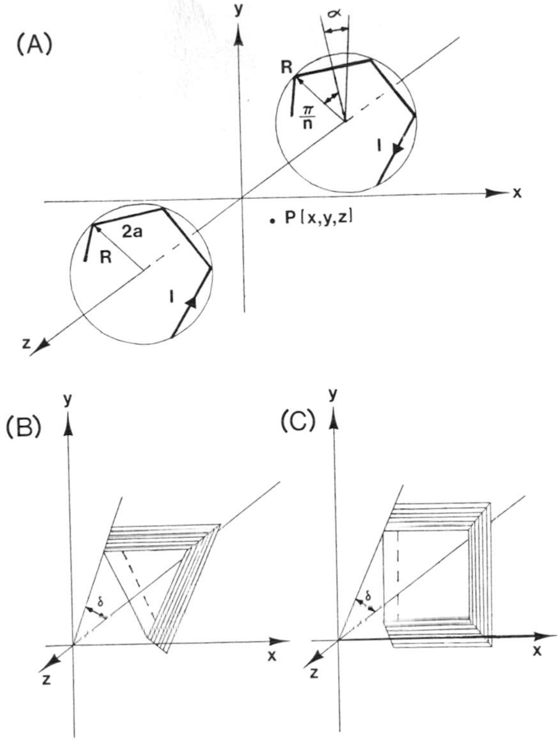

(A)

(B)

(C)

Figure 71–9. Polygonal x gradient coils.[16,17] A, A general schematic illustrating the geometrical configuration for inscribed polygonal gradient coils. B, An example of one segment of a triangular coil pair (D3h group symmetry). C, An example of one segment of a rectangular coil pair (D4h group symmetry).

constraints on the allowable axial positioning of the coils and the resultant requirements on the relative diameters.[17]

TRANSVERSE X AND Y GRADIENT COILS

Independent, orthogonal, linear gradient fields G_x and G_y are required also in the x and y directions, respectively, as discussed in the introduction. From symmetry considerations, it is clear that any coil set assembly designed to provide G_y may be physically rotated through 90 degrees to produce G_x. Therefore, the discussion need develop only the concepts relating to one direction. The following will address aspects of y gradient coils.

One method of producing a transverse gradient is through the use of four straight, parallel conductors located at the corners of a rectangle, each carrying a current of equal magnitude flowing in the same direction (Fig. 71–10A). This type of gradient coil design has been described by a number of authors[9,24] following the methods of Zupancic and Pirs[25] in which the magnetic field at a point (y, z) due to a current in a single infinite conductor oriented parallel to the x axis at location (y_ℓ, z_ℓ) is given as the real part of the complex function representing the solution of the Biot-Savart law. (See the Appendix to this chapter for mathematical details.) For the four-conductor configuration of Figure 71–10A, in which all currents are in the same direction, the contributions for each wire at point (y, z) combined such that all even powers in the expression cancel. The y gradient is given as: $G_y = \partial B_z(y, z)/\partial y$ evaluated at $z = 0$. The third order term that would represent the first dominant contaminant and restrict the region of linearity may be made zero under the condition that $\phi = \pi(1/2 + m)/4$, $m = 0, 1, 2, 3 \ldots$ Two angles of interest fulfilling this criteria are $\phi = 22.5$ degrees and $\phi = 67.5$. If the four conductors lie on a circle of radius r_o with $\phi = 22.5$ degrees, the

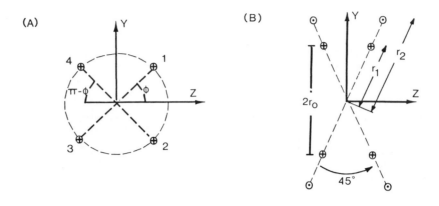

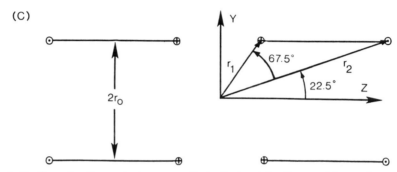

Figure 71–10. *A*, Configuration for producing a *y* gradient, G_y, involving four straight conductors. *B* and *C*, Return path options that maintain the "purity" of the gradient field. (Modified from reference 9.)

gradient up to the fourth order in the expansion coefficient will be[9]:

$$G_y = \partial B(y, z)/\partial y = 1.414\mu_o I/(\pi r_o^2) \tag{6}$$

whereas for $\phi = 67.5$ the gradient will be:

$$G_y = -1.414\mu_o I/(\pi r_o^2) \tag{7}$$

As discussed by Mansfield and Morris,[9] these results suggest methods of addressing the requirement for providing a return current path (closed loop) for any real coil configuration. Two possible arrangements are indicated schematically in Figure 71–10*B* and *C*. In effect, the return path is constrained to a greater radius and would contribute a component of G_y having a smaller magnitude. In Figure 71–10*B*, this contribution is negative and the net gradient strength would be reduced; whereas in Figure 71–10*C*, the contribution is additive. In either case, the linearity characteristics would not be compromised because, with the conditions for the specified values maintained, the return conductors generate a gradient field with contaminating terms of the same order as those produced by the primary wires. In addition, for the latter option, with all four conductor pairs lying in parallel planes as shown, the field from the end connecting wires that are oriented parallel to the *z* axis would not contribute to G_y. In general, however, the coil dimensions required for whole body MRI systems are somewhat too large to be practical for the latter option.

Up to this point, the discussion has been concerned with the theory for infinite parallel conductors. Obviously, in practice, coils of finite size must be employed with the appropriate return paths provided. The infinite length model may at best be used only as a guide to the optimum real world design. Bangert and Mansfield[24] described their gradient coil system, which is comprised of four trapezium loops exhibiting a relatively low inductance suitable for switched field applications.

Another approach to the design of transverse gradient coils involves analysis of the spherical harmonic description under the cylindrical symmetry outlined in the Appendix to this chapter for z gradient coils. To produce a transverse field, the coils must be designed such that A_{11}^s is the predominent coefficient for the y gradient set (with A_{11}^c predominant for the x gradient). (See the Appendix to this chapter for an explanation of the A^s and A^c coefficients.) Figure 71–11 shows the configuration for a single coil made from two opposed circular arcs, one running from ϕ_o to $\pi - \phi_o$ and the other from $\pi + \phi_o$ to $2\pi - \phi_o$. With the current oppositely directed in each arc, the angular variation of the surface current density $f_\phi(\phi_o)$ equals 1 for ϕ_o to $\pi - \phi_o$, -1 for $\pi + \phi_o$ to $2\pi - \phi_o$, and 0 everywhere else. This configuration produces fields that vary only as $\cos m\phi$ with m odd. The coefficients $A_{nm}^c = 0$ for all n and m while $A_{nm}^s = 0$ for m even.

If the shape function is even such that $\sigma_\phi(-Z_o) = \sigma_\phi(Z_o)$, all coefficients A_{nm}^s with n even are made equal to zero. Thus, through the use of circular arcs with the symmetry properties discussed above, a y gradient field will be produced that has A_{11}^s as the leading term and various contaminants of the form A_{31}^s, A_{32}^s, A_{51}^s, A_{53}^s, A_{55}^s, A_{71}^s, etc.

A common design for transverse gradient coils utilizes arrays of circular arcs in the saddle coil configuration (Figs. 71–5B and 71–6). Four arcs are required to provide the necessary symmetry to establish the transverse gradient with four additional arcs required for the return current paths. In addition, a total of eight interconnecting paths parallel to the z direction are required which do not contribute to the B_z field but do substantially increase the inductance and resistance of the coil. The design considerations now center on techniques to reduce some of the contaminating terms to zero. The terms A_{31}^s and A_{32}^s have the most severe effect upon the linearity. They may be eliminated by the judicious selection of the coil geometry. The term A_{33}^s, which is proportional to $\cos 3(\phi_o + \pi/2)$, may be made zero by choosing $\phi_o = \pi/3$, which indicates that each arc should subtend an angle of 120 degrees.

The term A_{31}^s may be eliminated through the appropriate relative positioning of

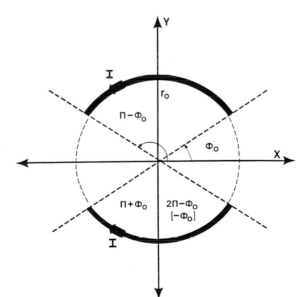

Figure 71–11. Two opposed arcs situated at ϕ_0 to $\pi - \phi_0$ and $\pi + \phi_0$ to $2\pi - \phi_0$ with current directions as shown. This configuration will produce a y gradient, G_y.

these arcs along the z axis. Golay[26] showed that this condition would be satisfied if the arcs were placed at the roots of the equation $4Z_o^4 - 27Z_o^2 + 4 = 0$, which yields $Z_o = \pm 0.39$ and ± 2.57. However, coils built with these dimensions would be quite long, with the total length almost three times the diameter, and consequently would exhibit large values for L and R. The requirement that $A_{31}^s = 0$ may still be met if the outer arc is brought much closer to the origin and the inner arc is moved only slightly outward. In practice it is common also to modify the basic saddle coil design by adding an additional inner arc to each segment (providing three instead of two arcs per segment at the same radius), which is adjusted both geometrically and with regard to its current load to improve the gradient linearity characteristics.

A photograph of the saddle coils constructed at the University of Cincinnati for the 0.15 tesla whole body MRI unit, which used Z_o values of ± 0.39 and ± 1.39, is shown in Figure 71–5B. An experimental plot of the y gradient characteristics for the $z = 0$ plane is shown in Figure 71–7B.

Other styles of gradient coils have been utilized, including those suitable for use with transverse geometry in which the main magnetic field is oriented perpendicular to the patient axis. Hutchinson has described quadrupole sets and distributed winding configurations.[27] The latter consists of straight wires running on the surface of and parallel to the axis of the supporting cylinder with the density of conductors (number per radian) proportional to the sine of twice the angular position around the circumference ($\sin 2\phi$). These coils provide an acceptable linear gradient over a region extending to nearly 90 percent of the cylinder radius.

ELECTRONIC CIRCUITS FOR DRIVING GRADIENT COILS

As NMR imaging techniques have evolved, so too have the complexity and capabilities of the electronics used to drive the gradient coils. The electronics required to energize the gradient coils of an NMR imaging system depend upon a number of factors, e.g., pulse protocol, type of imaging (projection or 2DFT), electrical characteristics of the gradient coils, and so on. In this section, a brief overview of the evolution of gradient coil electronics is provided by discussing static and pulsed gradients. A detailed description of a modern gradient drive design for arbitrary gradient manipulation is given. Examples of gradient waveforms generated and typical operating characteristics are provided.

Static Gradients

Early imaging experiments were performed using a partial saturation pulse sequence, projection reconstruction,[28] and no slice selection. The gradients needed to produce a projection of an object in the x–y plane are provided by a steady state current in each of the x and y gradient coils. The magnitude of these currents is related simply to the angle of the projection, ϕ, by, $I_x = G \sin \phi$, and $I_y = G \cos \phi$, where G is the gradient strength. These currents are independent of time and need not be changed until data at a new projection angle is required. The circuits used to provide these currents could be as simple as a variable DC power supply; however, the circuit shown in Figure 71–12A, more typical of those actually used, provides computer control of the gradient fields. Two digital to analog converters (DAC) are supplied with a stable voltage reference and digital data representing the sine and cosine of the projection angle θ. The computer or other logic source (e.g., PROMS) is used to supply the digital information. The DACs are followed by multiplying digital to analog converters

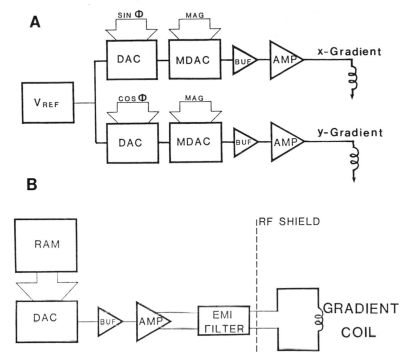

Figure 71–12. *A*, Block diagram of a system utilized for control of static field gradients used in projection reconstruction. The digital data controlling the DACs determine the direction of the projection and the data controlling the MDACs determine the strength of the gradient. *B*, Block diagram of a system used to generate an arbitrarily shaped current waveform in the gradient coil. Digital information in the RAM together with the bandpass characteristics of the AMP and EMI filters determines the temporal response of the gradient field.

(MDAC), which provide direct control of the magnitude of the gradient G. The outputs of the MDACs are buffered and routed through amplifiers capable of providing 2 to 10 amps for a typical set of saddle coils as discussed previously.

Time Varying Gradients

The first method devised for localizing the observed NMR signal to a thin slice within a three-dimensional object was based upon the use of oscillating field gradients.[29] The gradients used were linear functions of space and oscillatory functions of time. Typical frequencies used for gradient oscillation were 10 to 100 Hz. By recording the NMR signal and averaging a number of FIDs, which occur at random times with respect to the period, a signal representative of the spins in a plane could be obtained. For oscillating gradient applications, the power amplifiers used had to be capable of operating in a current controlled feedback mode and have a usable bandwidth greater than the maximum audio frequency used for gradient oscillation (generally 500 Hz). Recently, Macovski[30] has described an extension of this sensitive point technique that provides volumetric NMR imaging with more complex time varying gradients. The stated advantages of this method are (1) that all points in the volume are imaged simultaneously with image quality being immune to magnetic field inhomogeneity and chemical shift artifacts, and (2) that spectroscopic information is available also for each point.

More common forms of NMR imaging make use of the spin echo phenomenon and rely on pulsed field gradients. The pulsed field gradients provide slice selection capability and are needed also for preparing the spin system for echo formation.

The early forms of pulsed field gradient circuits made use of "tuned" circuit designs. Charge storage, switching components, and pulse shaping networks were used to drive the gradient coils. This approach was taken to avoid the cost of high power,

A) Analog Circuit for Generating Pulsed Field Gradients

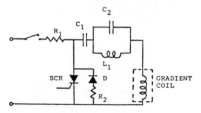

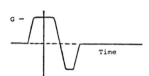

B) Typical Waveform Used for Slice Selection

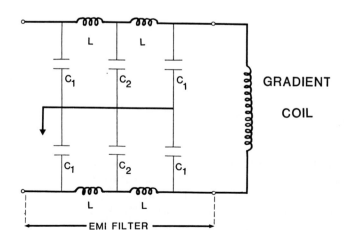

Figure 71–13. Pulsed field gradients used for slice selection. *A* shows the analog circuit used to generate the typical waveform presented in *B*. (From Hutchinson JMS: NMR proton imaging techniques. *In* Foster MA [ed]: Magnetic Resonance in Medicine and Biology. New York, Pergamon Press, 1986. Used by permission.)

wide bandwidth linear amplifier systems. Figure 71–13 illustrates the type of circuit used for pulsed gradient applications. Panel A shows a schematic of the circuit and panel B shows the type of waveform produced. The design details are documented elsewhere.[31] This design allows the large inductive load of the gradient coil, L1, to be incorporated into the design of the driving circuit. The high transient current needed to energize the coil is provided by the charge stored on the capacitors. A modest DC power supply is sufficient to energize the entire system because of the relatively long recycle delay period.

Modern NMR imaging systems use gradient drive electronics that incorporate complete digital control of every aspect of the current waveforms to the gradient coils. The block diagram of a typical circuit is shown in Figure 71–12*B*. A DAC is used to generate the analog voltage corresponding to an arbitrary gradient current waveform stored in a random access memory (RAM). This signal is buffered, amplified, and applied to the

Figure 71–14. Detail of the multiple-pole PI filter, which can be used to suppress electromagnetic interference (EMI) in the gradient fields. For the University of Cincinnati gradient coil systems $L = 44$ H, $C_1 = 0.0047$ μF and $C_2 = 0.0068$ μF. The inductance of the coils themselves was 8 mH, with a resistance of 1.5 ohms.

Table 71–1. CHARACTERISTICS OF A TYPICAL SADDLE GRADIENT COIL AND DRIVE SYSTEM OF A RESISTIVE WHOLE BODY NMR IMAGING SYSTEM

Coil impedance	
L	~10 millihenries
R	~1 ohm
Power amplifier	
Bandwidth	20 KHz
DC output	4 KVA (20 A @ 200 V)
Output impedance	<0.1 ohm

gradient coil. Normally, some type of electromagnetic interference (EMI) filtering is incorporated in the circuit so that stray radio frequency signals are not fed into the immediate vicinity of the magnet. A circuit used for EMI filtering is shown in Figure 71–14.

Modern imaging techniques require a gradient drive that can produce rapidly switched or shaped currents. Figure 71–2 shows four different pulse sequences that are commonly used in projection reconstruction, 2DFT, 3DFT, and gradient echo imaging techniques and the relations of the required gradient currents to the rf pulses. Using this approach requires wide bandwidth and high current drive capability of the gradient power amplifiers. For example, the switching needed to produce the slice selection gradient may require changes of approximately 20 amps in a 1 ms time interval. Power amplifiers used must have current controlled feedback, wide bandwidth, and stable operating characteristics when driving inductive loads.

In most instances, gradient amplifiers can be cooled by convection or forced air. In some designs, however, the gradient amplifiers may need to dissipate as much as 10 kilowatts of power. Water cooling may be required to dissipate the heat generated under these operating conditions.

METHODS FOR CORRECTING GRADIENT NONLINEARITIES

The ideal spatial variation of field gradients used for NMR imaging encoding is thought to be linear. This results from a number of factors, such as ease of signal processing and reconstruction, uniformity of resolution over the image plane, and freedom from geometric distortion. For this reason, the traditional approach for imaging systems has been to design gradient coils to produce field gradients with spatial variations as close to the linear "ideal" as possible. Any effects of residual nonlinearities were either tolerated or ignored.

Recently the mathematical formalism to correct for gradient field nonlinearities has been developed for projection reconstruction[32,33] and 2DFT[8] imaging methods. The potential advantages of using these correction techniques are (i) that more accurate NMR images can be produced by existing imaging systems and (ii) that more power efficient and space efficient gradient coil designs can be developed if the requirement of perfect gradient linearity is relaxed.

In this section an overview of the correction techniques for projection and 2DFT imaging is presented. Only the two-dimensional imaging case is discussed; however, both techniques are applicable to three-dimensional imaging for correction of smoothly varying, minor gradient nonlinearities. For a complete description of the techniques presented, the reader is encouraged to see the Appendix to this chapter for more details and to review the original articles.

Projection Reconstruction

In conventional two-dimensional NMR projection reconstruction, the projection, P, relates the object density function $F(r)$ and the magnitude field as

$$P_\phi(\beta) = 1/\gamma \int F(\bar{r})\delta(B_g - \beta)\, d\bar{r} \qquad (8)$$

where β is the observed angular frequency ω divided by the gyromagnetic ratio γ, δ is the dirac delta function and B_g is the functional form of the field gradients. Under ideal circumstances, the field gradients are linear functions of space and can be specified by a single angle, ϕ. Under these conditions, Equation (8) can be rewritten to express P_ϕ in terms of line integrals over straight line paths through the object density function. Image reconstruction then consists of inverting a series of these projection measurements made at many different angles ϕ in order to obtain an estimate of the original object density function.

In general the field gradients used to measure the projections of the object density function are not perfectly linear functions of space. Figure 71–15 illustrates this more general situation and shows the effect of nonlinear field gradients upon the standard methods of projection reconstruction. When the gradients are not linear functions of

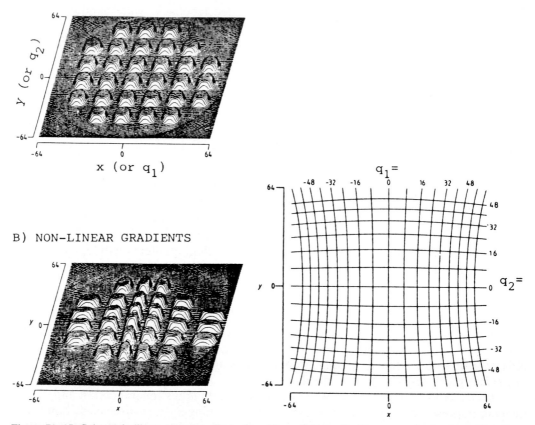

A) LINEAR GRADIENTS

B) NON–LINEAR GRADIENTS

Figure 71–15. Schematic illustrating the effect of nonlinear field gradients upon projection reconstruction. *A* shows a phantom image reconstructed using ideal data taken with linear field gradients. *B* shows the same phantom reconstructed from data taken with nonlinear gradients. The degree of nonlinearity and the curvilinear coordinate system used for image correction is shown in the plot on the right of *B* (From Lai CM: J Phys E: Sci Instrum *11*:217, 1978, and Phys Med Biol *28*:925, 1983.)

space, the measured projections remain line integrals of the object density function; however, now the integrals must be evaluated over bent or curved paths through the object density function.

Lai[32,33] has shown that it is possible to accommodate nonlinear field gradients in the formalism of projection reconstruction by introducing a curvilinear coordinate system. The effect of this coordinate system is to linearize the effects of nonlinear field gradients, i.e., transform the line integrals over curved paths back into straight line paths. Use of a curved coordinate system allows a rectilinear projection of the object to be measured and conventional image reconstruction to be used. The true image in the (x, y) coordinate system can be obtained from the image in the curved system by conventional (Jacobian) coordinate transformation techniques (see the Appendix to this chapter). Lai has shown that this correction technique allows geometrically accurate images to be formed using nonlinear field gradients. Image resolution, however, has been shown to be nonuniform and anisotropic. Resolution is better in regions of higher gradient strength.

The curvilinear coordinate system needed to perform this correction may be calculated analytically for a particular gradient coil design or may be derived numerically from an experimentally determined map of the field gradients.

Two-dimensional Fourier Transform Image Reconstruction

The effects of nonlinear field gradients and an inhomogeneous main field upon the two-dimensional Fourier transform (2DFT) imaging technique have been discussed recently.[8] The raw data used in this technique can be thought of as the two-dimensional Fourier transform of the desired image, sampled in a rectangular coordinate system. The coordinate system is defined by the direction, u, of the read out gradient and the direction, v, of the phase encoding gradient. The image produced can be expressed as $A(u, v)$.

The effect of gradient nonlinearities is to produce a geometric distortion of the image $A(u, v)$. The coordinate u is shifted to a new location $u + \epsilon u$ and the coordinate v is shifted to $v + \epsilon v$. The quantities ϵu and ϵv are maps of the departure from linearity of the read-out and phase encoding gradient fields over the image plane.

Image correction for gradient nonlinearities consists of forming a new image $A'(u, v)$ by repositioning pixels from the original image $A(u, v)$. The amount of repositioning has been shown to be proportional to the local gradient field nonlinearities. Additional intensity correction factors related to the rate of change of the field gradient must also be applied (see the Appendix to this chapter).

The nonlinearity factors, ϵ, can be measured experimentally or estimated from theoretical calculations based upon gradient coil geometry. Use of slightly nonlinear field gradients with the 2DFT imaging method has no adverse effect upon resolution as long as the ϵ factors are reasonable approximations of the true nonlinearities present.

APPENDIX: MATHEMATICAL DETAILS OF GRADIENT COIL DESCRIPTION

General Considerations

The spin system–gradient field interaction may be expressed in terms of second rank tensor[9] where the gradient tensor, written in Cartesian coordinates as a dyadic is:

$$\mathbf{G} = \begin{bmatrix} \overline{ii} \dfrac{\partial B_x}{\partial x} & \overline{ij} \dfrac{\partial B_x}{\partial y} & \overline{ik} \dfrac{\partial B_x}{\partial z} \\[2mm] \overline{ji} \dfrac{\partial B_y}{\partial x} & \overline{jj} \dfrac{\partial B_y}{\partial y} & \overline{jk} \dfrac{\partial B_y}{\partial z} \\[2mm] \overline{ki} \dfrac{\partial B_z}{\partial x} & \overline{kj} \dfrac{\partial B_z}{\partial y} & \overline{kk} \dfrac{\partial B_z}{\partial z} \end{bmatrix} \tag{9}$$

The Hamiltonian for an isolated spin, $\overline{I}$, at position $\overline{r}$ within a magnetic field, including the gradient, component is

$$\mathbf{H} = \hbar(\omega_o I_z + \gamma \overline{I} \cdot \mathbf{G} \cdot \overline{r}) \tag{10}$$

where I_z is the component of the spin parallel to the static magnetic field defined in the z direction. Under conditions of a small gradient magnetic field strength ΔB relative to a large static field B_0 defining the z axis of the spin system, the vector tensor product may be approximated as[9]:

$$\overline{I} \cdot \mathbf{G} \simeq I_z \overline{G} \tag{11}$$

where the gradient vector $\overline{G}$ has three independent orthogonal components:

$$G_x = \frac{\partial B_z}{\partial x} , \; G_y = \frac{\partial B_z}{\partial y} , \; G_z = \frac{\partial B_z}{\partial z} \tag{12}$$

Expansion of the vector product form of the Biot-Savart law provides the components of $\overline{B}$; for example:

$$B_z(x, y, z) = \frac{\mu_o I}{4\pi} \left[\int_\ell \frac{(x - x_\ell)}{|r - r_\ell|^3} d\ell_y - \int_\ell \frac{(y - y_\ell)}{|r - r_\ell|^3} d\ell_x \right] \tag{13}$$

In general, it is possible to expand any function $f(x, y, z)$ that satisfies Laplace's equation, $\nabla^2 f = 0$, in terms of an infinite set of solid spherical harmonics. Because $\nabla^2 B_z = 0$ at all points within the image volume of interest, one may write

$$B_z = \sum_{n=0}^{\infty} \sum_{m=0}^{n} [A_{nm}^c r^n P_n^m(\cos \theta) \cos m\phi + A_{nm}^s r^n P_n^m(\cos \theta) \sin m\phi] \tag{14}$$

where $P_n^m(\cos \theta)$ are the associated Legendre polynomials and A_{nm}^c and A_{nm}^s are appropriate constants determined by the shape of the coils and the strength of the currents in them. In the most important case for gradient coil design consideration, the current carrying conductors will be located on a cylinder surrounding the imaging region. Under these conditions the general coefficients may be given by the simplified expressions:

$$A_{nm}^c = \frac{\mu_o}{4\pi r_o^{n+2}} \iint \lambda_\phi(\phi_o, z_o) f_{nm}(Z_o) \cos m\phi_o \, dA \tag{15}$$

and

$$A_{nm}^s = \frac{\mu_o}{4\pi r_o^{n+2}} \iint \lambda_\phi(\phi_o, z_o) f_{nm}(Z_o) \sin m\phi_o \, dA \tag{16}$$

where the normalized location of the winding along the cylinder surface (i.e., normalized axial position is $Z_o = z_o/r_o$ with the radius of the cylinder r_o and the element of surface area given by $dA = r_o^2 d\phi_o Z_o$). In most situations of interest, the surface current density $\lambda_\phi(\phi_o, a_o)$ may be expressed as the product of two functions, one depending on ϕ_o and one depending only on Z_o such that:

$$\lambda_\phi(\phi_o, z_o) = c f_\phi(\phi_o) \sigma_\phi(Z_o) \tag{17}$$

where c is a constant of proportionality, $f_\phi(\phi_o)$ expresses the angular variation of the surface current density and $\sigma_\phi(Z_o)$ expresses the variation along the cylindrical axis (z direction).

Axial Z Gradient Coils

The current density in the ϕ direction on the surface of a cylinder is given by the simplified expression:

$$\lambda_\phi = c\sigma_\phi(Z_o) \tag{18}$$

with the antisymmetry condition that $\sigma_\phi(-Z_o) = -\sigma_\phi(Z_o)$ and $c = N_t I/r_o w_{r_o}$ where N_t is the total number of turns without regard to sign and r_o is the cylinder radius. The dimensionless parameter w_{r_o} involves the shape function through the relationship

$$w_{r_o} = \int_{-Z_m}^{Z_m} | \sigma_\phi(Z_o) | \, dZ_o \tag{19}$$

where Z_m is defined with respect to the total length of the coil (i.e., extent in the z direction, $2r_o Z_m$). Thus when the shape function $\sigma_\phi(Z_o)$ (which specifies the winding density as a function of position) and the radius are fixed, c is proportional to the total number of ampere-turns on the coil. For this configuration, the magnetic field produced by the coil may be expressed as an expansion in solid spherical harmonics about the center of the coil involving only odd terms (the even terms cancel as a consequence of the antisymmetric cylindrical geometry):

$$B_z = \sum_{n=1,3,5\ldots}^{\infty} A_n r^n P_n(\cos\theta) \tag{20}$$

with the expansion coefficients given by:[19,20]

$$A_n = \frac{\mu_o c}{2r_o^n} \int_{-Z_m}^{Z_m} \sigma_\phi(Z_o) f_n(Z_o) \, dZ_o \tag{21}$$

$$= \frac{\mu_o c \gamma_n}{2r_o^n} = \mu_o N_t I \gamma_n (2r_o^{n+1} w_{r_o})^{-1} \tag{22}$$

where

$$\gamma_n = \int_{-Z_m}^{Z_m} \sigma_\phi(Z_o) f_n(Z_o) \, dZ_o \tag{23}$$

with

$$f_n(Z_o) = P_{n+1}^1(\cos\theta_o)/(1 + Z_o^2)^{(2n+3)/2} \tag{24}$$

One of the primary design objectives is to determine the current distribution, $\sigma_\phi(Z_o)$, for a given order of homogeneity of magnetic field under the constraint that the energy stored in the coil is a minimum. It can be shown that the inductance, L, is given by:

$$L = \frac{2\mu_o N_t^2 r_o}{w_{r_o}^2} S \tag{25}$$

and that the stored energy, W, in the magnetic field is given by:

$$W = \frac{4r_o^{2n+3}}{\mu_o} \frac{A_n^2}{2\gamma n^2} S \tag{26}$$

where the dimensionless factor S is defined as:

$$S = \int_{-Z_m}^{Z_m} \int_{-Z_m}^{Z_m} \frac{1}{k} \left[\left(1 - \frac{k^2}{2}\right) K(k) - E(k) \right] \sigma(Z_o)\sigma(Z_o') dZ_o' dZ_o \tag{27}$$

with the modulus, k, defined by:

$$k^2 = 4/(4 + (Z_o - Z_o')^2) \tag{28}$$

and $K(k)$, $E(k)$ are complete elliptical integrals of the first and second kind.

An expression for the z gradient G_z may be obtained by differentiating the expression for B_z and setting $z = 0$,

$$G_z = (dB_z/dz) \mid = A_1 = \frac{\mu_o c \gamma_1}{2r_o} \tag{29}$$

For $n = 1$, the stored energy would be given as:

$$W = \frac{4r_o^5}{\mu_o} G_z^2 \frac{S}{\gamma_1^2} \tag{30}$$

Therefore, for a specified value of G_z, the stored energy can be minimized by choosing the shape function $\sigma_\phi(Z_o)$ such that S is minimized subject to the normalization constraint that $\gamma_1 = 1$. The terms γ_3, γ_5, γ_7, etc., represent contaminants that limit the gradient field linearity. Design of more sophisticated gradient coils with progressively improved linearity requires additional constraints on $\sigma_\phi(Z_o)$ to achieve conditions such that

$$\gamma_3 = 0, \gamma_5 = 0, \gamma_7 = 0 \ldots, \text{ etc.} \tag{31}$$

Transverse X and Y Gradient Coils

Following the methods of Zupancic and Pirs,[25] the magnetic field at a point (y, z) due to a current in a single infinite conductor oriented parallel to the x axis at location (y_ℓ, Z_ℓ) may be expressed as the real part of the complex function representing the solution of the Biot-Savart law. For the component of the field in the z direction, this expression would be:

$$B_z(y, z) = \frac{\mu_o I}{2\pi} Re[((y_\ell + iz_\ell) - (y + iz))^{-1}] \tag{32}$$

Letting $y + iz = \xi$ and $y_\ell + iz_\ell = ie^{i\phi}$, the above expression for B_z may be expanded as a Taylor series under the condition that $|\xi| < r_\ell$ (where r_ℓ and ϕ are the polar coordinates of the wire) giving:

$$B_z(y, z) = \frac{\mu_o I}{2\pi} Re \sum_{n=0}^{\infty} (\xi/r)^n e^{-i(n+1)\phi} \tag{33}$$

Methods for Correcting Gradient Nonlinearities

PROJECTION RECONSTRUCTION

Normally the angle ϕ of the projection is defined by a linear field gradient of magnitude G and is of the form

$$B_g(\bar{r}, \bar{u}) = G(\bar{r} \cdot \bar{u})$$
$$= G(x \cos \phi + y \sin \phi) \tag{34}$$

where u is a unit vector pointing in the direction of ϕ.

Under these conditions the equation (n) for $P_\phi(\beta)$ above can be written as a line integral of $F(\bar{r})$ over a straight line path $\bar{r}\cdot\bar{u} = \beta/G$

$$P_\phi(\beta) = (1/\gamma) \int F(\bar{r})\delta(\bar{r}\cdot\bar{u} - \beta/G)d\bar{r} \tag{35}$$

For nonlinear field gradients, Lai[32,33] has defined a curvilinear coordinate system that is directly related to the gradient field.

$$q_1 = Gb_x(x, y) \tag{36}$$
$$q_2 = Gb_y(x, y)$$

This coordinate transformation is used to linearize the effect of the nonlinear field gradients. In the curvilinear coordinate system the gradient field becomes

$$B_g(\bar{q}, \bar{u}) = \bar{q}\cdot\bar{u} \tag{37}$$

$$P_\phi(\beta) = 1/\gamma \int F(\bar{r}(\bar{q}))\delta(\bar{q}\cdot\bar{u} - \beta)/ \mid J(\bar{q}) \mid d\bar{q} \tag{38}$$

where $J(\bar{q})$ is the Jacobian of the transformation from object coordinates (x, y) to gradient field coordinates (q_1, q_2). In this curved coordinate system, $P_\phi(\beta)$ is the "rectilinear" projection of the object

$$H(\bar{q}) = F(\bar{r}(\bar{q})) \mid J(\bar{q}) \mid \tag{39}$$

Conventional back projection techniques allow the image of $H(\bar{q})$ to be formed in the curvilinear coordinate system. The true image in the (x, y) coordinate system can be simply derived as

$$F(\bar{r}) = H(\bar{q}(r)) \mid j(\bar{r}) \mid \tag{40}$$

where $j(\bar{r})$ is the inverse transformation Jacobian

$$j(\bar{r}) = \begin{vmatrix} \partial q_1/\partial x & \partial q_1/\partial y \\ \partial q_2/\partial x & \partial q_2/\partial y \end{vmatrix} \tag{41}$$

Two-dimensional Fourier Transform Image Reconstruction

$$\epsilon_u(u, v) = \frac{B_u(u, v) - G_o\Delta d}{G_o\Delta d} \tag{42}$$

$$\epsilon_v(u, v) = \frac{B_v(u, v) - G_o\Delta d}{G_o\Delta d} \tag{43}$$

In these expressions, $B_u(u, v)$ is the field produced by the read-out gradient at the point (u, v), and $B_v(u, v)$ is the field produced by the maximum phase encoding gradient at the point (u, v). G_o represents the assumed linear field gradient and Δd is the pixel spacing. Image correction for gradient nonlinearities consists of constructing a new image $A'(u, v)$.

$$A'(u, v) = K_u(u, v)K_v(u, v)A[u - \epsilon_u(u, v), v - \epsilon_v(u, v)] \tag{44}$$

The K_u and K_v factors are needed for intensity correction.

$$K_u(u, v) = 1/[1 + \partial\epsilon_u/\partial u\Delta d]$$
$$K_v(u, v) = 1/[1 + \partial\epsilon_v/\partial v\Delta d] \tag{45}$$

References

1. Bottomley PA: Instrumentation for whole-body NMR imaging. *In* Witcofski RL, Karstaedt N, Partain CL (eds): NMR Imaging: Proceedings of an International Symposium on Nuclear Magnetic Resonance Imaging. Winston-Salem, N.C., The Bowman Gray School of Medicine, 1982, pp 25–31.

2. Thomas SR, Ackerman JL: The instrumentation of nuclear magnetic resonance imaging. *In* Gerhard GC, Miller WT (eds): Frontiers of Engineering and Computing in Health Care, 1983. Proceedings, Fifth Annual Conference IEEE Engineering in Medicine and Biology Society, 1983, pp 25–31.

3. Pykett IL, Buonanno FS, Brady TJ et al: Techniques and approaches to proton NMR imaging of the head. Comput Radiol *27*:1–17, 1983.

4. Lai CM, Lauterbur PC: True three-dimensional image reconstruction by nuclear magnetic resonance zeugmatography. Phys Med Biol *26*:851–856, 1975.

5. Haase A, Frahm J, Matthaei D et al: Rapid images and NMR movies. (Abstract). Society of Magnetic Resonance in Medicine. 4th Annual Meeting, August 19–23, 1986. London, England, pp 980–981.

6. Holland GN: Systems engineering of a whole-body proton magnetic resonance imaging system. *In* Partain CL, James AE, Rollo FD, Price RR (eds): Nuclear Magnetic Resonance (NMR) Imaging. Philadelphia, W.B. Saunders Company, 1984, pp 128–151.

7. Edelstein WA, Bottomley PA, Hart HR et al: NMR imaging at 5.1. MHz: Work in progress. *In* Witcofski RL, Karstaedt N, Partain CL (eds): NMR Imaging: Proceedings of an International Symposium on Nuclear Magnetic Resonance Imaging. Winston-Salem, N.C., The Bowman Gray School of Medicine, 1982, pp 139–145.

8. O'Donnell M, Edelstein WA: NMR imaging in the presence of magnetic field inhomogeneities and gradient field nonlinearities. Med Phys *12*:20–26, 1985.

9. Mansfield P, Morris PG: NMR imaging in biomedicine. New York, Academic Press, 1982.

10. Golay MJ: Field homogenizing coils for nuclear spin resonance instrumentation. Rev Sci Inst *29*:313–315, 1968.

11. Anderson WA: Electrical current shims for correcting magnetic fields. Rev Sci Inst *32*:241–250, 1961.

12. Tanner JE: Pulsed field gradients for NMR spin-echo diffusion measurements. Rev Sci Inst *36*:1086–1087, 1965.

13. Ginsberg DM, Melchner MJ: Optimum geometry of saddle coils for generating a uniform magnetic field. Rev Sci Inst *41*:122–123, 1970.

14. Parker RS, Zupancic I, Pirs J: Coil system to produce orthogonal, linear magnetic field gradients. J Phys E: Sci Instr *6*:899–900, 1973.

15. Odbery G, Odbert L: On the use of a quadrupole coil for NMR spin-echo diffusion studies. J Magn Reson *16*:342–347, 1974.

16. Blicharski JS, Sobel WT: A new type of magnetic field gradient coil for NMR measurements. J Magn Reson *46*:1–8, 1982.

17. Sobol WT, Blicharski JS: Triangular pyramidal magnetic field gradient coils for NMR diffusion measurements. J Magn Reson *60*:83–90, 1984.

18. Romeo F, Hoult DI: Magnetic field profiling: Analysis and correcting coil design. Magn Reson Med *1*:44–65, 1984.

19. Schenck JG, Hussain MA, Edelstein WA, Noble G: An integral equation for the design of magnetic field coils. Proceedings of the 1982 Army Numerical Analysis and Computers Conference. ARO Report 82-3. Research Triangle Park, North Carolina, U.S. Army Research Office, pp 397–409.

20. Schenck JF, Hussain MA: Formulation of design rules for NMR imaging coils by using symbolic manipulation. Proceedings of the 1981 ACM Symposium on Symbolic and Algebraic Computations, Association for Computing Machinery, New York, New York, pp 85–93.

21. Bottomley PA: A versatile magnetic field gradient control system for NMR imaging. J Phys E: Sci Instr *14*:1081–1087, 1981.

22. Thomas SR, Ackerman JL, Kereiakes JG: Practical aspects involved in the design and set up of a 0.15T, 6-Coil resistive magnet whole body NMR imaging facility. Magn Res Imag *2*:341–348, 1984.

23. Saint-Jalmes H, Taquin J, Barjhoux Y: Design data for efficient axial gradient coils: Application to NMR imaging. Magn Reson Med *2*:245–252, 1985.

24. Bangert V, Mansfield P: Magnetic field gradient coils for NMR imaging. J Phys E: Sci Instr *15*:235–239, 1982.

25. Zupancic I, Pirs J: Coils producing a magnetic field gradient for diffusion measurements with NMR. J Phys E: Sci Instr *9*:79–80, 1976.

26. Golay MJ: Homogenizing coils for NMR apparatus. US Patent 3,622,869, 1971.

27. Hutchison JMS: NMR proton imaging techniques. *In* Foster MA (ed): Magnetic Resonance in Medicine and Biology. New York, Pergamon Press, 1986, pp 173–190.

28. Lauterbur PC: Image formation by induced local interactions: Examples employing NMR. Nature *242*:190–191, 1973.

29. Hinshaw WS: Spin mapping: The application of moving gradients to NMR. Phys Lett A *48*:87–88, 1974.

30. Macovski A: Volumetric NMR imaging with time-varying gradients. Magn Reson Med *2*:29–40, 1985.

31. Hutchinson JMS, Sutherland RJ, Mallard JR: NMR imaging: Image recovery under magnetic fields with large non-uniformities. J Phys E: Sci Instr *11*:217–221, 1978.

32. Lai CM: Reconstructing NMR images under non-linear field gradients. J Phys E: Sci Instr *16*:34–38, 1983.

33. Lai CM: Reconstructing NMR images from projections under inhomogeneous magnetic fields and nonlinear field gradients. Phys Med Biol *28*:925–938, 1983.

72

Radio Frequency Resonators

CECIL E. HAYES
WILLIAM A. EDELSTEIN
JOHN F. SCHENCK

In this chapter we provide background information needed to design and evaluate the radio frequency (rf) resonators used in biomedical applications of NMR. The emphasis is on the large structures required for head and whole body imaging. We cover briefly the fundamentals of resonant circuits followed by a more detailed treatment of the signal-to-noise performance of resonators. We give a general discussion of the relevant design considerations, including coil inductance, stray electric fields, shielding, quadrature excitation and reception, and rf field homogeneity. We review the principal types of imaging resonators, such as the solenoid, the saddle coil, the slotted tube resonator, the "birdcage" resonator, and the crossed ellipse coil. We then describe the interfacing of the rf resonator to the transmitter and receiver sections of the spectrometer. We conclude with a brief discussion of surface coils.

In a conventional nuclear magnetic resonance (NMR) spectrometer a radio frequency coil provides the interface between the magnetic moments of the nuclei and the electronics of the spectrometer. The coil assembly has two primary functions: the excitation of nuclear spins and the detection of the resulting nuclear precession. During excitation, the rf coil serves as a transducer that converts rf power into a transverse rotating rf magnetic field B_1 in the imaging volume. High efficiency for this transmit mode of operation corresponds to maximum B_1 in the sample volume for minimum rf power. By tuning the rf coil with a capacitor to create a resonant circuit, the rf energy can be recycled many times. The rf energy is stored alternatively as magnetic field energy in the coil and electric field energy in the capacitor. During reception, the rf coil and its associated reamplifier serve as a transducer that converts a precessing nuclear magnetization into an electrical signal suitable for further signal processing. High efficiency for this reception mode corresponds to minimal degradation of the inherent signal-to-noise ratio of the sample volume. A well-designed coil with low losses can be highly efficient as both a transmitter and receiver.

In this chapter we will often use the term "rf resonator" instead of the more traditional term "rf coil" in order to emphasize the changes of design needed to meet the requirements of a large-bore imaging system compared to those of the more traditional small bore NMR spectrometer. The definitive design parameter is the size of the sample relative to the wavelength of the rf radiation used. In conventional NMR spectroscopy, the sample volume is small compared to the wavelength. Hence a multiple-turn coil and a discrete capacitor can be used for frequencies below 100 MHz. The magnetic field and electric field energy storage occurs separately in two physically distinct components of the resonant circuit. The coil is the inductive component, and the capacitor is the capacitive component. At microwave frequencies, where the relevant sizes are comparable to the wavelength, a cavity resonator is appropriate. In this

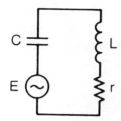

Figure 72–1. Simple LCR circuit.

case the magnetic and electric energy storage overlaps in the same volume. The cavity resonator provides both the inductive capacitive functions in a single structure. For whole body imaging, the sample volume is only slightly smaller than the wavelength. Neither the multiple-turn coil nor the cavity resonator is appropriate. Both the inductive and capacitive functions should be integrated into a single structure, but only the magnetic energy storage should occur in the sample volume. Electric field energy storage, which should not occur in the sample volume, can be confined to discrete capacitors. Hence for whole body imaging, the appropriate resonator is a hybrid of lumped and distributed elements.

NMR rf resonators differ significantly in function from traditional antenna designs. In particular an rf transmitting antenna is designed to radiate a large fraction of its input power into its far field region. In contrast, an NMR resonator needs to store magnetic energy during transmit mode in its near field region with minimal dissipation and preferably no radiation. Although the sample material may absorb significant rf energy, only a miniscule fraction of it is actually absorbed by the nuclear spins. Likewise, the NMR resonator detects the rotating nuclear magnetization during receive mode without extracting any significant energy from the nuclear spins. Such a transfer of energy from the spins to the rf resonator would cause a shortening of the free induction decay.

For whole body imaging it is desirable for the excitation and reception to be spatially uniform in the imaging volume. Unfortunately, spatial uniformity and high efficiency cannot be optimized simultaneously. Increasing the spatial uniformity will increase the rf power required and decrease the signal-to-noise ratio. The improved signal-to-noise performance of surface coils is a direct consequence of their poorer spatial uniformity.

In the following sections we treat first the fundamentals of LCR circuits and their signal-to-noise performance. Then we enumerate some general resonator design principles and apply them to a discussion of several specific geometries. Next we show how resonators are interfaced to the rf power amplifier and the preamplifier. Finally, we describe surface coils and how their design requirements differ from whole body or head-sized resonators.

RESONANT CIRCUIT FUNDAMENTALS

The simple series LCR circuit of Figure 72–1 can serve as an equivalent circuit for most NMR coils. If the frequency of the voltage source $E = E_0 e^{i\omega t}$ is varied. The maximum peak current occurs for

$$\omega = \frac{1}{\sqrt{LC}} \tag{1}$$

provided $r \ll \omega L$. At resonance, energy is alternately stored as magnetic energy in the inductor, L, and then as electrostatic energy in the capacitor, C. During the transfer of this stored energy, some is dissipated in the series resistor, r. The resonant circuit quality factor, Q, is a measure of the circuit's energy storage efficiency. Q is defined as

$$Q = \frac{\text{maximum energy stored}}{\text{average energy dissipated per radian}} \tag{2}$$

Q may be determined by measuring the resonant frequency and the full 3 dB bandwidth $\Delta\omega$:

$$Q = \frac{\omega}{\Delta\omega} \tag{3}$$

Q is also given by

$$Q = \frac{1}{r\omega C} = \frac{\omega L}{r} \tag{4}$$

Equating the right sides of Equations (3) and (4) yields

$$r = \Delta\omega L \tag{5}$$

If L is known, a rather straightforward measurement of bandwidth can be substituted for a more difficult measurement of the small, frequency-dependent quantity r. If L is not known, it can be deduced by increasing r by a known increment δr and observing the incremental change in bandwidth $\delta\omega$:

$$L = \frac{\delta r}{\delta\omega} \tag{6}$$

The δr must be inserted into the circuit at a point where all the current passes through it. It is often more practical to deduce the value of L from its resonant frequency when connected to a known capacitor. This procedure eliminates the lead inductance that may occur when making a direct measurement of L with an impedance meter. Resonant frequencies and bandwidths can be observed by exciting the resonance with a variable frequency signal source coupled via a small inductive loop placed on one side of the resonant circuit. The circuit's response is monitored on a scope or spectrum analyzer by way of a second small inductive loop placed on the opposite side of the resonant circuit. For high Q circuits, weak coupling must be used to prevent extraneous loading the source impedance or scope's input impedance. A frequency counter may be needed to measure small bandwidths accurately.

SIGNAL–TO–NOISE CONSIDERATIONS

A precessing set of nuclear spins will induce a voltage in a rf coil that is proportional to frequency of precession, the number of spins, the degree of spin polarization, and the strength of coupling between the nuclei and the coil. The number of spins will be proportional to the sample volume, V_s. The spin polarization is proportional to the static magnetic field B_0, which also determines the frequency of precession, ω. The degree of coupling between the spins and the coil is a function of geometry, which is delineated by the Principle of Reciprocity.[1] The latter states that a time varying magnetic dipole, $\overline{m}$, induces a voltage

$$\epsilon = -\frac{\partial}{\partial t}(\overline{m}\cdot\overline{B}_1) \tag{7}$$

where $\overline{B}_1$ is the magnetic field at the position of $\overline{m}$ due to a unit current in the coil. Note that only the component of B_1 that is parallel to the precessing component of $\overline{m}$

is important. That is, the coil sensitivity is proportional to $(B_1)_{xy}$, the component of B_1 perpendicular to B_0, which is usually taken to be along the z axis. Hence the induced signal in the coil is given by

$$\text{Signal} \propto V_s\omega^2(B_1)_{xy} \tag{8}$$

The signal can be represented as a series voltage source in the LCR circuit of Figure 72–1.

The fluctuation-dissipation theorem indicates that there is a direct relationship between electrical resistance and noise. The thermally activated motions of the charge carriers in dissipative media produce random electric and magnetic fields, which can be detected as noise. A resistance, r, produces an rms noise voltage, V_n, given by

$$V_n = \sqrt{4kTr\,\Delta f} \tag{9}$$

where k is the Boltzmann's constant, T is absolute temperature of the resistance, and Δf is the bandwidth set by the data acquisition system. For the LCR circuit, another series voltage source with magnitude given by Equation (9) should be included in Figure 72–1 to account for the noise voltage generated by r.

Equations (8) and (9) can be combined to obtain an expression for the signal-to-noise ratio (SNR)

$$SNR \propto \frac{V_s\omega^2(B_1)_{xy}}{\sqrt{r}} \tag{10}$$

For the special case of small solenoidal coils used in early NMR spectrometers, Equation (10) can be rearranged[1] to give

$$SNR \propto \eta\omega^{3/2}Q^{1/2}V_c^{1/2} \tag{11}$$

where V_c is the volume of the solenoid and η is the filling factor defined as the ratio of rf magnetic energy stored in the sample volume to the total rf magnetic energy stored by the coil. Hence, for conventional spectroscopy, one desired a high Q coil with good filling factor for as large a sample volume as would fit in the homogeneous region of the magnet. For in vivo NMR imaging, a slightly modified Equation (10) is more applicable, since coil Q and filling factor play a less direct role in SNR. The factor V_s in Equation (10) must be divided out because imaging is concerned with SNR per unit volume or SNR for a fixed voxel size, which is determined by the desired resolution and not by the total sample volume. Hoult and Lauterbur[2] extended Equation (10) to whole body imaging by including both coil losses and patient losses in the resistance r. The patient losses may be due to dielectric effects and magnetically induced eddy currents. Magnetic losses are unavoidable, since the coil responds to magnetic fields generated by the nuclear spins as well as by the random thermally activated currents in the patient. Dielectric losses arise from electric fields in the patient due to stray capacitance between patient and coil. They should be minimized because electric field effects carry no useful information. Hoult and Lauterbur[2] estimated the equivalent resistance of a patient by calculating the magnetically induced eddy current losses in a sphere of radius b with conductivity σ exposed to an rf field $(B_1)_{xy}$ due to a unit current in the coil. They found

$$r_{\text{patient}} \propto \sigma\omega^2(B_1)_{xy}b^5 \tag{12}$$

the resistance of the coil r_{coil} is proportional to the square root of the frequency due to the rf skin effect.[1] Replacing the r in Equation (10) with the sum of r_{coil} and r_{patient} leads to the expression

$$SNR \propto \frac{\omega^2(B_1)_{xy}}{\sqrt{\alpha\omega^{1/2} + \beta\sigma\omega^2(B_1)_{xy}^2 b^5}} \tag{13}$$

Assuming the coil's dimensions are determined by the sample radius b, $(B_1)_{xy}$ will decrease and the coil resistance will increase with increasing sample size. However, the term for patient losses will increase more rapidly than the coil losses when either ω or b are increased. For a low-loss high Q body coil at 6.4 MHz, the coil losses r_{coil} can be approximately equal to the patient losses $r_{patient}$.[3] Hence at higher frequencies,

$$r_{patient} \gg r_{coil} \tag{14}$$

is possible. In the limit of high frequencies, Equation (13) reduces to

$$SNR \propto \frac{\omega}{b^{5/2}} \tag{15}$$

Here, in contrast to Equation (11), the signal-to-noise ratio increases linearly with frequency and is apparently independent of filling factor η and coil Q. In fact the SNR for a fixed voxel size decreases as sample size b is increased. Due to the spatial discrimination of the imaging process, the tissue outside the voxel adds to the noise but not to the signal. The coil Q and filling factor effects have dropped out of Equation (15) only because both are sufficiently large to satisfy Equation (14). A high Q corresponds to a small r_{coil} and a high filling factor provides a large value of $(B_1)_{xy}$ in $r_{patient}$. The relative values of r_{coil} and $r_{patient}$ can be determined by measuring Q when the coil is empty and when it is loaded by a patient. The best indicator of coil sensitivity is the ratio

$$\frac{Q_{empty}}{Q_{loaded}} = \frac{r_{coil} + r_{patient}}{r_{coil}} \tag{16}$$

provided dielectric losses do not contribute to $r_{patient}$. At 1.5 tesla, this ratio can be 5 or more. This implies that coil losses contribute less than 11 percent of the observed noise voltage.

RADIO FREQUENCY COIL DESIGN CONSIDERATIONS

We begin by listing some obvious and less obvious requirements for the rf coil assembly in an MR imaging system. The rf coil should resonate at the desired operating frequency, be large enough to accommodate the imaging volume, produce a homogeneous B_1 field, have a good filling factor, have minimum coil losses, be able to withstand the applied voltages, produce minimal electric fields in the sample, have minimum interaction with the rest of the system, and permit quadrature excitation and reception. We will discuss these issues and their inter-relationships in the following paragraphs.

There is a strong linkage between coil volume and its resonance frequency. Making a body-sized resonant circuit using conventional LCR circuit techniques becomes increasingly difficult as the desired resonant frequency (or static magnetic field B_0) is increased. If a simple multiple-turn solenoidal coil is scaled up in size, its inductance increases proportional to its linear dimension. The capacitance needed for a given resonant frequency varies inversely with the inductance. The lower limit of capacitance is determined by the stray capacitance of the coil, which also depends on its size. Hence the upper bound on the operating frequency is set by the inductance and stray capacitance of the coil. Since the inductance of a simple solenoid increases as the square of its number of turns, one can obviously increase the resonant frequency by minimizing the number of turns. Unfortunately, as the number of turns is decreased, the B_1 field homogeneity can also suffer. Thus, for frequencies over about 15 MHz, body-sized wire wound coils are inappropriate. At high frequencies it is conceptually useful to think in terms of rf resonators instead of rf coils. This transition from lumped element circuits to distributed element resonators occurs at a much lower frequency for whole body imaging than for small sample NMR spectroscopy.

Designing high frequency resonators requires reduction of both the inductance and the stray capacitance. Using a single wide conductor in place of multiple turns of discrete wire reduces the inductance. The wider conductor permits a lower surface current density, which corresponds to a lower inductance. The rf field near the conductor, which has only a tangential component, is proportional to the surface current density. Thus, the magnetic energy density, which is proportional to the field squared, is less near the surface of a wide conductor than a smaller wire. High energy storage near the conductors but outside of the sample volume degrades the filling factor. Wide sheet conductors are opaque to rf flux and can also be used to manipulate the flux distribution within the sample volume. A good filling factor requires that all inductive elements contribute to the B_1 field in the sample. Hence the capacitors should be located as close to the coil as possible to minimize extraneous magnet energy storage and energy dissipation in the capacitor leads. Similarly, placing several small valued capacitors across the break in a wide conductor instead of a single larger valued one will reduce surface current density and lead inductance. The resonator's inductive elements should be connected in parallel rather than in series if possible.

Minimizing the inductance has two advantages in addition to permitting higher resonant frequencies. Lowering the inductance lowers the voltage developed during the transmit pulses. For a fixed magnetic flux the voltage increases linearly with frequency and proportional to the square root of the inductance. Hence during transmit, higher inductances produce higher voltages, which can lead to corona discharge. Lowering the inductance also reduces the stray electric fields in the sample, which correspond to dielectric losses in the sample. At low frequencies, the electric field can be screened from the sample with a Faraday shield.[4] The screen works on the principle of imposing a grounded grid between the coil and the sample. The grid shunts to ground the electric field lines that would otherwise pass through the sample. The screen is unusable at high frequencies for two reasons. The screen introduces a large stray capacitance to ground, which limits the maximum resonant frequency. At high frequencies, the self-inductance of the grid prevents it from defining a ground plane. At higher frequencies, electric fields can be reduced by using coil symmetry to introduce virtual ground planes.[5] For example, the balanced circuit in Figure 72–2 has a virtual ground at the center of the coil. The maximum voltage in the coil with respect to ground is one half what it would be if one end of the coil were grounded.

The fringe field of a coil extends outside the coil for a distance comparable to one or so diameters. Thus the coil may interact strongly with the surrounding environment. Such interactions with the gradient or shim coils, for example, can produce spurious resonances or extraneous losses in the coil. The usual solution is to surround the coil with a shield opaque to rf fields. The shield develops image currents that concentrate the fringe field between the coil and shield and reduce the field strength in the sample volume. Such distortion of the field distribution increases as the spacing between shield and coil decreases. Thus a tightly fitted shield can reduce the filling factor and add to the resistive coil losses.

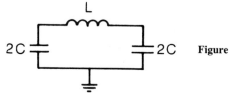

Figure 72–2. Balanced circuit.

Another desirable design feature for an rf resonator that should find increasing utility in the future is the ability to implement quadrature excitation and reception.[6] Such a structure should have two geometrically and electrically orthogonal resonant modes tuned to the same resonant frequency. Exciting both modes with equal magnitudes but with phases differing by 90 degrees develops a constant magnitude B_1 rotating in the same direction as the nuclear spin precession. It requires half as much rf power to generate such a rotating B_1 field compared to the more conventional oscillating linear B_1 field. The signal received in each of the two resonant modes can be summed after phase shifting one channel by 90 degrees. The signal-to-noise ratio will be increased by a factor of the square root of 2, since the two signals are coherent but the two noises are not coherent. Quadrature excitation and reception have the additional advantage of reducing rf penetration artifacts when imaging at high fields.[7] Quadrature operation will be possible in a resonator that possesses a fourfold axis of rotation along the B_0 field directions, but this is not a necessary condition.

The homogeneity of the rf field $B_1(\bar{r})$ determines the spatial uniformity of the image intensity. The signal will be proportional to the transverse component of magnetization $M_{xy}(\bar{r})$ developed by the transmit excitation. $M_{xy}(\bar{r})$ depends strongly on the flip angle, θ, which is proportional to $B_1(\bar{r})$. For a $\theta - \tau - 2\theta$ spin-echo pulse sequence, $M_{xy}(\bar{r})$ is proportional to $\sin^3 \theta(\bar{r})$.[6] The coupling of $M_{xy}(\bar{r})$ to the coil during signal reception is also proportional to $B_1(\bar{r})$. As noted before, improvements in B_1 within the imaging volume can be increased by enlarging the rf coil. However, this approach increases the coil losses, decreases the filling factor, and adds extra tissue losses by including greater tissue volume within the coil. An alternative is to use separate transmit and receive coils. In this case, the transmit coil is enlarged, since transmit flip angle inhomogeneity has the stronger effect on image uniformity. The receiver coil is smaller to minimize tissue losses. However, this approach precludes the use of quadrature excitation and reception. On the other hand, there are single coil designs with adequate B_1 homogeneity that also permit quadrature operation (see Fig. 72–3).

Whole body imaging requires a homogeneous B_1 field in a cylindrical volume. The B_1 field may be parallel or transverse to the cylinder's axis. The axial rf field is useful in iron core magnets or some air core magnets that produce a transverse B_0 field. The transverse B_1 field is applicable to the more common solenoidal magnets. A perfectly homogeneous axial field can be generated in an infinitely long cylinder with a uniform surface current density directed around the cylinder. This corresponds to an infinite solenoid. A perfectly homogeneous transverse field can be generated in an infinitely long cylinder by surface currents parallel to the cylinder's axis. In this case, the current density is not uniform but is proportional to the sine (or cosine) of the azimuthal angle, ϕ. For the sin ϕ distribution, a positive current flows on the top of the cylinder and a negative current flows on the bottom of the cylinder to give a horizontal transverse field. If the two cylinders have equal non-zero surface resistivities, then it requires twice as much power per unit length to generate a unit transverse field as to generate a unit axial field. The infinite solenoid may be more efficient because it stores all its magnetic energy within the cylinder, whereas for the transverse field configuration,

Figure 72–3. Single turn solenoid.

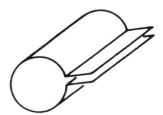

flux must also exist outside the cylinder. Perfect homogeneity is destroyed when the two cylinders are cut down to finite lengths. For a coil length equal to the diameter, the field on the axis at the end of the cylinder is about one half the strength at the center of the coil. For the sin ϕ current distribution, conductive end rings must be added to convey currents between the top and bottom halves of the cylindrical surface. These end rings conduct current proportional to cos ϕ. These added current paths, which are not needed in the finite solenoid, contribute additional coil losses for the transverse field configuration. Thus, the nearly ideal axial field coil has inherently fewer losses than the nearly ideal transverse field coil, but perhaps to a lesser degree than Hoult and Richards' findings for solenoid and saddle coils.[1]

RADIO FREQUENCY COIL REVIEW

In this section we describe a number of coil designs that are currently being used or developed for body and head imaging.

The multiple turn solenoid has been widely used in lower frequency NMR spectrometers that employ an iron core magnet. A long solenoid is a good approximation to the ideal current distribution required for a uniform axial rf field. Hoult[8] has suggested that the length of the optimum solenoid for imaging should be only about 80 percent of the coil's diameter. Here he has sacrificed some B_1 homogeneity to improve signal sensitivity by reducing patient losses. He also found that increasing coil losses due to the "proximity effect" requires that space between adjacent turns should equal about one half the diameter of the copper tubing used to wind it. The operating frequency of the multiple turn solenoid is limited by its high inductance and stray capacitance. Cook and Lowe suggest a modification that allows a solenoid to operate at a much higher frequency.[9] They insert a capacitor in series between each turn of a multiple turn solenoid. Each capacitor cancels the inductive reactance of a single turn of the solenoid. For example, an N turn solenoid with inductance L might require a very small capacitor, C, to resonate at a high frequency $\omega = 1/\sqrt{LC}$. Instead of a single small capacitor, N capacitors of value NC each are used; $N - 1$ of them are inserted between turns of the solenoid and the last capacitor is connected between the end terminals of the inductor. The net effective inductance of the composite coil appears to be L/N, since it resonates with an external capacitor equal to NC.

An alternate means of reducing the inductance of a solenoid is to wind a single turn from a wide sheet of conductor. The homogeneity is maintained by making the width of the conducting sheet equal to the desired length of the solenoid. Because the sheet is opaque to rf, it forms a "flux pipe," which channels the magnetic flux in one end of the cylinder and out the other. The presence of a uniform rf magnetic field adjacent to the inner surface of the conducting sheet implies that there must also be a uniform surface current flowing around the inner surface of the cylinder. To maintain this current distribution and the corresponding field homogeneity and low inductance, the tuning capacitor must be distributed evenly along the whole width of the sheet. Figure 72–3 shows how the conducting sheet can be extended to form the capacitor.[10]

There are a number of resonant devices for producing transverse rf fields in a cylinder. We will consider several in terms of how well they approximate the ideal sinusoidally weighted surface current distribution. We will deal with the case where the current density is proportional to sin ϕ. If $\phi = 0$ corresponds to the x axis, then the transverse field generated is parallel to the x axis. The simplest approximation to sin ϕ is a two point fit with wires running on the surface parallel to the z axis at $\phi = $ 90 degrees and $\phi = 270$ degrees. Figure 72–4 shows this surface current distribution and the corresponding coil. The two end rings complete the current path in a symmetric

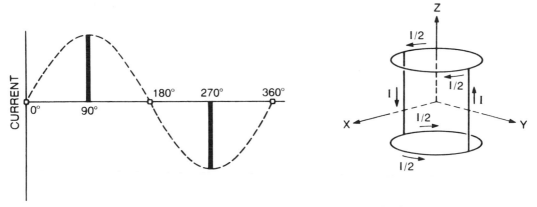

Figure 72–4. Four point fit to a sinusoidal current distribution.

manner, which permits access along the cylindrical axis. This could also be considered a four point fit to sin φ, where the zero currents at φ = 0 degrees and 180 degrees require no wires. The next simplest approximation to sin φ is a six point fit shown in Figure 72–5. This is the saddle coil configuration with two equal positive currents at φ = 60 degrees and 120 degrees and two equal negative currents at φ = 240 degrees and 300 degrees. The wires at φ = 0 degrees and 180 degrees and parts of the end ring can be omitted because they carry no current. The inductance of the saddle coil can be reduced by connecting both turns in parallel and by widening both conductors until they merge along φ = 90 degrees and 180 degrees. In the limit of very wide conductors, the saddle coil reduces to the topologically equivalent single turn coil in Figure 72–4. Alderman and Grant[5] used symmetry arguments to determine preferred locations for capacitance on the single turn coil in Figure 72–4. Assuming a single capacitor, C, tunes the coil when placed in the straight segment at φ = 90 degrees, they found they could replace it with capacitors equal to C at φ = 0 degrees and 180 degrees on each of the two end rings (Fig. 72–6). The centers of these four capacitors define a virtual ground plane, the x-z plane. To shield the sample from the electric fields developed in the vicinity of the capacitors, they added a guard ring inside each of the two end rings. The guard rings float with a ground potential at φ = 0 degrees and 180 degrees and develop much smaller potentials than the voltage drop across the capacitors. The transverse midplane (z = 0) is a mirror plane of symmetry, which implies it is also a virtual ground plane. Thus the sample volume is exposed to greatly reduced stray electric

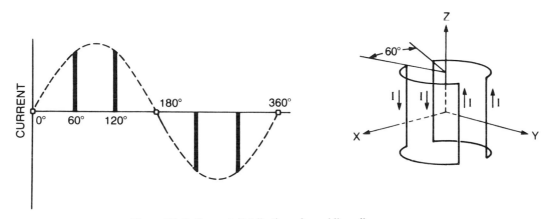

Figure 72–5. Current distribution of a saddle coil.

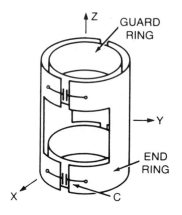

Figure 72–6. Alderman-Grant coil.

fields. This structure, originally intended for high frequency spectroscopy, has been extended to head imaging at 64 MHz by Bottomley et al.[11] More detailed descriptions of this resonator design as applied to imaging have been published recently.[12,13]

The Alderman and Grant design is closely related to the slotted tube resonator of Schneider and Dullenkopf.[14] Consider a transmission line made of two parallel conductors of length ℓ separated by an air space. This line has a standing wave resonance whenever ℓ is equal to an integer number of half wavelengths. For the one half wavelength resonance, there are high voltages at each end where electrostatic energy is stored in the capacitance between conductors and high currents in the middle region where magnetic energy is concentrated between the lines. Schneider and Dullenkopf[14] made their transmission line by cutting a slot along both sides of a conducting tube. They enclosed the slotted tube transmission line in a cylindrical conducting shield. They adjusted the angular width of the slots ϕ and the ratio of the shield radius to transmission line radius b/a to optimize the rf magnetic field homogeneity (Fig. 72–7). To avoid electric fields in the sample, the useful sample volume of a half wavelength line would have to be restricted to a small length at the center of the line. This restraint would lead to a poor filling factor, since there is a large overlap of electric and magnetic energy storage volumes. At imaging frequencies, a half wavelength line would also be awkwardly long. This resonant line length can be greatly shortened if each end of the shortened line is terminated by a lumped capacitance to replace the distributed capacitance so removed. Furthermore, fitting half the terminating capacitance on each side of the cylinder produces the Alderman-Grant configuration (less the guard ring). Shorting out one end of a transmission line produces resonances corresponding to odd multiples of a quarter wavelength. The quarter wavelength resonator can likewise be reduced to a convenient length by capacitively terminating the open end. If the slotted tube is shorted with a transverse sheet across the cylinder, as Alderman has suggested, field homogeneity is improved.[12] The conducting sheet behaves as a flux mirror, which

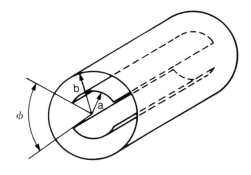

Figure 72–7. Slotted tube resonator.

effectively doubles the length of the coil. Such a coil, with access from only one end, has been built for head imaging.[12]

The slotted tube resonator develops a current distribution that is peaked near the edges of the conductors adjacent to the slots. In this respect it resembles the current distribution of the four wires of the saddle coil in Figure 72–5. But there is an important difference. The conducting sheets of the slotted tube resonator are opaque to rf field and divert all the flux through the two slots. Hence the ideal slot aperture angle, ϕ, is significantly different from the 120 degree angle found in the saddle coil. A sinusoidally weighted surface current density produces optimum field homogeneity only if the cylinder's surface not only conducts current but is also transparent to rf magnetic flux. Such a surface can be approximated by a large number of parallel conductors spaced apart to allow the flux to pass between them. To improve on the saddle coil approximation to the ideal current distribution with more conductors requires a means of developing unequal, sinusoidally weighted currents in adjacent conductors (Fig. 72–8). A standing wave in a one wavelength transmission line generates the needed sinusoidal current distribution. Hinshaw and Gauss[15] wound a one wavelength coaxial cable evenly spaced onto a toroidal form. They removed the coaxial shielding from the cable lying on the inner diameter of the toroid. The exposed center conductor of the coax has the sinusoidal current weighting needed to produce a homogeneous transverse field in the inner bore of the toroid. This structure is limited to low frequencies by the need to wind a many turn toroid from a single wavelength of cable. Roeschmann[16] has built a one turn version of this concept to operate at 85 MHz by exposing the center conductor at only two places. His rf field homogeneity is similar to that of a saddle coil.

We have applied the resonant transmission line in a different way to generate a sinusoidal surface current. Consider a transmission line made from two parallel wires, each formed into a closed circle (Fig. 72–9). Such a transmission line closed on itself can support standing wave resonances consisting of an integer number of wavelengths. For the single wavelength resonance, if the voltage is proportional to sin ϕ, then the current is proportional to cos ϕ in the upper circle and $-\cos \phi$ in the lower circle. This current tends to produce a transverse field along the x axis. At 64 MHz (1.5 T), the circle's diameter would be about 1.5 meters, which is too large for a body or head coil. We shorten the resonant wavelength by adding many evenly spaced, equal, lumped-element capacitors between the two lines of the transmission. We call the result a "birdcage" resonator (Fig. 72–10).[17] The transmission line forms the two end rings with a voltage difference across the capacitors proportional to sin ϕ. Hence the currents in the capacitors are also proportional to sin ϕ. The long leads of the capacitors carry the desired approximation to a sinusoidal surface current density. This circuit is essentially a lumped-element balanced delay line joined on itself. It can also be thought

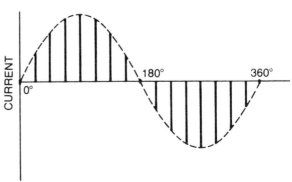

Figure 72–8. Multiple point fit to a sinusoidal current distribution.

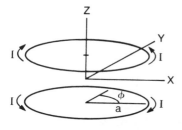

Figure 72–9. Closed loop transmission line.

of as an N segment low pass filter. Each segment produces a phase shift of $2\pi/N$ at resonance. We have also built a high pass version of the birdcage resonator in which the capacitors are evenly spaced around both end rings and the straight segments between end rings are purely inductive (Fig. 72–11). We believe the birdcage resonator incorporates a number of the design guidelines discussed in the preceding section. The large number of wires can accurately simulate the desired sinusoidal surface current. Radio frequency field homogeneity is limited only by the finite length of the structure. The multiple turns of the coil are effectively wired in parallel to reduce the inductance to that of a single turn coil or less. The distributed currents lower the coil losses and prevent the development of high concentrations of magnetic field close to the conductors. Thus the uniformity of the field improves the filling factor. The lead inductance of the capacitors is fully utilized to create the desired B_1 field. The high symmetry of the resonator facilitates the use of quadrature excitation and reception. When the birdcage has fourfold symmetry, the fundamental homogeneous mode is doubly degenerate. The two modes, corresponding to surface current densities proportional to $\sin\phi$ and $\cos\phi$, are geometrically and electrically orthogonal. Both modes are excited simultaneously but with a relative phase shift of 90 degrees to produce a rotating B_1 field.

The crossed-ellipse coil[18-20] also possesses a fourfold symmetry axis. The two ellipses are generated at the intersection of two orthogonal, equal radii cylinders. If each ellipse carries an equal current, the field generated is parallel to the axis of one of the cylinders. Reversing the polarity of current in only one ellipse switches the field to be parallel to the axis of the other cylinder. These two modes are orthogonal and permit quadrature operation if the static magnetic field B_0 is perpendicular to the axes of both cylinders. Redpath[21] has pointed out that the two ellipses can be wired in parallel with both modes tuned and driven independently (Fig. 72–12). Capacitor C_1 tunes the mode corresponding to currents I_1, and C_2 tunes the mode with currents I_2. Modes 1

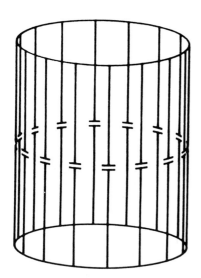

Figure 72–10. Low pass birdcage resonator.

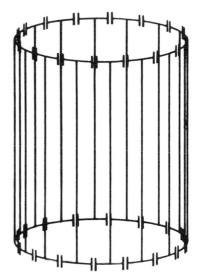

Figure 72–11. High pass birdcage resonator.

and 2 can be at the same frequency but 90 degrees out of phase for quadrature or at different frequencies for double resonance experiments.

A uniform azimuthal current density on the surface of a sphere creates a homogeneous field within a spherical volume. Bydder et al.[22] fabricated spherical head coils by spiraling four or five turns of copper tube on the surface of each hemisphere. The two half coils were connected in parallel with enough space between them to provide access for the face and neck. Elsewhere there was only 1 or 2 centimeters spacing between the coil and the patient's head. The empty Q to loaded Q ratio was about 4 for operation at the relatively low frequency of 6.4 MHz. Hence patient-induced noise is dominant even at 0.15 tesla. The more uniform field and lower current density of the spherical configuration produced a higher filling factor and lower coil losses than a standard sized saddle coil.

INTERFACING THE RADIO FREQUENCY COIL TO THE SPECTROMETER

The design requirements for connecting the rf coil to the transmitter differ somewhat from those for connecting the rf coil to the receiver. The coil serves as the load for the transmitter as the signal source for the preamplifier. In the transmit mode, one desired to deliver power from the transmitter to the rf coil as efficiently as possible. In the receive mode, one wishes to extract a signal from the coil while minimizing the

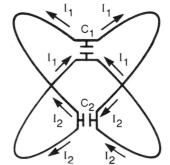

Figure 72–12. Crossed ellipses coil.

noise contribution from the preamplifier. Additional requirements are the protection of the preamplifier during the rf power pulses and the elimination of any noise contribution from the transmitter during signal acquisition.

We will consider the transmitter-to-coil interface first. In general the transmitter is located some distance (tens of meters) from the rf coil and is connected to it by an rf transmission line. The transmission line conveys power most efficiently when both the source impedance and the load impedance match (or equal) the characteristic impedance Z_0 of the transmission line. Typically Z_0 is a real quantity in the range of 50 to 100 Ω. Transmitter circuits usually incorporate output impedance matching networks to generate the needed match to Z_0. Another matching network is needed at the interconnection of the transmission line and the rf coil. The resistance, r, in the LCR circuit of Figure 72–1 is usually quite small compared to Z_0. For a reasonably high Q circuit, the voltage drop across L or C is substantially larger than that across r. Tapping into a fraction of this larger voltage drop is equivalent to performing an impedance transformation from r up to Z_0. The coil matching network will be most efficient if it introduces a minimum number of additional components and is located in close proximity to the coil.

Two popular capacitive matching schemes for coupling a source impedance Z_0 to the coil resistances r are pictured in Figure 72–13A and B. Both circuits can be analyzed by converting the network consisting of E_{source}, Z_0, C_1, and C_2 into a series equivalent network consisting of an equivalent voltage, e', an equivalent resistor, r', and an equivalent capacitance, C_{12}, as shown in Figure 72–13C. Resonance occurs when $\omega^2 L C_{12} = 1$, and power matching occurs when $r' = r$. Note the latter condition implies that proper matching of the source impedance doubles the effective series resistance of the LC circuit and therefore halves the Q. The matching process may also be thought of as converting the whole LCR circuit into a single load resistor $R_L = Z_0$, which replaces the coil assembly (Fig. 72–13D). The impedance matching condition and resonant frequency are given approximately by

$$Z_0 \cong \frac{1}{r(\omega C_2)^2} \qquad \omega^2 \cong \frac{1}{L}\left(\frac{1}{C_1} + \frac{1}{C_2}\right) \tag{17}$$

for the network in Figure 72–13A and

$$Z_0 \cong r\left(1 + \frac{C_1}{C_2}\right)^2 \qquad \omega^2 \cong \frac{1}{L(C_1 + C_2)} \tag{18}$$

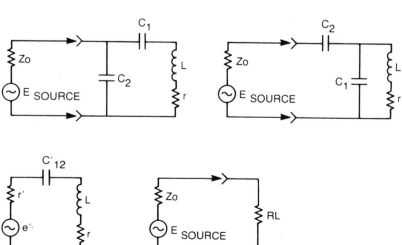

Figure 72–13. Capacitive matching networks.

for the network in Figure 72–13*B*. Inductive coupling provides an alternative matching technique. A second inductor can serve as the primary winding and the rf coil as the secondary of air core transformer. Input impedance is adjusted by varying the spatial separation between the two inductors. The input impedance, R_L, of the coil is also its output impedance when used as a source for the preamplifier.

As stated before, the primary goal of interfacing the rf coil to the preamplifier is not optimum power transfer but optimum noise performance. The ideal preamplifier would amplify both the signal and the source noise but would add no extra noise of its own. A preamplifier is characterized by its noise figure, *NF*, which specifies how much excess noise it adds to the noise generated by a specified source impedance. An amplifier's *NF*, expressed in decibels, is defined by

$$NF = 10 \log \left(\frac{\text{total output noise power}}{\text{output noise power due to sources}} \right) \qquad (19)$$

An equivalent definition for *NF* uses the ratio of square of the SNR in the coil without the preamplifier attached to the square of the SNR at the preamplifier output. Individual active components such as transistors are also characterized by an *NF*. The *NF* of a transistor is a function of the signal source impedance. There is an optimum source impedance R_{opt}, which minimizes the transistor's *NF*. R_{opt} will not, in general, equal either the input impedance of the transistor or the source impedance of the rf coil (assumed to be Z_0). For optimum noise performance, the front end of the preamplifier must include a matching network that transforms the coil's source impedance Z_0 to equal R_{opt} at the transistor, but the resulting input impedance Z_{in} at the front of the preamplifier will not, in general, equal the coil's source impedance Z_0. If Z_{in} is grossly different from Z_0, some detuning of the coil may occur during the receive mode if the coil was tuned for the transmitter's Z_0. Additional feedback network components can be added to the preamplifier to make its input impedance equal its optimum source impedance. (There are numerous vendors who supply low noise preamplifiers optimized in this manner for 50 Ω operation). For the case $Z_{in} = Z_0$, the preamplifier loads the rf coil the same amount as the transmitter did. Hence, the preamplifier adds an effective series resistance $r' = r$ in the coil and would also double the noise power if the series resistor r' contributed the normal Johnson noise given in Equation (9). Doubling the noise power corresponds to an *NF* of 3 dB for the preamplifier. For a preamplifier with *NF* less than 3 dB, the added series resistor r' can be thought of as cooled below room temperature. Hoult[23,24] has manipulated the preamplifier's loading of the coil to damp out ringing in high Q, low frequency rf imaging coils to increase their bandwidth and reduce their recovery time after the transmitter pulse.

The linear rf power amplifiers commonly used in MR imaging generate white noise at their output, which can seriously degrade the SNR if they are connected to the rf coil during signal reception. Turning off or blanking the power amplifier during signal acquisition will eliminate this active noise source. But the long transmission line leading from the coil to the inactive amplifier must also be disconnected from the coil to prevent unnecessary loading and detuning effects on the coil during data acquisition. A simple series diode switch D_1 can be added into the transmission line where it connects to the coil input (Fig. 72–14). The diode switch is made of one or more pairs of crossed low-capacitance switching diodes. During the high power rf pulse, the diodes conduct with a relatively small "on" resistance. During the low-level signal acquisition, the diodes are off and exhibit a high resistance shunted by their junction capacitance. The nonlinear operation of passive diodes distorts the transmitter waveform somewhat at low levels. An alternative is to replace the crossed diodes with a single pin diode which is biased on during transmit to give a low linear resistance.

The protection of the preamplifier during the transmit pulse is achieved in Figure

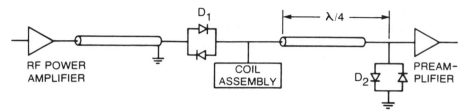

Figure 72–14. Interface of coil with rf power amplifier and preamplifier.

72–14 by using the special properties of a quarter wavelength ($\lambda/4$) transmission line.[25] The input impedance Z_{in} of a quarter wavelength line terminated by impedance Z_L is given in terms of its characteristic impedance Z_o by $Z_{in} = Z_o^2/Z_L$. During the transmit pulse, crossed diodes D_2 have an "on" resistance small compared to Z_o so the cable's input impedance at the coil appears high. The clipping diodes D_2 limit the voltage at the preamplifier during transmit but effectively drop out of the circuit during the low level signal acquisition. If the input impedance of the preamplifier equals Z_o, the quarter wavelength line has little effect on preamplifier performance. At lower frequencies, where a quarter wavelength would be awkward, a lumped element equivalent such as in Figure 72–15 can be substituted.

Surface Coils

Surface coils, as the name implies, do not enclose the sample but instead are placed on the surface of the sample material. Their greatest signal sensitivity is limited to a superficial region whose dimensions are comparable to the coil size. Surface coils were used initially for in vivo spectroscopy, where their localized response permits acquisition of spectra predominantly from a particular organ or tissue type.[26] More recently, surface coils have been applied to imaging to achieve greatly improved signal-to-noise performance within the local region compared to whole body or head coil imaging.[27–29] The enhanced signal strength may be used to reduce signal averaging or to improve image resolution by decreasing the voxel size.

The simplest surface coil is a single circular loop of radius a, which has been tuned and matched for the desired operating frequency. This coil may be thought of as a very short solenoid which stores about half of its magnetic energy in the sample. Hence it has a fairly high filling factor and couples strongly to sample. Lengthening the solenoid would decrease the filling factor because additional field energy would be concentrated outside the sample. The B_1 field and the corresponding signal sensitivity for the short solenoid are highly inhomogeneous. Peak values of B_1 occur adjacent to the conductor. Along the axis of the coil (taken as the x axis), the field per unit current varies as

$$B_1 \propto \frac{1}{a \left(1 + \dfrac{x^2}{a^2} \right)^{3/2}} \tag{20}$$

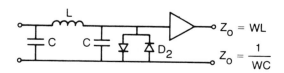

Figure 72–15. Lumped element preamplifier protection.

The noise performance of this coil as a function of coil radius can be understood in terms of Equation (13). The signal sensitivity, B_1, at the center of the coil ($x = 0$) is inversely proportional to the coil radius, a. The coil resistance will be approximately proportional to a. The tissue losses, which arise mainly from the region tightly coupled to the coil, vary approximately as a^3 (based on dimensional analysis). Hence at the sample surface, SNR for a fixed voxel size is proportional to a^{-n}, where $n > 1.5$. Smaller coils produce better SNR at the surface, but their SNR decreases more rapidly with depth because the coil radius is also the scaling factor for the sensitivity rolloff in Equation (20). Figure 72–16 illustrates the observed depth dependence of SNR at 1.5 T in a lossy head-size phantom for three different surface coils and a birdcage style head coil.[30] In this case, the spins were initially excited by a uniform rf field from a body coil. The spatial dependence of SNR along the coil axis is therefore given by Equation (20). Note that for depths greater than about 6 cm the head coil outperforms all three surface coils. The price of improving the SNR with surface coil imaging is a great loss in signal strength uniformity within the image. The surface coil is insensitive to both the signal and the noise originating from distant regions of the sample.

When a surface coil is used as both transmitter and receiver coil, an even greater spatial variation in signal strength occurs.[31,32] The spin flip angle of the transmitter pulse varies with spatial position and rf power level. Different parts of the sample may be flipped 90 degrees, 180 degrees, 270 degrees or more. An image would show dark bands of signal intensity corresponding to nulls created by spin flips of 180 or 360 degrees instead of 90 or 270 degrees. Bendall and coworkers[33,34] have exploited the spatial variation in flip angle to achieve spatial selectivity for in vivo spectroscopy without applying field gradients. They apply a series of pulses that cause cancellation of the signal except in a narrow zone of the sample. Grist and Hyde[35] have recently described the construction and performance of a single turn rf surface coil for ^{31}P spectroscopy.

Figure 72–16. SNR versus depth for surface coils and head coil.

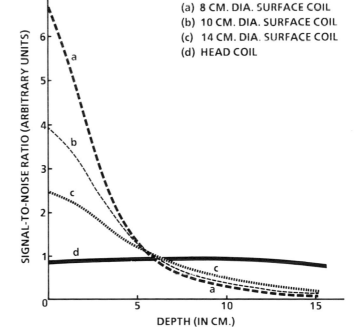

(a) 8 CM. DIA. SURFACE COIL
(b) 10 CM. DIA. SURFACE COIL
(c) 14 CM. DIA. SURFACE COIL
(d) HEAD COIL

References

1. Hoult DI, Richards RE: Signal-to-noise ratio of nuclear magnetic resonance experiment. J Magn Reson 24:71–85, 1976.
2. Hoult DI, Lauterbur PC: The sensitivity of the zeugmatographic experiment involving human samples. J Magn Reson 34:425, 1979.
3. Easton E, Flugan D, Hinshaw W, Salmon R, Zinger J, Floyd MF: Superiority of MRI in the detection of avascular necrosis of femoral head. 3rd Annual Meeting, Society for Magnetic Resonance in Medicine, 1984, p. 200.
4. Pandey L, Hughes DG: Electrostatic shield for the suppression of piezoelectric ringing in pulsed NMR. J Magn Reson 56:443–447, 1984.
5. Alderman DW, Grant DM: An efficient decoupler coil design which reduces heating in conductive samples in superconducting spectrometers. J Magn Reson 36:447–451, 1979.
6. Chen C-N, Hoult DI, Sank VJ: Quadrature detection coils. A further improvement in sensitivity. J Magn Reson 54:324–327, 1983.
7. Glover GH, Hayes CE, Pelc NJ, Edelstein WA, Mueller OM, Hart HR, Hardy CJ, O'Donnell M, Barber WD: Comparison of linear and circular polarization for magnetic resonance imaging. J Magn Reson 64:255–270, 1985.
8. Hoult DI: Radiofrequency coil technology in NMR scanning. In Witcofski R, Karstaedt N, Partain CL (eds): NMR Imaging. Winston-Salem, NC, Bowman Gray School of Medicine, 1982, p 33.
9. Cook B, Lowe IJ: A large-inductance, high-frequency, high-Q series-tuned coil for NMR. J Magn Reson 49:346–349, 1982.
10. Hoult DI: The NMR receiver: a description and analysis of design. Prog NMR Spectrosc 12:41–77, 1978.
11. Bottomley PA, Hart HR, Edelstein WA, Schenck JF, Smith LS, Leue WM, Mueller OM, Redington RW: Anatomy and metabolism of the normal human brain studied by magnetic resonance at 1.5 Tesla. Radiology 150:441–444, 1984.
12. Leroy-Willig A, Darrasse L, Taquin J, Sauzade M: The slotted cylinder: An efficient probe for NMR imaging. Magn Reson Med 2:20–28, 1985.
13. Cross TA, Mueller S, Aue WP: Radiofrequency resonators for high-field imaging and double-resonance spectroscopy. J Magn Reson 62:87–98, 1985.
14. Schneider HJ, Dullenkopf P: Slotted tube resonator: a new NMR probe head at high observing frequencies. Rev Sci Instrum 48:68–73, 1977.
15. Hinshaw WS, Gauss RC: U.S. Patent No. 4,429,733, 1984.
16. Roeschmann P: Ring resonator RF: Probes for proton imaging above 1 Tesla. 3rd Annual Meeting, Society of Magnetic Resonance in Medicine, 1984, p 634.
17. Hayes CE, Edelstein WA, Schenck JF, Mueller OM, Eash M: An efficient, highly homogeneous radio frequency coil for whole-body NMR imaging at 1.5 T. J Magn Reson 63:622–628, 1985.
18. Hoult DI, Richards R: Critical factors in the design of sensitive high resolution nuclear magnetic resonance spectrometers. Proc R Soc Lond A 344:311–340, 1975.
19. Moore WS, Holland GN: Experimental considerations in implementing a whole-body multiple sensitive point nuclear magnetic resonance imaging system. Phil Trans R Soc Lond B 289:511–518, 1980.
20. Redpath TW, Selbie RD: A crossed ellipse RF coil for NMR imaging of the head and neck. Phys Med Biol 29:739–744, 1984.
21. Redpath TW: Crossed ellipse coils for NMR imaging of the head and neck. 2nd Annual Meeting, Society of Magnetic Resonance in Medicine, 1983, p. 293.
22. Bydder GM, Butsen PC, Harman RR, Gilderdale DJ, Young IR: Use of spherical receiver coils in MR imaging of the brain. JCAT 9:413–414, 1985.
23. Hoult DI: Fast recovery, high sensitivity NMR probe and preamplifier for low frequencies. Rev Sci Instrum 50:193–200, 1979.
24. Hoult DI: Fast recovery with a conventional probe. J Magn Reson 57:394–403, 1984.
25. Lowe IJ, Tarr CE: A fast recovery probe and receiver for pulsed nuclear magnetic resonance spectroscopy. J Phys E, Ser. 2, 1:320–322, 1968.
26. Ackerman JJH, Grove GH, Wong GG, Gadian DG, Radda GK: Mapping of metabolites in whole animals by 31-P NMR using surface coils. Nature 283:167–170, 1980.
27. Axel L: Surface coil magnetic resonance imaging. JCAT 8:381–384, 1984.
28. El Yousef SJ, Duchesneau RJ, Hubay CA, Haaga JR, Bryan PJ, LiPuma JP, Ament AE: Initial experience with nuclear magnetic resonance (NMR) imaging of the human breast. JCAT 7:215–218, 1983.
29. Schenck JF, Foster TH, Henkes JL, Adams WJ, Hayes CE, Hart HR, Edelstein WA, Bottomley PA, Wehrli FW: High-field surface coil MR imaging of localized anatomy. AJNR 6:181, 1985.
30. Hayes CE, Axel L: Noise performance of surface coils for magnetic resonance imaging at 1.5 Tesla. Med Phys 12:604, 1985.
31. Haase A, Hanicke W, Frahm J: The influence of experimental parameters in surface-coil NMR. J Magn Reson 56:401–412, 1984.
32. Evelhoch JL, Crowley MG, Ackerman JJH: Signal-to-noise optimization and observed volume localizations with circular surface coils. J Magn Reson 56:110–124, 1984.
33. Bendall MR, Gordon RE: Depth and refocusing pulses designed for multipulse NMR with surface coils. J Magn Reson 53:365–385, 1983.
34. Bendall MR, Aue WP: Experimental verification of depth pulses applied with surface coils. J Magn Reson 54:149–152, 1983.
35. Grist TM, Hyde JS: Resonators for in vivo 31-P NMR at 1.5 T. J Magn Reson 61:571–578, 1985.

73

Surface Coil Technology

M. ROBIN BENDALL

In in-vivo nuclear magnetic resonance (NMR) spectroscopy the two major technical problems are sensitivity and localization. This chapter predominantly addresses the problem of sensitive-volume localization while continually recognizing that the sensitivity of the NMR experiment must be kept at a maximum.

Metabolites are generally present at the millimolar level and so provide weak signals. Although it may be possible to relax the criterion of maximum sensitivity for some ^1H experiments, maximum sensitivity is of paramount importance for other nuclei. A small flat surface coil, placed on the surface of an animal or human subject, is the most sensitive way of obtaining spectra from tissues close to the surface. As a consequence, most physiological data from intact animals or humans have been obtained in this way. The sensitivity of the surface coil decreases rapidly with depth into the subject, and at some depth it becomes more efficient to use a whole-body or whole-head coil to detect more remote tissues or organs. However, at the present early stage of development of in-vivo NMR spectroscopy it is sensible to establish sound biochemical and physiological results by concentrating on those regions that can be detected with greatest sensitivity. Today's research using surface coil technology will provide the basis for routine in-vivo spectroscopy of the future.

The rapid decrease of the sensitivity of the surface coil to regions at increasing distance from the coil provides a crude form of sample localization. However, the sensitive volume does not have hard boundaries and its detailed shape (which is explored in the section the Radio Frequency Field of the Surface Coil) is quite complex and dependent on the experimental variables selected. The spatial variation of sensitivity throughout the sample is directly related to the spatial variation of the rf field produced by the surface coil. This property of rf inhomogeneity displayed by all surface-type coils may be contrasted with whole-body or whole-head coils that are designed to optimize rf uniformity across the body or head. Rf inhomogeneity is of central importance in this chapter.

It is always dangerous to assume that the crude localization provided by the surface coil is sufficient, though this may be valid in some cases. A common problem is the intense signals from the intervening tissue between the surface coil and the tissue of interest. Consider a few examples. Bottomley et al.[1] have reported surface coil ^{31}P spectra of the human brain, yet Pettegrew et al.[2] have shown that these spectra mostly represented extracranial muscle tissue. Conversely, ^1H NMR showing lactate in abnormal brain tissue would probably not be compromised by ^1H signals from the skull. The reverse situation applies to the human limbs, where ^1H lactate signals from within ischemic muscle would be swamped by lipid signals from the intervening fat layer, but the fat layer produces no significant ^{31}P signals to invalidate the ^{31}P spectrum. For the liver, the intervening muscle wall and fat layer would compromise both the ^{31}P and the ^1H spectrum, respectively. Another common problem is the diffuse boundary of the sensitive volume, which may, for example, extend into nonexercised muscle in the case of human limb studies or into normal brain tissue in the case of surface brain tumor or stroke investigations. Clearly, in general, additional means of sensitive-volume localization are required so that it can be stated with certainty that, say, 80 to 90 percent of the signal for a particular metabolite originates from the region of interest. Such a criterion could be relaxed if changes in the level of a particular metabolite were measured in a set of routine experiments and if it were known that such changes were only occurring in the tissue of interest, but this would have to be proved by complete localization prior to the set of routine experiments. While these remarks are simple common sense, such a basic knowledge of the problems of using rf coils for in-vivo studies is not universal (there has even been a report [thankfully unpublished] of 'rat heart spectra' obtained using a simple pulse/acquire experiment and an rf coil wrapped around the rat thorax).

The major part of this chapter is devoted to additional techniques for localizing the sensitive volume. These fall into two main classes: methods that require magnetic field gradients (see Localization Using Pulsed Field Gradients) and methods that utilize rf inhomogeneity (see Localization Using Radio Frequency Inhomogeneity). A third class combines these two methods (see Localization by Combining the Methods of Pulsed Field Gradients and Radio Frequency Inhomogeneity) and a fourth class uses multiple rf coils, one of which will be a surface coil (Localization Using Multiple Radio Frequency Coils). Throughout, most emphasis will be placed on surface-type coils, but the generalization of some methods to three-dimensional localization as would be appropriate for a whole-head or whole-body coil will be discussed.

In traditional NMR spectroscopy, the simplification of spectra by relaying information between two J-coupled nuclei has been a very important area of research for the last decade. There are also important applications to in-vivo spectroscopy, and this is explored in later sections, Heteronuclear Methods with Surface Coils, and ^{1}H Spectral Simplifications with Surface Coils.

The J-coupled experiments and the localization methods all require the application of two or more discrete rf pulses rather than a single pulse as in the simplest NMR experiment. Such multipulse sequences are composed of two simple types of pulse sequences. To facilitate an understanding of the various multipulse experiments described in this chapter, these two types of pulse sequences are described in the next section.

This chapter is written as a review of recent developments with additional information for some new techniques that had not been published in detail at the time of writing.

INVERSION–RECOVERY AND SPIN–ECHO SEQUENCES IN INHOMOGENEOUS RADIO FREQUENCY FIELDS

The rf pulse sequences that are useful for in-vivo spectroscopy and that are discussed in this chapter may, in virtual entirety, be considered to be made up of two simpler two-pulse sequences known as inversion-recovery and spin-echo sequences. Inversion-recovery and spin-echo sequences have enjoyed widespread use in conventional NMR spectroscopy throughout the last 15 years, the present era of pulsed NMR. Their prime use is for the measurement of *T1* and *T2* times, respectively, and this is discussed in detail in relation to imaging by Jones et al. in Chapter 61.

Pulsed NMR experiments may be readily understood by description in terms of a straightforward, but rigorous, vector model. This vector model begins with the total detectable NMR signal for each chemically distinct nucleus being represented by a single magnetization vector aligned with the axis (z axis) of the external magnetic field as in Figure 73–1. Only the vector component of magnetization at right angles to the magnetic field z axis can ever be detected, so maximum signal intensity is obtained by rotating the magnetization through 90 degrees using a single 90 degree rf pulse, for example. In general, as shown in Figure 73–1, a θ pulse will provide a component of detectable transverse magnetization which is proportional to sin θ.

In its simplest form, the inversion-recovery sequence is

$$180° - \tau - 90°; \text{ acquire signal} \tag{1}$$

An rf pulse that is twice as long as a 90 degree pulse will rotate the z, or longitudinal magnetization, through 180 degrees, i.e., net inversion of longitudinal magnetization, leading to no measurable signal intensity just as before the pulse. However, after the 180 degree pulse in Sequence [1], the inverted magnetization will decay exponentially with a time constant $T1$, i.e., it will relax back towards the initial equilibrium magnetization. The inverted magnetization decreases, and the equilibrium magnetization grows. In the inversion-recovery sequence, after the τ recovery period, a 90 degree pulse will permit signal detection of the partially recovered longitudinal magnetization and thus permit calculation of $T1$.

In simplest form, the spin-echo sequence is

$$90° - \tau/2 - 180° - \tau/2 - \text{acquire signal} \tag{2}$$

After the 90 degree pulse, the magnetization is transverse to the z axis; and the individual nuclear spins, which make up the total transverse magnetization vector, rotate at different rates in the transverse plane around the z axis, i.e., they dephase; and the magnetization (and the detectable signal) rapidly decays away. The individual nuclear spins rotate in the xy plane at the difference between their natural NMR frequency and the rf pulse frequency. This difference is the "resonance offset" frequency. There can be a variety of reasons for a spread of resonance offset frequencies and thus the dephasing observed for chemically identical nuclear spins, but in in-vivo spectroscopy it is predominantly caused by poor homogeneity of the external magnetic field, which can never be perfect, especially at the cellular level, where there are changes in magnetic susceptibility across the cell. The 180 degree pulse would invert any z axis magnetization if there were any, but in the spin-echo sequence it has a different purpose. It reverses the dephasing of the nuclear spins so that they are rephased after the second $\tau/2$ time and a maximum signal intensity can be detected once more, hence the term spin-echo, where the top of the echo occurs at the end of the two $\tau/2$ times. This type of 180 degree pulse is called a refocusing pulse. During τ the rephaseable magnetization decays experimentally via $T2$ relaxation and so the spin-echo signal is less than the

Figure 73–1. The initial magnetization vector, M_0, is rotated on angle of θ degrees around the x axis by a θ pulse of x phase (i.e., $\theta[x]$). After the pulse, a component equal to M_0 cos θ remains along the z axis and a component equal to M_0 sin θ is in the transverse plane and provides a detectable NMR signal. This is the on-resonance situation, which for simplicity of discussion, is presented in the text. The x and y axes in the figure are properly the transverse axes of the rotating reference frame (rotating around z at the Larmor frequency relative to the laboratory frame). In the text, again for simplicity, we make no distinction between the rotating frame and the laboratory frame; this does not introduce any contradiction into our present discussion.

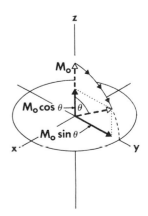

signal detectable directly after the 90 degree pulse, thus enabling measurement of the relaxation time *T2*.

For rf coils that produce a grossly inhomogeneous rf field, such as a surface coil, the above pulse sequences are a great oversimplification of reality. Because pulse angles are proportional to the strength of the rf field, actual pulse angles vary continuously and widely throughout sample space, from, say, 1000 degrees close to the coil wire down to ~1 degree at two coil diameters away. Thus the above pulse sequences must be written in terms of a general angle θ, becoming

$$2\theta - \tau - \theta; \text{ acquire signal} \tag{3}$$

and

$$\theta - \tau/2 : 2\theta - \tau/2 : \text{acquire signal} \tag{4}$$

respectively. It is well known that large artefacts result from the use of pulse sequences when pulse angles differ markedly from the ideal 90 degree and 180 degree angles, which would lead to large errors in the measurement of *T1* and *T2*, for example. Consequently it has been widely believed that these sequences cannot be used with a surface coil.[3-5] However, other authors have recognized that both pulse sequences will function perfectly well if one of the pulses is phase cycled during a series of transients.

The phase cycling appropriate for the inversion-recovery sequence is either

$$2\theta - \tau - \theta[\pm x]; \text{ acquire signal, receiver}[\pm] \tag{5}$$

or

$$2\theta[\pm x] - \tau - \theta; \text{ acquire signal} \tag{6}$$

where $[\pm]$ means the phase of the pulse is alternated between $+x$ and $-x$ during successive transients. Any phase may be chosen for those pulses that are not phase cycled, provided the selected phase is maintained throughout the experiment, of course. Receiver phase alternation, i.e., $[\pm]$ in Sequence [5], simply means addition and subtraction of the acquired signal. The phase alternation in Sequence [5] was proposed by Demco et al.[6] to improve the accuracy of *T1* measurements in traditional chemical spectroscopy, and it was independently recognized by us[7,8] and by Evelhoch and Ackerman[9] that this phase alternation was sufficient to eliminate the error introduced by nonideal pulse angles. It was subsequently recognized by us[10] and independently by Evanochko et al.[11] that if the pulse phases and the receiver phase are both inverted for the second transient of Sequence [5], the equivalent Sequence [6] is generated,

i.e., $2\theta[x] - \tau - \theta[-x]$; receiver$[-]$ becomes $2\theta[-x] - \tau - \theta[x]$; receiver$[+]$.

For a number of reasons that will become apparent, Sequence [6] is more generally useful in practice (and more useful for our discussion of this topic) and will be assumed from now on. Thus, for an inhomogeneous rf coil, such as a surface coil, the equivalent of an ideal 180 degree inversion pulse is a $2\theta[\pm x]$ phase-alternated pulse. It can easily be shown using simple vector diagrams like that of Figure 73–1[7,12] that a $\underline{2\theta[\pm x] \text{ pulse}}$ reduces initial unit z magnetization (and thus the final signal) to an amount given by

$$z \text{ magnetization} = \cos 2\theta \tag{1}$$

after the pulse. When $2\theta = 180$ degrees, $\cos 2\theta = -1$, i.e., correspondence with inverted longitudinal magnetization. The loss of signal intensity in some sample regions where 2θ is close to 90 degrees, 270 degrees, and so on is not necessarily a problem and can be used to discriminate against unwanted sample regions, a method explored in later sections.

The phase cycling necessary when applying a spin-echo sequence with a surface coil is

$$\theta - \tau/2 - 2\theta[\pm x, \pm y] - \tau/2 : \text{acquire signal, receiver}[+, -] \tag{7}$$

Thus four successive transients are required with the 2θ refocusing pulse cycled through all four phases. The receiver phase is inverted when the 2θ phase is $\pm y$. This form of phase cycling was introduced by Bodenhausen et al.[13] for use in two-dimensional variants of conventional NMR spectroscopy to eliminate artefact signals when the pulse angles differed from ideal 90 degree and 180 degree values. We were able to show quite simply in terms of the pictorial vector model[7,12] that this phase cycling permitted the use of any spin-echo method with inhomogeneous rf coils, and that existing unit transverse or xy magnetization after the initial pulse is reduced by the $2\theta[\pm x, \pm y]$ pulse to an amount given by

$$xy \text{ magnetization} = \sin^2 \theta, \tag{2}$$

(in the absence of $T2$ relaxation). This transverse magnetization is refocused at the end of the τ period.

The θ pulse has the same purpose in both the inversion-recovery Sequence [6] and the spin-echo Sequence [7], as it converts longitudinal (z) magnetization, which does not produce a measurable signal, to transverse (xy) magnetization, which does produce an NMR signal. The other pulses in these sequences do not convert z magnetization to xy magnetization. Indeed it is the phase cycling of these pulses that prevents the conversion. We will call the θ pulse the "excitation" pulse (we cannot call it the "90 degree pulse" as in the ideal case), and we will normally assume it to have x phase. From Figure 73–1 a $\theta[x]$ excitation pulse converts unit z magnetization to an amount of transverse magnetization given by

$$y \text{ magnetization} = \sin \theta \tag{3}$$

Note that the transverse magnetization is pure "absorption-mode" or y phase rather than nonideal x phase or "dispersion-mode" signal.

In summary, in this chapter we will be concerned with three types of rf pulse in any pulse sequence when using an inhomogeneous rf coil: a phase-cycled inversion pulse or $2\theta[\pm x]$ pulse; an excitation or θ pulse; and a phase-cycled refocusing pulse or $2\theta[\pm x, \pm y]$ pulse. One and only one excitation pulse is used in any pulse sequence, but any number of $2\theta[\pm x]$ or $2\theta[\pm x, \pm y]$ pulses can be used and the overall signal intensity is given by multiplying together the various factors given in Equations (1) to (3). For example, if two $2\theta[\pm x]$ pulses were used prior to θ and one $2\theta[\pm x, \pm y]$ pulse after θ, signal intensity would be proportional to $\cos^2 2\theta \sin^3 \theta$.

Equations (1) to (3) are exact when the rf pulse frequency is the same as the Larmor frequency of the nuclear spins, i.e., on resonance. However, in spectroscopy we are concerned with a spread of frequencies, and although these equations are virtually exact across normal spectral widths when using strong pulses, in in-vivo spectroscopy, rf pulses will often be weak enough for these equations to no longer hold true off resonance. In the pictorial vector model of pulsed NMR experiments, strong pulses of x and y phase act along the x or y axis of the usual frame of reference. For example, in Figure 73–1 the magnetization rotates around the rf field which is acting along the x axis. However, weak pulses act along axes that are tilted by an angle, α, towards the z axis. Experimentally, the strength of a radio frequency pulse is best expressed in terms of the length of pulse required for a 90 degree rotation on resonance; i.e., the 90 degree pulse time or t_{90}: the stronger the pulse, the shorter the t_{90} time. The tilt angle α and t_{90} are related by:

$$\tan \alpha = 4 \, \Delta H t_{90} \tag{4}$$

where ΔH is the frequency offset in H_z and the units of t_{90} are seconds. For any pulse θ, the rotation off resonance is increased to θ' given by

$$\theta' = \theta \sec \alpha \qquad (5)$$

A $2\theta[\pm x]$ pulse off resonance converts unit z magnetization to

$$z \text{ magnetization} = 1 - 2 \cos^2 \alpha \sin^2 \theta' \qquad (6)$$

A θ excitation pulse converts unit z magnetization to

$$y \text{ magnetization} = \cos \alpha \sin \theta' \qquad (7)$$

and

$$x \text{ magnetization} = \sin 2\alpha \sin^2(\theta'/2) \qquad (8)$$

Note here that off-resonance dispersion-mode signals are generated unlike the on-resonance case (Equation 3). A $2\theta[\pm x, \pm y]$ pulse converts unit xy magnetization to

$$xy \text{ magnetization} = \pm \cos^2 \alpha \sin^2 \theta' \qquad (9)$$

where the $\pm$ sign is plus for x magnetization and minus for y magnetization. Off-resonance Equations (6), (7), (8), and (9) take the place of Equations (1), (3), and (2), respectively, and reduce to these equations when t_{90} is small, i.e., when $\alpha \cong 0$. Equations (1) to (3) are sufficient to appreciate the methods described in the following sections, but Equations (6) to (9) are necessary for detailed calculation.

Equations (6) to (9) were determined using the pictorial vector model[12] and confirmed using a more abstract description in terms of rotation matrices.[14] For newcomers, the vector model is by far the quickest way of gaining a sound understanding of NMR pulse sequences, and contrary to some belief, the vector model is a completely accurate description. An introduction to this pictorial model can be found in Chapter 61 and for more relevance to the surface coil, reference 12 is appropriate.

THE RADIO FREQUENCY FIELD OF THE SURFACE COIL

The Shape of the Radio Frequency Field

A surface coil is one or more circular turns of wire connected to a tune and match network (see Fig. 73–21A). During an rf pulse a large oscillating current is induced in

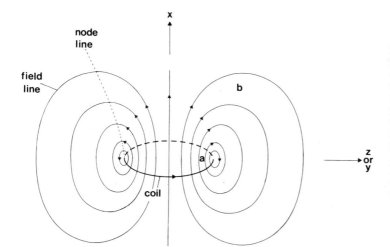

Figure 73–2. A direct current in a coil produces magnetic field lines of force in one direction through the coil center. An alternating current induces an alternating magnetic field along the same lines of force. If the plane displayed is the zx plane, there will be node lines where the rf field lines are parallel to z, the external magnetic field direction. (From Bendall MR: *In* James TL, Margulis AR [eds]: Biomedical Magnetic Resonance. San Francisco, Radiology Research and Education Foundation, 1984. Used by permission.)

the wire. Just as a direct current in a circular coil produces the magnetic field depicted in Figure 73–2, so too an alternating current will induce an oscillating magnetic field along the same field lines. The strength of the oscillating or rf field is proportioned to the density of the field lines in Figure 73–2, so the rf field is weaker at point b than point a. Obviously the rf field gets weaker along a line from the coil to its center, or from its center perpendicular to the coil, or outwards from the coil in the plane of the coil. This leads to a complicated distribution of pulse angles.

The pulse angle θ, at any point in space relative to the surface coil, is proportional to the strength of the rf field. By a reciprocal relation, the sensitivity of the coil to a signal excited at any point in space, is also proportional to the strength of the rf field that can be generated at that point by the coil, and so sensitivity is proportional to θ. From Equation (3), the transverse magnetization generated by a single rf pulse is proportional to $\sin \theta$, so overall the signal intensity from any volume element after a single pulse is proportional to $\theta \sin \theta$. This expression is valid for any coil, but for a coil that provides homogeneous rf across a sample, θ, and thus signal intensity, is constant throughout the sample.

The distribution of signal intensity relative to an rf coil can be conveniently revealed experimentally by using a slice phantom and a standard imaging method:

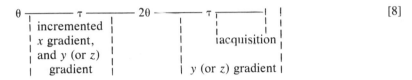 [8]

The incremented x field gradient provides the x spatial dimension by the usual Fourier transform imaging technique, and the y (or z) read gradient during acquisition of the complete signal echo provides the y (or z) dimension, a common imaging practice. Note that although the pulse sequence is a spin-echo sequence, the phase cycling of the 2θ pulse introduced in the last section, i.e., $2\theta[\pm x, \pm y]$, has been omitted. When using a homogeneous phantom sample (e.g., H_2O or H_3PO_4), the normal error signals from different parts of the sample are dephased relative to each other by the field gradients and so eliminated anyway without need for the $[\pm x, \pm y]$ phase cycling. For Sequence [8], the expression for the distribution of signal intensity is given by combining the θ sensitivity factor with the factors in Equations (3) and (2), giving $\theta \sin^3 \theta$.

The expression $\theta \sin^3 \theta$ has similar dependence on θ to the expression for a single pulse, $\theta \sin \theta$, with the difference that signal intensity is suppressed for θ values close to 0 degrees, 180 degrees, 360 degrees, and so on. This produces the convenient banded results illustrated in Figure 73–3, which were obtained for a slice phantom of H_2O placed in the xy plane of the surface coil in the manner shown in Figure 73–4. These images were obtained by increasing the θ pulse length in increments from frame 1 to frame 12. In frame 4 of Figure 73–3, for example, a curved line tracing the center of the large curved bright high intensity region corresponds to $\theta = 90$ degrees. A similar curve through the middle of the two bright regions just above the coil wire corresponds to $\theta = 270$ degrees. The dark region in between corresponds to $\theta = 180$ degrees. In frame 12, 90 degree, 270 degree, 450 degree, and 630 degree regions of signal intensity can all be observed. We will call the 270 degree and 450 degree regions ''high flux'' regions. Because of the θ sensitivity term, the 270 degree region provides three times more signal per unit volume than the 90 degree region; the 450 degree region provides five times more signal; and so on. However, because the volumes of the high flux regions become smaller with increasing pulse angle, their total contribution is of a similar magnitude to that of the 90 degree region, so we will normally omit the θ term from expressions such as $\theta \sin^3 \theta$. Note that 270 degree and 630 degree signals are

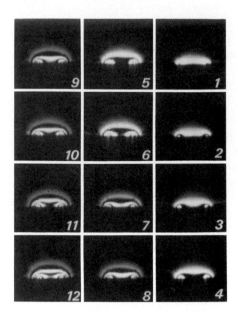

Figure 73–3. Images of the sensitive volume in the xy plane of a surface coil, as a function of a linear increase in pulse length, obtained using sequence [8] and a layer phantom as in Figure 73–4. The coil wire is just below the small bright regions (270 degree signals), in frame 4, for example. (Measurements were made by R. J. Ordidge, and the results are reproduced with the permission of Oxford Research Systems Limited.)

negative compared to 90 degree signals. Thus, as shown in Figure 73–5, overall signal intensity from the complete phantom obtained using a single θ pulse passes through a maximum when increasing the pulse length and then decreases as the 270 degree regions are pushed into the sample and subtract from the total. Note also that reasonable penetration of the sample, as in frames 5 and 6 of Figure 73–3, already corresponds to a considerable overall loss of signal. It is clearly necessary to tidy up the distribution of signal intensity if detection of tissue at some depth into the sample is required.

The rf field produced by any coil consisting of continuous wire may be calculated by using the Biot-Savart law to determine the magnetic field produced by direct current in the coil. Our results of such a calculation for a surface coil[7] correctly predict the experimental findings shown in Figure 73–3. The calculated field for the xy plane is illustrated in Figure 73–6a. In the figure, θ is assumed to be 90 degrees at one radius depth along the coil's axis, but any other pulse angle could be assumed with all other pulse angles scaled accordingly. With the pulse angles as given in Figure 73–6a, the figure corresponds to frame 7 of Figure 73–3. In an NMR experiment, the active component of the rf field is the oscillating component at right angles to the external field axis (z). For the xy plane displayed in Figures 73–3 and 73–6a the rf field is always transverse to the z axis. However, from Figure 73–2 it can be seen that in the xz plane there is a node line where the rf field is parallel to z and no NMR signal can be excited or detected. The calculated result for the xz plane is shown in Figure 73–6b, where it can be seen that this further complicates the shape of the sensitive volume for an rf

LAYER PHANTOM

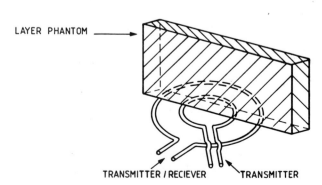

TRANSMITTER / RECIEVER   TRANSMITTER

Figure 73–4. Layer or slice phantom of H_2O or H_3PO_4 placed across a surface coil to obtain images of the sensitive volume. In our convention, the x axis is the coil axis, so the phantom can be placed in the xy or xz plane. The second, smaller coaxial coplanar transmit coil is relevant to the discussion in the section Localization Using Multiple Radio Frequency Coils.

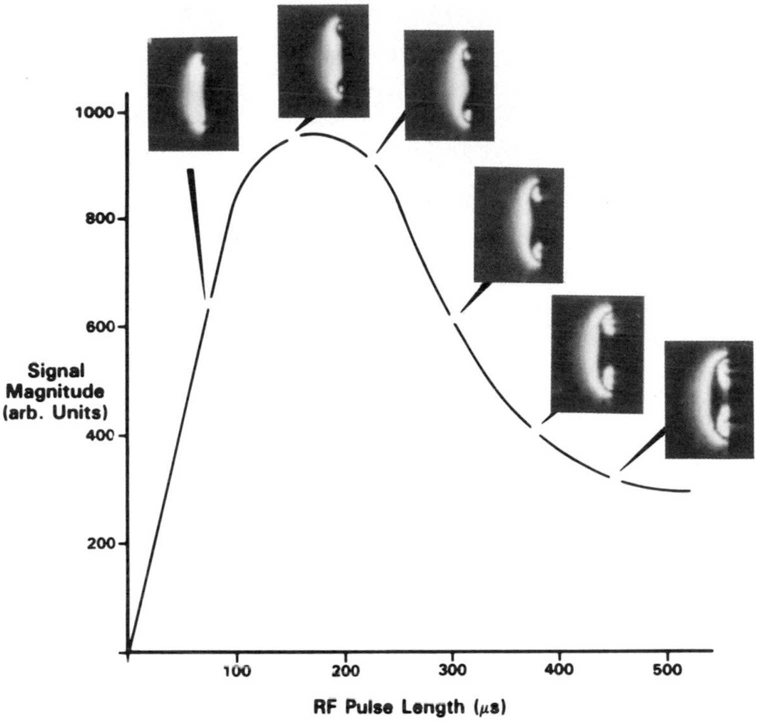

Figure 73–5. Plot of signal magnitude versus rf pulse length for a single loop surface coil and a layer phantom of H_2O as depicted in Figure 73–4. The images correspond to the frames in Figure 73–3. (Measurements were made by R. J. Ordidge, and the results are reproduced with the permission of Oxford Research Systems Limited.)

coil. Obviously, additional means of sensitive volume localization are required whenever it is necessary to study a sample region beneath a surface layer.

More recently, Haase et al.[15] and Evelhoch et al.[16] have extended the theoretical calculation of distribution of signal intensity to include the relaxation time $T1$ and the repetition time for each transient, TR. These calculations are complex, and the reasons for the particular results cannot be explained in a few words; interested readers are advised to consult the relevant references. However, their main conclusions are as follows: Our Figures 73–3 and 73–6 are accurate at fairly slow repetition rates, for example, TR equal to 2 to 5 times $T1$. At high repetition rates, for example, $TR = 0.05$ $T1$, and reduced pulse lengths, the distribution of signal intensity is significantly altered with less high flux signals near the surface and more signal intensity at one radius depth, i.e., a more uniform distribution of signal. Evelhoch et al., who were mostly concerned with maximizing overall signal-to-noise and not with localization, found that total signal intensity was doubled for optimum pulse lengths at these high repetition rates. A major concern of Haase et al. (and the central theme of this chapter) was the simulation of the detection of an inner organ. They found that despite the improvements at higher repetition rate, the signals from the intervening surface layer would still swamp the inner organ by a factor of 3 to 9 times. Additional localization methods are definitely required. A further interesting conclusion of Evelhoch et al., which might be guessed from Figure 73–5, is that if the sample is moved away from the coil by 0.4 coil radius, for example, longer pulse lengths will again provide a more uniform distribution of signal into the sample with only a minor loss in sensitivity.

Signal-to-Noise Maximization

In maximizing total signal-to-noise, the approach of Evelhoch et al.[16] is valid for experiments in which a thick surface layer is to be detected or in which an underlying

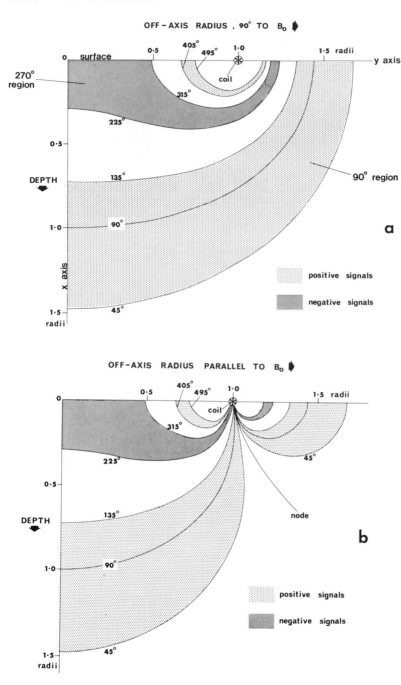

Figure 73–6. Plots of pulse angle contours for a surface coil assuming $\theta = 90$ degrees at 1.0 radius depth. One half of a plane through the center of the coil is given with the vertical axis being the coil axis, or x axis. The plane is the xy plane (transverse to the external magnetic field) (*a*) or the xz plane (parallel to the external magnetic field) (*b*). The shaded regions correspond to regions from which signal would be detected when using an appropriate depth pulse sequence (e.g., sequence [29]). The signal responses in the images of Figure 73–3 correspond to $\theta \sin^3 \theta$ and give the same banded results but with much more diffuse boundaries to the signal regions. The signal response after a single θ pulse would be zero only at $\theta = 180$ degrees, 360 degrees, 540 degrees, . . . , but the sign of the signal would alternate as shown in the figures. The signal response from the regions where $\theta \sim 270$ degrees and 450 degrees can be entirely removed and the 90 degree region can be expanded or narrowed using various depth pulse sequences. These pulse angle contours also correspond to sensitivity contours. (From Bendall MR: J Magn Reson *59*:406, 1984. Used with permission.)

layer is detected but the intervening surface layer does not contribute any interfering signals. Improvements can also be obtained in the signal-to-noise ratio without increasing the repetition rate of the experiment (and disturbing the normal ratio of spectral peak lines) by using a composite excitation pulse θ. Composite pulses are a succession of single pulses of different phases, as first described by Levitt and Freeman.[17] Freeman et al.[18] described the first composite 90 degree pulse, written in our terminology $\Theta = \theta[x]; \theta[y]$, which rotates more magnetization into the transverse plane when θ differs from 90 degrees than does the single θ pulse illustrated in Figure 73–1. For example, when $\theta = 45$ degrees or 135 degrees, the single pulse produces a transverse component of 0.707 M_0, whereas the composite pulse gives a 0.866 M_0 component in the xy plane.

Unfortunately a $\theta[x]$; $\theta[y]$ pulse does not yield pure absorption mode magnetization but introduces a dispersion mode component as well. For example at $\theta = 45$ degrees the xy component is 35 degrees to the y axis and at $\theta = 135$ degrees the phase error is -35 degrees. Considering Figure 6a for example, this means that the signal from a region where $\theta = 45$ degrees will not add coherently to the signal from a region where $\theta = 135$ degrees and the potential gain in signal-to-noise by using $\theta[x]$; $\theta[y]$ is not achieved (despite claims to the contrary[5]). Recently Tycko et al.[19] have described two composite excitation pulses that have a much reduced phase problem. These are $\theta[0°]$; $2\theta[105°]$; $2\theta[315°]$ and $3\theta[0°]$; $4\theta[169°]$; $2\theta[33°]$; $2\theta[178°]$. Both give a high degree of compensation for variation of θ from 90 degrees, for example, generating a transverse component of $0.96\,M_0$ when $\theta = 45$ degrees or 135 degrees, but equal phase errors at $\theta = 45$ degrees and 135 degrees of 34 degrees for the first pulse and 6 degrees for the second.

Hetherington et al.[20] have used the $\theta[y]$; $\theta[x]$; $\theta[-y]$; $\theta[x]$ composite pulse of Levitt and Ernst[21] and have achieved a 20 percent increase in signal-to-noise in surface coil studies of the rat brain. Although this composite 90 degree pulse does produce dispersive components, Hetherington et al. eliminated these by using the phase-cycled equivalent, $0[-y]$; $\theta[x]$; $\theta[y]$; $\theta[x]$ for alternate transients. Hetherington et al. have also extended the use of composite pulses to spin-echo sequences and surface coils, with both the θ excitation pulse and the 2θ refocusing pulse replaced by composite pulses, and achieved a 40 percent increase in signal-to-noise over simple pulses. This, however, requires a more complex but nevertheless general phase cycling scheme of the 2θ refocusing pulse than that shown in Sequence [7], as determined by Hetherington and Rothman.[22]

Most recently we have developed a complex excitation pulse where amplitude and frequency are continuously modulated during the pulse as sine and cosine functions. This "sin/cos" pulse operates under conditions known as "adiabatic half passage" in traditional NMR, and our preliminary results[23] show that it can be used under practical conditions with surface coils and that it will excite more than 90 percent of z magnetization to give pure absorption-mode signal across a variation of at least a factor of 10 in the strength of the rf field. This should be superior to any existing composite excitation pulses, and related adiabatic inversion pulses can also be used.[24] Adiabatic refocusing pulses have recently been developed, and it is now possible to obtain images using the surface coil as both transmitter and receiver.[146]

This short section was concerned with methods for obtaining as much signal as possible from as large a sample region as possible using a surface coil. The remainder of this chapter is primarily concerned with limiting the acquired signal to a known localized sample region.

LOCALIZATION USING PULSED FIELD GRADIENTS

From Figure 73–6 it is clear that when using a surface coil to detect a region below the surface, it is necessary to discriminate against the surface layer. This may be achieved by applying a selective pulse in a pulsed field gradient, where the gradient axis is the surface coil or x axis, so generating a selected slice that is parallel to the plane of the coil. The center of the slice should closely coincide with $\theta = 90$ degrees on the coil's axis, in which case the rf inhomogeneity of the coil will limit the lateral dimensions of the selected slice to approximately the diameter of the surface coil, depending on the detail of the method used. The sensitive volume thus generated would be disc shaped, centered on the coil's axis and flattened along the z dimension. Given calculations of the type illustrated in Figure 73–6, this general method is rather obvious;

the earliest example used a phase-cycled selective excitation pulse (a "depth pulse").[10,25,26]

There are three possible ways of using selective pulses for this purpose: a selective excitation pulse, a selective refocusing pulse, and a selective inversion pulse. The following discussion is divided accordingly. The various types of shaped soft pulses, which may be used in a pulsed field gradient to excite a slice within the sample, as commonly employed in NMR imaging, will not be discussed. The interested reader is referred to recent articles and references cited therein.[27-31] In the following discussion we will denote a selective pulse in an x gradient by Θ_{SX}. The selective pulse may be Gaussian, sinc, or any other shape.

When assessing selective pulse/field gradient methods, it is necessary to be aware of two fundamental problems. The first is the eddy currents induced by the pulsed field gradients. Subsequent to a selective pulse in a field gradient, the gradient must be switched off to enable the natural chemical shifts of the various nuclear species to be detected during acquisition of the NMR signal. However, switching of magnetic fields creates eddy currents in surrounding metal whose magnetic fields die away exponentially, thus slowing down the switching process. These eddy currents may be compensated electronically by generating exponentially decaying currents of the opposite sense in the gradient coils, but a short delay of up to 10 ms is still required for the switching process before signal acquisition. During this delay a means must be employed for preserving the magnetization in the selected slice, and this is discussed below in more detail for each of the three ways of using selective pulses. Technical improvements should improve field gradient switching, possibly to the point where it is not an important problem in spectroscopy. However, because of commercial competition, this area has received little attention in the literature so it is difficult to make an informed discussion.

The second basic limitation of selective pulses in a field gradient is that the spatial frequency limits of the slice, $\pm S$, is added to any natural chemical shift, ω, so that the slice boundaries become $\pm(S/g) + \omega/g$, thus shifting the selected slice a distance ω/g cm (where g is the gradient strength in gauss/cm) along the gradient axis relative to an on-resonance species. To limit this spread of localized regions, S may be increased relative to ω, but the gradient g will have to be proportionately increased to maintain the same separation ($2S/g$) of the boundaries. The current that can be applied to the field gradient coils, and thus g, is the limiting factor. Field gradients are presently limited to 2 gauss cm^{-1} at a 40 cm bore, or 3 gauss cm^{-1} if water cooled (with attendant loss of bore access size because of the water jacket). At a 1 meter bore size the present maximum is 1.5 gauss cm^{-1}. In a 40 cm bore, 2.3 tesla magnet, this translates to a maximum gradient g of 120 ppm cm^{-1} and about half this for a 1 meter bore, 2.3 tesla magnet, or for a 40 cm bore, 4.7 tesla magnet. Thus good localization can be obtained for 2.3 tesla, 40 cm bore systems for ^{31}P NMR (spectrum width ± 15 ppm; maximum localization error at 3 gauss cm^{-1} is ± 0.1 cm) or for ^{1}H NMR (± 4 ppm; equivalent error is ± 0.03 cm), but only a portion of a ^{13}C spectrum (± 100 ppm) can be satisfactorily localized at any one time. However, as the above figures show, this problem gets worse for increasing magnet field strength and increasing bore size and can be expected to be serious for a whole-body 4.7 tesla magnet. Furthermore, as field gradients are increased, the problems of eddy currents, and field gradient rise times, increase proportionately.

Another common method of using pulsed field gradients in imaging is to use an incremented field gradient in one half of a spin-echo sequence, called a phase-encoding gradient, and this method is known as the two-dimensional Fourier transform (2DFT) method. The use of this technique for localization in spectroscopy provides a fourth method discussed below. The earliest accounts of its use in spectroscopy were given by Maudsley et al.[32] and Haselgrove et al.[33] and it has a considerable advantage over the slice selection method because the natural chemical shift is not mixed with the spatial frequency shift and so does not impair localization. As a further consequence, much weaker field gradients can be used and so eddy current compensation is easier. Note that the third common method of using pulsed field gradients in NMR imaging, the use of "frequency-encoding" or "read-out" gradients during signal acquisition (see Jones et al., Chapter 61), should not be used for spectroscopy because this completely mixes spatial information with chemical shift information.

A further field gradient method, which has been proposed for localization in NMR spectroscopy, utilizes rf pulses with a rapid repetition rate during the application of slowly alternating field gradients. This is called the sensitive point steady-state free precession method. The present author is unfamiliar with the practicalities of the sensitive point method and refers the interested reader to the original literature,[34–36] a review of that literature,[37] and recent improvements[38,39]. However, in the context of this chapter it is relevant to point out that complete localization could be obtained using the sensitive point method with a surface coil by generating a selected slice parallel to the surface coil with a single alternating field gradient along the coil's axis.

Selective Excitation Pulse in a Field Gradient

In simplest form, the pulse sequence required for selective excitation of a slice at some depth into the sample is

$$\Theta_{SX}; \text{acquire signal} \qquad [9]$$

However, in general, use of Sequence [9] would mean acquisition of the NMR signal during the decay of the field gradient eddy currents, i.e., while the total magnetic field is changing, and this will lead to an unacceptable broadening of the NMR signals. It is insufficient to merely insert a τ delay after the Θ_{SX} pulse because the selected nuclear spins are in the transverse plane and will rapidly dephase under the influence of the changing field gradients across the sample (caused by the eddy currents) and because of the static field inhomogeneity. A $2\theta[\pm x, \pm y]$ refocusing pulse could be inserted at the middle of τ, and this would refocus the dephasing by the static field inhomogeneity but would only partially correct the exponentially decaying gradients, whose effect is greater in the first half of τ than in the second half. If the refocusing pulse is moved forward by experimental adjustment to part way through the first half of τ, the effect of the decaying gradients could be removed but now the dephasing effect of the static field inhomogeneity would not be fully refocused. A satisfactory compromise may be achievable by experimental trial and error, but such an adjustment would probably be required for every new sample (as for shimming) and the method is far from ideal.

One solution to the eddy current problem is to freeze the nuclear spins in the transverse plane by application of spin locking (SL) during the τ delay period. The SL pulse must be applied along the axis of the transverse magnetization because any component at right angles to the SL field rotates rapidly around the SL axis at a rate determined by the strength of the SL field. Because of rf inhomogeneity the strength will vary substantially within the excited slice and the rotating orthogonal component rapidly dephases and is lost. If an ideal selective pulse had overall x phase, the transverse magnetization would be aligned with the y axis after the pulse (see Figure 73–1), so the SL pulse should be of y phase, i.e.,

$$\Theta_{SX}[x]; SL[y]; \text{acquire signal} \qquad [10]$$

Unfortunately, there are no such ideal selective pulses. The nuclear spins dephase during a soft shaped pulse because of a spread of frequencies, which is the sum of their natural chemical shift and the frequency shift imposed by the field gradient, and are left spread out in the transverse plane. In imaging it is standard procedure to rephase the nuclear spins by reversing the field gradient for a short period after the pulse, but this only refocuses the spatial frequency shift and not the natural chemical shift. Both frequency shifts can be refocused along the y axis using a hard pulse,[30,40] which will be of magnitude 2θ for a surface coil. The pulsed field gradient must be left on for the short spin-echo, giving $(\Theta_S - t - 2\theta - t -)_x$, where the first t period begins at the midpoint of Θ_S and is half the length of Θ_S. However, the hard 2θ pulse will affect spins outside the selected slice and must be phase alternated. In addition, the tilt of the SL field in the presence of the field gradient (given by Equation 4) will spin-lock some z magnetization, which must be removed by a further alternation, giving overall

$$(\Theta_S[x] - t - 2\theta[\pm x] - t -)_x; \; SL[\pm y] \; ; \; \text{acquire signal}, \qquad [11]$$

and the method becomes too cumbersome to be generally useful, compared with the better selective refocusing and selective inversion methods described below.

Despite the shortcomings for general use, we have used spin-locking successfully with depth pulses.[10,12,25,26] The latter are composed of a series of phase-cycled hard pulses (described in Localization Using Radio Frequency Inhomogeneity) and are frequency selective without introducing the dephasing problem in the transverse plane. In consequence, depth pulses can simply take the place of Θ_S in Sequence [10]. Some results are described in Localization by Combining the Methods of Pulsed Field Gradients and Radio Frequency Inhomogeneity.

Surprisingly, Bottomley et al.[41,42] have obtained good results from the human brain by applying a sinc 90 degree pulse in a field gradient (x axis) and then acquiring the NMR signal immediately after (or slightly before) the nuclear spins are rephased by a reverse gradient. Thus no τ delay period was used to allow eddy currents to decay. Although not stated in their publications, the present author understands that the eddy current problem was avoided by Bottomley et al. by the use of a 0.6 meter diameter field gradient coils in their 1.5 tesla/1 meter bore magnet. This substantially eliminates the usual coupling between the gradient coils and the surrounding metal magnet. This is a proper solution but is not generally applicable to smaller bore magnets as used for animal systems or for higher field systems. The gradient strength was not recorded in these references so the error in localization across the spectrum is unknown. Note that the effects of natural chemical shift occurring during the sinc 90 degree pulse and the reversed gradient are not refocused in this method, and the final spectrum will have a large phase roll, which when corrected can lead to considerable spectral distortions. Bottomley et al. used a cylindrical NMR transmit coil and a surface receive coil, and this aspect of their work is discussed further in Localization Using Multiple Radio Frequency Coils. However, as can be appreciated from Figure 73–6a, the extent of the slices parallel to the surface coil depends only on the sensitivity of the surface coil as a receiver, and this sensitivity decreases gradually in the y direction, giving poor localization in this direction.

Selective Refocusing Pulse in a Field Gradient

Like selective excitation pulses, selective refocusing pulses are commonly used in imaging to generate a slice. The relevant experiment for a surface coil is

$$\theta - \tau/2 - 2\Theta_{SX}[\pm x, \; \pm y] - \tau/2 - \text{acquire signal, receiver}[+, \; -] \qquad [12]$$

where the initial pulse is a hard pulse as written. The second $\tau/2$ time should be adjusted to a sufficient length for eddy currrents to dissipate, e.g., 10 ms. The pulsed x gradient will be switched on just before the selective pulse $2\Theta_S$, and switched off immediately after. The switching on time should be adjusted to give maximum echo signal, and because of the substantial rise and fall times of the gradient it will be found that the pulsed gradient will need to be switched on a short time before $2\Theta_S$. This will ensure that the integrated effect of the gradient at the end of the first $\tau/2$ time (total dephasing) is mirrored by the integrated effect in the second $\tau/2$ time (total rephasing).

The phase cycling of the $2\Theta_S$ refocusing pulse and the receiver has been included in Sequence [12] even though such phase cycling is not normally used in imaging applications. As we noted in Inversion Recovery and Spin Echo Sequences in Inhomogeneous RF Fields, this phase cycling eliminates error signals, which arise from unwanted transverse magnetization components when $2\Theta_S$ is not the ideal value of 180 degrees. From Figure 73–1, after the θ pulse a z magnetization component equal to $M_0 \cos \theta$ remains. Again from Figure 73–1, the $2\Theta_S$ pulse rotates a part of the z magnetization into the transverse plane giving an unwanted error component equal to $M_0 \sin 2\theta \cos \theta$. When $2\Theta_S$ differs from 180 degrees, there is a second unwanted transverse component equal to $M_0 \sin \theta \cos^2 \theta$ which is not refocused at the end of the τ period.[7] The first error component is dephased by the field gradient at the beginning of the second $\tau/2$ period, and the second error component is dephased during the total period of the pulsed field gradient. The statement that such components *are* dephased and therefore eliminated is dangerous without relevant calculations, because such dephasing is only efficient across a homogeneous sample. The proportion of unwanted signal component left is given by $\sin \delta/\delta$ where δ is half the angle through which the nuclear spins have dephased. Thus the spins must dephase through three revolutions (or 6π) for the errors to fall to less than 10 percent of their initial value, or seven revolutions to fall to less than 5 percent. As an example, consider a heterogeneous sample that has a 0.2 cm thick fat layer in the gradient direction. For ^{1}H NMR with a gradient of 1.5 gauss/cm, the frequency gradient is 1300 Hz across the fat layer, thus requiring 2.3 ms for dephasing through three revolutions. This problem is proportionately worse at lower field strength, where lower field gradients are normally used, or for nuclei other than ^{1}H which have a lower gyromagnetic ratio. For imaging with homogeneous coils it may sometimes be satisfactory to discount the problem if pulse angles are close to ideal, because the error components will be small. However, for surface coils where the pulse angle θ takes all values there is a serious difficulty. The field gradient pulse could be lengthened to ensure efficient dephasing. However, for spectroscopy there is no good reason why the phase cycling should not be included. Adequate spectrometers/imagers *must* have appropriate software/hardware. Unlike imaging, where it is important timewise not to have repeated transients at each field gradient setting, in spectroscopy a four transient cycle is quite acceptable.

To further strengthen the above arguments concerning phase cycling, note that spins outside the selected slice experience the sequence $\theta - \tau -$ acquire. This will create an error signal many times larger than the selected slice signal, which in the absence of phase cycling is only reduced by dephasing in the pulsed field gradient. Even in imaging with homogeneous coils this will be a problem, though the minimal phase cycling necessary to remove it,

$$90° - \tau/2 - 180°[x, y] - \tau/2 - \text{acquire, receiver}[+, -], \qquad [13]$$

is sometimes used. For surface coils the phase cycling is a necessity.

It is interesting to note that a simple square refocusing pulse, rather than a shaped pulse, may give satisfactory results. Equation (9) for a $2\theta[\pm x, \pm y]$ pulse is plotted in Figure 73–7 for $\theta = 90$ degrees, and this shows that the pulse would be reasonably selective in a field gradient.[14] This would considerably simplify Sequence [12] as only

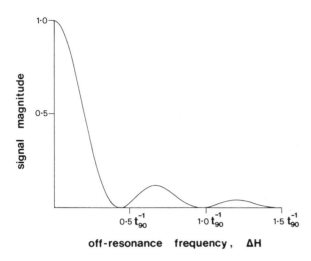

Figure 73–7. Plot of refocused signal intensity against frequency offset for a $2\theta[\pm x, \pm y]$ hard pulse, when $\theta = 90$ degrees on resonance. (Modified from Bendall MR, Pegg DT: Magn Reson Med 2:91, 1985.)

pulses at one power level would be required rather than the need to separately calibrate a hard and a soft pulse.

We are unaware of any reports of the application of the Sequence [12] method with surface coils, but Ordidge[43,44] has used a two-dimensional and a three-dimensional extension of it with a cylindrical homogeneous coil. The two-dimensional variation used a selective 90 degree pulse in addition to the selective 180 degree pulse of Sequence [12];

$$90°_{SY} - \tau/2 - 180°_{SX} - \tau/2 - \text{acquire signal,} \qquad [14]$$

to generate a selected column in the z direction. The three-dimensional method used a second selective 180 degree pulse for the z dimension:

$$90°_{SY} - \tau/2 - 180°_{SX} - \tau - 180°_{SZ} - \tau/2 - \text{acquire signal} \qquad [15]$$

Sequences [14] and [15] suffer from the difficulty, noted above in our discussion of selective excitation pulses, of adjusting the position of the refocusing pulses to rephase the eddy current effects as well as the static field inhomogeneity. This problem is compounded by the need to correctly position the pulsed field gradients around the 180 degree pulses so that in practice it is difficult to obtain a spin-echo at the ideal time. Furthermore, the total delay time has again been doubled, which would lead to a further signal loss via relaxation. Sequences [13] and [14] are not recommended, especially when compared to the selective inversion methods now described below.

Selective Inversion Pulses in a Field Gradient

Selective inversion pulses have not found any use in NMR imaging, but as proposed independently by Ordidge et al.[44,45] and by Roos et al.,[46] they are extremely useful for localization in in-vivo spectroscopy. Consider a selective inversion-recovery sequence alternated with a normal pulse/acquire experiment:

$$180°_{SX} - \tau - 90°; \text{acquire, receiver}[+] \qquad [16]$$
$$90°; \text{acquire, receiver}[-]$$

Subtraction of alternate transients eliminates signals from outside the selected slice but sums the signals from within the slice because here the nuclear spins are alternately inverted. Generalizing this to a surface coil and including the relevant phase alternation of the inversion-recovery Sequence [6] yields

$$2\Theta_{SX}[\pm x, \bar{0}] - \tau - \theta; \text{ acquire} \tag{17}$$

where the notation $[\pm x, \bar{0}]$ means that the pulse is applied with $+x$ and $-x$ phase for two transients and then not at all for two transients, with the bar over the zero implying that the receiver phase is inverted for the second pair of transients. For a $2\Theta_{SX}$ pulse, transverse magnetization given by $M_0 \sin 2\theta$ is created (see Figure 73–1) and our previous discussion in relation to selective refocusing pulses and the dephasing of transverse components is also applicable here. For applications with surface coils it is preferable to include the $\pm x$ phase alternation to eliminate the transverse component. When using a homogeneous rf coil, the phase alternation can be omitted as in Sequence [16].

One advantage of this method over selective refocusing is that no particular care is required with the timing of the pulsed field gradient because the selected spins are only affected by the gradient during the $2\Theta_{SX}$ pulse. A second advantage is that the eddy current delay period (τ) is half that required for selective refocusing, because eddy currents occur only in the second half of the spin-echo for the latter method. Furthermore, signal intensity is lost via $T1$ relaxation, which is slower than $T2$ relaxation as occurs during spin-echo sequences.

Subtracting 1 from Equation (6) and dividing by 2 shows that a hard $2\theta[\pm x, 0]$ pulse converts unit z magnetization to

$$z \text{ magnetization} = -\cos^2 \alpha \sin^2 \theta' \tag{10}$$

This is the same expression as plotted in Figure 73–7, so a hard 2θ pulse rather than a soft 2θ pulse may again provide reasonable slice selection while substantially simplifying the experiment. This also suggests that the slice selective sequence $2\Theta_S[\pm x, 0]$; θ gives exactly the same spatial response in a field gradient as the previous one using a selective refocusing pulse, i.e., θ; $2\Theta_S[\pm x, \pm y]$. Indeed, this can be shown to be formally true using rotation matrices.[47] This equivalence curtails the theoretical calculations necessary to separately establish the response of selective inversion and refocusing pulses.

Ordidge et al.[44,45] have obtained ^{31}P human brain spectra using selective inversion pulses with a surface coil. They have also extended the Sequence [16] method to selection in three dimensions and have obtained ^1H and ^{31}P localized arm spectra using a homogeneous cylindrical coil.

The three-dimensional extension of the general Sequence [17] method can be developed quickly by a consideration of formal theory. The effect of an rf pulse on $x, y,$ and z magnetization can always be written down as a rotation matrix. If all other aspects of a pulse sequence are held constant, the overall result for a phase-cycled pulse is a linear combination of the rotation matrices for each pulse phase, which we have called a "cycle matrix."[14] The cycle matrix for a $2\theta[\pm x, \bar{0}]$ pulse, where θ may be hard, soft, or composite, shows that z magnetization is not interconverted with transverse magnetization by the pulse.[47] Thus, if there is no transverse magnetization before the pulse, and the pulse is selective, the overall effect of the pulse is to preserve a slice of z magnetization and destroy z magnetization everywhere else. The cycle matrix is applicable to any number of sequential phase-cycled pulses, provided that the phase cycling is independent for each such pulse, i.e., provided that all other aspects of a pulse sequence are held constant during the cycle of each pulse. Thus Sequence [17] can be extended to three dimensions by applying one $2\Theta_S[\pm x, \bar{0}]$ pulse for each dimension:

$$2\Theta_{SX}[\pm x, \bar{0}]; 2\Theta_{SY}[\pm x, \bar{0}]; 2\Theta_{SZ}[\pm x, \bar{0}] - \tau - \theta; \text{ acquire} \tag{18}$$

Because the cycling for each pulse must be independent, Sequence [18] requires 64 transients for a complete cycle with receiver phase inversion whenever an odd number of the $2\Theta_S$ pulses are not applied. Given the ability to control the length of each selected dimension, the selected volume from a complete cycle will be a rectangular cuboid. For a surface coil, this cuboid will be superimposed on the inhomogeneous signal response typified in Figure 73–6.

For a homogeneous coil with well-adjusted pulses it may be assumed that the small transverse components generated by each $2\theta_S$ pulse are dephased by the field gradients between the pulses and the $\pm x$ phase alternation may be omitted, leaving

$$180°_{SX}[x, \bar{0}]; \ 180°_{SY}[x, \bar{0}]; \ 180°_{SZ}[x, \bar{0}] - \tau - 90°; \ \text{acquire} \qquad [19]$$

The $[x, \bar{0}]$ cycling must still be independent for each pulse so the complete cycle requires eight transients. This is the three-dimensional method used by Ordidge et al.[45] Some typical results are shown in Figure 73–8.

When using any of the selective inversion methods represented by Sequences [16] to [19], the nuclear spins outside the selected region will experience the pulse sequence θ; acquire, receiver[$\pm$], where $\theta = 90$ degrees for a homogeneous coil. Thus elimination of these unwanted signals depends entirely on the addition and subtraction of alternate transients. This situation is most critical for a homogeneous coil where maximum signal is generated from the whole sample. It is a common experimental observation that when the transients from two identical NMR experiments are subtracted, the cancellation error is generally of the order of 1 percent. This is a random effect that is caused by the variation of virtually any instrumental parameter that controls the experiment between transients. These parameters include the pulse amplitudes, phases and frequencies, the receiver phase and frequency, the signal amplification and the constancy of the magnet field and its homogeneity (or inhomogeneity). For relevant in-vivo experiments we must add variability arising from the mechanical vibration of field gradient coils, but most importantly motion of the sample arising from blood flow, respiration,

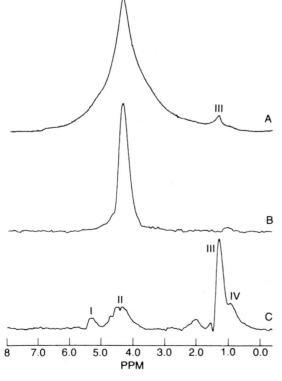

Figure 73–8. ^{1}H spectra obtained at 80 MHz using a cylindrical coil around the lower human leg. *A*, Total spectrum. *B* and *C*, Spectra obtained using sequence [19] from a cubic sensitive volume (4.1 cm^3) positioned within the soleus muscle and the bone marrow of the tibia, respectively. *B* and *C* are plotted at a scale that is two orders of magnitude greater than *A*. (From Ordidge et al.: J Magn Reson 66:283, 1986. Used with permission.)

digestion, and local muscle contraction. Being usually random, the error will average out like noise. That is, if the average error is 1 percent after two transients, it will be 0.5 percent after eight transients and 0.25 percent after 32 transients. This effect is well described by the term "subtraction noise" and has defeated many NMR experiments that rely on the subtraction of large signals to reveal small ones[48] (and has even occasioned parables of God decreeing that NMR spectroscopists shall always walk on thorns[49]). Subtraction noise is a disadvantage of selective inversion pulses compared with selective refocusing pulses, where the equivalent large signals are substantially dephased by the pulsed field gradient. Subtraction noise will be less serious when sensitive volumes near the sample surface are detected with a surface coil, with a consequent increase in the volume ratio of the localized region compared to the total field of view.

It is possible that the problem of subtraction noise can be reduced using other methods. Consider a selective $90°_s[x]$ excitation pulse again. The selected spins could be returned to the z axis using a hard $90°[-x]$ pulse and re-excited after an eddy current delay period, i.e.,

$$(90°_s[x]; 90°[-x])_x - \tau - 90°; \text{acquire.} \tag{20}$$

The symbolism is meant to indicate that the x pulsed field gradient is on until after the $90°[-x]$ pulse so that signals from spins outside the selected slice are predominantly dephased in the transverse plane and eliminated prior to any subtraction. Of course, pulses cannot be exact, and there will be relaxation during τ, so some z magnetization outside the selected slice will exist before the last 90 degree pulse. To prevent any error signal, the result of the corresponding inversion sequence,

$$(90°_s[-x]; 90°[-x])_x - \tau - 90°; \text{acquire,} \tag{21}$$

should be subtracted, but there will be much less subtraction error compared to Sequence [16]. This method has been proposed by Young,[50] but it suffers from the problem outlined earlier for selective excitation pulses:[40] the selected spins are left spread out in the transverse plane by 90°, and must be refocused with a 180 degree hard pulse, giving overall, by combining [20] and [21]:

$$(90°_s[\pm x] - t - 180° - t - 90°[-x])_x - \tau - 90°; \text{acquire, receiver}[\pm] \tag{22}$$

This can be extended to three dimensions as for Sequence [19], but the generalization to surface coils with θ and 2θ pulses is too complicated. The use of the sequence [22] method has recently been described in the literature, where it has been called the SPACE technique.[147] SPACE is a varient of another recent method called SPARS, which has the $90°_s$ pulse last in the spin-echo sequence rather than first as in sequence [22]. SPARS has an advantage over SPACE in that the field gradient is off during the hard pulses and thus does not impair their effectiveness.[148]

Sequence [20] is formally equivalent to that used by Aue et al.[51] for localization in spectroscopy (and derived from the imaging method of Post et al.[52]):

$$(45°_s[x]; 90°[-x]; 45°_s[x])_x - \tau - 90°; \text{acquire.} \tag{23}$$

However, although the spins spread out as usual during the first selective pulse, this is exactly reversed after the hard 90 degrees during the second $45°_s$ pulse. Aue et al. have used the three-dimensional extension of Sequence [23] for localization, but this has to be fairly unsatisfactory because some z magnetization will exist outside the selected volume just prior to the last 90 degree pulse, and so generate a substantial error signal. The obvious solution is to use the pulse sandwich equivalent to $90°_s[-x]$; $90°[-x]$ as in sequence [21], i.e.,

$$(45°_s[-x]; 90°[-x]; 45°_s[-x])_x - \tau - 90°; \text{acquire,} \tag{24}$$

but unfortunately for this pulse sandwich the dephasing of spins during the selective pulses is not refocused. There does not seem to be a simultaneous solution to all the problems using this method. Nevertheless, recently Müller et al.[53] have described some reasonable results using this method with surface coils, but their work raises further questions additional to the dephasing problem just noted. Having realized the problem caused by residual z magnetization, they introduced phase cycling but used $45°_S[x]$; $90°[x]$; $45°_S[x]$ instead of the pulse sandwich in Sequence [21]. This cannot function properly, which probably explains their observation that "optimum canceling of signals arising from outside of the selected slice may require somewhat different amplitudes of the x and $-x$ pulses." Furthermore, only a two transient phase cycle was used for the extension of the method to three dimensions, but clearly an eight transient experiment is required, based on independent cycling for each pulse sandwich, and this should probably be extended to a full 64 transient cycle when using surface coils. Calculations show that another problem occurs when the 90 degree pulse in the sandwich is not very hard (say >50 μs) as significant signal is then generated outside the selected volume.[54] Finally, for surface coils, sample regions outside of the selected region experience the sequence $\theta - \tau - \theta$ and $\theta - \tau - \theta - \tau - \theta - \tau - \theta$ for each transient for the one- and three-dimensional methods respectively. This leads to signal equal to $M_0 \sin \theta \cos \theta$ and $M_0 \sin \theta \cos 3\theta$ respectively as compared to $M_0 \sin \theta$ for Sequences [17] and [18]. Thus when using surface coils, subtraction noise is only reduced by a factor of 2 and 4, respectively, for the one- and three-dimensional methods compared to that for Sequences [17] and [18].

When considering general three-dimensional methods, there is another means of reducing subtraction noise. Having derived Equation (10) we noted that a $2\Theta_S[\pm x, \overline{0}]$ pulse before θ is formally equivalent to $2\Theta_S[\pm x, \pm y]$ after θ. Thus Sequence [18] converts to

$$\theta - \tau/2 - 2\Theta_{SX}[\pm x, \pm y]; 2\Theta_{SY}[\pm x, \pm y]; 2\Theta_{SZ}[\pm x, \pm y] - \tau/2 - \text{acquire} \qquad [25]$$

Subtraction noise is avoided because the large transverse signals from spins outside the selected region after the θ pulse are predominantly dephased by the pulsed field gradients. Compared to Sequence [18] this method will suffer more from loss of signal via relaxation during the delay periods. However, for homogeneous rf coils only one phase alternation need be retained to eliminate residuals from the large transverse signals after the initial 90 degree pulse:

$$90° - \tau/2 - 180°_{SX}[x, y]; 180°_{SY}; 180°_{SZ} - \tau/2 - \text{acquire, receiver}[+, -] \qquad [26]$$

This two transient cycle should prove useful.

Summary of Selective Pulse Methods

It is difficult to assess the likelihood of success of the numerous possible methods given the various sources of error signals and the present lack of comparative experiments. However, some major points can be listed to direct the user. Selective excitation pulses are not generally useful. Selective inversion pulses yield one-, two-, or three-dimensional methods with a minimal loss of signal from relaxation, and the problem of subtraction noise can be reduced for homogeneous coils. Selective refocusing pulses also yield multidimensional methods that avoid subtraction noise, but the problem of loss of signal from rapidly relaxing species is at its worst. The two-transient three-dimensional procedure for homogeneous coils (Sequence 26) is noteworthy.

In introducing the first three-dimensional localization method using selective pulses in field gradients, Aue et al.[51] described some general principles. From the proton image of the object under investigation, the region of interest can be defined relative to the zero crossing-point of the field gradients. The center of the sensitive volume can then be positioned appropriately by changing the frequency (and thus the spatial position) of each selective pulse. The cuboid shape of the sensitive volume is adjusted using the inverse proportionality of each dimension with the length of the selective pulses. The NMR spectrum can then be obtained for any nucleus. For surface coil studies, the y and z field gradients may be abandoned, but the link back to the proton image is still valuable. That image could best be obtained using a whole-body coil already in place.

Spatially selective pulses have been proposed and calculated using the assumption that rf fields are homogeneous and that the pulses are 90°s or 180°s. In this section we have not so far considered the detailed behavior of such selective pulses in inhomogeneous fields as provided by surface coils. Undoubtedly this will modify the ideal cuboid shape of the sensitive volume and may in some cases permit large spurious regions of signal intensity (e.g., high flux regions[53]) outside the preferred regions of interest. The outcome of selective pulses as a function of θ pulse angle can be calculated[29–31,55,56] and combined with the theoretical distribution of rf field for an inhomogeneous coil. There is a great need for such lengthy calculations to optimize surface coil experiments, but in their absence we can proceed on the basis that selective pulses will function properly and that their spatial behavior will be superimposed on the expected signal response illustrated in Figure 73–6. Some relevant calculations have recently been made.[149] Experimentally, this assumption can be tested by imaging the sensitive volume. The selected volumes generated by any of the above methods can be imaged by combining them with the Sequence [8] slice phantom method, and this method has successfully shown that Sequence [17] functions well with a surface coil when using a sinc-shaped pulse.[44,45] There is a good probability that much better selective pulses will be found. Indeed, Silver et al.[24,30] have already described a selective 180 degree pulse that is insensitive to rf power above a critical threshold.

Two-Dimensional Fourier Transform Localization

The two-dimensional Fourier transform (2DFT) technique utilizes an incremented field gradient in one half of a spin-echo sequence, which for an inhomogeneous rf coil may be written

$$\theta \text{———} \tau/2 \text{———} 2\theta[\pm x, \pm y] \text{———} \tau/2 \text{———} \text{acquire} \qquad [27]$$

incremented x
field gradient

In a normal imaging experiment this incremented gradient provides spatial information for one of the three dimensions. It is a valuable method for spectroscopy because whereas natural chemical shift is refocused because it is present in both $\tau/2$ periods, the x field gradient imposes a phase shift on all nuclear spins during the first $\tau/2$ period which cannot be refocused because it is omitted in the second $\tau/2$ period. This phase shift is incremented with the x field gradient and after Fourier transformation yields pure spatial information in one dimension with no contribution from the natural chemical shift. The latter is detected by the normal acquisition of signal in the absence of field gradients and so chemical shift information is cleanly separated from spatial information in the second dimension. This is clearly explained by Haselgrove et al.,[33] and an earlier presentation of the technique by Maudsley et al.[32] showed that a second and third spatial dimension could be added using additional incremented gradients. Brown et al.,[57] in an earlier report, described some basic principles of this form of chemical shift imaging but did not realize the separability of spatial information from chemical shift information by the spin-echo.

This prior work was entirely concerned with homogeneous coils as normally used in NMR imaging. Sequence [27] takes into account the spatial variability of pulse angles when using a surface coil. Note that the transverse error components of magnitudes $M_0 \sin 2\theta \cos \theta$ and $M_0 \sin \theta \cos {}^2\theta$ (discussed under selective refocusing pulses) are not dephased at all in Sequence [27] (except by external field inhomogeneity) and must be removed using the $[\pm x, \pm y]$ phase cycling.

In a normal imaging experiment with a homogeneous coil, the gradient is incremented a large number of times (e.g., 64), so generating the same number of slices orthogonal to the gradient axis. For a surface coil, as depicted in Figure 73–6, it would seem that only a few gradient incrementations would be necessary along the x axis to generate a few slices parallel with the coil with one centered on 1.0 radius depth, for example. The unwanted slices near the surface and at greater depth could be discarded leaving a well-shaped sensitive volume at the chosen depth of 1.0 radius. Off axis, the boundaries of the localized region are given by $\theta \sin 3\theta$ as displayed in Figure 73–3. This simple method has been suggested previously by us,[10,12] but there is a fundamental difficulty, which is apparent from a detailed consideration of sampling theory.

Fourier transformation of the data obtained for an equal number of transients at each gradient setting does not yield, as might be expected, the signal response from a series of pixels that are completely resolved from each other. As illustrated in Figure 73–9, the signal response from any one pixel contains contributions from surrounding pixels as given by a continuous $\sin x/x$ distribution.[58] Thus after a coarse incrementation yielding a pixel size of, for example, 0.3 coil radius thickness (a suitable slice thickness for a surface coil), surface regions would make large contributions to a pixel (slice) centered on 0.75 radius depth, especially considering the higher sensitivity of the coil to the surface regions.

This resolution problem could be solved by using a larger number of gradient increments, thus generating smaller pixels. The signal response from several of these pixels can then be summed to give a well-resolved thick slice. However, Mareci and Brooker have noted that this summation results in a decrease in the signal-to-noise ratio.[59,60] Indeed, Edelstein[61] has suggested that when the signal from N pixels are summed there is a $N^{1/2}$ loss of signal-to-noise compared with obtaining the signal from the larger pixel using a coarser incrementation, and this is supported by some detailed calculations by Rothman.[62] One way of explaining this is that it is impossible to generate a pixel with square edges and obtain maximum signal-to-noise at the center of the pixel. Thus resolution trades against signal-to-noise.

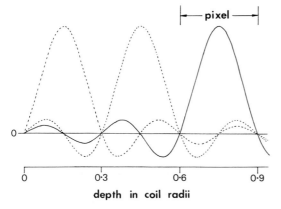

Figure 73–9. The continuous line shows the fractional contribution of signal, from each sample point, to the total signal that is associated with the pixel centered at 0.75 radius depth. The contribution from surface regions needs to be scaled upwards because of the higher sensitivity of the coil to these regions. The broken lines show the signal distribution for adjacent pixels.

Mareci and Brooker[59,60] have proposed a method designed to alleviate the resolution problem and maximize the signal-to-noise ratio. Instead of obtaining equal numbers of transients at each gradient setting, g_x, they obtain a variable number as determined by a calculated weighting function $P(g_x)$. If the weighting function is Gaussian, the spatial response function is also Gaussian, as in Figure 73–10, rather than sinc, as in Figure 73–9. The calculations provided by Mareci and Brooker and reproduced in Figure 73–10 give slices that are up to a factor of 2 too thin for our purposes; or in other words, the field of view of the two-dimensional Fourier transform method is a factor of 2 too large. The latter can be halved by halving the number of field gradient settings specified in Figure 73–10, leaving eight. Mareci and Booker are able to move the spatial response, i.e., sensitive volume, anywhere within the field of view relative to the zero crossing point of the field gradient by data manipulation after signal acquisition. We have mimicked this in Figure 73–10 by inserting a scale in terms of coil radii so that 0.75 radius depth coincides with the selected slice. It can be seen that with the field of view halved, corresponding to eight gradient settings, good suppression of surface signals will be achieved. Brooker and Mareci intend to provide a complete theoretical treatment of their selective Fourier transformation method.[63] Though it was initially designed for use with homogeneous coils, Mareci et al.[64] have extended this technique to surface coils in a very similar way to that described above. This is discussed further in Localization by Combining the Methods of Pulsed Field Gradients and Radio Frequency Inhomogeneity.

It is worth considering the maximum gradient required for this method. The width

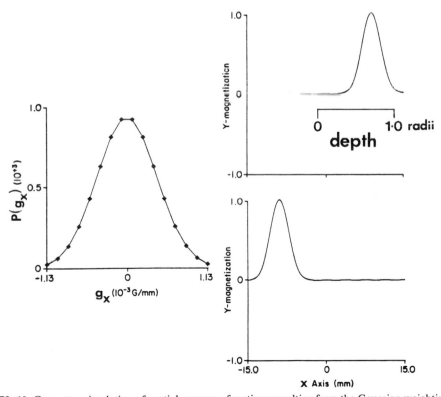

Figure 73–10. Computer simulation of spatial response functions resulting from the Gaussian weighting function on the left. The simulations assume signal acquisition at 16 gradient settings. By subsequent data manipulation, the spatial response can be moved anywhere in the field of view as indicated on the right. This positioning might be relative to a surface coil as depicted by the added scale giving depth in units of coil radii. (From Marcel TH, Brooker HR: J Magn Reson *57*:157, 1984. Used by permission.)

of the field of view is given by

$$V = (\gamma \, \Delta gt)^{-1} \tag{11}$$

where Δg is the field gradient increment in gauss cm^{-1} and t is the length of the pulsed field gradient. If an equal number of positive and negative gradient settings are used, and N is the number of settings, the maximum gradient required is

$$g_{max} = \Delta gN/2 \tag{12}$$

For ^{13}C NMR (γ = 1070 Hz gauss^{-1}), using a 7.5 cm diameter coil ($V \sim 7.5$ cm) with N = 8, g_{max} is only 0.25 gauss cm^{-1} for t = 2 ms. Considering the small gradient required, and thus less eddy currents, this would indicate a total spin-echo τ delay of about 5 ms, which should be kept as small as possible to reduce signal loss from $T2$ relaxation. Under equivalent conditions, g_{max} for ^{31}P is 0.16 gauss cm^{-1}. Note that the field gradient pulse does not need to be square, but just incrementable, and the eddy currents may continue into the second half of the spin-echo without any deleterious effect if they are also incremented by the main gradient as they should be. Note also that the selective Fourier transformation method of Brooker and Mareci enables the use of a small number of gradient increments, which in turn minimizes g_{max}. There are clear advantages in keeping field gradients as low as possible to minimize eddy currents.

The strength of this selective 2DFT/surface coil method is that chemical shift and spatial information are not mixed. It is consequently suitable for ^{13}C NMR, unlike selective pulses, and has advantages for ^{31}P NMR. It may not be convenient for some ^{1}H NMR applications considering the fairly large number of transients required to obtain a spectrum. However, it can be extended to simultaneously generate multiple slices from the surface inwards by using good composite pulses[19] in place of θ and 2θ, and this would increase its suitability for all nuclei.

LOCALIZATION USING RADIO FREQUENCY INHOMOGENEITY

Hoult[65] first suggested the use of an rf field gradient for imaging, and he called his technique "rotating frame zeugmatography." A version of Hoult's general method using incremented rf pulse lengths was applied by Cox and Styles[66] and others, and further detail of the application is given below. In contrast to this imaging method, we have developed a family of phase-cycled pulse sequences, called depth pulses, which select sample regions bounded by particular pulse angle limits chosen before the experiment.[7,8,10,12,14,25,26,67–69] This work is reviewed below, and in a third subsection a comparison is made with more recent depth pulse sequences, introduced by Shaka et al.[70,71] and by Tycko and Pines,[72] in which some of the pulses are composite pulses. Most recently, Garwood et al.[73] have used a Fourier series subset of the incremented rf pulses used in rotating frame zeugmatography to generate single pulse angle slices that are similar to those obtained with depth pulses. This Fourier series method is described in a fourth subsection.

All the above methods will provide sensitive volumes in the form of pulse angle slices, i.e., a sample region bounded by selected pulse angle values. Referring to Figure 73–6 and assuming pulse angle limits of 45 degrees and 135 degrees, it is clear that the slice obtained is not conveniently shaped, and in most cases an additional means of localization is required. Such combined methods are described in Localization by Combining the Methods of Pulsed Field Gradients and Radio Frequency Inhomogeneity, and Localization Using Multiple Radio Frequency Coils.

Rotating Frame Zeugmatography

Hoult[65] described some techniques under the title "rotating frame zeugmatography" which require the use of an rf field gradient. He employed a saddle transmitter coil with three turns on one side and a single opposed turn on the other side to generate a linear rf gradient. Cox and Styles[66] used a similar probe and showed that by incrementing a single excitation pulse length and applying a two-dimensional Fourier transform to the two-dimensional data set, then the NMR spectrum is produced in one dimension (Fourier transform of acquired signal) and spatial information is obtained in the second dimension (Fourier transform with respect to incremented pulse). The method is analogous to the normal 2DFT imaging method (e.g., Sequence 27) with the difference that the incremented magnetic field gradient is replaced with an incremented rf field gradient. The experiments of Cox and Styles were conducted using a small bore magnet, but the method could be extended to the head or body with larger rf gradient coils. Bolton has just discovered this imaging method.[74]

However, our prime interest is with surface coils that provide rf field gradients. Though these are nonlinear, the rf field gradient along the coil's axis is approximately linear from the center of the coil to 1.0 radius depth. Haase et al.[75] introduced this rotating frame zeugmatography technique to surface coils and convincingly demonstrated spatial resolution of phantoms by ^{31}P NMR, and Garwood et al.[76] have further extended the method with surface coils. They also demonstrated good spatial resolution of phantoms to 1.0 coil radius depth, but beyond that depth, resolution was defeated by the shallower slope of the rf field gradient. Garwood et al.[76] showed that use of an efficient presaturation pulse eliminated smearing in the spatial dimension, which otherwise appears when the recycle time of the experiment, *TR*, is short compared to $5T1$, and obtained ^{31}P metabolite maps of freshly enucleated bovine eyes, as illustrated in Figure 73–11. These experiments on an intact organ required 9h at 4.7 tesla. The contour map in Figure 73–11 indicates fluctuating amplitudes of GPC and UDPG from different

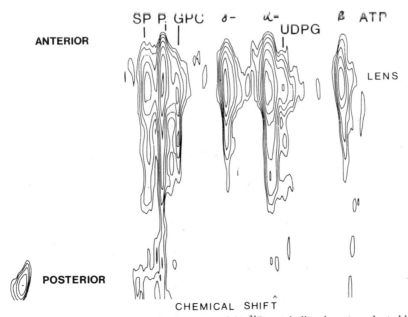

Figure 73–11. Contour plot of spatially localized spectra of the ^{31}P metabolites in an enucleated bovine eye. Distance is vertical, and chemical shift is horizontal. The signal in the bottom left-hand corner is a position marker placed on the optic nerve. (From Garwood et al.: J Magn Reson *60*:268, 1984. Used by permission.)

lens anatomical regions and shows that P_i is absent from the vitreous but present in the retina and choroid.

In this imaging method each pixel corresponds to a curved slice whose shape is given by the curved rf field isocontours in Figure 73–6. To obtain nearly planar slices through the lens region of the eye, Garwood et al. used a two-turn surface coil with the second turn (distal to the sample) 0.9 times the diameter of the first and spaced 0.25 times the large radius away. This improved the shape of the rf field for these studies with isolated samples, and although there may be some applications in vivo (e.g., by proptosing the eye), this imaging method is limited by the gross curvature of the rf field off axis beyond the diameter of the surface coil.

The close analogy with the 2DFT localization method indicates that each pixel will show poor resolution (as in Figure 73–9), and their summation will lead to much less signal-to-noise than can be obtained by other methods (e.g., depth pulse sequences). However, analogous improvements can be made corresponding to the selective 2DFT method and this leads to the Fourier series window method described at the end of this section.

Depth Pulse Sequences[7,8,10,12,14,25,26,67–69]

Details of these pulse sequences have been recently reviewed,[12] so here we will only be concerned to summarize the major features.

The basis of depth pulse sequences, phase-cycled pulses, have already been introduced in this chapter. Depth pulse sequences are derived from the phase-cycled pulses required to eliminate error signals (or transverse magnetization error components) when using the inversion-recovery or spin-echo sequences with inhomogeneous rf coils (described in Inversion Recovery and Spin Echo Sequences in Inhomogeneous Radio Frequency Fields). As we have already seen in preceding sections, such phase cycling is needed whenever there is more than one pulse (the excitation pulse) in a pulse sequence. So far we have seen that complex pulse sequences can be built up using just the phase-cycled inversion pulse $2\theta[\pm x]$, the excitation pulse θ, and the phase-cycled refocusing pulse $2\theta[\pm x, \pm y]$. This is indeed also true for depth pulse sequences and remains true for the remainder of the methods considered in this chapter.

Equations (1), (3), and (2) express the effect of the pulses $2\theta[\pm x]$, θ, and $2\theta[\pm x, \pm y]$, respectively, on the final detected signal intensity. These on-resonance factors are $\cos 2\theta$, $\sin \theta$ and $\sin^2\theta$ respectively and the overall effect for any phase-cycled pulse sequence made up of these pulses can be obtained by multiplying these factors together. A single excitation pulse ($\sin \theta$) yields signal from all points in the sample, except where $\theta = 180$ degrees, 360 degrees. . . . As shown in Figure 73–12, depth pulses are designed to restrict signal response to within chosen ranges of pulse angles, and Sequence [28] expresses a general form for a convenient family of depth pulse sequences:

$$(m \times 2\theta[\pm x])_n; \{\Sigma\ell \times \theta\}; 2\theta[\pm x, \pm y]; \text{acquire} \qquad [28]$$

Useful variations of Sequence [28] are summarized in Figure 73–13. Though any number of $2\theta[\pm x, \pm y]$ pulses could be used, one is normally sufficient for suppressing signals wherever θ is close to 0 degrees, 180 degrees, 360 degrees. . . . The usual θ pulse can of course be used (i.e., $\ell = 1$), but setting $\ell = 2/3$ gives zero signal when $\theta = 270$ degrees. Even better suppression of these high flux signals, for θ values around 270 degrees, can be achieved by applying any depth pulse twice with $\ell = 2/3$ and then for a third transient with $\ell = 4/3$. This is signified by the notation $\{2 \times 2\theta/3 + 4\theta/3\}$.

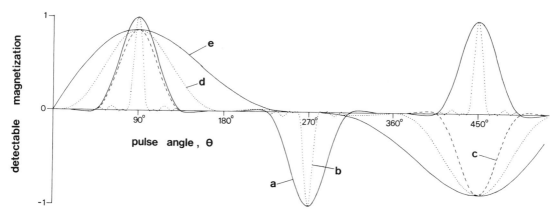

Figure 73–12. Plots of signal magnitude versus pulse angle θ for depth pulse schemes that limit signals to regions where (*a*) θ is within 90 ± 40 degrees, 270 ± 40 degrees, 450 ± 40 degrees, . . . (e.g., sequence [29]); (*b*) θ is within 90 ± 10 degrees, 270 ± 10 degrees, 450 ± 10 degrees, . . . (e.g., sequence [30]); (*c*) signals are limited as for *a* but 270 degree signals are suppressed (e.g., sequences [31] and [32]). In *d* and *e*, 270 degree signals are suppressed with little or no reduction of pulse angle limits around 90 degrees, as would be obtained with sequences [33] and [34]. (Modified from Bendall MR: *In* James TL, Margulis AR [eds]: Biomedical Magnetic Resonance. San Francisco, Radiology Research and Education Foundation, 1984.)

A more complex summation, shown in Figure 73–13, eliminates both 270 degree and 450 degree signals. As an alternative, high flux signals can be reduced using variations of the $2\theta[\pm x]$ pulse with $m = 1/6$ to eliminate 270 degree signals and $m = 1/10$ to reduce 450 degree signals. Thus it may be useful to use more than one $2\theta[\pm x]$ type pulse in any one sequence as expressed by the subscript n.

For a $m \times 2\theta[\pm x]$ pulse, the on-resonance factor is $\cos m \times 2\theta$, which is zero at $\theta = 45$ degree when $m = 1$. For $m = 2, 3, 4$ additional zeros are obtained between $\theta = 0$ degree and 90 degrees as listed in Figure 73–13 and these zeros are repeated at 180 degrees, 360 degrees, . . . plus or minus the listed values. Further zeros in the final signal can be generated by repeating a depth pulse sequence with the excitation pulse θ changed to an odd multiple, $3\theta, 5\theta, \ldots$, and subtracting or adding the result again as listed in Figure 73–13. Using one $2\theta[\pm x]$ pulse and an odd multiple as in Sequence [29],

$$2\theta[\pm x]; \{\theta - 3\theta\}; 2\theta[\pm x, \pm y]; \text{acquire,} \qquad [29]$$

signals are efficiently restricted to within the ranges 90 degrees ± 40 degrees, 270 degrees ± 40 degrees, . . . , as shown in Figure 73–12*a*. By choosing in each case an even spread of zeros from those listed in Figure 73–13, these limits can be successively reduced to 90 ± 28 degrees ([H]), 90 ± 21 degrees ([I]), 90 ± 17 degrees ([J]), using more extensive sequences and finally 90 ± 10 degrees ([K]) using Sequence [30], which is illustrated in Figure 73–12*b*:

$$4\theta[\pm x]; 6\theta[\pm x]; 8\theta[\pm x]; \{\theta - 3\theta + 5\theta - 7\theta + 9\theta\}; 2\theta[\pm x, \pm y]; \text{acquire} \qquad [30]$$

(The letters [H] to [K] refer to the depth pulse sequences listed in references 12, 14). Shaka and Freeman[77,78] have recently discovered the utility of these $m \times 2\theta[\pm x]$ pulses both to eliminate high flux signals (which they called harmonics[77]) and to reduce the pulse angle limits around 90 degrees.[78] Though Shaka and Freeman described these "prepulses" as a "new concept," they were already established in the literature.[12,69]

The methods for eliminating high flux signals may be combined with the methods for reducing the pulse angle limits around 90 degrees. For example, elimination of 270 degree signals can be added to Sequence [29] as in [31] or a Sequence equivalent to

$$(m \times 2\theta[\pm x])_n ; \{\Sigma\ell \times \theta\}; 2\theta[\pm x, \pm y]; \text{acquire}$$

CYCLED PULSE	EFFECT

$m \times 2\theta[\pm x]$

$m = 1/6$	$\frac{\theta}{3}[\pm x]$	Signal zero at $\theta = 270°$. Cancellation near $270°$ is efficient if two $\theta/3[\pm x]$ pulses are used.
$m = 1/10$	$\frac{\theta}{5}[\pm x]$	Signal zero at $\theta = 450°$. One $\theta/3[\pm x]$ and one $\theta/5[\pm x]$ pulse gives reasonable cancellation for $\theta \sim 270°$ & $450°$.

$m = 1$	$2\theta[\pm x]$	Introduces zeroes at: $\quad 45°$
$m = 2$	$4\theta[\pm x]$	$22.5° \qquad 67.5°$
$m = 3$	$6\theta[\pm x]$	$15° \qquad 45° \qquad 75°$
$m = 4$	$8\theta[\pm x]$	$11.25° \quad 33.75° \quad 56.25° \quad 78.75°$

$\{\Sigma\ell \times \theta\}$

$\{2 \times \frac{2\theta}{3} + \frac{4\theta}{3}\}$	Efficient cancellation for $\theta \sim 270°$.
$\{2.18 \times 0.489\theta + 1.75 \times 1.082\theta$ $+ 0.831\theta + 0.796 \times 1.561\theta\}$	Efficient cancellation for $\theta \sim 270°$ & $450°$.

$\{\theta - 3\theta\}$	Introduces zeroes at: $\quad 45°$
$\{\theta - 3\theta + 5\theta\}$	$30° \qquad 60°$
$\{\theta - 3\theta + 5\theta - 7\theta\}$	$22.5° \quad 45° \quad 67.5°$
$\{\theta - 3\theta + 5\theta - 7\theta + 9\theta\}$	$18° \quad 36° \quad 54° \quad 72°$

$\{c_0 \times \theta + c_1 \times 3\theta + c_2 \times 5\theta + ..\}$	Fourier series window reduction of limits of $90°$ signals using coefficients given in Table 1.

$2\theta[\pm x, \pm y]$	Reduces signal for $\theta \sim 180°, 360°, \dots$.
$2\theta[\pm x, \bar{0}]$	Reduces signal for $\theta \sim 180°, 360°, \dots$. May be used before $\{\Sigma\ell \times \theta\}$ in substitution for $2\theta[\pm x, \pm y]$. Eliminates dispersion signals by alternation with $2\theta[\pm x, \pm y]$.

Figure 73–13. Summary of the effects of various cycled pulses that may be used in a depth pulse sequence. The pulses, $m \times 2\theta[\pm x]$ and $\sum \ell \times \theta$ are generalized inversion and excitation pulses, respectively.

[29] as in [32]:[12,14]

$$(\theta/3[\pm x])_2; 2\theta[\pm x]; \{\theta - 3\theta\}; 2\theta[\pm x, \pm y]; \text{acquire} \qquad [31]$$

$$(2\theta[\pm x])_2; \{2 \times 2\theta/3 + 4\theta/3\}; 2\theta[\pm x, \pm y]; \text{acquire} \qquad [32]$$

This is illustrated by Figure 73–12c. Of course, high flux signals may be eliminated with only a small reduction in pulse angle limits around 90 degrees by using, for example,

$$\{2 \times 2\theta/3 + 4\theta/3\}; 2\theta[\pm x, \pm y]; \text{acquire}, \qquad [33]$$

or no reduction at all using just

$$\{2 \times 2\theta/3 + 4\theta/3\}; \text{acquire} \qquad [34]$$

The excellent suppression of negative 270 degree signals by Sequence [33] and [34] is shown in Figure 73–12d and e. Clearly, using this family of depth pulses, the 90 degree signal region, of Figure 73–6, for example, can be narrowed at will, with or without elimination of 270 degree and 450 degree signals at the same time.

This family of depth pulse sequences was developed in terms of the simple on-resonance trigonometric factors of Equations (1) to (3) and thoroughly tested with phantom samples and surface coils.[7,8,10,67] For in-vivo spectroscopy we must also consider the off-resonance characteristics, which are determined by multiplying together the more complicated factors given in Equations (6) to (9). This has been studied in detail for the whole family of depth pulses, both theoretically and experimentally,[10,12,14] and a contour plot of signal intensity against pulse angle θ and frequency offset for Sequence [29] is given in Figure 73–14a. This contour plot is typical of those already published, and although perfectly accurate, we now advise that such plots can be misleading. Such a graph represents the signal intensity that would be obtained from a small phantom by incrementing the pulse angle and resonance offset assuming a constant 90 degree pulse time on resonance (t_{90}). However, with a surface coil we are concerned with an extensive sample, and given a particular t_{90} at one radius depth, for example, along the coil's axis, at positions where $\theta = 30$ degrees for example, t_{90} is three times as long (rf field down to a third) and where $\theta - 270$ degrees, t_{90} is down to a third. Consequently, to compare the same resonance offset at different positions in an extensive sample it is necessary to superimpose rectangular hyperbolae as in Figure 73–14a. This is not convenient, and it is better to regraph the data as in Figure 73–14b and c, so that these rectangular hyperbolae become horizontal lines, by using in Equation (4) a variable t_{90}^{θ} in place of a constant t_{90}, where

$$t_{90}^{\theta} = t_{\theta} \times 90/\theta \tag{13}$$

t_{θ} is simply the actual length of the θ pulse used for any sequence, and it is of course equal to t_{90} at $\theta = 90$ degrees. Such figures are applicable to any inhomogeneous coil and directly provide an estimate of off-resonance signal intensity at any value of θ in an extensive sample and thus at any spatial point (by referring to rf field maps like Figure 73–6). For example, it is reasonable to suggest that depth pulses are useable across a spectral width to where 90 degree signals fall to 50 percent of their on-resonance intensity. By drawing a horizontal line tangential to the 50 percent intensity contour, as in Figure 73–14b and c, it can be seen that this line does not intersect any unexpected regions of signal intensity and so the rf discrimination predicted on resonance using the simple Equations (1) to (3) is retained off resonance in these cases. This is typical of depth pulses, with the 50 percent contour reaching $0.1 \, t_{\theta}^{-1}$ off resonance.

Apart from the decrease in signal intensity off resonance, which is common to all spectroscopic techniques, the only significant problem arises from the generation of dispersion signals by the θ excitation pulse as given by Equation (8). This causes no serious difficulty except when using the $\{2 \times 2\theta/3 + 4\theta/3\}$ type method for eliminating high flux signals, where it is found that large dispersion signals occur off resonance for θ values around 270 degrees. The removal of these error signals is easy for sequences that contain a $2\theta[\pm x, \pm y]$ pulse, such as Sequence [33], once it is realized that a $2\theta[\pm x, \pm y]$ pulse changes the sign of y magnetization but not x magnetization (see Equation 9), whereas a $2\theta[\pm x, \overline{0}]$ pulse has the same quantitative effect on the final signal but does not distinguish between x and y magnetization (see Equation 10). Thus dispersion signals (x) are removed by repeating a sequence with $2\theta[\pm x, \overline{0}]$ in place of $2\theta[\perp x, \pm y]$ and summing the results. For example, Sequence [33] becomes

$$\{2 \times 2\theta/3 + 4\theta/3\}; \, 2\theta[\pm x, \pm y]; \text{ acquire} \tag{35}$$
$$+ \, 2\theta[\pm x, \overline{0}]; \, \{2 \times 2\theta/3 + 4\theta/3\}; \text{ acquire}$$

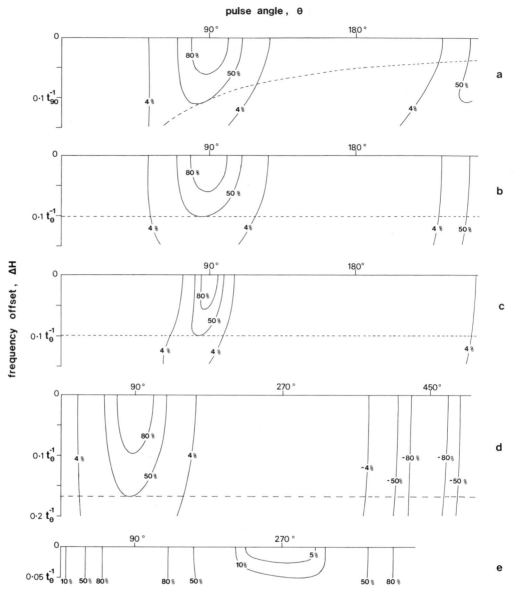

Figure 73–14. Contour plots of signal magnitude against pulse angle θ and frequency offset. Percentages are relative to 100 percent on resonance at θ = 90 degrees. *a*, Plot for sequence [29]. Resonance offsets are given in terms of t_{90} (seconds), which must be known for each point in the sample. The rectangular hyperbola tangential to the 50 percent contour allows for the inverse variation of t_{90} with actual pulse angle throughout a sample. *b*, Replot for sequence [29] assuming a constant length, $t_θ$ (seconds), for the θ pulse and allowing for variation of t_{90} in an inhomogeneous field. The usable frequency limit given by the horizontal line tangential to the 50 percent contour may be obtained by dividing the offset scale (0.1) by the actual $t_θ$ used. *c*, As for (*b*) for depth pulse [J] of references,[12,14] i.e., 2θ[±x]; 4θ[±x]; {θ − 3θ + 5θ − 7θ + 9θ}; 2θ[±x, ±y] which has limits of 90 ± 17 degrees. *d*, As for (*b*) for sequence [35]. The usable frequency limit is much greater at $0.17t_θ^{-1}$. *e*, As for (*b*) for sequence [34].

This method cannot be applied to Sequence [34], which is consequently limited to a range of 0.025 $t_θ^{-1}$ off resonance. The off-resonance characteristics of Sequences [35] and [34] are graphed in Figure 73–14*d* and *e*, respectively.

A convenient tabular summary of most of the useful depth pulse sequences is given in the recent review article.[12] Note that for any published sequence containing 2θ[±x,

$\pm y$], an equivalent depth pulse can be obtained by replacing $2\theta[\pm x, \pm y]$ after θ by $2\theta[\pm x, \bar{0}]$ before θ.

Like the rotating frame zeugmatography method, without another means of localization, depth pulse sequences are of limited use because we are restricted to the shape of the sensitive volume like that given in Figure 73–6. The 270 degree and 450 degree signal regions can be eliminated, and the 90 degree signal region can be narrowed or expanded, or pushed to various depths in the sample by altering t_θ or pulse power, but the 90 degree signal region will always curve back towards the sample surface and intersect the surface outside the diameter of the surface coil. Nevertheless, there are important applications for depth pulses when they are used on their own without other localization means.

The signal response depicted in Figure 73–6 is representative of Sequence [29] and is typical of most depth pulse sequences (except Sequence [34]) in that a hard boundary is imposed on the sensitive volume at some depth into the sample beyond which $\theta < 45$ degrees (or some other selected pulse angle). This contrasts with the single pulse/acquire experiment, where quite large signals are contributed from a thick diffuse boundary region; although both sensitivity and pulse angle ($\theta \sin \theta$) are small for, say, $\theta < 45$ degrees, the sample volume represented by each decrement of θ (the range θ to $\theta - \delta\theta$) increases in approximate proportionality to the cube of the distance from the coil center. It is often necessary to detect regions at moderate depth but avoid sampling deeper regions. This can be readily achieved with a depth pulse, and in many cases interfering signals from an intervening surface layer (e.g., skin, muscle wall, skull) may be weak enough from the region where the 90 degree sensitive volume cuts the surface that these are unimportant. Ng et al.[8,68] demonstrated these principles, as shown in Figure 73–15a and b, by detecting the gross necrotic region of a subcutaneously implanted tumor substantially separate from muscle and viable tumor regions. Interestingly, Ng et al.[8,68] were able to substantially null the phosphocreatine signal from the intervening muscle wall when attempting to detect just rat liver using a depth pulse and a surface coil against the rat chest. It is likely that the negative 270 degree signal region (as in Fig. 73–6) penetrated the muscle wall and subtracted from the positive 90 degree signals arising from outside the coil circumference. The results are shown

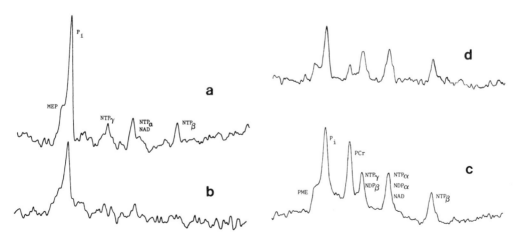

Figure 73–15. In-vivo ^{31}P NMR spectra obtained with a 2 cm two-turn surface coil at 81 MHz and a 3 s repetition rate, (a) of a Dunn osteosarcoma, subcutaneously implanted in a mouse, using a single 25 μs θ pulse (corresponding to maximal signal intensity), 512 scans; (b) using a depth pulse sequence similar to sequence [29] with a 55 μs θ pulse width, 640 scans; and (c) of a rat thorax using a single 25 μs θ pulse, 128 scans; (d) using a depth pulse similar to sequence [29] with a 55 μs θ pulse width, 192 scans. (From Ng TC et al.: Magn Reson Med *1*:450, 1984. Used with permission.)

in Figure 73–15c and d. Although this procedure may seem like cheating, it is nevertheless valid if the intervening surface layer is uniform and remains so during the experiment. Further applications have been described by James and co-workers,[79,80] and depth pulse methods have compared favorably with rival techniques.[79]

In our discussion of depth pulse sequences we have made no mention of τ delay periods because none are required for spatial localization on the basis of rf inhomogeneity (unlike the field gradient methods of the preceding section). If inversion-recovery $T1$ measurements or any spin-echo method is required, it is merely necessary to insert a τ delay after an initial $2\theta[\pm x]$ pulse or symmetrically around a final $2\theta[\pm x, \pm y]$ pulse, respectively.[7,8,12] Most depth pulses already contain one pulse of each type, but if the sequence in use does not, then, of course, a $2\theta[\pm x]$ or a $2\theta[\pm x, \pm y]$ pulse can simply be added. Gadian et al.[81] and Decorps et al.[82] have utilized the extra localization provided by a $2\theta[\pm x, \pm y]$ pulse in spin-echo sequences.

One important aspect that has received little attention to date is the reduction of recycle time, TR, to speed up signal acquisition. At some point, as TR is reduced compared to $T1$, the initial z magnetization will begin to fluctuate from transient to transient, and the selectivity of the depth pulse may break down. A careful study of the problem requires an enormous computational task, considering the number of variables: depth pulse sequence, pulse angle θ, resonance offset, order of phase cycle, and TR. Experimentally we generally use $TR \geqq 2T1$ and have experienced no difficulty. Recent results using one complete localization method showed no loss of localization at short recycle times.[150] One solution is to use a saturation pulse at the end of each acquisition as proposed by Garwood et al.[76] for rotating frame zeugmatography. Decorps et al.[83] have just studied this presaturation method in detail and have found that it does not change the spatial selectivity of any surface coil method when compared to the same method at long TR ($\geqq 5T1$), i.e., it functions properly. They further found that maximum signal was obtained at $TR \sim T1$, and although there was little gain over $TR \sim$ (2 to 3) $\times T1$ without presaturation, the presaturation method of course allows for a large range of $T1$ values as occurs for in-vivo ^{31}P species. Presaturation is probably an adequate solution for depth pulses.

Composite Pulse Depth Pulses

Subsequent to the publication and/or presentation of a considerable body of depth pulse research[7,25,28,67,68,84] Shaka et al.[70,71] and Tycko and Pines[72] recently introduced composite pulses for the same purpose. Considering that these composite pulse schemes are designed to limit signal response to regions where the θ pulse angle is within particular values, we will add these methods to the general class of "depth pulse" schemes rather than generate a new name and refer to them in particular as "composite depth pulses." The composite pulses[70–72] that have been proposed for spatial localization are narrow band inversion pulses; i.e., they invert z magnetization for a narrow band of 2θ values around 180 degrees. In consequence, they cannot be used on their own but must be inserted into a phase-cycled sequence. This situation is analogous to the use of spatially selective inversion pulses (discussed in Localization Using Pulsed Field Gradients), and by analogy with Sequence [17] an appropriate method is

$$2\Theta_C[\pm x, \bar{0}]; \theta; \text{acquire} \qquad [36]$$

where $2\Theta_C$ is the composite narrow band inversion pulse. (A τ delay is not required as in Sequence [17] because there are no eddy currents.) This is the method proposed by Tycko and Pines.[72] As we have shown,[47] and already noted in the previous section, $2\Theta[\pm x, \bar{0}]$ in front of θ is equivalent to $2\Theta[\pm x, \pm y]$ after θ, independently of whether

2Θ is hard, soft, shaped or composite. Consequently the equivalent Sequence to [36] is

$$\theta; \ 2\Theta_C[\pm x, \ \pm y]; \ \text{acquire} \tag{37}$$

and this is the procedure chosen by Shaka et al.[70,71] Sequence [37] is an example of the simplest original phase-cycled depth pulse scheme,[7] with a hard 2θ pulse replaced by a composite $2\Theta_C$ pulse. The reader should now be familiar with the purpose of the phase cycling so it only remains to analyze the quantitative effect of each type of composite pulse. Fortunately the coincidence between the methods of Shaka et al. and Tycko and Pines allows us to discuss their methods simultaneously.

Both groups of authors omitted to make a quantitative comparison between their composite depth pulses and our existing phase-cycled depth pulses. Using rotation matrices we have determined the degree of inversion, f_{zz}, for each $2\Theta_C$ pulse as a function of θ and resonance offset which enables us to determine the overall effect of Sequence [36] or [37] using[47]

$$xy \text{ magnetization} = \tfrac{1}{2}(1 - f_{zz})(\sin^2 2\alpha \sin^4(\theta'/2) + \cos^2 \alpha \sin^2 \theta')^{1/2}M_0 \tag{14}$$

The trigonometric terms in Equation (14) represent the θ pulse and correspond to $(x^2 + y^2)^{1/2}$ as given by Equations (7) and (8). It was found that for each proposed composite pulse, there is an existing phase-cycled depth pulse that gives similar rf discrimination on resonance ($\alpha = 0$). The comparison is shown in Figure 73–16. Q^1, Q^2 and Δ is the nomenclature used by Shaka and Freeman for their suggested $2\Theta_C$ pulses and T^3 is the 27-pulse composite pulse proposed by Tycko and Pines.[72] Shaka and Freeman also suggested the use of one of their composite pulses twice in the one sequence, i.e., $0; (Q^2[\pm x, \pm y])_2$ as in Figure 73–16d, which is the same principle of multiple use of phase-cycled pulses as proposed in the previously published original depth pulse papers.[7,84]

Although similar to phase-cycled depth pulses on resonance, in all cases these composite depth pulses are considerably inferior off resonance. As initially proposed,[70,71] the composite pulses give different results for positive and negative fre-

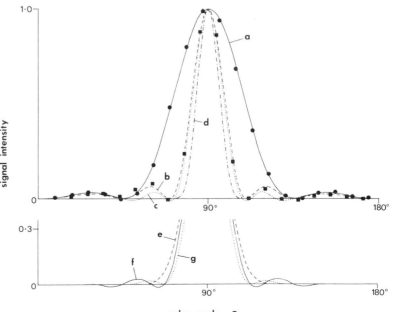

Figure 73–16. Theoretical curves of signal magnitude as a function of pulse angle θ on resonance for (a) depth pulse sequence [29] or the Q^1 composite in sequences [36] or [37], (b) the Q^2 composite in sequences [36] or [37], (c) depth pulse [J] of references 12 and 14 $(2\theta[\pm x]; \ 4\theta[\pm x]; \{\theta - 3\theta + 5\theta - 7\theta + 9\theta\}; \ 2\theta[\pm x, \pm y])$, (d) $(Q^2)_2$ in sequences [36] or [37] (this curve is still less discriminatory than that of sequence [30] drawn in Fig. 73–12b), (e) the Δ composite in sequences [36] or [37], (f) depth pulse [I] of references 12 and 14 $(2\theta[\pm x]; \ 4\theta[\pm x]; \{\theta - 3\theta + 5\theta\}; \ 2\theta[\pm x, \pm y])$, (g) the T^3 composite in sequences [36] or [37]. One percent, or less, deviations of theoretical curves from zero are not drawn. The points are experimental measurements. (From Bendall MR, Pegg DT: J Magn Reson 63:494, 1985. Used by permission.)

quency offsets. This represents a fundamental flaw for a localization technique because it would lead to the selection of different sample regions as a function of resonance offset. One solution to this problem of asymmetry about zero offset is to re-run each cycle with the phase of each pulse in the composite pulse changed from β to 360 degrees − β, a procedure denoted by $2\Theta_{\bar{C}}^{\pm}$.[47] The off-resonance characteristics for some representative composite depth pulses are shown in Figure 73–17. These are directly comparable to Figure 73–14b and c for depth pulses. Clearly the composite depth pulses have a much more limited range of usefulness off-resonance than phase-cycled depth pulses, either because of loss of selectivity or decrease in signal intensity or both.

Recently Shaka et al.[71] have acknowledged the problem of asymmetry about zero offset and have proposed a different solution, the use of the composite twice in the same sequence with the phase reversed for the repeated pulse, i.e., θ; $2\Theta_{\bar{C}}^{+}[\pm x, \pm y]$; $2\Theta_{\bar{C}}^{-}[\pm x, \pm y]$ in our nomenclature. Examples are given in Figure 73–17b and e, and as can be seen, Figure 73–17e corresponds to the best off-resonance result found for these composite pulses. This θ; $Q^{+1}[\pm x, \pm y]$; $Q^{-1}[\pm x, \pm y]$ sequence requires 16 transients for a complete cycle as compared to 24 transients for phase-cycled depth pulse [H] of references 12 and 14 (plotted in Figure 73–18a), which gives a little better rf discrimination. However, the composite depth pulse is only useful off resonance to $0.045\ t_{\theta}^{-1}$ compared to $0.1\ t_{\theta}^{-1}$ for the phase-cycled depth pulse. Since pulse times are proportional to the square root of pulse power, the composite depth pulse requires five times more power to cover the same spectral width.

Tycko and Pines[72] claim that composite depth pulses have a significant advantage

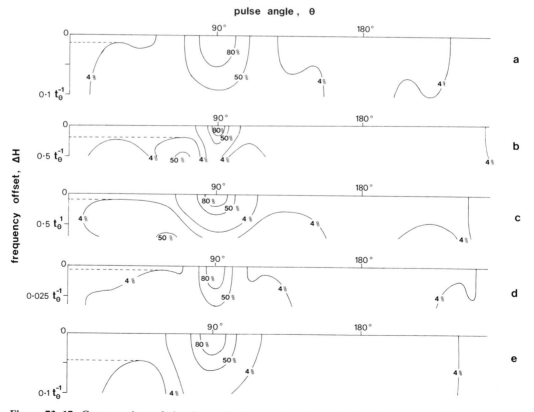

Figure 73–17. Contour plots of signal magnitude against pulse angle θ and resonance offset for various composite depth pulses used in sequences [36] or [37]. Plots drawn as for Figure 73–14b to e. a, $Q^{\pm 1}$. b, $(Q^{+2})(Q^{-2})$. c, $\Delta^{\pm}$. d, $T^{\pm 3}$. e, $(Q^{+1})(Q^{-1})$. For b and e, the phase-cycled composite pulse is used twice in the same sequence with phase reversal for the repeated pulse.

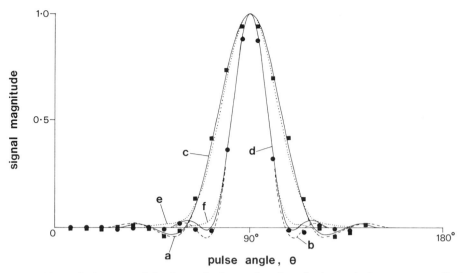

Figure 73–18. Theoretical curves of signal magnitude as a function of pulse angle θ on resonance for the 5 term (*a*) and the 9 term (*b*) square FSW of Table 73–1 (dashed curves); for depth pulse [*H*] (*c*) and the depth pulse [*J*] (*d*) of references 12 and 14 (continuous curves); and for the 6 term (*e*) and the 10 term (*f*) Gaussian FSW of Table 73–1 (dotted curves). The same experimental data was used for both *a* and *b* (and for similar experimental points for *e* and *f*, which are not shown), so illustrating the "zoom" feature. (From Garwood et al.: J Magn Reson 65:510, 1985.)

over phase-cycled depth pulses because the former require less transients for a complete cycle, up to five times less for the known examples. But for localized in-vivo spectroscopy of millimolar metabolites, a large number of transients will be needed for a reasonable spectrum anyway. The question of pulse power required to cover the spectrum is much more important. Because rf coils are often large, or of low Q, or the sensitive volume is remote from the inhomogeneous rf coil used, t_θ pulse times are usually long for in vivo applications. These pulse times cannot be reduced indefinitely by increasing pulse power because eventually arcing into the air occurs even if rf circuit components do not break down before this limit. The best of these composite depth pulses requires five times more pulse power with a minimal reduction in the number of transients as compared to the equivalent phase-cycled depth pulse. The $(Q^{\pm 2})_2$ method saves a factor of five in transients but is a factor of 50 worse off for pulse power. The T^3 composite pulse method of Tycko and Pines requires a factor of 900 times more pulse power. These composite depth pulses are not competitive with phase-cycled depth pulses.

Tycko and Pines[72] suggested the use of a τ period after the $2\Theta_C$ pulse and a pulsed field gradient to dephase transverse error components so that the $\pm x$ alternation would not be required. This runs completely counter to a commonsense approach. Both Tycko and Pines[72] and Shaka et al.[71] propose the use of 2θ/3 in place of the θ excitation pulse to suppress 270 degree signals. This is the crudest variant of a previously published[84] general method for eliminating high flux signals and a simplification of the specific previously presented[25,26] {2 × 2θ/3 + 4θ/3} method. A 2θ/3 excitation pulse leaves approximately 10 percent residual signals at θ = 255 degrees and 285 degrees, and large dispersion signals are introduced off resonance at θ' = 270 degrees beyond 0.02 t_θ^{-1}, which must then be removed using the Sequence [35] procedure.

Most recently Shaka and Freeman[78] have sought to improve the limited range of offset frequencies over which composite depth pulses are useful. However, in doing so, they have moved completely away from obtaining rf discrimination using composite narrow band inversion pulses, and instead this is achieved entirely by phase-cycled pulses as in our original depth pulse schemes. In deriving a large family of such schemes we noted that we have by no means listed all possible ways of obtaining any one result, and Shaka and Freeman[78] have proposed such an equivalent pulse sequence. Their new phase-cycled pulse can be written as $4\Theta[\pm x(2/3), 0(1/3)]$ in our nomenclature, where 2/3 and 1/3 imply that the pulse is not applied for 1/3 of transients (with retention of receiver phase), and this gives zeros at θ = 30 degrees and 60 degrees like $\{\theta - 3\theta + 5\theta\}$ (see Figure 73–13). Indeed, the sequence $\{\theta - 3\theta + 5\theta\}$ is exactly equivalent to $4\theta[\pm x(2/3), 0(1/3)]$; θ on resonance. Since $2\theta[\pm x, \overline{0}]$ is also equivalent to $2\theta[\pm x, \pm y]$, Shaka and Freeman's sequence, $2\Theta_C[\pm x]$; $2\Theta_C[\pm x, \overline{0}]$; $4\Theta_C[\pm x(2/3), 0(1/3)]$; θ, is exactly equivalent to our sequence [H] (of reference 12 and 14), $2\theta[\pm x]$; $\{\theta - 3\theta + 5\theta\}$; $2\theta[\pm x, \pm y]$, on resonance. The valuable new addition made by Shaka and Freeman was to substitute Θ_C composite pulses as written, which were designed to operate across an increased frequency bandwidth and thus extend the useable limits of the depth pulse to $0.25 \, t_\theta^{-1}$. However, these particular composite pulses are exactly equivalent to simple pulses on resonance and do not "enhance the sensitivity to rf inhomogeneity," as was maintained by Shaka and Freeman. In many cases the value of the improved offset range is illusory because the overall composite depth pulse is 2.7 times as long as the equivalent simple depth pulse. Thus, for in-vivo imagers/spectrometers that have large rf amplifiers (e.g., $\gtrsim 1$ kW) it is better to turn up the pulse power by $(2.7)^2$ times and use the shorter simple sequence. The same overall rf power is deposited and the same frequency range is achieved using a shorter pulse sequence. Note also that the offset range of our simple depth pulses can often be improved by avoiding the use of $2\theta[\pm x]$ pulses. Thus, $4\theta[\pm x(2/3), 0(1/3)]$; $\{\theta - 3\theta\}$; $2\theta[\pm x, \pm y]$ is also equivalent to depth pulse [H] on resonance but has an improved offset range similar to that shown for Sequence [35] in Figure 73–14*d*.

Composite depth pulses may well be improved to rival simple depth pulses. However, to gain a significant advantage, an rf selective 90 degree composite pulse is required, i.e., a pulse that requires *no* phase cycling at all. This would avoid the potential problem of fluctuation of initial *z* magnetization for *TR* small compared to *T1* and avoid the effects of experimental parameters varying between transients.

The simplest narrow band inversion pulse of Shaka and Freeman,[70] the Q^1 pulse, could be useful for the multiple coil/depth pulse technique described in the section Localization Using Multiple Radio Frequency Coils or the spin echo heteronuclear method detailed in the section Heteronuclear Methods With Surface Coils. The poor off-resonance behavior of the longer composite pulses would seem to rule out their application there too.

Fourier Series Windows

Garwood et al.[73] have looked at simplifications and improvements of the rotating frame zeugmatography experiment, which they have called the Fourier series window (FSW) method, and we have recently made further improvements.[85] The object is to obtain spectra from a well-resolved but thick slice bounded by isocontours of the rf field, in a similar fashion to depth pulses, and indeed this method is competitive with depth pulses and more convenient in some cases. Various window functions may be used for this rotating frame experiment, and this is exactly analogous to the use of various weighting functions for the selective Fourier imaging method of Mareci and Brooker[59,60] (described in Localization Using Pulsed Field Gradients), with the difference that the θ pulse is incremented in an rf gradient instead of a magnetic field being incremented.

The Fourier series for a square window of width δ centered on θ = 90 degrees, and repeated at $\theta = 270$ degrees, 450 degrees, . . . , is

$$\sum_{m=1}^{M} \frac{(-1)^m}{(1-2m)} \sin(2m-1)\delta \, \sin(2m-1)\theta = \sum_{m=1}^{M} C_m \sin(2m-1)\theta, \tag{15}$$

where M is the number of terms in the series. Written out, the series is

$$\sin \delta \sin \theta - \tfrac{1}{3} \sin 3\delta \sin 3\theta + \tfrac{1}{5} \sin 5\delta \sin 5\theta - \ldots \tag{16}$$

In practice, if used for localization, signal transients are obtained using three to twenty-odd multiples of the basic pulse angle θ, i.e., θ; acquire, 3θ; acquire, 5θ; acquire, and so on. The signal intensity from each of these transients provides the $\sin(2m-1)\theta$ term in Equation (16), and the summation is completed by multiplying each transient by the C_m coefficients in the formula. However, the window is only square for very large M. When the series is truncated, as is necessary in practice, wobbles of positive and negative signal intensity occur on either side of the square window, the sides of the window become less abrupt, and the flat top is distorted. This is illustrated by the simulations of Garwood et al.[73] To obtain good localization, it is important to minimize the wobbles outside the window, hopefully to a level that is insignificant relative to the spectral noise. There are particular values of the width parameter δ for which the wobbles are a minimum, the smallest being $\pi/2M$.[83] Examples of such windows are compared to similar depth pulses windows in Figure 73–18, and C_m coefficients for selected values of M are listed in Table 73–1. The wobbles for these and other values of M decrease from a minimum intensity of -4.7 percent to $+2$ percent, and then less than ± 1 percent on either side of the window.

It is also vitally important to maximize signal-to-noise, the major problem with rotating frame zeugmatography. At the center of the window where $\theta = 90$ degrees, $\sin(2m-1)\theta = (-1)^m$, which gives unity when multiplied by the existing $(-1)^m$ term in Equation (15). When $\delta = \pi/2M$, the $\sin(2m-1)\delta$ term ranges from $\sin \pi/2M$ to $\sin(1 - (1/2M))\pi$, and is consequently always positive. Thus the signals from sample regions where $\theta = 90$ degrees, obtained using each odd multiple of the basic θ pulse length, contribute maximally to the final summation. The only loss of signal-to-noise

Table 73–1. EXAMPLES OF FOURIER COEFFICIENTS FOR THE TRUNCATED SERIES C_0 SIN θ + C_1 SIN 3θ − C_2 SIN 5θ + . . . , WHICH PROVIDE AN OPTIMIZED FOURIER SERIES WINDOW GIVING SIMILAR RADIO FREQUENCY DISCRIMINATION TO DEPTH PULSES

Window Origin	p	Coefficients, C_m or C_n*						Pulse† Angle Limits
Square	1		0.536,	−0.357,	0.107 (M = 3)			90 ± 48°
Square	1	0.333,	−0.290,	0.215,	−0.124,	0.037 (M = 5)		90 ± 30°
Square	1	0.187,	−0.180,	0.165,	−0.145,	0.120,	−0.092,	90 ± 16°
		0.064,	−0.036,	0.011 (M = 9)				
Gaussian	1	0.330,	−0.277,	0.196,	−0.116,	0.058,	−0.024,	90 ± 30°
Gaussian	1	0.201,	−0.188,	0.166,	−0.138,	0.107,	0.078,	90 ± 16°
		0.054,	−0.035,	0.021,	−0.012			
Square	2/3	0.194,	0.190,	−0.173,	−0.162,	0.132,	0.116,	90 ± 30°
		−0.081,	−0.064,	0.029,	0.014 (N = 15)			
Square	1/2	0.120,	0.167,	0.115,	−0.108,	−0.145,	−0.097,	90 ± 30°
		0.084,	0.108,	0.068,	−0.052,	−0.062,	−0.036,	
		0.020,	0.018,	0.006 (N = 20)				

* Coefficients are normalized, i.e., $\Sigma \, C_n \sin(np \times 90°) = 1$. For C_n coefficients ($p \neq 1$), zero coefficients are not listed, and these occur between C_n's of opposite sign.
† For square windows, the limits correspond to pulse angles at which signal intensity crosses zero on either side of the window. For Gaussian windows, the listed limits correspond to the similar window of square origin. For $p = 2/3$, 270 degree signals are eliminated and for $p = 1/2$, both 270 degree and 450 degree signals are eliminated.

comes from summing transients, which have equal noise levels, with unequal weightings. The signal-to-noise as a fraction of the maximum possible is given by

$$\left(\sum_{m=1}^{M} | C_m | \right) \Big/ \left(M \sum_{m=1}^{M} C_m^2 \right)^{1/2} \tag{17}$$

which for all values of M between 3 to 20 is 88 percent of the maximum possible using the equivalent depth pulse for example.

Just like the depth pulse windows, when $\delta = \pi/2M$ for the FSW, the result is no longer square. The squareness is improved by increasing δ to π/M, where the wobbles outside the window are once again minimized. However, negative terms appear in the summation of Equation (15), and as a result, signal-to-noise is markedly reduced at $\theta = 90$ degrees. This second source of possible loss of signal-to-noise is a general phenomenon which accounts for the large loss for the complete rotating frame zeugmatography method when a number of adjacent pixels are summed to form a square window; signal-to-noise is traded against increased resolution at the window edges. A promising possibility, however, is to sum the coefficients for $\delta = \pi/2M$ with those for $\delta = \pi/M$ in a predetermined ratio because the wobbles for these two cases are 180 degrees out of phase.[86] Thus, the wobbles can be further reduced while increasing signal-to-noise over the $\delta = \pi/M$ case, but with the retention of reasonable squareness.

The wobbles of signal intensity, known mathematically as "Gibbs overshoot," induced by truncation of the Fourier series for an extreme square shape, can be reduced by moving away from the square shape in other ways, for example by using a Gaussian window, and some representative coefficients are listed in Table 73–1. Comparative plots, shown in Figure 73–18, indicate that the cutoff at zero intensity is a little less sharp than the equivalent depth pulse or square FSW, as might be expected, and the Gaussian window requires more terms in the Fourier series. There is neither gain or loss in terms of signal-to-noise.

A generalized form of Equation (15) may be derived from the equations of Garwood et al.[73] (by setting $\omega T = p\theta$):

$$\sum_{n=1}^{N} \frac{1}{n} \sin np \frac{\pi}{2} \sin n\delta \sin np\theta \tag{18}$$

where N is the number of terms in the series. The first window is centered at $\theta = 90$ degrees as usual, but the next window at large θ is centered at $\theta = ((4/p) - 1)\pi/2$. If $p = 2/3$, the next window is at $\theta = 450$ degrees, and if $p = 1/2$, the next window is at $\theta = 630$ degrees. This corresponds to elimination of the 270 degree and 450 degree high flux signals, respectively. When $p \neq 1$, less than maximum signal is obtained from the sample region where $\theta = 90$ degree, according to the $\sin np\theta$ term in Equation (18). This third source of a signal-to-noise loss is also common to rotating frame zeugmatography, where on average only 0.707 times the available magnetization is detected from any sample point. When $p = 1$, as in Equation (15), $\sin n\theta$ is zero for n even and unity for n odd. Thus, transients are not acquired for n even, and there is no loss of signal-to-noise, as already mentioned, though for the full rotating frame zeugmatography experiment a 50 percent loss would be obtained in this case. When $p = 2/3$ or $1/2$, the efficiency can also be maintained above the average 0.707 mark at 0.866 and 0.803, respectively, because again $\sin np\theta$ is zero for some values of n. Note that equivalent depth pulse methods for eliminating high flux signals also lead to some loss of signal-to-noise, so the loss for the FSWs because of the $\sin np\theta$ terms is not a comparative disadvantage for $p = 2/3$ or 1/2. The discussion above concerning Equation (15) and the minimization of wobbles outside the selected window also holds for Equation (18), and so minimum wobbles occur when $\delta = \pi/N$ (when $p = 1$, $N = 2M$), and some typically useful coefficients are listed in Table 73–1.

Another vital comparison with phase-cycled depth pulses is the off-resonance properties of the Fourier series windows. This can be readily calculated using Equations (7) and (8), which become for the Fourier series (from Equation 15, for example)

$$y \text{ magnetization} = \cos \alpha \sum_{m=0}^{M} C_m \sin[(2m + 1)\theta'] \qquad (19)$$

$$x \text{ magnetization} = \sin 2\alpha \sum_{m=0}^{M} C_m \sin^2[(2m + 1)\theta'/2] \qquad (20)$$

where C_m represents the coefficients in Table 73–1. Two examples are given in Figure 73–19a and d, and it is immediately clear that there is a problem off-resonance as rf discrimination is badly impaired for shifts greater than $0.05\ t_\theta^{-1}$. This problem results entirely from the dispersion magnetization, which is given by Equation (20). From our knowledge of depth pulses this can be dramatically reduced for θ' values around 180 degrees by adding a $2\theta[\pm x, \pm y]$ pulse, i.e., the Fourier series cycle, $\{\sum (2m + 1) \times \theta\}$; acquire (using the Figure 73–13 notation) becomes $\{\sum (2m + 1) \times \theta\}$; $2\theta[\pm x, \pm y]$;

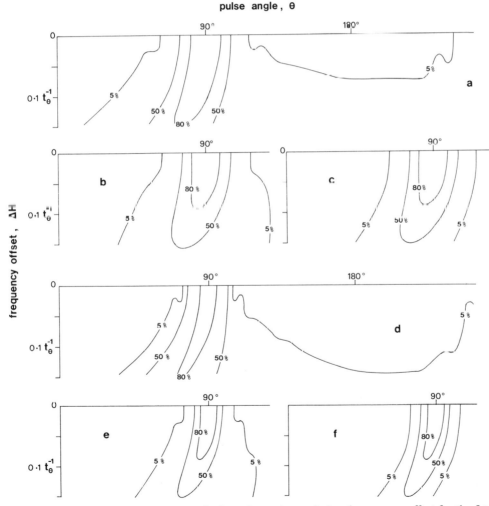

Figure 73–19. Contour plots of signal magnitude against pulse angle θ and resonance offset for the 5 term FSW of Table 73–1 ($\sum (2m + 1) \times \theta$; acquire) ($a$); the 5 term FSW with an added $2\theta[\pm x, \pm y]$ pulse ($\sum (2m + 1) \times \theta$; $2\theta[\pm x, \pm y]$; acquire) (b); the 5 term FSW with complete elimination of dispersion signals ($\sum (2m + 1) \times \theta$; $2\theta[\pm x, \pm y]$; acquire + $2\theta[\pm x, 0]$; $\sum (2m + 1) \times \theta$; acquire) ($c$); The same plots for the 9 term FSW of Table 73–1 are shown in d, e, and f.

acquire. This needs four times more transients than the straight FSW, but the off-resonance properties are much improved as shown in Figure 73–19b and e. There is still some loss of resolution because of the remaining dispersion signals, which also lead to large phase errors across the sensitive volume, but these dispersion signals can be totally removed by alternating $2\theta[\pm x, \pm y]$ with $2\theta[\pm x, \bar{0}]$ as described earlier for depth pulse Sequence [35], which further doubles the total number of transients required for a complete cycle. Examples are given in Figure 73–19c and f. This final result would be particularly dramatic if it were not for the curvature of the selected region as in Figures 73–19c and f, because signal intensity is maintained 50 percent further off-resonance than the corresponding phase-cycled depth pulse (see Figures 73–14b and c). However, this curvature, which arises from the increased pulse angle θ' off-resonance, cannot be avoided and restricts the use of the Fourier series depth pulses to less than about $0.1\ t_\theta^{-1}$. Beyond this, signals are from a substantially different localized region to those on-resonance. The curvature becomes proportionately more serious for increasing rf discrimination; compare Figures 73–14d and 73–19c and f, where the proportion of signal at $0.15\ t_\theta^{-1}$ that arises from outside the on-resonance localized region is approximately 0 percent, 30 percent and 75 percent, respectively. Note that the parent technique of rotating frame zeugmatography also suffers from the same off-resonance defects, and needs to be similarly corrected for routine use.

Comparing the Fourier series depth pulses in Figure 73–19c and f to similar phase-cycled depth pulses in Figure 73–14b and c, the Fourier series provides similar localization with a similar number of transients in a complete cycle and only a modest reduction in signal-to-noise of about 12 percent. One advantage of the Fourier series method is that the phase-cycled pulses can be omitted if t_θ is short, or if the NMR signals of interest are moved close to resonance, thus returning to the simple FSW procedure. A second feature not possible using depth pulse techniques is the ability after data collection to "zoom" in from a broad window, as in Figure 73–18a, to a narrower window, as in Figure 73–18b. Although this zoom feature implies that the spectra obtained for large values of n (or m) are not used for the broad windows, this loss of signal-to-noise can be minimized by obtaining more transients for small n (in rough proportion to the corresponding C_n), and, of course, maximum signal-to-noise is retained for the narrowest window, where it is most critical. This aspect will be useful for determining when the degree of localization is sufficient to eliminate signals from surrounding tissues. Just as depth pulse methods can be used to solve the off-resonance problems of the basic FSWs, so too FSWs can take the place of some or all of the phase-cycled pulses in established depth pulse applications described in this chapter. It is merely necessary to replace the excitation pulse in the depth pulse sequence by $\{\sum np \times \theta\}$, and then omit whatever phase-cycled pulses are no longer necessary. Indeed, existing depth pulse sequences already include truncated Fourier series with unit coefficients (C_m) in substitution for the θ excitation pulse. In this regard, FSWs can be considered as a valuable addition to the existing range of depth pulse possibilities.

Metz and Briggs[87] have also described some of the above features of Fourier series windows. While they have correctly concluded that it is possible to move the selected region by data processing after signal detection, note that this involves large penalties in signal-to-noise compared to depth pulses or the particular FSWs described above— up to a 50 percent loss in signal-to-noise (or an equivalent 4 times increase in signal acquisition time). Perhaps the earliest extension of rotating frame zeugmatography to Fourier series windows is that recently described by Pekar et al.,[88] but unfortunately they chose to mimic depth pulse sequences of the form $\theta; (2\theta[\pm x, \pm y])_n$, the most inefficient depth pulses which were superseded in the first depth pulse article.[7] The new "very fast" methods of Pekar and co-workers[89,90] are also impractical because they require a prior knowledge of *T1* times, which must be uniform across the sample and the same for each chemical species.

LOCALIZATION BY COMBINING THE METHODS OF PULSED FIELD GRADIENTS AND RADIO FREQUENCY INHOMOGENEITY

A primary motivation for continuing research into localization techniques is to develop methods that do not require pulsed field gradients and consequently avoid the problems of field gradient eddy currents and the mixing of spatial and chemical information. Thus it would seem counterproductive to add pulsed field gradients to the rf methods described in the preceding section. However, there will be many occasions when it is appropriate to do so. For example, the localization that can be achieved using a depth pulse (illustrated in Figure 73–6) may be good enough for a particular metabolic time-course study, but unless this can be proved, the data obtained is meaningless. Obviously, it would be valuable to filter out the intervening surface signals using a pulsed field gradient method. If this showed that the proposed experiment was not prejudiced by these surface signals, then a time-course study could proceed at maximum efficiency without the field gradient.

Although at this time no relevant experiments have been reported, the rotating frame imaging experiment and the related Fourier series windows can also be easily combined with pulsed field gradient methods. Expressing these experiments as θ_I; acquire where θ_I is the incremented imaging pulse, or takes particular values for the Fourier series method, then θ_I can simply replace θ in the selective inversion Sequence [17], or the selective refocusing Sequence [12], or the two-dimensional Fourier transform Sequence [27], which then becomes three-dimensional Fourier transform (3DFT). Unfortunately, adding spatially selective pulses to θ_I; acquire will also change those boundaries of the sensitive volume that are set by rf inhomogeneity, unless a selective 180 degree pulse such as that proposed by Silver et al.[30] which is insensitive to rf power variation, is used. Adding a hard $2\theta[\pm x, \pm y]$ pulse as required for the 2DFT method adds a $\sin^2 \theta$ term (or $\cos^2 \alpha \sin^2 \theta'$ term off resonance) and so also modifies the rf discrimination. For the scenario described above, where it is better to simply add a pulsed field gradient without changing the pulse sequence, phase-cycled depth pulses, which might be Fourier series depth pulses, have advantages.

Most useful phase-cycled depth pulses contain a $2\theta[\pm x, \pm y]$ pulse after the θ excitation pulse (see Figure 73–13), and this pulse can always be replaced by $2\theta[\pm x, \overline{0}]$ before θ to give an equivalent sequence (apart from a trivial sign change for any dispersion signal). We have already noted, as in Figure 73–7, that these phase-cycled hard pulses give reasonable slice selection. Because these phase-cycled pulses were derived from spin-echo and inversion-recovery sequences, necessary τ delays for gradient switching can be inserted. Signifying the remainder of the depth pulse in use by $DP(\theta)$, the combined method becomes

$$DP(\theta) - \tau/2 - 2\theta[\pm x, \pm y]_X - \tau/2 - \text{acquire} \qquad [37]$$

or

$$2\theta[\pm x, \overline{0}]_X - \tau - DP(\theta); \text{acquire} \qquad [38]$$

with the pulsed *x* field gradient on during $2\theta[\pm x, \pm y]$ or $2\theta[\pm x, \overline{0}]$ (as for Sequences [12] and [17], respectively). These combined methods have not yet been exploited.

If the spatial selectivity imposed by $2\theta[\pm x, \pm y]$ or $2\theta[\pm x, \overline{0}]$ in a field gradient is insufficient, the whole depth pulse, $DP(\theta)$, can be treated as a selective excitation pulse and applied in a pulsed field gradient,

$$DP(\theta[\pm x])_X; \; SL[y]; \; \text{acquire}, \tag{39}$$

which is the Sequence [10] method. (There are sufficient alternations in a depth pulse to make the additional alternation of Sequence [11] unnecessary). All phase-cycled depth pulses, which contain a $2\theta[\pm x, \; \pm y]$ pulse, show good frequency selectivity, being similar in this regard to a Gaussian shaped pulse, and this has been illustrated in Figure 73–14. There are no significant regions of signal intensity off resonance beyond the 4 percent contour. This combined localization method has been proved by phantom studies,[10,25,26] and some results are shown in Figure 73–20.

The third method possible with phase-cycled depth pulses is the 2DFT method (Sequence [27]), where an incremented pulsed field gradient (x) is used in the first $\tau/2$ period of

$$DP(\theta) - \tau/2 - 2\theta[\pm x, \; \pm y] - \tau/2 - \text{acquire} \tag{40}$$

The usual advantages of less eddy currents and no mixing of chemical and spatial information accrue. If $DP(\theta)$ is just θ, we have the simplest depth pulse θ; $2\theta[\pm x, \; \pm y]$; acquire, and Sequence [40] is identical to Sequence [27], which we have discussed in detail. It will be common to filter out the surface signals using an incremented x gradient, but it is also possible to divide up the 90 degree signal region into voxels using incremented gradients in both the y and z dimensions.[10,12] Mareci et al.[64] have also proposed the combination of depth pulses/surface coils/incremented field gradients in these ways and have demonstrated the viability of the techniques with phantom samples and their selective Fourier transform method. If imaging in the y and z dimensions is used, a quick look at Figure 73–6 shows that at least the 270 degree signals should be eliminated by using depth pulse [33] for example. A reasonable image can then be obtained for a region extending transaxially almost one coil diameter, after which the sensitive volume curves sharply into the sample surface.

Because depth pulses give some control over the transaxial extent of the sensitive volume, these combined methods may be credited with some value as localization methods in their own right, even when compared to field gradient methods alone. For example, Sequences [37] and [38] could be extended to slice selection in the x and y dimensions or slice selection in one dimension and imaging in the second. The node line in the z dimension (Figure 73–6b) ensures a sharp cutoff, and so a good cuboid sensitive volume can be generated without a z field gradient. Generally, pulsed z gradients induce the worst eddy currents because of coupling with the main magnetic field, so it is an advantage to eliminate them.

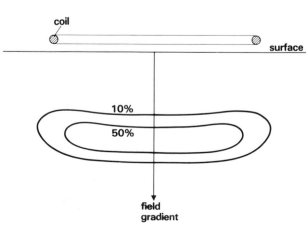

Figure 73–20. Experimental results obtained using a small phantom sample, which was moved relative to the coil, and a depth pulse (similar to sequence [29]) applied in a field gradient. A spin-lock pulse was applied during the eddy current delay period. The plane displayed is 45 degrees to the main field (z) axis. The intensity contours have been extrapolated from the results given in reference 10.

Finally we note that composite depth pulses could be used with the 2DFT method (Sequence 40) but not with any of the selective methods, Sequences [37] to [39], because none of the narrow band inversion composite pulses are frequency selective (see Figure 73–17).

LOCALIZATION USING MULTIPLE RADIO FREQUENCY COILS

For a simple surface coil, the 90 degree region of signal intensity must always curve back into the surface outside the circumference of the coil. This is true of any planar coil (including the "flux concentrator"[91–93]). It is possible that a three-dimensional coil could be developed such that within the perimeter of the coil there is an isolated minimum, maximum, or plateau region of fairly uniform rf field strength. This would enable complete localization using a depth pulse, but no such coil has yet been described. Recent reasoning indicates that it is impossible to design such a coil.[150] Thus, despite the ability to limit signal response to that part of the sample that experiences some intermediate range of rf field strengths (described in Localization Using Radio Frequency Inhomogeneity), we are unable to obtain complete localization using the rf inhomogeneity of a single coil.

The only localization methods presently employed use main field gradients or rf field gradients. To avoid the former, and thus eddy currents, we need to introduce at least a second rf field gradient, i.e., a second coil that produces an inhomogeneous rf field. There are two ways in which the rf response of a second coil can be used for enhancing localization.

First, the additional coil may be used to detect the signal excited by the first coil. The first coil becomes the transmitter and the second the receiver. This method uses the reciprocal relation between rf field strength and sensitivity (see The Radio Frequency Field of the Surface Coil). The shape of the rf field of a coil can be revealed by experiment (e.g., Sequence [8]) or predicted by calculation (at least for a coil manufactured from continuous wire). Thus, the sensitivity of a coil to three-dimensional space can be estimated, and a receive coil can be designed to discriminate against unwanted signal regions. This transmitter/receiver technique was introduced by us for localization and first demonstrated using two coaxial coplanar surface coils.[84] Styles et al.[94] have recently used this double-surface coil method for rotating frame imaging and obtained reasonable localization.

Second, some rf pulses may be applied with one coil and some with the second so that signal is only obtained from the region where the sensitive volumes of the two coils overlap. The principles of this multiple transmit coil method were also introduced by us[84] and recently proved by experiment.[95] Once again Shaka et al.[70,71] have shown a conspicuous inability to cite (sight) the literature by proposing in their recent papers the use of multiple coils as an original idea. We note that the use of more than one coil to provide rf field gradients is not a new concept, as it was proposed by Hoult[65] for imaging.

A popular idea in recent times is to use a transmit coil that provides a homogeneous rf field and a surface receive coil to obtain maximum signal-to-noise. A usual reason given or assumed for this procedure is that many multipulse techniques[5,96] or localization techniques[41,42] cannot be applied using the inhomogeneous rf pulses of the surface coil. From previous sections we know this is untrue, as these methods can be applied with appropriate phase cycling of pulses. However, for ¹H NMR the homogeneous rf coil can provide a convenient proton image on which the sensitive volume for spectroscopy may be located. Again, although it is assumed that the surface coil is used to optimize signal-to-noise, the surface coil also enhances localization because it is most sensitive to regions close to it. Indeed, if it were not for this fact, the slices generated by Bottomley et al.[41,42] for spectroscopy of the brain would have extended through the skull. For convenience, we include the homogeneous-transmit/surface-receive coil within the broad definition of the first method described above.

Before contemplating the detail of multiple-coil localization methods it is necessary to solve the problems of electrical/magnetic interactions between such coils.

Elimination of Multiple-Coil Coupling

Whenever two or more rf coils are used in close proximity, they interact or couple. In simple terms, the rf field of one coil induces an alternating current in the second coil, which in turn generates an rf field, which opposes the first rf field. In the extreme case of coaxial coplanar surface coils it is impossible, having first tuned the first coil to a particular frequency, to tune the second coil to this frequency. It is even dangerous to assume (as is normal) that coils arranged orthogonally do not interact. As we will see below, an orthogonal surface receive coil easily destroys the rf homogeneity of a larger cylindrical transmit coil.

The usual configuration for a rf coil is depicted in Figure 73–21a. The typical tuning and matching capacitors fulfill the resonant condition for an alternating current circuit and enable the input energy to generate a large alternating current in the coil and thus a large alternating magnetic and electric field, i.e., radiation of electromagnetic waves. This works in reverse for a receive coil. The resonant frequency is given by

$$f = 1/2\pi L^{1/2}C^{1/2} \tag{21}$$

where L is the inductance of the coil and C is the capacitance of the circuit, which is the sum of the coil capacitance, the tune capacitance (C_T), and most of the match capacitance (C_M).

We substantially eliminated the coupling between two coaxial coplanar receive and transmit surface coils by using crossed diodes in parallel with the receive coil (Figure 73–21b) and in series with transmit coil (Figure 73–21c).[84] Crossed diodes have high impedance at low voltages but short out under rf power. Thus during rf pulses, the diodes short in both circuits. The transmit coil acts normally, but the receive coil is detuned because the short eliminates $C_T + C_M$ from the total resonant capacity C. During acquisition of signal, the rf signal from the sample is very small and the crossed diodes are unaffected by the rf current induced in the receive coil, which responds normally. The diodes in the transmit circuit prevent any current being induced at all in that circuit. Unfortunately, commercial diodes have magnetic leads, which degrade the main field homogeneity when used in the receive circuit close to the sample. This is not usually a problem for the transmit coil if it is large, but the small impedance of the diodes when shorted will decrease the Q of the coil. Again, this was not found to be serious for surface coils,[84,96] but we have found the use of diodes for some large cylindrical transmit coils to be impossible. However, there are other solutions. We will consider the receive coil first.

Haase[97] has recently described the use of a quarter-wavelength ($\lambda/4$) coaxial cable between the receiver preamplifier and the coil, as drawn in Figure 73–21d. A $\lambda/4$ cable that is shorted at one end is open, or high impedance, at the other end. During pulses in the transmit coil the diodes short and the cable is open at the receive coil end. Haase claimed that this arrangement minimized the interaction of a surface receive coil with a surrounding saddle coil by preventing current from being induced in the surface coil. The coils were arranged in parallel orientation to maximize coupling when tuned. We[98]

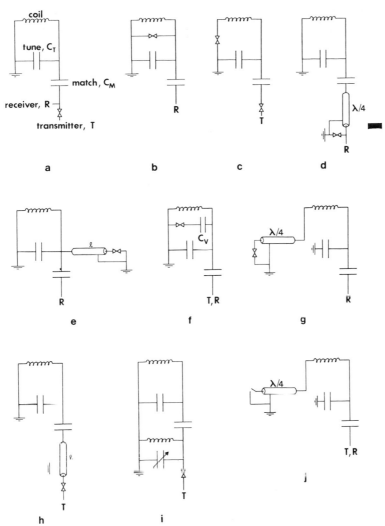

Figure 73 21. *a*, Circuit diagram for a normal coil that employs variable tune and match capacitors and that is connected directly to the receiver preamplifier and via crossed diodes (to reduce input noise during signal acquisition) to the spectrometer transmitter. *b*, Crossed diodes in parallel with a receive coil. *c*, Crossed diodes in series with a transmit coil. *d*, λ/4 Cable and crossed diodes to ground between the receiver preamplifier and the match capacitor of the coil circuit as employed by Haase[97] for a receive coil. *e*, Coaxial cable of variable length *l* and crossed diodes to ground inserted at the high voltage point of the circuit as used by Styles et al.[96] for a receive coil. *f*, Variable capacitor C_V and crossed diodes in parallel with the coil. During rf pulses, C_V can be adjusted to move the tuning point a few MHz off frequency for a receive coil, or to move the tuning point a few MHz onto the correct frequency for a transmit coil. *g*, λ/4 Cable and crossed diodes to ground inserted between the coil and ground for a receive coil. *h*, Coaxial cable of variable length between the normal crossed diodes in the transmitter line and the match capacitor of a transmit coil circuit, as devised by Styles.[99] *i*, Additional calculated inductance and trimming capacitance between ground and the input line to give an equivalent circuit to *h*, as developed by Styles.[99] *j*, λ/4 Cable with active switch to ground inserted between the coil and ground for a transmit or receive coil as used by Bendall et al.[98]

have been unable to repeat the success of Haase. In simple terms, the effect of the open cable at the coil end is to remove C_M from the total capacitance of the coil and thus shift the tuning point of the coil a small amount, of the order of 1 to 2 MHz in our experience for some typical surface coils, which is generally insufficient. Furthermore, because a complete circuit remains via the coil and the tune capacitance, current *will* be induced in the coil. This current can only be zero when $C_T = 0$, i.e., open circuit.

Styles et al.[96] have devised the circuit shown in Figure 73–21*e* so that the current in the coil is less than half the short-circuited current obtained just with crossed diodes as in Figure 73–21*b*. This condition is obtained by varying the length ℓ of the coaxial cable, by experimentation/calculation, up to a maximum length of $\lambda/8$. A similar result can be obtained using an additional capacitance C_V as in Figure 73–21*f*. If C_V was very large the circuit would be equivalent to Figure 73–21*b*, so C_V should be chosen small enough to move the resonant tuning point a few MHz off frequency, so that only a fraction of the short-circuited current can be induced in the coil. However, this configuration retains the magnetic diodes near the sample, unlike that of Styles et al.

Although the receive coil is detuned during transmit pulses by using the arrangements of Figures 73–21*b*, *e*, or *f*, it is left as a broad band coil, i.e., significant current can be induced in it by an rf field of any frequency. Thus the receive coil will modify the shape of the rf field of the transmit coil. But the rf fields of surface coils are already grossly inhomogeneous, so moderate changes to the shape of such fields is not usually important; indeed, such changes can be useful. Hence circuits of Figure 73–21*b* and *e* have been used successfully with coaxial surface coils.[84,96] However, such moderate changes cannot be tolerated when using a surface receive coil in the presence of a homogeneous cylindrical transmit coil. This is illustrated in Figure 73–22, where, in comparison to a good image of a homogeneous H_2O phantom in Figure 73–22*a*, the images in the presence of a detuned surface coil shown in Figure 73–22*b* and *c* are unacceptable. These represent fairly extreme conditions with the surface coil terminated with too much and too little capacitance, respectively, to tune at the NMR frequency. The detuning methods depicted in Figures 73–21*b* to *f* give similar or even

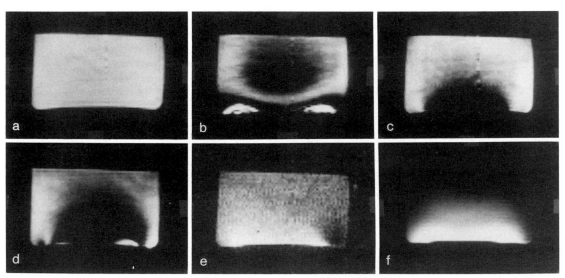

Figure 73–22. ^1H slice images obtained at 80 MHz from a 7.3 cm diameter cylinder of H_2O sitting on top of a 4.7 cm diameter surface coil within a large 15 cm diameter cylindrical transmit coil using sequence [8] ($\theta = 90$ degrees) with a slice selective refocusing pulse. The two coils are in parallel relation except for *d*. *a*, Surface coil open circuit (disconnected from ground and the tune capacitor); large coil receive. An identical result was obtained with the surface coil tuned (and terminated with 50Ω) but having a $\lambda/4$ cable and diodes to ground as in Fig. 73–21*g*. *b*, Surface coil tuning point shifted to 70 MHz; large coil receive. *c*, Surface coil tuning point shifted to 96 MHz; large coil receive. *d*, The coils orthogonal; surface coil tuned to 80 MHz; large coil receive. *e*, Surface coil receive employing Figure 73–21*g* circuitry. The crossed diodes were removed from the transmitter input to the large coil, thus increasing the noise input during signal acquisiton but preventing the chance detuning of the transmit coil during signal acquisition. A similar result, with less noise, was obtained with the diodes reinserted at a particular value of *l* that was known not to affect the tuning of the large coil. In both cases, the surface receive coil detects signals remote from it via the tuned transmit coil. *f*, Surface coil receive, employing Figure 73–21*g* circuitry and large coil transmit using Figure 73–21*h* circuitry. The nuclear spins are uniformly excited by the transmit coil, so the image depends only on the sensitivity of the surface receive coil, which is proportional to its expected rf field strength. (From Bendall et al.: Magn Reson Med *3*:157, 1986. Used by permission.)

worse results.[98] It is necessary to entirely prevent current from being induced in the receive coil by making it open circuit or by at least inserting a high impedance point within the circuit. The only method we have found to do this is shown in Figure 73–21g, which is a modification of a proven active detuning method discussed below.[95] During pulses by the transmit coil the diodes short, so the λ/4 cable is open at the point of insertion in the receive coil circuit with the result that the coil is no longer connected to ground and no current can flow in it. The effectiveness of this was demonstrated by obtaining an identical image to Figure 73–22a when the surface coil was tuned under low rf power using the circuitry of Figure 73–21g. Such λ/4 cables may reduce the Q of the receive coil, but we have found that such losses are insignificant when using good cable and when the coil is loaded with a biological sample.[98] The circuit depicted in Figure 73–21g provides a general method for any surface receive coil.

Orthogonality of coils is generally assumed to prevent coupling, but while the problem is greatly decreased, Figure 73–22d shows that this assumption is untrue. In addition, for in-vivo spectroscopy where it will be necessary to move the surface receive coil relative to the sample, good orthogonality is difficult to ensure, so at least one of the methods shown in Figures 73–21b, e to g should be used for orthogonal homogeneous-transmit/surface-receive coils. For example, Bottomley et al.[41,42] used parallel diodes as in Figure 73–21h.

Turning to the transmit coil, the potential problem is that during acquisition of NMR signal the nuclear spins will induce current in both the receive coil and the transmit coil if they are tuned. In simple terms, the receive coil will detect these spins plus the current in the transmit coil. It is sometimes assumed[96] that if the transmit coil is large, and therefore remote from the receive coil, this effect is small. Although it can be ignored for orthogonal coils, it cannot be disregarded for tightly coupled parallel systems such as coaxial coplanar surface coils, or for a surface receive coil and a parallel cylindrical transmit coil which gives the poor result shown in Figure 73–22e. The loss of Q using diodes as in Figure 73–21c can be mitigated using the modification in Figure 73–21f with C_V kept as small as possible to just achieve the required degree of detuning. However, in our experience this is still unsatisfactory for some large cylindrical coils.

A satisfactory alternative has been developed by Styles[99] and this is shown in Figure 73–21h. Haase[97] recently suggested this circuit with $\ell = \lambda/2$, but during signal reception both ends of the cable are open and this just removes C_M from the resonant circuit (as for Figure 73–21d) so detuning the circuit by only a small amount (e.g., 1 to 2 MHz). We find that if ℓ is correctly adjusted (e.g., using a trombone) to 5 to 20 percent less than λ/2, then when the diodes are open, the cable is brought into resonance with C_M, and the overall network is detuned to two points a few MHz either side of the original tuned frequency.[98] As illustrated in Figure 73–22f, this gives excellent results even for our worst case of parallel homogeneous-transmit/surface-receive coils. With the diodes shorted or removed, the cable has no effect and the transmit coil can be tuned normally with the receive coil open circuit (λ/4 cable shorted in Figure 73–21g). The diodes can then be replaced for both coils and the receive coil tuned. If during tuning, reflected power is observed using a wobble facility, the receive coil will also detect the two tuning points of the transmit coil, which can be adjusted using ℓ for equidistance from the central frequency. Experimentally, this is a simple procedure for an otherwise complicated coupled system. Styles[99] has also proposed the equivalent circuit in Figure 73–21i, and we find that when the diodes are not shorted and the trimming capacitance is minimum (inductance maximum), the detuned frequency split is 2.6 times that obtained with the Figure 73–21h circuitry. Thus the detuning is even more efficient with this variation.

We believe the arrangements depicted in Figure 73–21e and g to i adequately solve the coupling problem between separate transmit and receive coils for the range of situations that will arise when exploiting our first use of multiple coils for localization. There remains the problem of removing the interactions of two transmit coils, which is necessary for our second type of use of multiple coils. The transmit/receive methods are all passive: they rely on the shorting of crossed diodes during rf pulses. For multiple transmit coils a passive method cannot be used. Active switches are necessary.

To establish the use of multiple transmit coils for localization, we devised the switched coils illustrated in Figure 73–21*j*.[95] The principle is the same as that for the receive coil in Figure 73–21*g*, except that active switches are used at the end of the λ/4 cable. We used small rapid reed relays. At a ^{31}P frequency of 32 MHz, the λ/4 cables were long enough to be able to enclose the relays in a small steel box (to protect them from the main field), which was located outside the 30 cm bore magnet. The method is not general, because the cables would not be long enough at ^{1}H frequencies, or for a whole-body magnet. Multiples such as 3λ/4 and 5λ/4 could be used, but this might lower the *Q*s of the coils. This may not matter for transmit coils, and a third high *Q* receive coil could be added using the Figure 73–21*g* circuitry. The real difficulty is that there are no known switches that can replace the crossed diodes in the circuits of Figure 73–21*b* to *g*. Such switches would have to operate quickly (e.g., 1 ms), in a magnetic field, and withstand high voltages/currents, yet have low impedance when closed. Present research by us is focused on the circuits of Figure 73–21*h* and *i* because the crossed diodes are not located in the resonant circuitry and are thus subjected to much lower voltages (hundreds rather than kilovolts), and so may be replaced by actively switched PIN diodes. This research showed that the circuits in Figure 73–21*h* and *i* were inadequate but that of Figure 73–21*j* with PIN diodes in place of the reed relays has been very successful.[150] Hedges and Hoult[100] have also proposed this solution to the problem.

Localization Applications with Multiple Coils

We have demonstrated transmit/receive localization using coaxial coplanar surface coils as depicted in Figure 73–23.[10,84] The method depends on the shape of the rf field generated by the surface coil. In particular, the rate of decrease of the rf field with depth along the coil's axis is much slower than the rate of decrease with increasing

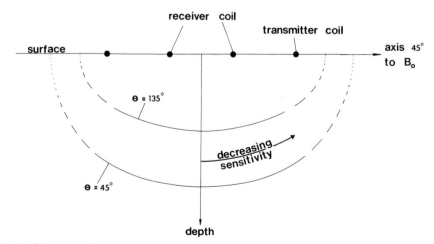

Figure 73–23. Schematic illustration of a transmit/receive system using two surface coils with a 3:1 ratio of diameters. For increasing off-axis distances, there is a gradual decrease in sensitivity of the receive coil to the sensitive volume generated by the transmit coil. (From Bendall MR: *In* James TL, Margulis AR [eds]: Biomedical Magnetic Resonance. San Francisco, Radiology Research and Education Foundation, 1984.)

radius on the surface outside the circumference of the coil. Compare the thickness of the 90 degree signal region along the coil's axis in Figure 73–6 with the thickness of the region where it intersects the surface. As indicated in Figure 73–23, 90 degree signals excited near the surface outside the circumference of the transmitter coil are discriminated against by the lower sensitivity of the smaller receive coil to these sample regions as compared with regions closer to the coil along the coil's axis. The viability of this method has been proved with depth pulses using ^{31}P phantom samples and a 3:1 ratio of coil radii. Pulse angle θ was set at 90 degrees at 0.6 to 0.8 radius (of the large coil) depth, and as shown in Figure 73–24, the 90 degree signals at the surface were reduced to about 10 percent of their normal intensity. It was found that depth pulse schemes that suppress high flux signals should be used, as expected from Figure 73–6, and the ratio of coil sizes should preferably be greater than 3:1. The technique has two major limitations: the 90 degree signals cannot be perfectly suppressed as they gradually decrease in intensity nearer the surface; the small coil is used as receiver, but this has lower sensitivity than the large coil to the remote sensitive volume. Nevertheless, this experiment is a first demonstration of localization for spectroscopy without field gradients.

Styles et al.[94] have used a similar probe for rotating frame imaging and have acknowledged the limitations of the method by restricting their spectra to a depth of about 1.5 radii of the small coil. Results obtained from the double coil placed over the lower rib cage are shown in Figure 73–25 and clearly resolve the liver spectra from the intervening muscle spectra. These results were obtained in 45 minutes, an acceptable time for patient examination. Further improvements can be expected with more available pulse power. It is now clear that in our introductory experiment we attempted to sample a region that was too far from the probe. The depth should be limited to about the radius of the small coil. Referring to Figure 73–23, this will greatly increase the sensitivity of the receive coil to the region near the coil's axis without much increase in the surface signals, thus gaining better discrimination overall.

When using separate transmit and receive coils, there is a potential phase problem. From Figure 73–2 it is clear that the rf lines of force take different directions in the laboratory xy plane at different points in sample space. These different directions are directly transferred to the NMR experiment as phase shifts in the NMR signal coming from any point in the sample. For a single coil we ignore these shifts because there is an exactly reverse shift when the NMR signal induces current back in the coil. However, for a separate receive coil the phase shift is not exactly reversed, and the signal induced in the coil will have a phase error equal to the difference in direction in the laboratory xy plane of the lines of force resulting from direct currents in the two coils. Thus, along the common axis of the two coaxial coils in Figure 73–23 there is no error, nor are there errors in the xz plane where active components are only in the x direction. How-

Figure 73–24. Experimental results obtained using a small phantom sample, which was moved relative to the transmit/receive coils, and a depth pulse (similar in rf discrimination to sequence [29] but utilizing the {2 × 2θ/3 + 4θ/3} procedure to suppress 270 degree signals). The intensity contours have been extrapolated from the results given in reference.[10] The plane displayed is the xy plane. Results obtained for the xz plane showed better suppression of signals close to the surface while results for a plane at 45 degrees to the main field axis showed ~15 degree signals at the surface.

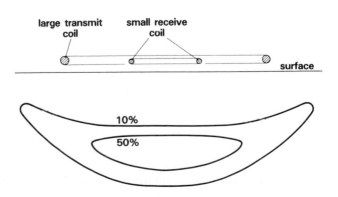

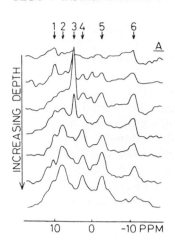

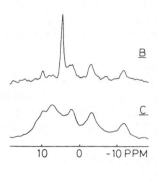

Figure 73–25. *A,* A set of spatially localized ^{31}P spectra from the thorax of a human subject obtained by rotating frame zeumatography using a 15 cm diameter transmit surface coil and a 6 cm diameter coaxial (nearly coplanar) receive coil. Each spectrum represents a slice of ~8 mm thickness. Peak assignments: 1, inorganic phosphate; 2, phosphodiesters; 3, phosphocreatine; 4, 5, and 6, adenosine triphosphate. *B,* A spectrum of human skeletal muscle obtained with a surface coil. *C,* A spectrum of human liver obtained with a surface coil in conjunction with the method of field profiling. (From Styles et al.: Magn Reson Med 2:402, 1985.)

ever, errors up to ±20 degrees were measured across the sensitive volume in the laboratory *xy* plane for the 3:1 ratio of coil size,[84] a variation that is not large and would hardly affect the coherent addition of signals.

Nevertheless, this potential phase problem must be borne in mind when other multiple coil arrangements are used. In particular, when using homogeneous-transmit/surface-receive coils, the rf lines of force of the homogeneous rf coil in the *xy* plane can be superimposed as parallel lines on those of the surface coil in Figure 73–2. Thus identical signals will cancel from two sample points where the surface coil lines of force are pointing in opposite directions.[101] This is not a problem if the localized region is kept small compared to the surface coil, but is otherwise a powerful argument *against* using large cylindrical coils and *for* using surface coils alone with any of the localization methods presented in this chapter. It has been argued that the cancellation of signal because of phase difference does itself enhance localization, but this is only true for a homogeneous sample (which is not interesting to an in-vivo spectroscopist). These problems represent a further limitation of the method of Bottomley et al.[41,42]

A potentially better method is to generate more than one sensitive volume using multiple transmit coils. This can be achieved by applying different pulses in a depth pulse scheme with different coils. Because the functions for each pulse given in Equations (1) to (3) are multiplied together, significant signal intensity will only be acquired from sample regions where the sensitive volumes overlap.

A fairly simple scheme utilizes two coaxial surface coils as in the previous example, and the overlapping sensitive volumes are depicted in Figure 73–26. There may be several reasonable ways of achieving the desired result, but one is to use the large coil, which we label the Θ coil, for excitation (θ pulse) and as receiver (better sensitivity to deep regions). Depending on the depth of penetration it may be necessary to eliminate the 270 degree signals excited by the Θ coil, but the ratio of coil sizes can be chosen so that the sensitive volumes do not overlap where θ ~ 450 degrees. Various depth pulse schemes *DP*(θ) would be appropriate for the Θ coil. Labeling the second coil, Φ, two 2φ[±*x'*, ±*y'*] pulses should adequately define the φ-sensitive volume after the *DP*(θ) pulse:

$$DP(\theta) - \tau - 2\phi[\pm x', \pm y'] - 2\tau - 2\phi[\pm x', \pm y'] - \tau - \text{acquire with } \Theta \text{ coil} \qquad [41]$$

From Figure 73–26 it is clear that the outer edge of the φ-sensitive region is important in eliminating the 90 degree signals at shallow depth, and on-resonance this is defined by $\sin^4 \phi$ (see Equation 3), which drops to 10 percent at φ = 35 degrees and 5 percent at φ = 28 degrees.

The spin-echo delays are included to allow time for the Θ coil to be detuned and

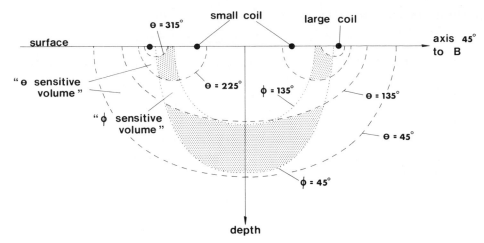

Figure 73–26. Schematic illustration of two sensitive volumes, designated θ and φ, generated using two transmitter coils. The limits have been nominally set at 90 ± 45 degrees, and 270 ± 45 degrees. Magnetization will be detected from the shaded regions where the sensitive volumes overlap, so the θ ∼ 270 degree region should be suppressed. For the discussion in the section on polarization transfer, the two coils correspond to irradiation of two different heteronuclei, ^{13}C (large coil) and ^{1}H (small coil). (From Bendall MR: *In* James TL, Margulis AR [eds]: Biomedical Magnetic Resonance. San Francisco, Radiology Research and Education Foundation, 1984. Used by permission.)

the Φ coil tuned after $DP(0)$, and vice versa just before signal acquisition. When using reed relays as in Figure 73–21*j*, τ can be as little as 1 ms. The central 2τ period is added to allow the 2φ pulses to refocus chemical shift and magnetic field inhomogeneity, i.e., two spin-echoes are necessary. The phases of the 2φ pulses are denoted as ±*x'* and ±*y'*. Because the two coils form two different rf circuits, the phase of the alternating current in the coils will be different. This generates a phase shift that is constant throughout sample space and is unimportant. However, as just described above, there will be a phase shift, β, which varies in the *xy* plane because of the different curvature of the rf lines of force from the two coils. Although one 2φ[±*x'*, ∓*y'*] pulse will impose this phase error on the final signal as 2β, two such pulses reverse the effect and there is no error. Furthermore, because the NMR signal is excited and detected by the same coil, the Θ coil, there is no phase problem as arises for separate transmit/receive coils.

We have proved this localization technique experimentally, again a first example of complete localization using the overlapping sensitive volumes of two rf coils.[95] The results are shown in Figure 73–27. Sequence [41] and the particular depth pulse scheme, $DP(\theta) \equiv 2\theta[\pm x]; \{2 \times 2\theta/3 + 4\theta/3\}; 2\theta[\pm x, \pm y]$, was used. The experimental images displayed in Figure 73–27 were obtained by inserting field gradients in the second spin-echo of Sequence [41] according to the scheme in Sequence [8].

There is, of course, need for much more experience with inanimate and live samples to discover idiosyncrasies and solve problems, such as routine pulse length calibration, before this multiple transmit coil method is established as routinely viable. From the aspect of the pulse sequence used, some improvements are already obvious. From the known equivalence between $2\theta[\pm x, \overline{0}]$ and $2\theta[\pm x, \pm y]$ before and after θ, Sequence [41] can be recast to the equivalent sequence:

$$(2\phi[\pm x, \overline{0}])_2 - \tau - DP(\theta); \text{ acquire with } \Theta \text{ coil} \qquad [42]$$

The problem of refocusing β phase shifts, which needed two spin-echoes in Sequence [41], is avoided in Sequence [42], and the tuning of the coils need only be switched once during the sequence. Provided there is sufficient rf power to cover the spectrum, the selectivity of the φ-sensitive volume can be increased using a single composite pulse (e.g., Q^1 pulse of Shaka and Freeman[70]) without increasing the number of transients for a complete phase cycle, i.e.:

$$2\phi_{\bar{C}}^{\mp}[\pm x, \bar{0}] - \tau - DP(\theta); \text{ acquire with } \Theta \text{ coil} \qquad [43]$$

Better control of the shape of the localized volume recently has been obtained using further improved versions of sequence [42], and the method has been proved by achieving localization on the liver of a rat.[150]

One disadvantage of the double surface coil probe is that the sensitive volume curves towards the surface, which is usually convex. This is true of the transmit/receive method (Figure 73–24) and the double transmit coil method (Figure 73–27). However, these techniques are general ones, and there are good prospects for improved modeling of localized regions. For example, as depicted in Figure 73–28, a surface coil can be used on either side of the head, with the large coil producing a depth pulse sensitive volume just inside the skull. A smaller surface receive coil can then detect localized signals, uncontaminated by the skull, by positioning over various parts of the large sensitive volume. Alternatively, the second coil can be an active transmit coil to gain better localization, and if of similar size, the overlapped sensitive volume could be positioned anywhere in the head between the two coils, as illustrated in Figure 73–29. There is also a vast range of possibilities for using coils which are differently shaped to the flat surface coil. Preliminary results have been described for the saddle surface coil[102] and "floppy" surface coils,[103] and various groups are calculating rf field profiles for various shapes.[46,102,104] The sectorial loop-gap resonator looks promising.[105] As a further example, using an array of four mutually orthogonal surface coils (with a common intersection point like an open four-petaled flower) as the Θ coil, and a fifth surface

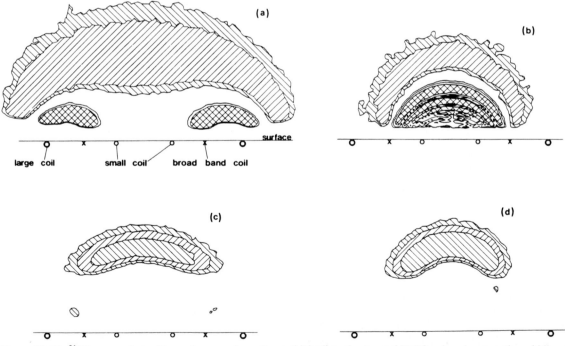

Figure 73–27. [31]P images of sensitive volumes using a 9 mm thick slice phantom of H_3PO_4 placed across the middle of the coil array as depicted in Figure 73–4. Intensity contours of arbitrary magnitude are shown. Image of the large coil (*a*) and small coil (*b*) sensitive volumes with the other coil deactivated using the circuit in Figure 73–21*j*. The cross-hatched regions correspond to high flux signal regions. Image of the sensitive volume in the *xy* plane (*c*) and the *xz* plane (*d*) using sequence [41]. The broad band coil indicated in the figure was a continuous circle of wire that couples with the transmit coils, so forcing the 90 degree region of the large coil outwards and that of the small coil inwards to enhance the difference in shape of the two sensitive volumes, which are otherwise too similar at the depth indicated. At shallower depths this passive coil was unnecessary. (From Bendall et al.: J Magn Reson *60*:473, 1984. Used by permission.)

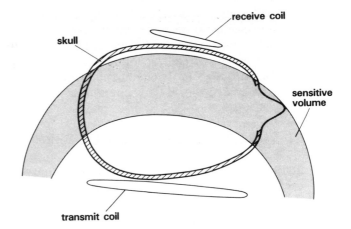

Figure 73–28. Illustration of the possible use of separate transmit/receive coils on opposite sides of the head in conjunction with depth pulses. A small phantom sample placed close to the receive coil against the skull would act as a control signal if the sensitive volume penetrated through the skull.

coil within and equally disposed to the four (toward the bottom of the flower) as the Φ coil, a discrete sensitive volume that curves away from the surface can be obtained.[106] Rf fields may also be shaped by introducing passive coils which couple with the transmit coils. An example is the circle of wire indicated in Figure 73–27, and Holcomb and Gore[103] have also made use of ''satellite'' coils to modify rf fields.

In relation to the use of multiple transmitter coils, Doddrell and co-workers[107] have described a new means of sample localization, the principles of which are confused. First, these authors went to considerable trouble to obtain ''phase coherence'' between a homogeneous rf coil (saddle) and a surface coil. Although such coherence is possible in the xz plane, we have already noted in this section that in the xy plane the relative phases of such coils can be visualized by superimposing parallel lines (representing the lines of force of the homogeneous coil) on the curved lines for the surface coil in Figure 73–2. Thus if the phases are coherent along the surface coil's axis, coherence is also obtained at the sample surface and in the xz plane, but nowhere else. Second, the effectiveness of the achieved ''phase coherence'' was demonstrated using a phase-alternated inversion-recovery sequence like Sequence [5] except that the inversion pulse was applied with the homogeneous rf coil and the excitation pulse with the surface coil. However, the phase of inversion pulses in such alternated sequences is immaterial, since no transverse magnetization is generated by them; yet, impossibly, these authors generated a substantial ''out-of-phase'' error in the final signal. Third, the ''volume-selection capabilities'' of their method was achieved primarily by matching the surface

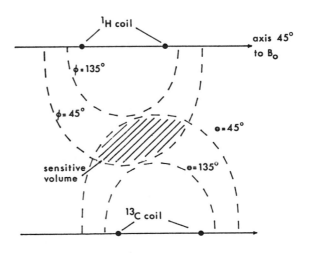

Figure 73–29. Schematic representation of the use of two transmit surface coils on either side of the sample. The shaded region defines the final sensitive volume. High flux regions do not overlap, and these do not need to be suppressed. The application could be a heteronuclear one, as described in the next section and as indicated by the ^{1}H and ^{13}C coil labels. (From Pegg DT, Bendall MR: Magn Reson Med 2:453, 1985. Used by permission.)

coil θ pulse to average 180 degrees over one of two small phantom samples, the first and crudest surface-coil localization procedure ever used.[108] Fourth, "excellent volume selection" was achieved by adding a "purging" 90 degree pulse applied with the homogeneous rf coil. Such a pulse can have no effect in the xz plane (as in Figure 73–6b) but imposes a node line in the xy plane of Figure 73–6a like that in Figure 73–6b. This improvement does not appear to be particularly worthwhile.

HETERONUCLEAR METHODS WITH SURFACE COILS

In recent years, NMR spectroscopists have invested a huge effort in the area of heteronuclear multipulse NMR, some of which is very relevant for in-vivo work. A sequence of rf pulses are applied to two J-coupled heteronuclei, and this causes a transfer of information or properties from one nucleus to its J-coupled neighbor. For in-vivo NMR, the most important applications are to ^1H–^{13}C systems, especially when using ^{13}C-enriched compounds. There are, however, other possibilities, e.g., ^1H–^{15}N systems and ^1H–^{19}F systems as exist in anesthetics. A vital aspect of the ^1H–^{13}C methods is that the weak ^{13}C signal can be enhanced, or the properties of the ^{13}C nucleus can be transferred to the ^1H nucleus and the ^1H signal can be detected with much greater sensitivity. The various pulse sequences fall into one of two classes, polarization transfer and spin-echo methods. It is impossible to convey a reasonable understanding of the mechanism of the various methods in the space available. Once again, vector descriptions provide the quickest way of gaining this understanding, and such descriptions are included in the cited literature (or references contained therein). A recent finding, additional to our knowledge of these heteronuclear methods within mainstream NMR, is that both the polarization transfer and the spin-echo sequences may be used for localization using depth pulse principles.[109,110]

Polarization Transfer

In an NMR experiment, only the excess of nuclei aligned in the magnetic field direction over those aligned in the opposite direction can be detected. This is known as the polarization of the nuclei. For coupled heteronuclear systems such as ^1H–^{13}C systems, the polarization of one set of nuclei, ^1H say, can be transferred via the spin-spin coupling (J) between the nuclei to the other set, ^{13}C, using a series of pulses known as a polarization transfer sequence. After such a sequence, the same excess number of ^{13}C nuclei can be detected as there were excess ^1H nuclei initially. For this example, because the natural ^1H polarization is four times greater than the natural ^{13}C polarization, the final ^{13}C signal will be enhanced by a factor of 4. The natural ^{13}C signal can be readily suppressed by phase alternation so that a signal will only be observed if polarization transfer occurs, and this may be used to enable signal detection from a particular sensitive volume. To obtain maximum signal-to-noise, ^1H decoupling need only be on during signal acquisition, which lowers the danger of rf heating compared to normal ^{13}C NMR (there is no need to generate a nuclear Overhauser enhancement by continuous decoupling).

The most conservative way, in terms of numbers of pulses, to achieve polarization transfer across a complete ^{13}C spectrum is to use the distortionless enhancement by polarization transfer (DEPT) sequence,[111,112] which, for homogeneous rf coils, is

$$^1H \quad 90°[x] - (2J)^{-1} - 180° - (2J)^{-1} - \quad 45°[\pm y] - (2J)^{-1} - \text{decouple}$$

$$^{13}C \qquad\qquad\qquad\qquad 90° \qquad\qquad 180° \qquad\qquad \text{acquire, receiver}[\pm] \qquad [44]$$

$(2J)^{-1}$ signifies delay periods, where the coupling constant J is about 125 to 140 Hz for aliphatic moieties. A description of the mechanism of DEPT would be too lengthy to elaborate here. However, to discuss the use of DEPT for localization using inhomogeneous rf fields, it is sufficient to note that the first two ^{1}H pulses form a spin-echo sequence, $90° - (2J)^{-1} - 180° - (2J)^{-1} -$ as do the two ^{13}C pulses. Thus, our knowledge of spin-echo sequences (see Inversion-Recovery and Spin-Echo Sequences in Inhomogeneous Radio Frequency Fields) must be applied twice here, and the phase-cycling required for application of DEPT with surface coils is

$$^1\text{H} \quad \phi[x] - (2J)^{-1} - 2\phi[\pm x, \ \pm y] - (2J)^{-1} - \frac{\phi}{2}\,[y] - (2J)^{-1} - \text{decouple}$$
$$^{13}\text{C} \qquad\qquad\qquad\quad \theta \qquad\qquad\qquad 2\theta[x, y] \qquad\quad \text{acquire} \tag{45}$$

We have applied DEPT with surface coils using the full $2\theta[\pm x, \pm y]$ cycling[109] but have since found that half this phase cycling is redundant as written in Sequence [45].[113]

If applied with a double-tuned surface coil with $\phi = \theta$ for maximum signal, on-resonance signal intensity will be given by $\theta \sin^6 \theta \, f(\theta)$ where $f(\theta)$ is $\sin(\theta/2)$ for methine (CH) groups, $\sin \theta$ for methylene (CH$_2$) groups, and $0.75[\sin(\theta/2) + \sin(3\theta/2)]$ for methyl groups.[111,112] Consequently, the spatial distribution of signal intensity will be similar to that depicted in Figure 73–6. If applied with two coaxial coplanar surface coils, signal intensity is given by $\theta \sin^3 \theta \sin^3 \phi \, f(\phi)$ and the situation shown in Figure 73–26 applies where the larger Θ coil is the ^{13}C transmit/receive coil and the Φ coil is the ^{1}H transmit coil. To enhance localization, depth pulse schemes can be applied separately to each of the ^{1}H and ^{13}C parts of the DEPT sequence. For coaxial coplanar surface coils, Sequence [46] will be good enough:

$$^1\text{H} \quad 2\phi[\pm x]; \phi[x] - (2J)^{-1} - 2\phi[\pm x, \ \pm y] - (2J)^{-1} - \frac{\phi}{2}\,[y] - (2J)^{-1} - \text{decouple}$$

$$^{13}\text{C} \qquad (2\theta[\pm x])_2; \left\{2 \times \frac{2\theta}{3} + \frac{4\theta}{3}\right\} \quad 2\theta[x, y] \qquad\quad \text{acquire} \tag{46}$$

The $\{2 \times 2\theta/3 + 4\theta/3\}$ variation is needed to eliminate the signal at $\theta \sim 270$ degrees, but the second $2\theta[\pm x]$ pulse is probably unnecessary. For coils on opposite sides of an object, as shown in Figure 73–29, the 8-transient Sequence [45] is likely to be sufficient. The different $f(\phi)$ dependencies for different CH$_n$ groups will change the dimensions of the final sensitive volume, but calculations show that the differences are marginal.[113]

Although this technique has not yet been used for in-vivo work, excellent localization, as depicted in Figure 73–26, has been confirmed by phantom studies with surface coils using a sequence similar to Sequence [46].[109] Sequence [46] requires 192 transients for a complete cycle, which is not too large for low sensitivity ^{13}C spectroscopy. Off-resonance effects have been studied, theoretically and experimentally, and found to be similar to those of ordinary phase-cycled depth pulses.[113] Of course, relaxation times of the species under investigation need to be greater than the total delay time in the DEPT sequence, which is 12 ms.

In mainstream NMR, a major use of DEPT is to edit a ^{13}C spectrum into separate CH, CH$_2$, and CH$_3$ spectra.[114] We have applied this successfully to dissected organs of a ^{13}C enriched rabbit using homogeneous rf coils.[115] Although this editing can be applied with surface coils, the present methods[116] involve a signal-to-noise penalty that may not be acceptable, so the spin-echo method mentioned below is probably the better choice.

Polarization may be transferred in the reverse direction from ^{13}C to ^{1}H using the inverse DEPT sequence,[117] which is similar to DEPT with the ^{1}H and ^{13}C labels interchanged. Inverse DEPT may be modified for application with surface coils in a similar fashion to the modification of DEPT above,[113] to give localized ^{1}H spectra of ^{13}C enriched metabolites, with a sensitivity gain over ordinary ^{13}C NMR of up to a factor of 16. Although the spin-echo methods described below provide a greater sensitivity gain, this polarization transfer method is useful for ^{1}H resonances close to the H_2O resonance.[48]

If necessary, imaging methods can be combined with polarization transfer. For example, an incremented field gradient can be inserted into the first $(2J)^{-1}$ period of Sequence [44] or [45] for the 2DFT method. (If the $(2J)^{-1}$ period is not long enough, it may be increased using principles previously described for two-dimensional DEPT spectroscopy[118]). Recently, Aue et al.[119] pointed out a clever general principle. If a selective pulse is applied to the ^{1}H spins and polarization is transferred to ^{13}C, the small spread of ^{1}H chemical shifts does not cause a significant spread of localization regions as would result from a selective ^{13}C pulse. Thus a well-localized ^{13}C spectrum is obtained despite the large spectral width. The selective ^{1}H pulse should be a selective inversion pulse prior to the DEPT sequence; i.e., DEPT takes the place of θ in Sequence [17]. Thus for example, using either method, a well-localized ^{13}C spectrum can be obtained with maximum signal-to-noise using a homogeneous cylindrical ^{1}H coil (in place for ^{1}H imaging) and a ^{13}C surface coil, with a single pulsed field gradient along the surface coil's axis. There are, as usual, several other permutations.

Heteronuclear Spin-Echo Techniques

Without exception, any of the pulse sequences given in this chapter are already spin-echo sequences or can be converted to spin-echo sequences suitable for inhomogeneous rf coils by the addition of $- \tau - 2\theta[\pm x, \pm y] - \tau -$.[7] The well-known gated-decoupled spin-echo experiment for a coupled AX system can be set up in two very general ways, either gated on:

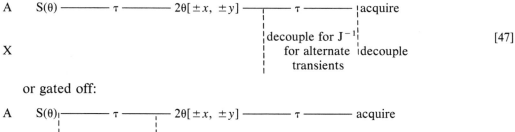

$S(\theta)$ is the rest of the pulse sequence and may be just θ or any depth pulse (phase-cycled, composite, or Fourier series window), or a selective pulse sequence utilizing a pulsed field gradient. The $2\theta[\pm x, \pm y]$ refocusing pulse may be any sort of composite pulse or selective pulse in a pulsed field gradient. The spin-echo may be part of an imaging sequence using incremented field gradients for the 2DFT method. The gated-on or gated-off periods must be contained within one half of the spin-echo (i.e., $\tau \geqq J^{-1}$). The τ period may be much longer than J^{-1} to facilitate suppression of water and fat signals by $T2$ relaxation. Whereas the gated-off period may otherwise be anywhere in the pulse sequence, the alternative gated-on period must immediately precede decoupling during signal acquisition to avoid spin randomization[120,121] effects.

For in-vivo spectroscopy, the most important applications are in $^1H/^{13}C$ spectroscopy, but there is relevance to such coupled systems as $^1H/^{15}N$ and $^1H/^{19}F$. If $A \equiv {}^{13}C$ and $X \equiv {}^1H$ and alternate transients are accumulated into separate computer memory blocks, then addition of the two blocks yields a methylene/quaternary subspectrum and subtraction yields a methyl/methine subspectrum. This valuable simplification of the ^{13}C spectrum is obtained in the same time as a normal spectrum and has found widespread use in high resolution NMR.[122–124] The benefit to in-vivo spectroscopy has recently been established in a study of ^{13}C-enriched organs in a high resolution spectrometer.[115]

If $A \equiv {}^1H$ and $X \equiv {}^{13}C$, a spectrum of only those protons attached to ^{13}C nuclei can be obtained by subtraction of alternate transients. This has obvious applications in ^{13}C-enrichment studies and benefits from a large potential gain in signal-to-noise over conventional ^{13}C spectroscopy. The maximum possible gains are factors of 64, 128, and 192 for CH, CH_2, and CH_3 moieties. If maximum nuclear Overhauser enhancement is achievable for the conventional ^{13}C spectrum, these gains are a factor of three less. There will normally be a further loss of about a factor of two in achievable signal-to-noise because ^1H resonances are usually broader than ^{13}C resonances because of field inhomogeneity and homonuclear coupling. In practical use, the problem of suppressing the H_2O resonance (discussed in the next section) and eliminating the huge signals of $^{12}CH_n$ systems by alternate subtraction increases the noise because of subtraction inaccuracies (see "subtraction noise" in Localization Using Pulsed Field Gradients). Nevertheless, Rothman et al.[125] obtained an 11-fold increase in sensitivity for the CH_3 of lactate and a 6-fold increase for the CH_2 of glutamate in the rat brain in vivo during a continuous infusion with ^{13}C-labeled glucose. By comparing the ^1H resonance of just the $^{13}CH_n$ spectrum to the ordinary spectrum ($^{12}CH_n + {}^{13}CH_n$), the fractional enrichment can be determined. Some typical results are shown in Figure 73–30. With the aid of modern stable instrumentation it should be possible to routinely gain a substantial increase in sensitivity over normal ^{13}C NMR, in which case this will be a very important method.

The detection of only those protons attached to ^{13}C nuclei was first introduced by us[126] and by Freeman et al.[127] using a pulse on the ^{13}C nucleus rather than gated decoupling:

$$
{}^1H \quad 90° \text{——} J^{-1} \text{————} 180° \text{————} J^{-1} \text{————} \text{acquire, receiver}[+, -]
$$
$$
{}^{13}C \qquad\qquad\qquad 180°[x, 0] \qquad\qquad\qquad \text{decouple}
$$
$$[49]$$

Generalizing this to inhomogeneous coils and including a larger τ period suitable for various purposes gives

$$
{}^1H \quad DP(\theta) \text{————} \tau \text{————} 2\theta[\pm x, \pm y] \text{————} \tau \text{————} \text{acquire, receiver}[+, -]
$$
$$
{}^{13}C \qquad\qquad J^{-1} \text{——} 2\Phi_C[x, 0] \qquad\qquad\qquad\qquad \text{decouple}
$$
$$[50]$$

The $2\Phi_C[x, \bar{0}]$ pulse is a composite narrowband inversion pulse of the type described by Shaka et al.[70] or Tycko and Pines,[72] or simpler versions given by us[110] and is applied for alternate transients. $DP(\theta)$ is any depth pulse sequence, including a Fourier series. We recently proved, using phantom samples, that Sequence [50] allows complete sensitive volume localization when using separate ^1H and ^{13}C inhomogeneous rf coils as in Figures 73–26 and 73–29.[110] Thus, this important method of detecting only protons attached to ^{13}C can be applied with surface coils for partial localization, then combined

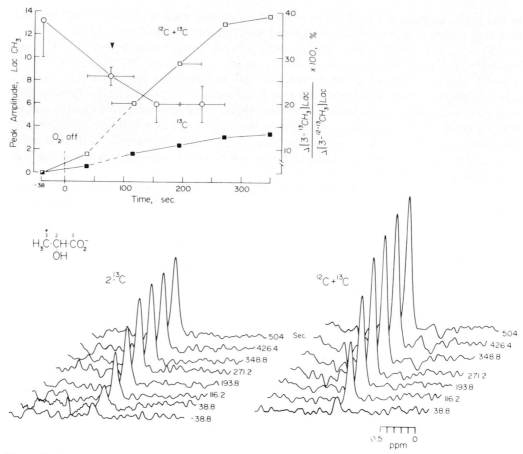

Figure 73–30. *Top,* Amplitudes (arbitrary units) of the proton resonances of [3-^{13}CH$_3$]lactate (■) and [3-$^{12+13}$CH$_3$]lactate (□) in the brain of an intact rat plotted as a function of time after the start of terminal anoxia. In addition, the fractional ^{13}C enrichment of newly formed lactate during ischemia is plotted (○). (*Bottom*) Stacked spectra of [3-^{13}CH$_3$] and [3-$^{12+13}$CH$_3$]lactate as plotted at top. The spectra were obtained with a doubly-tuned ^{13}C/^{1}H 14 mm diameter surface coil centered 6 mm posteriorly to the bregma. (From Rothman DL et al.: Proc Natl Acad Sci USA 82:1633, 1985. Used by permission.)

with pulsed field gradients (Sequences [47] and [48]) or with separate transmit coils (Sequence [50]) for complete localization.

Because of the small J values (long J^{-1} times) for ^{1}H–^{31}P coupling and the short *T2* times of relevant ^{31}P metabolites, the methods described in this section are unlikely to be very useful for ^{31}P NMR. However, Brindle et al.[128] have proposed a ^{1}H/^{31}P heteronuclear method, which was claimed to be related to Sequence [49], to null ^{1}H-coupled phosphomonoester and diester resonances in ^{31}P surface coil NMR of the human brain. This may be appropriate to more clearly reveal longer $-T2$ unprotonated resonances such as inorganic phosphate, but some aspects of this work are misleading or in error. There are two simple spin-echo methods for nulling protonated resonances, and for surface coils these may be written generally as

$$ \text{A} \qquad \theta \text{———} \tau \text{———} 2\theta[\pm x, \pm y] \text{———} \tau \text{———} | \text{acquire} $$
$$ ^1\text{H} \qquad\qquad\qquad\qquad\qquad \phi \qquad\qquad\qquad\qquad | \text{decouple} \qquad [51] $$

If φ is 180 degrees (as claimed by Brindle et al.), τ must be (4J)$^{-1}$ and ^{1}H decoupling must be used during signal acquisition as is well known from ^{1}H/^{13}C work.[129] However, Brindle et al. did not mention ^{1}H decoupling, in which case τ must be (2J)$^{-1}$ and φ must be 90 degrees. Although ^{1}H decoupling for the latter method is preferable, such a method will work without decoupling, as has been established again from ^{1}H/^{13}C studies.[114,130] Presumably Brindle et al. used this method (ϕ was adjusted experimentally), but note that for good cancellation, ϕ needs to be close to 90 degrees across the whole sensitive volume, and so for surface coils a good 90 degree composite pulse[19] is appropriate. Brindle et al. did not indicate that phase cycling of the 2θ pulse was used; as pointed out by Rothman et al.,[131] when using long spin-echoes this does not necessarily lead to errors if resonances are broad because of field inhomogeneity, since the error signals dephase in the field gradients. Nevertheless, when the aim is to localize on a small region with good field homogeneity, and the sample is heterogeneous, it is wise to include the phase cycling (if available) as a matter of course. Finally, Brindle et al. used $2\theta/3$ in place of θ to suppress 270 degree signals, which we have already noted is a crude version of the previously described $\{2 \times 2\theta/3 + 4\theta/3\}$ method.

^{1}H SPECTRAL SIMPLIFICATIONS WITH SURFACE COILS

^{1}H spectroscopy is a rapidly growing and very important part of in-vivo NMR. The purpose of this section is to briefly indicate the application of recent new methods using surface coils, and future possibilities in this area, which includes localization.

Water Suppression

The water resonance is a particular problem in in-vivo ^{1}H NMR, because it is so massive compared to millimolar metabolites that its base covers the whole ^{1}H spectrum. Presaturation with low power single frequency rf is commonly used, but while this is efficient at the center of the H_2O signal, a significant proportion of the broad wings remains. These wings can be removed with reasonable efficiency if the method in use includes receiver phase alternation[125] (as in Sequence [50] or [52], for example), but, as usual, this will lead to subtraction noise. Williams et al.[132] use a Carr-Purcell-Meiboom-Gill (CPMG) pulse train lasting several hundred milliseconds because they have shown that the true $T2$ of water in rat muscle (30 ms) is a factor of 10 less than many ^{1}H metabolites. But the CPMG requires a train of 180 degree pulses which cannot be applied with an inhomogeneous rf coil such as a surface coil, and it appears that the pseudo $T2$'s for H_2O and ^{1}H metabolites during a simple spin echo are much more similar.[132]

A recent innovation that shows great promise is that of binomial water suppression.[133–135] Instead of a θ pulse, a pulse train is applied, which may be $\theta/2 - \tau - \theta/2$, $\theta/4 - \tau - \theta/2 - \tau - \theta/4$, $\theta/8 - \tau - 3\theta/8 - \tau - 3\theta/8 - \tau - \theta/8$, abbreviated as 1–1, 1–2–1, 1–3–3–1, and so on. Essentially, the H_2O resonance is not excited at all and so the broad wings are avoided. If every other pulse has inverted phase, e.g., 1–$\bar{3}$–3–$\bar{1}$, the H_2O signal can be on resonance and so poor off-resonance suppression effects are avoided.[134] All these pulse sequences produce a window centered on H_2O which is not excited and a window on either side in which resonances are excited, i.e., they are broad selective pulses. The frequency difference between the middle of the excited and unexcited windows is $(2\tau)^{-1}$ Hz. The width of the excitation null (and thus the accuracy of H_2O suppression) increases as the length of the binomial series is increased.

Brindle et al.[136] have used binomial water suppression in a spin-echo as (1–$\bar{3}$–3–$\bar{1}$) $- \tau - (2$–$\bar{6}$–6–$\bar{2}) - \tau -$ acquire, i.e., by simply doubling the length of the pulses for the 180 degree refocusing pulse. Hetherington et al.[137] have shown that this can be used with a surface coil, and indeed it can be shown, using rotation matrices,[14] that any pulse in a depth pulse sequence may be split into a binomial sequence[138] so that H_2O is never excited. The usual phase cycling for each such pulse is, of course, retained. Just as the effects of various phase-cycled pulses in a pulse sequence, as in Equations (1) to (3), are multiplied together, so too the selective effects of each binomial pulse train in a pulse sequence must be multiplied together. Thus the selectivity is cumulative, and care must be taken with a depth pulse, or even a spin-echo, that the overall effect not be too selective, in which case a shorter binomial series should be used, e.g., $1-\bar{2}-1$ instead of $1-\bar{3}-3-\bar{1}$.

Recent experience shows that binomial water suppression is easily efficient enough for in-vivo ^1H NMR with surface coils, especially when further suppression is obtained via a spin echo as now described.[137,139]

^1H Spectral Editing

Despite the ability to suppress the H_2O resonance, the ^1H spectrum is still mostly intractable because of a large broad multicomponent fat resonance and numerous overlapping ^1H metabolites. No doubt, there will be important clinical uses for straight ^1H spectra showing the major fat and other resolvable components, but the greatest potential lies with millimolar metabolites such as lactate, which are obscured in the normal spectrum. Use of a spin-echo does assist in reducing the fat resonance, but at least part of it has a similar $T2$ to the ^1H metabolites of interest, and other suppression methods are necessary. Campbell and Dobson[140] have described a spin-echo double resonance method that they used to detect certain coupled resonances in vitro. This editing technique has been used by Rothman et al.[141] to separate resonances of alanine, lactate, glutamine, and glutamate from the large lipid resonances in excised leg muscles and heart of a rat and to observe alanine, β-hydroxybutyrate, glutamate, and glutamine in a perfused mouse liver. Williams et al.[132] have since used the same method to detect the build up of lactate in a rat leg during ischemia. Although these studies were done using homogeneous rf coils, Rothman et al.[142] have also used the method to reveal lactate in the in-vivo rat brain using a surface coil.

For a surface coil, the editing experiment is

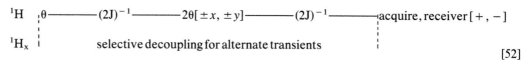

$$[52]$$

The method relies on the homonuclear coupling (J) between two adjacent protons in the metabolite, H_A and H_X, e.g., between the lactate CH_3 and CH protons. Single frequency decoupling is applied to H_X for alternate transients. The decoupling may be continued during signal acquisition, but there is little to be gained because the homonuclear coupling is usually not resolved ($1/J > T2^*$). The mechanism of the sequence is rather similar to that of the heteronuclear Sequences [47] and [48], the difference being that for the homonuclear case a hard 2θ pulse irradiates all protons, including H_X. If binomial water suppression is used and H_X lies in the unexcited window (as will be common when H_X is a CH proton and H_A are CH_2 or CH_3 protons), the method becomes exactly analogous to the heteronuclear case. Writing the binomial pulses as Θ_W, the method becomes

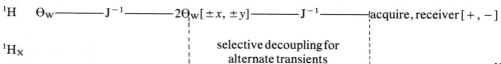

$$[53]$$

If necessary, the spin-echo delays may be extended for other purposes, as indicated in Sequences [47] and [48], though this will not usually be necessary, since J^{-1} is quite long (~130 ms). Indeed, although various ^{1}H metabolites have $T2$'s of a few hundred milliseconds, Sequence [53] cannot be favored because the spin-echo delays are twice those of Sequence [52], leading to greater signal loss via $T2$ relaxation. There are also difficulties with selective decoupling, which will perturb the lipid resonances to a small degree, on alternate transients, and so lead to subtraction errors. This effect can be greatly reduced by moving the decoupling frequency an equal distance to the other side of H_A instead of switching it off for alternate transients, but there are still some unavoidable errors, such as Bloch Sigart frequency shifts, when the decoupler is on in alternate transients.[143] This is especially true at low field strength, where frequency separations are less.

A better alternative to Sequence [53] is to use the exact equivalent of the heteronuclear Sequence [50]:

$$^1\text{H} \quad | \Theta_\text{w} \text{————} \tau \text{————} 2\Theta_\text{w}[\pm x, \pm y] \text{————} \tau \text{————} \text{acquire, receiver}[+, -]$$
$$^1\text{H}_\text{X} \quad | \text{————} J^{-1} \text{————} 2\Phi_\text{s}[x, 0]$$

$$[54]$$

$2\Phi_\text{S}$ is a chemical shift selective 180 degree pulse applied just to H_X, and since both H_A and H_X are separately irradiated in the sequence, it functions in the same way as Sequence [50]. Rather than not apply the pulse at all on alternate transients (as implied by [x, 0]), the pulse should be moved an equal frequency shift to the other side of H_A. For $2\Phi_\text{S}$ to be selective, it will be of a few milliseconds duration, so τ is set greater than J^{-1} to permit this. Hetherington et al.[137] have used this method to detect lactate and alanine in the rat brain post mortem using a surface coil. Some results are shown in Figure 73–31. We[139] have since attempted to use this same method on the human arm to measure lactate during ischemia but were defeated by a consistent error in suppression of the fat resonances. We have since traced this theoretically to a small off-resonance effect of the $2\Phi_\text{S}$ pulse on the lipid signals, which is magnified by the high rf field of the surface coil in the fat layer of a human arm adjacent to the coil. We believe the error can be eliminated by repeating the sequence as

$$^1\text{H} \quad \Theta_\text{w} \text{————} \tau \text{————} 2\Theta_\text{w}[\pm x, \pm y] \text{————} \tau \text{————} \text{acquire, receiver}[+, -]$$
$$^1\text{H}_\text{X} \quad 2\Phi_\text{s}[x, 0] \text{————} J^{-1} \text{————}|$$

$$[54]$$

Experiments are continuing. Lactate in human arm muscle has recently been observed by an extension of this technique.[151]

Apart from the crude localization afforded by the surface coil, ^{1}H editing has not been applied in conjunction with localization. Incremented field gradients could be included in one half of the spin-echo to achieve localization by the 2DFT method. Alternatively, these sequences could be substituted for the θ pulse in Sequences [17] or [18], or a selective refocusing pulse could be used in Sequence [52]. However, it seems to the present author that the effect of field gradient eddy currents will be at their worst during a long spin-echo. All that is necessary to completely destroy the final signal is a decaying field gradient that produces a frequency shift across the sensitive volume, which is on average 8 Hz greater in the first τ period (65 ms) than in the second. This is a difficult, maybe impossible, situation to avoid. The alternative is to use rf inhomogeneity for localization, and any of Sequences [52] to [55] can be combined with depth pulses, by substituting $DP(\theta)$ or $DP(\Theta_\text{w})$ for θ or Θ_w. This combined method has recently been proved by localized detection of lactate in the cat brain.[152] In theory, complete localization can be achieved with Sequence [54]/[55] by applying the $2\Phi_\text{S}[x, 0]$ pulse with a second transmit coil, a method that is again anal-

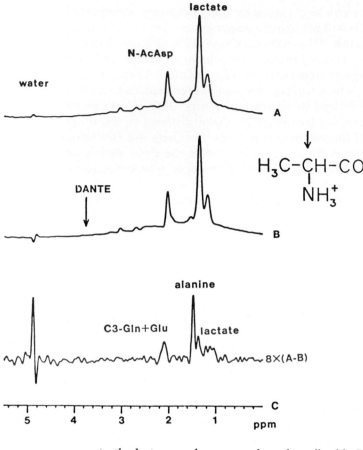

Figure 73–31. [1]H spectra of an intact rat brain, post mortem. A Dante pulse was used for $2\Phi_S[[x, 0)$ in sequence [54]. *A*, Dante pulse not applied. *B*, Dante pulse applied to the CH of alanine at 3.78 ppm. *C*, Difference spectrum between *A* and *B*, revealing the CH$_3$ protons of alanine with excellent suppression of overlapping lactate. The concentration of CH$_3$ alanine protons in the post-mortem rat brain has been estimated to be 1 to 2 mM. (From Hetherington HP et al.: Proc Natl Acad Sci *82*:3115, 1985. Used by permission.)

ogous to the heteronuclear procedure described in Heteronuclear Methods with Surface Coils.

CONCLUSION

Given the reality of large-bore high field strength magnets, and spectrometers that will deliver any sequence of hard or soft pulses with or without pulsed field gradients, the challenge is to optimize localization and sensitivity for in-vivo NMR spectroscopy. A plethora of different methods has resulted, and there are now real solutions to the problem of sensitive-volume localization, though none are in routine use; insufficient time has passed. Although we may now have a reasonable idea of the range of possible solutions, no doubt new solutions will be devised for some time to come, and the task of optimizing the present methods for routine application has hardly begun. By no means all of the possible localization methods have been discussed, e.g., the field profiling method of Topical NMR,[144] which is not now commercially popular, and spectroscopy using projection reconstruction, which is presently being developed.[145]

It is impossible to conclude that one method is best overall; that conclusion depends on the particular investigation in mind. However, in any one case it is possible to assess the sources of errors and judge whether a localization method is required or sufficient. Despite the pressures involved in seeking research grants, it is not good enough to ignore the pitfalls: to state that various errors dephase during pulsed field gradients without quantitative justification, or that they dephase because of field inhomogeneity while at the same time attempting to optimize this homogeneity; to ignore subtraction errors; to propose a localization method based on the axial properties of a surface coil and downplay the off-axis properties; to prove such a localization method using large disc-shaped phantoms that conveniently avoid the problems by not extending beyond the diameter of the coil; to consider only ideal pulses on resonance. In many cases the errors will not be obvious as errors in the final spectra, which may look very nice, but the conclusion of the study will be invalid.

The need for maximum sensitivity ensures the future importance of inhomogeneous rf coils. Taken as a whole the various questions that arise are complex and numerous. However, the present author has found it useful to consider the various methods as being composed of an excitation pulse and a few types of phase-cycled pulse; this permits a detailed but straightforward examination of each method in terms of the individual building blocks, and allows simplifications to be made, such as abandonment of the phase cycling, where appropriate. In combination with the physical picture of rf pulses in terms of magnetization vectors, the reader may find this approach worthwhile. During the next decade, as the various methods are pushed into routine applications, it will be wise to include one scientist, who has a detailed knowledge of the various methods, within each major research group.

ACKNOWLEDGMENT

The author acknowledges support In part by the Esther A. and Joseph Klingenstein Fund.

References

1. Bottomley PA, Hart HR, Edelstein WA, Schenck JF, Smith LS, Leue WM, Mueller OM, Redington RW: NMR imaging/spectroscopy system to study both anatomy and metabolism. Lancet *ii*:273–274, 1983.
2. Pettegrew JW, Minshew NJ, Diehl J, Smith T, Kopp SJ, Glorek T: Anatomical considerations for interpreting topical ^{31}P-NMR. Lancet *ii*:913, 1983.
3. Shoubridge EA, Briggs RW, Radda GK. ^{31}P NMR saturation transfer measurements of the steady-state rates of creatine kinase and ATP synthetase in the rat brain. FEBS Lett *140*:288, 1982.
4. Ackerman JJH, Evelhoch JL, Berkowitz BA, Kichura GM, Devel RK, Lown KS: Selective suppression of the cranial bone resonance from ^{31}P NMR experiments with rat brain in vivo. J Magn Reson *56*:318–322, 1984.
5. Crowley MG, Evelhoch JL, Ackerman JJH: Composite pulse and homogeneous (B_1) excitation: The surface coil antenna. Proceedings of the Third Annual Meeting of the Society of Magnetic Resonance in Medicine, New York, August 1984, pp 173–174.
6. Demco DE, Van Hecke P, Waugh JS: Phase-shifted pulse sequence for measurement of spin-lattice relaxation in complex systems. J Magn Reson *16*:467–470, 1974.
7. Bendall MR, Gordon RE: Depth and refocusing pulses designed for multipulse NMR with surface coils. J Magn Reson *53*:365–385, 1983; M.R. Bendall, U.S. Patent No. 4,486,709 (1984).
8. Ng TC, Glickson JD, Bendall MR: Depth pulse sequences for surface coils: Spatial localization and *T1* measurements. Magn Reson Med *1*:450–462, 1984.
9. Evelhoch JL, Ackerman JJH: NMR *T1* measurements in inhomogeneous B_1 with surface coils. J Magn Reson *53*:52–64, 1983.
10. Bendall MR: Elimination of high-flux signals near surface coils and field gradient sample localization using depth pulses. J Magn Reson *59*:406–429, 1984.
11. Evanochko WT, Ng TC, Sakai TT, Krishna NR, Glickson JD: Development of improved techniques for in vivo NMR studies of tumors and other intact tissues. Magn Reson Med *1*:149–150, 1984.
12. Bendall MR: Surface coils and depth resolution using the spatial variation of radiofrequency field. *In* James TL, Margulis AR (eds): Biomedical Magnetic Resonance. San Francisco, Radiology Research and Education Foundation, 1984, pp 99–126.
13. Bodenhausen G, Freeman R, Turner DL: Suppression of artifacts in two-dimensional J spectroscopy. J Magn Reson *27*:511–514, 1977.
14. Bendall MR, Pegg DT: Theoretical description of depth pulse sequences, on and off resonance, including improvements and extensions thereof. Magn Reson Med *2*:91–113, 1985.
15. Haase A, Hänicke W, Frahm J: The influence of experimental parameters in surface coil NMR. J Magn Reson *56*:401–412, 1984.
16. Evelhoch JL, Crowley MG, Ackerman JJH: Signal-to-noise optimization and observed volume localization with circular surface coils. J Magn Reson *56*:110–124, 1984.

17. Levitt MH, Freeman R: NMR population inversion using a composite pulse. J Magn Reson *33*:473–476, 1979.
18. Freeman R, Kempsell SP, Levitt MH: Radiofrequency pulse sequences which compensate their own imperfections. J Magn Reson *38*:453–479, 1980.
19. Tycko R, Cho HM, Schneider E, Pines A: Composite pulses without phase distortion. J Magn Reson *61*:90–101, 1985.
20. Hetherington HP, Wishart D, Fitzpatrick SM, Cole P, Shulman RG: The application of composite pulses to surface-coil NMR. J Magn Reson *66*:313–330, 1986.
21. Levitt MH, Ernst RR: Composite pulses constructed by a recursive expansion procedure. J Magn Reson *55*:247–254, 1983.
22. Hetherington HP, Rothman DL: Phase cycling of composite refocusing pulses to eliminate dispersive refocusing magnetization. J Magn Reson *65*:348–354, 1985.
23. Bendall MR, Pegg DT: Uniform sample excitation with surface coils for in vivo spectroscopy by adiabatic rapid half passage. J Magn Reson *67*:376–381, 1986.
24. Silver MS, Joseph RI, Hoult DI: Selective spin inversion in nuclear magnetic resonance and coherent optics through an exact solution of the Bloch-Riccati equation. Phys Rev A *31*:2753–2755, 1985.
25. Bendall MR: Sample localization using surface coils and multipulse sequences for high resolution NMR. International Society of Magnetic Resonance, Chicago, August, 1983. Bull Magn Reson *5*:191, 1983.
26. Bendall MR: Localized high-resolution spectroscopy with surface coils using multipulse sequences. Magn Reson Med *1*:105–106, 1984.
27. Hoult DI: The solution of the Bloch equations in the presence of a varying B_1 field: An approach to selective pulse analysis. J Magn Reson *35*:69–86, 1979.
28. Locher PR: Computer simulation of selective excitation in n.m.r. imaging. Phil Trans Roy Soc London Ser B *289*:537–543, 1980.
29. Bauer C, Freeman R, Frenkiel T, Keeler J, Shaka AJ: Gaussian pulses. J Magn Reson *58*:442–457, 1984.
30. Silver MS, Joseph RI, Hoult DI: Highly selective $\pi/2$ and π pulse generation. J Magn Reson *59*:347–351, 1984.
31. Frahm J, Hänicke W: Comparative study of pulse sequences for selective excitation in NMR imaging. J Magn Reson *60*:320–332, 1984.
32. Maudsley AA, Hilal SK, Perman WH, Simon HE: Spatially resolved high resolution spectroscopy by "four-dimensional" NMR. J Magn Reson *51*:147–152, 1983.
33. Haselgrove JC, Subramanian VH, Leigh JS, Gyulai L, Chance B: In vivo one-dimensional imaging of phosphorus metabolites by phosphorus-31 nuclear magnetic resonance. Science *220*:1170–1173, 1983.
34. Scott KN, Brooker HR, Fitzsimmons JR, Bennett HF, Mick RC: Spatial localization of ^{31}P nuclear magnetic resonance signal by the sensitive point method. J Magn Reson *50*:339–344, 1982.
35. Scott KN, Schurehaus RA, Mick RC, Bennett HF, Brooker HR: Experimental variables in spatial localization of ^{31}P nuclear magnetic resonance signal by the sensitive-point method. Magn Reson Med *1*:246–247, 1984.
36. Mick RC, Fitzsimmons JR, Scott KN, Schuerhaus RA: Computer modeling and experimental results on the sensitive-point method. Magn Reson Med *1*:203–204, 1984.
37. Scott KN: Localization techniques for nonproton imaging or nuclear magnetic resonance spectroscopy in vivo. *In* James TL, Margulis AR (eds): Biomedical Magnetic Resonance. San Francisco, Radiology Research and Education Foundation, 1984, pp 79–97.
38. Macovski A: Volumetric NMR imaging with time-varying gradients. Magn Reson Med *2*:29–40, 1985.
39. Shenberg I, Macovski A: Design considerations of an MRI system with time-varying gradients. Proceedings of the Fourth Annual Meeting of the Society of Magnetic Resonance in Medicine, London, August 1985, pp 1056–1057.
40. Ordidge RJ: Personal communication.
41. Bottomley PA, Foster TB, Darrow RD: Depth-resolved surface-coil spectroscopy (DRESS) for in vivo ^{1}H, ^{31}P, and ^{13}C NMR. J Magn Reson *59*:338–342, 1984.
42. Bottomley PA, Edelstein WA, Foster TH, Adams WA: In vivo solvent suppressed localized hydrogen nuclear magnet resonance (NMR): A new window to metabolism? Proc Nat Acad Sci USA *82*:2148–2152, 1985.
43. Gordon RE, Ordidge RJ: Volume selection for high resolution NMR studies. Proceedings of the Third Annual Meeting of the Society of Magnetic Resonance in Medicine, New York, August 1984, pp 272–273.
44. Ordidge RJ, Bendall MR, Gordon RE, Connelly A: Volume selection for in vivo biological spectroscopy. Proceedings of the Eleventh Biennial International Conference of Magnetic Resonance in Biological Systems, Goa, September 1984, pp 387–397.
45. Ordidge RJ, Connelly A, Lohman JAB: Image selected in vivo spectroscopy (ISIS) a new technique for spatially selective NMR spectroscopy. J Magn Reson *66*:283–290, 1986.
46. Roos MS, Hasenfeld A, Bendall MR, Huesman RH, Budinger TF: Simulations of spatial sensitivity for multiple pulse sequences and selective excitation in inhomogeneous B_1 fields. Proceedings of the Third Annual Meeting of the Society of Magnetic Resonance in Medicine, New York, August 1984, pp 632–633.
47. Bendall MR, Pegg DT: Comparison of depth pulse sequences with composite pulses for spatial selection in in vivo NMR. J Magn Reson *63*:494–503, 1985.

48. den Hollander JA, Rothman DL, Bendall MR: Unpublished positive and negative results.
49. Rothman DL: Edited excerpts of the sayings of JA den Hollander. Yale Literary Review 101:202–506, 1983.
50. Young IR: U.K. Patent application No. 2,122,753 A.
51. Aue WP, Müller S, Cross TA, Seelig J: Volume-selective excitation: A novel approach to topical NMR. J Magn Reson 56:350–354, 1984.
52. Post H, Brünner P, Ratzel D: Bruker Medizintechnik, Karlsruhe FRG, personal communication.
53. Müller S, Aue WP, Seelig J: NMR imaging and volume-selective spectroscopy with a single surface coil. J Magn Reson 63:530–543, 1985.
54. Garwood M: Personal communication.
55. Hasenfeld A: Design of amplitude and phase modulated rf pulses for selective region spectroscopy. Proceedings of the Third Annual Meeting of the Society of Magnetic Resonance in Medicine, New York, August 1984, pp 306–307.
56. Lurie D: A systematic approach to the optimisation of 90° and 180° selective excitation. Proceedings of the Third Annual Meeting of the Society of Magnetic Resonance in Medicine, New York, August 1984, pp 486–487.
57. Brown TR, Kincaid BM, Ugurbil K: NMR chemical shift imaging in three dimensions. Proc Nat Acad Sci USA 79:3523–3526, 1982.
58. Ordidge RJ: Personal communication.
59. Brooker HR, Mareci TH: High-resolution NMR spectra from a sensitive volume defined by pulsed field gradients. Magn Reson Med 1:118–119, 1984.
60. Mareci TH, Brooker HR: High-resolution magnetic resonance spectra from a sensitive region defined with pulsed field gradients. J Magn Reson 57:157–163, 1984.
61. Edelstein WA: Signal and noise considerations in NMR imaging and spectroscopy. Proceedings of the Third Annual Meeting of the Society of Magnetic Resonance in Medicine, New York, August 1984, pp 202–203.
62. Rothman DL: Personal communication.
63. Brooker HR, Mareci TH, Mao J: Magn Reson Med, in press.
64. Mareci TH, Thomas RG, Scott KN, Brooker HR: Combination of pulse gradient and surface coil localization of chemical shift resolved spectra. Proceedings of the Third Annual Meeting of the Society of Magnetic Resonance in Medicine, New York, August 1974, pp 493–494.
65. Hoult DI: Rotating frame zeugmatography. J Magn Reson 33:183–297, 1979.
66. Cox SJ, Styles P: Towards biochemical imaging. J Magn Reson 40:209–212, 1980.
67. Bendall MR, Aue WP: Experimental verification of depth pulses applied with surface coils. J Magn Reson 54:149–152, 1983.
68. Ng TC, Bendall MR: Depth pulse localization of surface-coil sensitive region. Magn Reson Med 1:216–217, 1984.
69. Bendall MR: The technology of the surface coil. General spectroscopic methods for any RF coil or coil array. Proceedings of the Third Annual Meeting of the Society of Magnetic Resonance in Medicine, New York, August 1984, p 41.
70. Shaka AJ, Freeman R: Spatially selective radiofrequency pulses. J Magn Reson 59:169–176, 1984.
71. Shaka AJ, Keeler J, Smith MB, Freeman R: Spatial localization of NMR signals in an inhomogeneous radiofrequency field. J Magn Reson 61:175–180, 1985.
72. Tycko R, Pines A: Spatial localization of NMR signals by narrowband inversion. J Magn Reson 60:156–160, 1984.
73. Garwood M, Schleich T, Ross BD, Matson GB, Winters WD: A modified rotating frame experiment based on a Fourier series window function. Application to in vivo spatially localized NMR spectroscopy. J Magn Reson 65:239–251, 1985.
74. Bolton PH: Magnetic resonance imaging using flip angle gradients. J Magn Reson 63:620–621, 1985.
75. Haase A, Malloy C, Radda GK: Spatial localization of high resolution ^{31}P spectra with a surface coil. J Magn Reson 55:164–169, 1983.
76. Garwood M, Schleich T, Matson GB, Acosta G: Spatial localization of tissue metabolites by phosphorus-31 NMR rotating-frame zeugmatography. J Magn Reson 60:268–279, 1984.
77. Shaka AJ, Freeman R: Spatially selective pulse sequences: Elimination of harmonic responses. J Magn Reson 62:340–345, 1985.
78. Shaka AJ, Freeman R: "Prepulses" for spatial localization. J Magn Reson 64:145–150, 1985.
79. Chew WM, Moseley ME, Nishimura MC, James TL: Comparison of localization techniques in vivo. Proceedings of the Fourth Annual Meeting of the Society of Magnetic Resonance in Medicine, London, August 1985, pp 952–953.
80. Gonzalez-Mendez R, Moseley ME, Murphy-Boesch J, Chew WM, Litt L, James TL: Selective inversion with surface coils: Use of depth pulses for the inversion transfer experiment in vivo. Proceedings of the Fourth Annual Meeting of the Society of Magnetic Resonance in Medicine, London, August 1985, pp 971–972.
81. Gadian DG, Proctor E, Williams SR, Cox IJ, Gardiner RM: Quantitation of brain metabolites in vivo using ^{1}H NMR. Proceedings of the Fourth Annual Meeting of the Society of Magnetic Resonance in Medicine, London, August 1985, pp 785–786.
82. Decorps M, Blondet P, Albrand JP: New water signal suppression sequence for in vivo ^{1}H NMR spectroscopy with surface coils. Proceedings of the Fourth Annual Meeting of the Society of Magnetic Resonance in Medicine, London, August 1985, pp 779–780.

83. Decorps M, Laval M, Confort A, Chaillout J-J: Signal to noise and spatial localization of NMR spectra with a surface coil and the saturation-recovery sequence. J Magn Reson *61*:418–425, 1985.

84. Bendall MR: Portable NMR sample localization method using inhomogeneous rf irradiation coils. Chem Phys Lett *99*:310–315, 1983.

85. Garwood M, Schleich T, Bendall MR, Pegg DT: Improved Fourier series windows for localization in in vivo NMR spectrocopy. J Magn Reson *65*:510–515, 1985.

86. Pegg DT: Personal communication.

87. Metz KR, Briggs RW: Spatial localization of NMR spectra using Fourier series analysis. J Magn Reson *64*:172–176, 1985.

88. Pekar J, Leigh JS, Chance B: Harmonically analyzed sensitivity profile. A novel approach to depth pulses for surface coils. J Magn Reson *64*:115–119, 1985.

89. Pekar J, Renshaw PF, Leigh JS: Rapid sensitivity profiling for surface coils: Very fast HASP. Proceedings of the Fourth Annual Meeting of the Society of Magnetic Resonance in Medicine, London, August 1985, pp 176–177.

90. Pekar J, Leigh JS: Very fast rotating-frame zeugmatography. Proceedings of the Fourth Annual Meeting of the Society of Magnetic Resonance in Medicine, London, August 1985, pp 178–179.

91. Radda GK: Clinical studies by ^{31}P NMR spectroscopy. Proceedings of the Third Annual Meeting of the Society of the Magnetic Resonance in Medicine, New York, August 1984, pp 605–608.

92. De Klerk D: Methods of decreasing the forces in the coil. *In* The Construction of High-field Electromagnets. Newport Instruments Ltd., Newport Pagnell, Bucks, 1965, pp 114–117.

93. Kim VB, Plattner ED: Flux concentrator for high-intensity pulsed magnetic fields. Rev Sci Instrum *30*:524–533, 1959.

94. Styles P, Scott CA, Radda GK: A method for localizing high resolution NMR spectra from human subjects. Magn Reson Med *2*:402–409, 1985.

95. Bendall MR, McKendry JM, Cresshull ID, Ordidge RJ: Active detune switch for complete sensitive-volume localization in in vivo spectroscopy using multiple rf coils and depth pulses. J Magn Reson *60*:473–478, 1984.

96. Styles P, Smith MB, Briggs RW, Radda GK: A concentric surface-coil probe for the production of homogeneous B_1 fields. J Magn Reson *62*:397–405, 1985.

97. Haase A: A new method for the decoupling of multiple-coil NMR probes. J Magn Reson *61*:130–136, 1985.

98. Bendall MR, Connelly A, McKendry JM: Elimination of coupling between cylindrical transmit coils and surface-receive coils for in vivo NMR. Magn Reson Med *3*:157–163, 1986.

99. Styles P: Personal communication.

100. Hedges LK, Hoult DI: Isolation of non-orthogonal radio-frequency coils for NMR. Proceedings of the Fourth Annual Meeting of the Society of Magnetic Resonance in Medicine, London, August 1985, pp 1096–1097.

101. Crawley MG, Evelhoch JL, Ackerman JJH: The surface-coil NMR receiver in the presence of homogeneous B_1 excitation. J Magn Reson *64*:20–31, 1985.

102. Clarke GD, Nunnally RL: Investigation of N.M.R. surface coil geometries. Proceedings of the Third Annual Meeting of the Society of Magnetic Resonance in Medicine, New York, August 1984, pp 161–162.

103. Holcomb WG, Gore JC: Novel designs for surface and intracavity coils for NMR imaging. Proceedings of the Third Annual Meeting of the Society of Magnetic Resonance in Medicine, New York, August 1984, p 333.

104. Schleich T: Personal communication.

105. Jesmanowicz A, Grist TM, Froncisz W, Hyde JS: Sectorial loop-gap resonator for ^{31}P NMR of the human liver. Proceedings of the Fourth Annual Meeting of the Society of Magnetic Resonance in Medicine, London, August 1985, pp 489–490.

106. Bendall MR: Unpublished experimental results.

107. Field J, Brooks WM, Bulsing JM, Irving MG, Doddrell DM: A strategy for performing volume-selected multipulse NMR spectroscopy in vivo. J Magn Reson *63*:612–619, 1985.

108. Balaban RS, Gadian DG, Radda GK: Phosphorus nuclear magnetic resonance study of the rat kidney in vivo. Kidney Int *20*:575–579, 1981.

109. Bendall MR, Pegg DT: DEPT at depth. Polarization transfer and sample localization combined using surface coils. J Magn Reson *57*:337–343, 1984.

110. Bendall MR, Pegg DT: Sensitive-volume localization for in vivo NMR using heteronuclear spin-echo pulse sequences. Magn Reson Med *2*:298–306, 1985.

111. Doddrell DM, Pegg DT, Bendall MR: Distortionless enhancement of NMR signals by polarization transfer. J Magn Reson *48*:323–327, 1982.

112. Pegg DT, Doddrell DM, Bendall MR: Proton-polarization transfer enhancement of a heteronuclear spin multiplet with preservation of phase coherency and relative component intensities. J Chem Phys *77*:2745–2752, 1982.

113. Pegg DT, Bendall MR: Theory of localized polarization transfer. Magn Reson Med *2*:453–468, 1985.

114. Bendall MR, Pegg DT: Complete accurate editing of decoupled ^{13}C spectra using DEPT and a quaternary-only sequence. J Magn Reson *53*:272–296, 1983.

115. Bendall MR, den Hollander JA, Arias-Mendoza F, Rothman DL, Behar KL, Shuman RG: Application of multipulse NMR to observe ^{13}C-labeled metabolites in biological systems. Magn Reson Med *2*:56–64, 1985.

116. Pegg DT, Bendall MR: Pulse-sequence cycles for editing ^{13}C spectra when using an inhomogeneous radiofrequency field. J Magn Reson *63*:556–572, 1985.

117. Bendall MR, Pegg DT, Doddrell DM, Field J: Inverse DEPT sequence. Polarization transfer from a spin-$\frac{1}{2}$ nucleus to n spin-$\frac{1}{2}$ heteronuclei via correlated motion in the doubly rotating reference frame. J Magn Reson *51*:520–526, 1983.

118. Pegg DT, Bendall MR: Two-dimensional DEPT NMR spectroscopy. J Magn Reson *55*:114–127, 1983.

119. Aue WP, Müller S, Seelig J: Localized ^{13}C NMR spectra with enhanced sensitivity obtained by volume-selective excitation. J Magn Reson *61*:392–395, 1985.

120. Bendall MR, Pegg DT, Doddrell DM: Comparison of decoupling and spatial randomization methods for use in editing ^{13}C spectra. J Magn Reson *52*:407–423, 1983.

121. Levitt MA, Bodenhausen G, Ernst RR: The illusions of spin decoupling. J Magn Reson *53*:443–461, 1983.

122. Cookson DJ, Smith BE: Improved methods for assignment of multiplicity in ^{13}C NMR spectroscopy with application to the analysis of mixtures. Org Magn Reson *16*:111–116, 1981.

123. Brown DW, Nakashima TT, Rabenstein DL: Simplification and assignment of carbon-13 NMR spectra with spin-echo Fourier transform techniques. J Magn Reson *45*:302–314, 1981.

124. Bendall MR, Pegg DT, Doddrell DM, Williams DH: Strategy for the generation of ^{13}C subspectra. Application to the analysis of the ^{13}C spectrum of the antibiotic ristocetin. J Org Chem *47*:3021–3023, 1982.

125. Rothman DL, Behar KL, Hetherington HP, den Hollander JA, Bendall MR, Petroff OAC, Shulman RG: H-Observe/^{13}C-decouple spectroscopic measurements of lactate and glutamate in the rat brain in vivo. Proc Natl Acad Sci USA *82*:1633–1637, 1985.

126. Bendall MR, Pegg DT, Doddrell DM, Field J: NMR of protons coupled to ^{13}C nuclei only. J Am Chem Soc *103*:934–936, 1981.

127. Freeman R, Mareci TH, Morris GA: Weak satellite signals in high-resolution NMR spectra. Separating the wheat from the chaff. J Magn Reson *42*:341–345, 1981.

128. Brindle KM, Smith MB, Rajagopalan B, Radda GK: Spectral editing in ^{31}P NMR spectra of human brain. J Magn Reson *61*:559–563, 1985.

129. Bendall MR, Doddrell DM, Pegg DT: Editing of ^{13}C NMR spectra. A pulse sequence for the generation of subspectra. J Am Chem Soc *103*:4603–4605, 1981.

130. Bendall MR, Pegg DT, Doddrell DM, Johns SR, Willing RI: Pulse sequence for the generation of a ^{13}C subspectrum of both aromatic and aliphatic quaternary carbons. JCS Chem Comm 1138–1140, 1982.

131. Rothman DL, Behar KL, den Hollander JA, Shulman RG: Surface coil spin-echo spectra without cycling the refocusing pulse through all four phases. J Magn Reson *59*:157–159, 1984.

132. Williams SR, Gadian DG, Proctor E, Sprague DB, Talbott DF, Young IR, Brown FF: Proton NMR studies of muscle metabolites in vivo. J Magn Reson *63*:406–412, 1985.

133. Sklenář V, Starčuk Z: 1 – 2 – 1 Pulse train: A new effective method of selective excitation for proton NMR in water. J Magn Reson *50*:495–501, 1982.

134. Hore PJ: Solvent suppression in Fourier transform nuclear magnetic resonance. J Magn Reson *55*:283–300, 1983.

135. Starčuk Z, Sklenář V: New hard pulse sequences for the solvent signal suppression in Fourier-transform NMR. J Magn Reson *61*:567–570, 1985, and references cited therein.

136. Brindle KM, Porteous R, Campbell ID: ^{1}H NMR measurements of enzyme-catalyzed ^{15}N-label exchange. J Magn Reson *56*:543–547, 1984.

137. Hetherington HP, Avison MJ, Shulman RG: ^{1}H Homonuclear editing of rat brain using semiselective pulses. Proc Natl Acad Sci *82*:3115–3118, 1985.

138. Bendall MR, Hetherington HP: Unpublished results.

139. Hetherington HP, Jue T, Bendall MR, Lohman JAB: Unpublished results.

140. Campbell ID, Dobson CM: Spin echo double resonance: A novel method for detecting decoupling in Fourier transform nuclear magnetic resonance. JCS Chem Comm 750–751, 1975.

141. Rothman DL, Arias-Mendoza F, Shulman GI, Shulman RG: A pulse sequence for simplifying hydrogen NMR spectra of biological tissues. J Magn Reson *60*:430–436, 1984.

142. Rothman DL, Behar KL, Hetherington HP, Shulman RG: Homonuclear ^{1}H double-resonance difference spectroscopy of the rat brain in vivo. Proc Natl Acad Sci USA *81*:6330–6334, 1984.

143. Rothman DL, Hetherington HP: Unpublished results.

144. Gordon RE, Hanley PE, Shaw D, Gadian DG, Radda GK, Styles, P, Bore PJ, Chan L: Localization of metabolites in animals using ^{31}P topical magnetic resonance. Nature *287*:736–738, 1980.

145. Lauterbur DC, Levin DN, Marr RB: Theory and simulation of NMR spectroscopic imaging and field plotting by projection reconstruction involving an intrinsic frequency dimension. J Magn Reson *59*:536–541, 1984.

146. Garwood M, Ugurbil K, Bendall MR, Rath AR, Foxall DL: NMR imaging with extremely inhomogeneous B_1 fields. Proceedings of the Sixth Annual Meeting of the Society of Magnetic Resonance in Medicine, New York, August 1987, p. 363.

147. Doddrell DM, Brooks WM, Bulsing JM, Field J, Irving MG, Baddely H: Spatial and chemical-shift-encoded-excitation. SPACE, a new technique for volume-selected NMR spectroscopy. J Magn Reson *68*:367–372, 1986.

148. Luyten PR, Marian JH, Sijtsma B, den Hollander JA: Solvent-suppressed spatially resolved spectroscopy. An approach to high-resolution NMR on a whole-body MR system. J Magn Reson *67*:148–155, 1986.

149. Garwood M, Schlich T, Bendall RM: Simulation of selective pulse techniques for localized NMR spectroscopy. J Magn Reson *73*:191–212, 1987.
150. Bendall RM, Foxall DL, Nichols BG, Schmidt JR: Complete localization of in vivo NMR spectra using two concentric surface coils and rf methods only. J Magn Reson *70*:181–186, 1986.
151. Hetherington HP, Hamm JR, Rothman DL, Pan JW, Shulman RG: Localized ^{1}H NMR of lactate in human arm muscle after ischemic exercise. Proceedings of the Sixth Annual Meeting of Magnetic Resonance in Medicine, New York, August, 1987, p 606.
152. Hanstock CC, Hetherington HP, Boisvert DP, Allen PS: Localized in vivo proton spectroscopy using depth-pulse spectral editing. J Magn Reson *71*:349–354, 1987.

74

Understanding Basic MR Pulse Sequences

MARK R. MITCHELL
ROBERT W. TARR
THOMAS E. CONTURO

To effectively plan and utilize magnetic resonance imaging (MRI), the MRI practitioner must thoroughly understand the pulse sequence options available. Multiple investigators have noted the apparently nonintuitive relationship between MR image intensity and technique.[1-8] As experience accumulated, it became apparent that many of these changes could be understood on the basis of mathematical models derived from the Bloch equations.[9-11] These models relate image pixel intensity (I) to the pulse sequence timing intervals and tissue parameters. Although initial results were somewhat imprecise,[3] improvements in the equations and tissue parameter measurements have increased the predictive value of these models to the point that they now represent one of the most valuable tools that the MRI practitioner has at his disposal for understanding and predicting the results of technique selection.[2,8,12,13]

This chapter will review the basic pulse sequence options available and explain the relationship between timing intervals and tissue parameters by breaking down the overall relationship into its component relationships; these relatively simpler components describe the interaction of individual timing intervals and tissue parameters and form the basis for understanding the more complex interactions. Guidelines that can be used by the MRI practitioner in a clinical setting have also been deduced from the analysis of these relationships for setting spin-echo and inverted spin-echo techniques.

The purpose of this chapter is to explain the relationships between the pulse sequences, timing intervals, and tissue parameters in terms of their relative N, $T1$, and $T2$ weighting (as defined below) so that the MRI practitioner can manipulate these variables to get the desired results. For a discussion of the newer "fast" sequences using limited tip angles and gradient echoes, see Chapter 96.

Pulse Sequence Nomenclature

A pulse sequence name should at the very least describe the type and order of the radio frequency (rf) pulses used; it can also convey information about the intended rate of repetition of the sequence. Unfortunately, pulse sequence names have frequently been used in an imprecise fashion, leading to confusion. Although the ACR MRI glossary was a major advance in standardizing MRI nomenclature,[14] the terminology continues to evolve as new pulse sequence variations develop. Most of the currently used pulse sequences are listed in Table 74–1; the names and abbreviations in the table have been chosen for their descriptive precision and indicate the order and type of rf pulses

Table 74–1. PULSE SEQUENCE NOMENCLATURE

Abbreviation	Pulse Sequence Name
SR	Saturation recovery
PS	Partial saturation
SE*	Spin echo
ME*	Multiecho
PSSE*	Partial saturation with spin echo
PSME*	Partial saturation with multiecho
IR†	Inversion recovery
PSIR†	Partial saturation with inversion recovery
ISE†	Inverted spin echo
IME†	Inverted multiecho
PSISE†	Partial saturation with inverted spin echo
PSIME†	Partial saturation with inverted multiecho
SSFP	Steady state free precession
GE or FE	Gradient echo or field echo

* All of these sequences are usually termed spin echo.
† All of these sequences are frequently labeled only as inversion recovery.

used and the length of time between the pulses relative to the $T1$ and $T2$ values being evaluated.

Throughout this chapter, specific MRI techniques will be indicated by specifying the pulse sequence by the abbreviation listed in Table 74–1, followed by the timing intervals in the following order: $TI/TE1–TEn/TR$, where $TE1$ indicates the TE of the first echo and TEn the TE of the nth echo in a multiecho series with equally spaced TE intervals; if the TE intervals are not equally spaced, the individual TE times will be separated by commas. Only the timing intervals used in the sequence will be included.

Three basic pulse sequences that were developed for evaluation of $T1$ and $T2$ in spectroscopy have been adapted to MR imaging. These include saturation recovery (SR), spin echo (SE), and inversion recovery (IR). Partial saturation (PS) is a special form of SR with equally spaced 90 degree rf pulses. The addition of multiple 180 degree pulses in the SE sequence produces the multiple echo (ME) sequence. An important hybrid technique that combines the effects of SE and IR is the inverted spin-echo (ISE) sequence; it uses a 180 degree initiating pulse that inverts the net magnetization vector followed by a spin echo. The inversion can also be followed by a multiecho sequence producing the inversion multiecho sequence (IME). All of these pulse sequences are diagrammed in Figure 74–1 with their appropriate timing interval designations.

The magnitude of the signal produced using the above pulse sequences is a function of the N, $T1$ and $T2$ of the tissues present. The degree of influence that a particular tissue parameter has on the resultant signal will be called weighting. The more weighting present, the more change there will be in I for a given change in that particular tissue parameter. N is a contributing factor in all images; the degree of $T1$ or $T2$ weighting depends upon both the technique selected and the tissue parameters of the tissues being examined. With appropriate timing intervals SR, PS, and IR can have N or N and $T1$ weighting, while SE and ISE can have N; N and $T2$; N and $T1$; or N, $T1$ and $T2$ weighting.

If the basic pulse sequences described above are repeated rapidly, with insufficient time for complete $T1$ relaxation, the three basic pulse sequences become partially saturated and can be spoken of as partial saturation variations of the original sequences,[6] i.e., partial saturation with spin echo (PSSE), partial saturation with inversion recovery (PSIR), and partial saturation with inverted spin echo (PSISE). In reality, since some tissues such as cerebrospinal fluid have very long $T1$ values that require exceedingly long TR intervals for complete $T1$ relaxation, virtually all imaging is performed in a

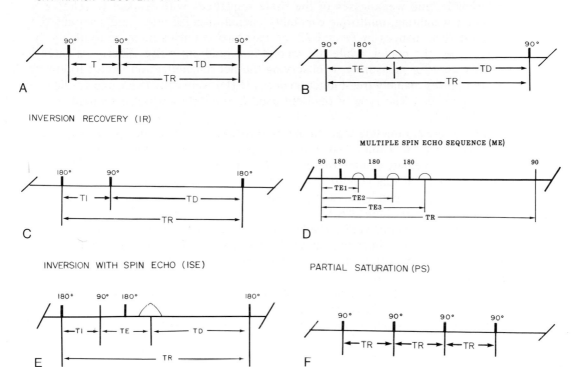

Figure 74–1. The order of rf pulses and timing intervals diagrammed for *A*, saturation recovery; *B*, spin echo; *C*, inversion recovery; *D*, multiple spin echo (multiecho), *E*, inverted spin echo; and *F*, partial saturation, where T = tau; TD = delay time; TR – repetition time; TE = echo time, and TI = inversion time.

partial saturation mode for at least some of the tissues in the image.[15] Although this fact is usually ignored when specifying the sequence name, it is extremely important to recognize the difference, since most or all of the *T1* weighting in some sequences is due to the fact that they are being used in a partial saturation mode; this partial saturation effect is what gives SE its *T1* weighting. Since the partial saturation component of the name is awkward and lengthy, it is probably not unreasonable to leave this portion of the name out in common usage, but the reader should understand the distinction.

A variation of PS is steady-state-free precession (SSFP); here the pulses are repeated very rapidly, in a time less than *T2*.[16] With 90 degree rf pulses, the SSFP sequence yields a very small signal-to-noise ratio; therefore, SSFP is usually performed with non–90 degree tip angle. SSFP is currently being combined with short *TR*'s to produce fast scanning techniques (see Chapter 96).

Table 74–2 lists the basic sequences with their partial saturation and multiecho variations. The relationship of the timing intervals to *T1* and *T2* that determine the

Table 74–2. PARTIAL SATURATION VARIATIONS

Standard Sequence Conditions	Partial Saturation Conditions
SR ($T \gg TI$, $TD \gg TI$)	PS ($TR \gg TI$ and $T = TD$)
	SSFP ($TR \gg T2$, $\theta \neq 90°$)
SE ($TR \gg TI$)	PSSE ($TR \gg TI$)
ME ($TR \gg TI$)	PSME ($TR \gg TI$)
IR ($TD \gg TI$)	PSIR ($TD \gg TI$)
ISE ($TD \gg TI$)	PSISE ($TD \gg TI$)

appropriate name for each sequence has also been indicated. Table 74–3 lists some of the strengths and weaknesses of the basic sequences with respect to relative tissue parameter weighting, multislice capability, signal-to-noise ratio, and scanning time.

To detect changes in $T1$ and $T2$, at least two rf pulses must be used; the first rf pulse excites the nuclei, while the second is a read-out pulse. There are three basic methods used for measuring or observing the net magnetization vector following the read-out pulses, namely free-induction decay (FID), spin echo (SE), and gradient echos (see Chapter 96). The type of read-out used in the different pulse sequences is listed in Table 74–4.

The tissue parameters that can be used to weight the various pulse sequences are also summarized in Table 74–4. For this discussion, it is assumed that the FID read-out begins immediately after the end of the rf pulse, or in a time that is very short compared to $T2$; if this condition is not met, the sequences with FID read-out begin to have some $T2$ dependence, and produce images similar to sequences with spin echo read-out with a very short TE.[17]

The pulse sequence names used in the literature sometimes fail to specify the read-out method used. For instance, an SE sequence with a short TE may be referred to as PS on the assumption that the TE used is sufficiently short to eliminate the effects of $T2$. When this assumption is valid, the SE sequence acts very much like PS, but the available TE intervals are usually not short enough to meet this criterion and the pulse sequence continues to have SE characteristics. Therefore, it seems advisable to use the more specific pulse sequence names whenever possible and practical to avoid ambiguity.

MRI Technique

Selecting an x-ray technique requires determination of the appropriate KVP and MAS for a particular application.[19] Similarly, MRI technique selection involves choosing the pulse sequence and timing intervals most suited to the clinical situation. To accomplish this, one must have a thorough understanding of the relationships between the timing intervals TI, TE, TD, and TR and tissue parameters N, $T1$, and $T2$, since these relationships can be used to achieve the desired image intensity characteristics and contrast.

A detailed analysis of the SE and ISE sequences will be used to develop a number of guidelines that can be used by the MRI practitioner for technique selection in a clinical setting. The spin-echo read-out variations were chosen, since one can easily convert the basic principles developed with these sequences into an understanding of the FID read-out sequences by simply dropping the $T2$ dependence added by the spin

Table 74–3. PULSE SEQUENCE STRENGTHS AND WEAKNESSES

Pulse Sequence	Sensitivity to:			Multislice Application	Signal-to-Noise Ratio*	Scanning Time
	N	$T1$	$T2$			
SE c̄ long TR	+ + +	0	+ + +	+ + +	+ + +	−
SE c̄ short TR	+	+ +	+	+	−	+ +
ISE	+ +	+ + +	+	+ + +	+	−
PS	+ +	+ + +	0	+	−	+ + +
SR	+	+ +	0	+ + +	+ + +	−
IR	+ +	+ + +	0	+ + +	+	−

* Sequence with short scanning times can be repeated and signal averaged to improve the signal to noise ratio, but this lengthens scanning time.

Table 74–4. PULSE SEQUENCE CHARACTERISTICS

Sequence	Read-Out	Tissue Parameters Measured*
SR and PS	FID	*N, T1*
PSSE and PSME	Echo	*N, T1, T2*
IR and PSIR	FID	*N, T1*
ISE and PSISE	Echo	*N, T1, T2*
SSFP	FID	*N, T1, T2*

* Assumes FID read-out is performed in a time ≪ *T2*. This may not always be the case, but it is correct in most situations.

echo. For the sake of simplicity, the partial saturation portion of the names will not be used further in this chapter. The reader should, however, be aware that the sequences being discussed are almost always being used in a partial saturation mode for at least some of the tissues in the image.

The apparently nonintuitive relationship between timing intervals and tissue parameters can be greatly simplified by separating and graphing the individual components involved. Graphing image pixel intensity (*I*) as a function of individual timing intervals while independently varying the tissue parameters permits visualization of the interaction of *TE* with *T2* and *TI, TD,* and *TR* with *T1*. Graphs based on the "parameter sensitivity" evaluation, described later, tie these individual interactions into an integrated whole by permitting visualization of the interdependence of the timing intervals. Armed with an understanding of these principles and a number of guidelines derived from this analysis, the MRI practitioner should be able to select pulse sequences and adjust timing intervals to achieve the desired imaging characteristics for screening or maximum tissue discrimination; this understanding also improves the ability to predict the pathologic tissue parameter changes responsible for the image intensity characteristics obtained with a particular technique.

MATERIALS AND METHODS

Image pixel intensity (*I*) for the SE and ISE techniques has been described as a function of *N, T1, T2, TI, TE, TD,* and *TR* in Equations (1) and (2).[9,11,18,20] These equations have been used to generate the pixel intensity curves in Figures 74–2 to 74–6 and 74–10 to 74–15. Slightly different equations are needed for precise description of ME and IME imaging characteristics, but the results are probably not important for this clinical discussion and the distinction will not be made here.

Spin-Echo Intensity Equation

$$I = Ne^{-TE/T2}(1 + e^{-TR/T1} - 2e^{-(TR - 1/2TE)/T1}) \tag{1}$$

Inverted Spin-Echo Intensity Equation

$$I = Ne^{-TE/T2}[1 + e^{-TI/T1}(2e^{-(TD + 1/2TE)/T1} - e^{-(TD + TE)/T1} - 2)] \tag{2}$$

Each of these intensity equations can be used to derive three additional equations that predict the rate of change in *I* expected for a small change in an individual tissue parameter by taking the partial derivative of *I* with respect to *N, T1,* and *T2* independently. The resulting equations form the basis of the "parameter sensitivity" evaluation[8,20] and define the sensitivity parameters SN (sensitivity to change in *N*), ST1 (sensitivity to change in *T1*), and ST2 (sensitivity to change in *T2*). (Equations 3 to 8):

Table 74–5. TISSUE PARAMETER VALUES

	N*	T1 (ms)	T2 (ms)
Cerebral White Matter	107	540	84
Hypothetical Tissue	100	500	100

* Units for N are relative and arbitrary.

Spin-Echo Parameter Sensitivity Equations

$$SN = e^{-TE/T2}(1 + e^{-TR/T1} - 2e^{-(TR - 1/2TE)/T1}) \tag{3}$$

$$ST1 = \frac{N}{(T1)^2} e^{-TE/T2}(TRe^{-TR/T1} - (2TR - TE)e^{-(TR - 1/2TE)/T1}) \tag{4}$$

$$ST2 = \frac{N}{(T2)^2} e^{-TE/T2}(1 + e^{-TR/T1} - 2e^{-(TR - 1/2TE)/T2}) \tag{5}$$

Inverted Spin-Echo Parameter Sensitivity Equations

$$SN = e^{-TE/T2}[1 + e^{-TI/T1}(2e^{-(TD + 1/2TE)/T1} - e^{-(TD + TE)/T1} - 2)] \tag{6}$$

$$ST1 = Ne^{-TE/T2}e^{-TI/T1}[-(TR + TD + TI)e^{-(TD + 1/2TE)/T1} + TRe^{-(TD + TE)/T1} + 2TI] \tag{7}$$

$$ST2 = -NTEe^{-TE/T2}[1 + e^{-TI/T1}(2e^{-(TD + 1/2TE)/T1} - e^{-(TD + TE)/T1} - 2)] \tag{8}$$

A set of hypothetical tissue parameter values have been selected to create the pixel intensity graphs. The hypothetical N, $T1$, and $T2$ values chosen approximate cerebral white matter values obtained at 0.5 tesla on a Technicare superconducting system (Table 74–5). Hypothetical values have been used in these graphs to simplify visual analysis of the relationships between individual timing intervals and their relevant tissue parameters. Actual white matter tissue values have been used for the parameter sensitivity plots, however, so that they can be compared with images acquired with a variety of pulse sequence timing intervals.

The parameter sensitivity plots are independently scaled so that 100 represents the largest value calculated for all combinations of the indicated timing intervals. Individual lines on these plots represent the set of timing interval combinations for which the sensitivity to the individual tissue parameter being examined is expected to be the same. An increased numerical value of the line indicates a relative increased parameter sensitivity for the set of timing intervals that define the line. Solid lines represent positive parameter sensitivity; dashed lines represent negative values. Positive values indicate that I increases when the tissue parameter increases while negative values indicate that I decreases when the corresponding tissue parameter increases.

Imaging was performed on a Technicare 0.5 tesla superconducting system using a variety of imaging techniques including multislice SE and ME sequences and single slice multiecho ISE and IME sequences.

RESULTS

Spin-Echo Graphs

The following line graphs of predicted I for SE were generated using Equation (1):
1. I vs. TE using linear and logarithmic x axes for TE (Fig. 74–2A and B).
2. I vs. TR using a logarithmic x axis (Fig. 74–3A).
3. I vs. TE and TR for two tissues with different N values (Fig. 74–4A and B).

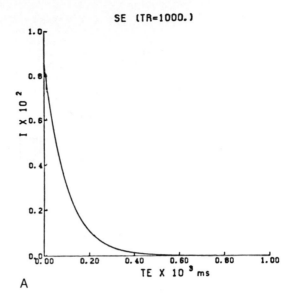

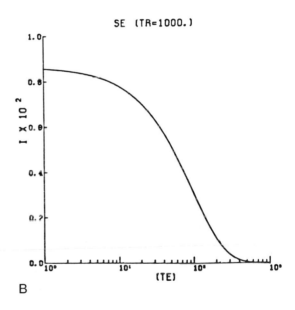

Figure 74–2. *A*, I versus TE spin-echo plot using linear *x* axis. Note the crowding of image intensity information toward the left portion of the graph ($N = 100$; $T1 = 500$ ms; $T2 = 100$ ms; $TR = 1000$ ms). *B*, I versus TE spin-echo plot using logarithmic *x* axis. Note that the image intensity information is distributed across the extent of the graph. A shoulder and toe portion of the graph is evident where changes in timing interval produce very little change in image intensity ($N = 100$; $T1 = 500$ ms; $T2 = 100$ ms; $TR = 1000$ ms).

4. *I* vs. *TE* and *TR* for two tissues with different *T1* values (Fig. 74–5*A* and *B*).
5. *I* vs. *TE* and *TR* for two tissues with different *T2* values (Fig. 74–6*A* and *B*).
The following isocontour plots of the sensitivity parameters for SE were created using Equations 3 to 5:
1. *ST2* vs. *T2* and *ST1* vs. *T1* (Fig. 74–7*A* and *B*).
2. *SN*, *ST1*, and *ST2* for all combinations of *TE* and *TR* (Fig. 74–8*A*, *B*, and *C*).
3. An overlay of the isocontour plots for *SN*, *ST1*, and *ST2* above (Fig. 74–9).

Inverted Spin-Echo Graphs

The following line graphs of predicted *I* for *ISE* were generated using Equation 2:
1. *I* vs. *TE*, *I* vs. *T1*, and *I* vs *TD*, for two tissues with different *N* values (Fig. 74–10*A*, *B*, and *C*).

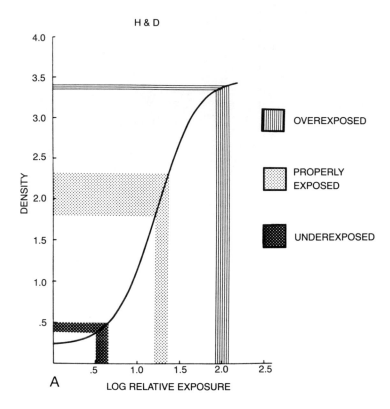

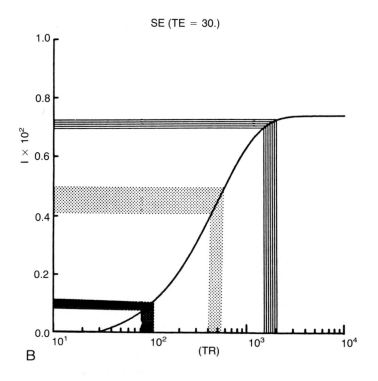

Figure 74–3. *A* and *B*, I versus TR spin-echo plot using logarithmic *x* axis compared with a standard H and D curve for radiographic film. Note in *A* that the greatest contrast on radiographic film occurs when an exposure level falls on the steep portion of the H and D curve. Overexposure, which falls on the shoulder of the curve, produces a uniformly black film, while underexposure, which falls on the toe of the curve, produces a uniformly white film. Similarly in *B*, selecting TR values that are relatively long or short compared to the *T1* values of the tissues being evaluated compresses the contrast into a narrow range of image pixel intensities. (From Mitchell MR et al.: RadioGraphics *6*:249, 1986. Used by permission.)

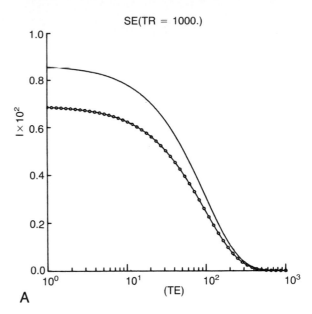

A

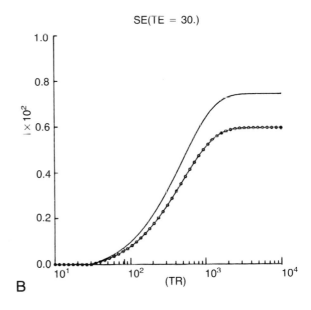

B

Figure 74–4. N effects in spin echo. *A*, I versus TE plot with *TR* = 1000 ms, and *B*, I versus TR plot with *TE* = 30 ms, for two hypothetical tissues with different N values. Note that a change in *N* produces a simple multiplicative change in I in both *A* and *B*. (Solid line: *N* = 100; *T1* = 500 ms; and *T2* = 100 ms. Open circles line: *N* = 80; *T1* = 500 ms; and *T2* = 100 ms; *TR* = 1000 ms.) (From Mitchell MR et al.: RadioGraphics 6:251, 1986. Used by permission.)

2. *I* vs. *TE*, *I* vs. *TI*, and *I* vs. *TD*, for two tissues with different *T1* values (Fig. 74–11*A*, *B*, and *C*).

3. *I* vs. *TI* for three tissues with different *T1* values using magnitude reconstruction (Fig. 74–12).

4. *I* vs. *TE* for two tissues with different *T2* values using varying *TI* values (Fig. 74–13*A*, *B*, and *C*).

5. *I* vs. *TI* for two tissues with different *T2* values (Fig. 74–14).

6. *I* vs. *TD* for two tissues with different *T2* values using varying *TI* values (Fig. 74–15*A* and *B*).

The following isocontour plots of parameter sensitivity for *ISE* were created using Equations 6 to 8:

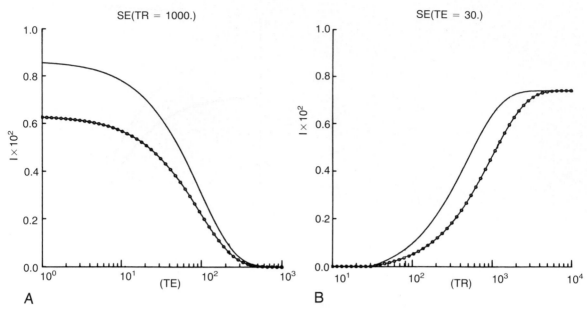

Figure 74–5. *T1* effects in spin echo. *A*, I versus TE plot for two hypothetical tissues with different *T1* values. Note that an increase in *T1* produces a diminished I due to a decrease in longitudinal (*T1*) relaxation. *B*, I versus TR the same two hypothetical tissues with different *T1* values. Note that an increase in *T1* shifts the intensity curve to the right without changing the maximum intensity. (Solid line: $N = 100$; $T1 = 500$ ms; $T2 = 100$ ms. Open circles line: $N = 100$; $T1 = 500$ ms; $T2 = 100$ ms; TE = 30 ms.) (From Mitchell MR et al.: RadioGraphics 6:251, 1986. Used by permission.)

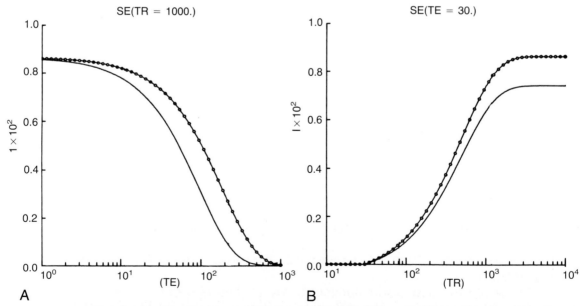

Figure 74–6. *T2* effects in spin echo. *A*, I versus TE for two hypothetical tissues with different *T2* values. Note that an increase in *T2* shifts the curve to the right without changing the maximum value of I. *B*, I versus TR for the same two hypothetical tissues with different *T2* values. Note that an increase in *T2* causes an increase in I for all values of TR, since less transverse (*T2*) relaxation occurs during the fixed TE interval. (Solid line: $N = 100$; $T1 = 500$ ms; $T2 = 100$ ms. Open circles line: $N = 100$; $T1 = 500$ ms; $T2 = 200$ ms; $TE = 30$ ms; $TR = 1000$ ms.) (From Mitchell MR et al.: RadioGraphics 6:251, 1986. Used by permission.)

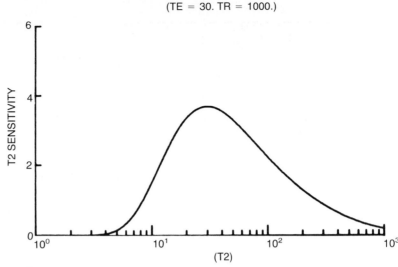

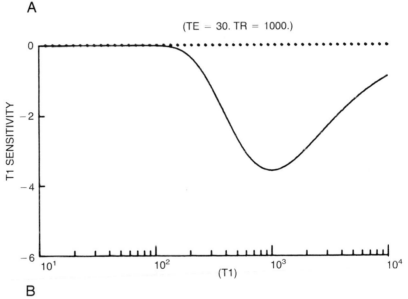

Figure 74–7. Spin echo rate of change graphs. *A,* Rate of change of I (*ST2*) versus *T2.* Note that the maximum *ST2* occurs when *T2* = *TE.* (*T1* = 500 ms; *TE* = 30 ms; and *TR* = 1000 ms.) *B,* Rate of change of I (*ST1*) vs. *T1.* Note that the maximum *ST1* occurs when *T1* = *TR.* (*T2* = 100 ms; *TE* = 30 ms; and *TR* = 1000 ms.) (From Mitchell MR et al.: RadioGraphics 6:252, 1986. Used by permission.)

1. *ST1* vs. *T1* (Fig. 74–16).

2. *ST2* vs. *T2* using varying *TI* values (Fig. 74–17*A,* *B* and *C*).

3. Isocontour plots for *SN* for multiple combinations of *TE, TI,* and *TD* (Fig. 74–18*A, B,* and *C*).

4. Isocontour plots for *ST1* for multiple combinations of *TE, TI,* and *TD,* respectively (Fig. 74–19*A, B,* and *C*).

5. Isocontour plots for *ST2* for multiple combinations of *TE, TI,* and *TD,* respectively (Fig. 74–20*A, B,* and *C*).

6. Overlays of the above isocontour plots of *SN, ST1,* and *ST2,* for multiple combinations of *TE, TI,* and *TD* (Fig. 74–21*A, B,* and *C*).

Images created in a normal volunteer and in patients with diffuse white matter disease, metastatic melanoma to the thyroid, a brainstem infarct, and a large subarachnoid cyst (Figs. 74–22 to 74–29) have been used to demonstrate the relationships indicated in the graphs.

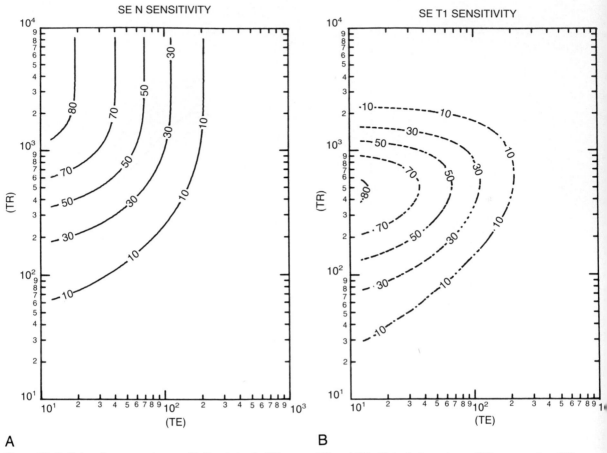

Figure 74–8. Spin echo parameter sensitivity plots. *A*, SN versus TE and TR. Note that maximum SN occurs when *TE* ≪ *T2*, and *TR* ≫ *T1*. *B*, ST1 versus TE and TR. Note that maximum ST1 occurs when *TE* ≪ *T2* and *TR* = *T1*.

DISCUSSION

Choice of Graphic Display

The utility of a graph displaying *I* as a function of timing interval plotted on a logarithmic *x* axis can be appreciated by comparing the results with the familiar H & D curve.[20] The use of a linear scale for *TE* in the SE, *I* vs. *TE* graph (Fig. 74–2*A*) crowds the region of rapid signal intensity change, a region of considerable interest, towards the left; using a logarithmic scale produces a shoulder on the curve with shorter *TE* intervals (Fig. 74–2*B*). The importance of this shoulder can be appreciated by noting the striking similarity between the *I* vs. *TR* graph using a logarithmic scale and a conventional H & D curve (Fig. 74–3*A* and *B*). Both curves have a shoulder and a toe. Near the toe of the curve, the signal will be lost in noise. On the shoulder, the relative variation in film density or image pixel intensity is compressed into a narrow range, decreasing image contrast.

When an exposure or MR technique falls on the steep portions of these curves, the film density difference due to inherent tissue contrast characteristics is maximized. The steep portion of the *I* vs. *TR* curve indicates the *TR* settings where small changes in *TR* or *T1* will produce the greatest difference in *I*. For a specific normal tissue of interest, selecting a *TR* interval that localizes *I* on the steep portion of the *I* vs. *TR* graph (Fig. 74–3*A*) produces maximum SE image contrast due to small changes in *T1*;

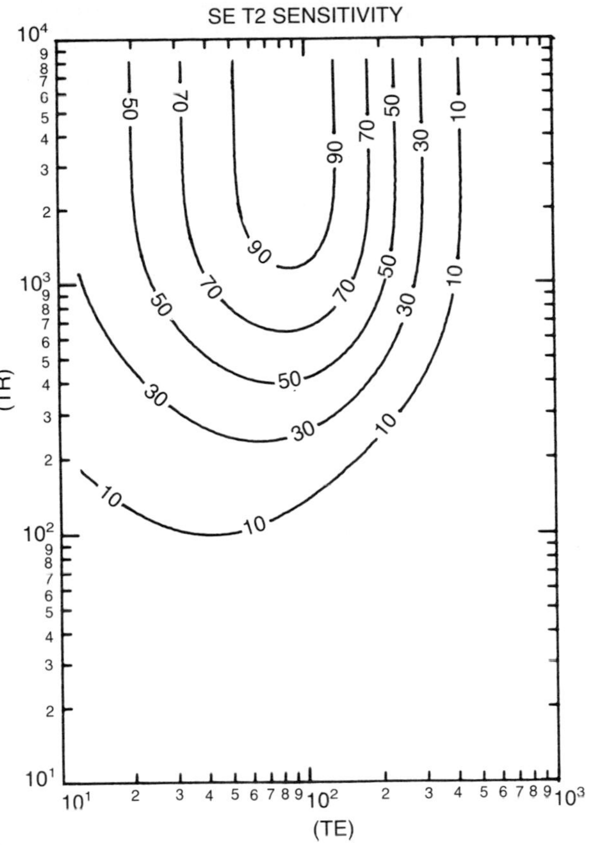

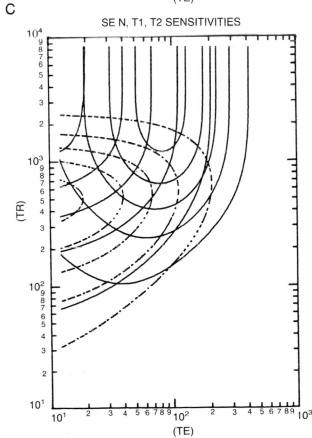

SE T2 SENSITIVITY

Figure 74–8 *Continued C*, ST2 versus TE and TR. Lines represent expected relative percentage change in I for a small change in *N*. Dashed lines indicate a decrease in I for an increase in *N*. Measured white matter tissue parameter values were used to create the plot. (From Mitchell MR et al.: RadioGraphics 6:253, 1986. Used by permission.)

C

SE N, T1, T2 SENSITIVITIES

Figure 74–9. Combined spin-echo parameter sensitivity plot. The individual parameter sensitivity graphs for SN, ST1, and ST2 for white matter are overlayed to show the competitive and complementary tissue parameter effects (regions with both solid and dashed lines indicate competition; areas with only solid or dashed lines indicate synergism.) (From Mitchell MR et al.: RadioGraphics 6:254, 1986. Used by permission.)

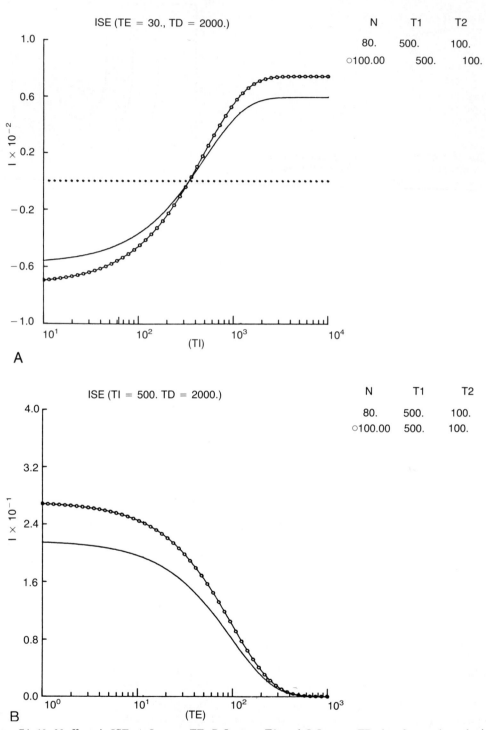

Figure 74–10. *N* effects in ISE. *A*, I versus TE; *B*, I versus T1; and *C*, I versus TD plots for two hypothetical tissues with different *N* values. Note that a change in N produces a simple multiplicative change in I in all three graphs. (Solid line: *N* = 80, *T1* = 500 ms; *T2* = 100 ms. Open circles line: *N* = 100; *T1* = 500 ms; and *T2* = 100 ms. *TI* = 500 ms and *TD* = 2000 ms.)

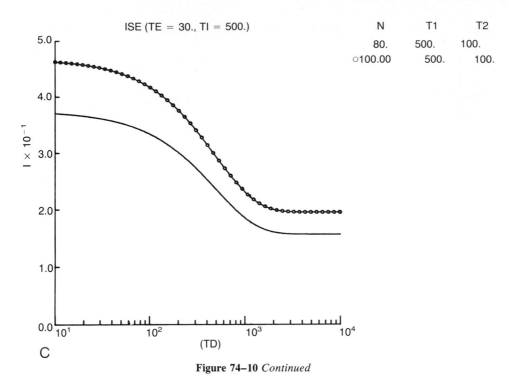

N	T1	T2
80.	500.	100.
○100.00	500.	100.

ISE (TE = 30., TI = 500.)

C

Figure 74–10 *Continued*

similarly, selecting a *TE* interval that falls on the steep portion of the *I* vs. *TE* graph (Fig. 74–2*B*) produces maximal contrast due to small changes in *T2*. Furthermore, selecting a *TI* interval on the steep portion of the *I* vs. *TI* graph (Fig. 74–10*B*) also enhances the contrast effects of small *T1* changes in the ISE sequence.

Spin-Echo Technique

BASIC SPIN-ECHO RELATIONSHIPS

Figures 74–4 to 74–6 demonstrate the effect on *I* of changes in each of the tissue parameters. In these graphs the hypothetical tissue parameter values listed in Table 74–5 were used to create a baseline curve, indicated by a solid line, that can be used as a reference point for observing the effects of independently changing *N*, *T1*, or *T2*. Intensity predictions for an altered hypothetical tissue are indicated on the graphs by a line with circles. Six basic relationships emerge from analysis of the image pixel intensity curves for the SE sequence:[20]

Relative Intensity

Maximal *I* in the SE sequence is produced when *TE* is short and *TR* is long, as demonstrated in Figures 74–2*B*, and 74–3*A*. This is due to the fact that transverse (*T2*) relaxation disperses the net magnetization vector in the *xy* plane, causing progressive diminution in *I* as *TE* increases relative to *T2*; on the other hand, longitudinal (*T1*) relaxation reestablishes the net magnetization vector, resulting in a progressive increase in *I* as *TR* lengthens compared to *T1*. Therefore, to get maximal *I*, one should minimize *T2* relaxation and maximize *T1* relaxation by using short *TE* and long *TR* intervals.

N Effects

Changes in *N* produce simple multiplicative changes in *I*. In Figure 74–4*A* and *B*, the non–baseline tissue has an *N* of 80 compared with the baseline *N* of 100. *T1* and

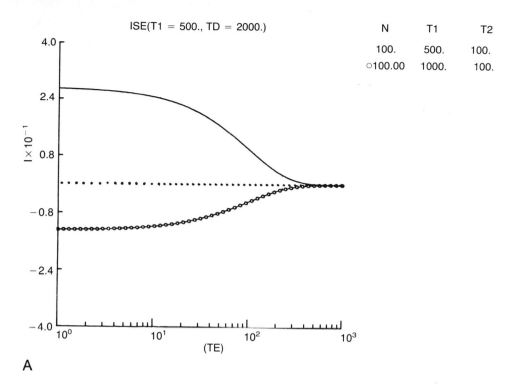

	N	T1	T2
	100.	500.	100.
○	100.00	1000.	100.

A

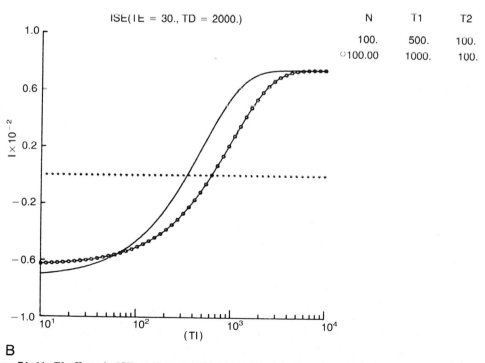

	N	T1	T2
	100.	500.	100.
○	100.00	1000.	100.

B

Figure 74–11. *T1* effects in ISE. *A*, I versus TE for two hypothetical tissues with different *T1* values using phase reconstruction. Note that the tissue with the greater *T1* value has a decreased maximum I, since less longitudinal relaxation is allowed to occur during the fixed *T1* and *TE* intervals. (*T1* = 500 ms and *TD* = 2000 ms.) *B*, I versus *T1* for two hypothetical tissues with different *T1* values using phase reconstruction. Note that an increase in *T1* shifts the curve and the zero intensity level to the right without changing the maximum intensity, since a longer *T1* requires a longer *T1* for an equivalent amount of longitudinal relaxation. (*TE* = 30 ms and *TD* = 2000 ms.)

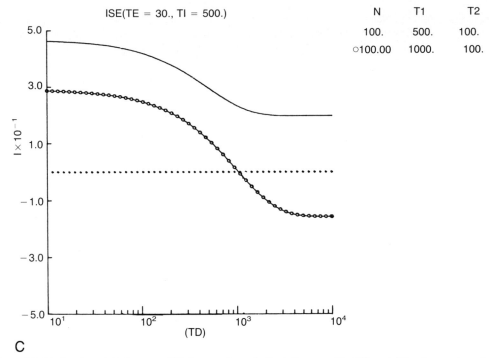

C

Figure 74–11 *Continued C,* I versus TD for two hypothetical tissues with different *T1* values using phase reconstruction. Note that an increase in *T1* decreases the maximum absolute intensity and decreases I for any given TD. (*TE* = 30 ms and *TI* = 500 ms.) (Solid line: *N* = 100; *T1* = 500 ms; *T2* = 100 ms. Open circles line: *N* = 100; *T1* = 1000 ms; *T2* = 100 ms.)

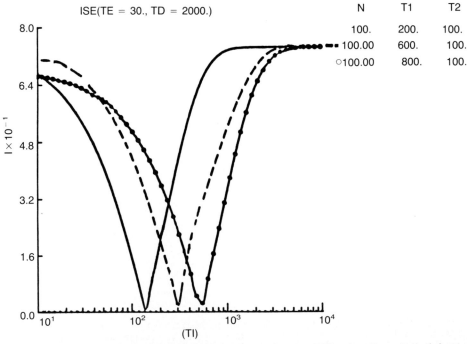

Figure 74–12. Magnitude reconstructed ISE pulse sequence. I versus TI for three hypothetical tissues with different *T1* values using magnitude reconstruction. Only the absolute value of image intensity is registered on the graph. The bounce-point occurs when *TI* = .693 × *T1* and therefore changes as T1 changes. (Solid line: *N* = 100; *T1* = 200 ms; *T2* = 100 ms. Dashed line: *N* = 100; *T1* = 600 ms; *T2* = 100 ms. Solid circles line: *N* = 100; *T1* = 800 ms; *T2* = 100 ms; *TE* = 30 ms; *TD* = 2000 ms.)

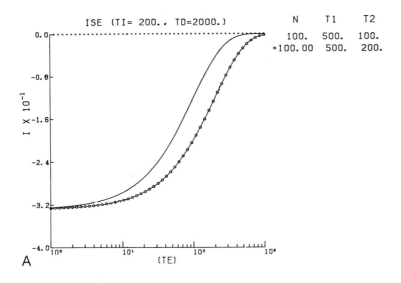

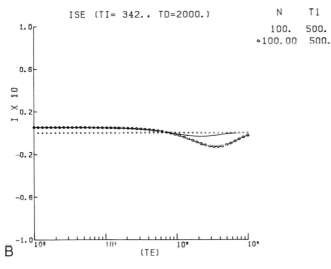

Figure 74–13. *T2* effects in ISE. *A*, I versus TE plot for two hypothetical tissues with different *T2* values. Increasing *T2* causes the image intensity curve to shift to the right, since a longer *T2* requires a longer TE for an equivalent amount of transverse relaxation. ($TE = 30$ ms and $TI = 200$ ms.) *B*, I versus TE plot for the same two hypothetical tissues with TI is increased to 342 ms. *C*, I versus TE plot for the same two hypothetical tissues with TI increased to 500 ms. Note that varying the TI interval changes the position of the graph in *A*, *B*, and *C*. When TI approaches .693 × *TI*, as in *B*, image intensity approaches zero for all TE values. When $TI <$ or $> 693 \times TI$, image intensity becomes negative, or positive, respectively. (Solid line: $N = 100$; $TI = 500$ ms; $T2 = 100$ ms. Open circles line: $N = 100$; $TI = 500$ ms; $T2 = 200$ ms.)

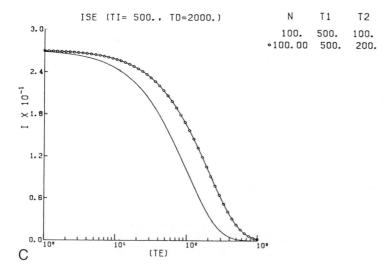

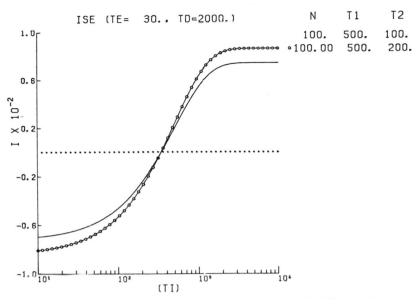

Figure 74–14. *T2* effects in ISE. I versus TI for two hypothetical tissues with different *T2* values. Note that increasing *T2* increases the maximum I, since less transverse relaxation occurs in the fixed TE interval. (Solid line: $N = 100$; $T1 = 500$ ms; $T2 = 100$ ms. Open circles line: $N = 100$; $T1 = 500$ ms; $T2 = 200$ ms. $TE = 30$ ms and $TD = 2000$ ms.)

T2 are the same for both tissues. This 20 percent decrease in *N* produces a uniform 20 percent decrease in *I* regardless of what timing intervals are used. The greatest absolute change in *I* occurs when *I* is maximal, however; therefore, maximum change in *I* due to a change in *N* will occur when *TE* is short and *TR* is long.

T1 Effects

Changes in *T1* produce varied effects on the intensity curves. In Figures 74–5A and *B*, the non–baseline tissue has a *T1* of 1000 ms, twice that of the baseline value, *N* and *T2* are the same for both tissues. On the *I* vs. *TE* plot (Fig. 74–5A), an increase in *T1* produces a decrease in *I* similar to that seen when *N* is diminished; this is due to the decrease in *T1* relaxation during the fixed *TR* interval.

On the *I* vs. *TR* plot (Fig. 74–5B), lengthening *T1* shifts the intensity curve to the right without changing the maximum intensity produced with a long *TR* interval. This is due to the fact that a longer *TR* interval is required to permit the same amount of *T1* relaxation.

T2 Effects

Changes in *T2* also have a variety of effects on *I*. In Fig. 74–6A and *B*, the non–baseline tissue has a *T2* of 200 ms, twice the baseline value; *N* and *T1* are the same for both tissues. Since *TR* is constant in the *I* vs. *TE* plot (Fig. 74–6A), the amount of *T1* relaxation is also constant. With very short *TE* intervals, that minimize *T2* relaxation, maximal *I* is not affected by changes in *T2*; therefore maximal *I* is unchanged on the *I* vs. *TE* plots. The curve is shifted to the right because longer *T2* values require longer *TE* intervals for an equivalent degree of *T2* relaxation. On the *I* vs. *TR* plot (Fig. 74–6B), an increase in *T2* produces an increase in *I* for all values of *TR*, similar to an increase in *N*. This is due to the fact that less transverse relaxation has occurred during the constant *TE* interval of 30 ms.

Rate of Change

The rate of change in *I* for a small percentage change in *T2* is maximal when *TE* = *T2* (Fig. 74–7A). Similarly, the greatest rate of change in *I* for a small percentage

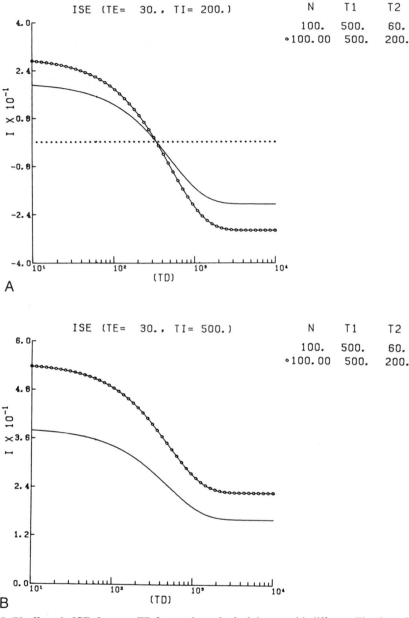

Figure 74–15. *T2* effects in ISE. I versus TD for two hypothetical tissues with different *T2* values. Note again that an increase in T2 increases the maximum I. *A*, *TI* = 200 ms. *B*, *TI* = 500 ms. (Solid line: *N* = 100; *T1* = 500 ms; *T2* = 60 ms. Open circles line: *N* = 100; *T1* = 500 ms; *T2* = 200 ms. *TE* = 30 ms.)

change in *T1* occurs when *TR* = *T1* (Fig. 74–7B). As *TR* and *TE* deviate from *T1* and *T2*, the rate of change in *I* for a given percentage change in *T1* or *T2* decreases significantly. When *T1* or *T2* are very long or very short compared to *TR* and *TE*, respectively, no significant change in *I* will be produced by a small change in these tissue parameters. Using these timing intervals makes the technique relatively insensitive to pathologic changes in *T1* or *T2* for the tissue of interest.

Signal-to-Noise

To maintain a good signal-to-noise ratio, avoid situations where *I* approaches 0, i.e., *TR* ≪ *T1* and/or *TE* ≫ *T2*.

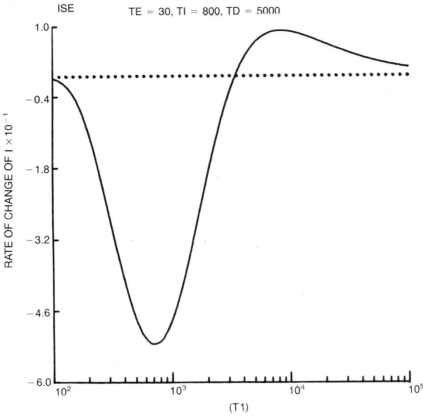

ISE   TE = 30, TI = 800, TD = 5000

Figure 74–16. Rate of change of I (*STI*) versus *TI* for ISE. *STI* is graphed as a function of *TI*. Note that the maximum *STI* occurs when *TI* = *TI*. A second peak, in the opposite direction, occurs when *TD* = *TI*. (*N* = 100; *T2* = 100 ms; *TE* = 30 ms; *TI* = 800 ms; and *TD* = 5000 ms.)

From the above discussions, it is obvious that changes in *N*, *T1*, and *T2* can produce a variety of changes in *I*. Therefore, one must use a variety of pulse sequences to deduce the appropriate cause and effect relationship. Fortunately, using imaging strategies that create images with a high degree of weighting for one parameter while minimizing weighting for other parameters can significantly simplify this deductive process. A method for selecting these selectively weighted sequences will be discussed below.

SPIN-ECHO PARAMETER SENSITIVITY EVALUATION

The parameter sensitivity evaluation is based on the idea that one can determine an optimal screening technique for a particular clinical situation by selecting a normal tissue of interest with known *T1* and *T2* values that is likely to contain the pathologic changes sought. Timing interval selection is designed to maximize image sensitivity to subtle deviations from normal in that tissue. Isocontour plots of the previously described parameter sensitivity terms, *SN*, *ST1*, and *ST2* (Fig. 74–8), permit visual evaluation of the interdependent effects of *TE* and *TR* on tissue parameter weighting for all combinations of timing intervals. Overlaying the plots for all three parameter sensitivity terms (Fig. 74–9) illustrates the synergistic effects of *N* and *T2* and the competitive effects of *T1* with *N* and *T2*. On these plots, the isocontour lines indicate the relative change in the parameter sensitivity value being graphed like hills or valleys on a topographic map. The highest sensitivity on the plot has been set to 100. Solid lines represent positive sensitivity parameter values while dashed lines represent negative

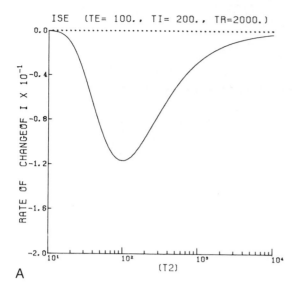

A

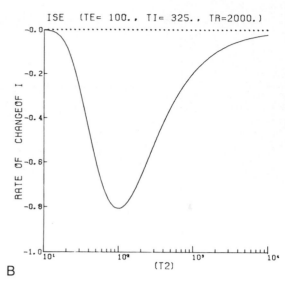

B

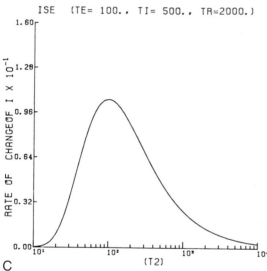

C

Figure 74–17. Rate of change of I (*ST2*) versus *TI* for ISE. *A*, *ST2* is graphed as a function of *T2* with *TI* = 200 ms. Note that maximum *ST2* occurs when *TE* = *T2*. *B*, The same graph with *TI* = 325 ms. Note that the peak ST2 has become less negative and approaches zero as TI approaches .693 × *TI*. *C*, The same graph with *TI* = 500 ms. Note that the peak *ST2* becomes positive as *TI* > .693 × *TI*. Note the different *y* axis scales in the three graphs. (*N* = 100 and *TI* = 500 ms. *TE* = 30 ms; *TI* = 200 ms; and *TR* = 2000 ms.).

values. Large positive or negative parameter sensitivity values indicate timing interval combinations where small changes in the tissue parameter should result in a relatively large percentage change in *I* compared to all other timing interval combinations on the plot. These combinations produce images with maximal weighting for that tissue parameter.

N, *T1*, and *T2* Sensitivity

On the sensitivity plots *SN* is maximal when *TE* ≪ *T2*, and *TR* ≫ *TI* (Fig. 74–8*A*), *ST1* is maximal when *TE* ≪ *T2* and *TR* = *TI* (Fig. 74–8*B*), and *ST2* is maximal when *TE* = *T2* and *TR* ≫ *TI* (Fig. 74–8*C*). Therefore, *TE* ≪ *T2* and *TR* ≫ *TI*, *TE* ≪ *T2* and *TR* = *TI*, and *TE* = *T2* and *TR* ≫ *TI* are combinations that produce good *N*, *T1*, and *T2* weighting, respectively. Unfortunately, looking at the isolated effects of different weighting factors is not enough; the interactions between *N*, *T1*, and *T2* must also be considered.

In most pathologic processes involving tissues with a predominance of water protons, *N*, *T1*, and *T2* generally move in the same direction.[21–24] A few exceptions to this rule include tissues with a significant contribution from lipid protons[21] and tissues

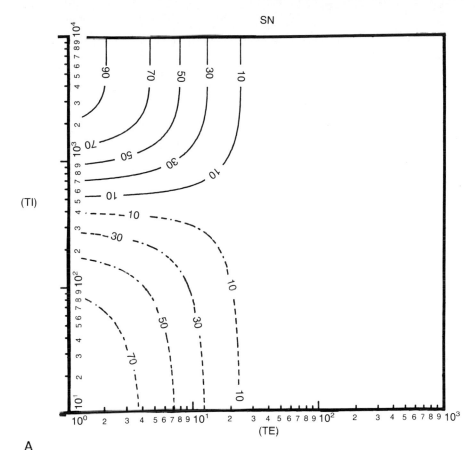

A

Figure 74–18. ISE parameter sensitivity plots for *N*. Using WM tissue parameter values, SN is plotted for (*A*) all combinations of TE and TI.

Illustration continued on following page

with paramagnetic effects such as hemolyzed blood.[25] Because of this general concordance in tissue parameter changes, and because an increase in *T1* causes a decrease in *I* while an increase in *N* or *T2* causes an increase in *I*, the effects of *T1* tend to counteract the effects of *N* and *T2* in many imaging situations.

Sensitivity Interactions

ST1 is negative for all combinations of *TE* and *TR*. This indicates that increasing *T1* in SE images always decreases *I*. *SN* and *ST2* are always positive, indicating that an increase in *N* or *T2* in SE images always increases *I*. Consequently, when all three tissue parameters move in the same direction, *T1* effects compete with *N* and *T2* effects. Superimposing the graphs of *SN*, *ST1*, and *ST2* on a single plot demonstrates the competitive effect of these sensitivities (Fig. 74–9). In regions where a high degree of sensitivity exists for more than one tissue parameter, the sensitivities complement each other if they are of similar sign and oppose each other if they are of opposite sign. The overlapping positive values of *SN* and *ST2* on the top of the plot indicate that *N* and *T2* effects are additive when *TR* is long; the overlapping negative *ST1* and positive *SN* and *ST2* isocontour lines at the left margin of the plot indicate the presence of competition between *T1* effects and *N* and *T2* effects that decreases the contrast due to *T1* changes.

Because of this competition, the spin-echo technique is not particularly efficient in obtaining *T1* weighted images unless *TE* is significantly less than the shortest *T2* of interest; if this condition is met, the SE sequence approximates the PS sequence, which

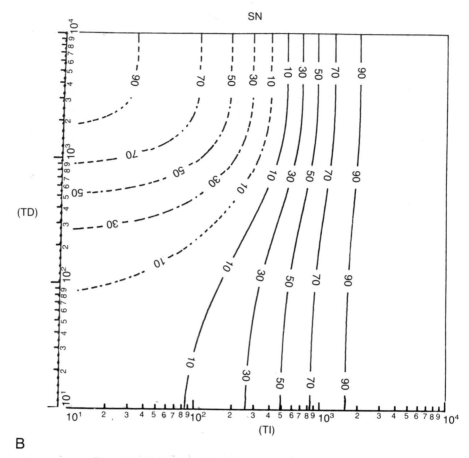

B

Figure 74–18 *Continued* (*B*) all combinations of TI and TD.

has no *T2* dependence; *T1* effects must still compete with *N* effects, however. Unfortunately, the commonly used *TE* values of 28 to 32 ms are usually not short enough to fulfill these criteria. Therefore, in most situations the SE sequence is not an optimal method for obtaining images with a high degree of *T1* weighting unless some form of image post-processing is used to eliminate or reverse this competition or short *TE*'s become more readily available. Techniques for improving *T1* weighting, including ratio and difference images, are promising. Unfortunately, these post-processing techniques are not presently available on standard instrumentation; they also tend to compound the noise in the images.[26]

In comparison, SE is excellent for obtaining *N* and *T2* contrast using long *TR* intervals that eliminate the competitive effects of *T1* for most normal tissues. The reader should be cautioned, however, that many pathologic processes have *T1* values that are longer than those found with normal tissues. If *T1* gets long enough, the *TR* interval is no longer ≫*T1* and *T1* again competes with *N* and *T2*. Cerebrospinal fluid (CSF) is a good example of this effect. Although an SE 60/2000 is a relatively *N* and *T2* weighted sequence for normal brain substance with *T1* and *T2* values of approximately 500 and 90 ms, respectively, it is a relatively *T1* weighted sequence for CSF that has *T1* and *T2* values closer to 2000 and 200 ms, respectively. That is why CSF does not appear white on a *T2* weighted SE 60/2000 sequence in spite of its very long *T2*; its long *T1* effectively competes with *T2* because the sequence has considerable *T1* weighting for a tissue with a *T1* of 2000 to 3000 ms. Therefore, the relative *N*, *T1*, or *T2* weighting of a particular imaging sequence is dependent upon the particular tissue being evaluated.

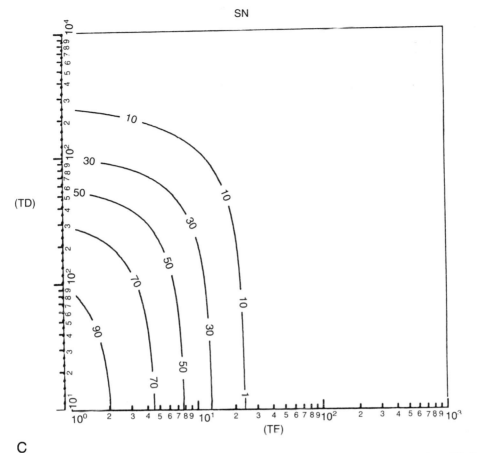

C

Figure 74–18 *Continued* (C) all combinations of TE and TD. Note that SN is maximal when *TI* ≪ *T1*, *TD* ≫ *T1*, and *TE* ≪ *T2*, or when *TI* ≫ *T1*, *TD* ≪ *T1*, and *TE* ≪ *T2*.

Using SE for *T1* weighting is also limited by the fact that short *TR* intervals can decrease the signal-to-noise (S:N) ratio considerably, requiring signal averaging or systems that have a high inherent S:N ratio. Short *TR* intervals also limit the number of slices that can be obtained in a multislice acquisition. In contrast, the long *TR* intervals used for *N* and *T2* weighting improve S:N and allow ample time for multislice-multiecho techniques. Short *TR* sequences do provide excellent contrast in situations in which *T1* decreases while *N* and *T2* stay the same or increase (hemorrhage, for example) since the tissue changes are inherently complementary in this situation.

Since competition between the tissue parameters can totally cancel the expected changes in *I* needed to produce image contrast, timing interval combinations should be selected so that they are relatively sensitive to complementary tissue parameters and insensitive to competing parameters. Thus, isolating the effects of *N* and *T2* from the effects of *T1* is one of the major objectives in SE technique selection.

GUIDELINES FOR SPIN-ECHO TECHNIQUE SELECTION

From the preceding discussion, the following guidelines can be stated for the SE sequence:
1. Use *TE* to control *T2* dependence.
2. Use *TR* to control *T1* dependence.
3. *T1* effects compete with *N* and *T2* effects.

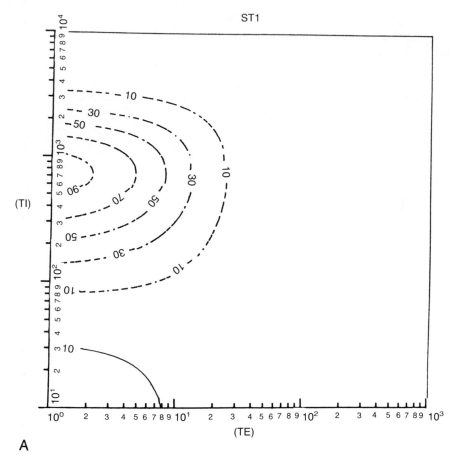

A

Figure 74–19. ISE parameter sensitivity plots for *T1*. Using WM tissue parameter values, *ST1* is plotted for (*A*) all combinations of TE and TI.

4. Using the *T1* and *T2* of a normal target tissue:
   a. Set *TE* ≪ *T2* and *TR* ≫ *T1* for maximal intensity and maximal *N* weighting.
   b. Set *TE* = *T2* and *TR* ≫ *T1* for maximal *T2* weighting.
   c. Set *TE* ≪ *T2* and *TR* = *T1* for maximal *T1* weighting.

Inverted Spin-Echo Technique

The ISE sequence is essentially a 180 degree inverting pulse followed by a spin-echo sequence; therefore, many of the relationships in ISE are similar to SE. The interaction of these effects can produce some unexpected results, including the potential for reversing the competitive effects of *T1* and *T2*, so that *N*, *T1*, and *T2* effects add together.

Magnitude Versus Phase Reconstruction

The negative signal produced by the ISE technique can be handled in one of two ways. The mathematical sign of the intensity can be retained, using "phase reconstruction," permitting both positive and negative image pixel intensity values, or the negative sign can be dropped, using "magnitude reconstruction" that employs the absolute magnitude of *I* to assign image pixel intensities. (Some manufacturers have

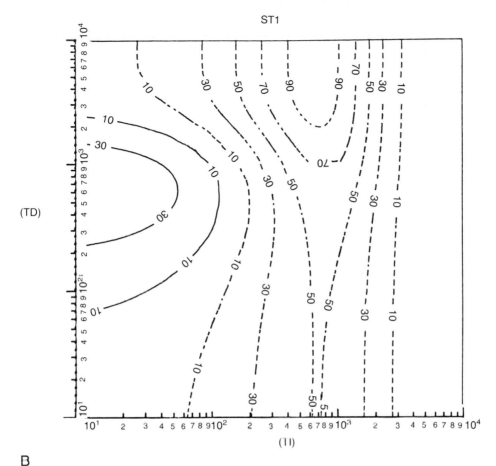

B

Figure 74–19 *Continued* (*B*) all combinations of TI and TD.

Illustration continued on following page

also assigned all negative values to zero; this option will not be discussed here.) These two methods produce markedly different results; therefore, the availability and selection of the reconstruction mode greatly influence ISE timing interval selection.

Phase reconstructed images usually have some tissues with long *T1* values, such as CSF, that have negative intensities; these tissues appear "blacker" than the surrounding air, which is set to zero. Other tissues with shorter *T1*'s will be brighter than the background. As one can see on the *I* vs. *TI* plots (Figs. 74–10*A* and 74–11*B*), using both positive and negative intensities doubles the dynamic range for variation in *I* compared to magnitude reconstruction where the negative values would be inverted (Fig. 74–12). This increased dynamic range is one of the main factors contributing to the high degree of *T1* sensitivity in the ISE technique.

Magnitude reconstruction assigns pixel values on the basis of magnitude only. This can produce a considerable amount of confusion by making the intensity of tissues with long and short *T1* values the same (Fig. 74–12). It also produces a "bounce-point" artifact, since $I = 0$ whenever $TI = 0.693 \times T1$ and $TD \gg T1$ of a tissue. One then has the peculiar situation of observing an increase in *I* as *T1* becomes either longer or shorter than the bounce-point value. Although the bounce-point artifact can be avoided by setting *TI* > the longest *T1* of the tissues of interest, the resulting image has less *T1* weighting and lacks some of the advantages of the ISE pulse sequence. In addition, the potential for additive tissue parameter effects, which will be discussed subsequently, is eliminated by the use of long *TI* intervals. Magnitude reconstruction also uses only

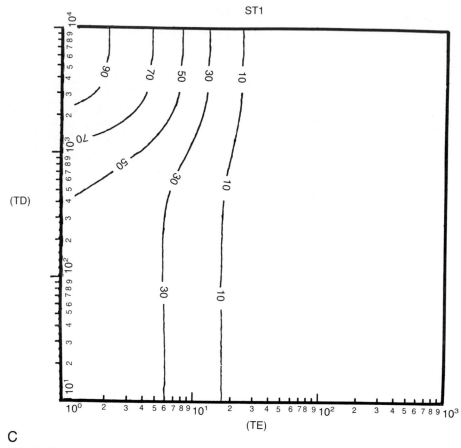

C

Figure 74–19 *Continued* (*C*) all combinations of TE and TD. Note that *STI* is maximal when *TI* = *T1*, *TD* ≫ *T1*, and *TE* ≪ *T2*.

one-half of the dynamic range available with phase reconstruction. In spite of these limitations, magnitude reconstruction may be the only method available for ISE on some scanning units. Used properly, magnitude reconstruction can produce valuable results, as will be explained subsequently. In summary:

Phase Reconstruction
1. *I* = 0 when *TI* = 0.693 × *T1* (*T1* = 1.44 × *TI*), and *TD* ≫ *T1*.
2. *I* > 0 when *TI* > 0.693 × *T1* (*T1* < 1.44 × *TI*) and *TD* ≫ *T1*.
3. *I* < 0 when *TI* < 0.693 × *T1* (*T1* > 1.44 × *TI*) and *TD* ≫ *T1*.
4. When *TD* is not ≫ *T1*, *I* = 0 at varying combinations of *TI* and *TD* even when *TI* < 0.693 × *T1*.

Magnitude Reconstruction
1. *I* is always positive.
2. Bounce-point artifact occurs when *TI* = 0.693 × *T1* (*T1* = 1.44 × *TI*), and *TD* ≫ *T1*. (Bounce-point artifact occurs at shorter *TI* values when *TD* is not ≫ *T1*.)
3. Uses one-half the potential dynamic range of phase reconstruction.

BASIC INVERTED SPIN-ECHO RELATIONSHIPS

Several basic relationships emerge from analysis of the ISE image intensity curves.
Relative Intensity
Maximum positive *I* occurs when *TI* is long and *TE* and *TD* are short. Maximum negative *I* occurs when *TD* is long and *TE* and *TI* are very short (Figs. 74–10*A*, *B*, and

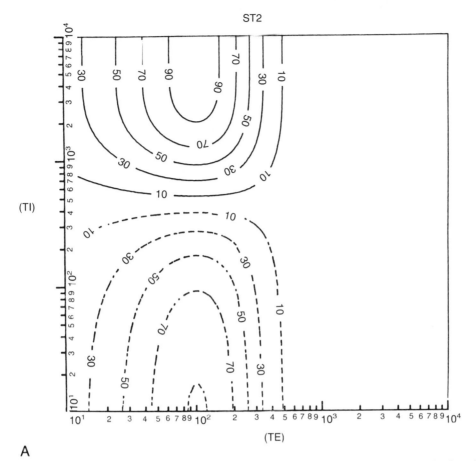

A

Figure 74–20. ISE parameter sensitivity plots for *T2*. Using WM tissue parameter values, *STI* is plotted for (*A*) all combinations of TE and TI.

Illustration continued on following page

C). Both of these situations produce images that are relatively independent of *TI* and *T2* effects due to the fact that long *TI* and *TD* intervals permit complete longitudinal relaxation, while a short *TE* minimizes transverse relaxation. A very short *TI* produces maximal negative *I* because the net magnetization vector is maximally negative immediately after the initial 180 degree pulse; if *TI* is short, the 90 degree read-out pulse measures this large negative vector before longitudinal relaxation can decrease its magnitude.

N Effects

A change in *N* produces a simple multiplicative change in *I* just as it does in the SE sequence. Consequently, differences due to *N* are proportional to the magnitude of *I* and are therefore maximal when *I* is maximal as described above (Figs. 75–10*A*, *B*, and *C*). If *N* increases, the absolute value of *I* increases; with phase reconstruction, if *I* is negative it becomes more negative; if *I* is positive it becomes more positive.

T1 Effects

Changes in *T1* produce a variety of effects (Fig. 74–11*A*, *B*, and *C*). On the *I* vs. *TI* plot (Fig. 74–11*B*), an increase in *T1* shifts the curve and the bounce-point artifact to the right without changing the absolute maximum intensity, since a longer *T1* requires a longer *TI* for an equivalent amount of longitudinal relaxation. On the *I* vs. *TE* plot (Fig. 74–11*A*), increasing *T1* decreases the maximum *I* obtained since less longitudinal relaxation occurs during the fixed *TI* and *TD* intervals.

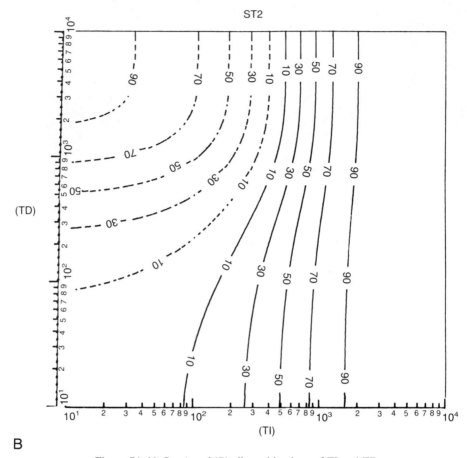

Figure 74–20 *Continued* (*B*) all combinations of TI and TD.

T2 **Effects**

Changes in *T2* also have characteristic effects on the intensity plots (Figs. 74–13*A*, 74–14, and 74–15*A*). On the *I* vs. *TE* plot (Fig. 74–13*A*), increasing *T2* shifts the curve to the right because a longer *T2* requires a longer *TE* for the same amount of transverse relaxation. Similarly, on the *I* vs. *TI* (Fig. 74–14) and *I* vs. *TD* plots (Fig. 74–15*A*), increasing *T2* simply increases the maximum *I*, since less transverse relaxation occurs during the fixed *TE* interval.

Rate of Change

The rate of change in *I* due to a small change in *TI* (Fig. 74–16) is greatest when *TI* = *T1*. It also reaches a peak of less magnitude when *TD* = *T1*. Since these two maxima are of opposite sign they compete; therefore they cannot be used synergistically. Consequently, *TD* should not be used to control *T1* dependence in the ISE sequence.

The rate of change in *I* due to a small change in *T2* (Figs. 74–17*A*, *B* and *C*) is maximal when *T2* = *TE*. This rate of change decreases as *T2* becomes larger or smaller than *TE*. This maximal rate of change is best appreciated when *TI* and *TD* are set to maximize *I*. If *I* is close to zero (for example, when *TI* = 0.693 × *T1*, and *TD* ≫ *T1*), the change in *I* will be small since *I* is small. The change is positive when *I* is positive with either phase or magnitude reconstruction, meaning that an increase in *T2* produces an increase in *I*. It is negative with phase reconstruction and positive with magnitude reconstruction when *I* is negative, however.

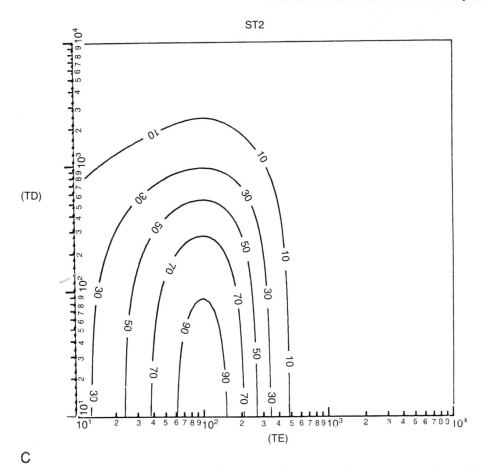

C

Figure 74–20 *Continued* (*C*) all combinations of TE and TD. Note that *ST2* is maximal when *TE* = *T2* and either *TI* ≪ *T1* and *TD* ≫ *T1* or *TI* ≫ *T1* and *TD* ≪ *T1*.

Reversing the Competition Between *N*, *T1* and *T2*

When *TI* < 0.693 × *T1* and *TD* ≫ *T1*, increasing *N*, *T1*, or *T2* with phase reconstruction produces a more negative *I*; magnitude reconstruction reverses this situation, producing a more positive *I*. In either case, the usual competition between *T1* and *T2* has been reversed and the effects of all three parameters will be synergistic if the tissue parameters change in the same direction.

Both reconstruction techniques provide the same basic information when *TI* < 0.693 × the shortest *T1*, and *TD* > the longest *T1* of the tissues of interest. Magnitude reconstruction may be easier to perform, and makes the pathologic changes appear as areas of increased signal intensity rather than decreased signal intensity when a short *TI* is used; this is usually preferred by clinicians. It has some limitations, however. Although a short *TI* generally eliminates bounce-point artifacts with magnitude reconstruction, if a pathologic tissue such as a resolving hematoma has a *T1* that is shorter than 1.44 × *TI*, a bounce-point artifact will surround this structure. Therefore, if phase reconstruction can be performed efficiently, it may be preferable to use phase reconstruction with a video reversal that would make the pathological lesions white but completely eliminate bounce-point artifacts.

Signal-to-Noise

To maintain a good signal-to-noise ratio, avoid situations where *I* approaches zero, i.e., *TI* = 0.693 × *T1* and *TD* ≫ *T1*, *TE* ≫ *T2*, and certain combinations of *TI* and *TD*

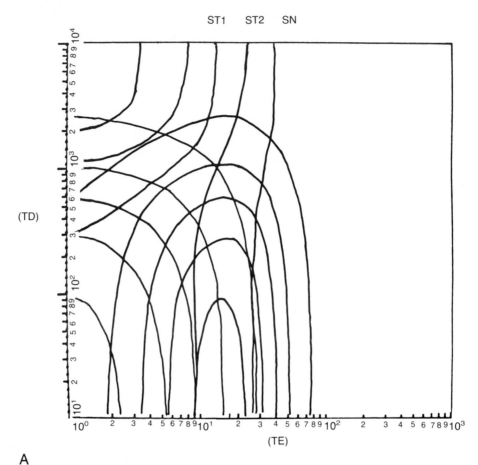

ST1   ST2   SN

(TD)

(TE)

A

Figure 74–21. Combined ISE parameter sensitivity plots. Overlayed SN, ST1, and ST2 plots for (A) all combinations of TE and TI.

when $TI < 0.693 \times T1$ and TD is not $\gg T1$. An exception to this rule is the use of short TI intervals with TI set approximately equal to $0.693 \times$ the $T1$ of fat. This sequence effectively cancels the image signal intensity of fat and is a useful adjustment for imaging the retroperitoneum, the pelvis, and the spinal column, since the abundance of fat in these areas can obscure pathological changes.[27–29]

INVERTED SPIN-ECHO PARAMETER SENSITIVITY EVALUATION

The "parameter sensitivity" plots demonstrate the interaction between pairs of timing intervals and the complementary or competitive effects of the tissue parameters. The following discussion assumes the use of phase reconstruction. When magnitude reconstruction is used, some negative parameter sensitivity values may become positive. Positive and negative sensitivity values indicate that I increases or decreases, respectively, as the plotted tissue parameter value increases.

N Sensitivity

Figures 74–18A, B and C demonstrate that SN is maximally negative when $TI \ll T1$, $TE \ll T2$ and $TD \gg T1$; SN is maximally positive when $TI \gg T1$, $TE \ll T2$, and $TD \ll T1$ (actually, TD can be almost any value when $TI \gg T1$ but there is a slight improvement in SN with shorter TD intervals). These combinations of timing intervals also produce maximum I, since the distribution of SN matches the distribution of rela-

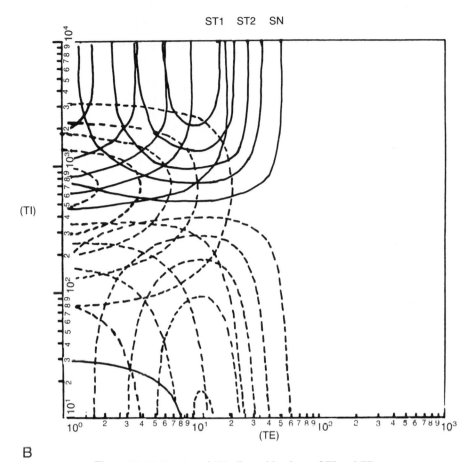

B

Figure 74–21 *Continued* (*B*) all combinations of TI and TD.

Illustration continued on following page

tive *I* for all timing interval combinations. SN is positive when *I* is positive and negative when *I* is negative.

T1 Sensitivity

Similarly, maximum *ST1* (Figs. 74–19*A*, *B* and *C*) occurs when *TI* = *T1*, *TD* ≫ *T1*, and *TE* ≪ *T2*. There is also a local maxima when *TD* = *T1*, and *TI* ≪ *T1*; the magnitude of *ST1* in this situation is significantly smaller than the maxima at *TI* = *T1*. This smaller maxima is due to spin-echo effects and moves *I* in the opposite direction from the larger maxima due to the inversion; therefore, these two *T1* maxima cannot be used in an additive manner and the spin-echo *T1* effect is probably not useful in ISE and will not be discussed further.

T2 Sensitivity

Maximal *ST2* (Figs. 74–20*A*, *B* and *C*) is observed when *TE* = *T2* and one of the following two conditions is met: *TI* ≪ *T1* and *TD* ≫ *T1* or *TI* ≫ *T1* and *TD* ≪ *T1* (again, when *TI* ≫ *T1*, the exact value of *TD* makes little difference, although shorter values yield slightly higher sensitivities). As with SN, *ST2* is positive when *I* is positive and negative when *I* is negative.

Sensitivity Interactions

Overlaying the ISE plots of SN, *ST1*, and *ST2* demonstrates the varied competitive or complementary effects of *N*, *T1*, and *T2* for varying combinations of *TI*, *TE*, and *TD* (Figs. 74–21*A*, *BB*, and *C*). Areas where the parameter sensitivity values are of opposite sign (mixed solid and dashed lines) are areas where the sensitivities compete if *N*, *T1*, and *T2* are moving in the same direction; this competition dampens the change

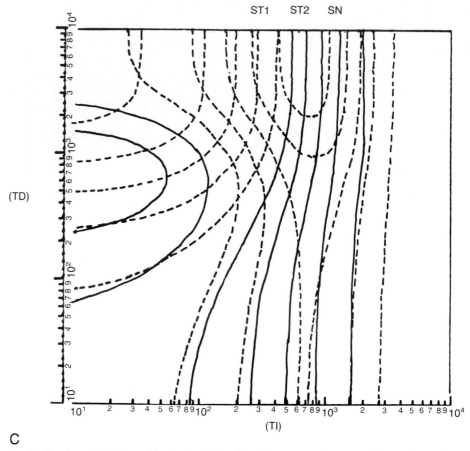

C

Figure 74–21 *Continued* (*C*) all combinations of TE and TI demonstrate the competitive and complementary effects between all three tissue parameters (regions with both solid and dashed lines indicate competition; areas with only solid or dashed lines indicate synergism.)

in *I* expected from an isolated change in one of the tissue parameters. Similarly, areas with all positive or all negative sensitivities indicate timing interval combinations where the effects of *N*, *T1*, and *T2* complement one another.

The plots demonstrate that SN, *ST1*, and *ST2* complement each other when *TI* < .693 × *T1*, *TD* ≫ *T1*, and *TE* < *T2*. If *TI* is kept below approximately 70 percent of the shortest *T1* of interest (white matter in the brain, for instance), all of the signal intensities will be negative. Under this condition, an increase in *N*, *T1*, or *T2* will produce a decrease in *I*. This allows the usually competing tissue parameter effects to act synergistically on *I*, creating a sequence with improved sensitivity to pathologic changes as long as *N*, *T1*, and *T2* move in the same direction and the signal-to-noise ratio is adequate.

Although both the phase and magnitude reconstruction techniques with *TI* < .693 × the shortest *T1* of interest produce an additive effect of SN, *ST1*, and *ST2*, it should be noted that *N*, *T1*, and *T2* effects are only synergistic when *N*, *T1*, and *T2* move in a parallel fashion. Although this is usually the case, some pathologic processes do not obey this generalization; a fatty tumor, for instance, may have an increase in *N* with a decrease in *T1*.[21] For an expected nonparallel change in tissue parameters, an ISE sequence with *TI* > *T1* or a *T2* weighted SE sequence would be better suited.

In summary, ISE has excellent *T1* sensitivity with phase reconstruction and the appropriate timing intervals; the signal-to-noise ratio can be a problem when *TI* = *T1*,

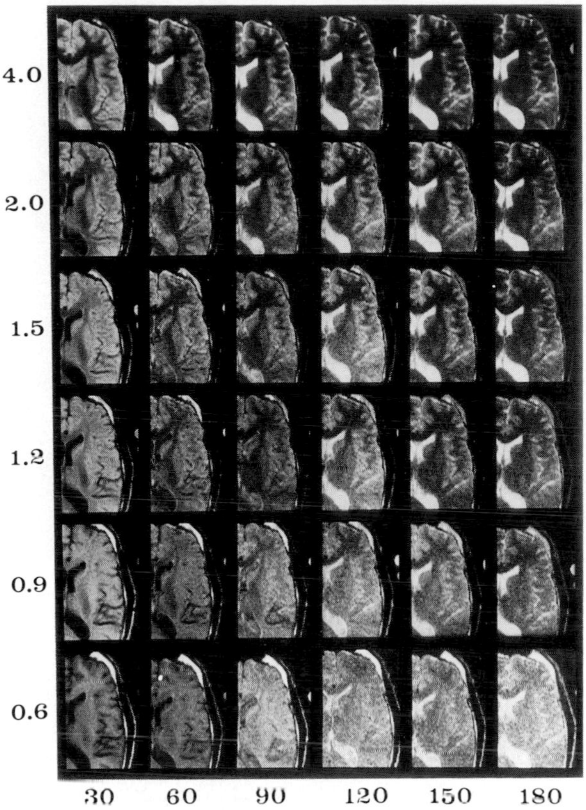

4.0

2.0

1.5

1.2

0.9

0.6

30 60 90 120 150 180

Figure 74–22. Multiecho SE image matrix. Images in a normal volunteer using the TE values indicated in milliseconds along the bottom of the matrix and the TR values indicated in seconds along the left-hand side of the matrix. Window setting 440, center varied. (From Mitchell MR et al.: RadioGraphics 56:255, 1986. Used by permission.)

however, since the increase in TI seen in many lesions may make TI close to 1.44 × TI where I is near zero. Additive N, $T1$, and $T2$ effects can be produced using a short TI; this makes ISE highly sensitive to parallel tissue parameter changes. Although ISE can be used to obtain N and $T2$ information, it has no inherent advantage over SE in this regard, and requires additional acquisition time. If the sequence is being used for

30/315   30/2000

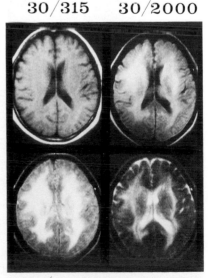

90/2000   240/2000

Figure 74–23. White matter disease using the SE pulse sequence. Images with timing intervals as indicated. Note that the white matter changes are not seen on the SE 30/315 image and are most evident on the ME 90/2000 image (see text for discussion). (From Mitchell MR et al.: RadioGraphics 6:257, 1986. Used by permission.)

45/1000   **90/1000**

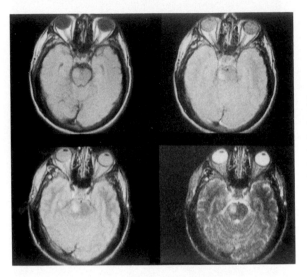

Figure 74–24. Brainstem infarct: Comparison of long and short TR intervals for the SE pulse sequence. Image matrix in a patient with a brainstem infarct. Note the increased image contrast on the long TR images (*bottom row*) as compared to the shorter TR images (*top row*). (*Top row, TR* = 1000 ms. *Bottom row, TR* = 2000 ms. TE as indicated. Window is set at 450 for all of the images; center is varied.)

90/2000   **210/2000**

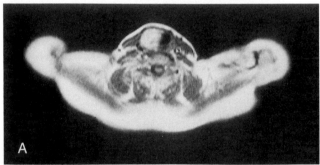

A

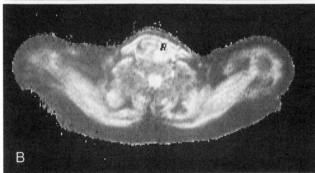

B

Figure 74–25. Metastatic melanoma of the thyroid using the SE pulse sequence. *A, T1* weighted 30/500 image. The lesion is seen as an area of increased signal intensity and appears to have a short *T1* using this *T1* weighted timing interval. *B,* Calculated *T1* (Technicare observed OT1) image. Note that the approximate *T1* of the lesion is greater than fat and is similar to muscle *T1* values. *C,* Calculated spin density image. Note that most of the increased signal intensity caused by the lesion is due to an increase in *N.*

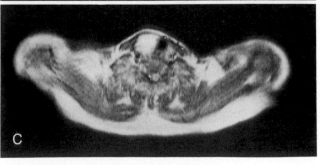

C

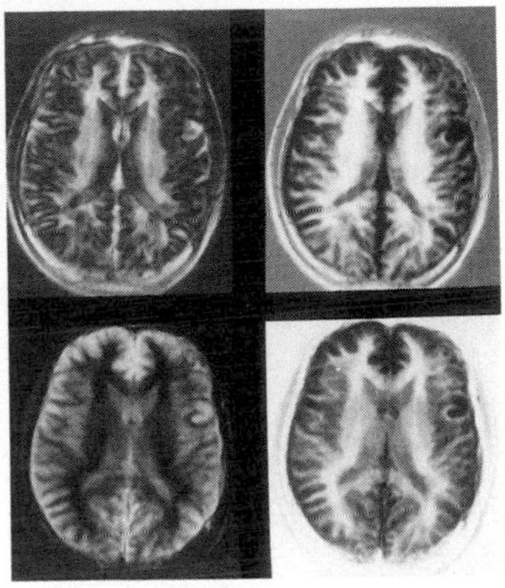

MAGNITUDE   PHASE

450/30/2450

250/30/2250

Figure 74–26. Phase and magnitude reconstruction ISE image matrix. Image matrix for a normal volunteer using phase and magnitude reconstructed ISE. TE, TI, and TR intervals for each horizontal row are as indicated. Magnitude reconstructed images are to the left in the matrix, and phase reconstructed images are to the right. (Window is set at 450 for all images, and the center is varied.)

its *T1* sensitivity, however, *T2* information can still be gleaned by using a multiecho technique with ISE; the signal-to-noise ratio in the later echos may be relatively poor, however.

Guidelines for Inverted Spin-Echo Technique Selection

ISE image contrast can be either enhanced or degraded by the selection of timing intervals. To select these intervals appropriately, the MRI practitioner must select a tissue of interest with known *T1* and *T2* values. Using this tissue as a target, the timing intervals are adjusted to maximize the signal intensity and minimize or reverse competition between the tissue parameters.

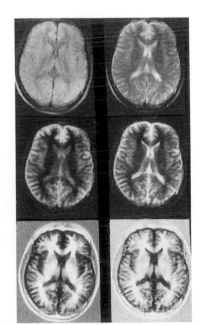

30   120

SE

2000

ISE

magnitude   250/2250

ISE

phase   450/2450

Figure 74–27. Image matrix for comparison of ME with optimized phase and magnitude reconstructed IME images. ME, magnitude reconstructed IME, and phase reconstructed IME image matrix from a normal volunteer. *Top row,* ME images. *Middle row,* Magnitude reconstructed IME images. *Bottom row,* Phase reconstructed IME images. TE intervals are indicated above each longitudinal row. TR and TI/TR intervals are indicated beside each horizontal row. Window is wet at 450, and center is varied for each image. *Top row,* Contrast in the ME images is due to additive *N* and *T2* effects. *Middle row,* Additive effects of all three tissue parameters contribute to image contrast when using optimized magnitude reconstructed IME technique. *Bottom row,* Most of the contrast is due to *T1* effects in optimized phase reconstructed IME images.

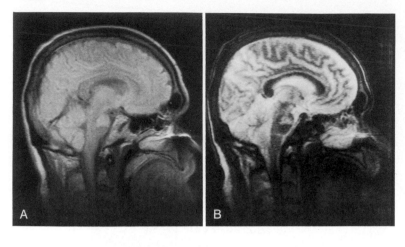

Figure 74–28. Brainstem infarct: Comparison of SE and magnitude reconstructed ISE. *A*, SE 30/2000 image. Note the suboptimal contrast between the lesion and the remaining brainstem on this relatively *N* weighted sequence. *B*, Magnitude reconstructed ISE 30/250/2250 image. Note the good image contrast due to the additive *N*, *T1*, and *T2* effects. The *T2* weighting is the same for both images. Window 450 for both images.

The following guidelines, summarized from the above description, should lead one in the proper direction in this selection process.

1. Use *TI* to control *T1* dependence.
2. Use *TE* to control *T2* dependence.
3. For the best *T1* weighting, use phase reconstruction with $TI = T1$, $TE \ll T2$, and $TD \gg T1$.
4. To avoid a bounce-point artifact when using magnitude reconstruction, keep $TI < 0.693$ times the shortest *T1* and $TD \gg$ the longest *T1* of any tissue in the region to be evaluated, or keep $TI > 0.693 \times$ the longest *T1*.
5. To reverse the normal competition between tissue parameters, set $TI < T1$, $TE < T2$, and $TD \gg T1$.
   a. If magnitude reconstruction is used, recognize that a bounce-point artifact will occur and confusing intensities will result if the pathologic process has a $T1 < 1.44 \times TI$.
   b. If phase reconstruction is used, realize that the desired complementary effects of tissue parameter changes become competitive if the pathologic $T1 < 1.44 \times TI$.

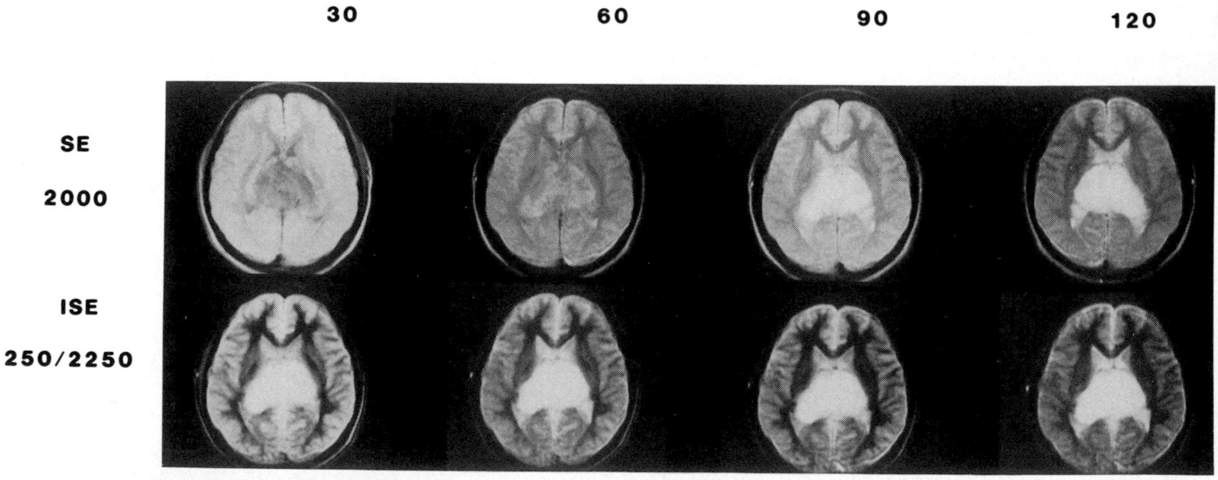

Figure 74–29. Subarachnoid cyst: Comparison of ME and magnitude reconstructed IME. Image matrix using ME and magnitude reconstructed IME pulse sequences. SE images are on the top row of the matrix; magnitude reconstructed IME images are on the bottom row. TE intervals are indicated above each longitudinal row. TR and TI/TR intervals are indicated adjacent to each horizontal row. Note the increased image contrast of the magnitude reconstructed IME images as compared to the ME images owing to the added *T1* effects. Window 450 for all images, center varied.

    c. Using this interval selection technique, the effects of tissue parameter changes are only additive when N, $T1$, and $T2$ all move in the same direction.

6. For maximal I and SN, set $TE \ll T2$ with $TI \ll T1$ and $TD \ll T1$ or $TI \gg T1$ and $TD \ll T1$.

7. For maximal $T2$ weighting, set $TE = T2$ with $TI \ll T1$ and $TD \gg T1$ or $TI \gg T1$ and $TD \ll T1$.

IMAGING EXAMPLES

An MRI image can be described as being N, $T1$, or $T2$ weighted on the basis of the expected change in I due to a small percentage change in each of the tissue parameters. The weighting for a particular technique indicates the relative sensitivity of the sequence compared to the other pulse sequence timing interval combinations that could be used. These descriptions are generalities, however, that are only accurate for tissues with a narrow range of $T1$ and $T2$ values close to those of the principal tissue of interest.

For example, an SE 30/2000 sequence is heavily N weighted for gray and white matter in a 0.5 tesla system where the $T1$ of these tissues is less than 500 to 600 ms and $T2$ is approximately 100 ms, making $TR \gg T1$, and $TE < T2$. A shorter TE, making $TE \ll T2$, would eliminate some of the $T2$ weight that is still present. If cerebrospinal fluid is considered the tissue of interest, however, the SE 30/2000 sequence should be considered $T1$ weighted since the $T1$ and $T2$ of cerebrospinal fluid are approximately 2000 to 3000 ms and 200 to 400 ms, respectively, making the TR approximately equal to $T1$ and $TE \ll T2$. Consequently, when talking about relative tissue parameter weighting for different MR techniques, it is necessary to keep in mind the relationship between the tissue parameter values and timing intervals that maintain that weighting description; as different tissues are considered, the relative weighting changes.

In most clinical situations the relative weighting of the images is not as clear cut as the above example; the differences in N, $T1$, and $T2$ between different tissues and between normal and pathologic tissues are usually more subtle than between brain matter and cerebrospinal and one must take into account both the relative weighting and competition between the different tissues. Still, this preliminary assignment of relative weighting for a tissue of interest is very helpful in setting up and discussing the image characteristics, and provides a basis for analyzing the tissue changes likely to produce a resultant image in a variety of lesions.

A matrix of multiecho images from a normal volunteer (Fig. 74–22) demonstrates the variety of tissue weighting described above. For white matter, maximal N weighting in this set of images occurs in the upper left corner, while maximal $T2$ weighting is present in the mid-upper portion on the matrix; $T1$ weighting increases toward the lower left corner. The lack of significant GM-WM contrast in the $T1$ weighted region is due to competition between $T1$ effects and N and $T2$ effects. Although the $T1$ weighting in this region is good, the minimum TE available (30 ms) is not short enough to eliminate $T2$ competitions; this together with competition from N cancels most of the contrast expected due to differences in $T1$.

A patient with diffuse white matter disease (Fig. 74–23) demonstrates the variable contrast characteristics available with the SE sequence. Note that the $T1$ weighted SE 30/315 image fails to demonstrate the diffuse white matter changes seen so clearly on the ME 30/2000 image even though the TE is the same for both images. The ME 30/2000 image has better contrast because the longer TR decreases noise and eliminates most of the competitive effects of $T1$, permitting better discrimination on the basis of N and $T2$ differences. As TE approaches the $T2$ of white matter in the ME 90/2000 image, the contrast between the normal brain substance and the diffuse white matter disease peaks. With a longer *TE*, 240 ms, there is some loss of contrast as the normal tissue intensity values approach the level of noise.

Another set of images (Fig. 74–24) from a patient with a brainstem infarct demonstrates the importance of using a relatively long *TR* when assessing *T2* effects. Although the area of pathology is seen on both the 45/1000 and 90/1000 images, some of the contrast between the lesion and the remaining normal brainstem is lost because the *TR* of 1000 ms is not sufficiently long to eliminate the competitive effects of *T1* on this relatively *T2* weighted pulse sequence. Lengthening the *TR* to 2000 ms improves the contrast between the infarct and the normal brainstem on the *T2* weighted images by suppressing this *T1* competition.

When analyzing pathologic signal intensity changes on an image, one must remember that a variety of tissue parameter changes can produce the same findings. For instance, in Figure 74–25, the high signal intensity of a metastatic melanoma in the thyroid on a relatively *T1* weighted SE 30/500 image might lead one to conclude that the lesion had a short *T1*, approaching the *T1* of fat. The calculated *T1* image (Technicare 0*T1* package) demonstrates that the approximate *T1* of the lesion is much longer than fat and more in the range of muscle. The calculated spin-density image indicates that most of the increased intensity is due to an increase in *N*. Therefore, one should consider all possible tissue parameter changes that might produce the resultant images and evaluate them with a variety of techniques before attempting to characterize a particular lesion.

A normal volunteer was selected to demonstrate the use of both magnitude and phase reconstruction with the ISE sequence in Figure 74–26. A magnitude reconstructed ISE 250/30/2250 image produces excellent tissue contrast due to the additive effects of *N*, *T1*, and *T2*. Image contrast on a phase reconstructed ISE 450/30/2250 image is also good due to the heavy *T1* weighting. With magnitude reconstruction, the ISE 450/30/2250 image has a bounce-point artifact at the WM-GM junction, resulting in inability to discriminate between WM and GM on the basis of image intensity.

ME images with optimal timing intervals and selected magnitude and phase reconstructed IME images from a normal volunteer are compared in Figure 74–27. The window setting has been kept constant for all of these images so that a direct comparison can be made. Tissue contrast in the ME images (top row) is primarily due to the additive effects of *N* and *T2*. The ME image on the top right (SE 120/2000) provides the most *T2* weighting, providing good WM-GM contrast. The magnitude reconstructed IME images (middle row) have more contrast than the ME images due to the additive effects of all three tissue parameters. There is some image degradation on the later IME echoes due to the poor signal-to-noise ratio. The phase reconstructed IME images (bottom row) use more *T1* weighting to produce image contrast. With a short *TE*, bottom left, there is good tissue discrimination because the short *TE* minimizes the competitive effects of *T2*. As *TE* is increased (bottom right) image contrast is degraded due to increasing *T2* competition and a decreasing signal-to-noise ratio.

A sagittal SE 30/2000 image of a patient with a brainstem infarct (Fig. 74–28) demonstrates suboptimal contrast between the lesion and the normal brainstem on a relatively *N* weighted image. A longer *TE* would provide considerably more contrast by adding more *T2* weighting. The magnitude reconstructed ISE 250/30/2250 image demonstrates good contrast between the infarct and the normal brainstem due to the additive effects of *N*, *T1*, and *T2*. Although increasing *TE* would increase contrast by adding more *T2* weighting, the image results would not be greatly improved due to the decreasing signal-to-noise ratio.

Images obtained in a patient with a large subarachnoid cyst using ME and IME (Fig. 74–29) demonstrate the differences between the ME and the magnitude IME techniques. *TR* was 2000 ms for all of the ME images (top row) and *TD* was 2000 ms for all of the magnitude IME images (bottom row). *TE* increases from left to right from 30 to 120 ms. All images were created with the same window settings to facilitate comparison. The magnitude IME images have more contrast between pathology and normal and between different normal tissues for every *TE* setting when compared to ME. This is due to the competitive effects of *T1* with *N* and *T2* in the SE sequence compared with the additive *N*, *T1*, and *T2* effects inherent to an optimized magnitude ISE technique.

In summary, these image examples illustrate that both SE and ISE pulse sequences have special attributes. Optimal SE techniques provide excellent *N* and *T2* weighting, although image contrast may be degraded by *T1* competition. Optimized short *T1* ISE techniques provide excellent image contrast due to the additive effects of *N*, *T1*, and *T2* with either magnitude or phrase reconstruction, assuming that the *N*, *T1*, and *T2* changes are correlated. Phase reconstructed ISE techniques optimized for *T1* weighting produce excellent results as long as *TE* is kept short enough to avoid significant *T2* competition.

Understanding MRI pulse sequence nomenclature and the effects of different pulse sequence techniques on MR images is essential for anyone planning optimal imaging protocols for clinical use.

Although the relationship between tissue parameters and timing intervals is complex, it can be simplified by separating the relationship into its component parts, permitting examination of the less complicated relationships between individual timing intervals and tissue parameters. These parts of the puzzle can then be woven into a meaningful pattern using the parameter sensitivity plots, where the effects of different timing interval combinations can be visualized.

From this analysis, it has been possible to generate several guidelines for setting up MRI techniques to maximize sensitivity to individual tissue parameters in specific normal tissues. These guidelines, listed in Table 74–6, provide a starting place for setting

Table 74–6. GUIDELINES FOR MAXIMIZING SENSITIVITY TO SUBTLE CHANGES IN SPECIFIC TISSUE PARAMETERS

Pulse Sequence	Desired Tissue Parameter Weighting*		
	N†	*T1*	*T2*
SR	$T \gg T1, TR \gg T1$	$T = T1, TR \gg T1$	—
PS	$TR \gg T1$	$TR - T1$	—
SE (PSSE)	$TE \ll T2, TR \gg T1$	$TE \ll T2, TR - T1$	$TE = T2, TR \gg T1$
IR (PSIR)	$TI \ll T1, TR \gg T1$ or $TI \gg T1, TD \ll T1$	$TI = T1, TD \gg T1$‡	—
ISE (PSISE)	$TI \ll T1, TE \ll T2, TR \gg T1$ or $TI \gg T1, TE \ll T2, TD \ll T1$	$TI = T1, TE \ll T2, TD \gg T1$†	$TI \ll T1, TE = T2, TR \gg T1$ or $TI \gg T1, TE = T2, TD \ll T1$

	Additive Tissue Parameter Effects§	
	Parameters Added	
IR (PSIR)	*N*, *T1*	$TI < 0.7 T1,^{\|} TD \gg T1$
ISE (PSISE)	*N*, *T1*, *T2*	$TI < 0.7 T1,^{\|} TE < T2, TD \gg T1$

* *T1* and *T2* are the relaxation times of the normal tissue most likely to harbor the pathology.
† Maximal sensitivity to *N* also produces maximal signal intensity.
‡ Phase reconstruction is required to preserve the appropriate positive and negative signals. All other IR and ISE sequences can be performed with either phase or magnitude reconstruction.
§ The tissue parameter effects only add when *N*, *T1*, and *T2* changes move in the same direction.
‖ *T1* in this case represents the shortest of *T1* of any tissue in the region of interest on the image.

up screening techniques that can then be modified to suit the user's preference as experience accumulates.

References

1. Bydder GM, Steiner RE, Young IR, et al: Clinical NMR imaging of the brain: 140 cases. AJR *139*:215–236, 1982.
2. Wehrli FW, MacFall JR, Shutts D, et al: Mechanism of contrast in NMR imaging. JCAT *8*:369–380, 1984.
3. Wehrli FW, MacFall JR, Clover GH, et al: The dependence of nuclear magnetic resonance (NMR) image contrast on magnetic resonance image interpretation. Noninvas Med Imag *1*:193–204, 1984.
4. Zeidses des Plantes BG, Falke THM, den Boer JA: Pulse sequences and contrast in magnetic resonance imaging. RadioGraphics. *4*:869, 1984.
5. Edelstein WA, Bottomley PA, Hart HR, et al: Signal noise and contrast in nuclear magnetic resonance. JCAT *7*:391, 1983.
6. Hendrick TR, Hendee N, Hendee WR: Optimizing contrast in magnetic resonance imaging. Magn Reson Imag *2*:23, 1984.
7. Crooks LE, Mills CM, Davis PL, et al: Visualization of cerebral and vascular abnormalities by NMR imaging. The effects of imaging parameters on contrast. Radiology *144*:843–852, 1982.
8. Mitchell MR, Gibbs SJ, Partain CL, et al: NMR imaging: Optimization times on magnetic image interpretation. Noninvas Med Imag *1*:193–204, 1984.
9. Mitchell MR, Conturo TE, Gruber TJ, et al: Two computer models for selection of optimal magnetic resonance imaging (MRI) pulse sequence timing. Invest Radiol *19*:350–360, 1984.
10. Hinshaw WS, Lent A: An introduction to NMR imaging; From Bloch equation to imaging equation. Proc IEEE *71*:338–350, 1983.
11. Farrar TC, Becker ED: Pulse and Fourier transform NMR. Introduction to Theory and Methods. The Bloch Equations. New York, Academic Press, 1971.
12. Kroeker RM, McVeigh ER, Hardy P, et al: In vivo measurement of NMR relaxation times. Magn Reson Med *2*:1–13, 1985.
13. Kjos BO, Ehman RL, Brant-Zawadzki M, et al: Reproducibility of relaxation times and spin density calculated from routine image sequences: Clinical study of the CNS. AJR *144*:1165–1170, 1985.
14. Axel L, Crooks LE, Luiten A, et al: Magnetic Resonance Glossary. Technicare, reprinted with permission of American College of Radiology, 1984.
15. Bradley WG, Crooks LE, Newton TH: *In* Newton TH, Potts DG (eds): Advanced Imaging Techniques. San Francisco, Clavadel Press, 1983.
16. Hinshaw WG: Image formation by nuclear magnetic resonance: The sensitive point method. J Appl Phys *47*:3709–3721, 1977.
17. Pykett IL, Buonanno FS, Brady TJ: Technique and approaches to proton NMR images of the head. Comput Radiol *7*:1–17, 1983.
18. Young IR, Bailes DR, Burl M, et al: Initial clinical evaluation of whole body nuclear magnetic resonance (NMR) tomography. JCAT *6*:1–18, 1982.
19. Christensen EE, Curry TS, Dowdey JE: Photographic characteristics of x-ray film. *In* Christensen EE, Curry TS, Dowdey JE (eds): An Introduction to the Physics of Diagnostic Radiology. Philadelphia, Lea & Febiger, 1978.
20. Mitchell MR, Tarr RW, Conturo TE, Partain CL, James AE: Spin echo technique selection: Basic principles for choosing MRI pulse sequence timing intervals. RadioGraphics *6*:245, 1986.
21. Davis PL, Kaufman L, Crooks LE: Tissue characterization. *In* Margulis AR, Higgins CB, Kaufman L, et al (eds): Clinical Magnetic Resonance Imaging. San Francisco, Radiology Research and Education Foundation, 1983.
22. Ortendahl DA: Analytical tools for magnetic resonance imaging. Radiology *153*:479–488, 1984.
23. Bovee W: Tumor detection and nuclear magnetic resonance. JNCI *52*:595–597, 1974.
24. Inch WR: Water content and proton spin relaxation time for neoplastic and non-neoplastic tissues from mice and humans. JNCI *52*:353–356, 1974.
25. Han JS, Kaufman B, Alfidi RJ, et al: Head trauma evaluated by magnetic resonance and computed tomography: A comparison. Radiology *150*:71–77, 1984.
26. Singh RP, Mitchell MR, Price RR, et al: MRI spin-echo ratio images. Abstract presented at the 33rd Annual Meeting of the Association of University Radiologists. Vanderbilt University, May, 1985.
27. Young IR, Payne JA, Khemia S, et al: Cancellation of tissue signals in inversion recovery and partial saturation sequencies. Abstract presented at the 4th Annual Meeting of the Society of Magnetic Resonance in Medicine, London, England, August 1985.
28. Steiner RE, Bydder GM, Young IR: Comparison of CT and short TI inversion recovery sequences in imaging the retroperitoneum and pelvis. Abstract presented at the 4th Annual Meeting of the Society of Magnetic Resonance in Medicine, London, England, August 1985.
29. Bydder GM: Recent developments in imaging of the central nervous system. Presented at the 4th Annual Meeting of the Society of Magnetic Resonance in Medicine, London, England, August 1985.
30. Bydder GM, Young IR: MR Imaging: Clinical use of the inversion recovery sequence. JCAT *9*:659–675, 1985.

75

T1 and T2 Measurement

JEROME P. JONES

Both the magnetic resonance (MR) signal intensity and contrast between tissues depend upon the local values of spin density (N), and the relationships between $T1$, $T2$, and the interpulse time intervals. Neglecting flow, these factors can be summarized in an equation of the form (1):

$$I = kNf(T1)g(T2) \tag{1}$$

where I is the signal intensity, k is a proportionality constant, and f and g are functions of the type of pulse sequence. For a spin-echo sequence of $(90° - TE/2 - 180° - TE/2 - \text{echo} - TD)_n$, f and g are given by (1):

$$f = 1 + e^{-TR/T1} - 2e^{-(TR - TE/2)/T1} \tag{2}$$

$$g = e^{-TE/T2} \tag{3}$$

where $TR = TE + TD$ is the time for one complete sequence. These equations suggest an immediate scheme for calculating $T1$: keep TE fixed while collecting images with different TR values. Then the ratio of signal intensities is

$$I_1/I_2 = [1 + e^{-TR_1/T1} - 2e^{-(TR_1 - TE_1/2)/T1}]/[1 + e^{-TR_2/T1} - 2e^{-(TR_2 - TE_1/2)/T1}],$$

which can be solved for $T1$. In practice, $TR \gg TE/2$, so this ratio can be shortened to

$$I_1/I_2 = [1 - e^{-TR_1/T1}]/[1 - e^{-TR_2/T1}] \tag{4}$$

and the value of $T1$ deduced by an iterative scheme. Similarly, using the approximation $TR \gg TE/2$, the value of $T2$ can be deduced by holding TR constant while varying TE. The ratio is then

$$I_1/I_3 = e^{-TE_1/T2}/e^{-TE_3/T2}$$

from which $T2$ directly follows as:

$$T2 = (TE_3 - TE_1)/\ell n(I_1/I_3). \tag{5}$$

Knowledge of $T1$ and $T2$ is not simply an academic curiosity. Many diseases are apparent with certain pulse sequences but not visible with others (e.g., multiple sclerosis plaques). The fact that lesions can be seen at all shows that they have different kN, $T1$, and/or $T2$ values from normal tissues, but the fact that they are not seen on some sequences means that an optimization scheme is needed to assure that the proper sequence is used without spending excessive time to find it. In one such scheme,[2] Mitchell et al. are able to optimize the contrast based upon a knowledge of $T1$ and $T2$. Further, there is the possibility that kN, $T1$, and $T2$ values may aid in the differential diagnosis of disease. Without knowledge of $T1$ and $T2$, MR imaging will remain a trial and error grope (though the gropings of others are very useful) with good sensitivity but low specificity. In short, some of its potential may be wasted.

The problem has been that $T1$ and $T2$ values calculated from Equations (4) and (5) have not proved to be reliable. There are many possible reasons for this, though most lack direct proof. For example, Equation (1) may not be valid for many tissues; certainly each tissue will contain many different compounds each contributing their own $T1$ and $T2$ relaxation to the signal. Using Equation (1) to represent this distribution of values by an effective $T1$, $T2$ pair may lead to the effective values depending upon the TR and TE values used. Another possibility is related to selective excitation of a "slice"; the slice is never sharply defined, so atoms near the "edge" of the slice are not tipped as far as those in the center of the slice, and make a contribution to the signal which is not described by Equation (1). These are both difficult problems which may ultimately limit the usefulness of computed $T1$ and $T2$ values, and they may certainly be responsible for the unreliability observed thus far.

However, there is another factor—noise. Environmental radio frequency (rf) noise, internal electronic rf noise, random phase shifts due to imager field nonuniformities (including mutual inductance between gradient and shim coils)—all contribute to uncertainty in the measured signal. Both Equations (4) and (5) show that this uncertainty is propagated into $T1$ and $T2$ uncertainty. Thus sequences that propagate small errors should be used; otherwise the problems of the previous paragraph will never be sensibly studied.

The remainder of this chapter will discuss error propagation and give two basic approaches for dealing with it. One obvious approach is to make more than two measurements and fit the data set to Equation (1) (with kN, $T1$, and $T2$ the fitting parameters). The other approach is to use only two measurements, but choose the sequences which propagate minimal error. Each approach has its own advantages and disadvantages.

THE BASIC PROBLEM

Formally, the problem is solving Equation (1) for the three unknowns kN, $T1$, and $T2$. This requires at least three independent pulse sequences:

$$I_1 = kNf_1(T1)g_1(T2) \tag{6a}$$

$$I_2 = kNf_2(T1)g_2(T2) \tag{6b}$$

$$I_3 = kNf_3(T1)g_3(T2) \tag{6c}$$

The error propagation through these equations can be found from the total differential of a function of three independent variables:

$$dI = \frac{\partial I}{\partial(kN)}\, d(kN) + \frac{\partial I}{\partial T1}\, dT1 + \frac{\partial I}{\partial T2}\, dT2$$

and when applied to these three sequences gives

$$dI_1/I_1 = d(kN)/kN + a_1(dT1/T1) + b_1(dT2/T2) \tag{7a}$$

$$dI_2/I_2 = d(kN)/kN + a_2(dT1/T1) + b_2(dT2/T2) \tag{7b}$$

$$dI_3/I_3 = d(kN)/kN + a_3(dT1/T1) + b_3(dT2/T2) \tag{7c}$$

where

$$a_i = (T1/f_i)(df_i/dT1) \qquad b_i = (T2/g_i)(dg_i/dT2), \tag{8}$$

and $i = 1, 2, 3$. Equation (7) shows directly how changes in kN, $T1$, and $T2$ affect the signal intensities, but these equations can be inverted to show how changes (errors) in

I_1, I_2, and I_3 affect kN, *T1*, and *T2*. Using Kramer's rule gives

$$\frac{d(kN)}{kN} = \frac{\begin{vmatrix} dI_1/I_1 & a_1 & b_1 \\ dI_2/I_2 & a_2 & b_2 \\ dI_3/I_3 & a_3 & b_3 \end{vmatrix}}{D} \qquad \frac{dT1}{T1} = \frac{\begin{vmatrix} 1 & dI_1/I_1 & b_1 \\ 1 & dI_2/I_2 & b_2 \\ 1 & dI_3/I_3 & b_3 \end{vmatrix}}{D}$$

$$\frac{dT2}{T2} = \frac{\begin{vmatrix} 1 & a_1 & dI_1/I_1 \\ 1 & a_2 & dI_2/I_2 \\ 1 & a_3 & dI_3/I_3 \end{vmatrix}}{D} \qquad D = \begin{vmatrix} 1 & a_1 & b_1 \\ 1 & a_2 & b_2 \\ 1 & a_3 & b_3 \end{vmatrix}.$$

These equations do show error propagation, but with a restriction. Differentials are *signed* quantities, whereas random errors are always unsigned quantities. For example, if two variables are to be subtracted, their signed error subtracts, while their random error adds. This must be accounted for, because in NMR imaging, systematic (signed) errors are rarely known, while random errors are easily deduced as the standard deviation of intensity in a region of interest.

Equation (7) is more general than Equations (4) or (5), but these latter two will follow from Equation (7) if

$$g_1 = g_2 \qquad (TE_1 = TE_2)$$
$$f_1 = f_3 \qquad (TR_1 = TR_3).$$

In the above error equations, this makes $b_1 = b_2$ and $a_1 = a_3$. These results simplify the *T1* and *T2* error equations more than is at first evident:

$$dT1/T1 = (dI_1/I_1 - dI_2/I_2)/(a_1 - a_2) \tag{9a}$$
$$dT2/T2 = (dI_1/I_1 - dI_3/I_3)/(b_1 - b_3). \tag{9b}$$

These equations show very clearly that they describe the propagation of signed errors only. To properly modify them for random errors would require a knowledge of the underlying error distributions of I_1 and I_2 and deduction of the standard deviation of their combined distribution. An easier alternative is to simply create a modification that is convenient but may not have a clear statistical interpretation (such as a precise confidence level). Analytically, the simplest choice is the sum of the error magnitudes:

$$S_{T1} \equiv (|\, dI_1/I_1\,| + |\, dI_2/I_2\,|)/|\, a_1 - a_2\,| \tag{10a}$$
$$S_{T2} \equiv (|\, dI_1/I_1\,| + |\, dI_3/I_3\,|)/|\, b_1 - b_3\,| \tag{10b}$$

These equations will be used to estimate the error levels and compare the error propagated by different sequence pairs. A root-mean-square combination (suggested by Gaussian statistics) could also be used but is far more complex for analytical treatment.

T2 ERROR

For the spin-echo sequence, $b_i = TE/T2$, and Equation (10b) becomes

$$S_{T2} = (|\, dI_1/I_1\,| + |\, dI_3/I_3\,|)/(|\, TE_3 - TE_1\,|T2) \tag{11a}$$
$$S_{T2} = (|\, dI_1/I_1\,| + |\, dI_3/I_3\,|)/|\, \ell n(I_1/I_3)\,|. \tag{11b}$$

These equations are instructive. First, the total signal error will be magnified unless TE_3 and TE_1 are chosen so that $I_1 \geq 2.71 I_3$ (or $\ell n(I_1/I_3) \geq 1$). If $I_1 \approx I_3$, the error will be unbounded. For example, Table 75–1 shows two sets of *T2* calculations each having

Table 75–1. TWO EXAMPLE *T2* CALCULATIONS

Reasonable	Unreasonable
1. True $T2 = 100$ ms	1. True $T2 = 100$ ms
2. $TE_1 = 30$ ms $TE_3 = 100$ ms	2. $TE_1 = 30$ ms $TE_3 = 60$ ms
3. True $I_1/I_3 = 2.01$	3. True $I_1/I_3 = 1.35$
4. Measured $I_1/I_3 = 2.21$ ($+10\%$)	4. Measured $I_1/I_3 = 1.48$ ($+10\%$)
5. Calculated $T2 = 88$ ms	5. Calculated $T2 = 77$ ms
6. Error = 12%	6. Error = 23%

a 10 percent error in I_1/I_3. The one for which TE_1 and TE_3 bracket the true $T2$ gives a similar $T2$ error, while the other pair give double the error. Thus, in the presence of minor signal errors, large $T2$ errors can occur if TE_1 and TE_3 are not properly chosen.

Equation (11a) suggests that TE_1 and TE_3 should be very different; the problem is that if one or the other is too large, there will be no signal, making the numerator unbounded. Thus TE_1 and TE_3 should be as different as possible without either signal becoming too small, and finding this condition requires a knowledge of $|\,dI/I\,|$ as a function of TE.

Figure 75–1 shows a graph of $|\,dI\,|$ versus I for an assortment of spin-echo images of various objects. Though somewhat scattered, the points follow a description of the form:

$$|\,dI\,| = u + vI \text{ if } u + vI \geq w \tag{12a}$$

$$|\,dI\,| = w \qquad \text{otherwise.} \tag{12b}$$

Here, w is the steady noise level in the system, while u and v also include the effects of field nonuniformities, digitizing errors, and other signal-dependent causes of error. Assuming that the small signal levels of Equation (12b) will be avoided, Equation (11a) becomes:

$$S_{T2} = \frac{(u/kNf_1)(e^{TE_3/T2} + e^{TE_1/T2})}{|\,TE_3 - TE_1\,|/T2} + \frac{2v}{|\,TE_3 - TE_1\,|/T2}.$$

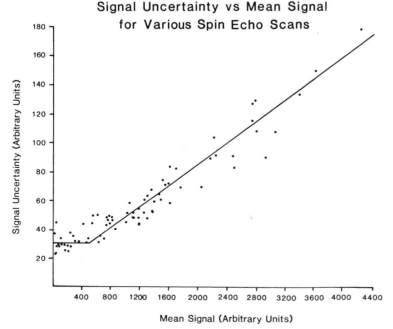

Signal Uncertainty vs Mean Signal for Various Spin Echo Scans

Signal Uncertainty (Arbitrary Units)

Mean Signal (Arbitrary Units)

Figure 75–1. A plot of the observed standard deviation of a structure ($|\,dI\,|$) versus the mean value of its intensity (I) for an assortment of phantoms and patients using spin-echo images.

Table 75–2. CONDITIONS FOR MINIMAL *T2* ERROR

1. Spin-rich sample (large N)
2. High sensitivity coil (large k)
3. Long *TR* (more signal; no *T1* weighting)
4. Smallest TE_1 possible (more signal; no *T2* weighting)
5. $TE_3 \geq 1.27\ T2$ (*T2* weighting without excessive noise)

The second term is readily minimized by making $|TE_3 - TE_1|$ as large as possible. The first term is only a little more difficult; assuming $TE_3 > TE_1$, one arrives at minimizing

$$e^{TE_1/T2}[e^{(TE_3-TE_1)/T2} + 1]/[(TE_3 - TE_1)/T2],$$

which requires that $TE_3 - TE_1 = 1.27\ T2$ and that TE_1 be as small as possible. Table 75–2 summarizes the requirements for best *T2* accuracy. Note that the examples of Table 75–1 are consistent with these results. Also note that the minimum *TE* with most MR imagers is about 30 ms, which eliminates all hope of accurate *T2* calculations in the range of 30 ms and smaller.

The inversion-recovery pulse sequence can also be used for *T2* calculations: this $(180° - TI - 90° - TE/2 - 180° - TE/2 - \text{echo} - TD)_n$ sequence has the functions

$$f = 1 - 2e^{-TI/T1} - e^{-TR/T1} + 2e^{-(TR-TE/2)/T1} \approx 1 - 2e^{-TI/T1} + e^{-TR/T1} \tag{13}$$

$$g = e^{-TE/T2} \tag{3}$$

Since its g is the same as for a spin-echo sequence, it gives the same *T2* results. Since $TR = TI + TE + TD$ is usually longer than the spin-echo $TR(= TE + TD)$, inversion recovery is seldom used for *T2* calculation.

T1 ERROR

When cleared of fractions, Equation (4) leads to

$$e^{-TR_1/T1} - re^{-TR_2/T1} + r - 1 = 0, \quad (r = I_1/I_2)$$

to solve iteratively for *T1*. However, some care is needed, since $T1 \to \infty$ is a "solution" for any r. This equation can be easier to solve if TR_1 is chosen to be an integer multiple of TR_2. Defining $s = TR_1/TR_2$ and $x = \exp(-TR_2/T1)$, this equation becomes the polynomial

$$x^s - rx + r - 1 = 0,$$

which has the extraneous "solution" of $x = 1$ for any r. Factoring out this "solution" leaves

$$x^{s-1} + x^{s-2} + \cdots x + 1 = r. \tag{14}$$

If $s = 2$ or $s = 3$, Equation (14) can be solved in closed form, with *T1* then deduced from this value of x. For larger s, an iterative scheme may still be needed, although Equation (14) will have only one real root in the range $0 < x < 1$. To see if this is a useful approach, the *T1* error will be analyzed in a fashion similar to the *T2* error analysis.

Table 75–3 shows a pair of calculations of *T1* assuming again a 10 percent error in r. The results show even larger errors than for *T2*. Noting that for a spin echo f, $a = -(TR/T1)/(e^{TR/T1} - 1)$, and Equation (10a) becomes

$$S_{T1} = (|dI_1/I_1| + |dI_2/I_2|)/|F(z_2) - F(z_1)|, \tag{15}$$

Table 75–3. TWO EXAMPLE SPIN–ECHO *T1* CALCULATIONS

Reasonable Try	Unreasonable Try
1. True $T1$ = 500 ms	1. True $T1$ = 500 ms
2. TR_1 = 2s TR = 500 ms	2. TR_1 = 1500 ms TR_2 = 750 ms
3. True I_1/I_2 = 1.55	3. True I_1/I_2 = 1.22
4. Measured I_1/I_2 = 1.71 (+10%)	4. Measured I_1/I_2 = 1.34 (+10%)
5. Calculated $T1$ = 600 ms	5. Calculated $T1$ = 695 ms
6. Error = 20%	6. Error = 39%

where

$$F(z) = -z/(e^2 - 1), \qquad z_2 = TR_2/T1, \qquad z_1 = TR_1/T1$$

Figure 75–2 is a sketch of $F(z)$ versus z; it has an initial value of -1 and monotonically approaches zero as z increases. Thus $|F(z)|$ is always between zero and unity, so that $|F(z_2) - F(z_1)|$ is likewise between zero and unity, and S_{T1} is always greater than the total signal error.

To find the conditions for minimum error, Equation (12a) is substituted into (15), giving

$$S_{T1} = [u/kNe^{-TE_1/T2}] \frac{\left[\dfrac{e^{z_1}}{e^{z_1} - 1} + \dfrac{e^{z_2}}{e^{z_2} - 1} \right]}{\left| \dfrac{z_1}{e^{z_1} - 1} - \dfrac{z_2}{e^{z_2} - 1} \right|} + \frac{2v}{|F(z_2) - F(z_1)|} \qquad (16)$$

The second term is readily minimized by making TR_1 and TR_2 as different as possible, but the first is a more difficult exercise. Minimizing it requires making the numerator as small as possible and the denominator as large as possible; assuming $z_1 > z_2$, this is achieved by making z_1 as large as possible ($e^{z_1}/(e^{z_1} - 1)$ equals its minimum value of 1 and $z_1(e^{z_1} - 1)$ equals its minimum value of zero). This leaves the expression

$$\left[1 + \frac{e^{z_2}}{e^{z_2} - 1} \right] \Big/ \left[\frac{z_2}{e^{z_2} - 1} \right]$$

to minimize, which results in the condition $z_2 = 0.77$. Thus large TR_1 is consistent with both terms, but TR_2 should be no more than 77 percent of the true $T1$, depending upon which term in Equation (16) predominates. The conditions for best $T1$ accuracy are summarized in Table 75–4.

Even under the best conditions, Equation (15) reveals that S_{T1} is still 51 percent greater than the total signal uncertainty. Thus $T1$ calculations with two spin-echo images require very low noise; a 10 percent total signal error (5 percent in each signal) becomes

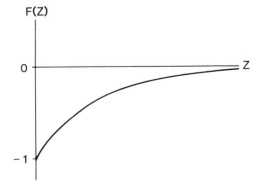

Figure 75–2. A sketch of the spin-echo sensitivty function for *TR* > 0.

Table 75–4. MINIMUM *T1* ERROR CONDITIONS FOR TWO SPIN–ECHO SEQUENCES

1. Spin-rich sample (large *N*)
2. High sensitivity coil (large k)
3. Short *TE* (more signal; no *T2* weighting)
4. Long TR_1 ($TR_1 > 2.5\ T1$) (more signal; no *T1* weighting)
5. $TR_2 \leqslant .77\ T1$ (*T1* weighting without excessive noise)

a 15 percent *T1* error at best. This leads one to examine other alternatives for *T1* calculation.

One combination used with some MR imagers is an inversion-recovery and spin-echo pair, each with the same *TE*. The ratio equation is

$$I_2/I_1 = (1 - 2e^{-TI_2/TI} + e^{-TR_2/TI})/(1 - e^{-TR_1/TI}),$$

which when cleared of fractions becomes

$$2e^{-TI_2/TI} - e^{-TR_2/TI} - re^{-TR_1/TI} + r - 1 = 0 \tag{17}$$

This equation has the trivial "solution" of $T1 \to \infty$ also, but its error propagation is more interesting. For the inversion recovery f,

$$a = \frac{(TR/TI)e^{-TR/TI} - 2(TI/TI)e^{-TI/TI}}{1 - 2e^{-TI/TI} + e^{-TR/TI}},$$

and Equation (10a) becomes

$$S_{TI} = (|\,dI_1/I_1\,| + |\,dI_2/I_2\,|)/|\,F(z_1) - G(y_2,\,z_2)\,| \tag{18}$$

where F and z_1 are defined under Equation (15) and

$$G(y,\,z) = \frac{ze^{-z} - 2ye^{-y}}{1 - 2e^{-y} + e^{-z}}, \qquad y_2 = TI_2/TI, \qquad z_2 = TR_2/TI.$$

Figure 75–3 is a sketch of $G(y,\,z)$ as a function of y with $z - y$ held constant. If $z = y$, $G(z,\,z)$ is the same as $F(z)$ in Figure 2. But for $z > y$, the sketch changes markedly because the denominator of $G(y,\,z)$ is zero when y has the value

$$y_o = \ell n(2 - e^{-(z-y_o)}) \tag{19}$$

For $0 < y < y_o$, G starts at a value between zero and -1, and increases without limit as y approaches y_o. G is undefined at $y = y_o$, but then switches sign and monotonically approaches zero as y further increases. The large magnitude of G at y near y_o helps make S_{TI} small, but I_2 is also near zero when y is near y_2. To deduce the behavior of S_{TI} in this region, Equation (12b) is applied for $|\,dI2/I2\,|$ (since $|\,I_2\,|$ is small). $F(z_1)$ can

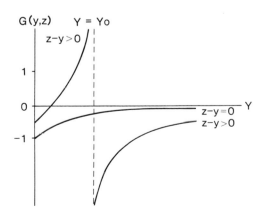

Figure 75–3. A sketch of the inversion-recovery sensitivity function, with $z - y$ held constant on each graph.

be neglected, leaving

$$S_{TI} = \frac{u/I_1 + v}{|G(y_2, z_2)|} + \frac{w}{kNe^{-TE_1/T2}} \frac{1}{|z_2 e^{-z_2} - 2y_2 e^{-1/2}|}. \tag{20}$$

The first term is minimized for I_1 as large as possible, which requires a long TR_1. Minimization of the second term leads to maximizing

$$|z_2 e^{-z_2} - 2y_2 e^{-y_2}|$$

The first term varies between zero and e^{-1}, while the second varies from zero to at most $2e^{-1}$ when $y_2 = 1$. However, the largest yo can be is 0.69 (from Equation (19)), so the above expression is maximized by a large z_2 and a y_o of 0.69. This may not be the minimum TI error, however. If $y_2 = 1$, the above expression equals $2e^{-1}$, but $y_2 = 1$ may make $|I_2|$ large enough that Equation (12b) will no longer apply. Then S_{TI} becomes

$$S_{TI} = \frac{u/I_1 + 2v}{|G(y_2, z_2)|} + \frac{u}{kNe^{-TE_1/T2}} \frac{1}{|z_2 e^{-z_2} - 2y_2 e^{-y_2}|} \tag{21}$$

Again, one concludes that TR_1 should be large, TR_2 should be large, and $TI_2 = TI$. One cannot tell whether Equation (20) or Equation (21) gives a smaller S_{TI} unless u, v, and w are all known, but evaluation of the known terms indicates that they are comparable. Even better, Equation (18) implies that S_{TI} is only 36 percent of the total signal error when $TR_2 \gg TI$ and $TI_2 = TI$, so the error is much smaller than that for two spin-echo sequences. Another advantage of having $TI_2 = TI$ is that since $I_2 > 0$, the structure of interest will be visible in the image. Table 75–5 gives a summary of the conditions for minimal TI error.

These results suggest that two inversion recovery sequences might be even more accurate. In principle, this could be true. If TI_1 were chosen to be slightly less than $TI_o (TI_o = y_o TI)$ and TI_2 to be somewhat greater, each G would have a large magnitude and opposite sign. Thus their magnitudes would add, but both $|I_1|$ and $|I_2|$ would be small. However, the worst problem is that TI would need to be known quite well a priori in order to bracket it very closely with TI_1 and TI_2. Other problems are that G_1 changes magnitude very quickly as TI_1 decreases from TI_o so that a bad guess at TI would lose this advantage, and $|I_1|$ could be so small that the object of interest might be difficult to identify. However, inversion recovery has another problem which could make this scheme useless in practice.

The problem is that the signal is negative whenever $TI < TI_o$; physically, this negative signal is detected as being 180 degrees out of phase. But because phase encoding is used to build the image, it is not easy to properly correct the negative signal (which is mixed in with positive signals). Some MR imagers do not even attempt it; they simply compute the signal magnitudes without regard for the sign. Others attempt it, but it is difficult to tell when the correction has been properly made, and the operator can easily make all the signals reconstruct as negative (the correction is like a constant subtraction whose proper magnitude is unclear). For the closely bracketed two inver-

Table 75–5. MINIMUM *TI* ERROR CONDITIONS FOR AN INVERSION–RECOVERY/SPIN–ECHO PAIR

---

1. Spin-rich sample (large N)
2. High sensitivity coil (large k)
3. Short *TE* (more signal; no *T2* weighting)
4. Long TR_1 ($TR_1 > 2.5$ *TI*) (spin echo; more signal; no *TI* weighting)
5. Long TR_2 ($TR_2 > 2.5$ *TI*) (inversion recovery; more signal)
6. Set $TI_2 \sim .7$ *TI* $- 1.0$ *TI* (small positive signal; heavy *TI* weighting)

---

sion-recovery images, it is possible that both TI_1 and TI_2 are greater than TI_o, or less than TI_o, making it difficult to sort out the proper sign. The inversion-recovery/spin-echo pair has much less problem here since TI_2 should exceed TI_o and therefore be a positive signal not requiring phase correction. As a result, the most workable and accurate two-point TI calculation method should be the inversion-recovery/spin-echo method as summarized in Table 75–5; at least one commercial MR system uses this method.

MULTIPLE POINTS T2 CALCULATION

This can be carried out by collecting numerous spin-echo images having the same TR and progressively longer TE values. If Equation (1) is valid, one should observe a single decaying exponential with time constant $T2$, with the effects of noise "averaged out" by the fitting process. However, collecting successive images at about 5 minutes per image requires a lot of time; this is a general problem with multiple point methods.

However, $T2$ calculation using anywhere from four to eight points can be made from a single multiecho data collection (about 5 minutes for the entire set). All have the same effective $T1$ dependence, so they can be analyzed in the same way as successively collected images.

The reason that all multiecho images have the same $T1$ dependence is that each 180 degree refocusing pulse inverts the recovered longitudinal magnetization. This effectively erases the $T1$ recovery since the previous 180 degree pulse, until after the last 180 degree pulse, $T1$ recovery continues until the end of the sequence. Because less time is required than even for a two-point determination, this is the preferred method for $T2$ calculations. It also allows a check on the validity of Equation (1); about its only drawback is that induced currents in the shim coils from the rapidly pulsed gradients may cause phase distortions in some of the later echoes. Thus the number of echo images is somewhat limited, but most MR imagers can collect at least four satisfactory images.

MULTIPLE POINTS T1 CALCULATION

There is no $T1$ analogue to a multiecho collection. Further, having to change TR from one image to another can easily lead to an hour or more of data collection. However, one commercial system uses the shortcut of not producing $T1$ images. A line is selected for analysis, and signals collected only from this line for several different TR values. This method is fast (about 2 minutes), since phase encoding is not used, though the exact localization procedure is not known to this author. However, in solving these problems, this method adds another problem: the line must be very accurately localized or else the $T1$ value(s) could be associated with the wrong position. Since many abnormal structures are very thin, localization must be very carefully checked. The accuracy of this procedure on a clinical basis has yet to be determined, but it is a promising method for $T1$ calculation in vivo.

Reliable $T1$ and $T2$ calculations have been very difficult to generate from MR imagers despite the interest in this data for tissue characterization and pulse sequence optimization studies. While these are compelling reasons to suggest that imaging $T1$ and $T2$ data are of limited use, simple noise propagation is not taken into account, and can easily cause a twofold or threefold increase in the error. In such a case, studies of more fundamental problems can never be conclusive because of the effects of uncorrected noise. To minimize noise propagation, one can use an optimized two-image set consisting of a spin density weighted image and a *T2* weighted spin-echo image (for *T2* calculations) or a *T1* weighted inversion recovery image (for *T1* calculation). Alternatively, one can use multiple data sets, with a multiecho image set very convenient for *T2* calculations, and a repeat study of a selected line for *T1* calculations. The optimum approach for *T2* calculations seems to be the multiecho method; it gives anywhere from four to eight echoes from which the presence of multiple *T2* components can be detected and analyzed, as well as reduce the effects of noise by curve fitting. In addition, all the images are collected in less time than two separate images. The optimum approach for *T1* calculations is less clear. The two point method can have problems with phase corrections and requiring a reasonable guess at the true *T1*, but it does result in a *T1* image. It also fails to check for the presence of multiple *T1* components. The multipoint method does give this check and requires little knowledge of the true *T1*, but proper registration to assure that the selected line is the one actually measured can be a problem. But at least the methods analyzed here should make one aware of the fundamental problems of *T1* and *T2* calculations, and serve as a guide for further investigations into the use of *T1* and *T2* values. One conclusion perhaps not evident was that two spin-echo images cannot be recommended for accurate *T1* calculation unless the total signal noise is very small. This is because the spin-echo sequence is not sufficiently sensitive to *T1* to keep it from propagating large errors into the *T1* calculation (or equivalently, two tissues of appreciably different *T1* can give the same signal intensity with spin-echo sequences).

ACKNOWLEDGMENT

The author wishes to acknowledge the assistance of the Medical Editing Department for typing and editorial assistance with this manuscript, Barbara Siede for the artwork, and Carroll Punte for photography of the figures.

References

1. Jones JP, Partain CL, Mitchell MR, et al.: Principles of magnetic resonance. *In* Kressel HY (ed): Magnetic Resonance Annal 1985. New York, Raven Press, 1985, pp 71–111.
2. Mitchell MR, Conturo TE, Gruber TJ, Jones JP: Two computer models for selection of optimal magnetic resonance imaging (MRI) pulse sequence timing. Invest Radiol *19*:350–360, 1984.

76

Artifacts in the Measurement of T1 and T2

I. R. YOUNG
J. A. PAYNE
D. J. BRYANT
D. R. BAILES
A. S. HALL
G. M. BYDDER

This chapter outlines some of the problems caused by artifacts in the measurement of tissue parameters in MR imaging. These are numerous and can be identified as coming from four major sources: (1) machine defects, (2) unpredictable bits of metal (ferromagnetic or conducting) associated with the patient, (3) sequence dependent errors, and (4) fundamental problems. The first two are not considered here. It is assumed, firstly, that the data from which parameters are being calculated are free of faults due to machine deficiencies such as incorrect and inconsistent gradient amplitudes, DC field drift and fluctuations in time and space; radio frequency (rf) design, implementation and stability problems; poor tuning and inadequate rf screening; truncation errors in data acquisition and handling; and computing defects. Secondly, it is assumed that there are no difficulties due to prosthetic devices, pieces of metal either known or otherwise, or life support or other patient monitoring equipment that contains either ferromagnetic material or enough conducting metal to distort the rf field. Many of these produce gross, though quite recognizable, artifacts.

Sequence dependent errors are genuinely under experimental control. These arise because changing one or more sequence timing parameters may have unexpected by-products, such as alterations in the slice shape,[1,2] while, unless care is taken with the rf pulses, other errors are introduced.[2,3] These artifacts arise even when the basic questions of forming the correctly shaped slice in the correct location, as analyzed most effectively by Hoult and his co-workers,[4,5] have been resolved.

Sequence design is also responsible for other errors. Artifacts can be introduced, for example, because not all the signals monitored were from magnetization that had been excited in the manner intended, as the signal detected is the sum of all those present at the time of acquisition no matter how produced. It is easy to create such problems, as will be suggested, particularly with more complicated sequences.

Equally, of course, good design can assist in minimizing errors. For example, errors in rf amplitude, either due to machine defects or due to patient coupling or absorption, can often be minimized by, for example, alteration of the direction of the pulses on successive acquisitions, as is common in spectroscopy.[6]

Fundamental problems are more comprehensible and in many ways more interesting to study. Thus, any measurement involves the risk of partial volume effects, where voxels contain bits from more than one tissue. In MR, however, unlike other modalities, it is possible to design procedures that help to resolve this problem. On the other hand, the great range of tissue parameters means that they may respond distinctly and differently to a sequence, resulting in variations in the quality of measurements across a single slice.

Phenomena, which may themselves be of interest, can also cause artifact. Flow, perfusion, and diffusion are examples of various magnitudes of motion; chemical shift, J-coupling, and chemical exchange are all things that are interesting in their own right but can cause errors in generating estimates, particularly of *T2*.

Genuine complications, such as the existence of multiexponential components, become almost secondary in comparison with other factors.

It is not possible in a short article to give more than a very sweeping outline of these difficulties and to try to indicate strategies that may be of some value in tackling them. It is easy to gain an impression that accurate measurement is hindered by so many difficulties as to be nearly impossible in the time available for a clinical examination. However, as long as individual studies are conducted in accordance with strict protocols, useful and repeatable numerical results may be obtained, even though it would be optimistic to describe them as the true values of *T1* and *T2*.

SEQUENCE DESIGN ARTIFACTS

None of the artifacts are totally independent of each other, so that in the discussion that follows it should be borne in mind that a beneficial change affecting one artifact might actually make another one worse.

When making measurements, it is clearly desirable to choose sequence timings which allow the maximum sensitivity to changes in the parameter being measured. Manipulation of the equations relating signals to the tissue parameters, using only the simplest theoretical models for the three main sequences, shows that in

a. partial saturation (PS) (or saturation recovery [SR]) $dS/dT1$ is a maximum where $TR = T1$ mean (where $T1$ mean is the average of those for the tissues to be resolved).

b. inversion recovery (IR) $dS/dT1$ is a maximum where $TI = T1$ (assuming $TR \gg T1$).

c. spin echo (SE), $dS/dT2$ is a maximum where $TE = T2$.

where dS/dx is the sensitivity of S with respect to a parameter x. In practice the inaccuracies of the models used (particularly for partial saturation) mean that the values given above may be significantly in error.

As Table 76–1 indicates, however, the range of tissue parameters is so great that it is necessary to choose the best sequence settings for the study that is being done. The reliability of computed images of complete sections, unless using parameters cal-

Table 76–1. TYPICAL VALUES OF BRAIN TISSUE PARAMETERS (USED IN MODELING CHARACTERISTICS)

Tissue	Proton Density Relative to Gray Matter	*T1* (ms)	*T2* (ms)
Gray matter	1.0	520	95
White matter	0.9	380	85
Typical edema or infarction	1.0	600	150
Malignant tumor	1.0	800	200
Fat	0.75	160	100
CSF	1.2	2000	1000

culated from a multiplicity of sequences, are necessarily influenced by the varying accuracies achieved in different tissues from a limited choice of sequences.

Table 76–1 shows typical values of some brain tissue parameters at 0.15 tesla to illustrate their very wide spread. Generally, the range is rather smaller in the body (which lacks the extreme represented by the cerebrospinal fluid values). Gray matter is taken as unity on the proton density scale, since studies involving cerebrospinal fluid numerical values tend to be much less common, so that it makes a poor reference.

Slice Shape Artifact

Calculations of $T1$ and $T2$ involve assumptions about the form and location of the magnetization that is detected. Implicit in the simple equations normally used is the assumption that the slice is rectangular, with all its magnetization rotated through the angle intended, and with no signal from anywhere outside it. In fact, slice form is complex and varies substantially with the sequence and timing in use. This topic has been described extensively in the literature[1,2,7,8] so that the consequences of the artifact will only be reviewed briefly here.

Its level and form are a function of the sequence in use[2] so that sequences such as IR and SE in which the inverting pulse is not selective are relatively immune to it. The artifact, while its form can be derived rigorously from the Bloch equations,[9] can be thought of empirically as arising from the variation in the effective precession angle of the magnetization between the center of the slice (90 degrees) and its extreme edges (nominally zero). Clearly, the change between these angles must involve a finite amount of magnetization, and, as was pointed out by Ernst and Anderson,[10] the signal-to-noise ratio of an experiment may be optimized by adjusting the precession angle. Since the edge of a slice is excited, in theory, by the range of precession angles up to 90 degrees, angles in the optimum range predicted by Anderson and Ernst will be found for any value of $T1$ of tissues in the slice.

The slice form in any system where slice selection is used at every rf excitation shows characteristic "peaking" of the edges as illustrated in Figures 76–1 and 76–2 which show the slice shape displayed by the method described in the legend for Figure 76–1. The size of the errors due to assuming that the simple models for the magnitude of the signals usually assumed are valid can be substantial, as indicated in Table 76–2. This shows the apparent $T1$ values that would be measured were the simple model for the signal used to compute $T1$ from images of a phantom with a $T1$ of about 300 ms.

Table 76–2 represents an experiment to illustrate the magnitude of errors to be expected from the calculation of $T1$ using an incorrect model. A sample with a $T1$ of 300 ms was placed in the field at 0.15 tesla and a series of PS images, with identical field echo data acquisition,[25] taken. Signal amplitude was measured, and the values of $T1$ calculated from the pairs of data values are shown in column 1, the simple model of the signal for the PS sequence ($M_y = M_0(1 - \exp(-TR/T1)) \exp(-TE/T2)$). The results are shown in column 2, which shows the tendency for the measured value of $T1$ to drop as quicker sequence pairs are used in the calculation; this is due to the "peaking" of the edges of the slice described in the text.

Of all the sequences, partial saturation (PS) (which most closely resembles the system studied by Ernst and Anderson, and is currently of interest because it is potentially quick) is the most vulnerable. It is this artifact, too, which makes numerical estimation of many other parameters difficult, including, for example, flow measurements by recording signal amplitudes[11,12] rather than phases.[13,14]

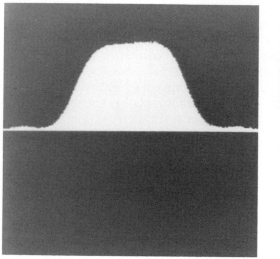

Figure 76–1

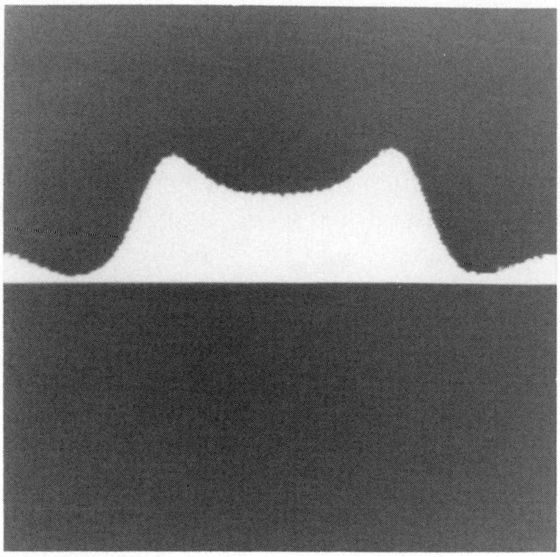

Figure 76–2

Figure 76–1. Image showing the form of slice when $TR \gg T1$ (in fact, $tR/T1 = 5.0$). The image was formed by using a relatively small object containing doped water with a $T1$ of about 600 ms. The sample was excited with a tR of 3 s by a 90 degree pulse in the presence of a slice selection gradient. Rephasing was performed with a reversed gradient, which was deliberately kept low so that the echo (optimal rephasing) was formed substantially later (about 10 ms) than usual, and the signal was sampled for 5 ms on either side of the echo. The data was then Fourier transformed and its magnitude displayed.

Figure 76–2. As for Figure 76–1 with the same experimental set-up except that TR was 120 ms ($TR/T1 = 0.20$).

Radio Frequency Amplitude Artifacts

Artifacts due to variations in rf amplitudes fall into two classes: (a) unintentional, which arise from defects in coil homogeneities, or errors in setting up and (b) deliberately induced to obtain an expected result. The former case is much the most common, and both its predictable consequences for image quality (lack of homogeneity) and simplest remedy (phase cycling of one form or another) are well known. (Phase cycling is much used in spectroscopy, for example in systems like CYCLOPS,[6] and is certainly used in imaging, although this is usually not mentioned explicitly in the literature.) One problem is that its use requires multiple acquisitions and extended scan times. In general, since the derivation of parameters involves taking the ratios of sets of data, use of identical sequences with different timing can often minimize the problem so that extracting $T1$ information from two single slice IR experiments with different values of TI and identical rf pulses minimizes errors due to rf inaccuracies. Extraction of $T2$

Table 76–2. APPARENT VALUES OF *T1* CALCULATED USING
A PAIR OF PS SEQUENCES AS GIVEN

Sequences for Calculation (All PS)		
Short (ms)	*Long (ms)*	*Apparent Value of T1 (ms)*
600	3000	372
600	1500	360
400	1000	297
300	600	243
200	400	163
100	1500	161
100	600	121
100	400	98

values from a pair of succeeding echoes is subject to error if alternating phases are not used for the two inverting pulses needed, leaving aside artifacts for example, due to flow.

Other rf manipulations can help resolve specific problems, but it is difficult to generalize. Thus, adiabatic fast passage[15,16] is an attractive method of inverting the magnetization accurately in inversion recovery, minimizing errors due to field inhomogeneity. However, it is not applicable to the inverting pulse in a spin echo nor to contiguous multislice experiments, although, in any case, better accuracy of measurement of tissue parameters is generally to be expected from single slice experiments.

An extreme case of the use of inhomogeneous rf transmitter fields is in the application of surface coils, in which the drop in rf field away from the coil can be used in defining a region of interest near the coil, and can be exploited in spatial encoding.[17] As has been shown, however, appropriate design of sequences permits good measurement using these coils.[18,19]

Deliberate variation of the pulse angle reflects the observation noted previously,[10] which predicts that the optimum signal-to-noise ratio for a simple partial saturation (90 – TR – 90 –) sequence is obtained where the precession angle $\propto$ is given by

$$\propto \; = \; \cos^{-1}(\exp(TR/T1)) \tag{1}$$

Methods of rapid imaging often exploit variations in precession angle to optimize the experiment, exemplified by the work of Waterton and his colleagues.[20] Optimization of precession angles at even relatively slow repetition rates can result in enhanced image contrast as shown in Figures 76–3 and 76–4, a pair of partial saturation images both acquired with a TR of 300 ms. Figure 76–3 was taken using a precession angle of 90 degrees, while Figure 76–4 was acquired using a pulse angle of 56 degrees. This is optimized for gray matter (T1 of about 520 ms at 0.15 T, the operating field of the machine used), and this, in conjunction with an improvement in slice shape, results in a substantial gain in differentiation between gray and white matter. However, it is

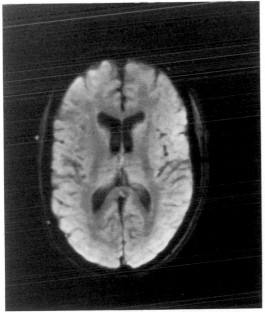

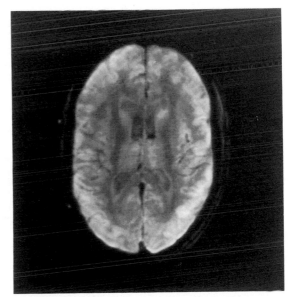

Figure 76–3   **Figure 76–4**

Figure 76–3. PS image of the brain of a volunteer (matrix 256 × 256, slice thickness 4 mm) taken with a TR of 300 ms, and rf precession angle of 90 degrees.

Figure 76–4. Image taken with the same parameters as for Figure 76–3, but with a precession angle of 56 degrees.

unlikely that such an image as Figure 76–4 could be used with others taken with appropriate, but different, settings of the rf precession angle to calculate image parameters, because the shape of the slice alters differently depending on the $T1$'s of the individual tissues.

Mixed Relaxation Mechanisms

The calculation of tissue parameters invariably assumes that all the magnetization available at the time of data acquisition has arisen using the method intended. This is not usually a problem with simple sequences except where the rf precession angle is so far from the expected value that the sequence does not seem to behave as predicted. (For example, the expression for inversion recovery assumes that the inversion angle is substantially 180 degrees whereas, if it deteriorates towards 90 degrees, the sequence degenerates towards partial saturation.)

Other sequences such as those based on stimulated echoes[21,22] introduce the possibility of the magnetization being measured having arisen by unintended processes. The sequence is illustrated in Figure 76–5, and it is apparent that if TB is extended, and TA is short, magnetization recovered by $T1$ relaxation will be excited at the third 90 degree pulse and overlap with magnetization being refocused by the same pulse. The results of such a problem are illustrated in Figure 76–6, whereas Figure 76–7 is an image of the same slice taken with the modification to the sequence indicated at the foot of Figure 76–5, which ensures that any relaxed magnetization excited at the third pulse is not rephased.

Both stimulated echo and IR systems with small values of TI (STIR sequences[23]) produce data in which contrast due to $T1$ and $T2$ is additive. Unfortunately, both have

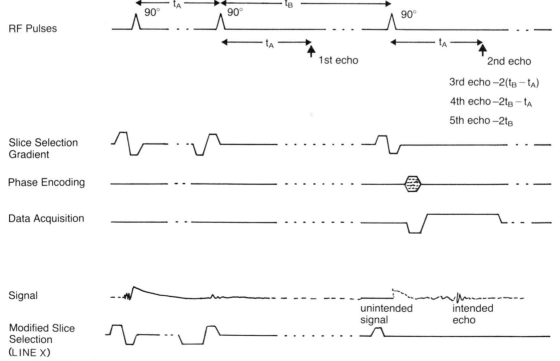

Figure 76–5. Diagram showing the form of the stimulated echo sequence, in its simplest, most direct form with slice selection of each rf pulse. The presence of wanted echo signals is indicated, as is the unwanted directly recovered signal. A number of ways exist to avoid this, including the method shown in line X where all the rephasing for the echo is completed before the final excitation.

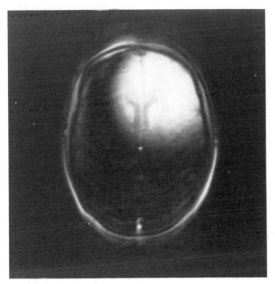
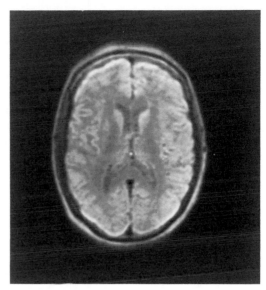

Figure 76–6   **Figure 76–7**

Figure 76–6. Image taken with a stimulated echo sequence with $TA = 22$ ms, $TB = 50$ ms (matrix 128×128, slice thickness 4 mm) showing gross artifact due to the mixing of signals.

Figure 76–7. Image as in Figure 76–6, but with the precaution indicated in Figure 76–5, to avoid mixing data.

reduced signal levels, as predicted theoretically in the case of the former[21,24] and as arises in the latter from the need to allow a suitable delay time for whatever signal manipulation is wanted. During the period of TI signal amplitudes fall. The short TI IR (STIR) sequence can be designed either with a field echo data acquisition[25] or spin echo with any length of TE, or, indeed, with multiple echoes.

Fundamental Factors

The range of tissue parameters poses a problem in MRI that is inescapable, particularly in the head. Because of the artifacts mentioned in the previous sections, there is no simple sequence from which optimum measurements for all parameters and tissues can be acquired.

The major problem is most obviously with $T1$, since the range of values for this in the head is 10:1 (Table 76–1), and all the artifacts mentioned before are consequently potential problems. On the other hand, while it appears that $T1$ shows little evidence of multiple components[26] and a single exponential model is adequate, $T2$ is quite likely to be multiexponential.[26,27] However, restrictions on the number of echoes that are possible because of the need to switch gradients, and acquire blocks of data using acceptable bandwidths, means that the accuracy with which multiple exponents can be recognized and measured is very limited. The adequacy of the number of echoes needed to ensure that diffusion is not a significant artifact is noted elsewhere (Flow and Motion Effects).

Partial Volume Effects

The likely inaccuracies that can occur from the mixing of tissues with quite different parameters in a single voxel are obvious. In magnetic resonance imaging, however, unlike the comparable situation with computed tomography, it is possible in many instances to design sequences to help delineate one from the other.

Three distinct methods can be employed:

(a) the use of any available excess signal-to-noise ratio to reduce slice thickness;

(b) adjustment of the timing of the data acquisition in sequences using field rather than conventional spin echoes. Correctly timed asymmetric spin echoes, analogous to the methods for chemical shift imaging developed by Dixon[28,29] and Sepponen et al.,[30] are another approach.

(c) adjustment of the value of *TI* in inversion recovery so as to result in zero signal from material with a *TI* intermediate between those of the tissues to be resolved. The STIR method[23] is a special case of this approach (being designed to cancel the signal from regions containing lipid only).

EXCESS AVAILABLE SIGNAL-TO-NOISE RATIO

The desirability of minimizing slice thickness relative to planar dimensions is apparent from examination of the shape of the voxels. When imaging the head with a matrix of 256 × 256 and a 5 mm slice, the face dimensions of the voxel are 1 mm, 20 percent of the depth. A more symmetrical voxel is less likely to contain more than one tissue without this being recognized, and any available unnecessary signal-to-noise ratio is usefully employed in reducing slice width (to which it is directly proportional).

DELINEATION BY CHEMICAL SHIFT CANCELLATION

The second method works by delaying data acquisition until the signals from tissues with different chemical shifts are reduced by relative dephasing. In practice, in proton imaging, only lipid and water are present in sufficient abundance and with a reasonable enough balance in magnitude between them for there to be useful effects in the images.

The method is applicable to field echo[25] or asymmetric spin echo[28] methods in which the delay time (Figure 76–8) is given by:

$$TD = \frac{\phi}{\gamma \delta B_0} \tag{2}$$

where B_0 is the main field; δ is the chemical shift; and the phase difference, ϕ, is π radians in the most useful case. While the mutual cancellation of signals has little real

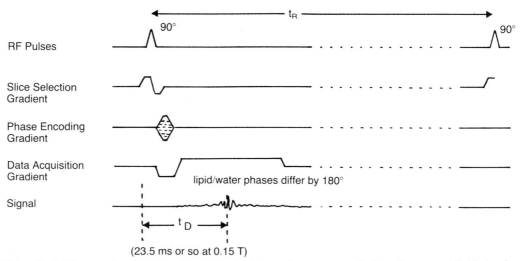

Figure 76–8. Diagram showing the pulse pattern leading to the cross cancellation of water and lipid signals in a field echo experiment. *TD* is the delay interval to the echo required.

analytical potential, its application in highlighting the presence of fat planes is considerable. Voxels containing such planes where, as is very likely, there is a mix of lipid and water signals can show markedly reduced signal intensity. This is shown in Figure 76–9, with typical boundaries marked.

DELINEATION BY CHOICE OF *TI* IN IR SEQUENCES

The method just described is not applicable to regions like the brain which lack any lipid component. The alternative IR technique is applicable to any pair of tissues as long as their *T1* values are significantly different (otherwise their signal levels in the final image are too low). Cancellation of signals in an IR sequence occurs when *TI* is chosen such that:

$$2 \exp(-TI/T1) = 1 + \exp(-TR/T1) \qquad (3)$$

By choosing *TI* to be intermediate between the two *TI*'s needed to eliminate signals from a pair of tissues, the boundaries of which are to be resolved, the relative signals for the two components (A and B) are then as shown in Figure 76–10. Magnitude reconstruction of the data results in an image like that in Figure 76–11, which was designed to differentiate between gray and white matter (although, incidentally, it does the same for white matter and cerebrospinal fluid (which has an even longer *T1*) and would do so with anything else with a *T1* greater than that for which the signal is zero).

Both methods produce images that can be used as part of the measurement procedure. Thus, the IR image can be used directly as one set of data for measuring *T1*, and using a spin echo data acquisition (with multiple echoes if necessary) as part of the measurement of *T2*. The chemical shift method can be used with IR as well as the PS and SR sequences—though, of course, multiple echoes are less practicable. On the other hand, resolution of several tissue pairs by the IR method may be a lengthy process, as each may require a separate image.

Patient Motion

The consequences of patient motion in two-dimensional Fourier transform imaging are familiar—repeated faint reflections of highly contrasting edges spread across the

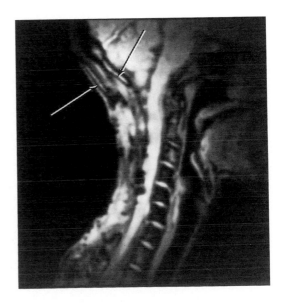

Figure 76–9. PS image (256 × 256 matrix, 4 mm slice thickness) with a *TD* (Fig. 76–8) of 22.5 ms (*T1* phase difference between lipid and water components at 0.15T) showing cancellation effects in fat planes between tissues (arrows).

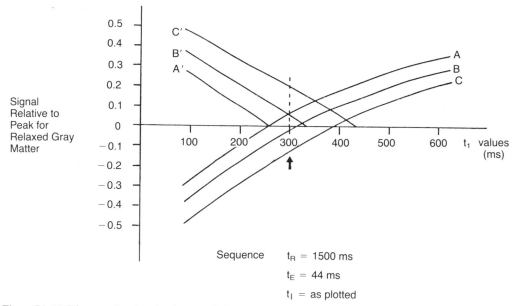

Sequence
t_R = 1500 ms
t_E = 44 ms
t_I = as plotted

Figure 76–10. Diagram showing the characteristics and indicating how the boundaries between tissues develop in an inversion recovery image (around the zero point). The reconstruction used in this configuration is by magnitude only, and the true characteristics are plotted, with *A* being white matter; *B*, gray matter; *C*, tumor. Dash superscript shows magnitude characteristic. If *TI* is as arrowed, amplitudes of gray and white are *y* (coincidentally the same) and tumor *z*.

image. From images such as Figure 76–12, it is intuitively obvious how bad their effect can be on the accuracy of any measurements of *T1* and *T2* which may be attempted, although this is equally difficult to predict theoretically. The rim of fat at the anterior of the abdomen is a major source of the artifact and has proved much more difficult to control than the apparently much greater motion of the heart. Heart motion is, however, much quicker, and simple EKG units supply good signals to which the scanning system may be locked. Time penalties resulting from this are acceptable, and images are good. However, the accuracy of *T2* measurements must be regarded with caution, as motion during the period between the 90 degree pulse and the data recovery

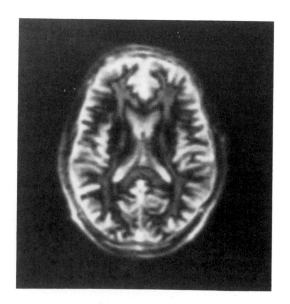

Figure 76–11. IR image with *TI* = 255 ms and *TR* = 1400 ms (128 × 128 matrix, 10 mm slice) showing the delineation of the boundaries between gray and white matter.

results in loss of signal, since the coherence of echo formation depends on the maintenance of the field pattern before and after the 180 degree pulse.

Control of abdominal motion can require all the available methods to obtain adequate control. Unfortunately, this can often extend imaging time, with conventional forms of respiratory gating potentially increasing it by a factor of 3 or more.

Techniques that show direct benefit include the STIR method,[23] aimed at canceling the signal from fatty tissue. Images produced by the method look substantially different from those from SE sequences, although they have a similarity of appearance with those from computed tomography. Since the form of data collection is at the user's discretion, both long and short *TE* spin echoes can be used.

Methods for minimizing the delays in conventional gating, such as respiratory ordered phase encoding (ROPE), can be employed at the same time. Discussion of this is not appropriate here, since that can be found in the literature,[31] but the effectiveness of the method is illustrated by Figures 76–12 and 76–13.

Other methods, such as phase alternation of the 180 degree pulses between successive data acquisitions, require a minimum of two averages for each data line, and thus take significantly longer to image, although signal-to-ratio is improved.

Flow and Motion Effects

There are many potential errors in all types of images due to flow and motion artifacts. Included in the latter are fundamental molecular level effects like diffusion and less basic artifacts with the same consequences, such as multidimensional perfused flow. The method used for resolving diffusion effects is the Carr-Purcell sequence and its variants,[32,33] although, in a whole body machine, there are a number of engineering constraints that mean that the sequence can only be implemented with a limited number of echoes.

Carr and Purcell[32] showed that reduction of diffusion effects, for example, to 0.25 percent of their presence in a single echo, required that the number of echoes in the same time should be in the region of 10. Two factors restrict the number of echoes and the rapidity of their repetition: the various safety regulations and the difficulty of operating a large machine very fast. The former are important because of rf dose levels

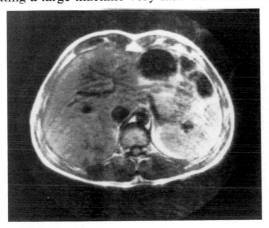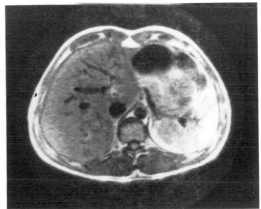

Figure 76–12   **Figure 76–13**

Figure 76–12. SE image (SE 544/44) of the abdomen of a volunteer (256 × 256 matrix, 5 mm slice) showing the successive faint hoops across the image that are characteristic of the motion artifact in the two-dimensional Fourier transform system.

Figure 76–13. Pair of the image in Figure 76–12, except that respiratory corrected phase encoding has been used to minimize motion artifact.

(from a large number of inverting pulses) and the possibility of high rates of change of field from the encoding gradients. Operating very quickly means that the gradient and rf powers needed may become very great, and the difficulty of designing gradient coils with a low enough inductance to allow very fast switching is substantial.

Particularly if an interleaved slice acquisition is employed, the need to form the slices means, firstly, that gradients other than those needed in generating the slice must be turned off, and secondly, that if short inverting pulses are used gradients must be large. If a single slice method is employed, the data acquisition gradient need not be switched, providing the rf pulses used are short enough.[34] Even with this simplification, it is hard to form echoes at intervals of less than 5 ms while maintaining adequately small bandwidth to generate worthwhile images. Since data can be acquired usefully for 200 to 250 ms in regions such as the brain, this means a maximum of 40 to 50 good quality echoes.

Whereas diffusion effects affect the amplitude of signals,[35] flow artifacts of all kinds modify their phase. If the flow is not transverse to the slice, phase errors can produce amplitude artifacts, even with magnitude reconstruction, independent of the sequence design. The effect is analogous to the chemical shift manipulation of signals described by Dixon[28] and Bydder.[36] The danger is then of unrecognized flow artifacts. The problem is illustrated by the pair of images in Figures 76–14 and 76–15. These are a pair of gated images, that in Figure 76–14 at systole and that in Figure 76–15 at diastole. Observation of the subarachnoid space (arrowed) shows significant differences in appearance due to flow in the cerebrospinal fluid.

It is not proposed to discuss the phase-based techniques used in measuring flow, as these are fully documented in the literature,[13,14] but the data in them can be generated from images that appear virtually identical.[37] In such circumstances, in order to be sure of what is happening, it may be necessary to take a second image with appropriate modification of the sequence and calculate a phase difference image so that locations where there is the possibility of the signal being artifacted by flow may be identified.

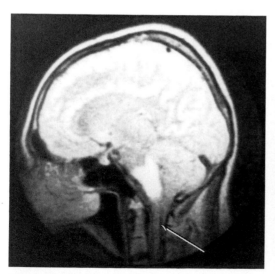 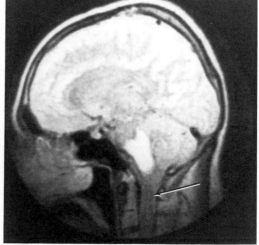

Figure 76–14   **Figure 76–15**

Figure 76–14. Gated sagittal SE image (SE 544/44) of the brain at systole. The matrix was 256 × 256 and the slice thickness 4 mm.

Figure 76–15. Image as in Figure 76–14, but at diastole. The arrows point to the subarachnoid space, which shows differences between the two images indicative of flow in the CSF. Without knowledge of what was happening, incorrect tissue parameters would be calculated in the region.

Biochemical and Multicomponent Effects

In practice, artifacts in the measurements due to the chemical characteristics and behavior of metabolites can be ignored. Their concentration in aggregate is much too low for them to contribute to the signal levels of a typical imaging experiment. In practice, only lipid and water signals are significant, and even the former can be regarded as having a single chemical line. There is then little likelihood of chemical based artifacts in *T1* and *T2* measurements.

The presence of multiple components with substantially different time constants has been discounted in the case of *T1*[26] but is recognized as being quite probable in the case of *T2*. This is not the same as saying that the experiments actually done are necessarily affected by their presence. Many of the short components of *T2* in normal tissue (typically on the order of 5 ms or less) are such that if the examination does not involve spin-echo times (*TE*) of less than 20 ms (at which the signal from a short *T2* component will be small, perhaps 2 percent of its original value), they can be regarded as not contributing significantly to the measurement. Generally, unless large numbers of echoes are acquired, it is unlikely that any useful assessment of possible multiple components in *T2* can be made, and, it is virtually impossible to allow enough time in an examination to evaluate any *T1* components properly.

It might seem that there are so many artifacts that the measurement of *T1* and *T2* can never be made with high accuracy inside the time available for a typical examination. However, this may not be a major disadvantage, since studies that track changes in the parameters in a single case or in a population can be completed in a relatively short time with consistency. The result is not the measurement of *T1* or *T2* but of parameters that can be reproduced as long as the experiments are done with care. This may well be adequate for the large majority of examinations.

Acknowledgments

We are grateful to the DHSS, and especially to Mr. G. R. Higson and Mr. J. L. Williams, for their continuing support and encouragement.

References

1. Rosen BR, Pykett IL, Brady TJ: Spin-lattice relaxation time measurements in two-dimensional nuclear magnetic resonance imaging. Corrections for plane selection and pulse sequence. J Comp Asst Tomogr 8:195–199, 1984.
2. Young IR, Bryant DJ, Payne JA: Variations in slice shape and absorption as artifacts in the determination of tissue parameters in NMR imaging. Magn Reson Med 2:355–389, 1985.
3. Foster MA: Examining the image slice. Proceedings of the Second Annual Congress of the European Society for Magnetic Resonance, Medicine, and Biology, Montreux, Switzerland, 1985, p 27.
4. Hoult DI: A criticism of the concept of a selective pulse in the presence of a field gradient. J Magn Reson 26:165–167, 1977.
5. Silver MS, Joseph RI, Hoult DI: Highly selective $\pi/2$ and π pulse generation. J Magn Reson 59:347, 1984.
6. Hoult DI, Richards RE: Critical factors in the design of sensitive high resolution nuclear magnetic resonance spectrometers. Proc R Soc Lond Ser A 344:311–340, 1975.
7. Bryant DJ, Payne JA, Young IR: Effect of slice distortion in MR imaging on accuracy of measurement. Proceedings of the Third Annual Meeting of the Society for Magnetic Resonance Medicine, New York, 1984, pp 109–110.
8. Young IR, Bydder GM: Some factors involving slice shape which affect contrast in nuclear magnetic resonance (NMR) imaging. Ann Radiol (Paris) 28:112–118, 1985.
9. Bloch F, Hansen WW, Packard ME: The nuclear induction experiment. Phys Rev 70:474–485, 1946.
10. Ernst RR, Anderson WA: Application of Fourier transform spectroscopy to magnetic resonance. Rev Sci Inst 37:93, 1966.
11. Singer JR, Crooks LE: Nuclear magnetic resonance blood flow measurements in the human brain. Science 221:654–656, 1983.

12. Singer JR: Blood flow measurements by NMR of the intact body. *In* Partain CL, et al (eds): Nuclear Magnetic Resonance (NMR) Imaging. Philadelphia, WB Saunders, 1983.
13. Moran PR: A flow velocity zeugmatographic interleave for NMR imaging in humans. Magn Reson Imaging *1*:197–203, 1982.
14. Bryant DJ, Payne JA, Firmin DN, Longmore DB: Measurement of flow with NMR imaging using a gradient pulse and phase difference technique. J Comp Asst Tomogr *8*:588, 1984.
15. Abragam A: The Principles of Nuclear Magnetism. Oxford, Clarenden Press, 1978, pp 35–37, 65 et seq.
16. Hardy CJ, Edelstein WA, Vatis D, Harms R, Adams WJ: Calculated *T1* images derived from a partial saturation-inversion recovery pulse sequence with adiabatic fast passage. Magn Reson Imaging *3*:107–116, 1985.
17. Cox SJ, Styles P: Towards biochemical imaging. J Magn Reson *40*:209–212, 1980.
18. Thulborn KR, Ackerman JJH: Absolute molar concentrations by NMR in inhomogeneous B1. A scheme for analysis of in vivo metabolites. J Magn Reson *55*:357–371, 1983.
19. Evelhoch JH, Ackerman JJH: NMR *T1* measurements in inhomogeneous B1 with surface coils. J Magn Reson *53*:52, 1983.
20. Waterton JC, Jenkins JPR, Zhu XP, Love HG, Isherwood I, Rowlands DJ: Magnetic resonance (MR) cine imaging of the human heart. Br J Radiol *58*:711–716, 1985.
21. Hahn EL: Spin echoes. Phys Rev *80*:580–594, 1950.
22. Frahm J, Morboldt KD, Hanicke W, Haase A: Stimulated echo imaging, J Magn Reson *64*:81–93, 1985.
23. Bydder GM, Young IR: MRI: Clinical use of the inversion recovery sequence. J Comp Asst Tomogr *9*:659–675, 1985.
24. Sattin W, Mareci TH, Scott KN: Exploiting the stimulated echo in nuclear magnetic resonance imaging. I. Method. J Magn Reson *64*:177–182, 1985.
25. Sutherland RJ, Hutchison JMS: Three dimension NMR imaging using selective excitation. J Phys E: Sci Instrum *11*:79, 1978.
26. Bottomley PA, Foster TH, Argersinger RE, Pfeifer LM: A review of normal tissue hydrogen NMR relaxation times and relaxation mechanisms form 1–100 MHz: Dependence on tissue type. Med Phys *11*:425, 1984.
27. Barnes D, MacDonald WI, Tofts P, Johnson G: Private communication, September, 1985.
28. Dixon WT: Simple proton spectroscopic imaging. Radiology *153*:189–194, 1984.
29. Dixon WT, Faul DD: Proton spectroscopic imaging at 0.35T. Proceedings of the Third Annual Meeting of the Society for Magnetic Resonance Medicine, New York, New York, 1984, p 193.
30. Sepponen RE, Sipponen JT, Tanttu JT: A method for chemical shift imaging. Demonstration of bone marrow involvement with proton chemical shift imaging. J Comp Asst Tomogr *8*:585, 1984.
31. Bailes DR, Gilderdale DJ, Bydder GM, Collins AG, Firmin DN: Respiratory ordered phase encoding (ROPE), a method for reducing respiratory motion artifact in magnetic resonance imaging. J Comp Asst Tomogr *9*:835–838, 1985.
32. Carr HY, Purcell EM: Effects of diffusion on free precession in nuclear magentic resonance experiments. Phys Rev *94*:630–638, 1958.
33. Meiboom S, Gill D: Modified spin echo method for measuring nuclear relaxation time. Rev Sci Instrum *29*:688, 1958.
34. Meves M, Schmidberger P, Bielke G, Higer HP, Meindl S, Skalej M, Pfannensteil P: Clinical utilization of multiecho-pulse-sequences in NMR imaging of the brain. *In* Hopf M-A, Bydder GM (eds): Magnetic Resonance Imaging and Spectroscopy. Geneva, European Society for Magnetic Resonance Medicine and Biology, 1985, pp 84–89.
35. Packer KJ: The study of slow coherent molecular motion by pulsed nuclear magnetic resonance. Mol Phys *17*:355, 1969.
36. Bydder GM, Young IR: Clinical use of the partial saturation and saturation recovery sequences in MR imaging. J Comp Asst Tomogr *9*:1020–1032, 1985.
37. Young IR, Payne JA, Bydder GM: Flow measurement by the development of phase differences during slice formation in MR imaging. Magn Reson Med *3* (1986) (in press).

77

Image Reconstruction

RODNEY A. BROOKS

Magnetic resonance image (MRI) reconstruction is not easy; every physicist who has worked in the field, if he is honest, will admit to frequent periods of confusion. Yet, as is usually the case, there are underlying simplicities that are accessible to any intelligent person who makes the effort. While the mathematics uses Fourier transforms, a rather advanced methodology, the physical interpretations can be given in nonmathematical terms.

Our presentation is based on the unifying approach that the MRI signal is the two-dimensional Fourier transform of the image.[6,10] To help maintain simplicity, we have limited our discussion to the two most commonly used methods: reconstruction from projections and two-dimensional Fourier reconstruction. The number of equations has been held to a minimum, and complexities, such as refocusing gradients, have been neglected. Nevertheless, the use of multiple integrals and complex notation may prove foreboding; the nonmathematical reader is urged to skip over the equations and concentrate on the figures and text. A summary of notation is given in Table 77–1. The reader looking for a more extensive mathematical treatment should refer to any of a number of recent review articles. Particularly recommended is the King and Moran article.[6]

Historical Note. Mathematical image reconstruction was first proposed by Bracewell for reconstructing images of solar microwave emission.[1] In Bracewell's method, one starts with line-integrals, or ray-sums, of the quantity being measured. (For solar radio emission, the line-integrals were measured with a linear array of microwave antennas; the position and orientation of the line varied with the rotation and revolution of the earth.) A set of parallel line-integrals is called a projection. Bracewell showed that the Fourier transforms of the projections are equivalent to the Fourier transforms of the image. Thus, by appropriate projection measurements, one can obtain a full set of transform data and then one can reconstruct the image by taking the inverse two-dimensional transform. However, because the Fourier transform values obtained from the projections are not distributed at regular increments, it is first necessary to interpolate to a rectangular array.[9] The entire procedure is illustrated in Figure 77–1.

Because of the necessity for two-dimensional interpolation, as well as computational difficulties in taking Fourier transforms at the time, Bracewell later developed an alternative inversion formula, now called filtered back-projection (FBP), which is better suited for the polar coordinate array of transform values that result from projection measurements.[2] This is the method now used almost universally for x-ray computed tomography and positron emission tomography. For our purposes, filtered back-projection may be thought of merely as an alternative way to invert a two-dimension Fourier transform, in effect, a polar coordinate version of the fast Fourier transform algorithm. The reader is referred to the Brooks and Di Chiro review[3] for a comparison of the two methods.

Table 77–1. SUMMARY OF NOTATION

B	Magnetic field strength (tesla)
c	Sensitivity of rf coil and amplifier (volts/tesla-cm^2)
d	Diameter of field of view (cm)
f	Precession frequency of nuclei (cycles/sec or Hz)
g	Strength of magnetic field gradient (tesla/cm)
k	Wave number, or spatial frequency (cycles/cm)
m	Transverse nuclear magnetization density at measurement time (Hz)
p	Line integral of m (tesla-cm). A set of line integrals at the same angle is called a projection.
M, P	Fourier Transforms of m and p (complex)
r, s	Cartesian image coordinates rotated by angle ϕ (cm)
t	Time (s). The time of peak echo signal is $t = 0$.
τ	Time duration of y gradient (s)
v	Detected voltage from spin echo (volts) (complex to include quadrature signals)
x, y	Cartesian image coordinates (cm)
ϕ	Projection angle (radians)
γ	Modified nuclear gyromagnetic ratio, (Hz/tesla)

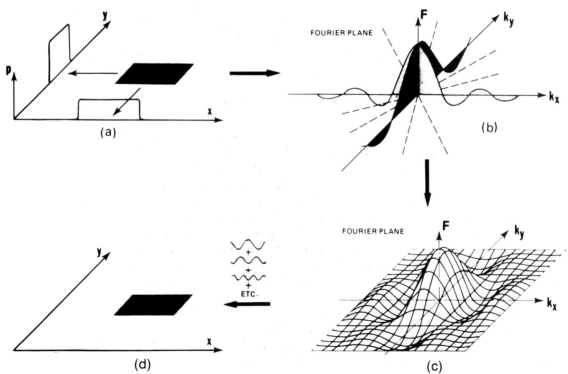

Figure 77–1. Illustration of two-dimensional Fourier reconstruction, as originally conceived by Bracewell.[1] For simplicity, a rectangle is chosen as the object being imaged. (a) Projections of the object are measured (only two are shown). (b) Fourier transforms of the projections are calculated (dashed lines suggest other transformed projections). (c) A rectangular array of transforms is interpolated from the polar data. (d) The image is reconstructed by taking the inverse two-dimensional transform. For MR tomography, step (b) is not needed, as transforms are measured directly. Also, the interpolation step (c) can be eliminated by using orthogonal field gradients and phase encoding. All that is required is the two-dimensional Fourier inversion (d). (From Brooks RA, Di Chiro G: Physics Med Biol *21*:689, 1976. Used by permission.)

MRI Historical Note. The development of MRI reconstruction[8] also began with the measurement of projections. In the first implementation the projections were measured one ray at a time using continuous excitation, in effect measuring the total NMR signal from those nuclei lying along a given ray. Pulse techniques were then introduced that enabled one to produce a parallel set of rays (i.e., one projection) following a single excitation pulse. After taking a full set of projection data, the image was reconstructed using filtered back-projection, for the reasons given above.

However, with MRI a unique capability exists that is not true of those methods that depend on the geometrical definition of rays by apertures. By phase-encoding the effect of field gradients,[4,7] one can generate directly the rectangular array of Fourier coefficients needed for use with the fast Fourier transform algorithm. This two-dimensional Fourier method is now the workhorse of MR imaging. Thus the 1956 approach of Bracewell has finally come to practical fruition.

Plan of Presentation. Our exposition begins with the basic two-dimensional Fourier reconstruction theorem (Eq. 1), along with some helpful interpretations of the Fourier integrals. The remainder of the chapter is an explanation of how this theorem is implemented—in particular, how the NMR signal is used to produce values of the Fourier coefficients of the image. A subsequent section, MR Signal Detection, is devoted to explaining the origin of the MR signal. However, the extraction of Fourier coefficients from the signal requires the use of magnetic field gradients. The simplest such method, involving one field gradient per measurement, is described in the section which follows, entitled Reconstruction from Projections. This method is very similar to x-ray computed tomography reconstruction. Finally, there is a section on Two-dimensional Fourier Reconstruction, the current method of choice in MRI tomography, which involves the use of two orthogonal field gradients per measurement. For each method it is shown how the detected MR signal is equivalent to the image Fourier transform, and therefore how the image can be synthesized by an inverse transform operation or equivalent. In each case, the explanation in terms of spatial Fourier transforms is augmented by an alternative interpretation, in which the MR signal is seen as a superposition of Larmor frequencies. An understanding that the superposition of Larmor frequencies in the MR signal is the same superposition needed for the two-dimensional spatial Fourier transform is the key to understanding MR image reconstruction.

THEORY OF IMAGE RECONSTRUCTION

The Inverse Two-Dimensional Fourier Transform

It is a well-known fact that any function can be built up from sine and cosine waves. This applies also to a function of two coordinates (x, y), such as the quantity depicted in a radiological image. For MR tomography, the quantity of interest is the net transverse magnetization density $m(x, y)$ that exists at the time of measurement. This in turn depends in a complicated manner on the excitation-measurement sequence and on the relaxation times of the tissue. Because of this the interpretation of NMR images is much more complex than x-ray or radionuclide images, but that is another question.

The equation that describes the synthesis of $m(x, y)$ from sinusoidal waves is the two-dimensional inverse Fourier transform:

$$m(x, y) = \iint M(k_x, k_y) \exp[2\pi i(k_x x + k_y y)] \, dk_x \, dk_y \text{*} \tag{1}$$

---

* All integrals in this chapter are definite integrals, extending from $-\infty$ to $+\infty$.

The variables k_x and k_y are the wave numbers, or spatial frequencies, of the sinusoidal waves in the x and y directions. The units of k_x and k_y are cycles/cm. An image with spatial resolution of 1 mm generally requires sinusoidal waves with wave numbers ranging from 0 to about 5 cycles/cm, so in practice the infinite integrals of Equation (1) can be replaced by finite summations.

In Equation (1) we have followed the capital letter convention for Fourier transform, so that $M(k_x, k_y)$ is the Fourier transform of $m(x, y)$, i.e., it represents the coefficients of the sine and cosine components. The reader may perhaps wonder where the sine and cosine functions are hiding. The answer is that, thanks to the magic of complex notation, they are both represented by the complex exponential; i.e., for any number a,

$$\text{Re exp}(ia) = \cos a$$

$$\text{Im exp}(ia) = \sin a$$

A complex number is nothing more than a way to encompass two real numbers simultaneously in a single expression. They are particularly useful in Fourier analysis, where sine and cosine contributions must both be included.

The Fourier coefficients $M(k_x, k_y)$ are also complex numbers. The real part of M gives the amplitude of the sine and cosine combinations that are symmetrical about the origin in the (x, y) plane, viz., $\cos(2\pi k_x x) \cos(2\pi k_y y)$ and $\sin(2\pi k_x x) \sin(2\pi k_y y)$. The imaginary part of M gives the amplitude of combinations that are antisymmetric about the origin, viz., $\cos(2\pi k_x x) \sin(2\pi k_y y)$ and $\sin(2\pi k_x x) \cos(2\pi k_y y)$. The power of complex notation is exhibited clearly in Equation (1) by its ability to compress a motley collection of products of sines and cosines into a simple formula.

It should also be noted that the integrals of Equation (1) extend over negative wave numbers. These, of course, are not physically meaningful but are merely a mathematical way to ensure that the result of the inverse transform, $m(x, y)$, is a real quantity. The values of M for negative wave numbers are redundant to the corresponding positive values. Specifically, the real part of M is symmetric about the origin in the Fourier plane (k_x, k_y), and the imaginary part is antisymmetric.

The reader not familiar with Fourier analysis should not worry about the details of Equation (1) but should simply understand that it represents a superposition of sine and cosine waves, with amplitudes, or coefficients, represented by M.

What is surprising is that Equation (1) is the only equation needed for MR image reconstruction. By appropriate pulse sequences and manipulation of field gradients, one can measure the Fourier coefficients $M(k_x, k_y)$ directly and then synthesize the image, using either Equation (1) or the filtered back-projection alternative. The remaining task of this chapter is to explain how the Fourier coefficients are obtained from the MR signals.

The Two-Dimension Fourier Transform

Fourier showed not only that any function can be synthesized from sines and cosines, but he also gave a formula for the coefficients in terms of the given function. The formula is called the Fourier transform and, surprisingly enough, is almost identical to the inverse transform:

$$M(k_x, k_y) = \iint m(x, y) \exp[-2\pi i(k_x x + k_y y)] \, dx \, dy \qquad (2)$$

It is necessary to understand this formula in order to understand how the coefficients are obtained from the MR signals. However, further discussion will be postponed until after the next few paragraphs, in which the one-dimensional transform is introduced. An intuitive understanding is easier when one has only one dimension to worry about.

Definition of Projection

The image Fourier transform is also closely related to the image projections, so it will be helpful to examine the concept of projections before proceeding. A projection, p, is defined as a set of parallel line-integrals across the image at a given angle φ:

$$p(r, \varphi) = \int m(x, y)\, ds \tag{3}$$

where the integral is taken along the ray defined by r and φ, as illustrated in Figure 77–2. In Equation (3) r gives the radial position of each ray, while s represents path length along the ray. A full set of parallel line integrals is called a projection, and φ is called the projection angle, or view angle.

To see the intimate relationship between the projection and the image, consider the one-dimensional Fourier transform of a projection with respect to r,

$$P(k, \varphi) = \int p(r, \varphi) \exp(-2\pi ikr)\, dr \tag{4}$$

Using Equation (3), and making an orthogonal coordinate transformation from (r, s) to (x, y), we obtain

$$P(k, \varphi) = \iint m(x, y) \exp(-2\pi i(k_x x + k_y y))\, dx\, dy = M(k_x, k_y) \tag{5}$$

where

$$k_x = k \cos \varphi$$

and

$$k_y = k \sin \varphi \tag{6}$$

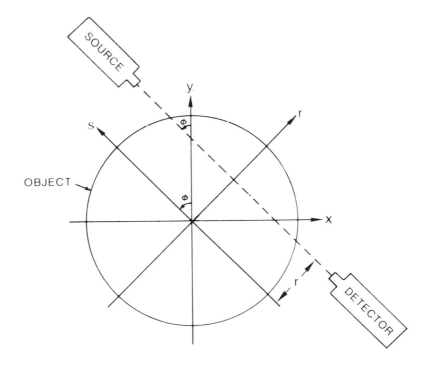

Figure 77–2. Illustration of image coordinate system (x, y) and projection coordinate system (r, s) rotated by the projection angle ϕ. The projection $p(r, \phi)$ is made up of line-integrals (dashed line) along parallel rays at different radial positions r. In this illustration, taken from an x-ray computed tomography article, the ray path is defined by an x-ray source and detector. In MR tomography the source and detector are not needed; instead the rays are defined by a magnetic field gradient in the r direction. This creates a different Larmor frequency along each ray path. Also in MR tomography all rays of a projection can be measured from a single pulse sequence. (From Brooks RA, Di Chiro G: Physics Med Biol *21*:689, 1976.)

are the components of k in the x and y directions. By comparing this result with Equation (2), we see that we have exactly the two-dimensional transform of m. In other words, the one-dimensional Fourier transform of a projection is equal to the subset of two-dimensional image transforms along a line in "k-space" that transects the origin at the projection angle φ, as suggested in Figure 77–1b.

Interpretation of the Inverse Fourier Transform

For those not familiar with Fourier analysis, the following descriptive explanation is offered. The inverse transform describes how any signal can be represented as a superposition of sinusoidal waves with proper amplitude and phase. The number that multiplies each component in the superposition, and hence determines its contribution (amplitude and phase), is called a Fourier coefficient. The most familiar example is in music, where it is well-known that any audio signal can be broken up into sinusoidal components. The ear itself is a kind of physiological Fourier transform computer, since different neural entities respond selectively to different frequency components of the sound.

A breakup into sinusoidal components is also possible for signals with a spatial, rather than temporal, variation, even when there are two or three spatial dimensions involved. The mathematics is the same, even though the equivalence of an image to a superposition of waves seems less intuitive to us (probably because the physiology of vision does not have a Fourier basis). The equivalence of a one-dimensional signal, e.g., a projection, to a sum of waves is illustrated in Figure 77–3. For a two-dimensional image the breakup into sinusoidal components requires waves extending in many dif-

FOUIER ANALYSIS OF PROJECTION

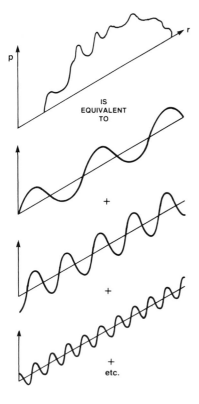

Figure 77–3. Illustration of how a one-dimensional spatial signal, such as a projection, can be expressed as a superposition of sinusoidal waves. The amplitude and phase of each component wave are expressed by a complex coefficient calculated with the Fourier transform formula. The superposition of sinusoidal waves to recreate the original signal is given by the inverse Fourier transform formula.

ferent directions, as shown in Figure 77–4. This picture is equivalent to, and much easier to draw than, products of waves in the x and y directions as in Equation (1). The difference between Figure 77–4 and the orthogonal wave picture (not shown) is tantamount to using polar coordinates, instead of rectangular coordinates, to describe the Fourier coefficients.

Interpretation of Fourier Transform

The formula for calculating Fourier coefficients is called the Fourier transform. To understand it better, we focus on the one-dimensional example shown in Equation (4), which consists of the integral of the ray-sums at each position r multiplied by a phase factor for that position. The phase factor, $\exp(-2\pi i k r)$, determines how much each ray will contribute to the cosine coefficient and how much to the sine coefficient. This may be seen better by writing the real and imaginary parts of the transform separately:

$$\text{Re } P(k, \varphi) = \int p(r, \varphi) \cos(-2\pi k r) \, dr \tag{7}$$

$$\text{Im } P(k, \varphi) = \int p(r, \varphi) \sin(-2\pi k r) \, dr$$

By examining the one-dimensional inverse transform,

$$p(r, \varphi) = \int P(k, \varphi) \exp(2\pi i k r) \, dk \tag{8}$$

it is easy to see that Re P is the coefficient of the cosine terms, and Im P is the coefficient of the sine terms. A similar interpretation has already been given for the two-dimensional transform $M(k_x, k_y)$.

FOURIER ANALYSIS OF IMAGE

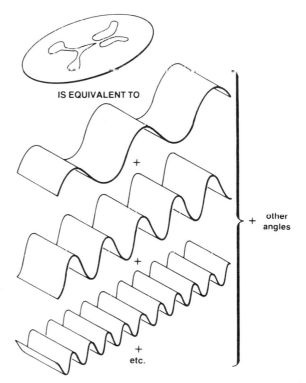

Figure 77–4. Illustration of how a two-dimensional image can be expressed as a superposition of sinusoidal waves. Note that waves in many different directions are needed.

The reader may ask: Why do Equations (2) and (4) produce the desired Fourier coefficients? The answer is that if the product of two sinusoidal waves is integrated from $-\infty$ to ∞, the result is zero, because of destructive interference, unless the frequencies and phases of the two waves are the same. Thus, multiplying an arbitrary signal by a sine or cosine, and integrating, selects out from the signal the Fourier component with the same wave number and phase as the multiplying factor, thereby producing the Fourier coefficient. It seems paradoxical that the transform and the inverse transform, which are identical mathematically (except for a minus sign), have opposite interpretations. In the transform, where the variable of integration is a spatial coordinate, the integral *selects out* the desired component. In the inverse transform, where the variable of integration is wave number, or spatial frequency, the same integral represents a *superposition* or *synthesis* of waves. The Fourier integral is like an optical illusion that changes its appearance, depending on how one looks at it.

In any event, it is important to understand that the Fourier coefficients are obtained by adding up contributions from magnetization at different points in space, each contributing with a different phase. Some regions of magnetization will contribute (negatively or positively) to the cosine coefficient, some to the sine coefficient, and some to both, depending on the phase angle $-2kr$ associated with that region.

SUMMARY

1. Any spatial signal, e.g., a one-dimensional projection or a two-dimensional image, can be built up from a series of sinusoidal waves of different wave numbers. The equation that describes the summation is called the inverse Fourier transform.

2. The coefficients needed for the above process are obtained by adding up contributions from the quantity of interest (magnetization) at all points, multiplied by a phase factor. This formula is called the Fourier transform.

3. The basic concept of present-day NMR tomography is to obtain the Fourier coefficients of the image from the NMR signal and to reconstruct the image by taking the inverse Fourier transform.

MR SIGNAL DETECTION

Slice Selection

The term tomography means literally "picture of a slice." In practice one images a thick "slab," as there would be no signal from a true slice of zero thickness (although the term slice is still commonly used). In x-ray and emission computed tomography, slice definition and selection are done with collimators that physically block off rays that do not traverse the desired slice. In MR imaging, detection is performed by electronic coils that cannot be shielded from out-of-slice magnetic radiation. Instead, slice definition is usually accomplished by selective excitation.

Excitation refers to the rotation of nuclear magnetization from its normal alignment with the static magnetic field B into the transverse plane. This is done by applying a burst of radio frequency (rf) current in a surrounding coil, whose axis is transverse to the field B. The rf frequency must be equal to the Larmor frequency of the nuclei:

$$f = \gamma B \qquad (9)$$

where γ is the nuclear gyromagnetic ratio. Following King and Moran, we incorporate $1/2\pi$ into the definition of γ, so that the units are Hz/tesla, in order to simplify our equations.

In practice the excitation pulse contains a range of frequencies, as specified by the bandwidth of the pulse. By simultaneously applying a gradient to the magnetic field in the z direction, the excitation may be limited only to those nuclei whose Larmor frequency falls within the bandwidth of the pulse. The location and thickness of the region of excitation are thus determined by the axial field gradient and the central frequency and bandwidth of the rf pulse. The axial gradient, of course, is removed after excitation is complete.

Slice Interleaving

After excitation and detection, it takes some time for the nuclear magnetization to realign itself with the static field—many seconds for some fluids such as cerebro-spinal fluid. Therefore a waiting time is necessary before repeating the excitation-detection sequence. It is now common practice to use this waiting time to excite other slices and detect the signals therefrom. This is accomplished by repeating the rf excitation pulse with a different central frequency relative to the axial field gradient.

Spin-Echo Detection

Immediately after excitation an rf voltage is induced in the receiving coil (usually the same as the excitation coil) as the nuclei precess at the Larmor frequency. This signal, however, dies away quickly as phase incoherence develops because of field inhomogeneity (deliberate or accidental). This process is called free induction decay.

The usual method of signal detection is the spin-echo technique. This method does not use the free induction decay; but instead an inverting, or 180 degree, pulse is applied to the coil, some time after excitation, which has the effect of reversing whatever phase differences have accumulated among the precessing nuclei. Provided the field inhomogenicities responsible for these phase differences remain the same, it follows that an equal time later phase coherence will be restored and an appreciable rf voltage will again be induced in the receiving coil. This signal is called the spin echo.

If the rf signal is simply rectified, the resulting voltage will reach a peak at the time of maximum phase coherence ($t = 0$) and then subside as dephasing occurs again. The peak voltage at $t = 0$ is proportional to the total transverse magnetization.

Phase-Sensitive Detection

In MR tomography, however, we are not interested in the total signal but in components at different frequencies, caused by the application of field gradients during the measurement. We will also need to measure any phase differences that have accumulated. These goals are accomplished by a technique called quadrature phase-sensitive detection, in which the induced rf voltage is multiplied by signals $\cos(2\pi f_0 t)$ and $\sin(2\pi f_0 t)$, generated by a reference oscillator at the nominal Larmor frequency f_0 corresponding to the nominal magnetic field B_0.

The result is two quadrature signals, which can be written as a single complex voltage

$$v(t) = c \iint m(x, y) \exp[2\pi i\{f(x, y) - f_0\}t] \, dx \, dy \qquad (10)$$

where $f(x, y)$ is the precession frequency for the magnetization component at coordinates (x, y), and c is the combined sensitivity of the coil and amplifiers. The real part of $v(t)$ gives the detected signal from the cosine multiplication and the imaginary part gives the detected signal from the sine multiplication.

While Equation (10) could be derived by expanding the trigonometric products, this derivation is omitted in favor of an intuitive interpretation. What happens is that the various Larmor frequencies $f(x, y)$ within the spin-echo signal "beat" against the reference frequency f_0, and produce "difference frequencies". Thus each element of magnetization contributes toward the detected signal according to its precession frequency. If the precession frequency is f_0, the contribution is nonalternating (DC), but in general each contribution alternates with a frequency equal to the difference between the actual precession frequency and that of the reference oscillator.

At this stage we can already see the appearance of a Fourier transform emerging in Equation (10) (cf. Eq. 2). All that remains is to apply field gradients to give the Larmor frequencies the proper spatial dependence, as will be shown in the next section.

SUMMARY

1. Slice selection is achieved by applying an axial field gradient during excitation, to excite only the slab of interest.

2. Signal detection is usually performed from the spin echo, using quadrature phase-sensitive detection. The resulting two signals contain contributions from all excited magnetization, multiplied by a phase factor that depends on the frequency of precession.

RECONSTRUCTION FROM PROJECTIONS
(Polar Coordinates)

Use of Field Gradient

The remaining task is to relate the frequency components of the detected signal linearly to spatial position. This may be done by applying a field gradient g in the direction of the r axis of Figure 77–1, so that the axial magnetic field is given by

$$B = B_0 + gr \tag{11}$$

Then the Larmor precession frequency will also be a function of r:

$$f(r) = \gamma B = f_0 + \gamma gr \tag{12}$$

If the gradient is present throughout the detection period (as well as for a symmetrical time before the reversing pulse, so as not to disturb the phase coherence of the spin echo), the detected signal (Eq. 10) becomes

$$v(t) = c \iint m(x, y) \exp(2\pi i\gamma grt)\, dx\, dy. \tag{13}$$

This is the key equation that relates the NMR signal to the image transform. By making the detecting frequencies correspond to position r, we have injected the position variable into the exponent in just the right way to make the detected signal coincide with the definition of the two-dimensional Fourier transform (Eq. 2). To see this mathematically, we identify the quantity $-\gamma gt$ with a wave number variable,

$$k = -\gamma gt \tag{14}$$

and define k_x and k_y as before (Eq. 6). Since $kr = k_x x + k_y y$, we can write

$$v(t) = c \iint m(x, y) \exp(2\pi i(k_x x + k_y y))\, dx\, dy = cM(k_x, k_y), \tag{15}$$

which, except for c, is equivalent to Eq. (2).

Alternatively, if we change the integration coordinates in Eq. (13) to (r, s) and use the definition of a projection (Eq. 3), we can write

$$v(t) = c \int p(r, \varphi) \exp(-2\pi ikr) \, dr = cP(k, \varphi), \qquad (16)$$

which is equivalent to Equation (4). In either interpretation, we see that the two quadrature MR signals measured at time t are proportional to the two-dimensional image transform value for wave number k, φ, (or, equivalently, k_x, k_y), and we see once again the equivalence of the image and projection transforms.

Image Reconstruction

One set of Fourier transforms, corresponding to a single projection, is not enough for image reconstruction. Therefore one repeats the above measurement procedure, after allowing enough time for nuclear realignment with the static field, with gradients applied in different directions, until a full set of data is acquired as shown in Figure 77–1*b* or Figure 77–5*a*. All that is needed now is to take the inverse two-dimensional transform. This can be done in one of two ways. On the one hand, we could interpolate to a rectangular array of coefficients and then use the two-dimensional fast Fourier transform algorithm (Fig. 77–1). On the other hand, we could proceed with filtered back-projection, which does not require a two-dimensional interpolation and so is better suited for inverting a polar data array. In practice, the second approach is usually followed.

Units of Reconstructed Image

If one knew the detector sensitivity, c, one could scale the reconstructed image in absolute units of magnetization. However, the sensitivity depends on, among other things, the size and structure of the subject, and so varies from image to image. In addition, the absolute value of $m(x, y)$ is not very useful, as it depends on the pulse sequence used. Therefore most manufacturers make no attempt to standardize on an image unit (as with the Hounsfield unit of x-ray computed tomography), but instead each image is usually scaled to an arbitrary maximum.

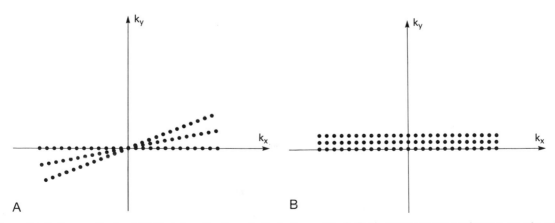

Figure 77–5. Two methods of NMR data collection. *A*, Projection method: Each measurement produces a set of coefficients along a "spoke" at the angle of the applied gradient. Three spokes are shown. *B* Two-dimensional Fourier method: Each measurement produces a row of Fourier coefficients in the direction of k_x, but with a different k_y offset. Three rows are shown.

Physical Interpretation of Signal

At this point we should stop and reflect, because a surprising thing has occurred. It is easy to understand that the detected signal contains many precession frequencies and that the amplitude of each frequency component depends on the total magnetization along the corresponding ray. After all, we applied a field gradient to achieve just this effect. In this sense the projection method is physically intuitive and very similar to the methods used in x-ray computed tomography.

What is surprising is that, as the detected signal evolves in time, it traces out the spatial Fourier transform of the projection. This is another example of the dual interpretation of the transform formula mentioned earlier. The formula for summing up Larmor frequencies to produce the total time-varying signal (Eq. 10), when looked at as a spatial integral, with proper field gradients present (Eq. 15 or 16), becomes a formula for selecting out a given spatial frequency. This is a consequence of the coupling between t and k (Eq. 14), made possible by the applied gradient. The superposition of sinusoidal waves in time that appears at the detector output is exactly the one needed to calculate the spatial Fourier transform of the magnetization for wave number $k = -\gamma g t$ and angle φ.

Alternative Interpretation

Equation (13) is a striking example of the dual personality of the Fourier integral. By identifying $-\gamma g t$ in the exponent with wave number k, we have seen the equation emerge as a Fourier transform which *selects out*, from the total magnetization density $m(x, y)$, the sinusoidal component with wave number k at direction φ.

But we also know that another grouping is possible in the exponent—the one used in deriving Equation (13), i.e., $\gamma g r$, which is the beat frequency, or difference frequency, emerging from the detector circuit. Under this interpretation, Equation (13) represents a *synthesis* of sinusoidally varying time functions, and the ray-sums $p(r, \varphi)$ are the coefficients. That is, each value of r corresponds to a different frequency, and the amplitude associated with that frequency is given by the corresponding ray-sum. (Remember that the frequencies encountered here are true frequencies in the time domain and not spatial frequencies.) Since real functions generally have complex Fourier coefficients, it follows that if the coefficients are real, the quantity being synthesized, $v(t)$, will be complex—hence the need for quadrature detection.

Under this alternate interpretation, one could easily obtain the projection, $p(r, \varphi)$ from the detected signal by taking its one-dimensional Fourier transform with respect to time. While such a possibility reveals the close connection of the MR signal to the ray-sums, it is not helpful for image reconstruction. What is needed to obtain the image function $m(x, y)$ is the two-dimensional inverse transform, not a one-dimensional transform that produces only the ray-sums.

Analogy with X-ray Computed Tomography

The MR projection method is similar to the reconstruction method used with "third generation" computed tomography scanners. These scanners contain an x-ray tube and a bank of detectors that rotate as a unit to different angular positions. At each position a measurement is made of x-ray attenuation along all the rays connecting the x-ray aperture with the individual detectors. This is analogous, in the MR case, to applying a field gradient in a given direction and measuring the detected signal at regular increments of time. The two principal differences are that the set of rays defined by the magnetic field gradient are parallel, rather than fan shaped, and the MR measurement gives directly the *transformed* projection, rather than the individual ray-sums.

Sampling Considerations

In practice, the integrals needed for reconstruction must be evaluated as discrete summations. That is, transform values are obtained for discrete values of k, at increments Δk, up to a maximum value k_m. Mathematically this represents a change from Fourier transforms to Fourier series, which is valid provided that Δk is less than the inverse diameter of the field of view, i.e., $\Delta k < 1/d$. However the imposition of a maximum wave number k_m implies a loss of fine detail or spatial smoothing. In fact, the choice of k_m dictates the picture element (pixel) width w needed to express the full picture detail. The relationship is

$$w = 1/(2k_m) \qquad (18)$$

For a typical head image, one might have a 25 cm field of view d and a 0.1 cm pixel width w. This would imply $\Delta k = 0.04$ cycles/cm and $k_m = 5$ cycles/cm, corresponding to 250 data measurements between $-k_m$ and $+k_m$ and to a picture matrix 250×250.

Another sampling consideration is the time needed to make the measurement, defined by t_m, where the measurement interval lies between $-t_m$ and $+t_m$. From Equations (14) and (18) we can write

$$t_m = k_m/(\gamma g) = 1/(2\gamma g w) = 1/(2\,\Delta f), \qquad (19)$$

where $\Delta f = \gamma g w$ is the change in Larmor frequency between two points separated by one pixel width along the field gradient.

Relation to Chemical Shift

It is a general requirement that Δf should be larger than the chemical shift, i.e., the difference in precession frequency between different chemical species, as well as frequency shifts caused by field inhomogeneities, in order to avoid artifactual mispositioning. For proton imaging in tissue, the two prevalent species are water protons and lipid protons, for which the fractional chemical shift is 3.5 ppm. This is also a typical magnitude for field inhomogeneity. With this as a criterion, and a field strength of 0.25 tesla ($f_0 = 10$ MHz), we have $\Delta f > 35$ Hz, corresponding to a measurement time $t_m < 10$ ms.

SUMMARY

By combining a spin-echo measurement with a linear field gradient, a special result happens.

1. The detected signal contains a superposition of frequencies, with each frequency component corresponding to a different parallel ray-sum. The total signal represents a full projection.

2. If we take the signal as it is, without separating it into frequency components, it traces out in time the spatial Fourier transform of the projection.

3. By digitizing the signal at regular time intervals, and repeating this for projections at different angles (determined by the field gradient), we can obtain a full set of Fourier coefficients. Because of the polar geometry of the projection data, the two-

dimensional inversion is generally done using filtered back-projection instead of the fast Fourier transform algorithm.

TWO–DIMENSIONAL FOURIER RECONSTRUCTION (Rectangular Coordinates)

Phase Encoding

Now consider a somewhat different sequence of events. Suppose we have applied a gradient g_x in the x direction and taken data as described for the projection angle $\varphi = 0$. This yields a set of Fourier coefficients for wave numbers

$$k_x = -k_m \, t_o + k_m$$

$$k_y = 0$$

Now instead of applying a gradient in a different direction, suppose we repeat the same sequence, but before the appearance of the spin-echo signal, we add a *second* gradient g_y in the y direction for a brief period of time, τ.

Of course g_y affects the spin precession while it is present, but one might suppose that the effect vanishes when g_y is removed. This is not true, because the circular position (phase) of each precessing nucleus is altered by the y gradient, and this phase difference is retained thereafter.

To see this mathematically, we note that during the application of g_y the precession frequency is

$$f(x, y) = f_0 + \gamma g_x x + \gamma g_y y. \tag{20}$$

Therefore, after the period τ the total signal is, from Equation (10),

$$v(t, \tau) = c \iint m(x, y) \exp[2\pi i(\gamma g_x xt + \gamma g_y y\tau)] \, dx \, dy, \tag{21}$$

where we have specifically included τ as an argument of v. Now if we define

$$k_x = -\gamma g_x t$$

and $\qquad\qquad\qquad\qquad\qquad\qquad\qquad\qquad\qquad\qquad\qquad\qquad\qquad\qquad$ (22)

$$k_y\tau = -\gamma g_y \tau,$$

we have

$$v(t, \tau) = c \iint m(x, y) \exp[-2\pi i(k_x x + k_y y)] \, dx \, dy = cM(k_x, k_y) \tag{23}$$

While Equation (23) is mathematically identical to Equation (15), the difference is that we now can vary k_x and k_y independently. Thus, by sampling the detected signal as before, we obtain a second set of Fourier coefficients—not at a different angle (since the applied gradient during the measurement is still in the x direction) but for a different k_y:

$$k_x = -k_m \, t_o + k_m$$

$$k_y = -\gamma g_y \tau$$

In other words, instead of building up a polar array of coefficients (Fig. 77–5a), as in the previous method, one "spoke" at a time, we are beginning to build up a rectangular array, one row at a time (Fig. 77–5b). This is exactly what is needed for direct Fourier inversion.

We can thus continue the procedure, changing τ (or, equivalently, g_y) for each measurement, until the full rectangular array of coefficients is obtained. From here it is very simple and computationally efficient to take the two-dimensional inverse fast Fourier transform to produce the image.

Physical Interpretation

The concept of phase encoding is not hard to understand; it is just a special case of the previous method. The general fact is that all regions of magnetization contribute toward the detected voltage, but the net signal depends on the phase of each contribution, and this is determined by the applied gradient. If the gradient is present during the measurement, the phase differences continue to accumulate as long as the signal lasts, and show up as different frequencies, but if it is present only temporarily, it leaves a set of phase differences that remain forever after (hence the term "phase encoding").

Since the phase factor associated with each magnetization element is also what determines which Fourier coefficient is being measured, we can generate Fourier coefficients at will. By keeping the x gradient during the measurement, we obtain a series of evolving phase factors "on the fly," corresponding to different k_x wave numbers. On the other hand, by applying a y gradient only before the measurement, we measure coefficients for a single k_y value at a time. Because of this, the direction of the continuous gradient is sometimes called the "free" direction, because one can acquire a set of values from one spin echo.

What is perhaps more confusing is that we have now abandoned the concept of a projection. It is only the set of values obtained without any y gradient that corresponds to a true projection at angle 0. The other data sets produce Fourier coefficients that correspond to a mixture of projection angles. Thus a helpful tool for visualization has been removed, and the process appears more abstract. Yet we can bring back a more direct physical insight by again invoking the dual interpretation of Fourier integrals.

Alternate Interpretation

We have seen that the signal $v(t, \tau)$ is a function of two different times, albeit t varies continuously during the measurement, while τ varies discretely between measurements. Since v varies with respect to both t and τ, each variation can be broken down into frequency components. To see this, let us rewrite the inverse transform (Eq. 1), using Equation (22) to change the variables of integration to t and τ:

$$m(x, y) = c' \iint v(t, \tau) \exp[-2\pi i(\gamma g_x xt + \gamma g_y y\tau)] \, dt \, d\tau, \tag{24}$$

where c' is a combination of constants.

We see that the formula that previously represented the superposition of spatial waves to build up the image now appears as a formula for selecting out from the total signal the component with a "t-frequency" $\gamma g_x x$ and a "τ-frequency" $\gamma g_y y$. In other words, by applying orthogonal gradients in such a way that the resulting shifts in Larmor frequency can be measured independently, we have assigned a unique pair of frequencies to each point.[5] This is analogous to the projection method in which a unique frequency was assigned to each ray. The reconstruction equation (Eq. 24) may thus be thought of as a way of measuring the contribution from a given point (x, y) by selecting the particular pair of frequencies involved.

SUMMARY

The two-dimensional Fourier method, which is now the workhorse of MR imaging, differs from the projection method in two ways.

1. Instead of rotating the direction of the field gradient between measurements, one applies a second orthogonal gradient for a brief period before each measurement. By repeating this many times, with different periods or gradient strengths, one obtains a rectangular array of Fourier image coefficients.

2. The image reconstruction is done by direct two-dimensional Fourier inversion, rather than filtered back-projection. The two-dimensional inversion formula may be thought of either as a summing up of spatial waves in many directions, or as a way of selecting out of the MR signal the Larmor frequencies associated with each point.

Conclusion

We have examined two closely related methods for MR image reconstruction. Of the two, the two-dimensional Fourier method is now more widely used. Both methods are based on the direct measurement of Fourier coefficients of the image, the essential difference being the geometry of the Fourier data, viz., polar vs. rectangular.

There are many other methods that have been used or proposed. For example, less efficient methods have been used in the past but are now discarded. Also, new methods have been proposed that may offer advantages beyond those presented here. For example, three-dimensional methods have been proposed wherein one excites a large volume, not just a single slice, and simultaneously acquires Fourier data from the entire volume.

Another example is chemical shift imaging, in which one may extract separate images of protons in different chemical environments, e.g., water (H_2O) and fat (CH_2). These two examples only scratch the surface of the endless "bag of tricks" that MR tomography appears to offer. It is hoped that this chapter will provide a foundation of understanding, not only for the two methods described, but for future variations as well.

In striving for simplicity and physical insight, we have omitted many experimental complications that require a modification of the simplified procedures presented herein. For example, the manner and exact times at which gradients are applied, the types of pulses used, the effect of field inhomogeneity, the effect of nuclear relaxation on detected signal, etc., require careful attention by the instrument designer, but may be neglected by the user who wants to understand basic principles.

References

1. Bracewell RN: Strip integration in radio astronomy. Aust J Phys 9:198–217, 1956.
2. Bracewell RN, Riddle AC: Inversion of fan-beam scans (in radio astronomy). Astrophys J *150*:427–434, 1967.
3. Brooks RA, Di Chiro G: Principles of computer assisted tomography (CAT) in radiographic and radioisotopic imaging. Phys Med Biol 21:689–732, 1976.
4. Edelstein WA, Hutchison JMS, Johnson G, Redpath T: Spin warp NMR imaging and applications to human whole-body imaging. Phys Med Biol 25:751–756, 1980.
5. Hoult DI: NMR imaging techniques. Br Med Bull 40:132–138, 1984.
6. King KF, Moran PR: A unified description of NMR imaging, data-collection strategies, and reconstruction. Med Phys *11*:1–14, 1984.
7. Kumar A, Welti D, Ernst RR: NMR Fourier zeugmatography. J Magn Reson *18*:69–83, 1975.
8. Lauterbur PC: Image formation by induced local interactions: Examples employing nuclear magnetic resonance. Nature *242*:190–191, 1973.
9. Thompson AR, Bracewell RN: Interpolation and Fourier transformation of fringe visibilities. Astronomical J *79*:11–24, 1974.
10. Twieg DB: The k-trajectory formulation of the NMR imaging process with applications in analysis and synthesis of imaging methods. Med Phys *10*:610–621, 1983.

78

Image Production and Display

JON J. ERICKSON
DAVID R. PICKENS

The use of the computer in magnetic resonance imaging (MRI) is generally similar to many other applications in medical imaging. However, there are some aspects that are unique to magnetic resonance imaging (MRI). The primary distinction is in the control of the imaging process. Although it is true that the computer is the primary data collection and analysis device for nuclear cardiology and digital subtraction angiography, it is also true that the clinical studies performed by these imaging techniques could be performed, albeit much more primitively, without the computer. Nuclear cardiology would still be using a series of analog images produced on a multi-imager by an EKG-gated camera, and the subtraction angiographer would still be dependent on analog film subtraction techniques. Although the computer plays an important role in these two examples, it is not required for the production of the clinical data. On the other hand, MRI could not exist in any form remotely resembling present systems were it not for the availability and capabilities of modern computer systems. The computer not only functions as an image analysis device, but also as a primary component in the production of the data.

The general thrust of the following discussion will be towards elucidating the technical aspects of the computer systems required for image production in MRI. The parts of the systems that are unique to this particular modality will be covered in more detail.

Three physical parameters are imaged by the MRI process. These are the concentration and distribution of the hydrogen nuclei in the patient's body and two "relaxation times" whose values depend upon the local chemical and physical state of the tissue being imaged. These MR phenomena allow the production of images that depict the distribution of hydrogen nuclei in the imaged region. By appropriate application of 90 degree and 180 degree pulses, it is also possible to produce images that depict the distribution of $T1$ and $T2$ relaxation times.

It is extremely difficult to produce images of a single parameter that are completely free of any contamination by the other two parameters. In most instances, the clinical images that are produced are complex combinations of proton distribution maps with $T1$ and $T2$ weighting.

All materials have characteristic $T1$ and $T2$ values. In living soft tissue, the value of $T1$ for protons (i.e., hydrogen) ranges from about 300 to 1500 ms. The value of $T2$ ranges from approximately 50 to 150 ms. The value of $T2$ is always smaller than the value of $T1$, and the relative values of $T1$ and $T2$ vary with the type of tissue being examined and with the physiological state of the tissue. Extensive discussion describing these parameters and their importance to diagnostic imaging can be found in other chapters.

The time frames in which measurements of $T1$ and $T2$ are made are very important, since these parameters have a direct impact on the length of time required to produce a map of the same parameters in the human body. The repetition time between the measurements can range from about 20 ms to several seconds. There also may be a delay of several seconds to allow the system to return to equilibrium if multiple measurements of the parameter are to be made.

Magnetic resonance images may be produced by a number of techniques that rely on the ability of the computer-controlled imaging system to modify the magnetic field of the imaging magnet selectively in the region of the object being imaged. The most primitive method of imaging is called the sensitive point method. It consists of driving the gradient field coils in such a way that there is only a single very small volume in the entire imaging volume that has the correct field strength to absorb radio frequency (rf) energy and radiate back a signal. The image is formed by stepping this sensitive point through the image plane and mapping out the image points pixel by pixel. This basis imaging technique was used early in the development of the technology, but it was replaced almost immediately by more sophisticated, faster data-gathering methods.

The change in resonance frequency with a change in magnetic field strength allows one to gather data about the desired MRI parameter simultaneously from multiple locations in the imaging plane. The so-called one-dimensional imaging technique modifies the magnetic field so that data are gathered along a line corresponding to a row or column in the final image. By knowing the magnetic field strength along the imaging line, one can transform the complex rf signal into its individual frequency components. The location of the source of each frequency component can be calculated from the Larmor equation (see Chapter 59). The magnitude of each component is directly related to the proton density at each point along the line. Thus, by a single excitation, one can reproduce the distribution of proton density (or MR parameter) along that image line. By successively stepping the sensitive line through the image plane it is possible to produce a complete two-dimensional image.

A more complex but still more efficient method of producing the MR image is possible using two-dimensional gradients so that the MR signal contains components of various frequencies with multiple phase angles. In this case, the frequency will determine the source of the signal along one axis of the image, and the phase will determine the location along the other axis. The total data-gathering process for the two-dimensional image reconstruction technique involves multiple excitation pulses and subsequent signal acquisitions. The production of an image with clinically useful spatial resolution normally requires 128, 256, or 512 individual pulse sequences. A slight modification of the gradient strengths with each of the pulse sequences provides the information needed for the image construction.

The delays in imaging that would normally result from having to wait for equilibrium to return after the application of the rf signal can be used for imaging other planes. Multiplanar imaging techniques are used by most commercial MR imaging systems and can significantly reduce the imaging time in patient applications. The two-dimensional imaging concept can be extended to a three-dimensional technique in which it is possible to produce a data set from which one can construct planar images of any desired orientation. Volume, or three-dimensional, imaging techniques are available on some commercial systems. These methods use an additional gradient and phase encoding technique which can result in a data set with a resolution or 256 by 256 by 256 points. The clinical utility of this technique is limited by the extended collection and processing time involved and the huge amount of data that the system has to store for each imaging procedure.

The extremely low signal intensity of the MRI measurement produces an unclear or noisy image. This is compensated for by making several measurements and averaging them into the final image. Imaging times of present instrumentation range from 20 seconds to several minutes for a single slice, depending on the number of measurements made, to as much as 20 minutes for a complete volume study. The final image is usually available within several seconds following the completion of the data gathering.

The picture element intensity in a magnetic resonance image is controlled by the relative values of proton density, *T1*, and *T2*. It is possible to alter the relative intensity of structures in a patient image by altering the timing of the measurements. The use of inappropriate pulse sequences may allow the presence of pathology to remain undetected owing to the fact that the image intensities of the normal and abnormal tissue are identical, whereas a slightly modified pulse sequence will clearly demonstrate the abnormality. This means that providing optimum sensitivity for the demonstration of a particular type of pathology will require a preliminary estimation of the pathology that may be present. The pulse sequence and timing are usually selected by the operator in an attempt to optimize the contrast in the structures of interest. The timing of the pulse sequences and the number of sample averages that are requested will determine the total imaging time for a clinical procedure. In some systems, it is also possible for the operator to select the spatial resolution desired and, thereby, to determine the number of separate measurements that are made to produce the image. This, too, will affect imaging time.

Since each procedure in MRI is controlled at all steps by the computer, the timing of the system operation is critically dependent on the ability of the computer to respond promptly. Although the information contained in the MR image data is very complex, the total volume of data for each MR image is relatively small when compared to other imaging modalities such as computed tomography (CT). As a result, using modern high speed minicomputers, it becomes possible to collect multiple images simultaneously by switching between images during the collection. Reconstruction of images from the raw data is done by equipment which is comparable to that used in CT scanners. Thus, complete multiplanar imaging studies can be performed in one or two imaging procedures in a short time.

SPECIAL FUNCTION HARDWARE

In all MRI installations, a large amount of special hardware is required to support the computer operation. In general, this is a combination of digital hardware, such as that found in computer systems, and analog hardware, such as that used to process the signals from the radio frequency (rf) receiver. This section will describe the special purpose hardware.

Analog-to-Digital Converter Systems

The signal induced in the receiver coils in an MR imager is a frequency and amplitude modulated rf wave. The carrier frequency is the Larmor frequency. Information from the proton distributions is expressed as deviations of several thousand cycles around the Larmor frequency. Thus, the Larmor frequency wave is modulated by the signal information. The receiver must process the modulated carrier so that the MR signal can be extracted.

After amplification, the radio frequency signal is mixed with a reference signal in a process called heterodyning, so that the received radio frequency MR signal (around 22 MHz for a 5 kilogauss proton imaging system) is transformed to a lower frequency while the signal information from the receiver is preserved. This is necessary because high resolution digitizers have relatively long conversion times and are not able to convert the high frequency MR signal directly.

The varying MR voltage is processed by detector circuits that preserve the phase and amplitude information. The phase information is extracted by a phase-sensitive detector circuit, called a quadrature detector, that separates the mathematical real and imaginary components of the MRI signal. A varying voltage representing the real part of the signal is digitized by one analog-to-digital converter (ADC) while another ADC simultaneously digitizes the imaginary component. The combined output is made up of two digital words. The real and imaginary signals contain phase and amplitude information and are stored in memory for later processing by the fast Fourier transform (FFT) reconstruction programs.

Information acquired by MR imaging devices is in the form of analog signals. Analog signals are those in which the information content is contained in the magnitude of the signal. Analog signals have a range of magnitudes through which the signal can vary in a continuous manner. In order to process the information with digital systems, the magnitude information must be converted to digital numbers. This is the function of the ADC (Fig. 78–1). There are a number of methods for accomplishing the analog-to-digital conversion. The choice for any particular application will depend on a number of factors, including conversion speed required, accuracy required, number of converters, type of analog signal, and resolution required.

The requirements for the ADCs used in MRI systems are wide dynamic range and minimum error. Usually, successive approximation ADCs are employed because of their good performance and low cost. These converters sample the incoming MR signal from the rf receiver, compare it to an internal reference voltage that is adjusted until a match is achieved, and produce a digital representation of the sampled voltage. The ADCs that are used in MRI have resolutions of 12 to 16 bits, giving them the capability of dividing the voltage into as many as 65,536 steps. This resolution is necessary to provide accurate digitizing and subsequent recovery of the MR information and to provide a wide range of signal handling capability.

Conversion speed and linearity are important characteristics of the ADCs. The ADCs must operate fast enough so that there is no loss of information. Signal processing mathematics show that the digitizer must operate at least twice as fast as the highest frequency in the sampled voltage to avoid serious distortion. Since MRI depends on

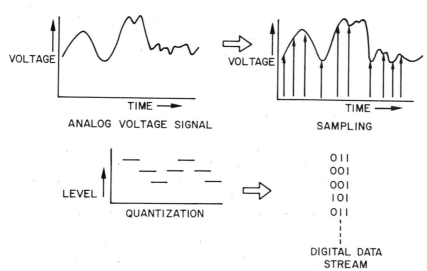

Figure 78–1. Analog-to-digital conversion (ADC). An analog voltage is one whose intensity varies continuously over a range of values. To convert an analog signal to digital form, three steps must be taken. (1) The signal must be sampled at a rate at least twice as fast as the highest frequency present. (2) A level must be assigned to the sample in a step called quantizing. (3) A digital level must be assigned to the quantized level. (From Pickens DR, Erickson JJ: Radiographics 5:31, 1985. Used by permission.)

converting signal frequency to spatial information using the FFT, any distortion in the digitized frequency resulting from inadequate ADCs shows up in the images as position shifts and spatial distortion of the image.

Digital-to-Analog Converters

A number of digital signals present in the computer system must be converted back to analog values to be used for image display or control operations. The digital-to-analog converter (DAC) is conceptually a simpler device than the ADC and is illustrated in Figure 78–2. In converting the digital number, each of the bits in the digital word is used to control an electrical current source. The amount of current supplied by any given source depends on the position of its controlling bit in the digital number. In the 4 bit converter illustrated in the figure, the least significant bit contributes one unit of current to the summing amplifier while the most significant bit contributes 8 units of current. The magnitude of the current produced by the summing amplifier will depend on which bits are "set" in the digital word.

The principle use for the DAC in MRI is in the operation of the image display. Images are stored in the computer as a series of digital values. They are presented on the video display or cathode ray tube (CRT) by synchronizing the reading of the computer memory with the raster scan of the electron beam in the CRT. At each picture element (pixel) location, the content of the corresponding memory word is transferred to a DAC. The output of the DAC is, in turn, used to control the brightness of the image point.

Digital-to-analog converters can be difficult to construct so that they do not introduce conversion errors. Two types of conversion errors are possible. Differential errors result from the inaccurate adjustment or insufficient stability of the individual current sources. Integral linearity errors may be present as a result of the inability of the analog current summing amplifier to operate satisfactorily over the entire current range. Differential linearity is probably a more serious defect in high quality image displays, since it can result in the generation of artificial contours in regions of the image in which the real intensity values vary slowly over wide areas. Integral nonlinearities will not significantly alter the image, except in severe cases, since they will appear only as alterations in the overall image contrast or brightness.

Array Processors

All but some very special purpose computers perform calculations in a serial fashion. If the reconstruction of data for a single point in an image requires a series of

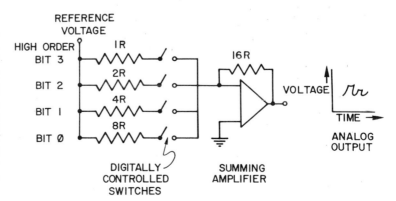

Figure 78–2. Digital-to-analog conversion (DAC). Digital numbers are sent to the digital-to-analog converter. Each bit in the digital number controls an electronic switch which, when closed, causes a current to be provided to a summing amplifier through a calibrated resistor. Each resistor is calibrated to reflect the value of the bit controlling it. The analog voltage appears on the output of the amplifier. Higher resolution DACs produce smoother analog output signals. (From Pickens DR, Erickson JJ: Radiographics 5:31, 1985. Used by permission.)

mathematical calculations, each of the calculations can be performed only after completion of the previous one. Similarly, the calculations for a second image point must wait upon the completion of the calculations for the previous image point. General purpose computers gain their power from the fact that they can be programmed to perform a wide variety of operations. However, this very versatility also works to the disadvantage of the system when extremely high speed or repetitive calculations are to be performed.

Many data processing procedures used in MRI consist of relatively long sequences of calculations that must be performed on every incoming data point. The repetitive nature of the calculation makes it feasible to use special hardware, i.e., array processors, to reduce the calculation time. Most array processors are constructed along the general form shown in the block diagram of Figure 78–3. The array processor is a special purpose computer. Communication between the array processor and the host computer is accomplished through the host interface, which is used to pass both data and commands between the host and the processor. In order to prevent the array processor from blocking the input-output circuits of the host computer, and to increase the possible calculation speed, the arithmetic operations are usually performed on data that are stored in the data memory of the array processor itself. Prior to the initiation of the calculation, a large number of data points, perhaps an entire image, is transferred to the array processor memory. Upon completion of the image manipulation, the modified data are passed back to the host machine for storage or display. This mechanism allows the host computer to perform other operations while the array processor is functioning.

The heart of the array processor is the pipeline arithmetic unit. This device is the source of much of the array processor's high speed. Consider the example of normalizing an image for display by subtraction of a background value followed by normalization (scaling) to some maximum value. The arithmetic sequence which must be performed on each image point consists of the following operations: *subtraction* (of background), *multiplication* (by display maximum), and *division* (by maximum value in image).

If this operation is to be performed by the host computer, each of these operations will have to be performed one after the other for each image point. Furthermore, the results of the intermediate calculations, i.e., subtraction and multiplication, will be stored in memory and then retrieved for the next calculation. In the pipeline processor,

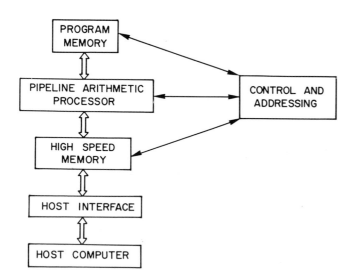

Figure 78–3. The array processor. A general purpose array processor has five important parts: (1) the program memory, which stores the instructions that tell the machine what to process; (2) the high speed memory, which stores data to be processed; (3) the control and addressing logic, which directs the operations of the array processor; (4) the pipeline arithmetic processor, which executes mathematical operations at high speed; and (5) the host interface, which communicates with the main computer. (From Pickens DR, Erickson JJ: Radiographics 5:31, 1985. Used by permission.)

the hardware performing each of the arithmetic operations is independent of the others, permitting multiple arithmetic operations to be performed simultaneously. Thus, the calculations of the example take place in the following manner. (1) The first image element is supplied to the subtraction circuit. (2) When the subtraction is complete, the result is passed to the multiplication circuit, (3) The second image element is fed to the subtraction circuit. If each operation requires 1 μs, the first normalized image point will emerge from the pipeline 3 μs after the operation is begun, but thereafter, a new point will emerge every microsecond. In general, a process requiring the performance of N operations with an average execution time of T microseconds on a data array of M elements will require $(N*M*T)$ microseconds in a standard serial calculation, but only $((N + M - 1)*T)$ microseconds in the pipeline calculation.

Array Processor Implementation

Array processors and other specialized computational hardware may be implemented in a number of ways. The actual design of the electronics to do the calculation will, in large part, determine the speed and versatility of the hardware. In CT, the array processor is used for the convolution calculations required by the filtered back projection algorithm and for the actual back projection itself. These calculations are relatively simple, but because of the large number of operations, the systems require extremely fast processing hardware. The limited versatility that is required permits the use of hard-wired convolvers and back projectors. These are analogous to computers that are wired to perform a specific program and can be changed only by changing the actual wiring in the machine.

The array processors used in newer, more recently developed hardware, such as are found in MRI equipment, are more versatile because their programming can be altered by the operating system in the computer. By using libraries of programs provided by the manufacturer, it is possible to completely redefine the function of the array processor. It can be used for the fast Fourier transforms required to produce spatial distribution information from the radio frequency information in MR imaging, or it can be programmed to perform the filtered back projection for CT images. Should a new reconstruction algorithm become available, the manufacturer of the MR imager need only send new programs which cause the programmable array processor to implement the new reconstruction technique.

Dedicated hardware array processors are faster and often less expensive than the more general purpose programmable systems, but they are restricted to the single function for which they were designed. The programmable systems are more versatile and better suited for use in less mature technologies such as MRI.

Image Processor/Video Display

Although MRI is based on computer processing and depends on its powerful image manipulation ability, the primary clinical diagnosis is made by a visual inspection of the displayed image. The success of the modality is heavily dependent on the quality of the image display and on the ability of the operator to interact with the image. In most clinical systems, the computer displays are used for two operations: the performance of the clinical study and the presentation of the final image. Usually these two functions require quite different capabilities. The former is primarily a matter of displaying textual information and numerical values, whereas the latter is a presentation of high resolution images with a large number of image points and a wide intensity range. For these reasons present-day MRI systems use dual displays, as shown in Figure 78–4.

The textual display is similar to the computer terminals that everyone has become familiar with in their daily interactions with airline reservation systems, computerized banking systems, and personal computers. The terminals communicate with the central computer through a serial line interface or a relatively low speed parallel interface. The terminals are capable of operating in two modes. The simplest mode is the "conversational" mode in which the computer asks the operator a single question at a time, and the operator must answer the question before the next is presented. The second mode is the "block" mode in which the computer displays a facsimile of a blank form on the terminal screen. The operator is able to fill in the form one space at a time in any order desired. When the form is filled, the entire set of data is transmitted to the computer. The operational mode used depends primarily on the application software. Either mode can be satisfactory, but block mode is often easier to use in a busy clinical situation, since it allows easier correction of data entry errors.

The quality of the diagnostic image display will depend on the number of pixels in the image and the number of intensity levels available. Current systems produce images in 256×256 and 512×512 arrays. In most cases, the images are actually reconstructed with the same resolution as they will be displayed. Some MRI systems produce images with asymmetric matrices. The original image matrix may be 256 pixels long and 128 pixels high. For display, this asymmetric image is interpolated in the vertical direction to produce a square 256×256 matrix. This usually does not cause problems with the clinician's ability to diagnose from the display, since the lower spatial resolution in the vertical direction is not visually distracting.

The effect of image matrix size on the ability of the imaging system to display anatomic detail can be easily calculated. MRI resolution depends on the strength of the magnetic field, design of the coils and electronics used for transmitting and receiving, and the pulse sequence employed. Typical resolution for a clinical imaging system is 1 mm with the head coil and 2 mm with the body coil. For a head coil 25 cm in diameter, a 256×256 display matrix produces pixels that are 1 mm square. A large image matrix would provide little or no advantage. Zooming the image at the display would not yield increased anatomic detail. However, a magnification during data collection can yield an image of a smaller region, with increased resolution. Similarly, a surface coil designed for high resolution imaging when used with acquisition magnification collection can yield spatial resolution of better than 1 mm. Figure 78–5 illustrates magnification, zoom, and the results expected using body, head, and surface coils. Magnification can be applied to any image collection to yield improved resolution.

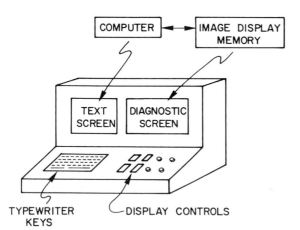

Figure 78–4. Control and diagnostic display. The control display is a video screen that displays text associated with entering commands into the imaging system and with receiving responses from the computer. Also, there is usually a typewriter-style keyboard and other controls on which to enter commands. The diagnostic video display is designed to display the processed images from the imaging system. These images are stored in a special image memory that is controlled by the computer. Various controls for window, level, and other functions are associated with the diagnostic display. (From Pickens DR, Erickson JJ: Radiographics 5:31, 1985. Used by permission.)

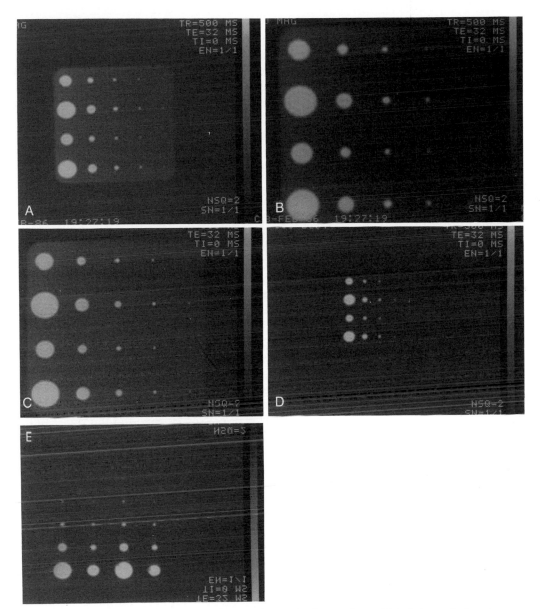

Figure 78–5. Magnification, zoom, and different coils. *A*, An image of a multiple hole resolution phantom using the head coil. No magnification or zoom was used. *B*, Zoom of 1.75 times of the image in *A*. Some blurring of the image can be seen. *C*, An image acquired using acquisition magnification of 50 percent. When compared with the images of *A* and *B*, this image shows finer detail without the blurring of *B*. *D*, The phantom was imaged with the body coil and with a surface coil (*E*). The surface coil image appears to produce the best overall image, which could have been acquired using magnification to produce very fine resolution.

Zoom can be applied to any image display to provide better visualization of information which was collected, though with no increase in resolution.

The 512 × 512 array is the maximum that is commonly used for the image because it can be displayed on a standard video system. In order to display higher resolution matrices, it is necessary to use nonstandard video systems. This entails special recording systems, monitors, and film camera systems. Currently, all commercially available MRI systems do not need more than a 512 by 512 display capability.

The numerical information representing the specific physical quantity of interest such as *T1* or proton density is displayed as changes in the intensity of the image. The range of numerical values in the image depends on the manufacturer of the particular system and on the specific parameter being displayed. MR images currently are displayed with a range of 1024 gray levels on some commercial instruments. The reduced intensity range of MRI systems compared to CT is indicative of the much higher noise levels found in these images and the more restricted dynamic range in the initial data. However, even this narrow range of values is greater than can be adequately displayed on the video screen of the video display.

In order to display the full dynamic range of the image, MRI uses a window and level method of displaying the image that is familiar to users of CT imaging systems. In this method, a narrower range of intensity information from the image is selected by the operator and this smaller range of values is presented on the screen using the entire intensity range of the video system (Fig. 78–6). Image intensity values above the selected range are presented as pure white, while values below the range are presented as black. In many systems, numerical ranges as small as one level can be selected. This provides an easily manipulated method for estimating numerical values in regions of the image.

Although MRI is used primarily for imaging nondynamic processes, that is, imaging structures rather than functions such as blood flow or the beating of the heart, there are some clinical procedures that produce images that benefit from dynamic, movie-type displays. This is fairly easy to accomplish in nuclear medicine systems because the image data can be compressed to only a few bits of gray per pixel and all of the images can be stored in memory at one time. For MRI, this is a more difficult problem because of the greater amount of data that must be presented. The ability of the system to sequentially play back a series of high resolution images will depend on a number of system parameters over which the operator has no control. The speed of the disk from which the image must be read, the size of the image matrix, and the speed of the memory all enter into the problem. The physical parameters, the exact design of the operating system, any simultaneous tasks, and the skill of the programmer will also affect the operation of the dynamic display.

Special Image Display Functions

A large number of image manipulation programs have been developed for obtaining quantitative information from the images produced by computer-based imaging devices. Parameters such as organ volume, linear dimensions, and dynamic function analyses are all of clinical interest. One of the most useful interactive capabilities is the ability

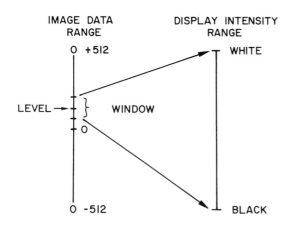

Figure 78–6. Window and level control. Window and level controls permit the physician to tailor the diagnostic display to his preference. In MRI systems, the number of densities available greatly exceeds the number that can be displayed on the screen at once, so the window control selects a range of gray levels to view, while the level controls where, in the entire range of the imager, the window will be positioned. Pixel values falling outside of the window are set to white if they are larger than the window levels or black if smaller. (From Pickens DR, Erickson JJ: Radiographics 5:31, 1985. Used by permission.)

to indicate regions of interest for subsequent processing. There are three principal devices that can be used to mark regions of interest. These are the lightpen, the joystick, and the trackball. The lightpen (Fig. 78–7A) is a light-sensing pointer that the user aims at the image in the region of interest. The output from the lightpen is timed to the display as the image is painted onto the screen. The place where the lightpen points can be marked on the screen by the computer and used to form an outline on the screen.

The joystick (Fig. 78–7B) contains two potentiometers, which the computer reads to determine the desired position in the image. A marker is placed in the image and is presented to the user. As the user moves the joystick, a new position is calculated and the marker moves accordingly in the image. When the position is as desired, the user indicates this by a pushbutton switch.

The trackball (Fig. 78–7C) consists of a smooth round ball mounted in the console table. The operator spins the ball freely in both the x and y direction. The trackball, in turn, is connected to two pulse generating devices that produce a stream of electrical pulses while the ball is moving. The pulses are counted by the display processor and are used to position the marker on the screen. Trackballs and joysticks can also be used to control image brightness and contrast or any other of a number of display features. The specific use of these devices depends solely on the software written to control the display.

Color is often used to provide an enhanced display. Since the images produced

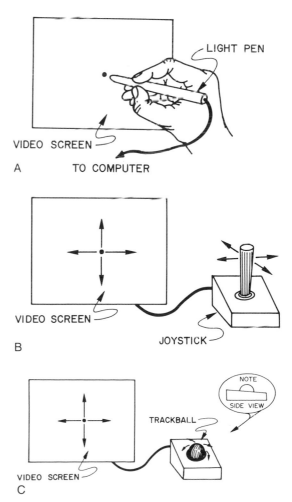

Figure 78–7. *A*, The light pen. The light pen is a hand-held device used to mark regions on the display screen. A photocell in the end detects light from the screen and is synchronized with the video signal so that when a point is selected with the light pen, the x-y position on the screen, as well as the intensity of the point, is provided to the computer. This information can be used to mark a region of interest. *B*, The joystick. The joystick is a small lever mounted so that it can move in any direction. The position of the joystick determines on what part of the screen a cursor is located. Like the light pen, x-y position and intensity are provided to the computer. *C*, The trackball. The trackball operates like the joystick in permitting the user to obtain x-y position and intensity on the screen. Some people prefer the trackball to either the light pen or the joystick because it often is capable of finer movement of a cursor. (From Pickens DR, Erickson JJ: Radiographics 5:31, 1985. Used by permission.)

by MRI do not have any inherent color, the color levels are assigned arbitrarily. The use of color provides the system with an ability to display many more intensity levels than the simple black and white display. Both hue and intensity can be altered to indicate changes in the numerical values of the image pixels. The effective use of color for the display of simple static images requires a very high quality color display, since limitations in the number of available colors or hues tend to introduce deceptive contours in the image.

In most clinical applications, there is a need for a hard copy of the images. The most common and preferred method of producing this copy is the use of a transparency camera, often referred to as a "multiformat camera." These cameras use a dedicated video monitor to produce an image transparency film. Each piece of film can carry multiple images and can be viewed like conventional x-ray film. There are some special photographic papers that can be used in the transparency cameras to produce photographic prints. These papers can be processed in the x-ray film rapid processors, so they are useful for creating high quality prints very rapidly. Nonphotographic printing systems are sometimes used to produce images on paper, but the results are usually not as good as with transparency cameras.

A magnetic resonance imaging system represents one of the most complicated and expensive instruments that a physician may have occasion to use for diagnosis of disease. The computer and mechanical engineering involved in designing a functioning system are impressive, as are the extremely complex programs that run the entire system and permit the elaborate display functions which are available. Understanding the interaction of the various functions of the system will help a diagnostician appreciate the complexities of the magnetic resonance phenomenon itself and the complex nature of the images which are produced.

Suggested Readings

Alexander P: Array processors in medical imaging. Computer 16:6:17–30, 1983.

Bronzino JD: Computer Applications for Patient Care. Reading, Massachusetts, Addison-Wesley, 1982.

Erickson JJ, Rollo FD: Digital Nuclear Medicine. Philadelphia, J.B. Lippincott, 1983.

Fukushima E, Roeder SBW: Experimental Pulse NMR: A Nuts and Bolts Approach. Reading, Massachusetts, Addison-Wesley, 1981.

Gonzales RC, Wintz P: Digital Image Processing. Reading, Massachusetts, Addison-Wesley, 1977.

Hoult DI: The NMR receiver: a description and analysis of design. Prog NMR Spectr *12*:41–77, 1978.

Lindon JD, Ferrige AG: Digitization and data processing in Fourier transform NMR. Prog NMR Spectr *14*:27–66, 1980.

Loriferne B: Analog-Digital and Digital-Analog Conversion. New York, John Wiley and Sons, 1983.

Newton TH, Potts DG (eds): Radiology of the Skull and Brain. Vol. 5: Technical Aspects of Computed Tomography. St. Louis, C.V. Mosby, 1981.

Partain CL, James AE, Rollo FD, Price RR: Nuclear Magnetic Resonance Imaging. Philadelphia, W.B. Saunders Company, 1983.

Pickens DR, Erickson JJ: Computers in computed tomography and magnetic resonance imaging in radiology. Radiographics *5*:31–50, 1985.

Spackman TJ, Bengman KW: Development of a useful picture archiving and communications system. AJR *148*:1025, 1987.

79

Computer Networks for Medical Image Management

GLENDON G. COX
ARCH W. TEMPLETON
WILLIAM H. ANDERSON
KENNETH S. HENSLEY
LARRY T. COOK
RICHARD L. LAWS
SAMUEL J. DWYER III

Digital technology has found numerous applications in the field of diagnostic radiology. Computed tomography (CT), nuclear medicine (NM) gamma cameras, ultrasound scanners (US), digital subtraction angiography (DSA), magnetic resonance imaging (MRI), and digital radiography (DR) are widely available imaging modalities that rely on digital technology. The use of these imaging modalities is increasing. Currently, between 15 and 28 percent of all radiographic imaging is performed using digitally formatted imaging equipment.[1-6] This could rapidly increase to over 60 percent should other modalities such as digital chest radiography find clinical acceptance.[7-10]

The successful management of digitally formatted image data is critical to any radiology department and its referring clinicians. At present, virtually all image management systems rely on conversion of digitally formatted data to analog images on radiographic film. The analog film images are produced following the interactive manipulation of the digital image at an interactive diagnostic display station (IDDS). The analog video signal from the display monitor of the IDDS is transmitted to a multiformat video camera, which records the image on film.[11] These films, together with a written interpretation, are placed in the patient's film jacket and stored in the department's film library. The original digital data are discarded as magnetic storage media are recycled to make room for new examinations.

The current method of managing image data and radiographic reports using patient film jackets provides the radiologist and referring physician with access to conventional radiographic films, multiformat film recordings of digital examinations, and written consultation reports. The departmental film library is indexed either by patient name or identification number. A given jacket is accessed by submitting the appropriate name or number to the department's film library personnel. Once the patient's film jacket is retrieved, view boxes located throughout the department and hospital offer an inexpensive means of viewing the contents of the film jacket. A single film jacket can store in excess of 50 sheets of conventional 14 × 17 inch radiographic film.

As the use of digital imaging devices increases and as radiology departments are required to service sites geographically remote from their central areas, the use of film jackets and central film files as a method of managing digital data will become unsatisfactory. The central problems of film jacket management are the conflict between the users' exclusive access and the increasing demand for use of image data. At any time, only one user has access to the contents of a particular film jacket. Owing to the geographic separation of imaging equipment, reading rooms, and various consultation areas within the hospital, the transfer of film jackets from user to user and location to location takes considerable time and effort. The integration of multiple examinations into a film jacket also takes time that could better be used by radiologists and their referring clinicians in patient management. Increased pressure from regulatory and reimbursement agencies to limit the number, type, and cost of radiographic examinations further intensifies the competition for the available radiographic data. Finally, the increase in the number of outpatient examinations relative to inpatient studies now being experienced by many departments necessitates more rapid location and transfer of patient files. These factors, in addition to the increasing number of digital examinations, have led to the search for more efficient, cost-effective methods of managing digital data.

Computer-based local area networks are being investigated and promoted as alternative management systems for digital image data.[12–21] The management functions to be performed by a local area radiology network include acquisition and formatting of image data from the various imaging modalities, interactive display of selected images and text, on-line and long-term archiving of data, generation of hard copy, and bridging to and from other information networks or terminal sites. This chapter reviews the general elements of digital radiographic image networks and the performance parameters that must be met. Analysis of system performance based on the mean throughput of the individual components provides a method for assessing a radiology network's ability to meet these requirements.

COMPONENTS OF RADIOLOGY IMAGE NETWORKS

The basic elements of a digital image network are shown in Figure 79–1. Points of data flow onto or from the network are termed nodes. Each imaging device is interfaced to the network through an image acquisition and formatting node. Display nodes providing the radiologist or referring clinician with the means for displaying digitally formatted images are called interactive diagnosis display stations (IDDS). The IDDS node is a computer work station with a high resolution, gray scale display, which allows interactive modification and display of desired images.[22–25] Computer storage for maintaining a patient's image data during periods of high demand is provided by on-line archiving nodes. Similarly, long-term archiving nodes provide for the storage and retrieval of digital data for extended periods of relatively low demand. Hard copy units on the network allow for reproduction of any desired hard copy image on media such as film or paper. Hard copy units are generally based upon raster gray scale cathode ray tube (CRT) cameras. However, devices based on laser film and paper graphics technologies are now becoming available.

From our experience in a medium-sized academic center of 540 beds, it is estimated that the digital image management network for the radiology department will acquire an average of 136 new digital examinations each day. This amounts to 949.8 megabytes of data each day (see Table 79–2). The rate of retrieval during the high demand period while data is stored in the on-line archival nodes is estimated to be 979.2 examinations per day. This average retrieval rate is based on an inpatient population accounting for 40 percent of the total daily examinations, with an average of 15.0 retrievals per day, and an outpatient population representing 60 percent of the new examinations acquired each day and having an average of two retrievals per day. The total number of ex-

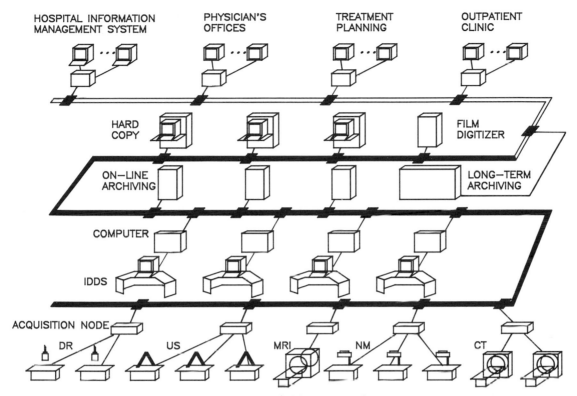

Figure 79–1. Digital image network.

aminations retrieved each day is given by 136 [.40 (15.0) + .60 (2)] = 979.2 examinations/day. Each retrieved examination will be displayed on an IDDS, and hard copy will be generated for 136 newly acquired examinations as well as for certain examinations from previous days.

In order to satisfy the requirements of the radiology network, operational characteristics are imposed upon each node type. Table 79–1 provides a summary of the tasks to be managed by each type of network node. The image acquisition and formatting nodes are required to acquire 136 new examinations per day via a variety of imaging device interfaces and to transmit all acquired images to the long-term archiving node at full spatial and contrast resolution. The acquisition and formatting node must also acquire, format, and transmit to the on-line archiving node the radiologist's consultation report along with a selected group of images whose spatial and contrast resolution have been modified to allow more rapid network transmission. After each operation, updated directories must be broadcast. Finally, the acquisition and formatting nodes must have the capability of reloading a small percentage of previous examinations in the event that questions arise concerning the examination.

The IDDS network nodes are required to receive 136 new digitally formatted examinations per day and broadcast their IDDS location. The IDDS node must also retrieve data from the on-line archiving nodes and display an average of 979.2 examinations per day. Finally, the IDDS must transmit to the hard copy node 136 new examinations per day.

The on-line archiving node is required to receive 136 new examinations per day from the acquisition and formatting nodes and to broadcast an updated location directory as each new examination is received. It must also retrieve an average of 979 previously acquired examinations, transmit them to an IDDS on the network, and

Table 79–1. REQUIREMENTS OF A RADIOLOGY IMAGE MANAGEMENT NETWORK

Overall Network Requirements

Acquire 136 digital examinations per day (949.82 megabytes) total. Retrieve 7.2 times 136 examinations each day (979.2 exams or a total of 6.83 gigabytes per day). All retrievals are displayed on network IDDSs. Hard copy recording of 136 examinations per day. Long-term archiving of all digital examinations.

Requirements of Specific Nodes

Acquisition and Formatting Node Requirements

Acquire 136 examinations per day. Transmit all 136 examinations to long-term archiving in their original format at full spatial and contract resolution. After display parameters are selected and a consultation report is generated the 136 examinations are transmitted to on-line archiving nodes. After each acquisition or transmission, broadcast updated directories.

IDDS Network Node Requirements

Receive from the acquisition and formatting nodes 136 new examinations per day for display and manipulation. Receive from the on-line archiving nodes a daily data average of 979.2 examinations for display and manipulation. Transmit 136 examinations to the hard copy generation nodes. After each reception, broadcast updated location directories.

On-Line Archiving Node Requirements

Receive 136 new examinations per day. Retrieve 979.2 examinations and transmit to IDDS network nodes. Transmit 136 exams/day that have not been retrieved in past 10 days to long-term archiving nodes. Broadcast dated directories after each reception or transmission.

Long-Term Archiving Node Requirements

Receive from the acquisition and formatting nodes 136 new examinations per day at full spatial and contrast resolution. After radiologist selects the images for on-line archiving and for display parameters, and generates the consultation, then transmit this data to the patient database. Daily retrieval of the long-term archiving nodes is estimated to be ten percent that of the on-line archiving nodes (97.9 examinations per day). Broadcast updated location directories.

Hard Copy Generation Node Requirements

Receive from the on-line archiving nodes 136 new examinations per day and generate analog hard copy recordings.

broadcast an updated location directory. The on-line archiving node also provides a back-up archival file for the 136 newly acquired examinations to improve the reliability of the network.

Each day, the long-term archiving node receives 136 new examinations from the acquisition and formatting node and stores them at full spatial and contrast resolution. It also receives 136 database directory messages identifying the images and display parameters selected by the radiologist to serve as documentation for his consultation report. The long-term archiving node maintains an intermediate and long-term database for two and five year periods, respectively. The hard copy node is required to generate hard copy images of 136 examinations per day as transmitted from the on-line archival files.

Image Acquisition and Formatting Nodes

Image acquisition and formatting nodes collect digital data from the various imaging modalities, reformat them into a network defined database format, and then notify all nodes on the network of their availability. Figure 79–2 is a block diagram of an image acquisition and formatting node. The node consists of a computer system (CPU, memory, disks, streaming tape drive, printer, terminals), interface hardware (network interface unit, image modality bus interface, and operator terminal), image disk, and software (operating system and application software). The node bus electrically connects the hardware within each node. The network interface unit (NIU) electrically connects the node bus to the local network cable and performs the protocols necessary to communicate over the multiaccess network channel.

Connection to a given imaging modality is accomplished through a modality-spe-

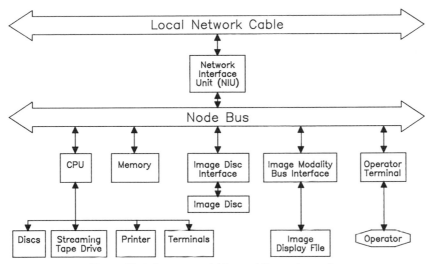

Figure 79–2. Image acquisition and formatting node.

cific bus interface. Manufacturers of imaging equipment offer and support a limited number of digital interfaces to their computer systems to allow access to a device's image display files.[26] Most of the available digital interfaces are intended for use with standard computer peripherals such as disk drives, printers, and modems. Due to the large amounts of image data and the high rate of data transfer necessary for network operation, a direct memory access (DMA) interface is required for transferring digital images to the network. Ideally these interfaces would be offered by each medical imaging manufacturer with hardware and software for new as well as older equipment.

The software required for an acquisition and formatting node includes computer operating system software, communications and database management programs, acquisition programs, and applications software. Acquisition programs are responsible for acquiring a patient's image data from the image display file of the imaging modality. Formatting programs are responsible for placing the image data into a standard image format for efficient network transmission. Database programs insure proper insertion of images and consultation reports into the network database structure using a sequence of headers and pointers. Once an examination is acquired, an updated location directory is broadcast throughout the network to inform other nodes of the availability of the new examination. The acquisition and formatting node is responsible for transmission of new examinations to an on-line archiving node, to a selected IDDS node, and to the long-term archiving node.

An estimate of the volume of digitally formatted data being generated by our department is provided in Table 79–2. As previously indicated, a total of 136 digitally formatted examinations are being generated each working day (253 working days per year). This amounts to a daily average of 2752 digital images of varying spatial and contrast resolution or a total of 949.82 megabytes of digital data to be handled by the image acquisition and formatting nodes.

The time available for data transfer from the imaging modality display file into the acquisition and formatting node is dependent upon the average time needed to acquire each examination. Table 79–3 provides the average examination times for each imaging modality. Ideally, transmission of a new examination onto the network should take place while the imaging device is acquiring the next examination. Thus, the acquisition and formatting of an examination by the network must be complete in the average 30 to 60 minute period required to examine each patient.

Table 79–2. DIGITAL DATA GENERATED DAILY BY AN ACADEMIC RADIOLOGY DEPARTMENT SERVING A 540 BED HOSPITAL POPULATION

Examinations	Patients	Display Images	Image Bytes (in Megabytes)	Nonimaging Bytes (in Kilobytes)	Total Bytes (in Megabytes)
		Average Number per Day			
Body CT*	16	20–40 (Avg = 26)	67.30	80†	67.38
Head CT*	18	16–20 (Avg = 18)	133.74	90	133.83
NM—static‡	24	8	12.77	120	12.89
NM—dynamic‡	8	15	7.98	40	8.02
Ultrasound‡	22	30–42 (Avg = 36)	208.4	110	208.5
DSA§	8	16	67.24	40	67.28
DR (estimated)‖	20	4	83.97	100	84.07
MR head (estimated)**	10	20	105.10	50	105.15
MR body (estimated)**	10	50	262.66	50	262.70

Total number of bytes generated per day: 949.82 Megabytes

* Each pixel of a CT display image has a possible contrast range of 10 ($2^{10} = 1024$ possible CT values) to 12 bits ($2^{12} = 4096$ possible CT values). Computer hardware and software systems used in CT scans usually require bytes of storage (8 bits/byte) per pixel. CT images are displayed in a circular format representing the circle of reconstruction. The diameter of this displayed circle is either 320 pixels for body scans (80,425 pixels/CT scan and 160,850 bytes of storage) or 512 pixels for head scans (205,887 pixels/CT scan and 411,775 bytes). An additional 1024 bytes are added to all digital images for header block information. Thus, each CT image generates a total of 161,874 bytes per 320 pixel diameter or 412,799 bytes per 512 pixel diameter.

† Each consultation report is assumed to average 500 words, each word averaging 10 characters in length. One character equals one byte.

‡ Each nuclear medicine gamma camera display image pixel has a contract range of eight bits ($2^8 = 256$ values). The digital array size for static image acquisition is 128 × 128 pixels (16,384 pixels). The digital array size for dynamic acquisition is 64 × 64 pixels (4096 pixels). However, owing to image viewing considerations all nuclear medicine images are now formatted as 256 × 256 × 8 bits (65,536 pixels). Each pixel of an ultrasound display usually has a contrast range of six bits ($2^6 = 64$ values). After postprocessing, the ultrasound digital display array is 512 × 512 pixels (262,144 pixels). An additional 1024 bytes are provided for each image's header block of information.

§ Each pixel of a DSA image currently has a contrast range of 10 bits. The digital array is either 512 × 512 pixels (262,144 pixels/image) or 1024 × 1024 pixels (1,048,576 pixels/image). Thus, including the 1024 bytes for header block information, there are 525,312 bytes per 512 × 512 × 10 bit image.

‖ Each pixel has a contrast range of eight bits as digitized from a high resolution 1023 line television camera with a signal-to-noise ratio of 1000:1. With the introduction of progressive scanning, each pixel will be digitized to 10 bits from a high resolution television camera with a signal-to-noise ratio of approximately 3000:1. The digital display array is 1024 × 1024 pixels. An additional 1024 bytes are used for header block informattion on each digitized image. Thus, there are 1,049,600 bytes per image for eight bit pixels and 2,098,176 bytes per image for 10 bit pixels.

** The digital data density for MR imaging is not yet standardized. Currently, each pixel has a contrast range betwen 10 and 12 bits. The digital display array is 512 × 512 pixels. With an additional 1024 bytes of header information, each MR image will have 262,144 pixels or 525,312 bytes of computer storage, assuming that each pixel is encoded into two bytes.

Table 79–3. AVERAGE TIME NEEDED TO ACQUIRE DIGITALLY FORMATTED EXAMINATIONS

Modality	To Complete Examination	To Display, Manipulate, and Generate Multiformat Film Recordings	To Generate Written Consultation
	Average Time (in Minutes) Needed per Patient		
Computed tomography	30	20–30	20
Nuclear medicine	60	20	15
Ultrasound	30–45	30	15
Digital subtraction angiography	45–90	30	30
Digital radiography (estimated)	30	15	20
Magnetic resonance (estimated)	60	30	15

To determine a system's ability to meet the demands imposed, estimates of system performance must be made. One such estimate is the mean system throughput, R, defined as the reciprocal of the time required by the system to complete a specified task. The mean throughput may be determined by summation of the times required for completion of each step performed in completing a task and taking the reciprocal such that:

$$R = 1/T$$

where:

$$T = \sum_1^{i=2} T_i$$

and T_i is the time required to complete the ith step in the task.

Table 79–4 summarizes the five step-by-step operations carried out by the acquisition and formatting node as modeled by Figure 79–2 during the acquisition of a new examination. For each step, certain components of the node are active while others remain inactive. For each step the active components are identified by placing a "1" in the appropriate column. The average time for completion of each step is shown in the rightmost column of Table 79–4.

In Step 1, the operator at the control console of the acquisition and formatting node enters the patient's name, ID number, date of examination, and other data. The operator then requests the transfer of the patient's images from a particular modality's display file. The resources active in Step 1 are the CPU, memory, operator terminal, and the operator. The mean time required to complete Step 1 is 20 seconds per examination. In Step 2 the patient's images are transferred from the image display file of the imaging device to the image disk via the node bus and image disk interface. The mean time to complete Step 2 is designated by $T_{transfer}$. $T_{transfer}$ is limited primarily by the speed of the various image modality interfaces available from the manufacturers (see first footnote, Table 79–4). The node bus is capable of transferring digital data at mean rate of 8 megabits per second and thus does not significantly contribute to $T_{transfer}$. In Step 3, the patient's examination data are reformatted into a standard network format such as $1024 \times 1024 \times 8$ bits, and stored on the image disk. In Steps 4 and 5 the operator is notified that the image acquisition and formatting are complete and broadcasts a message to all other network nodes indicating the availability and location of the newly acquired examination. The average total time for acquisition and formatting is given by the sum of the times required for completion of Steps 1 through 5.

The number of image acquisition and formatting nodes on a radiology network is determined by the number of digital imaging devices and the patient load in the department. In our department there are two CT units, six NM gamma cameras, six US units, two DSA units, one MRI unit, and one DR image intensifier system. One possible configuration for these devices, including six acquisition and formatting nodes, is illustrated in Figure 79–3.

An estimate of the average throughput for transmitting image data between the acquisition and formatting nodes and other nodes may be obtained with the aid of Figure 79–4 and Table 79–5. Figure 79–4 is a diagram illustrating the resources necessary for transferring image data between two nodes.[31–34] This figure includes the layered model of the software operating system for each node.[35–40] Assuming that one image of $1024 \times 1024 \times 8$ bits is to be transferred between nodes A and B, Table 79–5 identifies each processing step as well as the resources and time required for each step's completion.

Table 79–6 provides an analysis of the processing steps and average times required to transmit images from a variety of imaging devices at their full contrast and spatial

Table 79–4. PROCESSING TASKS AND RESOURCE ALLOCATION FOR ACQUISITION AND FORMATTING NODES

Step-by-Step Processing	Resource Allocation Map								Time (Seconds) per Patient Examination
	CPU	Memory	NIU	Image Disk	Image Modality Bus Interface	Image Display File	Operator Terminal	Operator	
1. Operator calls up display screen, enters data (name, ID number, date of exam, etc.), requests transfer of images from image modality to acquisition and formatting node.	1	1	0	0	0	0	1	1	20
2. Patient image file transferred from image display file on to image disk.	1	1	0	1	1	1	0	0	T_{transfer}*
3. Patient image file processed for formatting into standard 1K × 1K × 8 bit and stored on image disk.	1	1	0	1	0	0	0	0	$T_{\text{formatting}}$†
4. CPU notifies operator that patient image file is transferred, stored, and reformatted.	1	1	0	0	0	0	1	0	1.5
5. Acquisition node broadcasts a message to all other nodes that patient's image file is available. Address of patient's file and standard formatted file are included in message.	1	1	1	0	0	0	0	0	0.1

T_{transfer} times per patient examination are: CT body exam = 20.8 s; CT head exam = 36.9 s; NM static exam = 273.04 s; NM dynamic exam = 511.95 s; US exam = 93.6 s; DSA exam = 4,368 s; DR exam = 4,192 s; MRI head exam = 83.88 s; MRI body exam = 209.7 s.

$T_{\text{formatting}}$ times per patient examination are: CT body exam = 78 s; CT head exam = 54 s; NM static exam = 14.4 s; NM dynamic exam = 27 s; US exam = 180 s; DSA exam = 96 s; DR exam = 480 s; MRI head exam = 60 s; MRI body exam = 150 s.

* $T_{\text{transfer time}}$. For CT scanners, the data transfer rate from the image display file, through the image modality bus interface, to the image disc is 200,000 bytes/s (CT body = 0.80 s/image; CT head = 2.05 s/image), the transfer rate is 1920 bytes/s (19,200 bits per s; 8 bits + start bit + stop bit per byte) or 34.13 s/NM image. For ultrasound, the transfer rate is 100,000 bytes/s (2.6 s/US image). For DSA, the transfer rate is 1,920 bytes/s (512 × 512 × 16 bits = 524,288 bytes; 273 s/DSA image). For DR, the transfer rate is 1 megabyte/s (1024 × 1024 × 8 = 1,048,576 bytes/DR; 1.048 s/DR image). For MRI, the transfer rate is 125,000 bytes/s or 1 megabit/s (512 × 512 × 16 = 524,288 bytes/MRI image; 4.194 s/MRI image).

† $T_{\text{formatting time}}$. The time required for formatting images into a network standard of 1024 × 1024 × 8 bit format are the following. For CT body/head the formatting time averages 3 s per CT image or 12 s, since there will be 12 CT images per one standard network image. For nuclear medicine (256 × 256 × 8) images, the formatting time averages 1.8 s/image, or 16 × 1.8 = 28.8 s (16 NM images in one standard network image). For ultrasound (512 × 512 × 8) images, the formatting time averages 5 s/image, or 4 × 5 = 20 s (4 US images in one standard network image). For DSA (512 × 512 × 10) images, the formatting time averages 6 s/image, or 4 × 6 = 24 s. For digital radiography (1024 × 1024 × 8) images, the formatting time averages 120 s per DR image. For MRI (512 × 512 × 16) images, the formatting time averages 3 s per image or 4 × 3 = 12 s (4 MRI images in one standard network image).

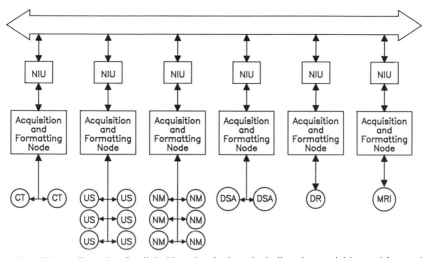

Figure 79–3. Possible configuration for digital imaging devices, including six acquisition and formatting nodes.

resolution. Table 79–7 extrapolates this data to give the average time each day that an acquisition and formatting node would be occupied with a particular task for each imaging modality.

Interactive Diagnosis Display Station

The function of the IDDS is to enable the radiologist to interactively display and manipulate the digitally formatted images available on the radiology network. Figure 79–5 is an illustration of the elements of this type of node. The node consists of a computer system, interface hardware, and software, including the operating system and interactive gray scale display software. An interactive device is used to signal the computer applications software that the radiologist wishes to modify the images on the display screen. The display computer services the signal by generating display commands that perform the desired modification of the displayed image.

Four groups of interactive computer display commands are required in the op-

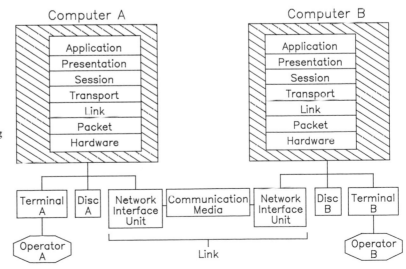

Figure 79–4. Model for transferring image data between two nodes.

Table 79–5. PROCESSING TASKS AND RESOURCE ALLOCATION FOR TRANSMITTING PATIENT EXAMINATIONS BETWEEN TWO NODES FOR PATIENT EXAMINATIONS FORMATTED INTO A 1024 × 1024 × 8 BIT STANDARD

Step-by-Step Process	Resource Allocation Map					Time (in Seconds) per Patient Examination
	Computer A	*Disk A*	*Link*	*Computer B*	*Disk B*	
1. Computer A requests a patient image file from Computer B.	1	0	1	1	0	0.001
2. Computer B retrieves patient image file from Disk B based upon an average 8 megabits/s throughput.	0	0	0	1	1	$T_{retrieval}$*
	$T_{retrieval}$ times per patient examination are: CT body exam = 7.34 s; CT head exam = 5.248 s; NM static exam = 1.0496 s; NM dynamic exam = 1.0496 s; US exam = 9.446 s; DSA exam = 4.198 s; DR exam = 4.198 s; MRI head exam = 5.248 s; MRI body exam = 13.64 s.					
3. Patient image examination is transmitted from Computer B to Computer A based upon an average 3 megabits/s throughput.	1	0	1	1	0	$T_{transmit}$†
	$T_{transmit}$ times per patient examination are: CT body exam = 19.59 s; CT head exam = 13.99 s; NM static exam = 2.798 s; NM dynamic exam = 2.798 s; NM dynamic exam = 2.798 s; US exam = 25.19 s; DSA exam = 11.195 s; DR exam = 11.195 s; MRI head exam = 13.99 s; MRI body exm = 36.386 s					
4. Computer A stores patient image examination on Disk A based upon an average 8 megabits/s throughput.	1	1	0	0	0	(same as $T_{retrieval}$ in step 2)
5. Computer A sends an acknowledgment back to Computer B.	1	0	1	1	0	0.001
6. Computer A notifies Operator A that file transfer is completed.	1	0	0	0	0	0.100

* $T_{retrieval}$. The retrieval times from disc per patient examination with the images formatted into 1024 × 1024 × 8 bit standard images are the following: CT head uses 7 standard images (26 average patient images/4 Ct head images per standard) and requires 7.34 s (7 × (1024 × 1024 × 8 + 1,024 × 8)/8 × 10⁶ = 7.34 s). CT body uses 5 standard images and requires 5.248 s. NM static and NM dynamic patient examinations use 1 standard image and require 1.0496 s. US uses 9 standard images and requires 9.446 s. DSA uses 4 standard images and requires 4.198 s. DR uses 4 standard images and requires 4.198 s. MRI head uses 5 standard images and requires 5.248 s. The MRI body uses 13 standard images and requires 13.64 s.

† $T_{transmit}$. The transmission times per patient examination using a standard format of 1024 × 1024 × 8 bits from Computer B to Computer A are calculated by the following: $T_{transmit}$ (s) = (number of standard images per exam) × (1,024 × 1,024 × 8 + 1,024 × 8)/(3 × 10⁶ bits/s). The number of standard images per exam is cited in preceding footnote.

eration of an IDDS. The first group of IDDS display commands are image formatting commands that provide for the selection, display formatting, and actual display of patient digital data. The second group of IDDS display commands are the image quantification functions, which provide the radiologist with an interactive means of quantifying the numerical data contained in an image. The third group of IDDS display commands are the image display parameter commands. These commands provide a means of rapidly and easily modifying the image display parameters. The fourth group of IDDS display commands are the image processing functions, which offer a means of applying image processing algorithms to the display images.

The capabilities of an IDDS depend on the location of the node within a department or hospital. At least three classes of IDDS are required, each with different display options and functions. One class would be IDDSs, whose operations are specific to a given imaging device, such as the IDDSs at the control consoles of CT or MRI scanners. A second type of IDDS would be used on the network within the radiology department. These would display images in the selected network-specific format, for example, 1K

Table 79–6. PROCESSING TASKS AND RESOURCE ALLOCATION FOR TRANSMITTING PATIENT EXAMINATIONS BETWEEN TWO NODES WITH FULL CONTRAST AND SPATIAL RESOLUTION

Step-by-Step Process	Resource Allocation Map					Time (in Seconds) per Patient Examination
	Computer A	*Disk A*	*Link*	*Computer B*	*Disk B*	
1. Computer A requests a patient image file from Computer B.	1	0	1	1	0	0.001
2. Computer B retrieves patient image file from Disk B based upon an average of 8 megabits/s throughput.	0	0	0	1	1	$T_{retrieval}$*
$T_{retrieval}$ times per patient examination are: CT body exam = 4.21 s; CT head exam = 7.43 s; NM static exam = 0.537 s; NM dynamic exam = 1.0 s; US exam = 9.477 s; DSA exam = 8.41 s; DR exam = 4.2 s; MRI head exam = 10.515 s; MRI body exam = 26.27 s.						
3. Patient image examination is transmitted from Computer B to Computer A based upon 3 megabits/s throughput.	1	0	1	1	0	$T_{transmit}$†
$T_{transmit}$ times per patient examination are: CT body exam = 11.23 s; CT head exam = 19.82 s; NM static exam = 1.43 s; NM dynamic exam = 2.67s; US exam = 25.27 s; DSA exam = 22.42 s; DR exam = 11.2 s; MRI head exam = 28.04 s; MRI body exam = 70.05 s.						
4. Computer A stores patient image examination on Disk A based upon an average of 8 megabits/throughput.	1	1	0	0	0	(same as $T_{retrieval}$ in Step 2)
5. Computer A sends an acknowledgment back to Computer B.	1	0	1	1	0	0.001
6. Computer A notifies Operator A that file transfer is completed.	1	0	0	0	0	0.100

* $T_{retrieval}$. The retrieval times from disc per patient examination with full contrast and spatial resolution for an average of 8 megabits/s throughput are calculated as follows: $T_{retrieval}$ (s) = total bits per patient examination (from Table 79–2)/(8 × 10⁶ bits/s).

† $T_{transmit}$. The transmit times from Computer B to Computer A per patient examination with full contrast and spatial resolution for an average of 3 megabits/s throughput are calculated as follows: $T_{transmit}$ (s) = total bits per patient examination (from Table 79–2)/(3 × 10⁶ bits/s).

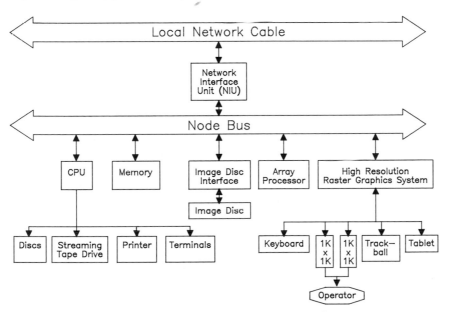

Figure 79–5. Diagram of elements of the IDDS.

Table 79–7. REQUIRED AVERAGE TIMES PER DAY IN SECONDS FOR ACQUISITION AND FORMATTING NODES

	CT Body	CT Head	NM Static	NM Dynamic	US	DSA	DR	MRI Head	MRI Body
Number of patients per day	16	18	24	8	22	8	20	10	10
Average number of images per patient	26	18	8	15	36	16	4	2	50
Time per day to acquire, format, and broadcast directory update	1,926.4* (seconds) (32.1 min)	2,025* (seconds) (33.5 min)	7,425.6* (seconds) (123.7 min)	4,484.4* (seconds) (74.74 min)	6,494.4* (seconds) (108.24 min)	35,886* (seconds) (598.1 min)	10,115.8* (seconds) (168.5 min)	1,654.8* (seconds) (27.58 min)	3,813* (seconds) (63.55 min)
Time per day to transmit all images to long-term archiving; broadcast update directory	316.02† (seconds)	626.07† (seconds)	62.54† (seconds)	38.176† (seconds)	975.17† (seconds)	314.7† (seconds)	394.04† (seconds)	491.7† (seconds)	1,226.92† (seconds)
Time per day to transmit formatted images once to on-line archiving node; broadcast update directory	549.95‡ (seconds)	442.58‡ (seconds)	119.98‡ (seconds)	39.99‡ (seconds)	972.04‡ (seconds)	157.5‡ (seconds)	393.86‡ (seconds)	225.92‡ (seconds)	637.68‡ (seconds)

* Total time in seconds per day to acquire, format into a network standard of $1K \times 1K \times 8$ bits, and broadcast a message identifying new patient image data is given by the following calculation (see Table 79–4): (number of patient examinations per day) $\times$ (20 s + $T_{transfer}$ + $T_{formatting}$ + 1.5 s + 0.2 s.)

† Total time in seconds per day to transmit all images in full contrast and spatial resolution one time to the long-term archiving node and to broadcast an updated directory is given by the following calculation (see Table 79–6): (number of patient examinations per day) $\times$ (0.001 second + $T_{retrieval}$ + $T_{transmit}$ + $T_{retrieval}$ + 0.001 + 0.100).

‡ Total time in seconds per day to transmit formatted ($1024 \times 1024 \times 8$ bits) images one time to the on-line archiving node and to broadcast an updated directory is given by the following calculation (see Table 79–5): (number of patient examinations per day) $\times$ (0.001 second + $T_{retrieval}$ + $T_{transmit}$ + $T_{retrieval}$ + 0.001 + 0.10).

× 1K × 8 bits, and would be capable of displaying multiple modality images on a single screen. They would also be capable of the full range of image manipulations. The third class of IDDS would be those outside the department in clinics, wards, and surgical suites. They would have only limited interactive capabilities and would function only to display image data.

The average utilization and display throughput rates for an IDDS are important in estimating the number of IDDSs required to serve a network. Table 79–8 presents a typical resource allocation table and the estimated average times required for each image displayed and manipulated on an IDDS. Table 79–9 provides an analysis of the average throughput times per day for the IDDSs related to various image modalities. These results illustrate the uneven utilization of the IDDS nodes between various modalities and suggest a distribution scheme that allocates relatively fewer nodes for certain modalities or combining nodes for less active IDDS sites.

On-Line Archiving Nodes

The function of the on-line archiving node is to maintain examination data during periods of high demand. Figure 79–6 is a block diagram of this type of node. A 9- to 20-day working period from the patient's most recent examination is generally selected as the period of on-line archiving. This period roughly corresponds to the average hospital stay for inpatients. At the end of the on-line archival period the patient's file is transferred to the long-term archiving nodes. Multiple copies of a patient's image file may be archived on the network in a combination of acquisition and formatting, IDDS, and on-line archiving nodes. When a node broadcasts a request for the file of a particular patient, the returned messages must be analyzed by the requesting node to select the proper file for transfer.

An estimate of the required amount of on-line storage may be obtained by considering the amount of data generated per day. Table 79–2 shows that during a typical working day 949.82 megabytes of digitally formatted data are generated. Satisfying a 10-day on-line requirement implies that the on-line archiving nodes must possess a storage capacity of 9.4982 gigabytes.

The retrieval rate from on-line archiving nodes is also an important parameter. An estimate of the retrieval rate can be obtained by analyzing the retrieval rate of film

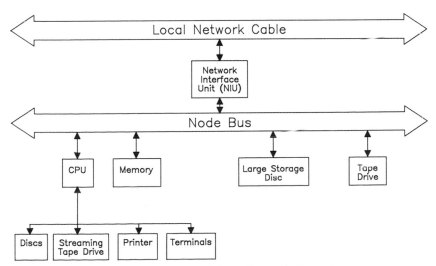

Figure 79–6. Diagram of the on-line achieving node.

Table 79–8. PROCESSING TASKS AND RESOURCE ALLOCATION FOR IDDS NODES

Step-by-Step Process	Resource Allocation Map								Time (Seconds) per Examination
	CPU	Memory	Disc	Raster Graphics System	Monitor 1 1K × 1K × 8	Monitor 2 1K × 1K × 8	Interactive Device	Operator	
1. Operator selects patient data by moving cursor over patient data listing.	1	1	0	1	1	0	1	1	T_{select} (0.5)
2. CPU searches database on disk for patient data file.	1	1	1	0	0	0	0	0	T_{search} (5.0)
3. CPU writes available patient database on screen of Monitor 1.	1	1	1	1	1	0	0	0	T_{write} (1.0)
4. Operator studies listing and selects patient desired with cursor.	1	1	0	1	1	0	1	1	T_{read} (10)
5. Operator selects which images to view by use of cursor on screen.	1	1	0	1	1	0	1	1	T_{select} (0.5)
6. CPU writes image data from disk to memory and then to display screen of Monitor 1.	1	1	1	1	1	0	0	0	$T_{\text{write screen}}$* (2.0)
7. Operator manipulates image on Monitor 1.	1	1	0	1	1	0	1	1	$T_{\text{display and manipulate}}$ (108)
8. Repeat Steps 3–7 for Monitor 2. (Repeat alternating between Monitors 1 and 2 until average number of images are displayed and manipulated).†	1	1	1	1	0	1	1	1	$T_{\text{display and manipulate remaining images}}$
9. Operator selects images to be hard copied.	1	1	1	1	1	1	1	1	$T_{\text{hard copy selection}}$ (100)

Times per patient examination are: CT body exam = 759 s; CT head exam = 506 s; NM exam = 0 s; US exam = 1,012 s; DSA exam = 379.5 s; DR exam = 379.5 s; MRI head exam = 253 s; MRI body exam = 379.5 s.

* $T_{\text{write screen}}$ is the time in seconds to write one display screen and is on the order of 2.0 s. The number of images written per display screen of size 1024 × 1024 pixels is the following: 4 CT images/screen; 16 NM images/screen; 4 US images/screen; 4 DSA images/screen; and 16 MRI images/screen. The times shown are the total times required to write groups of images alternating between Monitor 1 and Monitor 2 until all images have been displayed. These times represent the total times required to complete Steps 3 through 7 and are adequate so that all images are displayed only once.

† This assumes a display node incorporating two monitors.

Table 79–9. THE AVERAGE THROUGHPUT TIMES PER DAY FOR THE IDDS NODES

	CT Body	CT Head	NM Static	NM Dynamic	US	DSA	DR	MRI Head	MRI Body
Number of patients per day	16	18	24	8	22	8	20	10	10
Average number of images per patient	26	18	8	15	36	16	3	20	50
Number of images per screen	4	4	8	15	4	4	1	16	16
Average time per day (s) to display, manipulate, and select images for hard copy	15,776* (seconds) (4.38 hr)	13,194* (seconds) (3.665 hr)	5,448* (seconds) (1.51 hr)	1,816* (seconds) (0.504 hr)	27,258* (seconds) (7.57 hr)	4,852* (seconds) (1.34 hr)	12,130* (seconds) (3.36 hr)	4,800* (seconds) (1.33 hr)	6,065* (seconds) (1.68 hr)
Estimated average time per day to receive 136 standard formatted exams from the on-line archiving nodes and modified directory broadcast	549.95† (seconds)	442.58† (seconds)	119.98† (seconds)	39.99† (seconds)	972.04† (seconds)	157.5† (seconds)	393.86† (seconds)	225.92† (seconds)	637.68† (seconds)
Estimated average time per day to receive 7.2 × 136 examinations retrieved from the on-line archiving node and directory broadcast	3,959.64‡ (seconds)	3,186.576‡ (seconds)	863.85† (seconds)	287.51‡ (seconds)	6,998.6‡ (seconds)	1,134‡ (seconds)	2,835.8‡ (seconds)	1,626.62‡ (seconds)	4,591.3‡ (seconds)
Estimated average time per day to transmit 136 examinations to the hard copy node	549.95§ (seconds)	442.58§ (seconds)	119.98§ (seconds)	39.99§ (seconds)	972.04§ (seconds)	157.5§ (seconds)	393.86§ (seconds)	225.92§ (seconds)	637.68§ (seconds)

* Total time per day in seconds to display, manipulate, and select images for hard copy calculated as follows (see Table 79–8): (number of patient examinations per day) × (T_{select} + T_{search} + T_{write} + T_{read} + T_{select} + $T_{write screen}$ − $T_{write screen}$ − $T_{display and manipulate}$ + $T_{display and manipulate remaining images}$ + $T_{hard copy selection}$).

† Estimated average time per day to receive 136 examinations in a 1024 × 1024 × 8 bit standard format is taken from Table 79–7, time per day to transmit formatted images once to on-line archiving node.

‡ Estimated average time per day to receive 7.2 × 136 examinations as standard formatted images transmitted from the on-line archiving node (footnote †).

§ Estimated average time per day to transmit 136 examinations to the hard copy node (footnote †).

jackets containing multiformat film images from a department's film library. We have found that the peak retrieval demand for hospital inpatients averages 10 requests during the first three days of a patient's hospital stay (10/3 requests/day). During the remainder of a patient's hospital stay (6 days), there is an average peak retrieval demand of four requests (4/6 requests/day). There follows an average peak retrieval demand of three requests during the remainder of the first year following the patient's hospitalization (3/245 requests per day). The resultant data retrieval rate per day, R, for inpatients is given by:

$$R = X + \frac{10}{3} X + \frac{10}{3} X_{-1} + \frac{10}{3} X_{-2} + \frac{4}{6} X_{-3} + \cdots + \frac{4}{6} X_{-8} + \frac{3}{245} X_{-9},$$

where X is the number of inpatient bytes generated on a particular working day, X_{-1} bytes generated on the previous day, etc. If the number of bytes generated each working day is assumed to be equal to ($X = X_{-1} = X_{-2} = \cdots = X_{-9}$), then the retrieval rate per day, R, would be $15.01X$. Assuming that the outpatient retrieval is twice (once for the radiologist and once for the referring physician), then the outpatient retrieval rate per day would be $2X$. Since the ratio of inpatients to outpatients is currently 2 to 3, the estimated volume of data to be retrieved each day is given by the following: $[.40(15.01) + .60(2)][949.82 \text{ megabytes}] = 6.84$ gigabytes.

Assuming a uniform retrieval rate during the day, the average data throughput rate for on-line archiving nodes during a 12-hour workday is:

$$\frac{6.84 \text{ gigabytes} \times 8 \text{ bits/byte}}{12 \text{ hr} \times 3600 \text{ s/hr}} = 1.267 \text{ megabits/s}$$

Since this figure represents an average retrieval rate of image data, the actual retrieval rate is greater than this by a factor of approximately 5 to account for peak load and the transfer of nonimage data as well as system overhead and signaling necessary for the operation of the network communication protocol. Thus the actual mean throughput of the on-line archival node is approximately 6.34 megabits/s.

Table 79–10 presents the resource allocation table and the estimated average times required for the operation of each on-line archiving node. Table 79–11 presents the

Table 79–10. PROCESSING STEPS AND MEAN RESPONSE TIMES FOR ON-LINE ARCHIVING NODES

Step-by-Step Process	CPU	Memory	System Disk	NIU	Image Storage Disk	Tape Drive	Operator Terminal	Time (Seconds) per Patient Examination
1. Write/read image data into/from image storage discs based upon an average of megabits/sec throughput.	1	1	0	1	1	0	0	$T_{\text{write/read}}$*
			$T_{\text{write/read}}$ times per patient are: CT body exam = 7.34 s; CT head exam = 5.248 s; NM static exam = 1.0496 s; NM dynamic exam = 1.0496 s; US exam = 9.446 s; DSA exam = 4.198 s; DR exam = 4.198 s; MRI head exam = 5.248 s; MRI body exam = 13.64 s					
2. CPU broadcasts an updated directory.	1	1	1	1	0	0	0	$T_{\text{broadcast}} = 0.5$ s
3. CPU writes to tape drive the oldest patient examination file.	1	1	1	0	1	1	0	T_{write}†
4. CPU notifies operator terminal of directory update.	1	1	0	0	0	0	1	$T_{\text{notify}} = 0.1$ s

* Calculations same as first footnote (*), Table 79–5, assuming an 8×10^6 bit/s average throughput rate.
† T_{write} calculation is the same as first footnote (*) in this table, again assuming an average throughput rate of 8×10^6 bits/s.

Table 79–11. THE AVERAGE THROUGHPUT TIMES PER DAY FOR THE ON-LINE ARCHIVING NODES

	CT Body	CT Head	NM Static	NM Dynamic	US	DSA	DR	MRI Head	MRI Body
Number of patients per day	16	18	24	8	22	8	20	10	10
Averge number of images per patient	26	18	8	15	36	16	4	20	50
Number of images per screen	4	4	8	15	4	4	1	16	16
Average time per day to: (1) acquire and archive 136 new formatted exams from the acquisition and formatting nodes and broadcast an updated directory (Table 79–5); (2) retrieve and transmit to IDDS nodes 979.2 exams and broadcast an updated directory (Table 79–5).	4,509.6* (seconds) (1.25 hr)	3,629.156* (seconds) (1.0 hr)	982.5* (seconds) (0.27 hr)	327.9* (seconds) (0.09 hr)	7,970.7* (seconds) (2.2 hr)	1,291.5* (seconds) (0.36 hr)	3,229.6* (seconds) (0.89 hr)	1,852.5* (seconds) (0.51 hr)	5,228.9* (seconds) (1.45 hr)

* Calculation is as follows: (time per day to acquire and transmit formatted images once from archiving and formatting nodes to the on-line archiving nodes as shown in Table 79–7, line 5) + (7.2) × (time per day to acquire and transmit formatted images once from on-line archiving to IDDS nodes as shown in Table 79–9, line 5).

daily cumulative throughput times required on the on-line archiving nodes by each imaging modality. The average time per day to read/write one screen of image data is calculated by adding the average times for each step shown in Table 79–10.

Long-Term Archiving Node

The function of the long-term archiving node is to store digital image data for a 5- to 7-year period. The long-term archiving requirements for digital radiology networks are difficult to estimate. The difficulty in obtaining such estimates is due primarily to the recent increase in the use of digitally based imaging modalities and to the increasing ratio of outpatient to inpatient examinations. However, some estimates can be made based on a review of department statistics. For example, Table 79–12 shows the number of patients, total examinations, and percentage of the total examinations that were obtained from digital modalities in our department over the 9-year period from 1977 to 1985. Table 79–13 breaks these figures down by examination type for this period. The distribution of film jackets in our three library files is 2020 jackets in the 10-day file; 150,000 jackets in the 2-year intermediate file; and 409,600 in the 5-year long-term archiving file. During a typical 30-day period a total of 1030 film jackets are retrieved from the 5-year long-term file. Seventy-five percent of these are concurrent with acquisition of a new patient examination and are thereafter cycled into the 10-day high demand file. The remaining 25 percent are retrieved for outpatient clinics, retrospective clinical studies, and teaching activities. They are thereafter returned to the 5-year long-term archiving file.

Simulation models to aid in the estimation of long-term archiving requirements are being developed. One such model is a type of Markov chain.[51] A Markov chain predicts the probable outcome of a sequence of events based only on a knowledge of the outcome of the most recent events. Figure 79–7 illustrates a Markov chain model of the retrievals from the three files within the film library. Transition probabilities measure the likelihood of movement of a film jacket between the three files.

The transition probabilities, P_{ij}, shown in Figure 79–7, are for a single step of the Markov chain. For example, the transition probability P_{11} is defined as the probability of retrieving the patient's file from the 10-day file *on condition* that the last retrieval of the patient's file was from the 10-day file (written as P_{11} = Pr [retrieve from 10-day file | previously retrieved from 10 day file]). Likewise, P_{12} = Pr [retrieve from 2-

Table 79–12. A NINE-YEAR SURVEY SHOWING THE PERCENTAGE OF DIGITALLY FORMATTED EXAMINATIONS PERFORMED AT THE UNIVERSITY OF KANSAS COLLEGE OF HEALTH SCIENCES AND HOSPITAL

Fiscal Year	Number of Patients	Total Imaging Examinations	Digitally Formatted Examinations	Percentage of Digitally Formatted Examinations
1985	90,561	103,950	23,956	23.0
1984	84,218	99,207	23,121	23.3
1983	85,950	104,274	23,335	22.3
1982	89,280	108,648	21,954	20.2
1981	86,843	106,643	19,674	18.4
1980	80,507	102,271	18,901	19.2
1979	80,249	97,291	18,278	18.5
1978	80,701	97,828	17,498	17.9
1977	81,271	101,198	15,960	15.8

Table 79–13. NUMBER AND TYPES OF IMAGING EXAMINATIONS PERFORMED

Fiscal Year	Conventional Radiography	CT Body	CT Head	Mammography	Ultrasound	Special Procedures	Portable Surgery	Nuclear Medicine
1985	52,717	4,974	2,863	5,658	5,431	1,813	21,622	8,875
1984	53,786	4,783	2,986	4,800	5,523	1,878	17,500	7,951
1983	61,235	4,582	3,154	3,196	5,297	1,988	16,508	8,314
1982	66,826	4,400	3,216	2,882	5,019	1,973	16,986	7,346
1981	67,856	3,216	3,498	2,581	4,161	2,281	16,532	6,518
1980	70,032	2,333	1,380	1,781	4,087	1,972	11,557	9,129
1979	65,442	2,183	5,119	1,382	3,606	1,906	12,189	5,464
1978	68,873	1,630	4,103	700	3,768	2,022	10,757	5,975
1977	72,906	938	4,467	1,514	3,412	2,143	11,628	5,000

year file | previously retrieved from 10-day file] and $P_{31} = Pr$ [retrieve from 10-day file | previously retrieved from 5-year file]. Owing to the recycling of new examinations, it is clear that $P_{13} = P_{32} = 0$, since any new examinations require reinserting the file into the 10-day archiving file. The remaining transition probabilities for the initial step of the Markov chain may be determined by sampling retrievals from the film library for a period of time.

The Markov chain model for archiving provides a simple method for calculating the transition probabilities from state S_i to state S_j in exactly n steps. Let $P(n)$ denote the transition matrix with entries $P_{ij} = Pr$ (state j is attained after n transitions from starting state i). Then $P(1)^n = P(n)$. That is, multiply the matrix $P(1)$ by itself n times to obtain $P(n)$. If

$$P(1) = \begin{bmatrix} 0.75 & 0.25 & 0 \\ 0.60 & 0.30 & 0.10 \\ 0.75 & 0 & 0.25 \end{bmatrix}$$

then after eight steps ($n = 8$),

$$[P(n = 1)]^8 = \begin{bmatrix} 0.7119 & 0.2542 & 0.0339 \\ 0.7119 & 0.2542 & 0.0339 \\ 0.7119 & 0.2542 & 0.0339 \end{bmatrix}$$

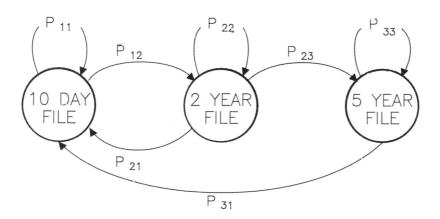

$$P_{ij} = \begin{bmatrix} P_{11} & P_{12} & P_{13} \\ P_{21} & P_{22} & P_{23} \\ P_{31} & P_{32} & P_{33} \end{bmatrix}$$

Figure 79–7. Markov chain model for retrieval from achieving files.

Note that after $n = 8$ steps, the transition probabilities in each column are equal. Furthermore, $P(n) = P(8)$ for $n > 8$, and the transition matrix has reached a steady state. Thus after eight steps the probability of retrieving a patient's file from the 10-day file is 71.19 percent, from the 2-year file is 25.42 percent, and from the 5-year file is 3.39 percent.

Mean throughput rates for long-term archiving of digitally formatted data can be estimated based on the following assumptions. First, the long-term archiving nodes will receive images from each acquisition and formatting node. At the completion of the 10-day archiving period, a message is sent to the long-term archiving nodes updating the patients' directory and detailing the display parameters used for transmission in the network format, here assumed to be 1K × 1K × 8 bits. Figure 79–8 is the block diagram for the long-term archiving node incorporating both the intermediate and long-term files. Tables 79–14 and 79–15 detail the various steps carried out by the long-term archiving node.

The Markov chain simulation predicts that 71.2 percent of film retrievals are from the 10-day file, 25.4 percent are from the 2-year file, and 3.4 percent are from the 5-year file. As previously described, the average number of retrievals each day is estimated to be 979.2 examinations. Thus, each day approximately 697.1 examinations will be retrieved from the 10-day on-line archiving node, 248.9 examinations will be retrieved from the 2-year file, and 33.2 examinations will be retrieved from the 5-year file. Table 79–16 summarizes the throughput times for various imaging modalities on the long-term archiving node.

Hard Copy Recording Nodes

Currently, any digital image management system must coexist with the conventional film jacket management system. For this reason, hard copy generation nodes must be incorporated into the radiologic network. Although such nodes may become obsolete for image management within a department should the "all digital department"

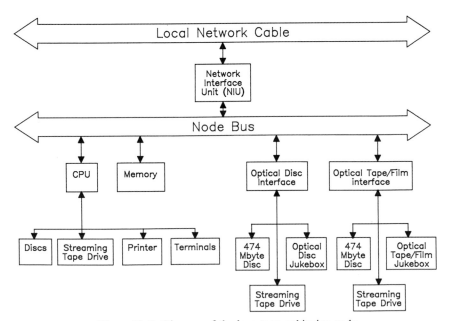

Figure 79–8. Diagram of the long-term achieving node.

Table 79–14. PROCESSING TASKS AND RESOURCE ALLOCATION FOR ACQUIRING EXAMINATION DATA FOR LONG-TERM ARCHIVING NODE

Step-by-Step Process	CPU	Memory	Disc	NIU	Optical Disk Interface	474 Mbyte Disc	Optical Disk Jukebox	Streaming Tape Drive	Operator Terminal	Time (Seconds) per Examination
1. Message received by CPU from acquisition and formatting nodes.	1	1	0	1	0	0	0	0	0	$T_1 = 0.1$
2. CPU acknowledges message and provides disk address for image data file.	1	1	1	1	0	0	0	0	0	$T_2 = 0.1$
3. Image data file transmitted from acquisition and formatting node to 474 Mbyte disk based upon 3 megabits/second throughput rate.	1	1	0	1	1	1	0	0	0	T_3^*
4. Data transfer from 474 Mbyte disc to optical disk based upon 8 megabits/second throughput rate. (transmit times same as second footnote (†), Table 79–6)	1	1	0	0	1	1	1	0	1	T_4†
5. Data transfer from 474 Mbyte disk to backup streaming tape drive based upon 8 megabits/second throughput rate. (transfer times same as first footnote (*), Table 79–6)	1	1	0	0	1	1	0	1	1	$T_5 = T_4$
6. Message received from on-line archiving node as to display parameters; added to data file.	1	1	1	1	1	0	0	0	1	$T_6 = 2.0$
7. A two year old file is transferred; from optical disk to 474 Mbyte disk on optical tape/film interface; to optical tape/film; backup streaming tape drive broadcast updated directory.	1	1	1	0	1	1	1	1	1	$T_7 = 3 \times T_4$

Table 79–15. PROCESSING TASKS AND RESOURCE ALLOCATION UTILIZATION FOR RETRIEVING IMAGE DATA FROM LONG-TERM ACHIVING NODE

Step-by-Step Process	Resource Allocation Map									Time (Seconds) per Examination
	CPU	Memory	Disk	NIU	Optical Disk Interface	474 Mbyte Disk	Optical Disk Jukebox	Streaming Tape Drive	Operator Terminal	
1. Message received by CPU for patient data retrieval.	1	1	0	1	0	0	0	0	1	$T_1 = 0.1$
2. Database directory searched for patient data files.	1	1	0	0	1	1	0	0	1	$T_2 = 15$
3. Patient data transferred from 2-year or 5-year archiving to 474 Mbyte disk based upon 8 megabits/second throughput.	1	1	0	1	1	1	0	0	0	T_3
(transfer times same as T_4, Table 79–14)										
4. Patient data transferred to requesting node and updated directory broadcast based upon 3 megabits/second throughput.	1	1	1	1	1	1	0	0	1	T_4
(transmit times sames as T_3, Table 79–14)										
5. Requesting node acknowledges receiving data.	1	1	1	1	0	0	0	0	1	$T_5 = 0.1$

Table 79–16. REQUIRED AVERAGE TIMES PER DAY IN SECONDS FOR LONG-TERM ARCHIVING NODE

	CT Body	CT Head	NM Static	NM Dynamic	US	DSA	DR	MRI Head	MRI Body
Number of patients per day	16	18	24	8	22	8	20	10	10
Average number of images per patient	26	18	8	15	36	16	4	20	50
Average time per day to acquire, archive, and broadcast updated directory (Table 79–14, sum of T_1 through T_7 times number of patients/day)	551.68 (seconds)	1,065.06 (seconds)	151.56 (seconds)	78.96 (seconds)	1,646.8 (seconds)	533.36 (seconds)	688 (seconds)	828.4 (seconds)	2,036 (seconds)
Average time per day to retrieve requested patient data files, transmit them to on-line archiving node, and broadcast updated directory	531.9* (seconds)	904.4* (seconds)	332.4* (seconds)	130.4* (seconds)	1,343.0* (seconds)	443.2* (seconds)	65.2* (seconds)	665.3* (seconds)	1,496.9* (seconds)

* The average time per day to retrieve requested patient image examination data, transmit them to the on-line archiving node, and broadcast an updated directory is calculated as follows: (7.2 × number of examinations per day) × (25.42 percent retrievals from 2 year file + 3.39 percent retrievals from 5 year file) × (total time of Table 79–15 + total time of Table 79–6).

Table 79–17. PROCESSING TASKS AND RESOURCE ALLOCATION UTILIZATION FOR THE HARD COPY GENERATION NODE

Step-by-Step Processing	Resource Allocation Map									Time (Seconds) per Examination
	CPU	Memory	Disc	NIU	Hard Copy Generation Interface	474 Mbyte Disk	Hard Copy Memory	Hard Copy Recorder Engine	Operator Terminal	
1. CPU receives message from a node wishing to generate hard copy recordings.	1	0	1	1	0	0	0	0	1	$T_1 = 0.1$
2. Image data transmitted from node to 474 Mbyte disk at 3 megabits/second throughput.	1	0	1	1	1	1	0	0	1	T_2
(transfer times same as second footnote (†), Table 79–6)										
3. Hard copy generation interface properly formats the image data for hard copy memory.	1	1	0	0	1	1	1	0	0	$T_3 = 1.0$
4. Hard copy generated by laser recorder engine (based on 20 seconds/1K × 1K × 8 bit formatted image).*	1	0	0	0	1	0	1	1	1	T_4
T_4 times per patients are: CT body exam = 140 s; CT head exam = 100 s; NM static exam = 20 s; NM dynamic exam = 20 s; US exam = 180 s; DSA exam = 80 s; DR exam = 80 s; MR head exam = 100 s; MR body exam = 260 s.										
5. Hard copy generator interface notifies CPU when recordings are completed.	1	0	0	0	1	0	0	1	0	$T_5 = 0.001$
6. CPU transmits message to requesting node that copies are completed.	1	0	1	1	0	0	0	0	1	$T_6 = 0.1$

* T_4 time calculated as follows: T_4 (seconds) = (average number of 1K × 1K × 8 bit images per patient examination) × (20 seconds for the laser film recorder to generate each 1K × 1K × 8 bit image). The average number of 1K × 1K × 8 bit images per patient for each imaging modality is shown in Table 79–18.

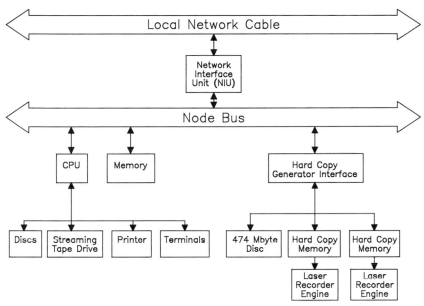

Figure 79–9. Diagram of the hard copy generation node.

become a reality, such devices will remain an important link in the communication of patient image data to sites not linked to the central radiology image management system.

Multiformat video cameras (MFVC) are now the most widely used devices for generating image hard copy. These cameras suffer from two major disadvantages. The first is the limitation of contrast image in the recorded images to less than 8 bits. This limit is imposed by the limited dynamic range of the light emitting phosphor of the camera's cathode ray tube by video noise attributable to either the CRT phosphor or electronic noise superimposed on the video signal. The second disadvantage of MFVCs is the necessity of incorporating either switched video equipment or broadband cable links into the network system to allow their continued use.

As a result of these difficulties with multiformat video cameras, various groups are evaluating devices that generate hard copy directly from digital signals. Most such devices are based on laser technology and may use a variety of media for hard copy generation, including conventional radiographic film, photographic film, and paper. Digitally formatted data is transferred directly to the laser controlling microcomputer. Currently, devices are capable of generating images of 300 pixels/inch spatial resolution. Local memory in the devices can hold up to 20 Mbytes. This local memory allows faster rates of image generation.

Figure 79–9 is a block diagram of a hard copy generation node. The resource allocation table and estimated throughput rate for each step in the processes of data transfer and image generation are presented in Table 79–17. Table 79–18 illustrates the average throughput times for a laser recorder generating 136 digital imaging examinations per day.

MEAN THROUGHPUT CALCULATIONS

The throughput of each node on the network is simply defined as the number of tasks completed by the node. It is designated by the symbol R. The time per task is designated by the symbol T. The throughput rate, designated by the symbol r, is defined as the instantaneous number of tasks completed per unit time. The relationship between

Table 79–18. ANALYSIS OF THE REQUIRED AVERAGE THROUGHPUT TIMES PER DAY IN SECONDS FOR HARD COPY GENERATION NODE

	CT Body	CT Head	NM Static	NM Dynamic	US	DSA	DR	MRI Head	MRI Body
Number of patients per day	16	18	24	8	22	8	20	10	10
Average number of images per patient	26	18	8	15	36	16	4	20	50
Average number of 1K × 1K × 8 bit analog hard copy images per patient	7	5	1	1	9	4	4	5	13
Average time per day to receive and generate hard copy images in the digital format of 1K × 1K × 8 bits	2,438* (seconds)	2,178* (seconds)	543* (seconds)	190.9* (seconds)	4,542* (seconds)	828.9* (seconds)	1,848* (seconds)	1,292.4* (seconds)	3,312.5* (seconds)

* Average time per day to receive and generate hard copy images for the image modalities is calculated as follows: (number of patients per day) × (time per examination) = $T_1 + T_2 + T_3 + T_4 + T_5 + T_6$ of Table 79–17.

r and *R* is given by

$$r = \frac{dR}{dt} \tag{1}$$

or

$$R(t') = \int_0^{t'} r\, dt \tag{2}$$

If one assumes that the throughput rate is constant, such that a simple reciprocal relationship exists between *r* and *T*,

$$r = 1/T \tag{3}$$

where *T* is the time to complete one task, then the throughput, *R*, is given by

$$R(t') = \int_0^{t'} 1/T\, dt$$
$$= t'/T$$

Thus the throughput, *R*, is a linear function of time. Figure 79–10A illustrates the assumed relationship of *r* to *T* as a function of time. Figure 79–10B shows the plot of *R* as a function of time to be linear with a slope of 1/*T*.

The time scale in Figure 79–10 may be changed from *t* in seconds to the number of tasks performed, *N*. If *T* is the time required to complete one task, then by plotting only those times, *t'*, for which $t' = NT$, we can plot graphs of $r(t')$ and $R(t')$ as illustrated in Figure 79–11. The interpretation of $R(NT)$ as a function of *NT* is that as *N* takes on the values $N = 1, 2, \ldots$, then $R(NT)$ is the throughput or the number of tasks accomplished in *NT* seconds when each task requires *T* seconds to complete.

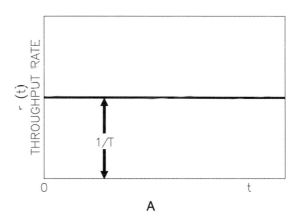

Figure 79–10. *A*, Assumed relationship of *r* to *T* as a function of time. *B*, Plot of *R* as a function of time to be linear with a slope of 1/*T*.

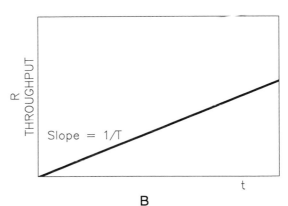

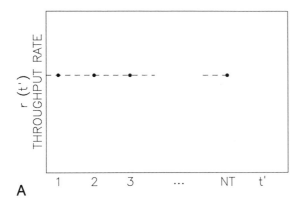

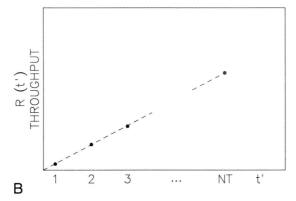

Figure 79–11. *A*, Relationship of γ to NT as a function of NT. *B*, Plot of R as a function of NT.

The calculation of throughput, *R*, for the network is difficult owing to the large number of possible situations that can arise. It is possible, however, to calculate the upper and lower bounds on *R* such that $R_{Lower} \leq R \leq R_{Upper}$. This provides an operating range for the actual throughput, *R*.

Calculation of Upper Bound of Throughput

Assume that the node for which we are attempting to calculate the throughput, *R*, operates for a period of *B* seconds. Clearly *B* is such that $0 \leq B \leq 24$ hours $\times$ 3600 s/hour. In most radiology networks the operating times are 12 hours/working day and 253 working days/year.

The upper bound of the throughput, R_{Upper}, is calculated by assuming that each patient examination to be processed by the network requires an average of *T* seconds. Then,

$$r(t) = 1/T$$

and

$$R(t') = t'/T$$

As the system task load (*N*) increases, the upper bound on the throughput, shown in Figure 79–11, also increases linearly until *B* seconds have been used in completing tasks. This occurs at the value $N = N'$ such that

$$N'T = B \text{ seconds}$$

or

$$N' = \frac{B}{T}$$

At this value of N, no further increase in the upper bound on throughput is possible and the system is said to be saturated. This situation is illustrated in Figure 79–12. The interpretation is that each task is executed at a throughput rate of $1/T$ seconds until all of the time available in the operating period of length B is utilized. At the value of $N = N'$, we have used all the time available in the operating period while executing each task uniformly at a throughput rate of $1/T$ tasks per second. Any further increase in system load delays completing the additional tasks. Under these conditions an upper bound, R_{Upper}, on system throughput is established such that the actual R system $\leq R_{Upper}$ throughput.

Calculation of Lower Bound of Throughput

The lower bound of the throughput, R_{Lower}, can be calculated by assuming that any patient examination to be processed by the network will be the last in line to be executed. Hence, if there are four patient examinations to be processed at any instant of time, then the lower bound on throughput is arrived at by calculating throughput for the last of the four execution requests. Thus, as the number of patients to be processed by the network increases, then the throughput rate declines. As an example, assume that the throughput rate is given by

$$r(t) = K\epsilon^{-\sigma t},$$

where $K = 1/T$ and $\sigma = 0.002$. Then

$$R(t') = \int_0^{t'} r(t)\, dt$$

$$= \int_0^{t'} K\epsilon^{-\alpha t}\, dt$$

$$= \frac{K}{\alpha}[1 - \epsilon^{-\alpha t'}]$$

The situation is shown in Figure 79–13. Figure 79–13A illustrates the throughput rate declining as a function of time, indicating that as the number of patients being processed increases, the instantaneous throughput rate decreases. The lower bound on throughput, R_{Lower}, increases to the point where there is no time remaining in the operating period of B seconds to process a patient's examinations successfully.

Figure 79–14 illustrates the operating region of the throughput, R, which is between the value of R_{Upper} and R_{Lower}.

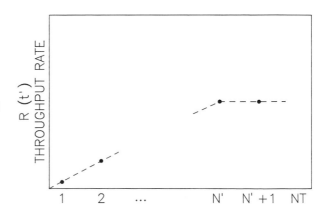

Figure 79–12. Plot of R versus NT, illustrating saturation.

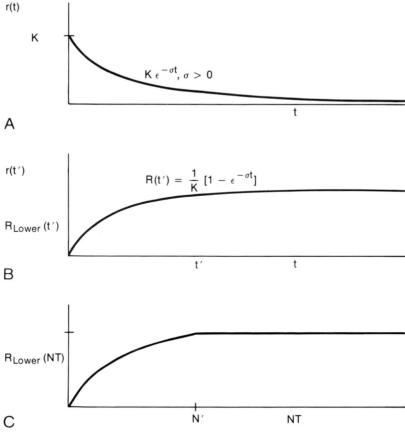

Figure 79–13. As the number of patients increases the throughput rate declines (*A*), and the lower bound on throughput increases to saturation (*B–C*).

Figure 79–15 provides a summary of the results of assuming several functions for the throughput rate, *r(t)*.

Acquisition and Formatting Node Throughputs

One possible distribution of acquisition and formatting nodes on a network is shown in Figure 79–3. Using the analysis to determine upper and lower bounds on throughput,

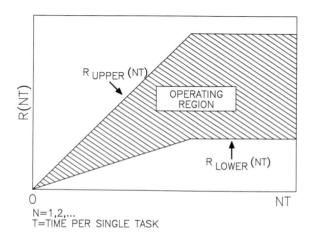

Figure 79–14. Operating region of the throughput, *R*.

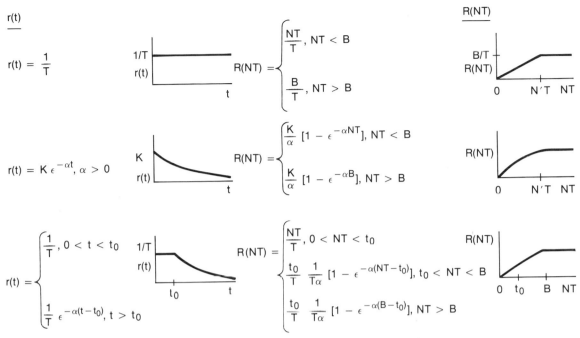

Figure 79–15. Mean throughput, $R(NT)$, for throughput rates, $r(t)$.

it is possible to show that this configuration is adequate for present system loads. Table 79–19 shows the average throughput requirements for each of the acquisition and formatting nodes. The average time per day that each acquisition and formatting node utilized is given by Table 79–7. The average time per patient, T, is calculated by dividing the average time per day that each node is in use by the average number of patients per day. The upper bound on throughput, R_{Upper}, is calculated by assuming that the throughput rate is $1/T$, where T is the average time per patient. The value at which the upper bound on throughput is saturated is given by $B = TN'$, where B is the available period of operation for each node and assuming that $B = 12$ hours, or 43,200 seconds. The value of R_{Upper} at N' is given by B/T.

Table 79–19. UPPER AND LOWER THROUGHPUT FOR ACQUISITION AND FORMATTING NODES

	CT Node	NM Node	US Node	DSA Node	DR Node	MRI Node
Average number of patients per day	34	32	22	8	20	20
Average time per day node in use	5,886.02* (seconds)	12,169.8* (seconds)	8,441.6* (seconds)	36,358.2* (seconds)	10,903.7* (seconds)	8,050.0* (seconds)
Average time per patient, T	173.1† (seconds)	380.3† (seconds)	383.7† (seconds)	4,544.8† (seconds)	545.18† (seconds)	402.5† (seconds)
Upper throughput, R_{Upper} at N' — saturation	249‡ patients	113‡ patients	112‡ patients	9‡ patients	79† patients	107‡ patients
Lower throughput, R_{Lower} at N' — saturation	51§ patients	22§ patients	22§ patients	1§ patients	15§ patients	21§ patients

* Calculations from Table 79–7.
† Calculations from: (average time per day node in use)/(average number of patients per day).
‡ Calculations for R_{Upper} from: (B seconds available)/(average time per patient, T).
§ Calculations for R_{Lower} at N'-saturation assuming that the throughput rate is given by: $r(t) = K \epsilon^{-\sigma t}$; $k = 1/T$, $\sigma = 1.155 \times 10^{-4}$.

The lower bound on the throughput, R_{Lower}, can be calculated in at least two ways. One way is to assume that each acquisition and formatting node is asked to process multiple cases simultaneously. If the average patient processing time is T seconds per patient and if 6 imaging devices are connected to a node, then the worst delay time will be $6T$. Since this is not a very tight lower bound on the throughput, an alternative method is to assure that the worst throughput rate will be given by $r(t) = K\epsilon^{-\sigma t}$. The lower throughput is then $R(t) = K/\sigma[1 - \epsilon^{-\sigma t}]$. The value shown for R_{Lower} in Table 79–19 are for $k = 1/T$ and $\sigma = 0.0001155$. Because there are only limited data available, the selection of an exponential function to represent the lower bound and the use of $\sigma = 1.155 \times 10^{-4}$ is necessarily arbitrary. For this reason, the calculated lower bound can be used only to assess relative limitations in node performance. Determination of actual lower bounds on node throughput must await further investigation.

IDDS Node Throughputs

The average throughput times per day for the IDDS nodes is shown in Table 79–9. A reasonable distribution and the number of these IDDS nodes are shown in Table 79–20. On the basis of this analysis, it would be possible to rearrange the distribution of IDDS nodes. The analysis presented by Table 79–20 does not imply that the IDDS user will have to travel to several IDDS nodes to view multiple imaging examinations on a specific patient.

The results from Table 79–20 suggest that the use of the six IDDS nodes will be extensive. The value of R_{Upper} is based upon the average time per patient, T. If the IDDS located in the CT reading area is used extensively for viewing CT examinations and a good portion of the US examinations, then the node will be unable to keep up with the utilization demand. A good procedure would be to identify those IDDSs that are available for use. An alternative is to add more IDDS nodes to the network.

On-Line Archiving Node Throughputs

The average throughput times per day for the on-line archiving nodes is shown in Table 79–11. A reasonable number of on-line archiving nodes is shown in Table 79–

Table 79–20. UPPER AND LOWER THROUGHPUT FOR IDDS NODES

	CT Area	NM Area	US Area	DSA Area	DR Area	MRI Area
Average number of patients per day	34	32	22	8	20	20
Average time per day node in use	38,100.63* (seconds)	8,735.7* (seconds)	36,200* (seconds)	6,301* (seconds)	15,753* (seconds)	18,810* (seconds)
Average time per patient, T	1,120† (seconds)	272.9† (seconds)	1,645† (seconds)	787.6† (seconds)	787.6† (seconds)	940.5† (seconds)
Upper throughput, R_{Upper} at N' − saturation	38‡ patients	158‡ patients	26‡ patients	54‡ patients	54‡ patients	45‡ patients
Lower throughput, R_{Lower} at N' − saturation	7§ patients	31§ patients	5§ patients	10§ patients	10§ patients	9§ patients

* Calculations from Table 79–9.
† Calculations from: (average time per day node in use)/(average number of patients per day).
‡ Calculations for R_{Upper} from: (B seconds available)/(average time per patient, T)
§ Calculations same as fourth footnote (§) Table 79–19.

21. This table does not imply that the six on-line archiving nodes are dedicated solely to the specific imaging modality archiving. Rather, the imaging data would be mixed. The columns of Table 79–21 are used to indicate the amount and source of imaging data.

The upper and lower throughput calculations shown in Table 79–21 suggest that four on-line archiving nodes will be adequate to serve the network.

Long-Term Archiving Node Throughput

The average throughput times per day for the long-term archiving node is shown in Table 79–19. Since only one long-term archiving node exists, then 136 patient examinations are handled per day. The average time per patient is the sum of the times calculated in Table 79–19 divided by 136 examinations (31,576.92 seconds). Hence, the average time per patient, T, is 31,576.92/136 = 232.18 seconds. The upper bound on the throughput, R_{Upper} at saturation is 186 patients (43,200/232.18). The lower bound on the throughput, R_{Lower}, at saturation is 37 patients. While the upper bound is more than satisfactory (186 patients > 136 patients), the lower bound is unacceptable (37 patients < 136 patients).

Hard Copy Node Throughput

The average throughput times per day for the hard copy generation node are shown in Table 79–21. The average time per patient, T, is given by 17,173.7/136 examinations = 126.2 seconds. Hence R_{Upper} at saturation is 342 patients and R_{Lower} at saturation is 68 patients.

Throughput for the Network

All calculations made for the upper and lower bounds on the throughput included the required transmission times on the network. By separating only those times for transmission, we find that the total time that two nodes are communicating between each other is 37,190 seconds. Owing to the use of concurrency programs, adequate time is available in the 12-hour period for node and network operations.

Table 79–21. UPPER AND LOWER THROUGHPUT FOR ON-LINE ARCHIVING NODES

	CT Area	NM Area	US Area	DSA Area	DR Area	MRI Area
Average number of patients per day	34	32	22	8	20	20
Average time per day node in use	8,138.7* (seconds)	1,310.4* (seconds)	7,970.7* (seconds)	1,291.5* (seconds)	3,229.6* (seconds)	7,081.4* (seconds)
Average time per patient, T	239.3† (seconds)	40.95† (seconds)	362.3† (seconds)	161.4† (seconds)	161.4† (seconds)	354.07† (seconds)
Upper throughput, R_{Upper} at N' – saturation	180‡ patients	1,054‡ patients	119‡ patients	267‡ patients	267‡ patients	122‡ patients
Lower throughput, R_{Lower} at N' – saturation	36§ patients	211§ patients	23§ patients	53§ patients	53§ patients	24§ patients

* † ‡ § All calculations are the same as those of Table 79–20 (using Table 79–11).

This chapter demonstrates the use of mean throughput, R, as a measure of the operational performance of a radiology network. The operational requirements are assumed to be those of a medium-sized state-supported academic radiology department serving an active 512 bed referral hospital. The difficulty with calculating the actual value of mean throughput is overcome by determining the upper and lower bounds of the mean throughput. Measurement of the mean time per patient examination, T seconds, is based upon an average network transmission throughput of 3 megabits/second and an average node bus throughput of 8 megabits/second.

The upper bound of the mean throughput, R_{Upper}, is based upon the throughput rate, $r(t)$, being assumed to be uniform such that $r(t) = 1/T$. The worst lower bound of the mean throughput, R_{Lower}, is based upon assuming that $r(t) = Ke^{-\sigma t}$, where $K = 1/T$ and $\sigma > 0$. Useful lower bounds on the mean throughput, R_{Lower}, have been obtained. However, these values do not represent actual lower bounds and are useful only for comparative purposes. Determination of actual lower bounds must await further evaluation of actual system performance under high load conditions.

Mean throughput analysis has shown that adequate performance can be obtained from the acquisition and formatting nodes. Initially it was believed that these nodes were the bottlenecks of the system. Such conclusions were based on the relatively slow data transfer interfaces available. However, our analysis indicates that by connecting multiple imaging modalities to each acquisition and formatting node, and by operating over a wide time window, an adequate mean throughput is possible. The acceptable mean throughput is, in part, due to the lengthy time required to acquire a patient examination (see Table 79–3). If there are six imaging units connected to a single acquisition and formatting node, and if T is the time required to process one patient, then the worst possible time for processing a patient will be $6T$. This can occur only when all six imaging modalities demand processing and the particular patient is always last to be serviced, or $T' = 6T$.

The bottleneck on the radiology network according to the mean throughput analysis seems to be the IDDS nodes. Six IDDS nodes are barely adequate to display the newly acquired image examinations plus the examinations retrieved from the on-line archiving nodes. Additional IDDS nodes will alleviate this bottleneck. This limitation is not perceived in the operation of today's radiology departments since analog hard copy recordings are extensively utilized.

According to the mean throughput analysis, the on-line and long-term archiving nodes are adequate as described in this chapter. However, if the number of digitally formatted examinations were to significantly increase, then these nodes would also become rate limiting.

The hard copy generation node is a departmental goal that could save time and significant resources. It would not be necessary to provide each imaging modality with its own hard copy node. The labor cost would be reduced by generating image recordings with preselected window and local values.

A mean throughput network transmission value of 3 megabits/second according to our analysis appears adequate to handle a radiology network with the operational parameters we have chosen. It is likely that the network communication links would become rate limiting if the number of active nodes were increased significantly.

References

1. Templeton AW, Dwyer SJ III, Johnson JA, Anderson WH, Hensley KS, Rosenthal SJ, Lee KR, Preston DF, Batnitzky S, Price HI: An on-line digital image management system. Radiology *152*:321, 1984.
2. Templeton AW, Dwyer SJ III, Johnson JA, Anderson WH, Hensley KS, Lee KR, Rosenthal SJ, Preston DF, Batnitzky S: Implementation of an on-line and long-term digital management system. RadioGraphics *5*:121, 1985.

3. Fischer HW: Radiology Departments: Planning, Operation, and Management. Ann Arbor, Edwards Brothers, 1982.
4. Macovski A: Medical Imaging Systems. Englewood Cliffs, New Jersey, Prentice-Hall, 1983.
5. Curry TS III, Dowdey JE, Murry RC: Christensen's Introduction to Physics of Diagnostic Radiology. 3rd ed. Philadelphia, Lea and Febiger, 1984.
6. Dwyer SJ III, Templeton AW, Martin NL, Lee KR, Levine E, Batnitzky S, Rosenthal SJ, Preston DF, Price HI, Faszold S, Anderson WH, Cook LT: The cost of managing digital diagnostic images. Radiology *144*:313, 1982.
7. Brody WR: Digital Radiography. New York, Raven Press, 1984.
8. Templeton AW, Johnson JA, Cox GG, Dwyer SJ III, Lee KR, Arnett GR, Anderson WH, Hensley KS, Scott CE, Fritz SL, Nelson DL: A 57cm x-ray image intensifier digital radiography system. *In* Lemke HU, Rhodes ML, Jaffee CC, Felix R (eds): Computer Assisted Radiology. Berlin, Springer-Verlag, 1985, p 276.
9. Sonoda M, Takano M, Miyahara J, Kato H: Computer radiography utilizing scanning laser stimulated luminescence. Radiology *148*:833, 1983.
10. Fraser RG, Breatnach E, Barnes GT: Digital radiography of the chest: Clinical experience with a prototype unit. Radiology *147*:1, 1983.
11. Elliott DO: Data recording and storage. *In* Newton TH, Potts DG (eds): Technical Aspects of Computer Tomography. St. Louis, C.V. Mosby, 1981.
12. Shoch JF, Dalal YK, Redell DD, Crane RC: Evolution of the Ethernet computer network. Computer *15*:10, 1982.
13. Stallings W: Local Networks, An Introduction. New York, Macmillan, 1984.
14. Kurose JF, Schwartz M, Yemini Y: Multiple-access protocols and time-constrained communication. ACM Computing Surveys *16*:43, 1984.
15. Stallings W: Local networks. ACM Computing Surveys *16*:3, 1984.
16. Tropper C: Local Computer Network Technologies. New York, Academic Press, 1981.
17. Martin J: Computer Networks and Distributed Processing. Englewood Cliffs, Prentice-Hall, 1981.
18. Tanenbaum AS: Computer Networks. Englewood Cliffs, Prentice-Hall, 1985.
19. Stuck BW, Arthurs E: A Computer and Communications Network Performance Analysis Primer. Englewood Cliffs, Prentice-Hall, 1985.
20. Bennett WR, Davey JR: Data Transmission. New York, McGraw-Hill, 1965.
21. Lathi BP: Modern Digital and Analog Communication Systems. New Jersey, Holt, Rinehart and Winston, 1983.
22. Newman WM, Sproull RF: Principles of Interactive Computer Graphics. 2nd ed. New York, McGraw-Hill, 1979.
23. Sherr S: Electronic Displays. New York, Wiley-Interscience Publication, 1979.
24. Templeton AW, Johnson JA, Anderson WH, Cook LT, Preston DF, Lee KR, Rosenthal SJ, Batnitzky S, Levine E, Tarlton M: Computer graphics for digitally formatted images. Radiology *151*:527, 1984.
25. Batnitzky S, Price HI, Cook PN, Cook LT, Dwyer SJ III: Three-dimensional computer reconstruction from surface contours for head CT examinations. J Comp Assist Tomogr *5*:60, 1981.
26. Lawrence GR: ACR/NEMA digital image interface standard. *In* Lemke HU, Rhodes ML, Jaffee CC, Felix R (eds): Computer Assisted Radiology. Berlin, Springer-Verlag, 1985, p 285.
27. Lo S-C, Huang HK: Radiological image compression: Full-frame bit-allocation technique. Radiology *155*:811, 1985.
28. Musmann HG, Pirsch P, Grallert H-J: Advances in picture coding. Proc IEEE *73*:523, 1985.
29. Jain AK: Image data compression: A review. Proc IEEE *68*:366, 1980.
30. Kunt M, Johnson O: Block coding of graphics: A tutorial review. Proc. IEEE *68*:770, 1980.
31. Cox GG, Templeton AW, Anderson WH, Cook LT, Hensley KS, Dwyer SJ III: Estimating digital information throughput rates for radiology networks. Invest. Radiol. *21*:162, 1986.
32. Conrad JW: Standards and Protocols for Communications Networks. Madison, New Jersey, Carnegie Press, 1982.
33. Green PE Jr (ed): Computer Network Architectures and Protocols. New York, Plenum Press, 1982.
34. Alisouskas VF, Tomasi W: Digital and Data Communications. Englewood Cliffs, New Jersey, Prentice-Hall, 1985.
35. Folts HD, des Jardins R (eds). Open systems interconnection (OSI)—standard architecture and protocols. Proc. IEEE *71*, 1983.
36. Day JD, Zimmermann H: The OSI reference model. Proc. IEEE *71*:1334, 1983.
37. McClelland FM: Services and protocols of the physical layer. Proc. III *71*:1372, 1983.
38. Conard JW: Services and protocols of the data link layer. Proc. IEEE *71*:1394, 1984.
39. Bartoli PD: The application layer of the reference model of open systems interconnection. Proc IEEE *71*:1404, 1983.
40. Massey JL: Random-access communications (special issue). IEEE Trans on Information Theory IT–31, 1985.
41. Pratt WK: Digital Image Processing. New Jersey, John Wiley and Sons, 1978.
42. Hall EL: Computer Image Processing and Recognition. New York, Academic Press, 1979.
43. Bracewell R: The Fourier Transform and Its Applications. New York, McGraw-Hill, 1965.
44. Otnes RK, Enochson L: Digital Time Series Analysis. New York, John Wiley and Sons, 1972.
45. Oppenheim AV, Schafer RW: Digital Signal Processing. Englewood Cliffs, New Jersey, Prentice-Hall, 1975.
46. Antoniou A: Digital Filters: Analysis and Design. New York, McGraw-Hill, 1979.

47. Dudgen DE, Mersereau RM: Multidimensional Digital Signal Processing. Englewood Cliffs, New Jersey, Prentice-Hall, 1984.
48. Alexandridis NA: Microprocessor System Design Concepts. Rockville, Maryland, Computer Science Press, 1984.
49. Duerinckx AJ, Dwyer SJ III, Prewitt JMS (eds): Digital image archiving in medicine, special issue. Computer 16, 1983.
50. Miller SW (ed): Mass storage systems, special issue. Computer 18, 1985.
51. Kemeny JG, Snell JL: Finite Markov Chains. Princeton, New Jersey, D. Van Nostrand Company, Inc., 1960.
52. Cox GG, Johnson JA, Templeton AW, Preston DF, Lee KR, Nelson DL, Hensley KS, Dwyer SJ III: Analog image recording using a laser printer and paper system. Invest Radiol 20:1003, 1985.
53. Cox GG, Templeton AW, Anderson WH, et al: Estimating digital information throughput rates for radiology networks model. Invest Radiol 21:162, 1986.

80

Gating: Cardiac and Respiratory

DAVID R. PICKENS

HISTORICAL PERSPECTIVE

Imaging the cardiovascular system has been a mainstay of diagnostic radiology for many years. In the mid-1960s nuclear medicine physicians discovered that it was possible to acquire images of the beating heart if the computer system collecting the image data was instructed to use information from the electrocardiographic (ECG) signal. This electrical signal can be detected on the surface of the body and can be used to control the collection process. Electrocardiographic information can be related to the relative position of the patient's heart in the chest. By detecting a prominent part of the ECG wave, the QRS complex, and using it as a reference to select slices of time for acquisition, it is possible to create an image of the heart without the usual blur from motion, as if the heart had been stopped during the imaging procedure.

Cardiac gating, as the technique is called, depends on detection of the QRS wave each time it occurs during a patient's cardiac cycle. The patient is connected by a conventional skin electrode arrangement to a cardiac monitor. The cardiac monitor is designed to detect the QRS complex and produces a pulse called an R-wave trigger, which corresponds to the presence of the cardiac wave. This pulse is sent via wire to the imaging computer, which uses it to time the cardiac cycle and collect information based on the cardiac cycle.

There are two types of collection procedures in nuclear medicine that use the ECG wave to control acquisition. They are in-core gated collection and list-mode collection. In the first method, the R-wave trigger provides a time reference for the collection program, which partitions the computer's memory into a preselected number of discrete areas into which image information can be placed. Each of these areas represents a segment of time during the R–R interval. At increasing times from the occurrence of the R-wave trigger, image information from a nuclear camera is summed into each storage area. This continues for each detected R-wave until a stopping criterion, such as a prespecified maximum number of counts or a time limit, has been reached. Thus, a series of images, which are windows in time of a part of the cardiac cycle, are built up in the computer's memory. When the acquisition is complete, the resulting images are summed composites of several minutes' worth of cardiac cycles. These images are written to disk for storage and can be displayed individually or played back in an endless loop or "movie" for viewing or processing. The dynamic nature of the playback provides considerable additional information about the condition of the heart in comparison to conventional static images.

Another technique from nuclear medicine involves cardiac acquisition by list-mode collection. This approach is a direct collection of image information to disk. Each detected event from the nuclear camera is recorded on disk as it occurs, along with time information and a gate indicator from the R-wave trigger signal. No attempt is made to use this information to create an image until the entire collection has been completed. Images are produced by reading the stored x-y coordinate information which is part of each detected event. During reconstruction of an image, counts are summed into the proper parts of the images based on the stored coordinates. The timing and gate information associated with each event determine into which image the event will be summed. In this scheme, images can be reconstructed in different matrix sizes and with different frame rates as desired. A major advantage of this type of gated collection is that irregular beats and counts associated with them can be rejected during the reconstruction procedure.[1]

Gating methods have also been used in other imaging modalities, such as digital radiography and computed tomography (CT). In digital subtraction angiography (DSA) of the coronary arteries, gating is used to reduce the motion that can occur between image acquisitions due to the physiologic activity of the heart. This motion can produce a significant artifact in conventional subtraction images, since the heart is unlikely to be in the same position during acquisition of the mask and the contrast images. By using a gated collection technique, acquisition of mask and contrast images can be synchronized with the cardiac motion so that the heart is in the same position when the x-ray generator fires each time. The R-wave trigger signal is used by the computer to start a timing cycle whose length can be specified. At the end of this cycle, the computer triggers the x-ray generator to acquire the first image. When the contrast is ready for injection, the same delay is used and the computer triggers the x-ray generator again, based on the occurrence of the R-wave trigger. The major function of gating in this application is to synchronize collection of data for the purpose of removing motion.

In CT a similar technique has been demonstrated. Dynamic CT studies of the heart have been used for determination of coronary arterty bypass patency and for the evaluation of the cardiac wall after a myocardial infarction.[2] In one set of experiments, ECG gate information was recorded along with eight 360 degree scans of a dog. All of the projection data were reorganized so that complete images could be reconstructed from all of the projection data, which corresponded to fixed narrow windows of time in the cardiac cycle. In this manner five images representing 100 ms of a 500 ms cardiac cycle were reconstructed. Thus, a series of images were formed that permitted the researchers to observe transaxial slices of the heart with the anatomy clearly visible without the usual motion artifact that is present without gating.

The techniques of gating that have been found to be useful in nuclear cardiology, DSA, and CT can be applied to magnetic resonance imaging (MRI). Considerable success has been noted in the literature using the ECG signal to control the acquisition phase of MR studies.[3,4,5,6-8] The goal is to reduce or eliminate the artifacts from the moving heart in a way analogous to digital radiography. Commercially available systems provide computer software and the necessary gating equipment to perform gated cardiac studies on a routine basis.

In any imaging procedure of the chest or abdomen in which the acquisition of data requires more than a few seconds, the respiratory motion from normal breathing can create artifacts in the images that are different from cardiac motion artifacts but that can also compromise the images. Methods similar to those used in accommodating cardiac motion can be used to suppress artifacts that result from respiration. Furthermore, combination approaches can reduce the effects of cardiac motion and respiration for those studies that require imaging the chest. These techniques are particularly important in MR imaging, since many imaging protocols take several minutes. However, respiratory gating has not been as successful as cardiac gating and may not be available at some installations.

MOTION

Motion effects in an MR image occur whenever a structure moves significantly during the acquisition phase of an imaging procedure.[9] The most serious artifacts are produced by periodic motion during the collection of raw MR signals, although sporadic patient motion can contribute artifacts. In general, motion can be expected to cause effects in an image that range from blurring of subtle details of an organ to the production of very prominent "ghosts" or secondary images that are overlaid on the real image and can be reflected to the edge of the image. The effects of motion that blurs structures are most often seen when imaging the heart. As shown in Figure 80–1, the inner details, such as the heart valves and the cardiac wall, are blurred together in an imaging procedure performed without cardiac gating. Since the heart beats relatively rapidly but does not move very much, the lack of gating does not produce significant ghosts.

When the chest and abdomen are imaged, the effects of respiration contribute to a ghost artifact that is often more severe than artifacts seen without cardiac gating.[8,9] Transverse images of the abdomen will often show not only a diffuse blurring but also secondary images that overlap the primary image and each other (Fig. 80–2). Depending on the individual's breathing habits, these effects can be more or less prominent. Deep or shallow breathing will tend to produce about the same amount of secondary image artifact with changes in the blur.

In imaging systems that use a two-dimensional Fourier transform imaging technique, the artifact is most often seen in the phase-encoding gradient direction. This is the direction in which a variable gradient pulse is active for a specified time during the acquisition of data. In phantom simulations Schultz and co-workers observed that at increased respiratory frequencies, the ghost artifacts that accompanied the motion were more widely separated than at lower frequencies.[9] Some blurring was observed, but the overwhelming degradation of the image was due to the ghost images, which seemed to reinforce themselves at some points in the image and cancel each other out in others. A similar effect was observed at increasing lengths of the repetition (*TR*) interval.

In computer simulation experiments and phantom studies of the motion from respiration, Wood and Henkelman evaluated motion artifacts and derived a mathematical description of the phenomenon.[10] They found that motion in the phase-encoding direction causes additional phase modulation in the signal that is reflected in image ar-

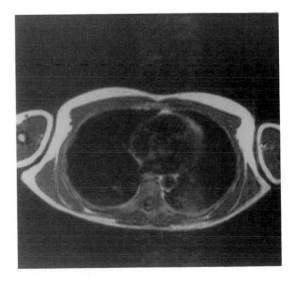

Figure 80–1. Ungated cardiac image. This transverse image of the heart (*TE* = 32 ms, *TR* = 500 ms) is a 1 cm thick section using four acquisitions. The aorta is clearly visible, but structural information within the heart is not visible. Also, an artifact is reflected above and below the heart due to the motion interaction with the phase-encoding gradients.

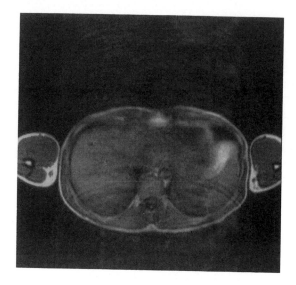

Figure 80–2. Ungated abdominal image. In this 1 cm 32/500 ms transverse section of the abdomen, no respiratory gating was used. The characteristic "ghosts," which are due to the motion in the direction of the phase-encoding gradients, can be seen above and below the image. Of special interest is the lack of any fine detail in the liver and spleen. There are no ghosts present over the arms, since they were not moving during imaging.

tifacts. The principal effect is from relocation of the magnetization from the moving structures that occurs between each application of the phase-encoding gradient. The ghosts that appear in the image are related to the frequency of respiration and the *TR* in use during the study. Motion in the direction of the frequency-encoding gradients was shown to produce image blurring and ghost artifacts perpendicular to the motion of the object. Motion in the *z* direction, perpendicular to the selected slice, would ordinarily be minimal during chest imaging because the slice selection pulses are very short when compared to the motion. However, oscillatory motion in the *z* direction can be reflected in ghost artifacts that also appear in the phase-encoding direction. This is due to modulation of the transverse magnetization by the motion that causes changes in the magnitude of the transverse magnetization.

CARDIAC GATING

Cardiac gating has enabled physicians to image the heart and see the details of the moving ventricular walls, valves, and vessels. Early development of gating the collection used nuclear medicine and CT as models for development of techniques and equipment. However, it was quickly recognized that the magnetic field gradients and radio frequency (rf) pulses would pose a potential problem, if not hazard, for traditional detection of the ECG electrical signal. Among the concerns were placement of metallic objects on the patient that might contribute to rf burns, overpowering of the very small ECG signal by the rf transmitter so that damage to the ECG system would result, and concerns over distortion of the image because of the proximity of metal in the ECG gating system to the receiving coils. By careful consideration of the design of the equipment and electrode placement, many of these concerns have been eliminated.

There are two types of motion present when the heart is imaged. The heart exhibits a contractile motion that causes it to change in volume. In so doing the walls of the atria and ventricles move in and out approximately radially from the centrum of the heart. Also, there is motion of the valve structures as different parts of the cycle are imaged. These activities cause the heart as a unit to rotate somewhat within the chest cavity. Secondarily, there are motion effects that are seen in the great vessels, especially the aorta, due to the pulse of blood during systole. Both of these motions contribute to the blurring of details in images of the heart and vessels in the chest.

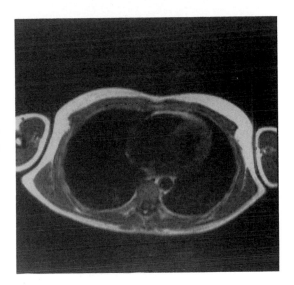

Figure 80–3. Ungated cardiac image. This is a 1 cm thick (32/ 500 ms) image that was acquired with no gating. As in Figure 80–1, there is little visible detail within the heart.

Cardiac gating seeks to control the acquisition of MR information so that it occurs only during the same phase of the cardiac cycle during an imaging procedure. Acquisition at the same phase of the cycle will find the heart in approximately the same position in the chest throughout the imaging session. The result of gating will be that the heart is "frozen" in time with the internal structures clearly visible. Figure 80–3 shows an ungated image of the heart. In this image the internal structure is not readily visible. This can be compared to the gated image in Figure 80–4, which shows the structural details clearly.

All motion artifacts cannot be eliminated by gating, however. Motion effects that are present during the interval after the excitation pulse but before read-out occurs can cause some image degradation. These effects are dependent on the particular pulse sequences in use. Inversion-recovery sequences with long inversion times (*TI*) are likely to be most susceptible to motion artifacts, while sequences having a few milliseconds between excitation and read-out will show little or no motion degradation.

Several different techniques have been investigated to permit the imaging system to acquire image information only during a specified part of the heart cycle. Among

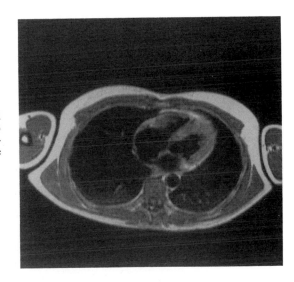

Figure 80–4. Gated cardiac image. This image was acquired with all the parameters identical to the image in Figure 80–3 except that cardiac gating was used. A comparison with Figure 80–3 shows that structural details of the left ventricle are clearly visible, as are additional details in the lungs.

the techniques that are available for providing a usable signal are plethysmography and ECG wave detection. A number of studies have been performed that indicate that using the ECG wave is the most convenient and most effective way of providing a trigger signal to the MR imager. Plethysmography methods, while appealing because of their simplicity, suffer from significant problems related to artifacts of various types and an inherent delay between the onset of the cardiac cycle and the detection of the trigger information in the peripheral vessel.[11] As a result, all manufacturers use ECG gating to trigger the imager during cardiac procedures.

ECG systems require that electrodes be placed on the body in order to detect the signal. Conventional low resistance skin electrodes are applied to prepared skin. The electrodes can be placed on either the forearms and one leg or on the subclavicular regions and right abdomen. Placement of electrodes on the limbs can be a potential source of artifacts. If the patient cannot lie still, electromyographic activity from the muscles can mask the ECG signal. In that situation the chest-abdomen electrode placement may be more reliable. In any event the signal is sent to an electronic module that converts it into a form that is usable by the imager.

A variety of designs have been described for use in conveying the EKG signal to the imaging system where it is converted into the appropriate trigger pulse. One system that is described in detail in the literature incorporates a battery-operated fiberoptic modulator, which converts the amplified EKG signal to modulated light.[12,13] The light travels in fiberoptic cable to an amplification and signal conditioning module, the output of which is the trigger signal used by the MR imager. This approach using fiberoptics insures that there is no possibility of injuring the patient with an electrical fault introduced through the ECG electrodes. The fiberoptic link fully insulates the patient and the imager from each other and from problems with ground loops. This system has been shown to perform very well in clinical situations. Other systems are similar and use conventional cable instead of fiberoptics to accomplish the same task.

Another fiberoptic system incorporates both respiratory and cardiac gating into a single unit.[14] The respiratory gate signal is obtained by a bellows system while the cardiac gate signal is obtained from conventional ECG electrodes. The battery-operated electronic package amplitude modulates the light signal so that a single fiberoptic cable can be used to transmit the combined gating signal to the image processor. The receiver at the image processor decodes the gating signals and detects the presence of the R wave of the ECG and the end-expiratory phase of the respiratory cycle. A combined gate signal is used to trigger the imager. Triggering occurs only on the R-wave peaks at those times when the patient's respiratory cycle is in the end-expiratory window.

An approach that has been used very successfully replaces the fiberoptic link with a radio telemetry system.[15] The advantage of a telemetry system is mostly one of convenience because there is no need for a connecting cable. However, the telemetry system must be selected so that there is no interference with the MR imager from the telemetry transmitter and no interference with the telemetry signal from the MR imager. In practice a conventional ECG telemetry system of the type used in cardiac care units has been used. The operating frequency of this system is 469 MHz, which is both a much higher frequency than the operating range of a .5 or .6 tesla magnet and is not a harmonic of the operating frequency, so no interference is experienced. Like the fiberoptic devices, full isolation from the power line voltages is provided by the telemetry system.

In any type of system designed to use the ECG wave as the trigger signal, considerable attention is necessary to prevent overload and damage to the amplifiers in the gating module and to provide signal conditioning for the ECG signal so that it is usable. Overload protection is designed into the electronics that protect them from any rf-induced signal or signal from the pulsed gradients during the imaging time. Additional circuitry may be present to filter the signal and to detect and exclude high amplitude information not associated with the ECG. Many manufacturers use extensive processing of the signal in order to arrive at an accurate, noise-free trigger pulse. A diagram of a gating system is shown in Figure 80–5.

Triggering is accomplished by detecting the R wave of the ECG waveform. This is accomplished after filtering and tailoring of the signal. Essentially, the operation is one of threshold detection: a voltage level is set that causes a circuit to operate when the voltage level is exceeded. The R wave is normally easy to detect in this manner. Once the presence of the R wave is established, a variable delay is introduced from detection of the R wave until the MR system is instructed to collect data. This delay is adjusted so that the appropriate phase of the cardiac cycle is selected. Thus, a short delay will provide an image that is close to end systole, while a relatively long delay will cause image information to be acquired during end diastole. Any delay can be selected so long as it is less than the R–R interval.

A potential problem might occur should a patient be experiencing premature beats. In this circumstance the R–R interval, which the computer expects to be regular, is actually varying from beat to beat. The system must be designed to accommodate variations in the lengths of beats by using some sort of window approach that permits the operator to select an operating range of the R–R interval. Figure 80–6 shows the timing of the ECG with respect to the trigger pulses. R waves that are detected and that fall within the defined window are permitted to trigger the scanner while beats that occur outside of the selected range are rejected. This bad beat rejection attempts to provide the imaging system with a constant R–R interval to minimize motion in the image.

While imaging with the ECG trigger operating, the effective repetition time, *TR*, is defined not by setting a parameter in the imager but by the heart rate of the patient. After detection of the QRS, there is a delay selected by the operator to produce images of a particular phase of the heart cycle. This delay defines the time between QRS detection and initiation of the imaging sequence. The imaging sequence will proceed in a normal fashion, having been triggered by the ECG. During this sequence, no other

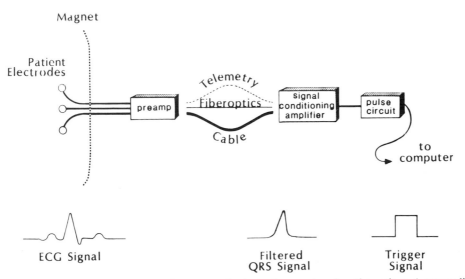

Figure 80–5. Cardiac trigger system. Nonferromagnetic electrodes are placed on the patient. A preamplifier, which is usually battery operated, performs preliminary signal processing and transmits the signal to the main processing system. Transmission is either by telemetry, fiberoptic cable, or conventional cable. The signal conditioner contains electronics that filter out noise in the signal and perform the threshold detection of the R wave peak. A pulse circuit produces the trigger that controls the computer.

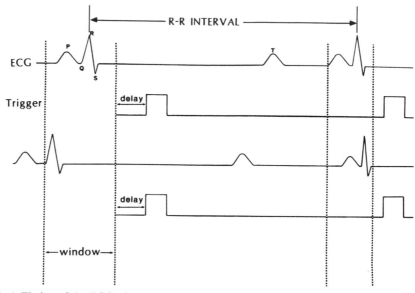

Figure 80–6. Timing of the ECG trigger. The system permits a window of acceptance to be defined so that any QRS wave that falls in the window is acceptable and results in a trigger pulse being produced. Thus, the R-R interval can vary somewhat, but the imager still collects data. The repetition rate corresponds to the average R-R interval. Bad beats, those where the QRS wave falls outside the defined window, do not trigger the system.

detected beats will trigger another imaging sequence. At the completion of the imaging sequence, a variable delay occurs during which the system awaits the next QRS wave to be detected. Since operation of the imager is dependent on the patient's heart rate, the study can be expected to take longer for patients with normal resting heart rates.

RESPIRATORY GATING

While a number of methods have been proposed to detect the respiratory cycle in order to develop a gating signal, there are two ways to determine the degree of inspiration or expiration. The inhaled or exhaled air stream can be monitored at the nose or mouth, or a mechanical sensor can be placed around the chest to detect the position of the chest. Both of these methods have been used in respiratory gating systems. Other methods that might be used to monitor the respiratory cycle, such as impedance plethysmography, have not been reported in the literature.

Producing a usable gate signal would seem to be a simple problem, but the practical implementation of the method has several difficulties associated with it. Ehman and his associates evaluated three different methods for producing a gate signal.[16] Two techniques involved monitoring the exhaled air from the patient, either through a respiratory mask such as those used for oxygen therapy or using a nasal-canula oxygen administration device. In each case a thermistor was used to detect air passing through the nose of the patient. Both of these techniques are workable and can provide the required information to develop a trigger signal, but they have been found to have drawbacks associated with them when actually used. The oxygen mask was found to be difficult to seal properly and was also reported to be uncomfortable when worn for long periods. The nasal-canula device was reported to be much more comfortable to wear for extended periods but was found to be very sensitive to small changes in airflow and position of the sensor, both of which caused problems with the gating signal.

A third method evaluated by Ehman used a mechanical displacement transducer

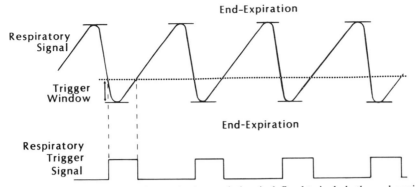

Figure 80–7. Timing of the respiratory trigger. A trigger window is defined to include the end-expiratory part of the respiratory cycle. End-expiration is chosen because its duration is longer than end-inspiration. The respiratory trigger pulse enables the imager to collect at the defined TR so long as the patient's respiratory cycle remains in the window. When the cycle is beyond the window level, no collection occurs.

consisting of a light source and modulator connected to a strap around the patient's abdomen or chest. As the patient breathes, the intensity of the light varies. The varying light travels by fiberoptic cable to a single processing circuit that produces an electrical signal proportional to the respiratory phase. The varying electrical signal is processed by a voltage level threshold circuit so that a part of the respiratory cycle can be selected. Only during the acceptance window is a trigger pulse produced (Fig. 80–7). This system was found to be very satisfactory in Ehman's studies. It exhibited low baseline drift and was found to be much more comfortable to use than the moving air systems.

Another type of mechanical displacement transducer system consists of a bellows and pressure transducer, which is described by Runge and his associates[15] and is diagrammed in Figure 80–8. This system uses a bellows connected to a piece of plastic tubing, which is in turn connected to a pressure transducer. The bellows is fastened around the chest or upper abdomen with a nonelastic strap or cord so that normal resting respiratory activity causes the bellows to stretch and retract. This results in very small pressure changes, which are detected by the pressure transducer and con-

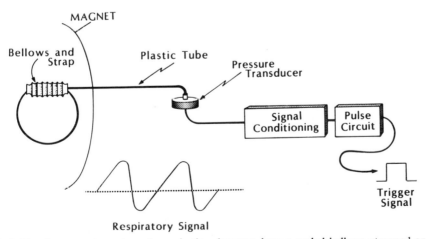

Figure 80–8. Respiratory gate system. A respiration detector, here a sealed bellows strapped around the patient's chest or abdomen, converts the mechanical motion of the chest into a signal that can be processed to produce a trigger. The signal in this design is a very small pressure change that is detected by a sensitive pressure transducer connected to the bellows by a plastic tube. The pressure transducer converts the pressure signal to a voltage that is conditioned and applied to a threshold circuit. The threshold circuit controls the pulse generator based on the selected window level. The pulses that result are applied to the computer to control collection.

verted into an electrical signal. This electrical signal from the pressure transducer is sent to the rest of the gating circuitry which conditions it and produces a trigger pulse. Figure 80–9 is an image that was acquired using this system that is notably free of the ghost artifacts present in Figure 80–2.

Baseline drift in which the average signal level may vary slowly as the respiratory activity continues, creating false triggers or failures to trigger, can interfere with operation of the trigger circuit. Many early simple respiratory gating systems exhibited this sort of defect. Proper signal conditioning and system design, however, can usually reduce or eliminate this difficulty.

Respiratory gating is different from cardiac gating in the way it affects image collection. With respiratory gating the imager uses the operator-specified *TR* interval to time the collection as is done without gating. However, the system also monitors the state of the respiratory cycle. When the respiratory cycle is within the window of acceptance, which is defined by the operator to be between end expiration and the beginning of inspiration, the imager is enabled for data acquisition. Thus, when the system is permitted to acquire data, the acquisition is timed by the computer. When the respiratory widow is not open, no acquisition occurs. Ehman and his associates call this technique respiratory gating without spin conditioning. They suggest that a somewhat more complex approach, using short *TR*s to keep the nuclei from relaxing between imaging collections, may yield images with less artifact. In the technique that they describe, the rf pulses and spin echoes continue to be evolved at the specified *TE/TR*, but the collection of information is only permitted to occur during the specified gating window. Consideration is given to collecting enough information at each gradient setting to reconstruct an image properly.

Respiratory gating has some limitations that affect its usefulness as a clinical technique. The most troublesome is the greatly extended collection times of 100 to 300 percent of the ungated time. This is because the window during which collection occurs is a fraction of the total respiratory cycle. When the patient breathes normally, much of the total time for the study is spent waiting for the next acceptable respiratory window. By asking a cooperative patient to control his breathing by taking fewer breaths, the length of time the respiratory window is open can be extended, which can shorten collection times.

Somewhat more cooperation from the patient is required in order to obtain a usable signal than with cardiac gating. With this in mind, a patient's anxiety must be reduced

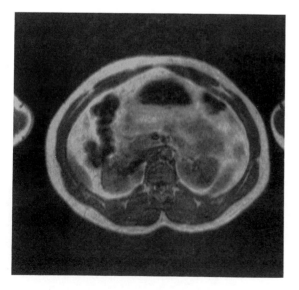

Figure 80–9. Respiratory gated image. This 1 cm image of the lower abdomen was acquired using the bellows gating system described in Figure 80–8. TE/TR was 32/500 ms with two acquisitions. While the typical respiratory artifacts are considerably reduced by gating, some motion artifact can be seen posteriorly in this image. Respiratory gating does not remove motion from peristalsis, which can cause degradation of abdominal images. (Courtesy of J. A. Clanton.)

as much as possible to insure stable breathing patterns. The adjustments of the gating trigger points require that the patient's respiratory patterns be consistent so that baseline drift can be minimized.

For imaging the heart, some workers have reported that combined respiratory and cardiac gating provides the best images. This might be expected in light of the types of motions that have been described as due to breathing and normal cardiac activity. When the MR system is collecting under combined gating, the ECG gate drives the system timing as has been described, but with the added condition that collection can only occur within the predetermined respiratory window. Runge and his associates have demonstrated a noticeable improvement in the appearance of the images using combination gating.[15]

An interesting technique has been proposed by Bailes and his associates that may eliminate a major problem with respiratory gating: greatly increased scan times.[17] Their approach is to devise a method of data acquisition that causes only the moving parts of the image to be blurred by the motion, rather than the entire image, as is the case with no gating at all. The method uses a specially designed respiratory sensor and permits acquisition to be performed at the normal imaging rates. The sensor output is used to control the application of the phase-encoding gradients so that only the moving parts of the image are blurred. Several manufacturers of MR scanners have implemented variations of this approach as alternatives to conventional gating.

While several methods have been described that can be used to produce a respiratory-gated image, the best method has not yet been determined. All of the approaches can produce images that show a substantial improvement when compared to ungated images. However, often very little improvement in image quality is seen while the collection times are greatly extended. Coupled with baseline drift and inconsistent triggering in some patients, respiratory gating is not as useful on a day-to-day basis when compared to cardiac gating. Nevertheless, with refinements in the design of gating systems, respiratory gating will contribute to improvements in abdominal and chest images in the future.

Cardiac gating provides a substantial improvement in the quality of cardiac images and is a useful clinical method in MR imaging. Gating permits visualization of details within the heart that would otherwise be obscured by blur from motion. Many laboratories are routinely performing cardiac gated imaging using a variety of instruments, all triggered from the ECG wave.

Respiratory gating has been demonstrated as a useful technique but the procedure itself suffers from some operational difficulties. It is often hard to adjust the gating apparatus on some instruments, and the time to perform an imaging study is greatly extended when using respiratory gating. While some techniques that may eliminate motion artifacts without gating are available, it remains to be determined how the respiratory motion artifact can best be removed, possibly this can be done with new ultrafast MRI scan techniques.[18]

References

1. Jones JP: Clinical imaging studies. In Erickson JJ, Rollo FD (eds): Philadelphia, J. B. Lippincott Company, 1983, pp 106–113.
2. Plewes DB, Violante MR, Morris TW: Intravenous contrast material and tissue enhancement in computed tomography. *In* Fullerton GD, Zagzebski JA (eds): Medical Physics of CT and Ultrasound: Tissue Imaging and Characterization. New York, American Institute of Physics, 1980, pp 213–214.
3. Go RT, MacIntyre JW, Kramer DM, Geisinger M, Chilcote W, George C, O'Donnell JK, Moodie DS, Meany TF: Volume and planar gated cardiac magnetic resonance imaging: A correlative study of normal anatomy with thallium-201 SPECT and cadaver sections. Radiology *150*:129–135, 1984.
4. Runge VM, Clanton JA, Wehr CJ, Partain CL, James AE Jr: Gated magnetic resonance imaging of acute myocardial ischemia in dogs: Application of multiecho techniques and contrast enhancement with GD-DTPA. Magn Reson Imaging *3*:255–266, 1985.

5. von Schulthess GK, Fisher M, Crooks LE, Higgins CB: Gated MR imaging of the heart: Intracardiac signals in patients and healthy subjects. Radiology *156*:125–132, 1985.
6. Stark DD, Higgins CB, Lanzer P, Lipton MJ, Schiller N, Crooks LE, Botvinick EB, Kaufman L: Magnetic resonance imaging of the pericardium: Normal and pathologic findings. Radiology *150*:469–474, 1984.
7. Higgins CB, Kaufman L, Crooks LE: Magnetic resonance imaging of the cardiovascular system. Am Heart J, January 1985, pp 136–151.
8. Steiner RE, Bydder GM, Selwyn A, Dearfield J, Longmore DB, Klipsten RH, Firmin D: Nuclear magnetic resonance imaging of the heart: Current status and future prospects. Br Heart J *50*:202–208, 1983.
9. Schultz CL, Alfidi RJ, Nelson AD, Kopiwoda SY, Clampitt ME: The effect of motion on two-dimensional Fourier transformation magnetic resonance images. Radiology *152*:117–121, 1984.
10. Wood ML, Henkelman RM: MR image artifacts from periodic motion. Med Phys *12*:143–151, 1985.
11. Fletcher BD, Jacobstein MD, Nelson AD, Riemenschneider TA, Alfidi RJ: Gated magnetic resonance imaging of congenital cardiac malformations. Radiology *150*:137–140, 1984.
12. Lanzer P, Barta C, Botvinick EH, Wiesendanger HUD, Modin G, Higgins CB: ECG-synchronized cardiac MR imaging: Method and evaluation. Radiology *155*:681–686, 1985.
13. Lanzer P, Botvinivk EH, Crooks LE, Arakawa M, Kaufman L, Davis PL, Herfkens R, Lipton MJ, Higgins CB: Cardiac imaging using gated magnetic resonance. Radiology *150*:121–127, 1984.
14. Blakeley DM, Gangarosa RE: Implementation of fiberoptic data link for cardiac and respiratory gating/monitoring. Abs Soc Magn Reson Med *2*:1073–1074, August 19–23, 1985 (London).
15. Runge VM, Clanton JA, Partain CL, James AE Jr: Respiratory gating in magnetic resonance imaging at 0.5 tesla. Radiology *151*:521–523, 1984.
16. Ehman RL, McNamara MT, Pallack M, Hricak H, Higgins CB: Magnetic resonance imaging with respiratory gating: Techniques and advantages. AJR *143*:1175–1182, 1984.
17. Bailes DR, Gilderdale DJ, Bydder GM, Collins AG, Firmin DN: Respiratory ordered phase encoding (ROPE): A method for reducing respiratory motion artifacts in MR imaging. J Comput Assist Tomogr *9*:835–838, 1985.
18. Rzedzian RR, Py Kett IL: Instant images of the human heart using a new, whole-body MR imaging system. AJR *149*:245, 1987.

81

Systems Engineering

G. NEIL HOLLAND

This chapter relates to the complex interaction of the many components that go into forming a magnetic resonance (MR) imaging system. It is one of the fascinations of the modality that the design of an MR system involves a multitude of different disciplines in physics and electrical engineering. In this chapter we discuss the design criteria of the basic system elements and show how system design is influenced by choice of nuclear magnetic resonance (NMR) techniques.

STATIC MAGNETIC FIELD GENERATION

The generation of the static magnetic field, B_0, is now accomplished primarily by superconducting magnets with the field coils immersed in liquid helium. Recent advances in superconducting research will probably yield magnets operating at liquid nitrogen temperatures in the next ten years and will further enhance the dominance of superconductive magnets for MR as utility is increased and cost is reduced.

Whole-body superconducting magnets have been developed that operate at as high a field as 4 tesla, the technology having risen from 0.15 tesla in less than ten years!

The rationale for increasing field strength is the same that has driven conventional NMR spectroscopy from 60 MHz to 470 MHz proton resonant frequencies in the last 20 years, namely improved signal-to-noise (S/N) and resolution. The conventional relationship, $S/N \propto B_0^{3/2}$, does not hold true, owing to dielectric and inductive losses within the human body; there is an approximately linear relationship between S/N and field strength for whole-body imaging systems.[1,2]

Field strength cannot continue to rise ad infinitum, even if improvements in magnet technology allow it to do so. Phase shift and absorption of the radio frequency (rf) field in body tissue ultimately limit resonant frequency, even though the early estimates at which these effects would become prohibitive has been found to be far below what can be attained in practice.

There are two principal characteristics of the B_0 field that are key to system performance, stability, and homogeneity. Short-term instability in the static field will cause random phase shifts in the NMR signal. In "spin warp" two-dimensional Fourier transform (2DFT) techniques this will lead to "ghosting" along the phase-encoding direction. In persistent mode superconducting magnets, the field is inherently stable at around 0.1 ppm per hour, although care must be taken to ensure that any resistive shimming coils have similar characteristics.

In resistive magnet technology, short-term field instability is one of the major technical problem areas, particularly in the design of the DC supply and cooling system.[3]

Field homogeneity requirements interact with the NMR techniques used, since certain ones are more susceptible to field variation than others, and with the operating field strength, since field variation is always quoted as a relative measure (in parts per million of the main field value) whereas the NMR experiment sees the absolute deviation, $\gamma \Delta B$, in proton hertz. It should be noted, therefore, that although two magnets operating at 0.5 tesla and 1.5 tesla might appear to have the same specification at, for example, 10 ppm, the higher field unit has a field that is three times poorer (640 Hz variation compared with 213 Hz at 0.5 tesla).

The principal technical reason that spin-echo 2DFT imaging with magnitude reconstruction has become the workhorse technique for routine clinical imaging is because of relative insensitivity to field inhomogeneity. Signal decay in the spin-echo sequence follows true $T2$, whereas in methods using field echoes, signals decay as $\exp - TE/T2*$ where $1/T2* = 1/T2 + \gamma \Delta B$ and $\gamma \Delta B$ is the inhomogeneity term.

Early systems used back projection as the reconstruction technique, which produces images with radial streak artifacts caused by miscentering of the projections due to field inhomogeneity. The 2DFT method avoids this effect, since each signal is "projected" onto a common axis, so that inhomogeneity only causes a distortion of the resultant image. Rapid changes in field do cause image artifacts if the real part of the complex Fourier transform alone is used. A so-called "real reconstruction" is employed when signals of both positive and negative sign are present, specifically in inversion-recovery techniques. It is possible to produce a phase map to correct for field related artifacts in real reconstructions, or the user can accept the contrast ambiguity that may occur when the magnitude image is displayed.

GRADIENT FIELD GENERATION

For spatial encoding of the NMR signal inherent to image formation it is necessary to produce three orthogonal gradient magnetic fields, G_x, G_y, G_z, where:

$$G_x = dB_z/dx$$

$$G_y = dB_z/dy$$

$$G_z = dB_z/dz$$

and B_z is the static field orientation.

Since the static field orientation in most systems is parallel to the patient axis, in superconducting solenoid systems gradient coils are affixed onto a cylindrical former into which the patient is inserted. Early systems used a simple Maxwell pair geometry for the generation of the G_z field, and so-called Golay coils consisting of four current arcs for each of G_x and G_y.[4] A set of Y coils is shown in Figure 81–1.

Newer designs have extended these basic geometries to improve linearity and efficiency by the incorporation of extra arcs or coil elements often distributed over the surface of the gradient tube to reduce inductance.

Gradient strength on whole body systems is often around 10 millitesla/meter to

Golay Coils
(4 current arcs) Y set shown

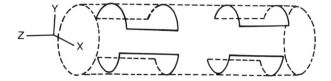

Figure 81–1. Golay gradient coil geometry.

accommodate the range of techniques and operating parameters in use today. For example, the gradient strength required for the slice select function is determined by the time length of the rf excitation, which should be kept as short as possible in order to prevent signal loss through T decay, since the slice selection function is essentially a field echo. Apodized sinc function rf waveforms are typically 5 to 10 ms in length, with bandwidths of a kilohertz or so, requiring a field of about 0.47 gauss for a 5 mm slice. The amplitude of the read gradient is dependent on the field of view, the total data sampling time, and the number of samples. For the phase gradient, its time duration, field of view, and number of phase encoding steps determine the amplitude. For a phase-encoding pulse about 4 ms in length, approximately 8 millitesla/meter is needed for a 12 cm field of view.

Gradient drive amplifier requirements to meet these gradient strengths are substantial. Current pulses of up to several hundred amperes are required, with rise times of less than 2 ms. In order to keep amplifier output voltage reasonable, at, for example, less than 300 volts, coil inductance must be less than a millihenry. Techniques like echo planar and its variants have even more extreme gradient system requirements because of the wider bandwidth pulses used.

The gradient system must also include some mechanism for counteracting the effect of eddy currents induced in surrounding conducting material when the gradients are pulsed. Generally, it is various parts of the magnet that are the conductors in question. Specifically, radiation shields formed of aluminum give rise to eddy currents with time constants of several hundred milliseconds, and some magnets with OFHC copper eddy current shields might exhibit eddy current time constants of greater than a second.

Eddy current correction takes one of two forms: (1) overshoot or "pre-emphasis" of the gradient drive waveform and (2) use of "active shield" gradient coils, which have an auxiliary set of coils outside the main gradient coils, which are designed to null the fields before they reach the eddy current surface.[5]

Correction of the first type is most common. Generally, the correction involves applying the desired waveform to a set of high pass filters connected in parallel, so that their outputs are summed. The filters are placed between waveform generator and gradient amplifier. Each filter has adjustable time constant and gain. By placing a search coil in the magnet and integrating its output, the gradient field can be monitored. By adjusting the filter parameters, the drive waveform can be modified so that the field profile closely matches the original unmodified waveform. The amount of overshoot required for eddy current compensation is dependent on the proximity of gradient coils to the eddy current surface and its conductivity. Typically an "overshoot" of up to 30 percent is required to compensate for eddy currents in a typical whole body magnet. Four filter time constants ranging from as short as 25 ms to as long as 1.5 s are typical.

RADIO FREQUENCY COILS

Radio frequency coils act as generators and detectors of the transmit and receive B_1 fields. For the transmit B_1 we want generally as homogeneous as field as possible in order to prevent significant flip angle variation within the imaged volume. Note that $\alpha = \gamma B_1 t_p$ where α is the flip angle and t_p is the pulse length. Since flip angle is used ever more to influence image contrast, particularly in fast field echo techniques, transmit homogeneity becomes more important than ever.

For the receive antenna we need as high a sensitivity as possible. This means achieving a high loaded quality factor (Q) and maximizing the B_1 field over the volume of interest. Techniques to aid the first of these requirements include operation of the coil in an electrically balanced configuration and/or the use of Faraday screening to reduce dielectric losses, minimizing resistive losses through careful construction and use of high Q electronic components (capacitors, varactors, etc.) To achieve the highest B_1 field, the use of circular polarization and/or close coupling of coil to sample are most appropriate.

Coil geometry is dependent primarily on frequency of operation and static field orientation. In standard superconducting systems, saddle coils formed from tube or wire are most often used for frequencies below 40 MHz. Above 40 MHz, such coils become self-resonant, and are therefore not effective as antennas. To increase self-resonant frequency, inductance must be reduced, for example, by using wide flat foil conductors or by using a lumped element scheme in which the inductance and capacitance are distributed around the coil. We tend to think of high frequency whole-body coils as transmission line resonators because of their distributed element properties.[6,7]

ANTENNA MATCHING

To efficiently couple rf energy into the transmit coil from the rf power amplifier, and from the receive coil into the preamplifier, matching schemes are required. These are probably the most tricky and sensitive electronic circuits in the MR system, especially when the same coil is used as both transmitter and receiver.

Power amplifiers are designed to drive a 50Ω resistive load at the operating frequency, whereas a simple parallel resonated coil might have an impedance on resonance of several thousand ohms. A matching network using series and parallel capacitance to transform the coil impedance to 50Ω is shown in Figure 81–2. Here the output impedance of the network is given by:

$$Z_0 = L_1/Q[1 + C_1/C_2]$$

Probe Matching Schemes

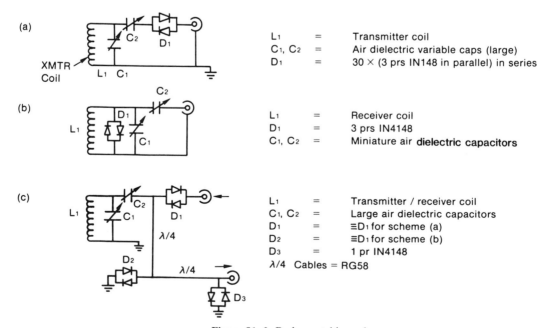

Figure 81–2. Probe matching schemes.

where Q is the coil quality factor; C_1 and C_2, the tune and match capacitors; and L, the coil inductance.

Note that output impedance is affected by coil Q and that loaded Q will vary from patient to patient quite significantly, especially at high frequencies (above 40 MHz). Consequently it is usually necessary to adjust the transmitter matching network for each patient exam. The capacitors used are large air or vacuum variables placed right at the coil, so adjustment requires mechanical coupling to the outside of the bore of the magnet, where, most often, electrical stepper motors are used to drive the capacitor rotors. Tuning is either manual, in which a power meter is observed while adjusting the network to minimize reflected power, or automatic, in which the motors are controlled by a microprocessor. In an automatic tuning system a patient tuning cycle can be accomplished in about 30 seconds.

The matching circuitry may also contain diodes to perform two functions: (1) to prevent noise coupling in from the power amplifier during the receive cycle and (2) to detune the transmit coil during receive, in order to reduce coupling between the receive coil and the transmit coil. This feature is essentially for surface coil operation, where electrical orthogonality is not easily achieved.

The diodes may be passively or actively switched. In passive switching the rf energy is used to turn on the diodes. Small fast switching types, such as 1N914, are used. The advantage of passive schemes is their simplicity; disadvantages include the large number of diodes needed to handle the power levels encountered and the possibility of clipping of the rf waveform, which directly impacts on the quality of selective excitation and hence slice profile. For these and other reasons, active decoupling is preferable, particularly in the more complex quadrature coil systems. Active decoupling uses high power PIN diodes (such as Unitrode UM4900 series) as the switching elements. These devices have an rf resistance that is inversely proportional to applied DC bias current. Several amperes of bias current are required at the power levels and frequencies encountered in whole-body imagers. The advantages of PIN diode schemes include low distortion switching, minimal Q damping, and the ability to use a single switching device. The disadvantages are the additional complexity and possibly the need to have fairly large DC current pulses applied to the rf coil.

Matching the receive coil to the preamplifier requires a type of circuitry similar to that described above for the transmitter. Since power levels are much lower, fully electronic tuning using varactor diodes is possible. These low power devices have a capacitance that varies with applied voltage (on the order of a few volts), thus allowing digital control of receiver coil tuning via a digital-to-analog converter (DAC). Many systems use preamplifiers with a 50Ω input impedance so that both tuning and matching are required. It is also possible to use preamplifiers with a high input impedance so that only coil tuning is required, and a simple parallel resonant circuit can be used. This scheme is particularly appropriate to surface coils with which a wide range of coil loading conditions occur. In addition to tuning and matching, the receive chain must include circuitry to protect the preamplifier during transmission of rf energy.[8] This takes two forms: (1) detuning of the coil using a diode switch circuit and (2) clamping diodes on the preamplifier input preceded by a quarter wavelength ($\lambda/4$) network. In fact, many of the circuits interfaced to the rf coils in an MR imager make use of the impedance inverting properties of $\lambda/4$ networks.

PREAMPLIFIERS

Preamplifiers by definition are the first amplification stage that the NMR signal is passed through. Usually separate preamplifiers are provided for head, body, and surface coils, with properties (gain, input impedance, etc.) tailored for the particular coil. As discussed earlier, preamplifiers are either 50Ω input or high input impedance. If 50Ω input is employed, the first stage transistors are most likely bipolar devices with very low noise voltage. Several individual transistors may be connected in parallel to improve noise figure. With careful construction, noise figures less than 1 dB are achievable. For those schemes in which the preamplifier has a high input impedance, the first stage uses JFET or MOSFET devices because of their very low noise currents.

All preamplifiers must have gain sufficient to overcome the noise contribution of subsequent amplification stages, which generally have poorer noise figures. The total noise figure of a cascaded amplifier chain can be determined from:

$$F_c = F_1 + \frac{F_2 - 1}{G_1} + \frac{F_3 - 1}{G_1 G_2} + \frac{F_n - 1}{G_1 G_2 \ldots G_{n-1}}$$

where F_1 to F_n are the noise figures in numeric form of the first to nth stages

$$\left(F = \log^{-1} \frac{NF_{dB}}{10} \right)$$

and G_1 to G_n are the numeric gains of the first to nth stages

$$\left(G = \log^{-1} \frac{G_{dB}}{10} \right)$$

Typically preamplifier gain is greater than 30 dB. The preamplifier must also have high dynamic range, since it must handle the full range of signal levels created by the different NMR techniques employed by the imager as well as the variation in signal from different body parts. Peak signal level might vary as much as 40 dB.

RADIO FREQUENCY POWER AMPLIFIER

The rf amplifier output power requirement is dependent on transmitter coil volume, type of B_1 field polarization, and operating frequency. For example, on low field imagers operating at frequencies below 15 MHz, a power output of 1 kW may suffice. On whole body systems with transmitter coil diameters of 55 to 60 cm operating at 64 MHz, greater than 15 kW power may be required. At the lower power level, the amplifier design is usually entirely solid state, using HF bipolar or power FET transistors rated at up to a few hundred watts each. For power levels greater than 1 or 2 kW, amplifier designs usually use vacuum tubes for the final output stage and a solid state driver stage. For example, a 15 kW amplifier can be constructed that uses a single 4CX 10,000 tube. The disadvantage of tube designs is that they are inherently narrow band, requiring a tuned output tank circuit. For systems operating at a specific frequency this is satisfactory. If more than one frequency of operation is required, either for operation at more than one field strength or for multinuclear studies, then output band switching and tuning are required. This usually takes the form of microprocessor controlled motor-driven capacitors, and switched inductors.

The key performance parameters of power amplifiers used in MR imagers are linearity and output stability (droop and drift). High linearity is required to faithfully reproduce the complex selective excitation waveforms. Generally, linearity of 1 dB over a dynamic range of greater than 40 dB is required. High stability is required because the rf pulse amplitude is precisely calibrated to give exact flip angles. The amplifier must have sufficient power supply capacity to prevent droop during the pulse (which may be as long as 10 ms) of less than 0.1 dB and to ensure pulse to pulse repeatability to within 0.1 dB. These are fairly exacting requirements, but they are necessary, since flip angle is used to influence image contrast and to prevent image artifacts due to improperly calibrated rf pulses.

THE SPECTROMETER

The spectrometer is defined as comprising a source of rf (crystal or synthesizer), a transmitter for providing modulated rf to the power amplifier, and a receiver that accepts incoming signals from the preamplifier and demodulates them to audio frequency baseband for digitization by analog-to-digital converters for subsequent image reconstruction.

The frequency source is required to have high temporal stability or low phase noise to prevent it being a cause of ghosting in 2DFT imaging. In multislice imaging, the rf frequency is moved from slice to slice for transmission and then returned to the center frequency for detection. The synthesizer used must maintain phase coherence during this switching process, which may cover as wide a range as $+/- 50$ kHz around the nominal center frequency. For this reason the frequency switching is usually accomplished by a digital low frequency synthesizer, the output of which is mixed in with the higher frequency rf section. The output frequency range required by the synthesizer is dependent on the magnetic field strength(s) the spectrometer is required to operate with and the frequency conversion scheme used within the spectrometer.

Most spectrometers use a heterodyned approach. That is, in the transmitter the output frequency is formed by mixing together two or more different frequencies, and in the receiver the incoming NMR signal is converted to an intermediate frequency before baseband demodulation. The reason for this conversion process is to allow for wider frequency coverage without performance compromise. In the transmitter this means amplitude modulation and phase switching at a fixed frequency independent of output frequency, which allows better control of amplitude linearity and phase accuracy. In the receiver, conversion and filtering allow image noise rejection to be tightly controlled.

The discussion of spectrometer performance parameters will be restricted therefore to heterodyned systems. Two schemes could be used: single conversion or multiple conversion. In single conversion, the output frequency is formed in one mixing step, whereas two or more are used in multiple conversion. Although more complex, the latter increases the useful frequency range of the spectrometer.

An example of a single conversion transmitter is shown in Figure 81–3. Here, the intermediate frequency is at 10 MHz, and the frequency synthesizer is set to $v_0 + 10$ MHz. When mixed together, sum and difference frequencies of the two inputs are produced. Filtering is used to pick out the appropriate component. Usually a low pass filter would be used to select the difference frequency, so that the useful frequency range of this design is from a few hundred kilohertz up to two times the IF of 10 MHz. For extension to higher frequency operation a higher frequency IF could be used, although care must be taken to ensure there are no unwanted mixer products at any desired output frequency.

The transmitter performs three functions: (1) gating of the rf to form pulses, (2) amplitude modulation to tailor the frequency content of the rf pulse, and (3) formation of discrete phases of rf: 0, 90, 180, and 270 degrees. The gating function requires high "off" isolation, so that during receive no leakage of the Larmor frequency occurs. This requires gates to be placed at several places in the transmitter to prevent formation of the output frequency, except when required.

Amplitude modulation for selective excitation requires tailoring of the frequency

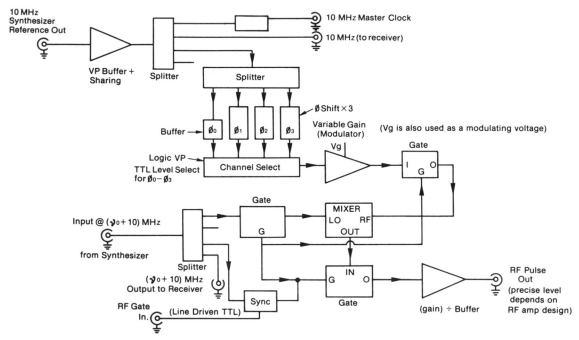

Figure 81–3. NMR imaging transmitter.

spectrum of the rf pulse in order to excite specific spins. The quality of modulation directly relates to slice profile in the image formation process. The modulation waveform comes from control electronics and is converted to an analog by a DAC. At least 12 bits are used, which gives a maximum dynamic range of 72 dB.

Many techniques require phase-shifting rf pulses. For example, phase alternation of successive 90 or 180 degree pulses during signal averaging allows the elimination of "out-of-slice" artifacts, those arising from imperfect rf pulse calibration. Consequently, the transmitter incorporates a scheme for providing pulses of four discrete phases. This may be accomplished, as shown in the diagram, by using delay lines as phase shifters with a set of gates to select the required phase signal under logic control. Alternatively, a "quadriphase modulator" can be used. Such devices are available commercially—they are used in communications—or they may be constructed from two double balanced mixers, a quadrature coupler and an in-phase power combiner.

The receiver accepts the incoming NMR signal and demodulates it to remove the rf carrier. Figure 81–4 shows a single conversion receiver again with an IF of 10 MHz. The first stage of the receiver contains a gain leveling device in the form of a variable attenuator, so that signals may be kept within the dynamic range of the ADCs. Attenuators are either adjustable in discrete (usually 1 dB) steps or continuously variable PIN diode types, where attenuation is proportional to a control voltage. The control voltage comes from a DAC to allow computer control of the receiver gain.

After the attenuator are a mixer and filter, which convert the signal to the IF. These two components are key to high performance. The mixer must have wide dynamic range, so a device with a high local oscillator (LO) level is used. The bandpass filter should have a passband bandwidth just wider than twice the highest NMR signal frequency. To attenuate unwanted components the filter should have high stopband attenuation. Such filters are usually multiple pole LC devices.

Following further gain the signal is passed to a pair of phase sensitive detectors. These are double mixers fed with an LO input at the IF. A 90 degree phase shift is introduced between the LO ports of first and second PSD so that the detectors operate

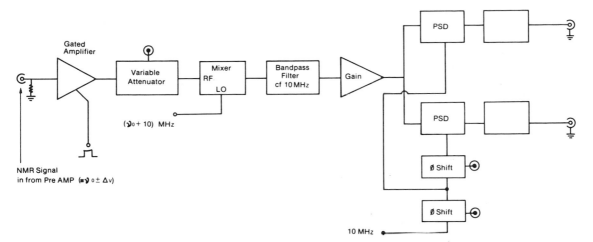

Figure 81–4. NMR imaging receiver.

in phase quadrature. Since the NMR signal is converted to be centered around the IF by the previous stage, mixing with IF in the PSDs results in the removal of the rf carrier to leave only the audio frequency difference signals. Image quality can be directly impacted by improper set-up of the PSDs. If the amplitude and phase relationship of the carrier are not tightly controlled, characteristic "mirror-image" artifacts result. If DC level in the PSDs is not carefully nulled, a central dot artifact results. After the PSDs there is usually additional audio frequency gain using operational amplifiers. Further details of spectrometer design can be found in the literature.[9,10]

THE DATA ACQUISITION SYSTEM

The basic data acquisition system (DAS) is shown in Figure 81–5. The analog signals entering the DAS are first passed through programmable low pass filters, which prevent noise aliasing occurring during digital sampling of the NMR signal. The band-

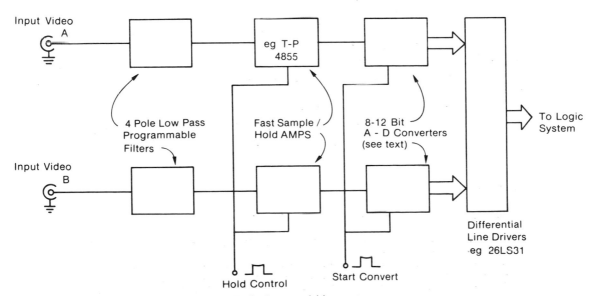

Figure 81–5. Basic data acquisition system.

width requirement is dependent on the choice of sampling time and so is method and field strength dependent. In general, shorter sampling time, hence wider bandwidth, is used at high field to reduce chemical shift artifact. For most techniques filter corner frequency is in the range of 5 to 30 kHz. Multiple pole filters with at least four poles are used, with Butterworth or Bessel types preferred. Following the filters are sample and hold amplifiers. These devices "instantaneously" sample the analog signal under logic control and hold it constant in a capacitor circuit for the duration of the acquisition period of the analog-to-digital converters (ADCs). The requirements on conversion rate are method dependent.[11] Some techniques, such as echo-planar imaging, require a conversion rate of greater than 300 kHz, whereas most 2DFT techniques use a rate of around 50 kHz. The ADC conversion time is dependent on word depth; the longer the word, the longer the conversion time. Here we have, however, been helped by technology. It is now possible to use ADCs that have a 16-bit word depth and a conversion time as short as 2 μs, which satisfy the needs of all conventional imaging techniques and provide resolution high enough for even the highest signal-to-noise systems.

CONTROL SYSTEM

All of the apparatus described in the preceeding sections has to be controlled in a coordinated manner. A significant amount of logic circuitry is required to do this, given the wide range of NMR techniques and operating parameters that are available on a contemporary whole-body imager.

The heart of the control system is the pulse programmer or scan controller. This is a computer or microprocessor driven device that provides the waveforms used for rf and gradient profiles and synchronizes the output of these profiles with data acquisition. Since profiles are repetitive slice to slice, loop instructions allow reduction in memory requirements. Even so, up to a megabyte of memory is required to control the more complex pulse sequences.

On the data acquisition side, again memory requirements are extensive. Note that a 64 slice 512 acquisition produces 128 kilobytes of data per view. The total amount of raw data for this sequence is 64 megabytes.

Control logic is also required to handle such system set-up functions as receiver gain adjustment, transmitter output level, and audio filter bandwidth. Static registers interfaced to the scan controller are usually used for this purpose. The system computer also plays a part in the control of the pulse sequence, usually in the form of operator entry of the pulse sequence parameters such as slice thickness, field of view, orientation, and so on.

The critical elements of an MR imaging system have been described in terms of their key performance requirements and operating parameters. Where appropriate the impact of NMR technique on subsystem design has been described.

References

1. Hoult DI, Richards RE: Signal-to-noise ratio of the nuclear magnetic resonance experiment. J Magn Reson 24:71–85, 1976.
2. Hoult DI, Lauterbur PC: The sensitivity of the zeugmatographic experiment involving human samples. J Magn Reson 34:425, 1979.
3. Thomas SR, Ackerman JL, Keriakes JG: Practical aspects involved in the design and set-up of a 0.15T, resistive magnet whole body NMR imaging facility. Magn Reson Imaging 2:341–348, 1984.
4. Golay MJ: Field homogenizing coils for nuclear spin resonance instrumentation. Rev Sci Instrum 29:313–315, 1958.

5. Mansfield P, Chapman B: Active magnetic screening of gradient coils in NMR imaging. J Magn Reson 66:573–576, 1986.
6. Schneider HJ, Dullenkopf P: The slotted tube resonator; A new NMR probe head at high observing frequencies. Rev Sci Instrum 48:68, 1977.
7. Leroy-Willig A, Darasse L, Taquin J, Sauzade M: The slotted cylinder, an efficient probe for NMR imaging. Magn Reson Med 2:20, 1985.
8. Bendall MR, Connelly A, McKendry JM: Elimination of coupling between cylindrical transmit coils and surface receive coils for in-vivo NMR. Magn Reson Med 3:157–163, 1986.
9. Holland GN, Misic GJ: Design concepts of pulsed Fourier transform NMR spectrometers. *In* Thomas SR, Dixon RL (eds): NMR In Medicine. AAPM Medical Physics Monographs No. 14. New York, AAPM, 1986, p 166.
10. Hoult DI: The NMR receiver: A description and analysis of design. Prog NMR Spectroscopy 12:41, 1978.
11. Pickens DR, Erickson JE: Computers in CT and MRI. *In* Keriakes JG, Simmons GH (eds): Special Monograph on Computers in Radiology. Radio Graphics 5:31–50, 1985.

82

Systems Optimization

WILFRIED LOEFFLER
ARNULF OPPELT

Over the past six to eight years magnetic resonance imaging (MRI) systems have undergone remarkable improvements in image quality. No single major change in technology accounted for most of this progress. Figure 82–1 shows a typical image for the first generation of systems built, either in university laboratories or in basic research departments of industrial firms. For comparison, Figure 82–2 is an image obtained only four years later using the same basic data acquisition and image reconstruction scheme. What made the difference was a steady process of improving the technology and performance of nearly every major component of the imaging system. This optimization is still ongoing, although the incremental improvements, as in any maturing technology, are becoming smaller and smaller. The various chapters of this book deal in depth with the technology and function of every component of an MRI system. Improvements and optimization of all of these components are of course essential for the performance of the total system. Since these improvements are very closely related to the technology of the specific components, they are described in detail in the corresponding chapters.

The objective of this chapter on systems optimization is to describe in a more generic way what the design parameters and operational modes of the system and its components ought to be for optimum performance. As an example, a well-designed system should be capable of running different data acquisition modes like driven equilibrium techniques or steady-state techniques as well as more commonly used methods like the spin-echo technique. A question of systems optimization then would be to find out the best way of operating for the highest signal-to-noise per unit time. Naturally this question might be answered differently if the optimization criterion was not signal-to-noise but, for example, contrast-to-noise for a certain pair of tissues. Therefore, it has to be clearly defined what the criteria for the optimization of the various operating parameters of the system ought to be. In order to limit and define this task, in each of the following paragraphs it will be clearly stated on which optimization criteria the evaluation is based. We tried to use our best judgment in picking the most reasonable and generally applicable criteria for each operational parameter. As mentioned above, specific design considerations for the optimization of critical components such as radio frequency (rf) coils are discussed in separate chapters. Here we will concentrate on the basic parameters for the design and operation of the total system: operating magnetic field strength, operating gradient field strength, imaging pulse sequence, and data acquisition mode. The optimization of pulse sequence parameters and data acquisition modes will be discussed here in terms of general physical criteria like signal-to-noise, spatial resolution, and imaging time. The optimization of certain contrast parameters for the optimum display of specific anatomical areas or pathologies using previous knowledge about the expected nuclear magnetic resonance (NMR) parameters like $T1$ and $T2$ is the subject of another chapter.

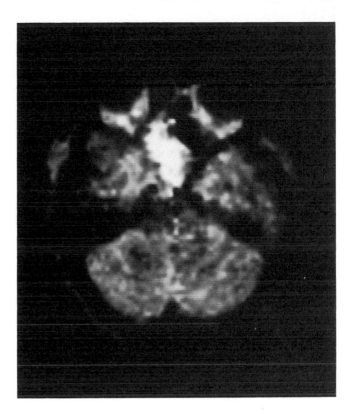

Figure 82–1. First patient image on a resistive MRI prototype system, 1980.

OPERATING FIELD STRENGTH FOR MRI AND SPECTROSCOPY

One of the reasons that there has been so much controversy over the question of the optimum magnetic field strength is that there are a number of distinct differences between analytical NMR or spectroscopy and proton imaging regarding the dependence of the operating performance on the field strength. There are three major differences. In analytical NMR the sample is quite small, while in imaging the sample is large and relatively more conductive. Second, in analytical NMR the signal is sampled in a field

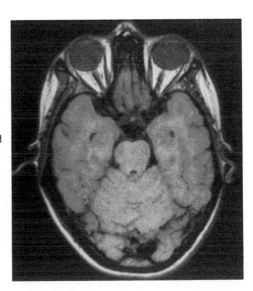

Figure 82–6. Selective excitation: Schematic plot of rf pulse shape and slice profile.

as homogeneous as possible; in imaging a field gradient is applied as the signal is sampled. And finally, the increasing chemical shift splitting at high field strengths is a help to analytical NMR but a hindrance to imaging.

The primary optimization criterion for the following analysis is the signal-to-noise (S/N) performance of an imaging system, since this is the basic image quality–related parameter that varies with the magnetic field strength. There will also be a discussion on the impact of the operating field strength on the rf power deposition into the patient and a brief discussion on siting requirements for the system, since those considerations might drastically limit the freedom in selecting the otherwise best field strength.

A simple way of assessing the question of the optimum field strength would be to evaluate the performance of existing systems at various operating fields. This can be highly misleading, since differences in engineering will be intermixed with differences due to the change in the operating field strength. In order to isolate the influence of the field strength, one, unfortunately, has to use a more theoretical approach and look at the frequency or field dependence of the parameters determining signal-to-noise and imaging speed.

The basic theory describing the frequency dependence of the signal-to-noise ratio in MRI has been developed by Hoult and Lauterbur.[1]

$$S/N = \text{const.} \frac{\nu^2}{\sqrt{\alpha\nu^{1/2} + \beta\nu^2}} \frac{1}{\sqrt{\Delta\nu}} \Delta V \tag{1}$$

where ν = NMR frequency = $\gamma/2\pi B_0$; $\Delta\nu$ = bandwidth of signal; α = "geometry" factor of rf coil; β = "geometry" factor of patient; and ΔV = voxel volume.

As is well known, the signal increases with the second power of the frequency or field. For the noise there are two contributions: the noise originating from the receiver coil increases only slightly with the frequency, while the noise introduced by the patient himself increases linearly with the frequency. Appropriate optimization of the rf coil allows a reduction of the first contribution to the noise. Therefore, at higher fields (above about 0.5 tesla), the coil contribution to the noise can be neglected,[1] leading to the following relationship for the frequency dependence of the S/N ratio:

$$S/N = \text{const.} \frac{\nu}{\sqrt{\Delta\nu}} \Delta V \tag{2}$$

In analytical NMR, because of the smaller sample size, one can usually neglect the sample contribution to the coil losses leading to a much stronger gain in signal-to-noise versus frequency.

The second factor that needs attention is the dependence of the signal-to-noise ratio on the bandwidth or frequency range over which the signal is spread. In imaging, the bandwidth can be varied by changing the gradient strength, whereas in analytical NMR it is determined by the line-width of the nucleus and compound being observed. The minimum gradient strength required for imaging is given by the natural line width or $T2$, the field inhomogeneity over one image element or voxel, and by the chemical shift difference between water and lipids.

$$ga > \frac{2}{\gamma T2} + \Delta B_0 + \frac{2\pi}{\gamma} \delta\nu \tag{3}$$

where g = gradient strength; a^2 = pixel area; ΔB_0 = field inhomogeneity over one voxel; and δ = chemical shift difference (lipid-water = 3.5 ppm).

The field inhomogeneity and chemical shift difference in absolute units increase with increasing field strength. As demonstrated by Table 82–1, the minimum required gradient strength is governed by the field inhomogeneity and chemical shift.

If the gradient is too small compared to the field inhomogeneity, the images will

Table 82–1. FACTORS DETERMINING MINIMUM REQUIRED GRADIENT STRENGTH*

Field in Tesla	Natural Line Width in Hz	ΔB_0/Voxel in Hz	Chemical Shift in Hz
0.35	13	37	45
0.5	13	52	65
1.0	13	105	130
1.5	13	160	190
2.0	13	210	250

*Values for $T2 = 25$ ms; $\Delta B_0 = 25$ ppm/10 cm; voxel size $= 1 \times 1 \times 10$ mm^3; $\delta = 3$ ppm.

become distorted. If the gradient is too small compared to the chemical shift difference between water and lipids, the relative positions of fatty and water-containing structures in the image will be shown incorrectly. This so-called chemical shift artifact shows up as a displacement of all fatty tissues with respect to primarily water-containing tissues in the images.[2] Figure 82–3 shows typical bright and black bands around the water-rich kidney tissue, which is embedded in surrounding fatty tissue.

The only reliable way to overcome the chemical shift artifact problem is to use sufficiently strong gradient fields, which have to be increased with the operating field strength. This increase in the gradient strength reduces the gain in signal-to-noise versus field strength. Whenever the gradient strength is determined by the chemical shift, which is increasingly the case at higher operating fields, the signal-to-noise ratio does not increase linearly with the field strength but rather with the square root of the operating field.[3,4]

$$S/N = \text{const.}\ \sqrt{v}\ \Delta V \qquad (4)$$

Since the objects to be imaged are biological tissues, one has to take into account the change of $T1$ values with the field strength[5] when assessing the imaging performance as a function of the field. Figure 82–4 shows a plot of $T1$ values for a couple of tissues against frequency. The values were obtained in vivo from images taken at different field strengths. In order to evaluate the consequences of these changes in $T1$ for a typical spin-echo image, one can combine the well-known saturation factor with the relationship of Equation 4.

$$S/N = \text{const.}\ \sqrt{v}\ (1 - e^{-TR/T1(v)})\ \Delta V \qquad (5)$$

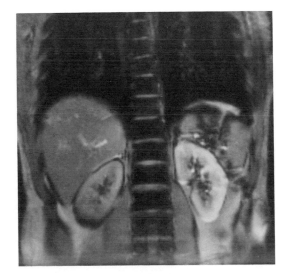

Figure 82–3. Coronal image through kidneys showing bright and black bands around kidneys due to chemical shift misregistration.

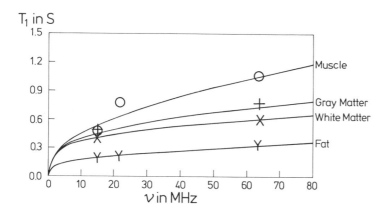

Figure 82–4. *T1* values for different tissues as function of NMR frequency.

Figure 82–5 shows the result. The plotted curves show the expected changes in signal-to-noise for spin-echo mode with a typical repetition time of 500 ms. The contrast-to-noise ratio that determines the detectability of tissue boundaries is given by the vertical distance between the curves.

With the exception of the curve for fat, all curves level out at about 1 tesla. The same is true for the vertical distance between the plots, which reflects the contrast-to-noise ratio for the different tissues. This means that there is still a gain in imaging performance at higher fields. However, the incremental benefit of increasing the operating field strength is becoming marginal and one has to evaluate if the increased system cost and other problems associated with operating at higher fields do not outweigh these benefits.

One of these problems is the increase in rf power deposition within the patient's body with increasing operating field. With otherwise unchanged pulse sequence parameters the power deposition in the patient increases with the square of the operating frequency.[6] While a final assessment of the maximum tolerable levels of rf power deposition at this time is probably premature, very closely spaced pulse sequences at frequencies of about 60 MHz will already more than double the heat dissipation within the body compared to the natural metabolic rate at rest.[7] While this is likely to have no adverse effects on healthy individuals, it probably puts a significant strain on the circulatory system of patients with severe heart disease.

Another point that has to be taken into consideration is the variety of problems associated with the siting of high field magnets (discussed in detail in Chapters 83 to 86). There seems to be a practical limit in the range of 1 to 2 tesla where the placing of an unshielded magnet becomes increasingly prohibitive or where the amount of iron needed for shielding exceeds the structural tolerance of most existing buildings.

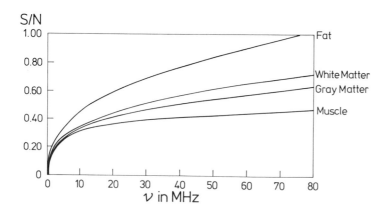

Figure 82–5. Signal/noise for various tissues as function of NMR frequency for spin-echo sequence with $T_R = 500$ ms.

In weighing the benefits of high field strengths against the problems associated with it, a reasonable way appears to be choosing a field strength at which the increase in performance begins to flatten out and the problems still appear controllable. A field strength in the range of 1 to 1.5 tesla for proton imaging makes optimum use of the performance increase without creating substantial problems in the areas of rf power deposition and magnet siting.

For systems to be used exclusively for spectroscopic research, on the other hand, the benefits of high fields predominate. For this application, the current judgment would be to use the highest field that can be accommodated from the point of view of cost and siting requirements. A final judgment, however, on where the best compromise for spectroscopy is to be found has to wait until the ongoing research has shown which nuclei and which procedures will be used for clinical applications.

GRADIENT FIELD STRENGTH FOR MRI

Slice Selection Gradient

Nearly all of the most widely used imaging sequences employ a combination of shaped rf pulses and magnetic field gradients for slice selection.[8] Although a variety of rf pulse shapes may be used, there are some general correlations that link the gradient strength used and the duration of the selective pulse with the sharpness of the slice profile and the amount of rf power deposition in the patient's body. In order to allow practical implementation, an ideally infinitely long rf pulse has to be truncated in time by a suitable apodization function. For a sin x/x shaped pulse, this means that the pulse has to be terminated after a finite number of side lobes. As a first order approximation it shall be assumed that the transverse magnetization produced by a shaped pulse follows the spectral shape of the pulse.[9] The sharpness or edge definition of the slice profile Δh as defined by Figure 82–6 depends on the number of contributing side lobes. Therefore, it shows the following dependence on the duration τ of the selective pulse.

$$\Delta h = \frac{4\pi}{\gamma\tau g} \tag{6}$$

The longer the selective pulse and stronger the slice selection gradient for a given slice thickness the better the sharpness of the slice profile will be and the easier the

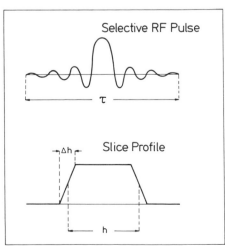

Figure 82–6. Selective excitation: Schematic plot of rf pulse shape and slice profile.

implementation of closely spaced multislice sequences will be. The power deposited in the patient's body by a selective rf pulse must also be considered. The energy deposition by a selective pulse is given by

$$P = \text{const. } A^2 \int_0^\tau s^2 \, dt \tag{7}$$

where A denotes an amplitude factor and $s(t)$ describes the shape of the pulse. With

$$S = \frac{1}{\tau} \int_0^\tau s^2 \, dt \tag{8}$$

this becomes

$$P = \text{const. } A^2 S \tau \tag{9}$$

To simplify the following considerations it shall be assumed that the normalized pulse integral S is kept independent of the slice width and gradient strength used. This means that by a variation in τ the pulse profile may be stretched in time but remains unchanged otherwise. The slice width, h, then, is related to the duration of the shaped pulse and the gradient strength

$$\tau^{-1} = \text{const. } gh \tag{10}$$

In order to keep the flip angle constant, $(A \cdot \tau)$ then has to be kept constant, leading to

$$P = \text{const. } S\tau^{-1} \tag{11}$$

$$P = \text{const. } Sgh \tag{12}$$

The rf power deposition for any given rf pulse shape like, for example, Gaussian or sin x/x pulses, therefore, increases linearly with the slice thickness and the gradient strength used.

The choice of the slice selection gradient strength has to be a compromise that does not exceed reasonable rf power limits while maintaining a sufficiently clean slice profile. Pulse profiles with only minimal negative side lobes generally help to keep the power deposition acceptably low by minimizing the power integral S. Some novel schemes for the optimization of rf pulse shapes recently have been reported.[10,11]

It is not possible to outline one simple optimization scheme resulting in an optimum strategy for slice selection gradient strength and pulse shape for all systems and each application. Instead one has to investigate for a specific system at a specific field strength what the relative importance of rf power deposition and sharpness of slice definition is, and thus find a suitable compromise. Generally slice selection gradients between 2 and 5 millitesla/meter have proved to be a reasonable choice.

Phase Encoding and Read-out Gradients

In the discussion of the signal-to-noise ratio as a function of field strength the minimum requirements for the read-out gradient strength have been evaluated. The three quantities determining the minimum tolerable read-out gradient strength are the natural line width $1/T2$, the magnet inhomogeneity, and the chemical shift difference between fat and water. At higher fields (above about 0.5 tesla) the chemical shift determines the minimum readout gradient. The magnitude of the chemical shift artifact δx, which is the displacement between waterlike and fatlike structures in an image, is given by

$$\delta x = \frac{\delta B_0}{g} \tag{13}$$

Table 82–2. MINIMUM GRADIENT STRENGTH AS FUNCTION OF FIELD STRENGTH AND SPATIAL RESOLUTION*

Field in Tesla	Minimum Gradient Strength in Millitesla/Meter for Pixel Dimensions			
	$a = 0.5\ mm$	$a = 1.0\ mm$	$a = 1.5\ mm$	$a = 2.0\ mm$
0.35	2	1	0.7	0.5
0.5	3	1.5	1	0.75
1.0	6	3	2	1.5
1.5	9	4.5	3	2.3
2.0	12	6	4	3

*Chemical shift misregistration shall not exceed pixel dimensions.

It is reasonable to limit the chemical shift displacement to less than the pixel size

$$a = \frac{2\pi}{\gamma T_s g} \tag{14}$$

where T_s = duration of the sampling interval. The resulting minimally tolerable gradient strength can be easily calculated and is given for a number of pixel sizes and field strength values in Table 82–2.

This consideration determines a lower limit for the read-out gradient strength. An upper limit may be given by the maximum capability of the gradient power supply. However, there is also a more fundamental reason not to use excessive read-out gradients. In order to evaluate this, one has to look at the relationship between the minimum possible echo time, *TE*, in a spin-echo sequence and the strength of the read-out gradient.

As detailed in Figure 82–7 the echo time, *TE*, is correlated with the sampling interval T_s through

$$TE = T_s + \tfrac{3}{2}\tau \tag{15}$$

where τ again denotes the duration of the selective rf pulses. As mentioned above, T_s and the desired spatial resolution determine the gradient strength.

$$g = \frac{2\pi}{\gamma T_s a} \tag{16}$$

As general optimization criteria for T_s or g the signal-to-noise ratio shall be used again.

Figure 82–7. Correlation between echo time, duration of selective pulses, and length of sampling interval in spin-echo imaging.

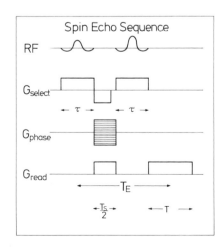

Since the bandwidth is given by T_s^{-1}, we obtain for the signal-to-noise ratio

$$S/N = \text{const. } e^{-TE/T2}\sqrt{TE - \tfrac{3}{2}\tau} \tag{17}$$

assuming all other sampling parameters remain constant. Equation 17 becomes maximum for

$$TE = \tfrac{1}{2}T2 + \tfrac{3}{2}\tau \tag{18}$$

or

$$T_s = \tfrac{1}{2}T2 \tag{19}$$

This means that short echo times and the associated strong read-out gradients are actually detrimental to the signal-to-noise ratio, a fact that is frequently disregarded when the optimum pulse sequence for the highest contrast between two specific tissues is being investigated. To do this properly the contrast-to-noise ratio has to be evaluated by taking the increase in noise for short echo times and large read-out gradients into account. Specific values for the optimum echo times then will depend on the tissue parameters *T1* and *T2* of the two tissues investigated as well as on the repetition time, *TR*.

LOW CONTRAST VERSUS SPATIAL RESOLUTION

Unlike all other diagnostic imaging modalities, MRI systems do not have inherent limits of their spatial resolution. There is no design parameter like the detector aperture of a computed tomography (CT) system, for example, which ultimately defines the maximum spatial resolution in MRI. Instead it is possible by varying the gradient strength and sampling speed of the analog-to-digital converter to control the spatial resolution or pixel size in MRI within wide limits. Finally, the practical limits for the spatial resolution in MRI are set by the signal-to-noise characteristics of the images rather than by any geometric limitations. With increasing spatial resolution and decreasing pixel size, the signal-to-noise ratio of the images decreases drastically. Therefore, in any given imaging situation, a compromise has to be found in order to obtain the required spatial resolution in an image with reasonable signal-to-noise characteristics, or, speaking in practical terms, the correct zoom factor has to be chosen depending on the diagnostic question, the rf coil being used, and the imaging time available.[12]

The quantity that suffers from a low signal-to-noise ratio when going to very small pixel sizes is the low contrast resolution. This is the ability of an observer to discriminate medium-sized objects from a uniform background with very little difference in gray level. The detection of fairly large lesions within uniform organs such as the liver depends critically on this parameter. It has been shown that the ability of an observer to identify objects showing little contrast is proportional to the diameter of the objects, *D*, and the difference in signal or gray level with respect to the background, ΔS, divided by the image noise, *N*.[13]

$$\text{Detection ratio} = \Delta = \frac{\Delta S}{N} D \tag{20}$$

In a pixeled image the diameter may be substituted by the square root of the number of pixels, *n*, within the object:

$$\Delta = \text{const. } \frac{\Delta S}{N} \sqrt{n} \tag{21}$$

Equation 21, therefore, just describes the ability of an observer to average the pixel values over certain areas in order to identify structures in an image.

For MRI the question now arises how the detection rate, Δ, for low contrast objects depends on the zoom factor or pixel size with otherwise unchanged conditions.

Assuming that the variation in pixel size is accomplished by varying the gradient strength and thus leaving the bandwidth per pixel constant, the signal-to-noise ratio in MRI depends linearly on the voxel volume.[1] If a^2 denotes the pixel area and h the slice thickness, this leads to

$$\Delta = \text{const.} \ (a^2 h)\sqrt{n} \tag{22}$$

The number of pixels in a certain structure, of course, is proportional to the inverse pixel area a^{-2}

$$\Delta = \text{const.} \ (a^2 h)\sqrt{a^{-2}} \tag{23}$$

$$\Delta = \text{const.} \ (ah) \tag{24}$$

The low contrast resolution, therefore, increases linearly with the pixel dimensions. This, unfortunately, means that the ability to identify low contrast objects in MRI suffers from an increase in spatial resolution if all other conditions, such as imaging time and receiver coil, remain unchanged. In order to demonstrate this behavior, a low contrast phantom was imaged twice with a different zoom factor but otherwise identical acquisition parameters. Figure 82–8 shows a comparison of the two images. The two upper rows of low contrast objects clearly are better visible in the image with inferior spatial resolution.

This behavior in MRI is in sharp contrast to x-ray CT. It has been shown that any improvement in detector or sampling geometry to upgrade spatial resolution in x-ray CT leaves the low contrast resolution unchanged.[14] The reason for this difference in the two modalities is, of course, the fact that x-ray CT measures the absorption parameters of objects with an external source of radiation, while the source of the signal in MRI is the object itself.

A suitable way to overcome the problems in low contrast resolution when imaging at a high spatial resolution is to use smaller rf receiver coils with inherently higher sensitivity. A natural way of doing so is the use of a head coil for higher resolution

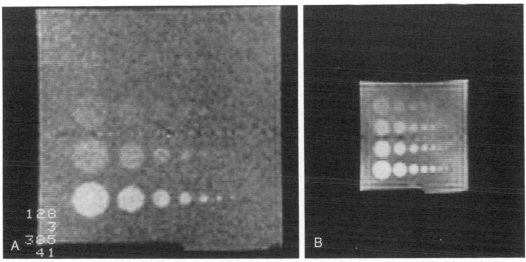

Figure 82–8. Images of low contrast phantom with different spatial resolution; otherwise unchanged acquisition parameters. A, Pixel size $(1.4 \text{ mm})^2$. B, Pixel size $(3.1 \text{ mm})^2$.

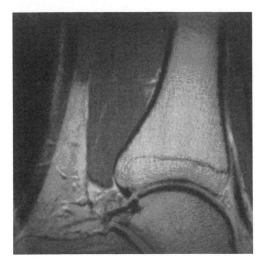

Figure 82–9. Surface coil image of ankle; pixel size $(0.4 \text{ mm})^2$; slice thickness 2 mm.

head imaging. For other organs, surface coils allow a further increase in sensitivity, provided that the penetration depth is sufficient for the specific organ. If the primary source of electrical losses in the rf coil is the resistance of the wire material, as is common in low field imaging, the sensitivity of the receiver coil increases about linearly with the inverse coil radius.[1] If, as in high field imaging, inductive coupling to the patient determines the electrical coil losses, the sensitivity increases with about the second power of the inverse coil radius.[1] Therefore, it is possible to at least partially compensate for the loss in low contrast resolution, if the coil being used can be adapted to the smaller field of view when zooming the image. Figure 82–9 shows a zoomed image of the ankle obtained with a surface coil. The contrast resolution is still excellent despite a pixel size of only $(0.37 \text{ mm})^2$ at a slice thickness of 2 mm.

Two conclusions can be drawn from the relationships outlined above. First, it is advisable to use the smallest receiver coil possible for any given anatomical area of interest. Second, one still has to find in each instance a reasonable compromise when choosing the zoom factor in order to obtain sufficient spatial resolution without an excessive loss in contrast resolution. The right choice of the zoom factor becomes specifically important when investigating regions deep inside the head or body where surface coils cannot be utilized.

OPTIMIZATION OF DATA ACQUISITION SCHEME

The influence of pulse sequence parameters like *TE* and *TR* on the contrast of MR images is discussed in great detail in Chapters 7, 8, and 74 . It is the purpose of this paragraph to describe the influence of these parameters or, more generally, of the data acquisition scheme on the effectiveness of the imaging method to obtain the highest signal-to-noise ratio in the shortest possible time. A way of quantifying the efficiency of an imaging method is by evaluating the signal-to-noise ratio of the images obtained divided by the square root of the acquisition time. The influence of different gradient strengths and sampling bandwidths on the signal-to-noise ratio of images has been investigated in the preceding paragraphs. For a relative comparison of different data acquisition schemes, the bandwidth and thus the noise can be held constant. Therefore, only the signal strength during data acquisition has to be compared:

$$Efficiency = \frac{Signal}{\sqrt{Measurement\ time}} \tag{25}$$

We will use Equation 25 to evaluate the relative efficiency of spin-echo imaging, echo-planar imaging, and a steady state free precession method for imaging. For this evaluation the NMR signal amplitude is normalized, such that maximum magnetization (e.g., spin echo with $TE \ll T2$ and $TR \gg T1$) would result in a signal of 1. Measurement time is the time needed to build up a complete N^2 image. Since a quadrature demodulator is usually used and both sides of the spin echo are sampled, it is possible to reconstruct an N^2 image by sampling only $N/2$ spin-echo signals.[15]

Spin-Echo Imaging

Spin-echo imaging is characterized by the acquisition parameters echo time, TE, and repetition time, TR. Even in multiecho imaging each image is reconstructed by using only data from a single echo with a fixed echo time. The signal amplitude is

$$S = e^{-TE/T2}(1 - 2e^{-(TR - TE/2)/T1} + e^{-TR/T1}) \tag{26}$$

The time to build up an N^2 image is $N/2\ TR$.

Echo-Planar Imaging

Echo-planar imaging has been introduced by Mansfield with the goal of allowing the reconstruction of a complete image with only one excitation.[16] The basic idea is to recall a number of echoes by repetitive gradient reversal and use a different gradient phase encoding for each echo. In contrast to the usual multiecho imaging, different echoes with different echo times are used to build up a single image faster. Because of very high demands on the gradient system it is frequently not possible to generate a sufficient number of echoes in a single excitation to allow the reconstruction of a complete image. Therefore, the idea of echo-planar imaging should be generalized to include all imaging schemes that use multiple echoes for the generation of a single image, even when more than one excitation is used to build up the image. In this sense a method recently developed and termed RARE[17] can be included in the discussion of general echo-planar imaging.

Since a number of echoes contribute to a single image, the signal amplitude in the image corresponds to an average over different $T2$ weighting factors:

$$S = \frac{1}{n} \sum_{k=1}^{n} (e^{-kTE/T2})(1 - e^{-(TR - nTE)/T1}) \tag{27}$$

$$S = \frac{e^{-TE/T2}}{n} \frac{1 - e^{nTE/T2}}{1 - e^{TE/T2}} (1 - e^{-(TR - nTE)/T1}) \tag{28}$$

It is assumed that n echoes with echo times of nTE are used and the repetition time is TR. The measurement time for an N^2 image then amounts to $NTR/(2n)$.

Steady State Free Precession Imaging

Introduced early in the development of MRI, this technique uses very closely spaced rf pulses to drive the magnetization into a steady state.[18] The basic difference between this and all other imaging modes is that transverse magnetization has to be retained from one excitation pulse to the next. A steady state will develop only if the spacing between successive excitation pulses, TR, is shorter than, or at least of the order of $T2$. Recently, steady state methods have been modified to allow Fourier reconstruction rather than the back projection method used earlier.[19] The signal amplitude depends on the flip angle of the rf excitation pulses φ and the $T1/T2$ ratio:

$$S = \frac{\sin \varphi}{\left(1 + \dfrac{T1}{T2}\right) + \left(1 - \dfrac{T1}{T2}\right) \cos \varphi} \tag{29}$$

The measurement time for an N^2 image again is $N/2 \, TR$.

Table 82–3 shows an evaluation of the relative efficiency of the data acquisition schemes mentioned when imaging different tissues. Also shown is the shortest possible imaging time for a 128^2 matrix. As described above, the efficiency parameter is a means of comparing the signal-to-noise ratio, which can be obtained with the various methods if the same total data acquisition time would be invested.

There are a number of conclusions that can be drawn from Table 82–3. First, comparing the short and long repetition time spin-echo sequence, it is obvious that for tissues with longer $T1$'s the signal loss when using short TR's cannot be compensated by using more acquisitions. From a pure signal-to-noise per unit time point of view, it does not make sense, therefore, to use repetition times much shorter than the $T1$ value of the tissue. The intrinsically faster echo-planar imaging and steady state free precession imaging methods also have a better signal-to-noise performance than spin-echo imaging if comparable data acquisition times are used. As expected, both fast imaging schemes are especially favorable for fairly short $T1$'s and long $T2$'s. However, as shown by Equations 28 and 29, the contrast mechanisms for these methods differ significantly from the usual relationship in spin-echo imaging (Eq. 26). Future experience will have to show if these different contrast relationships suit clinical needs well enough to allow fully utilizing the advantage in efficiency.

Of all diagnostic imaging modalities, MRI is probably the method that allows the greatest variation in the imaging result by using different acquisition parameters. Not only is it possible to use data acquisition methods that exhibit different contrast relationships, but parameters like TE and TR can be varied in a single acquisition scheme to vary the appearance of the image within wide limits. Some methods require imaging times almost exceeding the tolerance level of most patients, while others allow the generation of an image within seconds.

Many of the methods mentioned can actually be set up by relatively simple modifications to the software driving the system. Frequently it is even possible for the user to select among a large variety of different modes. In MRI, therefore, system optim-

Table 82–3. EFFICIENCY FOR DIFFERENT DATA ACQUISITION METHODS

Data Acquisition Method	Minimum Imaging Time for 128^2 Matrix	Fat $T1 = 0.3$ s $T2 = 0.1$ s	Efficiency for Muscle $T1 = 1$ s $T2 = 0.1$ s	Water $T1 = 2$ s $T2 = 2$ s
Spin-Echo Imaging				
$TE = 15$ ms $T_R = 3$ s	192 s	$0.062 \text{ s}^{-1/2}$	$0.059 \text{ s}^{-1/2}$	$0.055 \text{ s}^{-1/2}$
$TE = 15$ ms $T_R = 60$ ms	3.8 s	$0.062 \text{ s}^{-1/2}$	$0.019 \text{ s}^{-1/2}$	$0.011 \text{ s}^{-1/2}$
Echo-Planar Imaging				
$n = 12 \; T_E = 10$ ms $TR = 1$ s	5.3 s	$0.228 \text{ s}^{-1/2}$	$0.141 \text{ s}^{-1/2}$	$0.150 \text{ s}^{-1/2}$
$n = 12 \; T_E = 10$ ms $TR = 0.2$ s	1.1 s	$0.124 \text{ s}^{-1/2}$	$0.041 \text{ s}^{-1/2}$	$0.037 \text{ s}^{-1/2}$
Steady State Free Precession Imaging				
$\varphi = 90° \; T_R = 15$ ms	1 s	$0.255 \text{ s}^{-1/2}$	$0.093 \text{ s}^{-1/2}$	$0.510 \text{ s}^{-1/2}$

ization in the design stage can be only the first step to obtain the overall best imaging result. Since it is still fairly early in the clinical assessment of many of the various imaging schemes, the best system optimization is still for the hardware to allow a great amount of flexibility for the implementation of different methods.

Because of the unique flexibility of MRI, the user has to assume a great responsibility for obtaining optimum imaging results. The optimization criteria outlined in this chapter should help to find the right approach under different conditions. Together with the relationships described in Chapters 7 and 8 it should be possible to thoughtfully direct the development of clinical protocols. Practical experience is then essential for fine tuning. However, because of the great flexibility of the method and the many parameters involved, we can definitely look forward to an extended and exciting time of system design progress and even more protocol improvements.

References

1. Hoult DI, Lauterbur PC: The sensitivity of the zeugmatographic experiment involving human samples. J Magn Reson *34*:425, 1979.
2. Soila KP, Viamonte M Jr, Starewicz PM: Chemical shift misregistration effect in magnetic resonance imaging. Radiology *153*:819, 1984.
3. Loeffler W, Oppelt A, von Wulfen H, Zimmermann B: An approach for selecting the best field strength for proton imaging. Society of Magnetic Resonance in Medicine, Third Annual Meeting, Book of Abstracts, 1984, p 483.
4. Chen C-N, Sank VJ, Hoult DI: Probing image frequency dependence. Society of Magnetic Resonance in Medicine, Third Annual Meeting, Book of Abstracts, 1984, p 148.
5. Bottomley PA, Foster TH, Argersinger RE, Pfeifer LM: A review of normal tissue hydrogen NMR relaxation times and relaxation mechanisms from 1–100 MHz: Dependence on tissue type, NMR frequency, temperature, species, excision, and age. Med Phys *11*:425, 1984.
6. Bottomley PA, Andrew ER: RF magnetic field penetration, phase shift and power dissipation in biological tissue: Implications for NMR imaging. Phys Med Biol *23*:630, 1978.
7. Chen C-N, Sank VJ, Hoult DI: A study of RF power deposition in imaging. Society of Magnetic Resonance in Medicine, Fourth Annual Meeting, Book of Abstracts, 1985, p 918.
8. Garroway AN, Grannell PK, Mansfield P: Image formation in NMR by a selective irradiative process. J Phys C *7*:L457, 1974.
9. Loeffler W, Oppelt A, Faul D: Computer simulations of slice selection in NMR imaging. Magn Reson Med *1*:196, 1984.
10. Silver MS, Joseph RI, Hoult DI: Highly selective $\pi/2$ and π pulse generation. J Magn Reson *59*:347, 1984.
11. Conolly S, Macovski A: Selective pulse design via optimal control theory. Society of Magnetic Resonance in Medicine, Fourth Annual Meeting, Book of Abstracts, 1985, p 958.
12. Oppelt A, Stetter E, Loeffler W: Spatial and contrast resolution in NMR imaging. Society of Magnetic Resonance in Medicine, First Annual Meeting, Book of Abstracts, 1982, p 121.
13. Rose A: Vision: Human and Electronic. New York, Plenum Press, 1973.
14. Cohen G, DiBianca FA: Use of contrast-detail-dose evaluation of image quality in a CT scanner. J Comp Assist Tomogr *3*:189, 1979.
15. Margosian P: Faster imaging—imaging with half the data. Society of Magnetic Resonance in Medicine, Fourth Annual Meeting, Book of Abstract, 1985, p 1024.
16. Mansfield P: Multi-planar image formation using NMR spin echos. J Phys C *10*:55, 1977.
17. Hennig J: RARE-Imaging: A fast imaging method for clinical routine. Society of Magnetic Resonance in Medicine, Fourth Annual Meeting, Book of Abstracts, 1985, p 988.
18. Hinshaw WS: Image formation by nuclear magnetic resonance: The sensitive point method. J Appl Phys *47*:3709, 1976.
19. Haase A, Frahm J, Matthaei D, Haenike W, Merboldt K-D: Rapid images and NMR movies. Society of Magnetic Resonance in Medicine, Fourth Annual Meeting, Book of Abstracts, 1985, p 980.

XV

SITE PLANNING AND QUALITY ASSURANCE

83

Planning and Preparation

JOHN W. STEIDLEY
JANET D. COIL
STEVEN G. EINSTEIN

Site planning and site preparation for the installation of a magnetic resonance (MR) system are driven by two overriding sets of considerations.[1,2] First and foremost is the nature of the specific applications for which the system is intended. These applications dictate the field strength and operating frequency, or frequencies, of the system. The second set of considerations concerns the unique characteristics of the magnetic resonance system itself, namely, the type of magnet and its shielding if needed, the radio frequency subsystem and its screening, and cryogenics, if needed. Equally important, traditional siting considerations include system configuration, facility layout, structural requirements to address the potential problem of magnet weight, air conditioning, and equipment-related issues common to medical imaging systems. These considerations are, in general, not new to an institution's site planner. Thus, this chapter will focus on the key aspects of siting and preparation that are uncommon to the experienced hospital site planner.

The applications of an MR system include imaging and spectroscopy of protons or hydrogen (^{1}H), carbon (^{13}C), fluorine (^{19}F), sodium (^{23}Na), and phosphorus (^{31}P). All of these applications are described elsewhere in this book. In general, the magnetic field strength required for imaging of protons is in the range of 0.15 tesla to 2.0 tesla, where a tesla is a unit of magnetic field strength approximately 20,000 times the strength of the earth's magnetic field strength. As the strength of the magnet is increased, the signal-to-noise ratio of the system is improved; however, tradeoffs occur that ultimately limit the benefits of increased field strength. Of key concern to readers of this chapter are the restrictions that a high field system places on the site.[3,4] However, high field systems are generally required for the imaging of anything other than protons and for spectroscopy. Currently, most MR systems can be grouped as resistive of 0.15 tesla, mid-field of 0.3 to 0.6 tesla, or high field of 1.5 tesla or greater. At field strengths of 0.50 tesla and greater, superconducting technology requiring cryogenics is used.

The purpose of this chapter is to acquaint the reader with the concepts of magnetic shielding, radiofrequency screening, cryogenics, and other considerations unique to MR system site planning and preparation. The scope of the information presented in this chapter is intended to give the reader an overview of the concepts of MR site planning that will be addressed by a professional site planner. It is important to emphasize the words "addressed by a professional site planner," since the ultimate performance of an MR system may be dictated by the selected site, by the quality of magnetic shielding and radiofrequency screening which is chosen, and, at least in terms of financial performance, by cryogen considerations. Several representative site plans are shown to illustrate the general principles involved.

MAGNETIC SHIELDING

The strong magnetic field that is required for magnetic resonance imaging (MRI) presents site planning and preparation considerations unlike any posed by alternative imaging technologies. MR image quality and overall system performance can be adversely impacted by the surrounding environment, depending on the level, location, and motion of ferrous objects and structures. Structural steel, adjacent parking garages, and elevators can affect the diagnostic performance. Conversely, the fringe field of an MR system may affect magnet-sensitive devices such as pacemakers as well as equipment utilizing electron beams. The stray magnetic field, if not properly contained, can also impact magnetized devices such as computer memory banks, tapes, and credit cards.

Environmental Impact on Magnetic Resonance System Performance

Image quality and MR system performance depend on the stability and homogeneity of the magnetic field. If the uniformity of the magnetic field is disturbed during image acquisition, the image will be distorted and/or degraded by artifacts. For spectroscopic applications, an unstable or nonuniform field will scramble the resultant spectrum, producing uninterpretable results. For spectroscopy, a 1.5 tesla system must be maintained at a homogeneity of one part per million (ppm). For normal proton imaging, uniformity requirements are somewhat less demanding, with a specification of ± 10 ppm to ± 20 ppm (at 50 cm dsV). Generally, an unshielded magnet in a nonperturbing environment will provide these conditions; the objective of shielding is to preserve these conditions in an established medical environment (see Fig. 83–1 and Table 83–1). Moveable ferromagnetic objects in the vicinity of the magnet can cause image artifacts. Table 83–1 gives an indication of the field strength contour within which an object will induce a 0.1 ppm homogeneity shift in an imaging volume with a z axis 10 cm (4 inches) long.

Fringe Magnetic Effects on the Environment

MR site planning requires a careful analysis of the architecture, instrumentation, equipment, and human traffic flow in the vicinity of the MR suite. Field tolerances for sensitive equipment may require its own shielding. A fringe field standard of 0.5 millitesla or 5 gauss (ten times the earth's average magnetic field) has been established for unrestricted traffic areas (general population). This requirement stems from the concern of the fringe field's effect upon pacemaker operation. The magnetic field

Table 83–1. SENSITIVITY TO MOVEABLE OBJECTS

Object	Weight	Field Strength Contour (millitesla)
Medical instruments	0.2 lb	90
Hand tools	2 lb	45
Beds and stretchers	20 lb	5
Medium machinery	200 lb	0.9
Automobile	3000 lb	0.3
Elevator	10,000 lb	<0.1
Buses and trucks	25,000 lb	<0.1
Railway train	250,000 lb	≪0.1

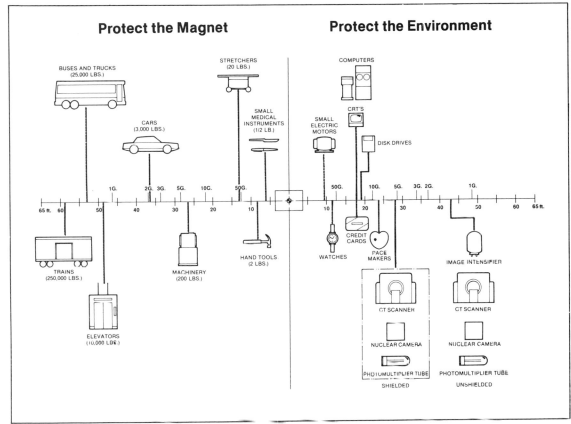

Figure 83–1. Recommended minimum distances between the center of a 0.5 tesla magnet and various objects. Distances increase for higher field strengths.

strength must be maintained at or below this level outside the marked "exclusion" or "controlled" zone of the equipment (see Fig. 83–1 and Table 83–2). Table 83–2 includes a sample of susceptible objects, or objects that are sensitive to magnetic fields. The maximum field strength in the table is the threshold field that can potentially distort or disrupt the operation of the given object.

Magnet Shielding Principles

Magnetism is often described as a series of lines of force (or flux) emanating from one pole and returning to the other pole. These poles are usually designated as north

Table 83–2. MAXIMUM PERMITTED FIELD STRENGTHS FOR SUSCEPTIBLE OBJECTS

Object	Maximum Field Strength (millitesla)
Watches	5.0
Magnetic data carrier (diskette, tape, credit card)	2.0
Video monitor, black/white	1.0
CRTs/Computers	1.0
Pacemaker	0.5
Metal detector	0.3
Image intensifier, gamma camera	0.1
CT scanner (unshielded)	0.1

and south. The lines of force make a kind of circuit, just as electric current must travel from the positive to negative terminal of a battery. While these lines of force cannot be absorbed, in the conventional sense as lead is used for x-ray shielding, the magnetic circuit can be channeled through certain materials (ferromagnetic materials). Steel is one of the best materials for redirecting the magnetic lines of force and one of the most cost effective.

The basic requirements of the magnetic shielding are that it maintain the circuit path or closed loop from one pole to the other and that it have sufficient capacity to channel the undesirable field. The closed loop property of magnetic shielding is complicated by the problem that the steel shielding, when placed too close to the magnet, will distort the central field. Symmetrical shielding will reduce this distortion. With the use of magnetic shielding, the field beyond the perimeter of the shield will be markedly reduced, while the field within this perimeter will increase. The increase will be most profound near the edges of the steel where the magnetic field will be concentrated. To ensure adequate magnetic flux carrying capacity, shielding mass can be added. Failure to maintain sufficient steel mass leads to the saturation of the shielding. The excess lines of force "spill-over" into the environment, increasing the fringe field.

Design of an effective magnetic shield requires an accurate determination of the strength of the magnetic field at different locations around the magnet. This is typically accomplished by means of a series of surveys. Measurements of effective field strengths are used in conjunction with theoretical calculations to provide an analysis of shielding requirements and constraints. Radial field plots are created, providing the basis for the design of the magnetic shielding for each site.

In general, there are three approaches to magnetic shielding that use passive iron shielding. Passive shielding is simply a scheme in which no energy is required, including self-shielding, prefabricated modular shielding, and custom room shielding. Alternatives (active shielding) include electrical shielding based on resistive or superconductive technology.

One prefabricated modular magnetic shielding approach, previously described as a case study in the American Hospital Association Guideline Report on MR, illustrates the principles of passive and active magnetic shielding.[5] The modular magnetic shielding dome was developed on the basis of on-site experience combined with theoretical and empirical research. The focus of the research was the creation of a shielding method to permit installation of MR systems in existing structures in a cost-effective manner.

The shielding system complements the MR system configuration through the use of a polygon-shaped dome construction shown in Figure 83–2. The dome's axis coincides with the magnet's axis; its shape follows the pattern of the magnetic force lines

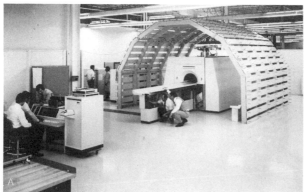
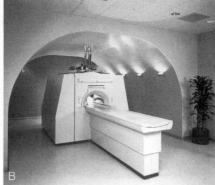

Figure 83–2. Dome shaped modular magnetic shielding before and after finish treatment.

to effectively redirect and contain them. The iron crossbars, which make up the dome, become magnetized and set up a weak counter field not only to contain but also to shape the effective magnetic fringe field. This configuration offers a high degree of symmetry, minimizing the corrections required to maintain homogeneity of the working internal field.

The size of the dome is designed to be compact, with a length of 5 to 7 meters and width measuring approximately 5 meters.[6] This is considered an optimal size because it provides enough distance from the magnet center to avoid disruption of homogeneity. Compared with the alternative shielding practice of full-room steel plating, the dome offers substantial savings in terms of construction costs and installation time. Compared with the alternative of self-shielding, floor loading is distributed over a much wider area.

The dome was also designed as a modular, flexible structure to accommodate the specific shielding requirements of the site. Time, labor, and materials are used economically to provide only the amount of shielding required for optimal system performance and acceptable environmental standards for the surrounding area (Fig. 83–3). The dome was prefabricated and then assembled on site in two days. Its modular design meant that flexibility was built into the shielding structure should future changes in magnet field strength or new construction require modifications in shielding. By recalculating new field patterns, the magnetic dome offered a means of reshielding for new requirements without extensive remodeling and construction costs.

The dome has also been installed with an active shield that utilizes a large peripheral coil at one end of the dome. By passing DC current through this coil, it is possible to provide additional, selective active magnetic shielding, which shapes the fringe field in at one end by another 20 percent. The dome itself reduces a fringe field by a factor of two or three. Because it does not completely surround the magnet (there is no dome underneath the magnet), its primary shielding effectiveness is above and around the magnet but not below. As both the medical community and system manufacturer become more bold in the placement of MRI systems, particularly high field systems, the suitability of the dome alone is called into question. It is now quite common to have large magnets in relatively small rooms on the upper floors of the hospital or clinic. This requires a more innovative solution, usually a hybrid or combination of two passive shielding schemes. The dome plus full-room shielding is often required. With this design, high field magnet systems can be placed in an area of approximately 1500 square feet. Unfortunately, this may require massive quantities of steel.

Alternatively, a self-shielded magnet with room shielding can be used. This may

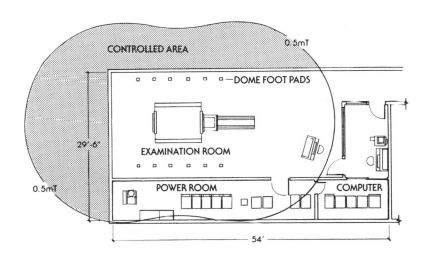

Figure 83–3. Modular magnetic shielding for a 0.5 tesla magnet used to control and shape the fringe magnetic fields.

reduce the overall weight of the installation, but the floor loading caused by the magnet is still high. Also, the issues of central field homogeneity and mechanical stability are raised.

Computerized Magnetic Field Analysis

The solution to the classical equations describing the distribution of a static magnetic field is simple only when the source of the field and the region of interest are also simple. For configurations of practical importance in actual magnetic resonance imaging installations, the equation needs to be solved numerically in light of boundaries, objects, and overall geometry, which require a three-dimensional treatment.

The typical procedure for performing the calculation to define the magnetic field consists of three phases: (1) preparation, (2) performing the calculation, and (3) evaluation of the results in terms of shielding requirements. Preparation consists of specifying an appropriate array of field points at which to calculate the magnetic intensity. This is generally a three-dimensional array that conforms as closely as possible to the geometry of the proposed shielding surface. For example, the polygonal shape of the magnetic dome is represented, as well as walls, floor, and ceiling of the room in which it is to be located.

Proper selection of field points is essential for cost-effective and accurate evaluation. The array of field points must incorporate locations at which the field changes rapidly with position, such as at iron boundaries, as well as areas that are particularly susceptible to magnetic interference (such as computer hardware). An unsuitable disposition of points will result in an inaccurate analysis and, consequently, inappropriate shielding, which will require modification. On the other hand, the number of field points must be minimized to limit the cost of the calculation, which can be considerable (requiring hours of computer time). As many as 60,000 field points have occasionally been used to evaluate complex installations, but generally the number is less. The calculation is finally peformed on a computer. The results of the calculation are evaluated by several criteria. These include the effectiveness of the shielding compared with the requirements of the surrounding environment, and the effect of the shielding upon the homogeneity of the central magnetic field.

Measurement of the Magnetic Fields

Two types of measurements are required for evaluation of MRI shielding: the external or "stray" field and the internal working field. Both are affected by the shielding configuration, and both must be evaluated to verify compliance with specifications. The two fields are measured quite differently and require different instrumentation. The "stray" or fringe field is the easiest to measure. It requires a high-quality Hall effect gauss meter and a tape measure. One must be careful to orient the probe in the direction of maximum value and record readings at all critical locations. It is advisable to obtain readings at several distances from the floor to establish vertical as well as horizontal gauss levels.

The internal working field of the magnet is measured with an NMR probe. This probe determines the resonant frequency of a sample at a fixed number of locations on the surface of an imaginary sphere (conventionally with a 50 cm diameter) at the center of the magnet. The locations of the measurements are conventionally at 12 equally spaced positions around the circumference of seven concentric circles for a total of 84 readings. The seven circles are coaxial with the magnet at 22.5 degree intervals of the polar angle. It is customary and desirable to employ a fixed structure to establish the detection geometry.

Data from the 84 readings make it possible to determine the uniformity coefficients, or Legendre expansion coefficients. These describe the field distribution within the working volume of the magnet. These coefficients are usually quoted in parts per million (ppm) of the central field. There is limited shimming capability incorporated into the magnet assembly to provide correction if one or more of the coefficients are excessively large. Internal magnet correction coils (shims) permit only relatively minor corrections, however, and it is essential that most field uniformity be provided by the shielding configuration and passive shimming design.

Effective magnetic shielding solutions are now available from MR system manufacturers that minimize the impact of the magnetic field on the environment and protect the sensitive imaging volume from distortions. Magnetic shielding channels the magnetic lines of force away from the environment. Computerized magnetic field analysis followed by measurement of the final fringe field and homogeneity within the magnet is used to verify performance.

RADIOFREQUENCY SCREENING

The actual data from which magnetic resonance images are constructed are radiofrequency (rf) signals. Therefore, the rf environment of the MR system must be carefully protected from extraneous and contaminating information. Because of this requirement, MR systems must be rf isolated from interference and environmental rf noise sources. Figure 83–4 shows several sources of transmitted interference. This consideration introduces a host of issues uncommon to any other diagnostic imaging modality.

The strategy for rf isolation, or screening, generally depends upon the field strength of the MR system and proposed long-term applications, i.e., the degree to which various

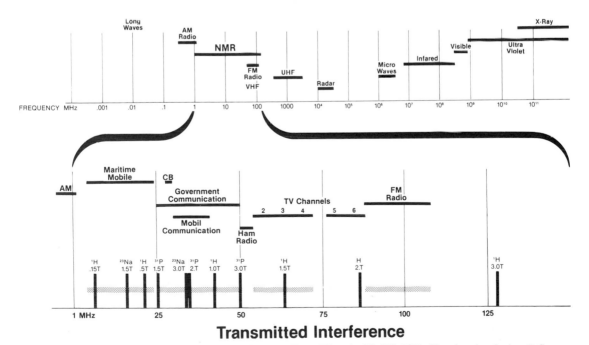

Figure 83–4. Typical sources of transmitted rf interference. (From Einstein SG, Hilal SK: Site planning design: Influences and implementation. *In* Kressel HY (ed): Magnetic Resonance Annual. New York, Raven Press, 1985.)

elements will be investigated. Because the resonant frequencies of ^1H, ^{13}C, ^{23}Na, ^{31}P, and ^{19}F are different, several frequency ranges need to be surveyed to determine the appropriate screening strategy for a given suite. The complexity of screening a site can range from requirements for installations of a single system used exclusively for hydrogen imaging to requirements for installations incorporating several systems, operating at different field strengths, with applications involving multiple elements.

The Radiofrequency Survey

Prior to final architectural planning or construction, the rf environment of the proposed MR site is typically evaluated with an rf survey. Usually, a survey can be arranged by the MR system manufacturer; alternately, the survey may be performed by private firms specializing in EMI/RFI testing services. The purpose of the rf survey is to characterize the environmental sources of rf interference in terms of frequency and strength. Using loop and dipole antennas, rf receiver, sweep generator, and recorder, the surveying engineer will develop a plot of rf signals in the immediate environment of the proposed system. The results of the survey will make it possible to categorize the environment as either moderate, isolated rf noise source, cluttered, or harsh. This information, combined with proposed clinical and research applications, will dictate the alternative approaches to rf screening.

Approaches to Radiofrequency Screening

There are several ways in which to protect the MR system from rf interference.[7] Internal system screening, full-room screening, magnetic field adjustment, or a com-

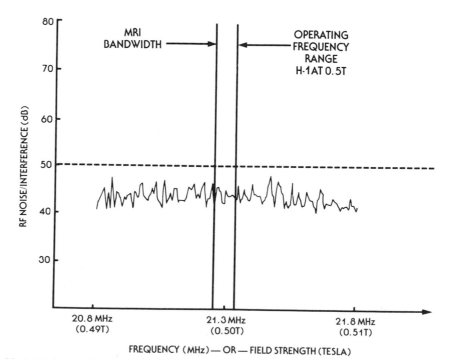

Figure 83–5. Moderate rf environment characterized by noise/interference below 50 dB. Shown above is a typical operating band width of a 0.5 tesla MR system.

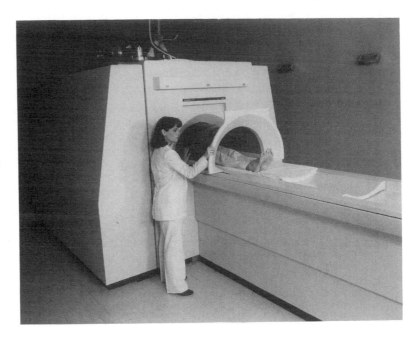

Figure 83–6. Internal rf screening used in moderate rf environments.

bination of two or more of these are options for the user; the choice can significantly affect overall system performance and cost.

In moderate rf environments (Fig. 83–5), internal screening of the MR images is sufficient to eliminate extraneous frequency bands. This type of screening is incorporated into the system itself and requires no further action by the user. Typically, this type of screening is composed of a copper mesh lining of the bore of the magnet and an extended mesh that pulls out over the table after the patient has been positioned. Figure 83–6 illustrates the pullout screen used for screening the two systems described in Table 83–3.

When interference includes narrow band sources, protection can be augmented by a minor adjustment in the system's magnetic field strength, to shift the resonant frequency of the element in question, usually hydrogen, away from the band of interference. This type of adjustment has no impact on clinical performance and provides a cost-effective, workable solution. It may be especially appropriate for 1.5 tesla systems operating in the vicinity of television transmitters. At 1.5 tesla, the resonant frequency for hydrogen is very close to channels 3 and 4 VHF television signals. A slight shift in magnetic field strength can often be sufficient to adjust the resonant frequency away from such interfering signals, as shown in Figure 83–7. When a potential site is cluttered with a wide range of narow band interference, appropriate rf screening may entail full-room shielding. Full-room screening requires a continuous network of screening on all surfaces, including the floor and ceiling. Special design of doors and windows is required

Table 83–3. RESONANT FREQUENCIES OF VARIOUS ELEMENTS AT TWO FIELD STRENGTHS

	0.5 Tesla	1.5 Tesla
Hydrogen	21.19 MHz	63.87 MHz
Carbon-13	*	16.06 MHz
Sodium-23	*	16.89 MHz
Phosphorus-31	*	25.84 MHz
Fluorine-19	*	60.07 MHz

* Imaging or spectroscopy for these elements is typically carried out only at field strengths of 1.5 tesla and above.

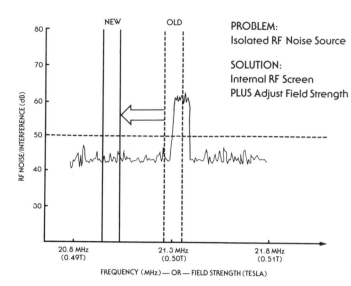

Figure 83–7. An isolated rf noise source can be avoided by a slight adjustment in the main magnetic field strength without impacting clinical performance.

to protect the integrity of the screening.[8] Figure 83–8 shows a schematic of the full-room shielding approach.

The effectiveness of full-room screening depends upon frequencies of importance, conductivity of the screening material, and the thickness of the material. One standard approach to full-room screening today utilizes aluminum or copper sheets laminated on both sides of particle board in 4 ft × 8 ft or 4 ft × 10 ft sections. Actual performance of the screening structure is critically dependent upon execution of joints, openings, and discontinuities. Of these, construction of the door is of utmost importance; improper design of the door can significantly degrade attenuation. In addition, ventilation lines, water pipes, and other mechanical devices must enter the screened area through wave guides constructed as an integral part of the modular rf panels.

Radiofrequency noise introduced by electric cables must be filtered with a filter rated equal to the overall room specification. One important specification must be added to full room screening. It is essential that the completed system be electrically isolated from the surrounding structure to avoid circulating currents. The completed room should be grounded only at one point to a positive earth ground.

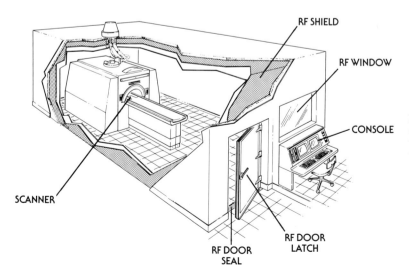

Figure 83–8. Full rf room screening entails rf door seal and latch, special windows, and filters on all electrical wiring going in or out of the room.

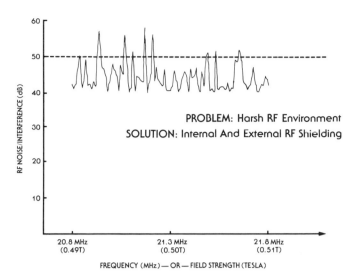

Figure 83–9. Radio frequency screening in unusually harsh rf environments.

The advantage of full-room screening is greater isolation of the system from outside interference. Disadvantages are high cost in terms of dollars and installation time and the "prisonlike" impression of a room with mesh-covered windows and a door with seals and heavy latch. The full-room screen is appropriate for cluttered rf environments where field strength adjustment does not offer the necessary flexibility to avoid all potential sources of transmitted interference. Finally, as shown in Figure 83–9, the combination of internal and external rf screening offers the most protection in harsh rf environments.

Depending on magnetic field strength and mix of ^{1}H, ^{13}C, ^{23}Na, ^{31}P, and ^{19}F applications, several frequency ranges need to be surveyed to determine an optimum radiofrequency screening strategy. In a moderate rf environment, internal rf screening of the patient is adequate. When additional rf interference includes narrow band sources, then adjustment in field strength can be used with internal screening. The advantages of the internal screen include lower cost and elimination of an rf door between operator and patient. In cluttered or harsh rf environments, total-room screening or total-room screening augmented with internal rf screening is desirable.

CRYOGENIC COOLING FOR SUPERCONDUCTING MAGNETS

Cryogens are a requirement unique to superconducting MR systems,[9] which make up the vast majority of imaging systems in use today. On installation, liquid helium, helium gas, and liquid nitrogen are required for filling and cooling the magnet. In addition, regular supplies of these liquids are required during operation for replacing evaporative losses. Use of a cryogenerator or reliquifier is an option that can reduce the consumption of liquid helium and eliminate the need for liquid nitrogen.

Cryogenic Effects

Care must be taken when handling cryogenic liquids. Helium boils at approximately 4.2° K (-452° F), and nitrogen at 77° K (-320° F). Any contact between these liquids, or their freshly evaporated vapors, and the skin must be absolutely avoided, since

Table 83–4. SOME PROPERTIES OF LIQUID NITROGEN AND LIQUID HELIUM

Physical Property	L Nitrogen	L Helium
Density (g/ml)	0.81	0.125
Boiling point at 1 bar		
degrees K	77	4.2
degrees F	−320	−452

severe frostbite will occur. Thus, cryogen use introduces a new dimension in staff training unless a service contract, obtained from the MR system manufacturer, is obtained.

In rare circumstances, superconducting magnets can "quench." The superconducting alloy of the magnet coil has no electrical resistance at its operating temperature (4.2° K). However, a very slight increase in temperature above the critical temperature results in the appearance of electrical resistance, causing the production of a large amount of heat. The magnet coils can withstand this heating, but the liquid helium will rapidly boil off and large volumes of cold helium vapors will be discharged. Separate venting pipes for boil-off and quench, connected to the outside, are required for safe venting of both helium and nitrogen gases.

Properties of Cryogenic Liquids

Some properties of liquid nitrogen and liquid helium are given in Table 83–4. Typical quantities of cryogens that are required for 0.5 tesla and 1.5 tesla magnets are given in Table 83–5. Liquid helium and liquid nitrogen must be obtained from a local supplier. It is usually distributed in well-insulated dewars with a capacity between 200 and 500 liters. Typical container properties for such dewars are given in Table 83–6. The nonmagnetic liquid helium dewar must be placed directly alongside the magnet for filling and top up so that site layout must include an access route from the delivery dock to the cryogen storage room to the examination room. Filing and top up of liquid cryogens are carried out with an insulated siphon as shown in Figure 83–10.

Quench Considerations

For safety reasons, helium and nitrogen gases released by normal evaporation must be vented to free air. As explained earlier, quenching of the magnet will result in the discharge of large quantities of helium and nitrogen gas. Separate venting for each is required. See Table 83–7 for typical gas venting system requirements. Venting must

Table 83–5. REQUIREMENTS FOR LIQUID NITROGEN AND LIQUID HELIUM

Cryogen Requirements	L Helium 0.5 Tesla/1.5 Tesla	L Nitrogen 0.5 Tesla/1.5 Tesla
Installation requirements	2000 L	2500 L
Capacity of tanks	750/1000 L	475/600 L
Minimum refill level	375/500 L	140/264 L
Evaporation rates		
Typical values	0.3 L/hr	1.1 L/hr
During gradient coil operation	0.4 L/hr	1.5 L/hr
Minimum refill interval	25–35 days	7 days
Atmospheric pressure range for safe operation	1013 millibars	±15%

Table 83–6. TYPICAL DEWAR PROPERTIES*

Container Properties	Liquid Helium		Liquid Nitrogen	
Capacity (liters)	275	500	160	220
Diameter	32 in	42 in	22 in	24 in
Height	59 in	72 in	52.5 in	57.5 in
Weight empty	450 lb	850 lb	187 lb	245 lb
Weight full	525 lb	999 lb	400 lb	676 lb
Loss rate percentage per day	1%	1%	1.4%	1.2%

* Note: These properties should be used for planning purposes only. Dimensions, weights, and other properties may vary by supplier.

also be provided in the cryogen storage room. Venting hardware between the cryostat turret and the outside of the building is required. All venting pipework and hardware should be insulated for safety purposes.

Cryogenerators and Reliquifiers

Installation of a cryogenerator (Fig. 83–11) or a helium refrigerator provides an electromechanical cooling element for the magnet, reducing consumption of liquid helium and eliminating liquid nitrogen. This approach minimizes down time associated with top-ups, which, without an electromechanical aid, would typically average 2 to 3 hours per week. The cryogenerator is typically located remotely from the system, connected to the magnet via a special vacuum-insulated transfer line. A reliquifier captures the boiled-off helium gas and reliquifies it. The liquid helium is returned to the magnet. Reliquifiers further reduce the demand for cryogens at the expense of increased electrical demands. Electromechanical systems to replace the continual need to supply cryogens is a rapidly developing trend. Financially, this reduces operating costs and labor but increases capital investment.

Superconducting magnet systems require low-temperature cryogenic fluids for cooling to maintain the superconducting properties of the magnet windings. Conven-

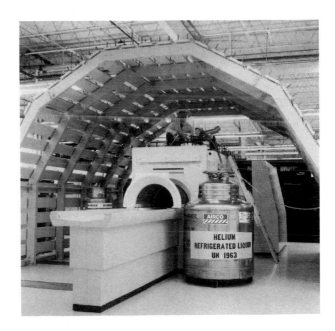

Figure 83–10. Filling or "top-up" of liquid cryogens requires expertise and approximately 2 hours per week for a typical superconducting MR system.

Table 83–7. TYPICAL CRYOGEN VENTING REQUIREMENTS*

Minimum Piping Dimensions
Helium
    4 inches ID for first 3 feet
    8 inches ID for next 21 feet
    12 inches ID for next 21 feet
Nitrogen
    2 inches ID for first 3 feet
    6 inches ID for next 21 feet
    10 inches ID for next 21 feet

* Note: Aluminum or stainless steel piping is required.

tionally, cryogens have been supplied on a refill basis following boil-off. Currently, the trend is to replace or reduce the operational cost in labor, down time, and materials with electromechanical cryogenerators and reqliquifiers. These cryogenic considerations often become a financial decision mitigated by logistics, risk management decisions, and operational needs.

MISCELLANEOUS CONSIDERATIONS INCLUDING SAFETY

There are several miscellaneous considerations, such as electric power requirements, magnet weights, air conditioning, water cooling of gradient power supplies and resistive magnet power supplies, and installation considerations, which are extremely important. It cannot be overemphasized that the variation between systems and manufacturers is significant; hence, an accurate description is only available from the Site Planning Guide supplied by the MR system manufacturer of interest. As an overview,

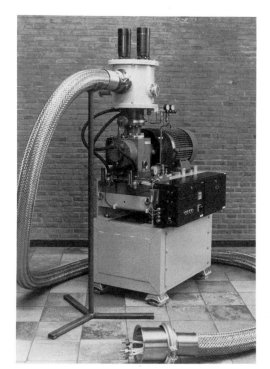

Figure 83–11. Commercially available cryogenerators reduce liquid helium consumption and eliminate liquid nitrogen consumption.

the AAPM has published a site planning checklist and planning form that identifies most topics that need to be considered.[10] This checklist is reproduced in Table 83–8.

There is a safety issue regarding the operation of MR systems due to a danger presented by inadvertent introduction of small ferromagnetic objects into the scanning room. Such objects can become dangerous projectiles, particularly if a patient is already

Table 83–8. SITE PLANNING CHECKLIST AND PLANNING FORM*

The following list identifies most topics to be considered in designing an MRI facility:

I. Functional Areas

Sq. Ft.

- The first group is normally required for an MRI facility:

  Scan room _____
  Control room _____
  Computer equipment room (include RF equipment and power supplies) _____
  Reading room (include physician's console) _____
  Cryogen storage _____

- The second group is required adjacent to the MRI facility but some areas can be shared with other imaging services when necessary or when spaces can be designed properly.

  Film processing _____
  Quality control and service _____
  Patient preparation, recovery, and emergency procedures area _____
  Patient reception and waiting _____
  Stretcher holding area _____
  Storage (supplies, magtapes, films, etc.) _____
  Washrooms _____
  Soiled utility _____
  Clean utility _____

- The third group lists additional functions, likely to be required, but which can be both remote from the MRI unit and shared with other services in extenuating circumstances.

  Secretarial and transcription services _____
  Conference area _____
  Additional storage (e.g. film library, magtapes) _____
  Offices _____

II. Construction and Access Considerations

Comments

Equipment transportation, unloading and
  installation access
Floor loading (including access routes)
Floor levelness
Ceiling heights (especially magnet room and
  access console)
Access for cryogens
Cryogen venting (normal and quench)
Controlled access to facility and well-controlled
  access to magnet room

III. Protecting the Magnetic Field

Possible Problems

Structural iron and steel (include reinforcing
  rod in concrete)
Other large ferrous structures or objects
Symmetrical location of ferrous structures
Moving ferrous objects (vehicles, lift trucks,
  elevators, carts, etc.)

IV. Protecting Surrounding Environment from Magnetic Fields

A three-dimensional survey of magnetically sensitive devices and equipment should be undertaken. Actual distance from the center of the magnet will depend on magnet field strength and design.

* From AAPM Site Planning for MRI Systems, Report 20, Task Group No. 2, Michael Bronskill, Chairman. Used with permission. Dec 1986.

in the magnet. Several MR system manufacturers recommend that the potential for a serious accident can be reduced significantly if metal detectors are installed at all points with direct access to the scanning room. These metal detectors can include both free-standing and hand-held models. An additional precaution is to minimize the number of access paths to the magnet.

REPRESENTATIVE SITE PLANS

A representative layout for a 1.5 tesla shielded magnet for a freestanding private diagnostic center incorporating MR, CT, and radiography and fluoroscopy is shown in Figure 83–12.[9] Such a center would require floor space of 4200 square feet. Figure 83–13 compares the installation of a 0.5 tesla and a 1.5 tesla magnet in an existing building.

The selection of a mobile or transportable MR system is a popular way to avoid many site planning issues, although new issues such as patient logistics, dealing with a remotely located imaging system, and restrictions on working floor space do emerge. A typical mobile MR system is shown in Figure 83–14. Offering more space is a transportable MR unit of somewhat larger dimensions than a mobile unit (60 ft × 12 ft versus 8 ft × 45 ft). Shown in Figure 83–15 is a site plan for one such transportable MR unit located in New York City, which is connected to an auxiliary trailer providing the added convenience of a patient waiting area, receptionist, dressing room, toilet, and physician's reading room. The transportable unit is designed to be relocated after one to two years of operation when space within the hospital becomes available for siting a new MR unit within the hospital.

Finally, more centers are now faced with the challenge of siting more than one MR unit at a given location. Figures 83–16 and 83–17 show actual solutions for the utilization of a 0.5 tesla and 1.5 tesla unit with a shared operators room and for the utilization of dual 1.5 tesla units.

The unique features of superconductive magnetic resonance imaging and spectroscopic systems that impact site planning and preparation include the magnetic fringe

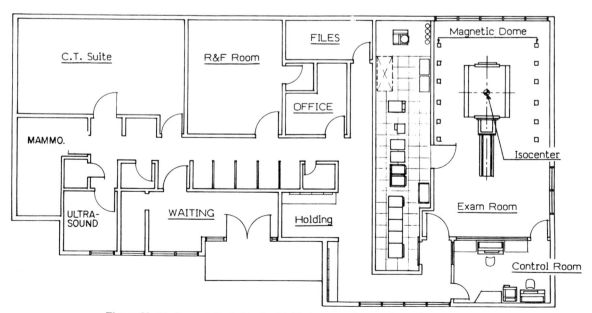

Figure 83–12. Layout for 1.5 tesla shielded magnet for a private diagnostic center.

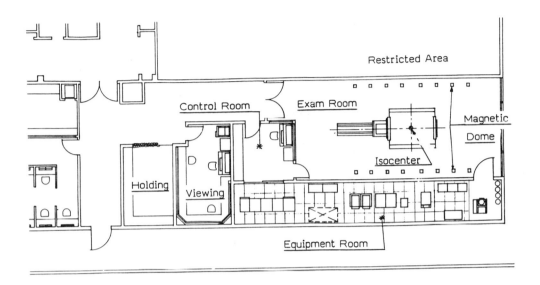

1.5T Shielded Layout

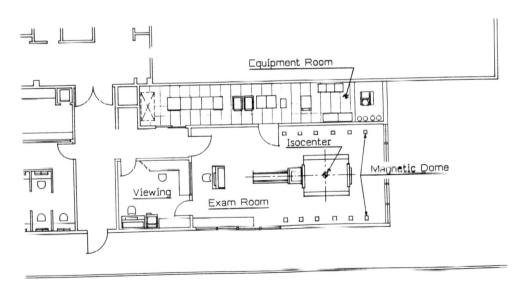

0.5T Shielded Layout

Figure 83–13. Layout for MR suite in an existing building with shielded 0.5 tesla magnet and 1.5 tesla magnet.

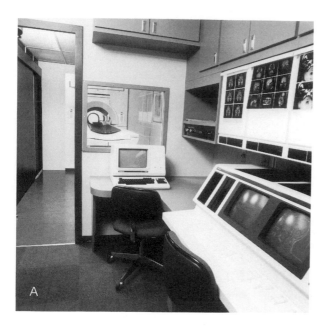

Figure 83–14. Interior view and floor plan of a 0.5 tesla Mobile MR system housed in a 8 ft × 45 ft van.

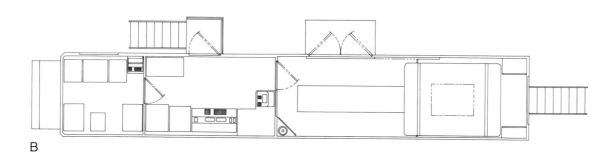

field, the system's reliance on a controlled radiofrequency environment, and the cryogenic cooling of the magnet. Although greatly oversimplified, the basic principle of MR site planning is to protect the system from the environment and the environment from the system. This requires magnetic shielding and radiofrequency screening, although the former requirement may be simply met by placement of the magnet far enough away from interfering environmental elements. Cryogenic considerations may be met by insuring that an appropriate supply of liquid nitrogen and liquid helium is always available. Alternatively, the use of liquid helium may be reduced and the use of liquid nitrogen may be totally eliminated with the use of cryogenerators at the site.

Since the performance of an MR system is dependent on the outcome of the successful site planning and preparation phase, it is extremely important to consult the aid of an experienced site planner. This consultive step should avoid any potential mistakes in the final facility layout, ensure an appropriate access route for the magnet, and help reduce costs. Further, reliance on and adherence to the recommendations of a site planner who is duly authorized by the system manufacturer that is finally selected may have important implications should anything go wrong during or after installation. Rather than dwell on negative issues it should be pointed out that in 1986 the key elements of site planning are well understood by reputable system manufacturers and

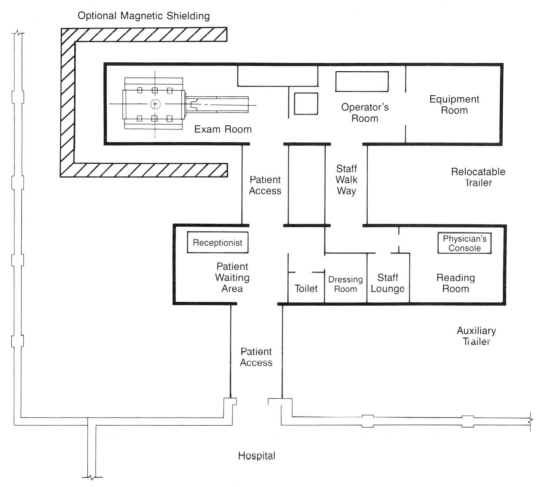

Figure 83–15. Actual site plan for a shielded, relocatable MR with auxiliary trailer for patients and physician's reading room.

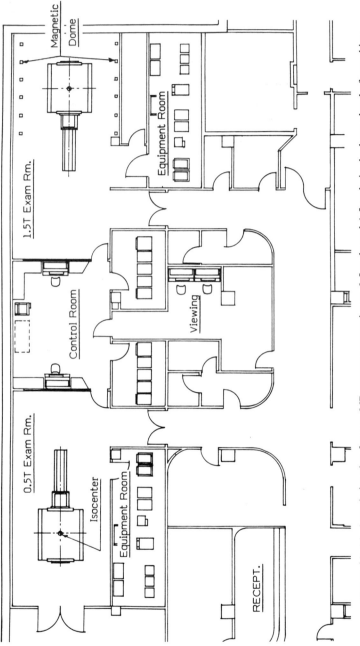

Figure 83–16. Actual site plan for two MR systems operating at 0.5 tesla and 1.5 tesla in the lower level of a parking ramp in New York City.

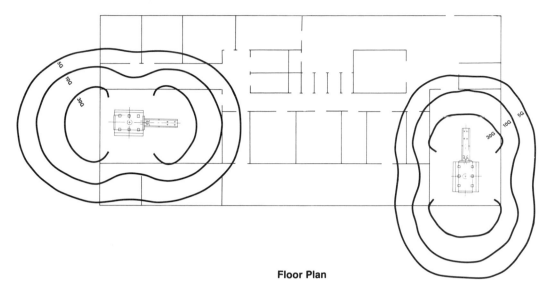

Floor Plan

Two 1.5 Tesla Systems

Figure 83–17. Actual site plan for dual 1.5 tesla MR systems operating in a freestanding facility in Zurich.

the key concerns for today include cost containment, efficient space utilization, and operational efficiency.[12]

Acknowledgments

The authors wish to thank the Site Planning Team at Philips Medical Systems, Inc. in Shelton, Connecticut, and at the N. V. Philips, Medical Systems Division, Best, The Netherlands, for help with this chapter. In addition, the support of Diane Ciaramella and Dan Zeno in the preparation of this manuscript was invaluable.

References

1. Einstein SG, Hilal SK: Site planning design: Influences and implementation. *In* Kressel HY (ed): Magnetic Resonance Annual 1984. New York, Raven Press.
2. Pavlicek W, MacIntyre WGR, O'Donnell J, Felglin D: Special architectural considerations in designing a magnetic resonance (MR) facility. *In* Esser P, Johnston RE (eds): Technology of Nuclear Magnetic Resonance. New York, The Society of Nuclear Medicine, pp 233–252.
3. Einstein S, Hilal SK, Maudsley A, Simon H, Sano R: Magnetic shielding for small room installation of a 1.5 Tesla NMR system. Magn Reson Med *1*:66, 1984.
4. Einstein S, Maudsley A, Mun SK, Simon H, Hilal SK, Sano R, Roeschmann P: Installation of high-field NMR systems into existing clinical facilities: Special considerations. *In* Esser P, Johnston RE (eds): Technology of Nuclear Magnetic Resonance. New York, The Society of Nuclear Medicine, pp 217–231.
5. American Hospital Association, Hospital Technology Series Guideline Report Vol. 4, Numbers 3 and 4. NMR—Issues for 1985 and Beyond, Richard diMonda, 1985.
6. Philips Medical Systems, Inc.: An innovative approach to magnetic shielding for MRI. Medical Applications News, November, 1984.
7. Steidley JW, Schlemm PJ, Conn W, Levsen H: A comparison of four approaches to radiofrequency shielding of MR imaging scanners. Radiology *156*:209, 1985.
8. The Keene Corporation: Ray Proof Division. Series 81. Catalog Number 812 (1983).
9. Philips Medical Systems, Inc.: MR Imaging Systems Site Planning Guide, 1985.
10. Bronskill M, et al: Site planning guide for MRI systems, Report 20, Task Group No. 2. Am Assoc Physicists Med, Dec 1980.
11. Einstein SG, Hilal SK: Site planning design: Influences and implementation. *In* Kressel HY (ed): Magnetic Resonance Annual, New York, Raven Press, 1985.
12. Patton JA, Kulkarni MV, Craig JK, Wolfe OH, Price RR, Partain CL, James AE Jr: Techniques, pitfalls and artifacts in magnetic resonance imaging. RadioGraphics *7*:505, 1987.

84

Bioeffects

S. JULIAN GIBBS
A. EVERETTE JAMES, JR.

There can be no doubt that effects are produced in tissue by the process of magnetic resonance imaging (MRI); without such effects there would be no signal and thus no possibility of creating an image. At present we have no conclusive evidence that these transient effects at the level of the atomic nucleus are in any way associated with the continued well-being of the exposed individual, at least at field strengths currently in clinical use. Many discussions may have considered the possibility of such adverse effects of MRI, but very little of substance has been written dealing specifically with such effects. A great deal, however, is known about biological effects of magnetic fields and of radio frequency (rf) irradiation. We are thus forced to rely on our knowledge of these components of the MRI process, and to speculate that the whole of any possible bioeffect is no greater than the sum of its parts.

This chapter will briefly review data detailing possible biological effects of static and time-varying magnetic fields and of rf radiation and the implications for MRI. This review is intended to be neither encyclopedic nor exhaustive. Furthermore, interactions with metallic implants, surgical clips, prosthetic devices, and pacemakers are not considered. This chapter is thus limited to consideration of biological effects in healthy tissue.

Concepts and approaches of traditional radiobiology are not necessarily appropriate for the study of the bioeffects of MRI. Biological effects of ionizing radiation, in the dose range of interest in diagnostic imaging, are stochastic in nature. They include induction of cancer, mutation, and perhaps certain congenital effects from exposure in utero, especially mental retardation. In an exposed individual, the probability of occurrence is a function of dose, which implies the absence of a threshold. That is, a stochastic effect is the result of an infrequent but catastrophic event resulting in the structural alteration of a molecule of biological importance (generally accepted to be DNA), such that the function of the gene or gene product is altered. This can occur, especially with sparsely ionizing radiation (x-rays or gamma rays), since a single interaction with tissue results in the deposition of a relatively large amount of energy in a very small volume. Thus, at the microscopic level, dose is very heterogeneous. The distribution of energy deposition with magnetic fields or rf irradiation is not of the nature of rare catastrophic effects on molecules. Thus bioeffects of MRI should be nonstochastic in nature: severity of the effect is proportional to "dose," implying the presence of a threshold of field strength or rf intensity, below which the level of effect is clinically insignificant. There is reasonable evidence supporting the concept that this "dose" from current MRI apparatus is below the biologically significant threshold. However, we must be cautious that future applications do not exceed it.

The confirmed effects that must be kept in mind when considering patient risks from MRI are electric currents induced by magnetic fields and tissue heating from rf

Table 84–1. CYTOGENETIC EFFECTS OF GAMMA RAYS AND MRI*

Effect	Control	Gamma Ray (0.28 Gy)	Gamma Ray (0.41 Gy)	MRI (2.2 T, 3 h)
Transformed foci (frequency $\times 10^5$)	5.0	4.2		1.8
Chromosome aberrations (per cell $\times 10^2$)	3.8		10†	0.3
Sister chromatid exchanges (per chromosome)	0.192		0.257†	0.173

* Data from Geard et al.[14]
† Significantly different from controls ($P < 0.05$).

irradiation. Literally hundreds of reports may be found in the literature dealing with other biological effects of magnetic fields and radio frequencies detected by physiologic, biochemical, or behavioral measurements. These are largely unsubstantiated. Virtually all reported positive findings are contradicted by negative reports under essentially equivalent circumstances. Review of all these reports is beyond the scope of this chapter. The interested reader is referred to recent reviews[25,31] or the nearest academic library for computer search of the world's literature. The persistent reader may find published reports that contradict many of the conclusions of this chapter.

One can find published support for the notion that virtually any possible biological effect of MRI exists and that it does not exist.[9] For example, using techniques of classical radiobiology, Malinin et al. reported in 1976 that exposure of L-929 and WI-38 cells in culture to static magnetic fields (0.5 tesla) for 4 to 8 hr induced a significant incidence of malignant transformations.[19] However, other investigators have not confirmed this observation. For example, Wolff et al. reported no induction of chromosome aberrations, sister chromatid exchanges, or suppression of DNA synthesis from exposure of Chinese hamster ovary or HeLa cells to MRI conditions (0.35 tesla) for 4 to 14 hr.[35] Thomas and Morris in 1981 reported no evidence of mutational or lethal events in bacteria exposed to static magnetic fields of 1 tesla for 1 or 5 hr or to MRI imaging conditions (0.094 tesla) for 40 m or 5 hr.[32] Also in 1981 Cooke and Morris reported no evidence of chromosome aberrations or sister chromatid exchanges from exposure of human lymphocytes in culture to static magnetic fields (0.5 and 1 tesla) for 1 hr or to conditions of MRI (not further specified).[11] Schwartz and Crooks reported in 1982 no increase in the frequency of mutant CHO cells determined by the hypoxanthine-guanine phosphoribosyl transferase assay from exposure to MRI conditions (0.35 tesla) for 24 hr.[29] Finally, Geard et al. found no evidence of malignant transformation, sister chromatid exchange, or chromosome aberrations (Table 84–1) from exposure of cultured mammalian cells to MRI conditions (up to 2.7 tesla) for up to 17 hr.[14] It should be emphasized that these are very sensitive assays of damage to the genetic apparatus of the cell. The absence of effect of MRI thus, although not conclusive proof of total safety, supports the notion that such effects are at most extremely unlikely.

STATIC MAGNETIC FIELDS

Potential health effects of static (or extremely low frequency) magnetic fields (SMF) have been investigated extensively for many years, principally in relation to occupational health for workers in industries that utilize such fields. Recent epidemiologic studies found increased incidence of leukemia and other cancers among aluminum workers and others occupationally exposed to SMFs up to 57 millitesla.[22,26] However, the workers were also exposed occupationally to a variety of chemicals, including hydrocarbon particulates, and it is not clear that exposure to magnetic fields was a contributing factor to the excess cancer.

Confirmed effects of SMF fall into two classes: (1) transient effects of no long-term significance, which disappear when the subject is removed from the field, and (2) effects that cannot be confirmed when other investigators attempt to repeat the experiments.[9]

The significant biological effect of SMF that has been demonstrated consistently and repeatably is induced electric current via flow,[28] which uses the well-known principle of induction of a current in a mass in motion in a magnetic field (consider the ordinary electric generator). Flow potential is given by

$$E = Bdv$$

where E = flow potential; B = flux density; d = vessel diameter; and v = flow velocity. Flow perpendicular to the magnetic field produces a potential across the diameter of the vessel. Since with conventional MRI systems the SMF is parallel to the long axis of the body, the major flow current would be induced across the diameter of the aortic arch, where it is about 16 mV/T in man. However, this level is across the diameter of the aorta. Across the dimensions of single cells, the electromagnetic field, EMF, can be regarded as insignificant. This effect is the most likely explanation for the electrocardiographic changes seen in experimental animals subjected to high SMF. In primates these effects have been shown to be transient; they disappear when the subject is removed from the magnetic field, and no biologically significant sequelae can be demonstrated.[30] It must be emphasized that these findings do not demonstrate an effect of magnetic fields on the conduction apparatus of the heart; they merely demonstrate an additional signal, induced in flowing blood by the magnetic field, that is detected by electrocardiography. However, there could be some concern regarding patients with arrhythmias.

In theory, the ionic currents of nerve conduction could be influenced in a manner similar to flow in a magnetic field. However, relatively simple calculations demonstrate that such interactions are very weak; fields of at least 24 tesla should be required to produce a 10 percent reduction in conductivity.[34] This conclusion has been verified, at least in part, experimentally; no measurable effect of a 2 tesla SMF on conduction or other bioelectric properties in isolated frog sciatic nerve has been detected.[31]

Some biological molecules and subcellular structures have diamagnetic susceptibility, which may vary with direction as compared to the axis of the magnetic field. If the field is of the order of 2 tesla or less, then the magnetization energy for these small structures is approximately 10^{-12} to 10^{-14} ergs, which is of the same order as thermal energy at body temperature.[9] Torque may be exerted on an organized structure containing a large number of such systems from magnetic fields currently in use in clinical MRI. Examples are seen in effects on retinal rod orientation[15] or alignment of sickled erythrocytes[24] in fields of 1 tesla. It is possible that orientation effects on bacteria,[7] animals,[23] and even man[2] may involve this mechanism.

TIME-VARYING MAGNETIC FIELDS

The major confirmed effect of time-varying magnetic fields (TVMF) is induction of electric fields in excitable tissue (muscle, nerve, sensory receptors) as[28]

$$E = \frac{r}{2} \frac{dB}{dt}$$

where E = electric field; r = inductive loop radius; and dB/dt = rate of change of magnetic field. Current density is given by

$$J = E\sigma$$

where J = current density and σ = tissue conductivity.

These effects (Table 84–2) are well documented in the literature dealing with biological effects of electric currents. Some are known to the author (and presumably the reader) from personal experience of accidental contact with electrodes. All of these effects exhibit clear thresholds and are highly frequency dependent, with maximum sensitivities at frequencies below 100 Hz. Current passing between electrodes is simple to measure; thus, thresholds are usually expressed in terms of electrode current. Induced currents within the body (such as from TVMF) are more difficult to measure and are generally expressed in terms of current density. Computation of threshold dB/dt for these effects can at best provide only a rather crude estimate, because of the complex interplay of pulse width and pulse frequency.[31]

From Table 84–2 it may be seen that phosphenes (the sensation of flashes of light) are the most sensitive of these effects, having been reported from AC currents as small as 10 μA RMS at 20 Hz.[1] The estimated tissue current density of 10 to 20 mA m^{-2} required at that frequency could be produced in an inductive loop of radius 10 cm (about the size of the adult human head) by a TVMF changing at the rate of about 2 tesla s^{-1}. It is important to note that field amplitude must be at least 10 millitesla, and pulse width at least 2 ms, for this effect.[4] Ventricular fibrillation requiring current density of 1 to 10 A m^{-2} might require magnetic field strength changing at more than 50 tesla s^{-1} at 60 Hz;[16] other estimates place this threshold at more than 100 and up to 1000 tesla s^{-1}.[9] Higher frequencies, such as those used in MRI, would require greater rate of change of field strength.

Recent reports of a possible health effect of exposure to power-frequency (60 Hz) TVMF have incited public concern, probably at an unwarranted emotional level.[31] These epidemiologic studies have purported to demonstrate an association between exposure to residential or occupational TVMF and increased cancer incidence.[33] Other similar studies have found no such association.[13] These studies are subject to question on grounds of small sample sizes, technical factors such as dosimetry, and statistical methods.

One additional effect is worthy of mention because of its clinical application. TVMFs were demonstrated in clinical reports in the 1970s to be of value in management of nonunion of bone fractures.[5] It has been recently suggested, however, that the immobilization required for the procedure may be at least a contributing factor.[3]

Table 84–2. THRESHOLDS FOR ELECTRICAL EFFECTS ON EXCITABLE TISSUES*

Effect	Threshold Electrode Current (mA)	Estimated Threshold Current Density (Am^{-2})	Frequency (Hz)	Approximate Threshold dB/dt ($T\ s^{-1}$)
Phosphene production	0.01	0.01–0.02	20	2
Cutaneous perception	0.5	1–10	60	
Release				
Female	6	1–10	60	
Male	9	1–10	60	
Thoracic tetany	18–22	1–10	60	60–1200
Ventricular fibrillation				
Child	30		60	
Adult	60–120	1–10	60	200–1000

* Data from Saunders and Orr.[28]

RADIO FREQUENCIES

It is well known that rf irradiation in the frequency range below about 100 MHz, such as commonly employed in MRI, deposits energy in tissue in the form of heat. Energy deposition in tissue is a function of rf frequency and power density; duration of the exposure; tissue properties such as conductivity, dielectric constant, and density; and coupling between the rf coils and the subject. Heating is also affected by rate of heat loss from tissue, principally by circulating blood in deep tissues. In the nineteenth century d'Arsonval demonstrated that such irradiation does not affect excitable tissue as do time-varying magnetic fields of much lower frequencies. The meaningful parameter is specific absorption rate (SAR), given by

$$SAR = \frac{\sigma E^2 D}{2\rho}$$

where σ = tissue conductivity; $E/\sqrt{2}$ = average induced electric field; D = duty cycle or ratio of pulse duration to repetition interval; and ρ = tissue density.

Since the average induced electric field is a function of frequency, SAR is directly proportional to frequency.[8] It is clear that the human body can dissipate heat indefinitely at the rate of about 1 W kg^{-1}, for that is average basal metabolic rate. SARs in this range should be well tolerated. Higher SARs might present problems in areas of poor blood supply (such as the testis) or no blood supply (such as the lens of the eye). Most other tissues are well equipped to dissipate excess heat. Because of the poor heat dissipation and recognized sensitivity to increased temperature, the testis (Table 84–3) and the optic lens have been used as models to study threshold effects. It has been shown by Saunders and Kowalczuk[27] that pathologic changes are induced in rodent testes from SARs of at least 20 W kg^{-1}. Dosimetric data for the lens are not adequate to specify thresholds. In man, acute lens opacification appears to involve thermal damage that occurs at exposure intensities of at least 100 mW cm^{-2}.[10] The expected temperature rise, in the absence of heat dissipation (e.g., blood flow), is then

$$\Delta T = \frac{SAR\ t}{h}$$

where t = time and h = specific heat.

Living cells can tolerate only a few degrees' increase in temperature and then only for brief exposures. Research in hyperthermia, now in widespread use for treatment of late-stage cancer, indicates that no mammalian cells can survive temperatures greater than 42° C for more than a few minutes.[12] Attainment of such temperature would require

Table 84–3. EFFECT OF MICROWAVE RADIATION IN THE TESTIS*

Effect	Spermatogonia Type B	Early Primary Spermatocytes	Late Primary and Secondary Spermatocytes
Microwave response			
Threshold SAR (W kg^{-1})	45	23	18
LD$_{50}$ SAR (W kg^{-1})	53	29	34
Temperature response			
Threshold (° C)	–	39	38
LD$_{50}$ (° C)	–	40	41

* Data from Saunders and Kowalczuk.[27]

a *SAR* of 20 W kg^{-1} for 20 minutes—in the absence of any heat dissipation—which must then be maintained for a sufficient time to produce the effect.

Heating of tissue produces the characteristic stress response, activating thermoregulatory mechanisms via neuroendocrine pathways.[21] At *SAR* > 3 W kg^{-1}, ACTH-mediated elevation of circulating steroids has been observed in rats.[17] There is also depression of circulating thyroid hormone levels, associated with decreased output of TSH from the pituitary.[18] The major result is alteration of blood flow in an attempt to dissipate the excess heat. Exposure of dogs to microwave frequencies with *SAR* > 4 W kg^{-1} leads to increasing body temperature followed by stabilization of temperature as the thermoregulatory response takes effect. Continued exposure, however, may lead to disruption of the thermoregulatory apparatus and death of the animal.[21]

It is clear that rf in sufficient intensity, appropriate frequency, and sufficient exposure time can produce a biological effect—heat—that is exploited clinically in oncology and in physical therapy. There are conflicting reports, however, as to threshold intensities for production of these effects.[21] Much of the conflict is thought to be the result of inadequate or inaccurate dosimetry. The issue is not resolved.

A few reported nonthermal effects are worthy of mention. Soviet scientists have accumulated over the last 30 years evidence that low-level rf fields in the microwave frequency range can alter neurological, cardiovascular, endocrine, and other systems.[20] Western scientists have not corroborated these findings, but collaborative efforts between scientists in the United States and the Union of Soviet Socialist Republics have confirmed some of them. A second nonthermal effect of considerable interest was the observation of altered binding of calcium to neuron surfaces by microwave irradiation with amplitude modulation at very low frequency.[6] These findings should provide impetus for further investigation of nonthermal effects of rf.

Conclusions

It seems reasonable to conclude that MRI, as presently practiced, carries negligible risk to the patient. Literally thousands of patients have undergone MRI examination, with no reports of adverse effects. It must be remembered, however, that cancer was not regarded as a risk of low-level ionizing radiation until excess leukemia was detected in Japanese atomic bomb survivors beginning about 1948. Long-term follow-up of patients subjected to MRI will not be available for several years. However, the following conclusions can be drawn for the present generation of MRI devices:[31]

1. No significant adverse affects have been found in mammals from exposure to SMF levels up to 2 tesla. Transient electrical effects are produced, but there are no serious sequelae from brief exposures at this level. Further investigation is required to assess the safety of possible future imaging systems operating at higher static field levels.

2. No significant harmful effects have been confirmed from time-varying fields that induce tissue current densities less than 10 mA m^{-2}, requiring time variations of 1 to 2 tesla s^{-1}. A few transient alterations have been reported, such as phosphenes at 1.3 tesla s^{-1}, but they are completely reversible.

3. It is clear that exposure to rf can lead to irreversible damage if heating exceeds normal heat dissipation capacity of the body as controlled by the thermoregulatory apparatus. Nonthermal effects of lower levels have been reported, but further investigation is required to assess the mechanism and the relationship to patient risk from MRI.

4. There is no consistent, confirmed epidemiologic evidence of adverse effects of either magnetic fields or rf in human populations.

References

1. Adrian DJ: Auditory and visual sensations stimulated by low-frequency electric currents. Radio Sci *12*:243, 1977.
2. Baker RR: Goal orientation by blindfolded humans after long-distance displacement: Possible involvement of a magnetic sense. Science *210*:555, 1980.
3. Barker AT, Dixon RA, Sharrard WJW, Sutcliffe ML: Pulsed magnetic field therapy for tibial non-union. Lancet *1*:994, 1984.
4. Barlow HB, Kohn HI, Walsh EG: Visual sensations aroused by magnetic fields. Am J Physiol *148*:372, 1947.
5. Bassett CAL, Pilla AA, Pawluk RJ: A non-operative salvage of surgically-resistant pseudoarthroses and non-unions by pulsing electromagnetic fields. Clin Orthoped *124*:128, 1977.
6. Bawin SM, Kaczmarek LK, Adey WR: Effects of modulated VHF fields on the central nervous system. Ann NY Acad Sci *247*:74, 1975.
7. Blakemore R: Magnetotactic bacteria. Science *190*:377, 1975.
8. Bottomley PA, Andrew ER: RF magnetic field penetration, phase shift, and power dissipation in biological tissue: Implications for NMR imaging. Phys Med Biol *23*:630, 1978.
9. Budinger TF: Nuclear magnetic resonance (NMR) in vivo studies: Known thresholds for health effects. J Comp Assist Tomogr *5*:800, 1981.
10. Cleary SF: Microwave cataractogenesis. Proc IEEE *68*:49, 1980.
11. Cooke P, Morris PG: The effects of NMR exposure on living organisms. II. A genetic study of human lymphocytes. Br J Radiol *54*:622, 1981.
12. Dewey WC, Hopwood LE, Sapareto SA, Gerweck LE: Cellular responses to combinations of hyperthermia and radiation. Radiology *123*:463, 1977.
13. Fulton JP, Cobb S, Preble L, Leone L, Forman E: Electrical wiring configurations and childhood leukemia in Rhode Island. Am J Epidemiol *111*:292, 1980.
14. Geard CR, Osmak RS, Hall EJ, Simon HE, Maudsley AA, Hilal SK: Magnetic resonance and ionizing radiation: A comparative evaluation in vitro of oncogenic and genotoxic potential. Radiology *152*:199, 1984.
15. Hong FT, Mauzerall D, Mauro A: Magnetic anisotropy and the orientation of retinal rods in a homogeneous magnetic field. Proc Natl Acad Sci US *68*:1283, 1971.
16. Kugelberg J: Electrical induction of ventricular fibrillation in the human heart. Scand J Thorac Cardiovasc Surg *10*:237, 1976.
17. Lotz WG, Michaelson SM: Temperature and corticosterone relationships in microwave-exposed rats. J Appl Physiol *44*:438, 1978.
18. Lu ST, Lotz WG, Michaelson SM: Advances in microwave-induced neuroendocrine effect: The concept of stress. Proc IEEE *68*:73, 1980.
19. Malanin GI, Gregory WD, Morelli L, Sharma VK, Houck JC: Evidence of morphological and physiological transformation of mammalian cells by strong magnetic fields. Science *194*:844, 1976.
20. McRee DI: Soviet and Eastern European research on biological effects of microwave radiation. Proc IEEE *68*:84, 1980.
21. Michaelson SM: Microwave biological effects: An overview. Proc IEEE *68*:40, 1980.
22. Milham S: Mortality from leukemia in workers exposed to electrical and magnetic fields. N Engl J Med *307*:249, 1982.
23. Moore BR: Is the homing pigeon's map geomagnetic? Nature *285*:69, 1982.
24. Murayama M: Orientation of sickled erythrocytes in a magnetic field. Nature *206*:420, 1965.
25. Persson BRR, Stahlberg F: Potential health hazards and safety aspects of clinical NMR examinations. Radiation Physics Department, Lasarettet, S221 85 Lund, Sweden, 1984.
26. Rockette HE, Arena VC: Mortality studies of aluminum reduction plant workers: Potroom and carbon department. J Occup Med *25*:549, 1983.
27. Saunders RD, Kowalczuk CI: Effects of 2.45 GHz microwave radiation and heat on mouse spermatogenic epithelium. Int J Radiat Biol *40*:623, 1981.
28. Saunders RD, Orr JS: Biologic effects of NMR. *In* Partain CL, James AE, Rollo FD, Price RR (eds): Nuclear Magnetic Resonance (NMR) Imaging. Philadelphia, W.B. Saunders Co., 1983. p 383–396.
29. Schwartz JL, Crooks, LE: NMR imaging produces no observable mutations or cytotoxicity in mammalian cells. Am J Roetgenol *139*:583, 1982.
30. Tenforde TS, Gaffey CT, Moyer BR, Budinger TF: Cardiovascular alterations in Macaca monkeys exposed to stationary magnetic fields: experimental observations and theoretical analysis. Bioelectromagnetics *4*:1, 1983.
31. Tenforde TS, Budinger TF: Biological effects and physical safety aspects of NMR imaging and in vivo spectroscopy. *In* Thomas SR, Dickson RL (eds): NMR in Medicine: Instrumentation and Clinical Applications. Proceedings of the American Association of Physicists in Medicine 1985 Summer School. American Association of Physicists in Medicine, 1986.
32. Thomas A, Morris PG: The effects of NMR exposure on living organisms. I. A microbial assay. Br J Radiol *54*:615, 1981.
33. Wertheimer N, Leeper E: Electrical wiring configurations and childhood cancer. Am J Epidemiol *109*:273, 1979.
34. Wikswo JP Jr, Barach JP: An estimate of the steady magnetic field strength required to influence nerve conduction. IEEE Trans Biomed Engr BME *27*:722, 1980.
35. Wolff S, Crooks LE, Brown P, Howard R, Painter RB: Tests for DNA and chromosomal damage induced by nuclear magnetic resonance imaging. Radiology *136*:707, 1980.

85

On the Safety of Nuclear Magnetic Resonance Imaging and Spectroscopy Systems

Successful magnetic resonance imaging (MRI) of the proton structure of living tissues requires the simultaneous exposure of a patient to intense static magnetic fields that align nuclei with a net magnetic moment in the direction of the applied field; to matched radio frequency (rf) magnetic fields that excite the aligned nuclei in a resonance state; and to rapidly changing (pulsed) magnetic fields that create a gradient of excitable nuclei with slightly different resonance frequencies so that they can be identified spatially in the plane of tissues being examined. The principles of imaging with magnetic resonance are discussed, for example, in recent reviews.[40,97]

Static magnetic field strengths in existing and planned systems vary from less than a hundred to a few thousand millitesla (mT); pulsed fields from a rate of change of a few hundred mT per second (mT s^{-1}) to a few tens of thousands of mT s^{-1}, involving a variety of waveforms, pulse widths, and repetition rates; and to rf fields in a frequency range of 1 to 100 megahertz (MHz), equivalent in the body to an absorbed averaged thermal energy of up to about 4 watts per kilogram (W kg^{-1}). Substantial portions of the body may be exposed during imaging for periods of a few tens of minutes if multiple exposure sequences are used; and it should be borne in mind that seriously ill patients may be exposed.

Topical magnetic resonance (TMR), otherwise referred to as magnetic resonance spectroscopy (MRS), is a technique for measuring the concentration of nuclei in molecules of living cells by the spectroscopic separation of images of their molecular "hosts." Nuclei heavier than the hydrogen nucleus (e.g., carbon-13, sodium-23, phosphorus-31) need more energy for excitation, and they are present in living tissue in much smaller concentrations than hydrogen-1. Phosphorus-31, for example, is two thousand times less abundant than hydrogen atoms, and magnetic fields in excess of about 2000 mT are required to excite nuclei to the point where relaxation can be detected. Because of the decreased sensitivity, the output and stability of the magnets need to be greater than for imaging, and more attention needs to be paid to designing equipment to avoid hazards.

In addition to measuring changes in the metabolism of phosphorus and carbon-containing molecules and the concentrations of electrolytes in living tissues, it is now becoming possible to study the metabolism of drugs in vivo. As an example, a non-invasive technique is being developed to "image" the uptake of fluorine-19–tagged anticancer drugs into tumor cells in order to gain insight into the drugs' clinical effectiveness.[68]

An indication of the progress being made in imaging and spectroscopy is given in a recent British Medical Bulletin[17] devoted to the clinical applications of MRI and MRS, and in abstracts of the proceedings of the 4th Annual Meeting of the Society of Magnetic Resonance in Medicine.[80]

POTENTIAL HEALTH HAZARDS WITH EXPOSURE TO MRI AND MRS

The photon energy exchanges that occur when nuclei are excited and relaxed are extremely small when compared with the photon energy released during ionization of atoms, and this has led some investigators to the view that the long-term risks of developing cancer or genetic damage as a result of cellular DNA damage following exposure are negligible.

There are certainly few positively identified effects that could be considered to be hazardous. Many of the early reported results on the effects of static, pulsed, and rf magnetic fields at the cellular and animal level of organization have not been confirmed by more recent experiments under carefully controlled conditions; the evidence of adverse effects in man is based largely upon anecdotal accounts and poorly conducted epidemiological surveys; and many thousands of patients have now been exposed without incident. Nevertheless it would seem premature to dismiss the possibility of long-term detrimental effects in our present state of knowledge.

Advice upon recommended levels of exposure must therefore be judged against this background. It can at best be provisional and should be revised as new and substantial facts become available. Guidelines have been issued by the National Radiological Protection Board (NRPB),[64,65] in which it is recommended that whole (or substantial) body exposure of patients should not exceed 2500 mT for static magnetic fields and 20,000 mT s^{-1} for time-varying magnetic fields for periods of magnetic field change longer than 10 ms. Exposure to rf magnetic fields should be such that the increase in body (core) temperature does not exceed 1° C. This is thought to be achievable by limiting the whole-body specific absorption rate to 0.4 W kg^{-1}. More relaxed limits can be used for time-varying magnetic fields when the periods of magnetic field change are shorter than 10 ms and an additional factor is introduced to prevent localized overheating of tissues from rf fields (i.e., 4 W kg^{-1} for any 1 g of tissue). Similar guidelines have been issued by the United States Bureau of Radiological Health[90] and the West German Federal Health Office;[33] the differences in limits, where they exist, are discussed later in this chapter. The basis for these guidelines is discussed in more depth in reviews by Budinger,[18] Saunders and Smith,[74] and Bernhardt and Kossel.[10] The NRPB guidelines additionally recommend that patients fitted with ferromagnetic aneurysm clips should be excluded; that it would be prudent to exclude women in the first three months of pregnancy; and that care should be taken when examining patients fitted with cardiac pacemakers or large metallic prostheses.

For operators of the equipment, the recommended limits of exposure to static magnetic fields are about one hundredth of those for exposure of patients; and the limits for rf magnetic fields are the same as those applied to patients.

In the absence of firm biological data, classic observations in electromagnetism initially provided a rational basis for assessing the potential hazards of magnetic resonance: namely that strong magnets attract ferromagnetic objects; that an electromotive force can be induced in a conducting wire if either the wire is moved in a static magnetic field or the magnetic field is pulsed while the wire remains stationary; and that absorbed rf radiation causes atoms in an absorber to oscillate more vigorously and that this energy can be released in the form of heat.

Classic physiological studies had demonstrated that electrical impulses pass rapidly along neurons by means of a localized, reversible depolarization of the nerve membrane. This was first demonstrated in isolated nerve preparations attached to muscle fibers by applying electrical currents directly to the nerve through miniature electrodes and by observing the muscle fibers contract. It is possible using this type of preparation to measure the threshold current density for neuromuscular irritability as a function of frequency, waveform, and pulse repetition.

A discussion of potentially harmful effects based upon a knowledge of these fundamental properties of electromagnetic radiations and of excitable tissues may conveniently be separated into three parts: the response of patients acutely exposed to intense field strengths; of staff who are exposed intermittently to much less intense field strengths; and of the occasional "passer-by" exposed to extremely low field strengths.

There are two important safety precautions that apply to both patients and staff. The first is to avoid the hazard of small ferromagnetic objects (screw drivers, spanners, scissors, and even paper clips) becoming dangerous projectiles in magnetic fields above about 10 mT.[16] They must therefore be excluded from the magnet room. In addition, patients at high risk are those who have ferromagnetic aneurysm clips inserted in tissues, particularly in the dural membranes.[24,47,63] No serious hemorrhages from displaced or overheated clips have yet been reported, but this may reflect careful screening of patients. It has been suggested that all patients should be screened for ferromagnetic clips with a metal detector or magnetometer,[34] and there is an obvious need for continuing vigilance in this area.

The other hazard is that superconducting magnets can suddenly "quench" owing to interruption of current flowing through the coil windings. The excess energy is dissipated as heat, and the liquid helium coolant surrounding the magnet begins to boil out of the cryostat. The consequences are that rapidly changing magnetic fields are induced in the patient's and operator's bodies and both are liable to be deprived of oxygen as room air is displaced by the escaping helium gas.

The only reported result of a deliberate quench showed that the rapid decay of the magnetic field over about 20 seconds was much less than expected.[15] It amounted to about 70 mT s^{-1}, which is equivalent to someone walking briskly away from the proximity of a 2000 mT magnet; the exposed subject (a 50 kg anesthetized pig) showed no harmful effects whatsoever. The authors nevertheless stressed that the results of this experiment do not necessarily apply to other superconducting magnets or to other magnetic resonance installations. Nor did the oxygen concentration in the room fall to dangerously low levels before staff were able to evacuate the room at a leisurely pace. The room housing the magnet was, however, large, and open high-level windows allowed the light helium gas to escape to the atmosphere. These design features would appear to be essential to provide adequate safety in the unlikely event of a "quench."[14]

PATIENT EXPOSURE

Acute Effects

High Intensity Static Magnetic Fields

As predicted from fundamental concepts, the flow of blood passing through a static magnetic field leads to induced electrical potentials, measurable on electrocardiogram recordings as an increase in the T-wave amplitude.[9,37,38] The potentials recorded from external electrodes placed on the chests of monkeys varied from about 0.1 to 0.4 mV in excess of the normal T wave potential in fields of 500 to 1500 mT respectively. It is thought that the potential across the aorta at peak blood flow is about twenty times higher than the externally recorded potential.[86] This would be equivalent to about 8 mV on a field of 1500 mT, well below the 40 mV considered to be the depolarization threshold for individual myocardial cells. The peak flow potential at 2500 mT is estimated by simple calculation to be about 40 mV across the aorta, but only a small fraction of this potential would be expressed across individual cells.[75]

Experiments conducted in healthy adult male monkeys have also shown that no measurable alterations in blood pressure resulted from exposure to static magnetic fields up to 1500 mT, even though an increase in the T-wave amplitude was observed.[86] In fact, mice chronically exposed to high field strengths (1000 mT for 750 days) showed no abnormalities whatsoever.[50] There is insufficient evidence, however, to conclude that the risks are negligible in exposing patients with failing myocardial muscle, although a cautious approach in one cardiology department has raised no undue alarm in adults, neonates, and fetuses examined for a variety of heart defects.[89]

Reports on the effects of static magnetic fields on isolated nerve preparations have provided conflicting information. To resolve this situation a carefully conducted experiment to measure the effect on the frog sciatic nerve has recently been carried out.[38] The action potential amplitude, conduction velocity, absolute refractory period, and relative refractory period were found to be unaffected by a continuous 4-hour exposure to 2000 mT fields; the conduction velocity remained unchanged after a 17-hour exposure; and the threshold for neural excitation remained unchanged in field strengths of 1000 mT. The authors suggest that previous contrasting results, where positive responses were obtained, could have been attributed to inadequate control of ambient temperature of the isolated nerve preparations.

Nevertheless, disruptive behavioral changes, as reflected in a transient suppressed response to a visual vigilance test, were consistently found in monkeys exposed for tens of minutes to field strengths in excess of about 5000 mT, some animals vomiting as the field strengths approached 10,000 mT.[87] The animals were restrained during behavioral testing, and this may have contributed to a generalized stress response.

This somewhat tentative evidence initially persuaded the ad hoc committee advising the NRPB to recommend a cautious approach in exposing epileptic patients, even though it was recognized that nerve conduction was unlikely to be influenced until the static field strengths reached a few tens of thousands of millitesla. Since 1981, two cases of epileptic patients who experienced a fit during exposure have been reported to the NRPB.[20] The patients had been exposed on previous occasions without incident, and the fits were probably fortuitous. While not advocating exclusion of epileptic patients there is still a need for caution and medical assessment of individual cases.

HIGH INTENSITY PULSED MAGNETIC FIELDS

Time-varying magnetic fields at the intensity used in imaging are considered capable of inducing electric currents in tissue that could be sufficiently large to interfere with the normal function of neuromuscular tissues. A typical nerve impulse is induced at a current density of about 30 A m^{-2} applied over a fraction of a millisecond. If additional pulses of similar amplitude are superimposed upon the physiological impulses, then adverse effects on the central nervous system (e.g., epileptiform type waves) and myocardial muscle (i.e., fibrillation) can be anticipated. The threshold for excitation, however, depends not only upon current density. It can be inferred from studies with nerve and muscle preparations that the myocardium is most susceptible to fibrillation when repeated pulses of greater than 10 ms duration are applied just before the period of muscle contraction.[72] But the response varies with the shape of the pulse (e.g., rectangular, sinusoidal, etc.), its amplitude, duration, and repetition rate.

The threshold for fibrillation has been reasonably well established for currents of short duration (e.g., shocks from 50 Hz sinusoidal mains-frequency electric current). The threshold was determined by placing electrodes of various sizes on the surface of the exposed heart of man and dogs during open-heart surgery. For continuous 50 Hz sinusoidal currents the threshold is about 3 A m^{-2} rms if the current is applied for 3 s or longer.[95] (The rms is the root mean square value of the current density represented by the effective [rise] time of the time-varying current.) It is also known that for pulsed currents this threshold increases as the pulse length shortens, and a conservation relaxation has been applied such that the quantity (current density)^2 × time is a constant.[46,72]

Another well-known response to applied electrical currents is the induction of visual light flashes (magnetic phosphenes) when current is applied through electrodes placed on the head. The threshold for this effect is about 0.2 A m^{-2} at 60 Hz, but it is frequency dependent.[2,5]

The problem is how to relate the intensity of pulsed magnetic fields to induced currents in the derivation of an acceptable limit of exposure, since the current strengths cannot be directly measured in tissue. As a working relationship Budinger[19] suggested that a rate of change of 1000 mT s^{-1} corresponds to a current strength of 0.01 A m^{-2}, recognizing that this value may be in error by an order of magnitude. Lövsund et al.[56] associated the threshold for magnetic phosphene induction with magnetic field strengths of 2000 to 5000 mT s^{-1} with the proviso that a minimum amplitude of about 10 mT was necessary at frequencies of about 30 Hz (i.e., the pulse should be applied in a particular direction for a minimum of 2 ms).

Using perception of the field when applied to the forearm as an endpoint, McRobbie and Foster[61] reported that human volunteers perceived strongly damped sinusoidal pulses of 0.3 ms duration above a threshold rate of change of about 2×10^6 mT s^{-1}, which they calculated as corresponding to a current density of 5 A m^{-2}.

Silny[79] has quantified the dose-response relationship for several endpoints, including magnetic phosphene induction, perception, and fibrillation, in several species using short periods of pulsed or sinusoidal magnetic fields. These data have confirmed that the most sensitive endpoint is magnetic phosphene induction at a threshold of about 2000 mT s^{-1} at 20 to 30 Hz with a minimum amplitude of 5 mT. Less sensitive endpoints included loss of visual concentration when the amplitude exceeded 20 mT, with headaches and visual evoked potentials occurring when the amplitude exceeded 60 mT. The stimulation thresholds for neuromuscular responses were associated with fields in excess of several hundred mT between frequencies of about 30 Hz and 1 MHz.

The decision on which of these endpoints to choose as acceptable in clinical imaging depends upon who is being exposed, i.e., patients or operators of equipment. Budinger recommends that because the complex relationships between waveform, amplitude, time duration, and repetition rate will vary with the conditions used for imaging, the safe threshold for all conditions of exposure is that which avoids magnetic phosphene induction.[19] This can be achieved by keeping the maximum rate of change below 5 mT in the frequency range 1 to 200 Hz for sinusoidal waveforms.

NRPB adopted a different approach based upon exposure of the patient. They recommended that the rate of change of the pulsed magnetic field should not induce a current density in myocardial muscle greater than one tenth of the threshold current known to produce fibrillation for pulses longer than 10 ms. This limit (0.3 A m^{-2}) could be relaxed for shorter pulses, provided that the square of the rate of change of magnetic flux density in the z gradient multiplied by the duration of the effective pulse length or half-period in ms did not exceed the numerical value of 4.

Simple calculation[75] suggests that these conditions can be achieved, assuming that the rate of change does not exceed 20,000 mT s^{-1} when the effective duration of magnetic field change exceeds 10 ms. The tentative nature of these assumptions is recognized, but it is assumed that perception of the field in peripheral tissues, where the largest current densities occur, will ensure adequate warning of more serious consequences in the myocardium before they occur.

McRobbie and Foster,[62] Polson et al.,[67] and Gore et al.[41] observed no adverse changes in the heart response during exposure of rodents to pulsed magnetic fields between 6×10^4 mT s^{-1} and about 2×10^6 mT s^{-1} with damped sinusoidal waveforms. The maximum current densities in heart muscle calculated from these rates of change correspond to 1.7 A m^{-2} in the experiment by McRobbie and Foster;[62] the current density in peripheral muscle was about 8 A m^{-2}, that is, well above the threshold (5 A m^{-2}) for peripheral muscle contraction. The threshold will, of course, be higher for shorter stimuli. These limited but valuable experiments confirm that the safety margin recommended by NRPB is adequate for their conditions of exposure.

On the other hand, Silny[79] did observe ectopic beats in the electrocardiogram in the dog during one period of exposure to a sinusoidal waveform at 50 Hz frequency at rates of change of 2×10^7 mT s^{-1}.

Still unresolved are the acute effects of exposure to pulsed magnetic fields in the central nervous system. One study[19] has shown no abnormalities on electroencephalograms in rats exposed for 10 minutes to rates of change of 2.4×10^4 mT s^{-1} at repetition rates of 30 s^{-1} with a rise time of 1 ms.

Despite these well-conducted experiments in recent years, it is considered prudent to take care in exposing patients with a history of cardiac and central nervous system abnormalities until more experience is gained in the handling of patients under a wide variety of conditions. Such advice need not inhibit the use of imaging equipment, but it introduces an element of caution that the clinician must weigh against the benefits of imaging.

RADIO FREQUENCY MAGNETIC FIELDS

Nearly all of the relevant research into the biological effects of rf and microwave radiation has been concentrated in a narrow frequency band between about 1000 and 4000 MHz. However, these data point to a thermal basis to explain most of the effects within the frequency range of interest in magnetic resonance imaging (viz., 10 to 100 MHz). The proposal is that energy deposition, and the consequent temperature rise, in a medium exposed to radiowaves occurs principally owing to the dielectric relaxation of polar molecules and increased motion of ions throughout the molecular lattice.

The biological effects of rf radiation are summarized in a recent draft report issued by the United States Environmental Protection Agency[30] and the National Council on Radiation Protection and Measurements.[98] The literature on cellular and subcellular effects points to irreversible damage in cells when their temperature reaches about 43° C and possibly to some irreversible damage if the temperature rises rapidly, even if it does not reach the critical temperature. Denaturation of DNA, base removal from DNA, and DNA mutation can all be expected to occur.

Partial or whole-body exposure of animals to rf radiation may lead to a variety of changes in bone marrow, endocrine and immune systems, the central nervous system, the gonads, and the developing fetus. One way of expressing the amount of energy absorbed during exposure to rf radiation is to relate the frequency and power density of the radiation to the dielectric properties of the tissue and the overall size of the exposed animal or man. This value, called the specific absorption rate (SAR), reflects the dose rate, usually referred to in W kg^{-1}. It is of limited use, however, because it is an estimate of the rate of absorbed energy averaged over the whole body mass and does not take into account the localized energy deposition or the thermoregulatory capacity of the animal or man to remove excess heat.

Despite these limitations it is a useful parameter for comparing effects in different tissues in different species. In general terms, adverse effects have been observed in laboratory animals exposed at SARs above 10 W kg^{-1}. These include damage to the fetus, sperm cells, and the lens of the eye. Effects reported at SARs below 10 W kg^{-1} include changes in bone marrow and blood cells, temporary infertility, immune and endocrine system stimulation, changes in the electrophysiological properties of neurons, and changes in behavior. But there are other reports of no effects in the same tissues at similar SARs.

After a critical review of the reported findings, the American National Standards Institute (ANSI) concluded that the most sensitive measure of biological effects was based upon behavioral changes; that despite considerable differences in frequency (600 MHz to 2450 MHz), species (rodents and primates), and mode of irradiation, reversible behavioral disruption was consistently found between 4 and 8 W kg^{-1} whole-body averaged SARs.[4] Behavioral changes, however, could be observed in animals at lower SARs (e.g., 1 W kg^{-1}) if they were already thermally stressed;[39] SARs of about 1 W kg^{-1} were associated with transient effects in the hematological, immune, and endocrine systems, while SARs of less than about 0.1 W kg^{-1} were associated with frequency-specific changes in cellular energy metabolism in brain tissue.[71] An alleged nonthermal effect that occurs at specific frequencies in the tens to a hundred Hz region is that of calcium ion efflux from brain tissue. The significance of this effect is unknown, but it has been observed in chick brain tissue at SARs as low as 0.0013 W kg^{-1} by Blackman et al.[11–13] and in cultured human brain cells at 0.5 W kg^{-1} by Dutta et al.[29]

With these findings in mind ANSI[4] considered that unacceptable reversible changes in behavior could occur after uniform whole-body exposure at SARs in excess of 4 W kg^{-1}. To ensure a wide margin of safety, a whole-body SAR of 0.4 W kg^{-1} averaged over any exposure period of six minutes was recommended. If localized exposure occurred, then the SAR should not exceed 8 W kg^{-1} averaged over any one gram of tissue.

The United States Food and Drug Administration subsequently issued guidelines to Institutional Review Boards that require an analysis of health effects if rf deposition during a magnetic resonance imaging exposure led to SAR greater than 0.4 W kg^{-1} averaged over the whole body. The NRPB considered that the exposure conditions used in imaging for both patient and operators should comply with the ANSI recommendations and by doing so felt that in both cases the core temperature would not rise by more than 1° C during exposure. There is now some evidence to support these recommendations.[76,91] For example, a 20-minute exposure to rf radiation (SAR 4 W kg^{-1}) using field strengths of 1500 mT and multiple imaging techniques produced an average core temperature rise of 0.3° C in healthy human volunteers. The highest increase in skin temperature was 3° C. Heart rate, respiratory rate, blood pressure, and blood and urine analysis remained unchanged; and a fundoscopic examination revealed no abnormalities. People with compromised cardiac function or with reduced thermoregulatory capability may, however, be less adaptable, and evidence of effects on such subjects is required. Studies with phantoms indicate that a core temperature rise sufficient to be uncomfortable in living persons might be anticipated after a 10-minute exposure at 2 W kg^{-1} in cardiac patients or in some infants and elderly patients with impaired thermoregulatory mechanisms.[19]

Prolonged elevation of the body (core) temperature (as reflected by temperature in the rectum or esophagus) to 5° C above normal is associated with heat stroke and brain damage, while a transient temperature rise of this magnitude after exposure for

3 hours caused a drop in the sperm count of healthy young men. As a general rule, a core temperature rise of less than about 0.5° C causes no detectable effects on reproduction, fetal weight, development in neonates, or hematological, immunological, and endocrine systems in laboratory animals. The American Conference of Governmental Industrial Hygienists considered the data and recommended that the threshold limit value for workers should be such that the average normal temperature rise for adult persons should not exceed 1° C (i.e., a core temperature of 38° C).[1]

The theoretical modeling of Guy et al.,[42] Spiegel et al.,[81] and Tell and Harlen[85] suggests that SARs of 1–4 W kg^{-1} for up to 1 hour will produce core temperature rises of up to 1° C at ambient temperatures of 25° to 30° C. These predictions have been confirmed experimentally in animals;[26,53,54] they do not, however, take account of the nonuniform distribution of energy in the body that could result in tissues in the head, neck, and chest experiencing several times more energy deposition than the lower abdomen. This situation has yet to be resolved in terms of magnetic resonance imaging and spectroscopy, although it could be argued from theoretical concepts that organs such as the eyes and testes lie outside the main body current loops, even though they are situated in parts where constriction of current paths occurs.

Delayed Effects

HIGH INTENSITY STATIC MAGNETIC AND PULSED MAGNETIC FIELDS

There are theoretical grounds for supposing that magnetic fields of high intensity could alter the rate of reactions involving radical intermediates,[60,73] thereby altering cell metabolism, but few quantitative studies have been made. This aspect is under consideration at present by the NRPB. In addition, cellular structures could be disorganized by re-orientation of strategically sited paramagnetic macromolecules, resulting in changes in the activity of membrane-bound enzymes. As one example, transient increases in thymidine kinase activity were observed at field strengths of 1400 mT following a 1-hour exposure of bone marrow cells,[32] but the significance of such effects is unknown.

Effects on cultured cells are equivocal. Respiratory activity was increased in cells from tumor and embryonic tissue,[31] and cloning ability decreased in fibroblasts exposed to fields of 350 mT.[58] But the changes in cloning ability were shown subsequently to be due to changes in the culture conditions rather than a genuine magnetic field–induced effect.[35] No cytotoxicity or increase in mutation incidence was observed in cells exposed to 350 mT static fields or 4600 mT s^{-1} pulsed fields,[77] supporting the previously reported results of Cooke and Morris[22] and Wolff et al.,[96] who reported no increased yields of chromosome aberration, sister chromatid exchange, or inhibition of DNA synthesis. The absence of gene mutation, however, is not in itself an indication of noncarcinogenicity.

Transient changes in blood cell counts and biochemical profiles in mice have been noted[6,7] but not confirmed in mice[50] or monkeys[8] exposed to 1000 mT and 2000 mT fields, respectively.

No significant changes were observed in the incidence of dominant lethal mutations in mouse sperm (1000 mT for 28 days),[57] or in the offspring of mice (1000 mT)[78] or rats (1000 mT)[48] exposed at various stages of pregnancy. Teratogenic effects were not observed when mice were exposed to 350 mT (15 MHz) or to 2300 mT (100 MHz) for 15 hours starting at the ninth day of pregnancy. A slight growth retardation, however, was noted, and this was related to a temporary weight loss of the mother.[44] In view of the known extreme sensitivity of the human embryo and fetus to mutagens when the central nervous system is developing, it is essential to confirm that no subtle damage is occurring as a result of exposure to electromagnetic radiations before concluding that it is safe to expose women in the first three months of pregnancy. In this respect the NRPB is planning a teratological and behavioral study on the offspring of exposed pregnant rats.

In a well-conducted experiment[49] in which rodents were exposed for up to 750 days to a 1000 mT static magnetic field or a 2000 mT m^{-1} gradient magnetic field, the results indicated no significant differences between exposed and sham-irradiated groups in terms of weight gain, heart rate and electrocardiograms, hematological and blood biochemistry profiles, prenatal development after exposure of pregnant animals, mortality rate, or the appearance of lesions (including tumors). There was a suggestion that exposure of animals already exposed to a known mutagen might exacerbate the effects of the mutagen as expressed in terms of damage to the developing sperm. The conclusion of this study was that exposure to magnetic fields did not result in a clearly identified pattern of change between exposed and sham-exposed groups, but some differences were noted that will require further analysis to determine whether they are related to exposure. It is important that carefully planned experiments to test for carcinogenicity be carried out in an appropriate species.

These cellular and animal studies on the whole confirm the view that delayed adverse effects are unlikely to occur, but it would be foolish to conclude the exposure to high intensity magnetic fields was completely harmless. Only a careful epidemiological survey of patients over many years may provide the final answer but such a study may prove to be impractical.

OPERATOR EXPOSURE

Acute and Delayed Effects

LOW INTENSITY STATIC MAGNETIC AND PULSED MAGNETIC FIELDS

While exposure of patients to magnetic fields is only temporary, operators may be exposed intermittently over periods of years. It is therefore necessary to consider the field conditions around the magnet. The "stray field" strength is proportional to the inverse of the cube of the distance from the center of the magnet. A person working six feet from the center of a 2000 mT magnet would be exposed to field strengths of about 10 mT; it is incumbent upon operators therefore that they should not work too closely to the magnet for longer than is necessary, particularly if larger magnets are to be used.

There is now substantial experience with workers exposed to high static fields (100 to 1000 mT) around experimental fusion reactors, superconducting energy storage devices, particle accelerators, superconducting spectrometers, and hydrogen bubble chambers. There have been anecdotal reports of transient, unpleasant responses (flicking light patterns in the eye [phosphene reaction] when workers turn their head sharply in static magnetic fields, nausea, disorientation, metallic taste in the mouth due to the effect on tooth fillings) during brief (tens of minutes) exposure to field strengths up to a few thousand mT, but no long-term detrimental effects have been reported. Based upon this experience, unofficial American standards have been proposed.[3] One such set of standards has been issued by the Stanford Linear Accelerator Center (SLAC), which recommends that the whole body or head of the workers should not be exposed for prolonged periods to more than 20 mT; this can be increased by a factor of 10 for periods of a few minutes and by a further factor of 10 if only the arms and hands are exposed. The National Accelerator Laboratory allows temporary exposure of the whole body to up to 10,000 mT for up to 15 minutes while operators are changing the film in bubble chambers; unofficial Russian recommendations allow up to 30 mT to the whole body during a continuous working day.

It would appear that the guidelines issued by SLAC have operated satisfactorily over many years and are applicable to the field conditions around magnetic resonance equipment. These findings led NRPB to recommend adoption of the SLAC standards for operators of nuclear magnetic resonance equipment.

There are some animal studies that lend support to the view that exposure to low intensity fields is harmless. No significant change in endocrine function was observed in monkeys chronically exposed to extra low frequency electric (20 vm^{-1} at 72 Hz) and magnetic (0.2 mT) fields[55] or to 1 mT fields at frequencies between 7 and 75 Hz.[27]

A recent American survey[59] of 320 workers exposed to up to 20 mT fields for prolonged periods concluded that there were no deleterious effects in this group compared to a matched control group of 186 nonexposed workers.

These findings were different from those of two Russian surveys[92,93] of workers exposed to average static or 50 Hz pulsed magnetic fields at around 0.5 mT with maximum exposures estimated to be 100 mT. General symptoms included headaches, chest pains, fatigue, blurred vision, dizziness, loss of appetite, and insomnia. Localized effects on the wrists and hands included itching and burning sensations, sweating, and moist desquamation; exposure was estimated to be in the range of 35 to 350 mT, but the workers also handled solvents and degreasing agents and were exposed to airborne metallic dusts and high ambient temperatures, so that it is difficult to separate the various potential causes of the skin irritation.

PRECAUTIONS FOR CARDIAC PACEMAKER WEARERS

Another effect to consider is that some types of cardiac pacemaker may be affected by stray fields.

Two types of effect on pacemakers are implicated, one in which the magnetic field induces current that mimics the natural electrical impulse of the heart muscle, thereby cutting out the pacemaker, and the other in which the magnetic field switches the pacemaker into activity to impose an additional impulse. The threshold for these pacemakers lies in the range of 0.05 to 0.17 mT[66,94] and it is the recommendation of a DHSS committee considering the effects of magnetic fields on pacemakers that passers-by wearing pacemakers should not enter an area where magnetic fields are in excess of 0.05 mT. This can be achieved by restricting access through security barriers or less satisfactorily by displaying warning notices outside the area of the magnet.

Some consideration may have to be given to less restrictive limits in the future as more experience is gained in the use of magnetic resonance techniques in medicine. It is known, for example, that pacemaker wearers are exposed in their domestic environment (public transport on the subway, phone headsets) to fields in excess of 0.05 mT without undue alarm.

LOW INTENSITY PULSED MAGNETIC FIELDS

There is some suggestion that weak electric currents, including those induced by magnetic fields, can affect the organization of embryonic mesodermal tissue. The abnormal development of chick embryo after exposure of fertilized eggs for 48 hours to weak (0.12 to 12 microtesla) 10 to 1000 Hz magnetic fields has been reported.[25] The effects were considered to depend strongly on the shape of the magnetic pulse and the orientation of the eggs relative to the earth's magnetic field;[88] the results have yet to be confirmed in other laboratories.

The poorly documented human epidemiological evidence for pulsed magnetic fields has been discussed in an earlier section of this chapter. It is concluded that there are no adverse effects at present that can be associated with exposure to low intensity pulsed fields, but the need for controlled epidemiological studies is stressed.

LOW INTENSITY RADIO FREQUENCY MAGNETIC FIELDS

While there is no conclusive evidence of long-term nonmalignant effects occurring, a more disturbing feature is a report that chronic exposure of rats to 2450 MHz radiation at an SAR of 0.4 W kg^{-1} resulted in increased activity in the adrenal glands and in the total malignant tumor incidence.[21] These results could be interpreted as reflecting a generalized stress reaction that provoked the tumors, but an analysis of the types of tumor found indicated that the incidence of each type of tumor in the irradiated group was not in itself significantly in excess when compared with the incidence of tumors in the control group. In fact, the total excess was due mainly to tumors of the endocrine system; no excess of other cancers actually occurred.

Other studies have been reported that claim to show a connection between cancer and rf/microwave exposure. An example of one of the earlier reports is an increased incidence of leukemia in mice exposed to 9270 MHz microwaves sufficient to cause a transient core temperature increase of 3° C;[69] but a critical reappraisal of the data seriously questioned the observation.[51] More recently, it was reported that daily exposure (2 hours per day, 6 days per week) for various periods up to 10 months at 2450 MHz radiation (SAR 2 to 8 W kg^{-1}) accelerated the appearance of spontaneous mammary tumors in female mice and of skin cancer in male mice treated with a cancer-promoting chemical during and after microwave exposure.[83,84] Thus the radiation may have been acting as a promoting agent, although other explanations could easily be a nonspecific stress reaction or a general effect on the immune response.

There are few data and no definitive studies on which to judge the long-term effects of rf radiation exposure on human survival. Two studies have evaluated the cause of death several years after exposure to rf radiation. In one study involving a comparison between employees stationed at the United States Embassy in Moscow who were allegedly chronically exposed to microwaves (7 × 10^{-4} W kg^{-1} maximum) and other United States embassies, no evidence was found that the Moscow group had experienced a higher mortality or any difference in specific causes of death.[52] In the other study the records of 20,000 United States naval personnel who were exposed to radar (0.05 W kg^{-1}) were compared with a similar matched group with no record of exposure. No apparent differences were found 20 years or more after exposure.[70]

In a 12-year survey of Polish workers exposed to microwaves for various periods, there were no additional adverse effects among those who worked at high levels (>8 × 10^{-3} W kg^{-1}) compared to those exposed to lower levels (<8 × 10^{-3} W kg^{-1}), but all had reversible functional disturbances of the central nervous system, gastrointestinal tract, and cardiovascular system.[23,82] Similar findings were reported by Djordjevic et al.[28] in groups of radar workers whose levels of maximum exposure were less than 0.2 W kg^{-1}.

A more recent survey was carried out among male physiotherapists who use rf, infrared, and ultrasound diathermy equipment.[43] The only significant finding in this preliminary study was that of association between ischemic heart disease and exposure to 27 MHz rf radiation.

Ocular effects and congenital abnormalities in offspring whose parents were exposed to rf radiation have also been described, but no causal relationship could be ascribed to rf radiation. It was the general conclusion from an extensive review on human health effects that the data are not adequate or sufficiently developed to be very useful in determining exposure limits for the general population.[45]

The biological bases for guidelines issued in 1983 by the National Radiological Protection Board are discussed in more depth in a 1984 review by Saunders and Smith in the British Medical Bulletin issue devoted to magnetic resonance and its clinical applications.[74]

The National Radiological Protection Board recommend that whole or substantial body exposure during clinical imaging should not exceed 2500 mT for static magnetic fields or 20,000 mT s^{-1} for a magnetic flux density change exceeding 10 ms. Whole or substantial body exposure to rf magnetic fields should not raise the body (core) temperature by more than 1° C, a condition that can be met if the whole body averaged SAR is restricted to below 0.4 W kg^{-1}. More relaxed limits can be applied for pulsed magnetic fields where the periods of magnetic field change are less than 10 ms. The guidelines additionally recommend that unacceptable localized overheating of tissues can be avoided by restricting the temperature rise to 1° C, or the SAR to 4 W kg^{-1}, in any 1 gram of tissue; that it would be prudent to exclude women in the first three months of pregnancy unless a planned abortion is anticipated; that patients with aneurysm clips should not be exposed; and that care should be taken when examining patients fitted with cardiac pacemakers or large metallic prostheses.

For staff, the recommended limits are about one-hundredth of those recommended for acute exposure of patients to static magnetic fields based upon the American National Standards Institute guidelines, and the limits for rf magnetic fields are the same as those recommended for patients.

However, these guidelines on staff exposure will be superceded by more general limits on occupational exposure and exposure of the public to ELF magnetic and electric fields and rf and microwave electromagnetic radiation, which are under consideration by the NRPB at present.[99]

The guidelines issued by the United States Bureau of Radiological Health are essentially similar to the above with the exception that exposure to pulsed magnetic fields be restricted to 3000 mT s^{-1}. This recommendation is based upon Budinger's advice in his 1981 review that exposure should be limited to the threshold for nonhazardous magnetic phosphene induction rather than the approach adopted by the National Radiological Protection Board in which a safety reduction factor of 10 is applied to the threshold for ventricular fibrillation. The Health Office in the Federal Republic of Germany issued a report in 1983 also recommending limiting pulsed magnetic fields on magnetic phosphene induction based upon a maximum body current density of 0.03 Am^{-2} or a field strength of 3 Vm^{-1} for pulses longer than 10 ms, with a relaxation for shorter pulses.

It is important at this stage of development of magnetic resonance techniques to achieve a balance between caution and the need to allow flexibility in order to explore the potential of the techniques. There appears to be a few potential hazards during exposure at the presently recommended limits, but the question of delayed effects remains open. The needs for further research are referred to in this chapter. However, some manufacturers are now designing the next generation of magnets that are capable of delivering more intense static magnetic fields (4000 mT) and rf fields (4 W kg^{-1}). Our knowledge of the effects of exposure to magnetic fields in excess of 2500 mT is extremely limited. Experimental data are required on the thresholds at which interruption of cardiac rhythm and impairment of the heart muscle excitability and the central nervous system occur during exposure to both static and pulsed magnetic fields; on the threshold at which demonstrable teratogenic effects may occur; and on the consequences of altering radical intermediate reaction rates in cells in the longer term.

More information is also required on the ability of exposed persons to dissipate heat, particularly those patients who may have elevated body temperature before they are exposed, or whose cardiac function is impaired, or who have a reduced thermoregulatory capacity.

It is suggested that careful consideration be given to these points before patients are exposed to these higher field conditions.

References

1. American Conferences of Governmental Industrial Hygienists: TLV's—Threshold limit values for chemical substances and physical agents in the workroom environment with intended changes for 1980. American Conference of Governmental Industrial Hygienists, Cincinnati, Ohio, 1983.
2. Adrian DJ: Auditory and visual sensations stimulated by low-frequency electric currents. Radio Science 12:243–250, 1977.
3. Alpen EL: Magnetic field exposure guidelines. In Tenforde TS (ed): Proceedings of the Biomagnetic Effects Workshop. Lawrence Berkeley Laboratory, LBL-7452, 1978, pp 19–26.
4. American National Standards Institute: Safety levels with respect to human exposure to radiofrequency electromagnetic fields, 300 kHz to 100 GJz. C95 Subcommittee (95.1–1982). New York, Institute of Electrical and Mechanical Engineers Inc., 1982.
5. Barlow HB, Kohn HI, Walsh EG: Visual sensations aroused by magnetic fields. Am J Physiol 148:372–375, 1947.
6. Barnothy MF: Haematological changes in mice. In Barnothy MF (ed): Biological Effects of Magnetic Fields. Vol. 1. New York, Plenum Press, 1964, pp 127–131.
7. Barnothy MF, Barnothy JM: Magnetic fields and the number of blood platelets. Nature 225:1146–1147, 1970.
8. Battocletti JH, Salles-Cunha S, Halbach RE, Nelson J, Sances A: Exposure to rhesus monkeys to 20,000 G steady magnetic field: Effect on blood parameters. Med Phys 8:115–118, 1981.
9. Beischer DE: Vectocardiogram and aortic blood flow of squirrel monkeys in a strong superconductive electromagnet. In Barnothy M (ed): Biological Effects of Magnetic Fields. Vol. 2. New York, Plenum Press, 1969, pp 241–259.
10. Bernhardt JH, Kossel F: Recommendations on the safe use of NMR equipment. Clin Phys Physiol Meas, 6:65, 1985.
11. Blackman CF, Elder JA et al: Induction of calcium-ion efflux from brain tissue by radiofrequency radiation: Effects of modulation frequency and field strengths. Radiol Sci 14:93–98, 1979.
12. Blackman CF, Bename SG et al: Induction of calcium-ion efflux from brain tissue by radiofrequency radiation: Effect of sample number and modulation frequency on the power-density window. Bioelectromagnetics 1:35–43, 1980.
13. Blackman CF, Bename SG et al: Calcium-ion efflux from brain tissue: Power-density versus internal field-intensity dependencies at 50 MHz RF radiation. Bioelectromagnetics 1:277–283, 1980.
14. Bore PJ, Timms WE: The installation of high-field NMR equipment in a hospital environment. Magn Reson Med 1:387–395, 1984.
15. Bore PJ, Galloway G et al: Are quenches dangerous? Society of Magnetic Resonance in Medicine, 1985. 4th Annual Meeting, London. Book of Abstracts, Vol. 2, pp 914–915, 1985.
16. Bore PJ: Safety of NMR (Letter). Lancet i:1107–1108, 1985.
17. Steiner, RE, Radda GK (eds): Nuclear magnetic resonance and its clinical applications. Br Med Bull 40:113, 1984.
18. Budinger TF: Nuclear magnetic resonance (NMR) in vivo studies: Known thresholds for health effects. J Comp Asst Tomogr 5:800–811, 1981.
19. Budinger TF, Pavllcek W et al: Society of Magnetic Resonance in Medicine, 1985. 4th Annual Meeting, London, Book of Abstracts, Vol. 2, 1985, pp 916–917.
20. Bydder GM: Personal communication, 1985.
21. Chou CK, Kunz L: Microwaves promote cancer. Results presented at the 1984 Meeting of the Bioelectromagnetics Society in Atlanta and discussed in more detail in Microwave News IV(6):3–6, 1984.
22. Cooke P, Morris PG: The effects of NMR exposure on living organisms. II. A genetic study of human lymphocytes. Br J Radiol 54:622–625, 1981.
23. Czerski P, Sierkierzynski M, Gidynski A: Health surveillance of personnel occupationally exposed to microwaves. I. Theoretical considerations and practical aspects. Aerospace Med 45:1137–1142, 1974.
24. Davis PL, Crooks L et al: Potential hazards in NMR imaging: Heating effects of changing magnetic fields and RF fields in small metallic implants. Am J Roentgenol 137:857–860, 1981.
25. Delgado JMR, Leal J et al: Embryological changes induced by weak extremely low frequency electromagnetic fields. J Anat 134:533–551, 1982.

26. de Lorge JD: The effects of microwave radiation on behaviour and temperature in rhesus monkeys. *In* Johnson ICC, Shore ML (eds): Biological Effects of Electromagnetic Waves. Vol. I. HEW Publication (FSA) 77-8010, Rockville, Maryland, 1976, pp 158–174.

27. de Lorge JD: Effects of magnetic fields on behavior in nonhuman primates. *In* Proceedings of the Biomagnetic Effects Workshop. Lawrence Berkeley Laboratory, LBL 7452, 1978, pp 32–33.

28. Djordjevic Z, Kolak A et al: A study of the health status of radar workers. Anat Space Environ Med *50*:396–398, 1979.

29. Dutta SK, Subramaniam A et al: Microwave radiation–induced calcium ion efflux from human neuroblastoma cells in culture. Bioelectromagnetics *5*:71–78, 1984.

30. Elder JA, Cahil DF (eds): Biological effects of radiofrequency radiation. Health Effects Research Laboratory, Office of Research and Development, United States Environmental Protection Agency, North Carolina. EPA-600/8–83-026A (Revised) April 1984, Final Draft.

31. Fardon JC, Poydock Sr ME, Basulto G: Effect of magnetic fields on the respiration of malignant embryonic and adult tissue. Nature *211*:433, 1966.

32. Feinendegen LE, Muhlensiepen H: Magnetic field effects thymidine kinase in vivo. Int J Radiat Biol *47*:723–730, 1985.

33. Federal Health Office of West Germany: Recommendations on avoiding health risks caused by magnetic and radiofrequency electromagnetic fields during nuclear magnetic resonance tomography and in vivo nuclear magnetic resonance spectroscopy. Bundesgesundheitsblatt *27*:92–96, 1984.

34. Finn E, Di Chiro G et al: Ferromagnetic materials in patients: Detection before NMR imaging. Radiology *156*:139–141, 1985.

35. Frazier ME, Andrews TK, Thompson BB: In vitro evaluations of static magnetic fields. *In* Biological Effects of Extremely Low Frequency Electromagnetic Fields. Proceedings of the 18th Hanford Life Sciences Symposium, Richland, Washington (1978), 1979, pp 417–435.

36. Gaffey CT, Tenforde TS, Dean EE: Alterations in electrocardiograms of baboons exposed to DC magnetic fields. Bioelectromagnetics *2*:209, 1980 (Abstract).

37. Gaffey CT, Tenforde TS: Alterations in the rat electrocardiogram induced by stationary electric fields. Bioelectromagnetics *2*:357–370, 1981.

38. Gaffey CT, Tenforde TS: Bioelectric properties of frog sciatic nerves during exposure to stationary magnetic fields. Radiat Environ Biophys *22*:61–73, 1983.

39. Gage MI: Microwave irradiation and ambient temperature interest to alter rat behavior following overnight exposure. J Microwave Power *14*:389–398, 1979.

40. Gordon RE: 1985. Magnets, molecules and medicine. Phys Med Biol *30*:741–770, 1985.

41. Gore JC, McDonnell JJ et al: An assessment of the safety of rapidly changing magnetic fields in the rabbit: Implications for NMR imaging. Magn Reson Imag *1*:191–195, 1982.

42. Guy AW, Webb MD et al: Determination of the average SAR and SAR patterns in man and simplified models of man and animals exposed to radiation fields of 50–2450 MHz and the thermal consequences (Abstract). Symposium on the Biological Effects of Electromagnetic Waves XIX General Assembly. International Union of Radio Sciences, Helsinki, Finland, 1978, p 13.

43. Hamburger S, Logue JN, Sternthal PM: Occupational exposure to non-ionizing radiation and an association with heart disease: An exploratory study. J Chron Dis *36*:791, 1983.

44. Heinrichs WL, Fong P et al: Analysis of teratogenesis and reproduction toxicity in BALB/C mice after mid frequency MRI and MRS exposure. Society of Magnetic Resonance in Medicine, 1985. 4th Annual Meeting, London. Book of Abstracts, Vol. 2, 1985, p 922.

45. Hill D: 1984. Human studies. *In* Elder JA, Cahill DA (eds): Biological Effects of Radiofrequency Radiation, Section 5-333-5-365. EPA-600/8–83-026A (revised) April 1984. Final draft. United States Environmental Protection Agency, North Carolina.

46. International Electrotechnical Commission: Effects of current passing through the body. IEC/TC64/WG4. Draft revision of publication 479 pt 5, Unidirectional impulse of short duration, 1983, pp 1–12.

47. Kean DM, Worthington BS et al: The effects of magnetic resonance imaging on different types of microsurgical clips. J Neurol Neurosurg Psych *48*:286–287, 1985.

48. Kelman BJ, Abernathy CS, Carlisle DW, Decker JR, Kalkwarf J: Biological effects of magnetic fields. *In* Pacific Northwest Laboratory Annual Report for 1982 to the DOE Office of Energy Research. Part I. Biomedical Sciences, PNL-4600 PT1 UC-48, 1983, pp 113–118.

49. Kelman BJ, Abernathy CS et al: 1984. Biological effects of magnetic fields. *In* Pacific Northwest Laboratory Annual Report for 1983 to the DOE Office of Energy Research. Part I. Biomedical Sciences, February 1984. PNL-5000 PTI VC-48, 1984 pp 83–85

50. Kelman BJ, Decker JR et al: Biological effects of magnetic fields. *In* Pacific Northwest Laboratory Annual Report for 1984 to the DOE Office of Energy Research, Part I. Biomedical Sciences February 1985, PNL-5500 PT1 VC-48, pp 79–81.

51. Kirk WP: Life Span and Carcinogenesis. *In* Elder JA, Cahill DA (eds): Biological Effects of Radiofrequency Radiation, Section 5-313-5332. EPA-600/8-83-026A (revised) April 1984. Final draft. United States Environmental Protection Agency, North Carolina.

52. Lilienfield AM, Tonascia J et al: Foreign service health status study: Evaluation of health status of foreign service and other employees from selected eastern European post. Final report Contract No. 6025-619073 (NTISPB-288163). Washington, D.C., State Department, 1978.

53. Lotz WG: Hyperthermia in rhesus monkeys exposed to a frequency (225 MHz) near whole body resonance. Naval Medical Research Development Commission MF58.524.02C-009. Pensacola, Florida, Naval Aerospace Medical Research Laboratory, 1982.

54. Lotz WG, Podgorski RP: Temperature and adrenocortical responses in rhesus monkeys exposed to microwaves. J Appl Physiol *53*:1565–1571, 1982.
55. Lotz WG, Saxton JL: Growth and sexual maturation of rhesus monkeys chronically exposed to ELF electric and magnetic fields. *In* Interaction of Biological Systems with Static and ELF Electric Magnetic Fields. 23rd Hanford Life Sciences Symposium, Washington, 1984. pp 347–364.
56. Lovsund P, Oberg PA, Nilsson SEG, Reuter T: Magnetophosphenes: A quantitative analysis of thresholds. Med Biol Eng Comput *18*:326–334, 1980.
57. Mahlum DD, Sikov MR, Decker JR: Dominant lethal studies in mice exposed to direct current magnetic fields. *In* Biological Effects of Extremely Low Frequency Electromagnetic Fields. Proceedings of the 18th Hanford Life Sciences Symposium, Richland, Washington (1978), 1979, pp 474–487.
58. Malanin GI, Gregory WD, Morelli L, Sharma VK, Houck JC: Evidence of morphological and physiological transformation of mammalian cells by strong magnetic fields. Science *194*:844–846, 1976.
59. Marsh JL, Armstrong TJ, Jacobson AP, Smith RC: Health effects of occupational exposure to steady magnetic fields. Am Ind Hyg Assoc J *43*:387–394, 1982.
60. McLauchlan KA: The effects of magnetic fields on chemical reactions. Sci Prog (Oxford) *67*:509–529, 1981.
61. McRobbie D, Foster MA: Thresholds for biological effects of time-varying magnetic fields. Clin Phys Physiol Meas *5*:67–78, 1984.
62. McRobbie D, Foster MA: Cardiac response to pulsed magnetic fields with regard to safety in NMR imaging. Phys Med Biol *30*:695, 1985.
63. New PJF, Rosen BR et al: Potential hazards and artifacts of ferromagnetic and ono-ferromagnetic surgical and dental materials and devices in nuclear magnetic resonance imaging. Radiology *147*:139–148, 1983.
64. National Radiological Protection Board: Exposure to nuclear magnetic resonance clinical imaging. Radiography *47*:258–260, 1981.
65. National Radiological Protection Board ad hoc Advisory Group on Nuclear Magnetic Resonance Clinical Imaging. Revised guidance on acceptable limits of exposure during nuclear magnetic resonance clinical imaging. Br J Radiol *56*:974–977, 1983.
66. Pavlicek W, Geisinger M et al: The effects of nuclear magnetic resonance on patients with cardiac pacemakers. Radiology *147*:149–153, 1983.
67. Polson MJR, Barker AT, Gardiner S: The effect of rapid rise-time magnetic fields on the ECG of the rat. Clin Phys Physiol Meas *3*:231–234, 1982.
68. Prior MJW, Maxwell RJ et al: The role of magnetic resonance spectroscopy in assessing drug delivery to tumors. Society of Magnetic Resonance in Medicine, 1985. 4th Annual Meeting, London. Book of Abstracts, Vol. 2, pp 740–741, 1985.
69. Prausmitz S, Sussking O: Effects of chronic microwave irradiation on mice. IRE Trans Biomed Electr *9*:104–108, 1962.
70. Robinnette CD, Silverman C, Jablon S: Effects upon health of occupational exposure to microwave radiation (radar). Am J Epidemiol *112*:39–53, 1980.
71. Sanders AP, Schaefer DJ, Joines WT: Microwave effects on energy metabolism of rat brain. Bioelectromagnetics *1*:171–181, 1980.
72. Saunders RD: Biological hazards of NMR. Proceedings of the International Symposium on Nuclear Magnetic Resonance Imaging, October 1–3, 1981. Bowman Gray School of Medicine, Wake Forest University, Winston-Salem, North Carolina, 1982, pp 65–71.
73. Saunders RD, Cass A: Magnetic field interactions with living systems. NRPB memorandum. NRPB-M96. National Radiological Protection Board, 1983.
74. Saunders RD, Smith H: Safety aspects of NMR clinical imaging. *In* Steiner RE, Radda GK (eds): Nuclear Magnetic Resonance and Its Clinical Application. Br Med Bull *40*:148–154, 1984.
75. Saunders RD, Orr JS: Biological effects of NMR. *In* Partain CL, James AE, Rollo FD, Price RR (eds): Nuclear Magnetic Resonance (NMR) Imaging. Philadelphia, W.B. Saunders Co., 1983, pp 383–396.
76. Schaefer DJ, Barber BJ et al: Society of Magnetic Resonance in Medicine, 1985. 4th Annual Meeting, London. Book of Abstracts, Vol. 2, 1985, pp 925–926.
77. Schwartz JL, Crooks LE: NMR imaging produces no observable mutation or cytotoxicity in mammalian cells. Am J Radiol *139*:583–585, 1982.
78. Sikov MR, Mahlum DD, Montgomery LD, Decker JR: Development of mice after intrauterine exposure to direct current magnetic fields. *In* Biological Effects of Extremely Low Frequency Electromagnetic Fields. Proceedings of the 18th Hanford Life Sciences Symposium, Richland, Washington, 1979, pp 462–473.
79. Silny J: Effects of low-frequency, high intensity magnetic field on the organism. *In* Proceedings of the International Conference of Electric and Magnetic Fields in Medicine and Biology. Institution of Electrical Engineers, London 1985, pp 103–107.
80. Society of Magnetic Resonance in Medicine. 4th Annual Meeting, London. Book of Abstracts, Vols. 1 and 2, 1985.
81. Spiegel RJ, Deffenbaugh DM, Mann JE: A thermal model of the human body exposed to an electromagnetic field. Bioelectromagnetics *1*:253–270, 1980.
82. Sierkierzynski M, Czerski P et al: Health surveillance of personnel occupationally exposed to microwaves. II. Functional disturbances. Aerospace Med *45*:1143–1145, 1974.
83. Szmigielski S, Szydzinksi A et al: Acceleration of cancer development in mice by long-term exposition to 2450 MHz microwave fields. *In* Berteaud AJ, Servantie B (eds): URSI International Symposium Proceedings, Ondes Electromagnetiques et Biologie, Paris, 1980, pp 165–169.

84. Szmigielski S, Szydzinski A et al: Accelerated development of spontaneous and benzopyrene-induced skin cancer in mice exposed to 2450 MHz microwave radiation. Bioelectromagnetics 3:179–191, 1982.
85. Tell RA, Harlen F: A review of selected biological effects and dosimetric data useful for development of radiofrequency safety standards for human exposure. J Microwave Power 14:405–424, 1979.
86. Tenforde RS, Gaffey CT et al: Cardiovascular alterations in Macaca monkeys exposed to stationary magnetic fields: Experimental observations and theoretical analysis. Bioelectromagnetics 4:1–9, 1983.
87. Thach JS: A behavioral effect of intense D-C electromagnetic fields. In Vatborg H (ed): Use of Non-human Primates in Drug Evaluation. Austin, University of Texas Press pp 347–356, 1968.
88. Ubeda A, Leal J, Trillo MA, Jimenez MA, Delgado JMR: Pulse shape of magnetic fields influences chick embryogenesis. J Anat 137:51H, 1983.
89. Underwood SR: Magnetic resonance in cardiology. RAD Magazine, July 1985, pp 25–26.
90. United States Bureau of Radiological Health: Guidelines for evaluating electromagnetic exposure risk for trials of clinical NMR systems.
91. Vogl T, Krimmel M, et al: Society of Magnetic Resonance in Medicine, 1985. 4th Annual Meeting, London. Book of Abstracts, Vol 2, pp 929–930.
92. Vyalov AM: Magnetic fields as a factor in an industrial environment. Vestwik 8: 52, 1967.
93. Vyalov AM: Clinico-hygienic and experimental data on the effects of magnetic fields under industrial conditions. In: Kholodov Y (ed): Influence of Magnetic Fields on Biological Objects. Natural Technical Information Service Rep, JPRS 63038, 1971, pp 20–35.
94. Watson AB, Wright JS, Loughman J: Electrical thresholds for ventricular fibrillation in man. Med J Aust 1:1179, 1973.
95. Williams JL, 1984. Personal communication.
96. Wolff S, Crooks LE, Brown P, Howard R, Painter RB: Tests for DNA and chromosomal damage induced by nuclear magnetic resonance imaging. Radiology 136:707, 1980.
97. Young I: Nuclear magnetic resonance imaging. Electronics and Power, March 1984, pp 205–210.
98. NCRP Report No. 86: Biological Effects and Exposure Criteria for Radiofrequency Electromagnetic fields. Recommendations of the National Council on Radiation Protection and Measurements. Bethesda, Maryland, 1986, pp 1–382.
99. NRPB: Advice on the protection of workers and members of the public from the possible hazards of electric and magnetic fields with frequencies below 300 GHz. A consultative document. Chilton, England, 1986.

86

Operational Guidelines: United States

ROGER H. SCHNEIDER
T. WHIT ATHEY
MARY P. ANDERSON
ROBERT A. PHILLIPS

In the United States, medical imaging devices are medical devices subject to the Medical Device Amendments of May 28, 1976, to the Food, Drug and Cosmetic Act. The purpose of this law is to assure that medical devices are safe and effective and properly labeled for their intended use. To accomplish this mandate, the Amendments provide the Food and Drug Administration (FDA) with authority to regulate devices during most phases of their development, testing, production, and distribution.

The Amendments provide for devices to be placed in three regulatory classes based upon the degree of control necessary for reasonable assurance of safety and effectiveness. The classifications of the preamendments devices, those on the market at the time of enactment of the Amendments (May 28, 1976), were recommended by panels of experts, composed of members from the research and medical communities, industry, and consumers.

Class I devices are subject only to general controls, e.g., mislabeling, adulteration, good manufacturing practice, and so on. They are not for use in supporting or sustaining life, are not of importance in preventing impairment to human health, and must not present a potential unreasonable risk of illness or injury.

Class II devices are those for which general controls are insufficient for reasonable assurance of safety and effectiveness and for which existing information is sufficient to establish a performance standard that provides such assurance. Until standards are established by regulation, general controls are the sole controls for such devices. No such performance standards have been established to date.

Class III devices are those for which insufficient information exists to assure that general controls and performance standards provide reasonable assurance of safety and effectiveness. Generally, these devices are represented to be life sustaining or life supporting, are implanted in the body, or present potential unreasonable risk of illness or injury. A postamendment device (introduced into the marketplace after the Amendments were enacted May 28, 1976) not "substantially equivalent" to a Class I or II preamendment device is automatically placed in Class III.

Marketing of a new Class III device may be permitted under two provisions of the law. The first is by approval of a Reclassification Petition, which asks that the classification of a device be changed to a lower class on the grounds that the premarket review requirements for Class III devices are not necessary to assure safety and effectiveness.

The second is the Premarket Approval Application (PMA), the normal route to market for Class III devices. This requires submission of scientific, technical and clinical data, and analyses that establish the reasonable safety and effectiveness of an individual device. NMR imagers are Class III devices by virtue of being postamendment devices not substantially equivalent to any preamendment device. No Reclassification Petition has been approved.

THE INVESTIGATIONAL DEVICE EXEMPTION

Class III devices may be used to obtain data from human patients for investigational purposes prior to premarket approval. This is permitted under an Investigational Device Exemption (IDE). The Institutional Review Board (IRB) (human research review committee) at the site of each proposed investigation must make a determination as to whether or not it would represent a "significant risk" to the experimental subjects. According to the IDE regulation, such a risk represents a "potential for serious risk to the health, safety or welfare of a subject." If the IRB determines that no significant risk is involved and approves the protocol, the investigation may proceed without notification to the FDA. If the IRB finds that significant risk exists, or if the FDA so requests, the sponsor of the investigation must apply to the FDA for an IDE.

Early on the FDA recognized that information on the biological effects of static, changing, and radiofrequency (rf) magnetic fields was limited and, perhaps, not readily accessible to IRBs. To assist them in making decisions on significant risk and to reduce the filing of unnecessary IDEs which might stem from excessively conservative attitudes, the FDA issued guidance[1] on significant risk in clinical MRI studies on February 25, 1982. This is quoted in part below.

Three areas of concern are addressed: (1) whole or partial body exposure to static magnetic fields, (2) whole or partial body exposure to time-varying magnetic fields, and (3) absorption of energy from radiofrequency (RF) electromagnetic fields. On the basis of current information the Bureau believes that a study which does not exceed these guidelines probably does not present an unacceptable risk in these three areas. Studies that expose patients above these guideline levels should be evaluated on an individual and more extensive basis to determine whether they should be considered to pose significant risk.

Guidelines:

(1) Static (DC) Magnetic Fields (B)—Whole or partial body exposures of 2 tesla.

(2) Time-Varying Magnetic Fields (dB/dt)—Whole or partial body exposures of 3 tesla/second.

(3) Radiofrequency Electromagnetic Fields—Exposure to RF fields that results in a specific absorption rate (SAR) that exceeds 0.4 W/kg as averaged over the whole body, or 2 W/kg as averaged over any one gram of tissue.

Static and Time-Varying Magnetic Fields

The guideline levels of exposure to DC and time-varying magnetic fields were determined after consideration of existing unofficial standards and recommendations[2-7] and their rationales and reports of biomagnetic effects.[7-17] The first three standards and recommendations (2, 3, and 4) (those of the National Accelerator Laboratory, the Stanford Linear Accelerator Center, and the Union of Soviet Socialist Republics) are for occupational situations where repeated or chronic exposures are expected. Some of the levels recommended are based on the maximum levels encountered in the installation rather than on biological risk assessment. The USSR recommendation has its origin in a clinical study of workers in engineering plants and in a human laboratory study. The effects reported in the laboratory study were primarily mild physiological changes that were rapidly reversible. The effects in the worker study were reported to be physiological and psychological and due to chronic exposure (years) to both DC and 50 Hz magnetic fields. In view of the applicability of these guidelines (clinical testing of a medical device under the supervision of an attending physician for short periods), and despite the findings reported by the USSR, exposures at levels within the Bureau's guidelines seem to pose acceptably low risk for human subjects.

Two recent advisories deal directly with medical NMR imaging—that of the British National Radiological Protection Board[6] and a paper by Thomas F. Budinger, M.D., Ph.D.[5] The Bureau concurs with the static and time-varying magnetic field limits recommended by Budinger. He supports his recommendations with a rather extensive review of the bioeffects literature and a discussion of the mechanisms of interaction.

Radiofrequency Electromagnetic Fields

The guideline for RF absorbed power (0.4 W/kg as averaged over the whole body) is identical to that recommended in the proposed ANSI C95.1 standard.[7] The guideline is in terms of the specific absorption rate (SAR) instead of field levels for three reasons: (1) the fields are primarily magnetic, (2) the fields are pulsed, and (3) the field level is not an independent variable of the system (a specific relationship must obtain for the field level, the pulse characteristics, and the frequency). The guideline allows an average power deposition which is about half the basal metabolic rate for adults and which should not result in significant elevations of local or core body temperature.

A dosimetric analysis of RF exposure in NMR systems by Bottomley and Edelstein[8] assumes that the RF magnetic field is parallel to the long axis of the subject's body, but similar considerations hold for the case of fields perpendicular to the subject. The RF magnetic fields are pulsed in NMR systems and the peak power (when the RF is on) is sometimes much higher than the average values to which the guidelines apply. The RF control system should be such that component failures do not allow continuous power to be delivered to the patient in excess of the guidelines. In cases where significant electric fields (RF) are present, their contribution to the power deposition must be considered.

A maximum SAR limit is also included in the guide because the heating of the body by NMR systems is uneven, being greatest near the surface and approaching zero at the center of the body (if the coil is concentric with the body). Partial body exposures are also possible with NMR systems. The proposed ANSI standard[7] permits an exclusion from its field strength limits when it can be shown that peak SAR is less than 8 W/kg (and average SAR is less than 0.4 W/kg). However, the value of 8 W/kg is based on the assumption that the far-field or near-field exposure produces a localized maximum in SAR. In the case of NMR coils, the peak SAR is deposited regionally in a layer of near-surface tissue that extends completely around the body. Therefore, a lower level of 2 W/kg was chosen as the limit on peak SAR to prevent overloading the thermoregulatory system in any region of the body.

In the ensuing months it became apparent that the agency's intent in issuing these guidelines was widely misunderstood. They were being taken as a regulatory expression of upper limits for human exposure. Accordingly, on December 28, 1982 FDA issued clarification in the form of a memorandum[18-19] to the medical NMR community. It stated, in part, the following:

A finding of 'significant risk' does not mean that a device is too hazardous for clinical studies. It does mean that a formal application must be made to the FDA for an IDE. The concepts of significant risk relevant to clinical NMR imaging are found in 21 CRF 812.3(m) (3) and (4). In summary a significant risk diagnostic device "(3) Is for a use of substantial importance in diagnosing, . . . and presents a potential for serious risk to the health, safety, or welfare of a subject, or (4) otherwise presents a potential for serious risk to the health, safety, or welfare of a subject."

Further,

Note that the definition of significant risk device contains the phrase ". . . presents a potential for serious risk . . .", that is, a significant risk device is not necessarily a device presenting a known risk to the human subject. The term significant risk device as used in the regulations is intended to differentiate between those devices which may be used with minimal initial and continuing review and those devices requiring more extensive review and the scrutiny of FDA before use on human subjects. I must emphasize the first paragraph of the guidelines which stated that "a finding of 'significant risk' does not mean that a device is too hazardous for clinical studies." Many medical devices meet the criterion "presents a potential for serious risk" but are accepted for widespread use in medical practice because the perceived benefits outweigh the associated risks.

Further,

It has been rather widely reported to us that the guidelines have been interpreted as limits for patient exposures in NMR imaging investigations as are conditions advised by the British National Radiological Protection Board (Radiography, Vol. XI, VII, No. 563). This is not our intent. To quote from the third paragraph of the guideline, "Studies that expose patients above the guideline levels should be evaluated on an individual and more extensive basis to determine whether they should be considered to pose 'significant risk.' "

PREMARKET APPROVAL

A second provision under which the agency has expressed limits for patient exposure governs the marketing of Class III devices. In the processing of PMA applications FDA reviews the specifications, safety, effectiveness, and labeling of each MRI device. The agency has taken the position that devices exposing patients to radiofrequency power deposition (SARs) in excess of 0.4 W/kg averaged over the entire body, or 8 W/kg locally, will not be approved unless significant clinical benefit to the patient, not available through less strenuous experience, can be demonstrated.

In addition, for premarket approval, the agency has required that the rate of change of time-varying magnetic fields not exceed 6 tesla per second in the region occupied by the patient's head or trunk for time intervals longer than ten milliseconds. For shorter time intervals, the time rate of change may be increased in proportion to the reciprocal of the interval length. These limits were chosen to assure patient safety in a conservative manner. They are not considered boundaries of definite risk.

The SARs are derived from the consensus represented by ANSI's C95.1 standard[7] as discussed above. The Scope and Purpose section of that standard states in part, "These recommendations are not intended to apply to the purposeful exposure of patients by or under the direction of practitioners of the healing arts." This statement does not, however, negate the validity of the supporting analysis for the population of medical patients. Indeed, prudence might suggest yet a lower exposure limit for those with impaired health.

FDA has taken this caveat on the application of C95.1 to mean that its framers did not intend their recommendations to be used as absolute limits on medical applications but rather that some comparison between potential risk and anticipated individual benefit should be made for each medical exposure situation. This is the requirement that the agency has imposed on manufacturers who request premarket approval for devices exceeding the above SARs. They are asked to demonstrate clinical benefit to the individual patient which justifies any such excess.

This approach is consistent with the intent of the law. The applicable regulation[20] states, in part, "In determining the safety and effectiveness of a device for purposes of . . . premarket approval of Class III devices the Commissioner and the classification panels will consider the following among other relevant factors . . . the probable benefit to health from the use of the device weighed against any probable injury or illness from such uses." And further, "There is reasonable assurance that a device is safe when it can be determined, based on valid scientific evidence, that the probable benefits to health from use of the device or its intended uses and conditions of use, when accompanied by adequate directions and warnings against unsafe use, and under conditions of use when accompanied by adequate directions and warnings against unsafe use, outweigh any probable risks."

The application of these general principles to the question of the safety of NMR imaging was discussed by one of the authors (RHS) at the meeting of the expert panel which reviewed the first three PMAs for these devices in July of 1983. Speaking as a representative of the Center, he said, in part,[20]

These devices expose the subject imaged to static magnetic fields, time-varying magnetic fields and radiofrequency magnetic fields, with a wide range of magnitudes and frequencies. The question of biological effects of such exposures is not completely understood at this time and is, in fact, a matter of increasing scientific interest and investigation.

It is not possible at this time to estimate the probability of occurrence of effects with associated latent periods, effects of chronic exposure . . . or effects of low incidence, that is, incidences on the order of those expected from diagnostic x-ray procedures for example. . . . The experience with these devices is, in time of observation and in number of subjects observed, inadequate to permit us to estimate the probability of occurrence of effects with associated latent periods, such as those associated with the cancer, effects of chronic exposure, . . . or effects of low incidence. Various analyses have concluded that no immediate acute effects are to be expected from the exposure conditions prevailing in the devices currently under investigation.

From available scientific information it is reasonable to assume that whatever risks may be associated with these exposures will be small compared to the benefits accruing to individual patients when it can be determined that use of the modality is medically indicated.

That is, in the face of the uncertainty about the scientific aspects of the health effects of these devices, it is our judgment that it is reasonable to assume that whatever risks there may be are small compared to the benefits accruing to the individual patients who need this modality in the diagnosis of their condition.

In light of this situation, we are assuming the responsibility of analyzing and integrating the information developed by the scientific community at large and the responsibility for developing guidelines and policies with respect to patient safety, while encouraging individual contributions from sponsors of these devices and independent investigators.

We recognize that the fundamental scientific uncertainties in this field will not be resolved by experiments of the type and size normally associated with medical device evaluation. Therefore in our communications with this industry we have not asked that each sponsor do a complete and thorough assessment of the safety of his device. Rather, we have asked that each sponsor provide a thorough assessment of the physical exposure conditions prevailing in his device.

The Center will continue to analyze new information from research on biological effects and clinical experience as it becomes available. We have, in fact, been active in this field for many years. Since the passage of the Radiation Control for Health and Safety Act in 1968 the Center and its predecessor, the Bureau of Radiological Health, have had a very active research program looking at the biological effects of non-ionizing radiation, including radiofrequency energy, microwave energy, ultrasound and so on.

We have been active participants in the establishment of the Bioelectromagnetic Society and safety assessments of such exposures by the World Health Organization. . . . We believe that we are on top of the scientific issues here and that they are too complex for us to require their resolution in the premarket approval of a medical device. We are accepting the responsibility for monitoring this field as it develops, and we will take whatever action is indicated by future events.

Given the state of our understanding of the possibility of the existence of risks associated with electromagnetic energies of the character employed in NMR imaging, these matters demand our continuing attention.

References

1. Bureau of Radiological Health: Guidelines for Evaluating Electromagnetic Exposure Risk for Trials of Clinical NMR Systems. Washington DC, Food and Drug Administration, February 25, 1982.
2. National Accelerator Laboratory: Interim Standards for Occupational Exposure to Magnetic Fields, July 1979.
3. Stanford Linear Accelerator Center: Limits on Human Exposure in Static Magnetic Field, May 1970.

4. Vyalov AM: 1971. Clinico-hygienic and experimental data on the effects of magnetic fields under industrial conditions. *In* Kholodov Y (ed): Influence of Magnetic Fields on Biological Objects. USSR, National Technical Information Service Report JPRS5303S, 1974.

5. Budinger TF: Nuclear magnetic resonance (NMR) in vivo studies: Known thresholds for health effects. J Comput Assist Tomogr 5:800–811, 1981.

6. National Radiological Protection Board (Great Britain): Exposure to nuclear magnetic resonance clinical imaging. Radiography 47:258–260, 1981.

7. American National Standards Institute (ANSI): Safety level with respect to human exposure to radio-frequency electromagnetic fields (300 kHz–100 GHz). Draft C95.1 Standard—February 1981. Text published in Microwave News 1, 1981.

8. Bottomley PA, Edelstein WA: Power deposition in whole-body NMR imaging. Med Phys 8:510–512, 1981.

9. Busby DE: Biomagnetics: Considerations Relevant to Manned Space Flight. NASA Contractor Report, NASA CR-889, 1967.

10. Ketchen EE, Porter WE, Bolton NE: The biological effects of magnetic fields on man. J Am Ind Hyg Assoc 39:1–11, 1978.

11. Kholodov YA: The Effect of Electromagnetic and Magnetic Field on the Central Nervous System. NASA Technical Translation NASA TT F-465, 1967.

12. Kholodov YA (ed): Influence of Magnetic Fields on Biological Objects. National Technical Information Service Report JPRS 6038, 1975.

13. Mahlum DD: Biomagnetic Effects: A Consideration in Fusion Reactor Developments, BNWL-1973, Battelle Pacific Northwest Laboratories, Richland, Washington, 1976.

14. Marino AA, Becker RO: Biological effects of extremely low frequency electric and magnetic fields: A review. Physiol Chem Phys 9:131–147, 1977.

15. St. Lorant SJ: Biomagnetism: A review. SLAC-PUB-1984, 1977.

16. Sheppard AR, Eisenbud M: Biological Effects of Electric and Magnetic Fields of Extremely Low Frequency. New York, New York University Press, 1977.

17. Tenforde TS (ed): Magnetic Field Effect on Biological Systems. New York, Plenum Press, 1979.

18. Office of Radiological Health, Division of Compliance: Memorandum on Guidelines for Evaluating Electromagnetic Risk for Trials of Clinical NMR Systems. National Center for Devices and Radiological Health. Washington DC, Food and Drug Administration, December 28, 1982.

19. Subchapter H—Medical devices, Medical device classification procedures, Determination of safety and effectiveness, 21CFR860.7.

20. Radiologic Devices Panel: Transcript of July 6 & 7, 1983 Meeting. Dockets Management Branch, FDA HFA-305, 5600 Fishers Lane, Rockville, Maryland, 20857.

87

Quality Assurance

JAMES A. PATTON
RONALD R. PRICE

Whenever a new imaging modality is introduced into the clinical environment, much effort must be devoted to establishing a quality assurance program that ensures the safety of the patient as well as the quality of the studies performed using that modality. Magnetic resonance imaging is certainly no exception to that rule, and in fact this modality poses new dilemmas because of the new technology associated with the performance of magnetic resonance imaging (MRI) procedures. In particular, the surrounding environment must be protected from the magnetic fields generated by the system and the system must be protected from external sources of radio frequency (rf) interference and metal objects that may alter the uniformity of the magnetic field. These problems must be dealt with carefully in the design and construction of an MRI facility, and manufacturers provide site planning guides illustrating the specific guidelines for site design recommended for each system.

PATIENT SCREENING, COMFORT, AND SAFETY

One of the exciting factors about MRI is that there appears to be little, if any, hazard associated with it because it does not make use of ionizing radiation. However, patient screening is important because there are certain situations in which patients cannot be imaged with the system. Because of the strong magnetic field necessary for MRI, patients must be imaged without ferromagnetic intravenous fluid stands, oxygen bottles, physiological monitors, and so on in close proximity to the magnet. An exception to this statement is the permanent magnet systems, which have a very limited field external to the magnet. Should a patient experience a cardiac arrest during an imaging procedure, it will probably be necessary to remove the patient from the vicinity of the magnet before resuscitation can begin. Emergency situations should be addressed by designating an emergency area adjacent to the imaging room and establishing emergency procedures to be followed in case a life-threatening situation should arise.

Certain categories of patients should be excluded from MRI studies altogether; these include those with cardiac pacemakers, specific surgical clips, and heart valves containing ferromagnetic materials (Fig. 87–1). It has been shown that pacemakers may actually move within the chest wall, change modes of operation, or cease functioning when placed in an MRI system.[1,2] Patients with any type of metal implant must be carefully screened before being studied. Heating of ferromagnetic implants due to the rf fields, one original cause for concern, has not proved to be of significant consequence at the present. The most serious effect is the fact that implanted ferromagnetic objects will experience a torque when placed in the magnet and try to align themselves with the magnetic field. This could be disastrous in the case of an aneurysm clip, for example.

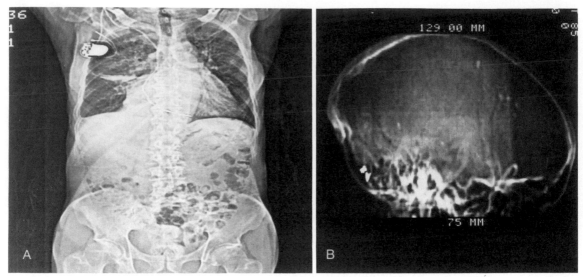

Figure 87–1. *A*, Computed tomography scout view of a patient with a pacemaker. *B*, Lateral skull film of a patient with surgical clips in the brain.

Some implants are nonmagnetic and present little cause for concern. However, unless there is very strong evidence to indicate that the implants are nonmagnetic or that movement of the implants present no hazard to the patient, it is suggested that those patients be excluded from MRI. It should also be stated that ferromagnetic metal implants, dental work, and so on will distort the magnetic fields in their vicinity and may severely degrade the image quality in that region, as described in the chapter on artifacts.

Currently available MRI systems are operating well below those levels at which patients should experience any physiological effects.[3] However, to ensure patient safety, specific guidelines for operating levels have been established by the Food and Drug Administration (FDA).[4] Specifically there are three different types of fields to which patients are exposed during an MRI study and which are potential causes for concern: static magnetic fields, changing magnetic fields, and rf fields.

In order to define a sensitive volume for the performance of an imaging procedure the patient is placed in a relatively strong, uniform static magnetic field. The FDA has stated that this field strength should not exceed 2 tesla because no cellular effects or significant changes in nerve conduction or ECG characteristics have been observed at or below this level.[4]

Specific regions of the patient are selected for imaging by changing the magnetic field at those regions through the use of pulsating gradient coils. The guideline established by the FDA is that the changing magnetic field associated with the gradient pulsations should not exceed 3 tesla per second. Although the actual change in field strength is only a few gauss, the change occurs in a few milliseconds so that the 3 tesla per second value could be reached or exceeded by current systems. No magnetic phosphenes, sensations of flashing light in the eyes, have been observed at or below this level, and ventricular fibrillations and alterations in bone healing have occurred only at higher levels. Thus these reported observations currently serve as the basis for this guideline.

The third cause for concern is the heating effects on body tissues as a result of exposure to rf fields. The current FDA guideline of 0.4 watts/kilogram over 1 gram of tissue is based on the theory that no more heating should be introduced into a body tissue than that which is normally produced by the body itself. Some investigators have reported data that suggest that this guideline is conservative,[5–7] and it may be raised in the future.

Careful attention to patient comfort must also be addressed. It is important to describe the procedure to patients before they enter the magnet to reduce their anxiety level. Some patients will still experience claustrophobia when placed in the magnet, especially when undergoing head imaging procedures. Therefore a pleasant environment is essential in order to make the patient feel at ease. Air flow directed through the patient tunnel, piped-in music, and continued patient contact during the study tend to relieve some of the anxiety. In addition, some installations have chosen to provide the patient with a ''panic button'' to be pressed when he feels that he needs attention. Infants and small children generally require sedation for MRI procedures. In some instances, adequate studies have been obtained by imaging patients in the prone position or imaging the head with the larger diameter body coil in order to decrease the anxiety level of the patients.

INSTRUMENTATION QUALITY CONTROL

As with any imaging modality, MRI requires routine quality control procedures to ensure the maintenance of high quality imaging performance. However, this is not a simple task because of the many different pulse sequences and techniques that are available with most imaging systems. Several investigators are currently involved in the development of phantoms and procedures for performing evaluations of MRI systems; however, there is not a consensus of opinion on optimum techniques at this time. The American Association of Physicists in Medicine and others are currently developing guidelines for quality assurance programs in magnetic resonance imaging with the goal of acquainting users with currently available phantoms and techniques for routine evaluations of image quality and equipment performance. The goal of the material presented here is to acquaint the reader with the various parameters that should be evaluated on a routine basis. Examples of phantoms and results are presented to demonstrate how these parameters can be examined.

Frequency Check

There are many parameters that warrant attention in a routine MRI quality assurance program. Daily measurements of operational frequency should be performed to evaluate the stability of the primary magnetic field and also to insure optimum image quality. This is accomplished by varying the frequency to tune the system for optimum signal using a phantom that produces a strong NMR signal. The Larmor equation can then be used to also calculate the operating field strength of the magnet.

Image Uniformity

Currently available MRI systems provide highly uniform magnetic fields with non-uniformities of only a few parts per million throughout the imaging volume. The use of specialized equipment is required to measure the uniformity of the magnetic field. Of more importance in imaging, however, is the uniformity of the images that are routinely obtained. Image uniformity can be evaluated subjectively on a regular basis by imaging a uniform disk phantom (Fig. 87–2A) containing propylene glycol or some other fluid that provides a strong NMR signal and visually inspecting the uniformity

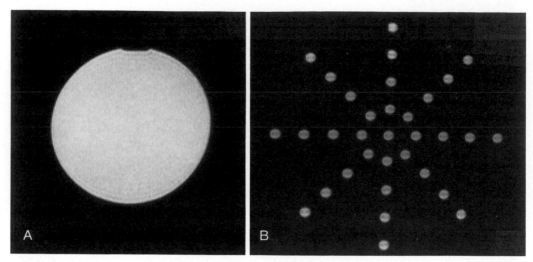

Figure 87–2. Images of a uniform disk phantom (*A*) and a phantom of discrete signal-producing cylinders (*B*) for uniformity measurements.

of the image obtained. Numerical data can be obtained by using a phantom containing discrete sources (Fig. 87–2*B*) and measuring the signal from each with region-of-interest capabilities that are available on most imagers. Routine measurements such as these should be performed using a reproducible geometry and a constant technique such as a spin-echo 30/500 pulse sequence. The qualitative data may then be plotted as shown in Figure 87–3 to assess image uniformity. These quantitative data illustrate a fall-off in signal intensity on either side of the center in the horizontal data set corresponding to the z direction along the long axis of the magnet. Patient positioning then becomes an important consideration when dealing with such nonuniformities as shown in Figure 87–4. Figure 87–4*B* is a transverse section through the body at the position of the cursor in the patient whose sagittal view is shown in Figure 87–4*A*. The image quality of the transverse view is poor due to the fall-off in signal intensity near the end of the coil as was shown in Figure 87–3. By positioning the patient such that the region of interest in at the center of the coil (Fig. 87–4*C*) improved image quality is obtained (Fig. 87–4*D*).

The measurement of operating frequency and image uniformity are the minimum recommendations for routine daily quality assurance. They do not begin to evaluate

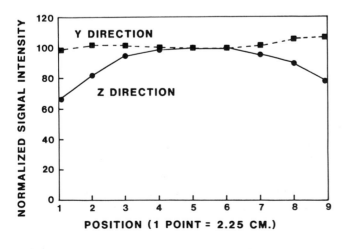

Figure 87–3. Plot of uniformity measurements in the vertical (*y*) and horizontal (*z*) directions obtained from an image of the phantom shown in Figure 87–2*B* (not the same data as in Figure 87–2*B*). Each data point represents a distance of 2.25 cm with point 5 corresponding to the center of the image.

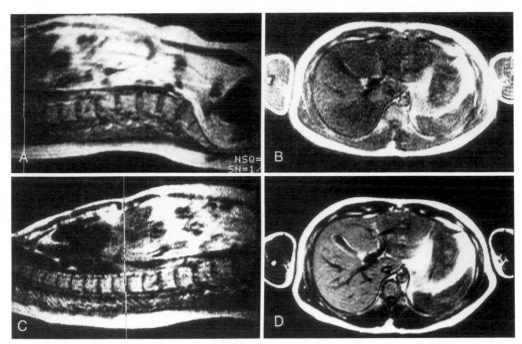

Figure 87–4. Sagittal view (*A*) and transverse view (*B*) corresponding to position of cursor in *A*. Note the improved image quality (*D*) obtained by positioning the patient such that the region of interest is at the center of the imaging volume (*C*).

all of the imaging capabilities of any instrument; however, they provide a quick analysis of the operational status of the system.

Signal-to-Noise

A parameter related to image uniformity that strongly affects image quality is the signal-to-noise. Signal is defined as the difference in the average signal intensity over a signal-producing area (S_v) and the average background signal intensity measured in air (S_a). A measure of noise (N) often used is the standard deviation of signal intensity over the background area (air). Signal-to-noise (S/N) is then calculated by dividing the signal value by the noise value.

$$S/N = (S_v - S_a)/N$$

Signal-to-noise can be calculated by using the disk phantom in Figure 87–2*A* to obtain an average S/N value or a series of vials yielding different strength NMR signals can be used to obtain a curve of S/N versus signal intensity. The latter measurement can be accomplished using vials containing increasing concentrations of deuterium oxide (D_2O) and distilled normal water (H_2O). The deuterium yields no NMR signal. Thus by linearly varying the concentration of deuterium a linear variation in proton density can be obtained with no variation in either *T1* or *T2*. A plot of S/N measured from 5 vials containing 100 percent, 75 percent, 50 percent, 25 percent, and 0 percent deuterium oxide is shown in Figure 87–5.

The measurement of signal-to-noise is very sensitive to variations in signal intensity and background noise and serves as an excellent technique for monitoring magnetic resonance image quality.

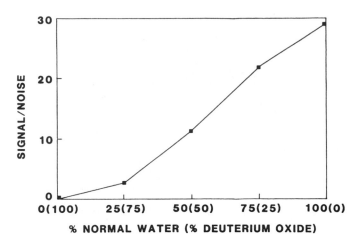

Figure 87–5. Plot of signal to noise (S/N) versus percent of normal water (percent deuterium oxide) as a measure of S/N linearity.

Signal Linearity

Signal linearity refers to the ability of an imaging system to accurately measure differences in signal intensity. This parameter can be measured using varying concentrations of deuterium oxide and distilled normal water as described in the previous section. In a perfect system the normalized signal intensity would correspond exactly to the percent of normal water in the sample. The linearity of a clinical system is assessed by evaluating the closeness of a series of measurements performed on the system to the identity line as shown in Figure 87–6.

Spatial Linearity

Spatial linearity evaluates the ability of an imaging system to precisely reproduce a distribution without geometric distortions. Suggested phantoms for evaluating this parameter center on the concept that images of straight line distributions should yield straight lines. Deviations from straight lines are documentations of spatial nonlinearities or distortions. Orthogonal holes, line grids, and bar patterns may be used to evaluate spatial linearity in both two-dimensional and three-dimensional imaging techniques. The aspect ratio (ratio of image field size in the horizontal and vertical directions)

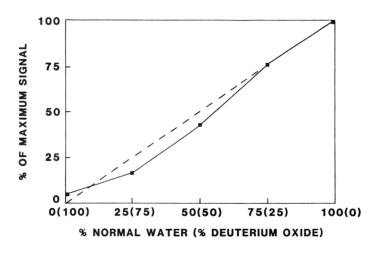

Figure 87–6. Plot of signal intensity normalized to the maximum intensity versus percent normal water (percent deuterium oxide) as a measure of signal linearity. The identity line is shown to represent the response for a perfect system.

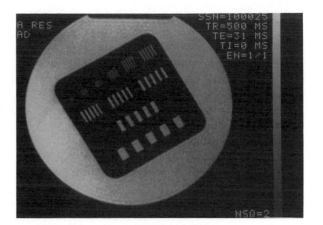

Figure 87–7. Measurement of line pair spatial resolution using a computed tomography phantom filled with propylene glycol to produce an NMR signal. The bars on the top row have thicknesses and spacings of 0.5, 0.6, 0.8, 1.0, 1.25, and 1.5 cm, left to right.

should also be evaluated. These measurements can be made at the same time spatial linearity is determined. Obviously, the aspect ratio of clinical systems should be 1.0.

Spatial Resolution

Spatial resolution refers to the ability of an imaging system to separate (resolve) small objects placed close together. Line pair spatial resolution can be measured using phantoms similar to those used in x-ray computed tomography with multiple signal producing cylinders or lines of varying sizes and separations as shown in Figure 87–7. The line pair spatial resolution is defined as the smallest objects that can be visually separated. One manufacturer (Technicare, Inc.) supplies a phantom for quantitative full width at half maximum (FWHM) spatial resolution measurements consisting of 10 cylinders containing signal producing material of diameters ranging from 0.8 to 19.1 mm. In practice region-of-interest measurements of signal intensity are measured from an image of this phantom and plotted as a function of cylinder diameter as shown in Figure 87–8. Spatial resolution (FWHM) is defined as the cylinder size at which the signal intensity drops to 50 percent of maximum.

Slice Thickness

Knowledge of accurate slice thickness in routine imaging is important in order to interpret patient studies and evaluate potential abnormalities. Variations of the slant

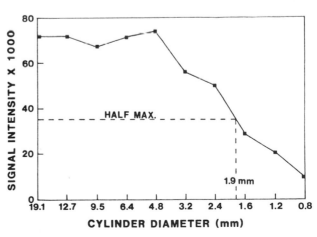

Figure 87–8. Measurement of FWHM spatial resolution by plotting signal intensity from a series of signal producing cylinders of varying diameter as a function of cylinder diameter.

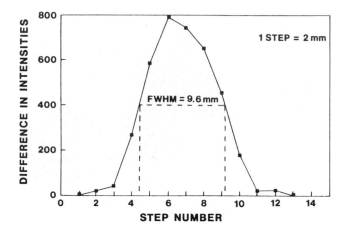

Figure 87–9. Measurement of slice thickness using a discrete step wedge phantom.

line, continuous wedge, and step wedge concepts have been used for these measurements. The step wedge measurement entails the imaging of a phantom containing incremental steps of a signal-producing material (2 mm steps for example) and plotting the difference in signal intensity between adjacent steps. The FWHM of this plot yields a measure of slice thickness as shown in Figure 87–9.

Slice Location

The accuracy of slice localization and distance between slices for multislice techniques is also of great importance for image interpretation. One method that has been used in nuclear medicine tomography as well as computed tomography for performing these measurements is the spiral line phantom shown in Figure 87–10. This phantom consists of a double helix formed with tubing containing signal producing material wound around a cylinder 18 cm in height. The helix is wound such that 10 degrees of arc corresponds to 1 cm of vertical distance. Two vertical lines are placed on opposite sides of the cylinder to serve as position references. A transverse section image through the phantom yields two high intensity spots corresponding to the point at which the image plane passes through the two arms of the helix as well as two additional spots corresponding to the intersection with the vertical lines (Fig. 87–11). In images of subsequent slices the line connecting the first two spots will rotate about the center in direct proportion to the displacement of each slice. The actual displacement of each slice is determined by measuring the amount of rotation and calculating the slice position from the known pitch (1 cm/10 degrees) of the phantom.

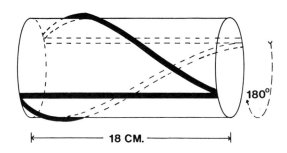

Figure 87–10. Spiral line phantom for slice localization measurements.

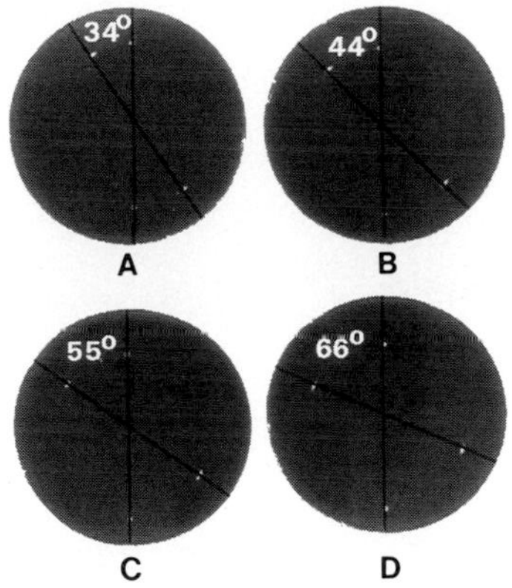

Figure 87–11. Four transverse slices through the spiral line phantom in Figure 87–10. The mean of the differences in angles of adjacent slices is 10.7 degrees. Since 10 degrees corresponds to 10 mm, the mean distance between slices for this acquisition was measured to be 10.7 mm.

Quantitative Measurements

As MRI technology becomes more advanced the need for accurate measurements of *T1* and *T2* will become more important. It will then become necessary to routinely measure phantoms containing standards with known values of *T1* and *T2* to assess the accuracy and reproducibility of these quantitative determinations.[8]

References

1. Budinger TF: Nuclear magnetic resonance (NMR) in vivo studies: Known thresholds for health effects. J Comput Assist Tomog *5*:800–811, 1981.
2. Pavlicek W, Geisinger M, Castle L, et al: The effects of nuclear magnetic resonance on patients with cardiac pacemakers. Radiology *147*:149–153, 1983.
3. BRH issue guidelines for NMR risks. Am Coll Radiol Bull *38*:9, 1982.
4. Saunders RD. Biologic effects of NMR imaging. Appl Radiol *11*:43–46, 1982.
5. Kanal E, Wolfe GL: Heat deposition effects in nuclear magnetic resonance imaging in 550 patients. Magn Reson Imag *4*:139, 1986.
6. Shellock FG, Schaefer DJ, Crues JV: Thermal response to different levels of radiofrequency power deposition during clinical magnetic resonance imaging at 1.5 Tesla. Magn Reson Imag *4*:94, 1986.
7. Shellock FG, Crues JV: Change in corneal temperature associated with high-field (1.5 Tesla) magnetic resonance imaging: Experience in 118 patients. Magn Reson Imag *4*:95, 1986.
8. Patton JA, Kulkarni MV, Craig JK, Wolfe OH, Price RR, Partain CL, James AE Jr: Techniques, pitfalls, and artifacts in magnetic resonance imaging. RadioGraphics *7*:505, 1987.

XVI

NMR SPECTROSCOPY

88

Phosphorus-31 Spectroscopy and Imaging

BRITTON CHANCE
JOHN S. LEIGH, Jr.
ALAN C. McLAUGHLIN
MITCH SCHNALL
TERESA SINNWELL

The possibility of continuous in-vivo monitoring of specific metabolites and physiologically important ions in organs and tissues affords an unparalleled opportunity for new overtures in medical research. The available technology of in-vivo nuclear magnetic resonance (NMR) is adequate for many of these goals, and great possibilities for future development exist. While medical research projects have often been characterized by incomplete information due to the invasiveness and discomfort of the particular tests and to radiation dose limitations, NMR provides, for the first time, a continuous and safe monitoring of the biochemistry of acute and chronic phases of disease and the response of patients to specific therapeutic protocols.

A number of cogent reasons have emerged for the direct measurement of cell biochemistry. The first is an obvious one. Invasion is required for classic biochemistry, while NMR spectoscopy provides an avenue to intercellular events without invasion. The second, equally important reason is that crucial energy metabolites, e.g., inorganic phosphate (P_i) and adenosine diphosphate (ADP), are often erroneously measured by analytical biochemical techniques. For example, P_i is often overestimated because of the degradation of phosphate esters during the extraction procedures, and the free ADP concentration is overestimated because of contributions from ADP bound to proteins. The latter problem is especially vexing because of the importance of the free ADP concentration in controlling the rate of intracellular oxidations.[1]

Other noninvasive methods are useful and under active development, particularly NADH fluorometry and cytochrome and hemoglobin spectrophotometry. In the latter case, deep transorgan illumination may be obtained in the near infrared region, while NADH fluorometry is a short range technique and usually requires exposure of the tissue surface. However, no optical method is available for the measurement of the functionality of tissue mitochondria in terms of ATP production, and phosphorus NMR is unique in that respect.

BACKGROUND

The emergence of NMR as a technique for the study of the chemical composition of living tissue has had an interesting history since the discovery of the principles of NMR by Purcell et al.[2] and Bloch et al.[3] nearly 40 years ago. In the beginning, NMR was a province of the physicists, but in the 1950s, with further development of high field NMR spectrometers, it became apparent that chemical bonding of the hydrogen atom with other elements slightly changed the resonant frequency of the protons, a phenomenon called the "chemical shift." This discovery attracted the interest of structural organic chemists, because of the opportunity it afforded them to identify and quantify specific compounds in solution. Interest spread rapidly, and NMR began to grow exponentially.

In 1959 Odeblad reported ^{1}H NMR studies of the chemical shift and relaxation times of water in human epithelial vaginal cells[4] and pointed out that ^{31}P, ^{13}C, and ^{23}Na NMR techniques could also be used to study human cells and tissues. He commented that "NMR really seems to possess extensive possibilities to help study, in a non-invasive way, many problems in biology and medicine," and predicted that "when instruments for NMR become more common and available at medical laboratories, we may expect direct routine clinical diagnosis with this new technique." In the last 10 years rapid advances in the application of NMR techniques to biochemical, physiological, and clinical problems have essentially confirmed this remarkable prediction.

NMR techniques utilize radiofrequency (rf) signals from physiologically important molecules and have the advantage that low-power rf magnetic fields are relatively harmless and can easily penetrate tissues. Perhaps the most striking advantage of the NMR technique is the wealth of metabolic information that is provided from a single spectrum. For example, the ^{31}P NMR spectrum from muscle or brain tissue contains signals from ATP, creatine phosphate, inorganic phosphate, and sugar phosphates and can be used to calculate the concentration of each of these components in the tissue. Also, the position of the ^{31}P NMR signal from inorganic phosphate can be used to calculate the intracellular pH of the tissue. Another advantage of the NMR technique is that spectra from a number of different nuclei can be observed. For example, while ^{31}P NMR techniques can be used to study phosphorylated metabolites, ^{1}H NMR techniques can be used to monitor intracellular lactate concentrations, ^{13}C NMR techniques can be used to follow the metabolism of ^{13}C-labeled substrates, and ^{23}Na and ^{39}K NMR techniques can be used to follow changes in transmembrane ionic gradients. Also, NMR techniques can be used to calculate steady-state rates of important physiological reactions in tissues and organs and have the potential to determine the three-dimensional localization of metabolites in specific tissues and organs. Each of these approaches is briefly discussed below.

^{31}P NMR Studies

MUSCLE

In 1974 Hoult et al.[5] demonstrated that ^{31}P NMR techniques could be used to follow changes in the creatine phosphate, ATP and inorganic phosphate concentrations, and the intracellular pH in excised muscle tissue from rat hind leg. In collaboration with Wilkie and his group, these experiments were soon expanded to study energy metabolism in toad and frog gastrocnemius muscle during periods of electrical stimulation and recovery,[6-8] and the results were interpreted in terms of the relationship between mechanical work performed by the muscle and transient changes in the levels of phosphorylated metabolites. In 1975–1976 Barany and his group reported a number of ^{31}P NMR studies on frog, toad, chicken, and rabbit muscle[9-12] and identified several hitherto "unknown" signals that were assigned to phosphodiester compounds, such as glycerophosphoryl choline and glycerophosphoryl ethanolamine. They also found that, compared to normal muscle tissue, the phosphodiester signals were higher in dystrophic chicken muscles and significantly decreased in human biopsy samples obtained from patients with Duchenne dystrophy.[10-13]

In 1978 the first horizontal bore superconductive magnet suitable for high resolution NMR spectroscopy in humans was commissioned, and ^{31}P studies on muscle were extended to intact human limbs. In 1980 and 1981 Chance et al.[14,15] published ^{31}P NMR studies of phosphorylated metabolites in human arm and calf muscle in the resting state, during exercise, and during recovery. The NMR techniques were used to determine the relationship between work output in the exercising human forearm and the steady-state capability of oxidative phosphorylation, as measured by the PCr/P_i ratio, and the results were explained in terms of metabolic control by the mitochondrial resting-to-active transition (state 3–state 4).[16]

A number of human myopathies have also been studied using ^{31}P NMR. For example, Ross et al.[17] studied a patient suspected of having McArdle's syndrome. They demonstrated that during exercise the decrease in PCr and the increase in P_i were more extensive than in controls, while the pH remained nearly constant or even increased; both of these findings were consistent with the suspected block in glycogen breakdown. Also, Chance et al.[18] studied a patient with a phosphofructokinase deficiency. They demonstrated that, in contrast to normal muscle, the P_i level remained low during exercise, while the sugar phosphate levels increased; both of these findings were consistent with a block in glycolysis.

HEART

In 1976 Gadian et al.[19] demonstrated that ^{31}P NMR techniques could be used to follow changes in phosphorylated metabolites in an ischemic excised heart. Further studies on perfused hearts followed the changes in PCr, ATP, sugar phosphates, and pH during partial[20-22] and global[23-26] ischemia and recovery. As expected, the PCr levels decreased and P_i levels increased rapidly after the onset of ischemia, while ATP levels did not appreciably decrease until PCr disappeared.[24] The effect of glycogen depletion on the pH change occurring during ischemia,[24] the effectiveness of drugs for treatment of myocardial infarction,[27] and the protective effect of preischemic additions of high KCl concentrations[21] have also been studied, and changes in the high-energy phosphate metabolites during the cardiac cycle of a free-running heart have been reported.[28]

KIDNEY

Sehr et al.[29] used ^{31}P NMR techniques to study the effect of cold ischemia and subsequent reperfusion of an isolated rat kidney under conditions chosen to mimic a kidney transplant operation. Radda et al.[30] and Ackerman et al.[31] also used ^{31}P NMR to monitor intracellular pH during acute renal acidosis in the perfused kidney.

LIVER

^{31}P NMR techniques have been used to study metabolism in hepatocytes[32] and perfused liver.[33-35] For example, McLaughlin et al.[33] studied the response of ATP and P_i to ischemia and recovery from ischemia. They also studied the effect of insulin on the ATP and P_i levels and showed that incubation with glucose and insulin decreased the rate of response of ATP and P_i to ischemia. Iles et al.[35] and Griffith et al.[36] also studied the response of a perfused liver to a "fructose load" and correlated the drop in ATP and phosphate levels with the rise in sugar phosphate levels.

BRAIN

Chance et al.[37] used ^{31}P NMR to study the effect of anoxia on the PCr/ATP ratios in the brain of an anesthetized mouse and introduced a new technique—"cryo-NMR"—to study the metabolic state of frozen brain tissue: at $-12°$ C phosphorylated metabolites are mobile enough to give observable ^{31}P NMR signals, and are stable enough in brain tissue that ^{31}P NMR spectra can be accumulated before substantial degradation of PCr occurs. In the last few years, a number of groups have reported ^{31}P NMR studies on brains of larger animals. For example Ackerman et al.[38] studied energy metabolism in the rat brain; Chance et al.[39] followed the brain energy states during and after periods of hypovolemia and ischemia in the cat brain; Prichard et al.[40] studied the effect of hypoglycemia, hypoxia, and experimental status epilepticus on the ATP and PCr levels and the intracellular pH in rabbit brain; and Wilkie et al.[41] and Younkin et al.[42] studied human neonatal brain.

TUMORS

In 1977 Navon et al.[43] reported ^{31}P NMR studies of Ehrlich ascites tumor cells and showed that the pH gradient across the cell membrane was very small, even under conditions of rapid glycolysis. ^{31}P NMR techniques have also been used to study metabolism in Walker carcinosarcoma tumors implanted in living rats[44] and to monitor changes in tumor metabolism during untreated growth and in response to treatment with various therapeutic modalities.[45–47] Phosphoethanolamine appears in high levels (~10 mM) in malignant neuroblastoma tumors in human infants[48] and decreases in remission and has been cited as a "fingerprint" of tumor invasiveness.[48]

KINETIC STUDIES

Saturation transfer techniques can be used to study steady-state unidirectional fluxes through enzyme-catalyzed reactions in cells and tissues. Brown et al.[49] used this approach to calculate the rate of ATP synthesis in *Escherichia coli* cells, and the technique was subsequently used to study the forward and reverse rates of the creatine kinase reaction in skeletal muscle,[50,51] heart,[52–54] and brain.[55]

METABOLIC CONTROL

Control of oxidative metabolism includes the delivery of ADP and P_i from the functional ATPases, the delivery of oxygen from the capillary circulation, and the delivery of substrates to form NADH, as indicated by Equation (1) (where the value of 3 is approximately):[56]

$$3ADP + 3P_i + NADH + H^+ + 1/2\ O_2 = 3ATP + NAD^+ + H_2O \tag{1}$$

A choice between ADP and P_i, or indeed ATP, as control chemicals for the rate of Equation (1) is equal insofar as the equations below are concerned, but P NMR has permitted a much more precise evaluation of this often vexing question.[57] Under various conditions, all of the substrates and products (except H_2O) might possibly serve as control chemicals. The control of respiration by ADP was first characterized by Chance and Williams;[16] however, biochemical assays of extracted tissues from various sources consistently revealed high ADP levels that changed by only small fractions when the tissue metabolic rates changed substantially. Metabolic control by inorganic phosphate has been favored in previous works[58,59] because analytical biochemistry showed large metabolism-linked variations of inorganic phosphate levels in ascites cells.[60] Recently, phosphorus NMR studies in vivo have begun to explain this old problem. Quantitative measurements in vitro showed the K_m for control of respiration in isolated mitochondria by inorganic phosphate to be about 1 mM, with significantly lower values for cardiac mitochondria (~0.2 mM).[61] NMR studies of human skeletal muscles show the resting (state 4) values of P_i to be in the range of 1 to 4 mM. By way of contrast, the values of ADP concentrations calculated from the P NMR data in the resting state are <10 μM, well below the K_m, consistent with ADP control of the respiration rate. In functional activity, in the transition from resting state 4 to the active state 3, the functional ATPase produces equal amounts of ADP and inorganic phosphate. Due to the hundredfold ratio of P_i/ADP, ADP levels rise 100 times more rapidly in proportion than does P_i, thus ensuring what amounts to ADP control of the transition from resting state 4 to the active state 3.

Metabolic control by NADH generating substrates is possible. For example, in insulin induced glucose deficiency,[62] the maximal capacity of ATP synthesis will decline. Under such conditions, the redox state of NADH shows oxidation well beyond that characteristic of the control state 4 or even the active state 3, a distinctive signal of deficiency of reducing substrate.[16]

Analytical biochemistry gives indirect support to the idea of P_i control, since ADP concentrations based on the analysis of total cell content give values that are manyfold K_m in ADP resting muscle[16] and in brain.[63] However, it is well known that a large fraction of the total cellular ADP is bound to various protein sites and thus unavailable for oxidative phosphorylation. This "bound" ADP is composed of two different classes of binding sites. Those ADP sites exchange with the pool of free ADP much more slowly than metabolic pool turnover times; i.e., >~1 min. This type of bound ADP is exemplified by the "structurally bound" ADP in actin and GDP in tubulin filaments. In skeletal muscle, heart, and brain this form may amount to 240, 160, and 320 n moles/g tissue.[64-67]

Other forms of "bound ADP" include that which is bound at enzyme active sites, e.g., creatine kinase, myosin, etc. While this form of ADP is in rapid equilibrium with the unbound pool, the equilibrium ratios of bound ATP/ADP are commonly near unity[68] and thus highly distorted from normal steady-state values for the unbound pools. Substantial portions of noncytoplasmic ADP are also identified with intraorganellar fractions. The intramitochondrial pool in heart and red skeletal muscle is particularly large due to the very high mitochondrial content. Bound ADP at allosteric control sites on various enzymes also accounts for a small fraction of the cellular ADP. The difficulties involved with properly delineating the various forms of metabolically active and nonmetabolically active ADP by biochemical extraction techniques are overwhelming but rarely fully appreciated. It is probably fair to say that this accounting has never yet been accomplished at a precision necessary for quantitative bioenergetic assessment.

The Mitochondrion as an ADP and P_i Indicator

Studies of isolated mitochondria showed that serial additions of increasing concentration of ADP resulted in a "Michaelis-Menten response"[69] of respiratory activity with a half maximal value of about 20 μm.[16] At the same time, it was found that NADH showed a half maximal oxidative response between the resting ADP deficient state 4 and fully activated, ADP saturated state 3.[70] By using the NADH response to ADP, as observed in vitro as an in-vivo ADP indicator in stimulated muscles, both perfused and in situ, a high sensitivity of mitochondria in vivo to ADP produced in single muscle twitches was demonstrated[70-72] and indicated that the mitochondria of the resting muscle are highly sensitive to ADP. These early observations identified free ADP in the cytosol as sensed by the mitochondrial translocase to be in the range of the K_m, only a small fraction of the bound plus free forms of ADP as measured by analytical biochemistry and consistent with that estimated by NADH fluorometry of the tissues. ^{31}P NMR results are especially relevant here, since the freely tumbling forms of P_i and PCr measured and the calculated values of ADP in the resting state are found to be much below the total ADP as measured by analytical biochemistry and consistent with that estimated by NADH fluorometry. Similar discrepancies of total and free ADP are found in brain.[73] Thus the free [ADP] is too small to be detected directly in the P NMR spectra; it must be computed from the creatine kinase equilibrium.

An In-Vitro Model

An in-vitro model portrays the steady state and thus simulates the physiological condition crucial to life.[74] In Figure 88–1, ATP synthesis must match ATP breakdown in a feedback loop involving ADP as the control chemical. Activation of the functional ATPase to break down ATP produces ADP and phosphate, which is translocated into the mitochondrial matrix to activate oxidative phosphorylation and to restore ATP, closing the feedback loop. The key feature of the system is that the ADP and phosphate concentrations regulate the rate of oxidative phosphorylation exactly to meet the needs of the functional ATPase so a homeostasis of the ATP level is obtained from this stable feedback loop. At the same time, the level of ATP is temporally and spatially buffered

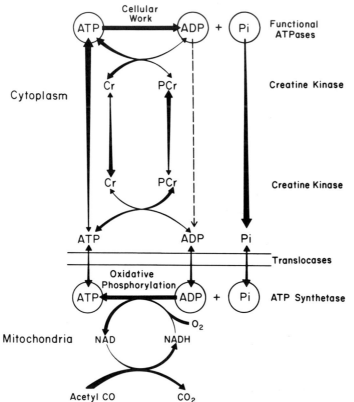

Figure 88–1. Illustration of the feedback interactions of the cytosolic and mitochondrial compartments of the muscle cell.

MD 731

by the creatine kinase equilibrium so that [ATP] and [ADP] are regulated and the variable parameters are PCr, P_i and Cr. As the levels of ADP and phosphate rise, glycolytic activity may be activated to further stabilize the ATP and ADP levels. As ATPase rates approach the maximal rate of oxidative phosphorylation, glycolysis takes over an increasing proportion of the metabolic burden, but the possibility of a stable metabolic state diminishes sharply. Thus, for each level of functional activity, there will be particular concentrations of PCr, P_i, and the control chemical, ADP.

The transfer function relates velocities or tissue work rates to the concentration of the control chemicals. There can be a transfer function for ADP, P_i, oxygen, substrate, or any of the parameters of Equation (1) or indeed for any combination of these. The intersection of the work or load line with the transfer function is termed the operating point. The operating point is confined to move along the transfer function as the work varies. We have determined the transfer function in vivo by an arm exercise protocol.

Derivation of Michaelis-Menten Relationship in Terms of NMR Parameters

It is apparent that the mechanisms by which ADP and phosphate react with the respiratory chain are through two different translocases; ADP reacts with the adenine nucleotide translocase, while P_i reacts with the phosphate transporter within the matrix space. ADP and P_i both come together to react at the matrix space ATP synthetase, but these species are probably not determinable by ^{31}P MRS (magnetic resonance spectroscopy) because of the high viscosity and multiple binding sites for ADP and P_i, especially as calcium phosphate. It is the change of the hydrogen ion gradient that "turns on" the mitochondrial respiratory chain and increases the velocity of mitochondrial oxidations, which in the steady state is equal to V of Equation (6) below. Since the adenine nucleotide translocases and the phosphate transporter have their own separate and independent K_m's, we would expect these to be noninteractive, since they are different membrane-bound enzymes. The cytosolic ADP and P_i concentrations control cell respiration according to our steady-state Michaelis-Menten formulation. We assume that the other substrates, NADH and O_2, and the product ATP are above their K_m's.

$$\frac{V}{V_m} = \frac{1}{1 + \dfrac{K'}{ADP} + \dfrac{K''}{P_i}} \qquad (2)$$

With ADP control and P_i in the range of its K_m, the P_i regulates the fraction of V_m that can be obtained at maximal ADP concentration. In the in-vivo case K'' is 1 mM or less and P_i may be 5 to 10 mM at $V = V_m/2$.

NMR perceives only indirectly the concentration of the control chemical, ADP, through the creatine kinase equilibrium and measures directly two major components of this equilibrium, namely, ATP and phosphocreatine.

$$PCr + ADP + H^+ \xrightarrow{K_{ck}} ATP + Cr \qquad (3)$$

$$[ADP] = \frac{[Cr] \times [ATP]}{[PCr] \times [H^+]} K_{ck} \qquad (4)$$

For this discussion, we shall assume a constant pH of 7.1, a temperature of 37°, a 1 mM free magnesium concentration, and a 5 mM ATP concentration giving $K_{cr}K \times [H^+] = 130^{63}$, K_m ADP $= 2 \times 10^{-5}$ M.[16]

Substituting these parameters in the Equation (2), we obtain

$$\frac{V}{V_{max}} = \frac{1}{1 + \dfrac{0.66}{[Cr]/[PCr]}} \tag{5}$$

However, it is useful for phosphorus NMR spectroscopy to measure the ratio of P_i/PCr, since this compensates for scale factors, differing relaxation times, etc. Under our conditions of steady-state exercise, we observe $PCr + P_i$ to be constant to approximately ± 10 percent.[75] Analytical data show $PCr + Cr$ is constant in a variety of studies.[76] Since the increments of Cr and P_i are necessarily equal in exercise over a range of 2 to 12 nM, relatively small inequalities of Cr and P_i are assumed to be negligible at higher work loads and large P_i values. Sensitive proton NMR can eventually afford the sum of PCr and Cr as well as the ratio. Replacement of Cr with P_i leads to the approximate expression:

$$\frac{V}{V_{max}} = \frac{1}{1 + \dfrac{0.66}{[P_i]/[PCr]}} \tag{6}$$

This simple and useful equation appears to be a very good approximation if P_i, NADH, and O_2 are above their K_m's and pH does not fall. Human arm exercise gives 0.65 ± 0.06[1], for a hyperbolic foot and 0.5 for a linearized Hanes plot.[75]

Control by ADP·P₁

For completeness two more general cases are included that cover the situation in which ADP and P_i are below their K_m's and the reversal of phosphorylation is significant.

The possibility that ATP, ADP, and P_i contribute to in-vivo metabolic control is suggested by our observation in isolated mitochondria that the reduction of NAD by succinate required ATP:

$$\text{Succinate} + \text{ATP} + \text{NAD}^+ \rightarrow \text{fumarate} + \text{NADH} + \text{ADP} + P_i + H^+ \tag{7}$$

It was further found that reduced cytochrome c was oxidized in anaerobic mitochondria by addition of ATP and that an ATP/ADP $\times$ P_i ratio of approximately 10^4 M^{-1} characterized the half-potential of this reaction. These results were confirmed and extended by Klingenberg[77] whose results suggested that respiration was governed by an ATP/ADP $\times$ P_i ratio of 1.6×10^4 M^{-1}. Thus it is important to recognize whether or not these results are of importance in exercised muscle as studied here.

A modification of Equation (2) to this point gives:

$$\frac{V}{V_{max}} = \frac{1}{1 + \dfrac{\text{ATP} \cdot 6.3 \times 10^{-5}}{P_i \cdot \text{ADP}}} \tag{8}$$

Substitution of the creatine kinase equilibrium then yields:

$$\frac{V}{V_{max}} = \frac{1}{1 + \dfrac{8.1 \times 10^{-3}/\text{Cr}}{P_i/\text{PCr}}} \tag{9}$$

For creatine concentration of 15 mM, this formulation predicts a P_i/PCr, "K_m" of 0.54.

Thus the transfer function between work, V/V_{max}, and biochemical response P_i/PCr is expected to approximate a rectangular hyperbola with "K_m" of 0.5 to 1. We have therefore explored this relation in detail over the past several years[75,78] in order to determine how well this simple equation fits the muscle exercise data and if so what the experimental value of "K'_m" may be.

Steady-State Exercise Protocol

Since the above relations apply to the steady state at constant pH and oxygen delivery, the subject performs graded levels of exercise, in a steady-state protocol from rest to approximately K_m; i.e., $P_i/PCr \sim 0.6$ (see Equation 6). The work is quantitatively evaluated by an ergometer coupled to the exercised limb, and the P_i/PCr value is measured by a surface coil placed upon the exercising muscle. Thus this is an essential aerobic exercise and contrasts with other exercise protocols that are carried out to the point of fatigue, lactic acidosis, etc. and generally non–steady-state conditions that also require a large pH correction to P_i/PCr.[79] Occasionally, we increase the work to near V_{max} to identify the maximal work capability but do not normally include this as part of the transfer function analysis.

Figure 88–2 illustrates a typical protocol for evaluation of steady-state,[75] endurance performance through the work P_i/PCr relationship. Each 5 min measurement interval is preceded by an interval of 3 min to ensure that a steady state is achieved that declines less than 10 percent during the 5 min measurement interval. This protocol also affords a "maximal bout" at the end of the steady-state interval in order to validate the V_{max} calculation.

Experimental Results

Figure 88–3 shows a typical transfer characteristic for an endurance performance test of a human arm where the work is varied from 10 to 35 J/min and the corresponding values of P_i/PCr increase from the resting value of 0.1 to a value slightly over 1. The

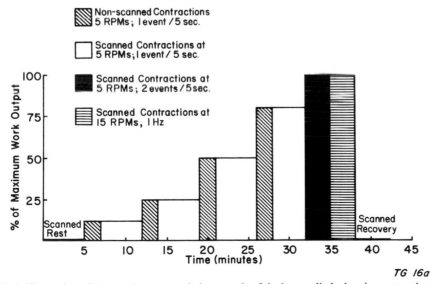

Figure 88–2. Illustration of the steady-state graded protocols of the human limb showing rest and contraction intervals. Each interval of measured performance preceded by a warmup interval.

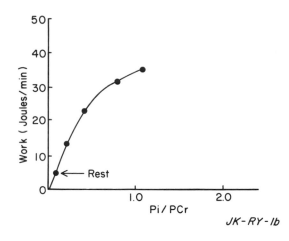

Figure 88–3. Illustration of the graded arm exercise protocol using the ergometer coupling.

form of the curve in this case approximates a rectangular hyperbola. The experimental data[1] are well fit to Equation 6 with a V_{max} of 59 J/min and a K_m of 0.65 + 0.06. This corresponds to K_m ADP = 25 μM. We can also use these values to calculate that the resting state value of V/V_{max} is approximately 0.1, which may not be the minimum value (see below).

The transfer function is also fit by Equation 9 with a V_{max} of 48.7 J/min assuming total creatine (Cr + PCr) concentration of 30 mM, and Cr = P_i + 10 mM. This yields a "K_m" of ~0.50.

Effect of Regulation of Oxygen Delivery on the Transfer Function

The decrease of inorganic phosphate in hyperemia following exercise has been attributed by us to a "luxury perfusion" of the organ in the hyperemic interval.[80] Radda[81] has suggested otherwise, proposing a sequestration of inorganic phosphate, perhaps in the mitochondrial matrix as calcium phosphate, indeed a plausible hypothesis. We have performed a simple exercise protocol that is described by Figure 88–3, in which an individual exhibiting a sigmoidal work/cost transfer characteristic has been instructed to exercise up to a particular point along the transfer characteristic 5, in the normal manner, to reduce the work level at point 6 to that corresponding to point 2 and continue with incremental work levels thereafter. The experimental data are telling. The initial slope of the transfer characteristic is very small, points 1 and 2, and steepens as the workload increases to form the limb of a rectangular hyperbola, which is usually observed under these conditions. During this exercise lasting approximately 15 min, the oxygen delivery to the limb increases and it "warms up" (both figuratively and literally). On returning to the lowest workload, the inorganic phosphate is considerably less and the phosphocreatine is greater. No evidence of a sigmoidal characteristic is observed; instead the limb of a rectangular hyperbola is seen, as would be expected for ADP (P_i/PCr) control. It is of note that the slope of the linear portion of the two transfer functions is identical, and thus it is only the initial portions of the transfer characteristic that are different.

An explanation is afforded by a simple form of the Michaelis-Menten transfer characteristic for both ADP and oxygen limitation.

$$\frac{V}{V_m} = \frac{1}{1 + \dfrac{K_1}{P_i/PCr} + \dfrac{K_2}{O_2}} \tag{10}$$

An oxygen limitation will necessitate an increase of ADP in order to maintain the particular velocity of the particular steady-state workload (V equal to the steady state ATP synthetase rate). If, however, the oxygen delivery is increased by the microcirculation so that it is no longer limiting, the simple form of Equation (6) holds true.

These results suggest that oxygen delivery to the limbs of certain individuals at rest is diminished to the point where its concentration is below the K_m for oxygen as determined in isolated mitochondria but that the microcirculation increases to deliver more than enough oxygen as the exercise is started. This parsimony of oxygen delivery is no doubt an important aspect of the body's economy, limiting cardiac output in the resting state to "minimal maintenance" values.

In this particular application, P phosphorus MRS is used as an "oxygen sensor"[82] and has been used to calculate directly the intracellular oxygen concentration. Thus, important information can be quantified not only on metabolic control phenomena and the velocity of intracellular oxidations but also on possible limitations by oxygen, as shown here, and in other cases, by NADH delivery.

Work-Cost Relations in Brain Metabolism

As one considers the locations in the cortical neuron where the energy-linked reactions occur (Fig. 88–4), the diagram shows dendrites, axons, and synapses.[83] In each of these, mitochondria are clearly delineated by cross striations. They make ATP from oxygen and glucose. ATP powers the ion pumps of synapses, axons, and dendrites. Oxygen lack in the neurons leads to the "electrical silence" of the anoxic brain, whether from stroke, head injury, aneurysm, or operative intervention. Following anoxia and

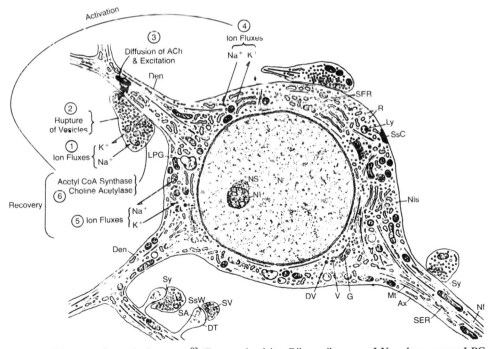

Figure 88–4. Diagram of a typical neuron.[83] (Den = dendrite; Rih = ribosome; LY = lysosomes; LPG = lipofuscin pigment granules; AX = axon; SER = endoplasmic reticulum; Nf = neurofilament; N = nucleus; NI = nucleolus; SsC = subsurface cisternae; DT = dendritic thorns; NS = nucleolar satellite; G = Golgi apparatus; Mt = microtubles; SsW = subsynaptic web; Nis = Nissl substance; DV = dense vesicles; Sy = axon terminals from synapse; SV = synaptic vesicles.)

Table 88–1. PROBES OF ENERGETICS OF CELL FUNCTION

(1) Neuronal Stimulation
$$K^+_{in} \rightarrow K^+_{out}$$
$$Na^+_{out} \leftarrow Na^+_{in}$$
(2) Ion Pumping
$$K^+_{out} \leftarrow K^+_{in}$$
$$Na^+_{in} \rightarrow Na^+_{out}$$
(3) Energy Cost Paid
$$ATP \rightarrow ADP + P_i$$
(4) Energy Recharge from PCr
$$ADP + PCr(\square) \leftrightarrow ATP(\square) + Cr$$
(5) Oxidative Phosphorylation
$$3ADP + 3P_i + NADH(\bigcirc) + \tfrac{1}{2}O_2(\triangle) + H^+ \rightarrow NAD^+ + H_2O + 3ATP$$
(6) Glycolytic Phosphorylation
$$Glucose + 2ADP + 2P_i + 2NAD^+ \rightarrow 2 \text{ Pyruvate} + 2ATP(\square) + 2NADH + 2H^+$$

Probes
$\square$ ^{31}P NMR
$\bigcirc$ Optical
$\triangle$ Tissue oxygen uptake

the loss of ion pumping activities are water movements into the cell, edema, further blockade of oxygen delivery, and eventual pathologic changes; physiologic derangement precedes histologic and anatomic changes.

NMR signals are fundamental to assessment of functional activity by measurements of ATP, PCr, and P_i, as noted by the chemical equations (Table 88–1). Electrical discharges following neuronal stimulation are the result of transmembrane sodium and potassium movements that require ion pumping to re-establish the ion gradients and membrane potentials. The energy is provided by the breakdown of ATP into ADP + P_i. Transient energy recharge from PCr restores ATP, indicated by a drop of PCr and an increase of P_i, both detectable by NMR. ATP is maintained in a steady state by oxidative phosphorylation supplemented to the extent of a few percent by the 36-fold less efficient glycolytic phosphorylation. When glycolysis rates of pyruvate production are greater than that which mitochondrial respiration is consuming, an undesirable production of lactate and intracellular acidosis ensues.

Another formulation assumes the ATP synthetase to be rate controlling and takes the matrix space ADP and P_i to be equal to the NMR determined cytosolic values.[84] For the reversible equilibrium of ADP + P_i and ATP, and including product inhibition a general equation is:[85]

$$\frac{V}{V_{max}} = \frac{[ADP][P_i] - ([ATP]/ke)}{\begin{array}{c} K_{ADP}K_{iPi} + K_{ADP}[P_i] + K_{Pi}[ADP] + (K_{Pi}/K_{iATP})[ATP][ADP] \\ + [ADP][Pi] + (K_{iADP}K_{Pi}/K_{iATP})[ATP] \end{array}} \tag{11}$$

where V_{max} is the maximal forward rate and ke is the equilibrium phosphorylation ratio.

Three assumptions are necessary to make the equation useful:

(1) $K_{iADP} \gg [ADP]$: This refers to the fact that ADP binding to an ATP-enzyme complex to form an inactive species is unlikely, since they would both occupy the same site on the ATP synthetase enzyme.

(2) $K_{ATP} \ll [ATP]$: The ATP binding site is occupied, and the back reaction is saturated.

(3) The binding of the substrates is interactive, as in the ATP synthetase. The resulting simplified equation is:

$$\frac{V}{V_{max}} = \frac{1 - (PR/Ke)}{1 + b(PR/ke)} \tag{12}$$

and

$$PR = [ATP/[ATP]$$

where b is the ratio of the maximal forward to maximal reverse rates. This expression also can be made to fit the in-vitro data of Gyulai et al.[86] for $b = 8$, which is in agreement with other measurements.[87] For PR $> Ke$, and for $b = 1$, this expression becomes identical to Equation (8).

This formulation has been applied to predict the response of the phosphorylation ratio (PR) in the brain to various levels of seizure activity. Figure 88–5 shows the relationship between the experimental results and theoretical prediction. Since ATP remained constant, this plot is of ADP·P_i.

Multinuclear Spectroscopy

Methods using frequency interleaved data acquisition can be used to simultaneously acquire information from several nuclei.[88,89] This technique is especially useful in the brain for monitoring simultaneously high energy phosphates and the intracellular pH through ^{31}P NMR; and lactate, the major product of anaerobic glycolysis, through ^{1}H NMR. Sample spectra from a cat brain under conditions of acute hypoxia with bilateral carotid occlusion are shown in Figure 88–6. These spectra clearly demonstrate the lactate increase that signifies an increase in the anaerobic metabolism associated with the decrease in the energy state of the brain during hypoxic-ischemic stress. Figure 88–7 shows the time course of the changes of the various metabolites in the cat brain during a protocol consisting of first, a 16 min hypoxic challenge followed, after a 50 min recovery period, by an 8 min challenge with hypoxia and bilateral carotid occlusion. During hypoxia and hypoxia/ischemia there was a decrease in the PCr level and an increase in P_i. There was also the development of an intracellular acidosis associated with lactate accumulation. ATP levels remained constant throughout the protocol. The lactate level and the pH are correlated, and a buffer capacity of 25.2 m·H$^+$/pH is calculated. The decrease of the lactate level accumulated during hypoxia and hypoxia/ischemia is zero-order in the lactate level, independent of the type or severity of the insult, and has a rate of 0.36 mM lac/min. With this slow rate of lactate clearance, it took up to 30 min to clear the acidosis.

ADP levels can be calculated through the creatine kinase equilibrium, assuming the K_{ck} of Veech.[90] Control values were found to be 13.4 ± 1.2 µM in five cats. This is an order of magnitude lower than extract results because in the extracts, ADP structurally bound to actin is also measured.[91] The calculated ADP levels show only a slight increase during hypoxia, with a marked rise during hypoxia with bilateral carotid occlusion (Fig. 88–8). The decrease in ADP during recovery is rapid (within 5 min), indicating that the more persistent decrease in PCr is due to the pH effect on the creatine kinase equilibrium stemming from the slow clearance of the lactate acidosis. The sig-

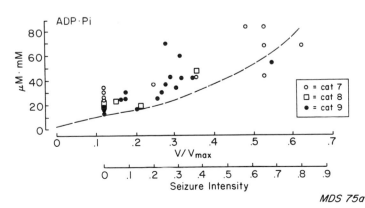

Figure 88–5. Plot of ADP·Pi as a function of brain work (quantified by serum intensity). Since ATP remained constant, this quantity is proportional to 1/PR.

MDS 75a

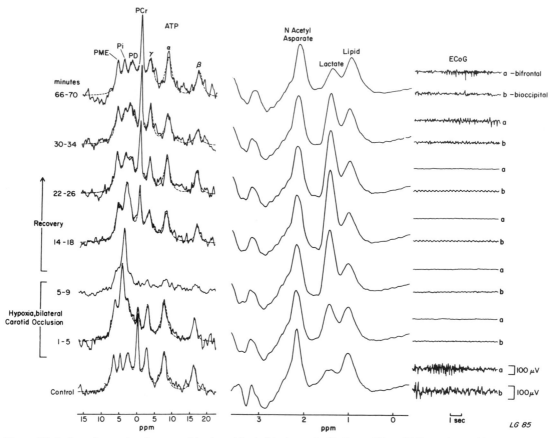

Figure 88–6. Sample spectra from a cat brain subjected to hypoxia (PaO$_2$ = 20) and bilateral carotid occlusion.

nificant decrease in PCr with little change in ADP during hypoxia alone also indicates that this effect is predominantly mediated by the H$^+$ effect on the creatine kinase equilibrium.

A protocol consisting of an intravenous injection of 2 to 6 mg/kg bicuculline to induce seizure activity has also been studied; but this time triple nuclear acquisition was used to also follow Na$^+$ in addition to lactate and high energy phosphates. Because of differences in NMR visibility of intra- and extracellular ^{23}Na, movement of the Na$^+$ into the cells is associated with a decrease in the intensity of the ^{23}Na peak.[92]

The injection of bicuculline was followed by the rapid onset of very high intensity rapid electrical activity that occurred continuously for approximately 4 to 5 min depending on the dose. After the initial phase of continuous seizure activity, the EEG showed a burst suppression pattern with the bursts getting shorter and the electrically silent period increasing in length as time progressed until there was a return of brain electrical activity to control. By analogy with the arm exercise protocol, the seizure activity was quantified as the percentage of time in a given period that there is high amplitude electrical activity. Decreases in PCr pH to approximately one half of control values were observed. The ^{23}Na signal decreased to approximately 85 to 90 percent of control values during the seizure and returned to normal with the cessation of the seizure. Figure 88–9 shows the time course of NMR changes during the protocol.

A plot of P$_i$/PCr as a function of seizure intensity is shown in Figure 88–10. During the seizure there is an increase in the energy usage of the brain, resulting in a greater rate of energy production. Since ATP and pH are not changing, Equation (6) indicates

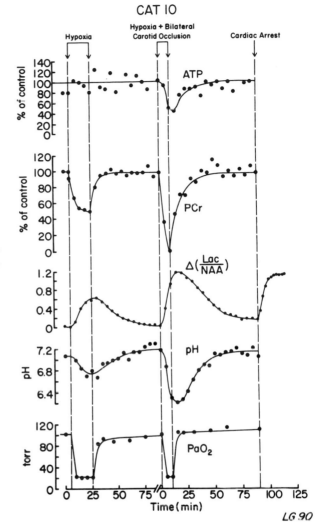

Figure 88–7. Time course of metabolic changes in the brain during hypoxia and hypoxia with bilateral carotid occlusion in the brain.

that the increase of P_i/PCr corresponds to an increase of V/V_m. There is also a correlation between the intensity of the Na signal and the seizure intensity (Fig. 88–11). During the seizure, there is known to be an influx of Na^+ and an efflux of K^+ from the cells. This could be expected to cause a decrease in the level of the ^{23}Na signal from the partial invisibility of the intracellular Na signal. It has been shown that the increase in extracellular K^+ is proportional to the seizure intensity.[93] Thus the correlation between the ^{23}Na signal intensity and the seizure intensity is consistent with

Figure 88–8. Time course of the response of the calculated ADP from the same cat as in Figure 88–7.

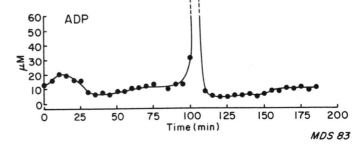

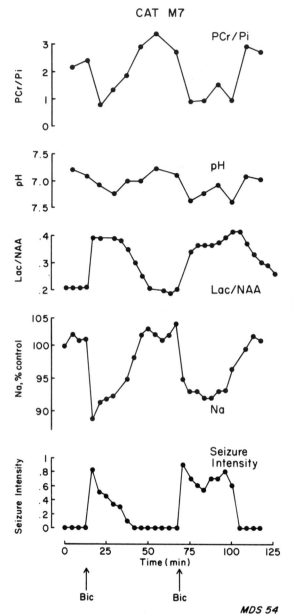

Figure 88–9. Time course of the metabolic response of a cat brain seizure.

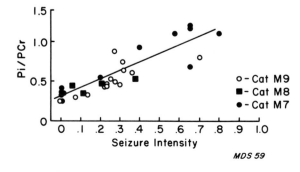

Figure 88–10. Plot of Pi/PCr as a function of seizure intensity.

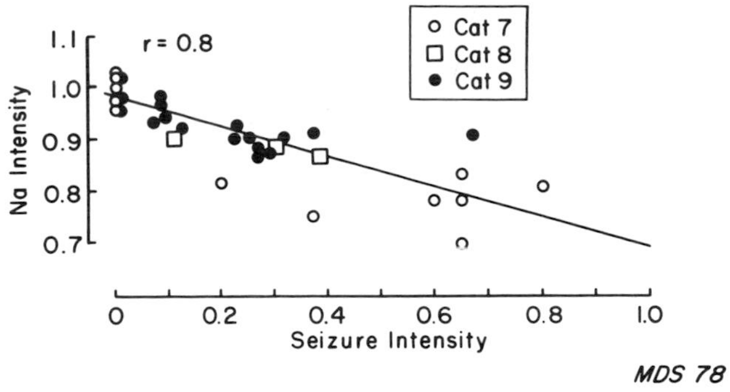

Figure 11. Plot of ^{23}Na intensity as a function of the seizure intensity. The decreased ^{23}Na intensity is from movement of Na into the intracellular space during seizure.

these measurements. A decrease in the ^{23}Na signal intensity has also been demonstrated during hypoxia and ischemia, when movement of Na$^+$ from the extracellular space to the intracellular space is known to occur.

ACKNOWLEDGMENTS

This work has been supported by NIH Grants RR 02305, AA 05662, NS 22881, HL 31934; the Benjamin Franklin Partnership's Advanced Technology Center of Southeastern Pennsylvania; and the Council for Tobacco Research 1493.

References

1. Chance, B, Leigh Jr JS, Clark BJ, Maris J, Kent J, Nioka S, Smith D: Control of oxidative metabolism and oxygen delivery in human skeletal muscle: A steady-state analysis of the work/energy cost transfer function. Proc Natl Acad Sci USA *82*:8384–8388, 1985.
2. Purcell EM, Torrey HC, Pound RV: Resonance absorption by nuclear magnetic moments in a solid. Phys Rev *69*:37–38, 1946.
3. Bloch F, Hansen WW, Packard M: The nuclear induction experiment. Phys Rev *70*:474–485, 1946.
4. Odeblad E: Research in obstetrics and gynecology with nuclear magnetic resonance. Acta Obstet Gynecol Scand *38*:599–617, 1959.
5. Hoult DI, Busby SJW, Gadian DG, Radda GK, Richards RE, Seeley PJ: Observation of tissue metabolites using ^{31}P NMR. Nature *252*:285–287, 1974.
6. Dawson MJ, Gadian DG, Wilkie DR: Contraction and recovery of living muscles studied by ^{31}P nuclear magnetic resonance. J Physiol *267*:703–735, 1977.
7. Dawson MJ, Gadian DG, Wilkie DR: Studies of living contracting muscle by ^{31}P nuclear magnetic resonance. In Dwck RA, Campbell ID, Richards RF, Williams RJP (eds): NMR in Biology. London, Academic Press, 1977, pp 289–321.
8. Dawson MJ, Gadian DG, Wilkie DR: Muscular fatigue investigated by phosphorus nuclear magnetic resonance. Nature *274*:861–866, 1978.
9. Barany M, Barany K, Burt CT, Glonek T, Meyers TC: Structural changes in myosin during contraction and the state of ATP in the intact frog muscle. J Supramol Struct *3*:125–140, 1975.
10. Burt CT, Glonek T, Barany M: Phosphorus-31 nuclear magnetic resonance detection of unexpected phosphodiesters in muscle. Biochemistry *15*:4850–4852, 1975.
11. Burt CT, Glonek T, Barany M: Analysis of phosphate metabolites in intracellular pH and the state of adenosine triphosphate in the intact muscle by phosphorus nuclear magnetic resonance. J Biol Chem *251*:2584–2591, 1976.
12. Glonek T, Burt CT, Meyers TC, Barany M: P^{31} NMR studies of dystrophic and normal muscle. Abstracts 170TL. Meeting of American Chemical Society, Chicago, No. 166, 1975.
13. Burt CT, Danon MJ, Millar EA, Homa FL, Vuolo MD, Barany M, Glonek T: Variation of phosphate metabolites in normal and duchenne human muscle. Biophys J *21*:184a, 1978.
14. Chance B, Eleff S, Leigh JL: Noninvasive, nondestructive approaches to all bioenergetics. Proc Nat Acad Sci USA *77*:7430–7434, 1980.
15. Chance B, Eleff S, Leigh JS, Sokolow D, Sapega A: Mitochondrial regulation of phosphocreatinal phosphate ratios in exercising human muscle: A gated 31-P NMR study. Proc Nat Acad Sci USA *78*:6714–6718, 1981.
16. Chance B, Williams G: Respiratory enzymes in oxidative phosphorylation. I. Kinetics of oxygen utilization. J Biol Chem *217*:383–393, 1955.
17. Ross BD, Radda GK, Gadian DG, Rocker G, Esiri M, Falconer-Smith J: Examination of a case of suspected McArdle's syndrome by ^{31}P NMR. N Engl J Med *304*:1338–1342, 1981.

18. Chance B, Eleff S, Bank W, Leigh JS, Warnell R: NMR Studies of control of mitochondrial function in phosphofructokinase deficient human skeletal muscle. Proc Nat Acad Sci USA 79:7714–7718, 1982.
19. Gadian DG, Hoult DI, Radda GK, Seeley PJ, Chance B, Barlow C: Phosphorus nuclear magnetic resonance studies on normoxic and ischemic cardiac tissue. Proc Nat Acad Sci USA 73:4446–4448, 1976.
20. Hollis DP, Nunnally RL, Jacobus WE, Taylor GJ: Detection of regional ischemia in perfused beating hearts by phosphorus nuclear magnetic resonance. Biochem Biophys Res Commun 75:1086–1091, 1977.
21. Hollis DP, Nunnally RL, Taylor GT, Weisfeldt ML, Jacobus WE: Phosphorus nuclear magnetic resonance. J Magn Reson 29:319–330, 1978.
22. Salhany JM, Stohs SJ, Reinice LA, Pieper GM, Hassing JM: ³¹P nuclear magnetic resonance of metabolic changes associated with cyanide intoxication in the perfused rat liver. Biochem Biophys Res Commun 86:1077–1083, 1979.
23. Garlick PB, Radda GK, Seeley PJ, Chance B: Phosphorus NMR studies on perfused heart. Biochem Biophys Res Commun 74:1256–1262, 1977.
24. Garlick PB, Radda GK, Seeley PJ: Studies of acidosis in the ischemic heart by phosphorus nuclear magnetic resonance. Biochem J 184:547–554, 1979.
25. Jacobus WE, Taylor EJ, Hollis DP, Nunnally R: Phosphorus nuclear magnetic resonance of perfused working rat hearts. Nature 265:756–758, 1977.
26. Bailey IA, Williams SR, Radda GK, Gadian DG: The activity of phosphorylase in total global ischaemia in the rat heart: A ³¹P NMR study. Biochem J 196:171–178, 1981.
27. Nunnally RL, Bottomly PA: Assessment of pharmacological treatment of myocardial infraction by phosphorus-31 NMR with surface coils. Science 211:177–180, 1981.
28. Fossel ET, Morgan HE, Ingwall JS: Measurement of changes in high-energy phosphates in the cardiac cycle by using gated ³¹P nuclear magnetic resonance. Proc Nat Acad Sci USA 77:3654–3658, 1980.
29. Radda GK, Sehr PB, Bore PJ, Sells RA: A model kidney transplant studied by phosphorus NMR. Biochem Biophys Res Commun 77:195–202, 1977.
30. Radda GK, Ackerman JJH, Bore P, Sehr P, Wong GG, Ross BD, Green Y, Bartlett S, Lowry M: ³¹P NMR studies on kidney: Intracellular pH in acute renal acidosis. Int J Biochem 12:277–281, 1980.
31. Ackerman JJH, Lowry M, Radda GK, Ross BD, Wong GG: The role of intra-renal pH in regulation of ammonia genesis. ³¹P NMR studies of the isolated perfused rat kidney. J Physiol 319:65–79, 1981.
32. Cohen SM, Ogawa S, Rottenberg H, Glynn P, Yamane Y, Brown TR, Shulman RG, Williamson JR: ³¹P nuclear magnetic resonance studies of isolated rat liver cells. Nature 273:554–556, 1978.
33. McLaughlin AC, Takeda H, Chance B: Rapid ATP assays in perfused mouse liver by 31-P NMR. Proc Nat Acad Sci USA 76:5445–5449, 1979.
34. Salhany JM, Stohls SJ, Reinke LA, Pieper GM, Hassing JM: Biochem Biophys Res Commun 86:1077–1083, 1979.
35. Iles RA, Griffiths JR, Stevens AN, Gadian DG, Porteous R: Effects of fructose on the energy metabolism and acid-base status of the perfused starved-rat liver: A ³¹phosphorus magnetic resonance study. Biochem J 192:191–202, 1980.
36. Griffiths JR, Stevens AN, Gadian GD, Iles RA, Porteous R: Hepatic fructose metabolism studied by ³¹P nuclear magnetic resonance in the anaesthetized rat. Biochem Soc Trans 8:641, 1980.
37. Chance B, Nakase Y, Bond M, Leigh JS, McDonald G: The detection of 31-P NMR signals in brain using in vivo and freeze-trapped tissues. Proc Nat Acad Sci USA 75:4925–4929, 1978.
38. Ackerman JJH, Grove TH, Wong GG, Gadian DG, Radda GK: Mapping of metabolites in whole animals by ³¹P NMR using surface coils. Nature 283:167–170, 1980.
39. Chance B, Eleff S, Leigh Jr JS, Barlow C, Ligetti L, Gyulai L: Phosphorus NMR. In Partain CL, James AE, Rollo FD, Price RR (eds): Nuclear Magnetic Resonance (NMR) Imaging. 1st ed. Philadelphia, W.B. Saunders Co., 1983, pp 399–415.
40. Prichard JW, Alger JR, Behar KL, Petroff OAC, Shulman RG: Cerebral metabolic studies in vivo by ³¹P NMR. Proc Nat Acad Sci USA 80:2748–2751, 1983.
41. Cady EB, Dawson MJ, Hope PL, Tofts PS, Costello AM, Wilkie DR: Non-invasive investigations of cerebral metabolism in newborn infants by phosphorus nuclear magnetic resonance spectroscopy. Lancet 1:1059–1062, 1983.
42. Younkin DP, Delivoria-Papadopoulos M, Wagerle LC, Chance B: In vivo 31-P NMR spectroscopy in neonatal neurological disorders. In Plum F, Pulsinelli W (eds): Cerebrovascular Diseases. New York, Raven Press, 1985, pp 149–159.
43. Navon G, Ogawa S, Shulman RG, Yamane T: ³¹P Nuclear magnetic resonance studies of Ehrlich ascites tumor cells. Proc Nat Acad Sci USA 74:87–91, 1977.
44. Griffiths JR, Stevens AN, Iles RA, Gordon RE, Shaw D: ³¹P NMR investigation of solid tumours in the living rat. Biosci Rep 1:319–325, 1981.
45. Evanochko WT, Ng TC, Lilly MB, Lawson AJ, Corbett TH, Durant JR, Glickson JD: In vivo ³¹P NMR study of the metabolism of murine mammary 16/C adenocarcinoma and its response to chemotherapy, x-radiation, and hypothermia. Proc Nat Acad Sci USA 80:334–338, 1983.
46. Evanochko WT, Ng TC, Glickson JD, Durant JR, Corbett TH: Human tumors as examined by in vivo ³¹P NMR in athymic mice. Biochem Biophys Res Commun 109:1346–1351, 1982.
47. Ng TC, Evanochko WT, Hiramoto RN, Ghanta VK, Lilly MB, Lawson AJ, Corbett TH, Durant JR, Glickson JD: ³¹P NMR spectroscopy of in vivo tumors. J Magn Reson 49:271–280, 1982.
48. Maris JM, Evans AE, McLaughlin AC, D'Angio GJ, Bolinger L, Manos H, Chance B: ³¹P nuclear magnetic resonance spectroscopic investigation of human neuroblastoma in situ. N Engl J Med 312:1500–1505, 1985.

49. Brown TR, Ugurbil K, Shulman RG: [31]P nuclear magnetic resonance measurements of ATPase kinetics in aerobic *Escherichia coli* cells. Proc Nat Acad Sci USA *74*:5551–5553, 1977.

50. Gadian DG, Radda GK, Brown T, Chance EM, Dawson MJ, Wilkie DR: The activity of creatine kinase in frog skeletal muscle studied by saturation transfer nuclear magnetic resonance. Biochem J *194*:215–228, 1981.

51. Meyer RA, Kushmerick M, Brown T: Application of ^{31}P NMR spectroscopy to the study of striated muscle metabolism. Am J Physiol *242*:C1–C11, 1982.

52. Nunnally RL, Hollis DP: Adenosine triphosphate compartmentation in living hearts: A phosphorus nuclear magnetic resonance saturation transfer study. Biochemistry *18*:3642–3646, 1979.

53. Matthews PM, Bland JL, Gadian DG, Radda GK: The steady state rate of ATP synthesis in the perfused rat heart measured by ^{31}P NMR saturation transfer. Biochem Biophys Res Commun *103*:1052–1059, 1981.

54. Bittl JA, Ingwall JS: Reaction rates of creatine kinase and ATP synthesis in the isolated rat heart. J Biol Chem *260*:3512–3517, 1985.

55. Shoubridge EA, Briggs RW, Radda GK: ^{31}P NMR saturation transfer measurements of the steady state rates of creatine kinase and ATP synthesis in the rat brain. FEBS Lett *140*:288–292, 1982.

56. LeMasters JJ: The ATP-to-oxygen stoichiometries of oxidative phosphorylation by rat liver mitochondria: An analysis of ADP-induced oxygen jumps by linear nonequilibrium thermodynamics. J Biol Chem *259*:13123–13130, 1984.

57. Chance B: Quantitative aspects of the control of oxygen utilization. *In* Wolstenhome GEW, O'Connor CM (eds): Ciba Foundation Symposium on the Regulation of Cell Metabolism. London, J. & A. Churchill, Ltd, 1959, pp 91–129.

58. Wu R, Racker E: Regulatory mechanisms in carbohydrate metabolism. IV. Pasteur effect and Crabtree effect in ascites tumor cells. J Biol Chem *234*:1036–1041, 1959.

59. Lynen F, Koenigsberger R: Zum Mechanismus der Pasteur'schen Reaktion: Der Phosphat-Kreislauf in der Hefe und seine Beeinflussung durch 2,4-Dinitrophenol. Liebig's Ann Chem *573*:60–84, 1951.

60. Chance B, Martin DK: Determination of the intracellular phosphate potential of ascites cells by reversed electron transfer. *In* Wright B (ed): Control Mechanisms in Respiration and in Fermentation. New York, The Ronald Press Co, 1963, pp 307–332.

61. Chance B, Hagihara B: Direct spectroscopic measurements of interaction of components of the respiratory chain with ATP, ADP, phosphates and uncoupling agents. *In* Proceedings of the Vth International Congress of Biochemistry. Vol. 5, New York, Pergamon Press, pp 3–37, 1963.

62. Behar KL, den Hollander JA, Petroff OAC, Hetherington HP, Prichard JW, Shulman RG: Effect of hypoglycemic encephalopathy upon amino acids, high energy phosphates and pH in the rat brain in vivo. Detection by sequential ^{1}H and ^{31}P NMR spectroscopy. J Neurochem *44*:1045–1055, 1985.

63. Lawson JWR, Veech RL: Effects of pH and free Mg^{2+} on the K_{eq} of the creatine kinase reactions and other phosphate hydrolyses and phosphate transfer reactions. J Biol Chem *254*:6528–6537, 1979.

64. Szent Gyorgyi AG, Prior G: Exchange of adenosine diphosphate bound to actin in superprecipitated actomyosin and contracted myofibrils. J Molec Biol *15*:515–538, 1966.

65. Weber A, Heiz R, Reiss I: The role of magnesium in the relaxation of myofibrils. Biochemistry *8*:2266–2270, 1969.

66. Maruyama K, Weber A: Binding of adenosine triphosphate to myofibrils during contraction and relaxation. Biochemistry *11*:2990–2998, 1972.

67. Watson WE: Cell Biology of Brain. New York, John Wiley & Sons, 1976.

68. Nageswara Rao BD, Cohn M: ^{31}P NMR of enzyme-bound substrates of rabbit muscle creatine kinase. J Biol Chem *256*:1716–1721, 1981.

69. Michaelis L, Menten M: Die Kinetik der Invertinwirkung. Biochem Z *49*:333, 1913.

70. Chance B: Reaction of oxygen with the respiratory chain in cells and tissues. J Gen Physiol *49*:163–188, 1965.

71. Chance B, Mauriello G, Aubert XM: ADP arrival at muscle mitochondria following a twitch. *In* Rodahl K, Horvath SM (eds): Muscle as a Tissue. New York, McGraw-Hill, 1962, pp 128–146.

72. Chance B: The response of mitochondria to muscular contraction. Ann NY Acad Sci *81*:477–489, 1959.

73. Granholm L, Siesjo BK: The effects of hypercapnia and hypocapnia upon the cerebrospinal fluid lactate and pyruvate concentrations and upon the lactate, pyruvate, ATP, ADP, phosphocreatine and creatine concentrations of cat brain tissue. Acta Physiol Scand *75*:257–266, 1969.

74. Burton A: The properties of the steady state compared to those of equilibrium as shown in characteristic biological behavior. J Cell Comp Physiol *14*:327–349, 1939.

75. Chance B, Leigh JS Jr, Kent J, McCully, K, Nioka S, Clark BJ, Mavis JM, Graham T: Multiple controls of oxidation metabolism in living tissues as studied by phosphorus magnetic resonance. Proc Natl Asso Sci USA *83*: 9458, 1986.

76. Duffy TE, Nelson SR, Lowry OH: Cerebral carbohydrate metabolism during acute hypoxia and recovery. J Neurochem *19*:959–977, 1972.

77. Klingenberg M: Respiratory control as a function of the phosphorylation potential. *In* Papa S, Tager JM, Quagliariello E, Slater EC (eds): The Energy Level and Metabolic Control in Mitochondria. Amsterdam, Adriatica Editrice, 1969, pp 189–193.

78. Kent J, Chance B, Leigh JS Jr, Maris J, O'Toole M, Hiller D: Muscle exercise performance evaluation of ^{31}P NMR. Fed Proc *44*:1371, 1985.

79. Arnold DL, Matthews PM, Radda GK: Metabolic recovery after exercises and the assessment of mi-

tochondrial function in vivo in human skeletal muscle by means of ^{31}P NMR. Magn Reson Med *1*:307–315, 1984.

80. Chance B, Leigh Jr JS, McCully K, Argov Z, Boden B: Evaluation of human exercise performance capability in human limbs. *In* Benzi G, Packer L (eds): Problems in the Biochemistry of Physical Exercise and Training. Amsterdam, Elsevier Science Publishers B.V., 491, 1986, pp 491–502.

81. Cresshull I, Dawson MJ, Edwards RHT, Gadian DG, Gordon RE, Radda GK, Shaw D, Wilkie DR: Human muscle analyzed by ^{31}P nuclear magnetic resonance in intact subjects. Proc J Physiol *317*:18P, 1985.

82. Chance B, Leigh Jr JS, Nioka S: P MRS as a sensor of oxygen in the heart or brain tissue. 5th Meeting of the Society for Magnetic Resonance in Medicine, Montreal, August. *4*:1368, 1986.

83. Lentz TL: Cell Fine Structure. An Atlas of Drawings of Whole Cell Structure. Philadelphia, W.B. Saunders Co., 1971, p 357.

84. Schnall MD: Simultaneous Multi-Nuclear NMR Studies of Brain Metabolism. Ph.D. Thesis, University of Pennsylvania, 1986.

85. Roberts DV: Enzyme Kinetics. Cambridge University Press, 1977, pp 107–134.

86. Gyulai L, Roth Z, Leigh Jr JS, Chance B: Bioenergetic studies of mitochondrial oxidative phosphorylation. J Biol Chem *260*:3947–3954, 1985.

87. Rottenberg H, Robertson DE, Rubin E: The effect of temperature and chronic ethanol feeding on the proton electrochemical potential and phosphate potential in rat liver mitochondria. Biochim Biophys Acta *809*:1–10, 1985.

88. Schnall MD, Subramanian HV, Leigh Jr JS, Gyulai L, McLaughlin A, Chance B: A technique for simultaneous ^{1}H and ^{31}P NMR at 2.2 T in vivo. J Magn Res *63*:401–405, 1985.

89. Styles P, Grathuchl C, Brown F: Simultaneous multinuclear NMR by alternate scan recording of ^{31}P and ^{13}C spectra. J Magn Res *35*:329, 1979.

90. Veech RL, Lawson JW, Krebs HA: Cytostolic phosphorylation potential. J Biol Chem *254*:6538, 1979.

91. Szent Gyorgyi AG, Prior G: Exchange of adenosine diphosphate bound to actin in superprecipitated actomyosin and contracted myofibrils. J Molec Biol *15*:515–538, 1966.

92. Civan MM, Shporer M: NMR of sodium and potassium-39 in biological systems. *In* Berlinger LJ, Ruben J (eds): Biological Magnetic Resonance. Vol. 1. New York, Plenum Press, 1–32, 1974.

93. Futamichi KJ, Mutani R, Price DA: Potassium activity in rabbit cortex. Brain Res *75*:5–25, 1974.

89

Carbon-13: NMR Spectroscopy

SHEILA M. COHEN

Over the last decade high-resolution nuclear magnetic resonance (NMR) spectroscopy has become an established technique in metabolic studies of living cells, isolated perfused organs, and whole animals. The rapid expansion of biomedical applications of ^{31}P NMR described in the preceding chapters of this volume has almost certainly been aided by the fact that 100 percent of the naturally occurring phosphorus is the spin $\frac{1}{2}$ isotope ^{31}P. The natural abundance of carbon-13 (^{13}C) nuclei is only 1.1 percent; consequently, only certain storage compounds, such as triacylglycerols or glycogen, which can have very high intracellular concentrations, are detectable at the natural abundance level by ^{13}C NMR. However, the low natural abundance of ^{13}C nuclei has proved to be advantageous for metabolic studies because it allows us to follow the flow of ^{13}C label introduced by specifically labeled substrates. Thus, in most of the applications of the ^{13}C NMR method discussed here, ^{13}C-enriched substrates are metabolized in the living cell, and signals from intermediates and end-products are observed; the distribution of the ^{13}C label in these metabolites is then used to elucidate pathways and kinetics. The ^{13}C NMR method has the particular advantage of simultaneously detecting the individual carbon atoms in all metabolites that have been adequately labeled. This property makes ^{13}C NMR especially useful in delineating changes in cellular metabolism occurring in different physiological or disease states and aids our understanding of the complex responses of the cell to hormonal stimulation or to direct challenges from specific enzyme inhibitors. Because, ultimately, the operation and regulation of the enzymes of intermediary metabolism must be understood within the context of the physiology of the whole cell, it is useful to exploit the nondestructive ^{13}C NMR method and its special properties to complement traditional in-vitro studies with purified enzymes or ^{14}C tracer investigations of metabolism.

The sensitivity of NMR is inherently low by comparison with optical spectroscopy or radiochemical methods. Fortunately, a series of significant technological advances in NMR instrumentation occurring over the last decade has made physiological ^{13}C NMR studies feasible. Despite the low sensitivity of the method, the advantages of ^{13}C NMR in metabolic studies are manyfold. First, no biopsies are required to follow carbohydrate metabolism in whole perfused organs or in vivo. Second, the method is repetitive, and metabolism can be followed in real time with a typical resolution of 5 to 10 min. Third, because ^{13}C NMR peaks in spectra of cells and perfused organs are in general sharp and because chemical shifts are fairly specific, a large number of metabolites usually can be distinguished and measured in a single spectrum. Fourth, because the chemical shifts of certain key metabolites, for example, citrate, are sensitive to such factors as pH and Mg^{2+} complexation, the spectra also can monitor intracellular conditions. Fifth, administration of certain combinations of ^{13}C-labeled substrates can introduce well-defined multiplet structure, due to ^{13}C-^{13}C scalar (J) coupling, into the NMR peaks of key metabolites; these multiplets contain, in effect, a composite history of the metabolite with respect to its sources of labeled precursors and the extent of contributions from unlabeled endogenous sources.[1] No counterpart of ^{13}C-^{13}C J coupling exists in the analogous ^{14}C isotopic experiment. Lastly, when highly enriched (>90 percent at a specific site) substrates are used, ^{13}C NMR usually has an effective sensitivity approaching that of ^{31}P NMR when factors such as the nuclear Overhauser effect[2] and sharpness of the peaks are considered. Several reviews have focused, at least in part, upon physiological ^{13}C NMR spectroscopy.[3–8]

^{13}C NMR SPECTROSCOPIC STUDIES OF LIVER

The liver is pivotal in carbohydrate, amino acid, and lipid metabolism. Thus, it is not surprising that physiological ^{13}C NMR techniques have been applied extensively to the study of hepatic metabolism.

Natural Abundance ^{13}C NMR Investigations of Endogenous Metabolites in Liver

Glycogen[9–13] and triacylglycerols[14–16] are typically the only endogenous compounds detectable at the natural abundance level of ^{13}C in liver. In liver from normal fasted animals, only the triacylglycerols are measured. The type of information obtainable under these conditions is exemplified by the spectra shown in Figure 89–1. The natural abundance background spectrum of perfused liver from a 24-hour fasted, genetically obese (ob/ob) mouse (Fig. 89–1*b*) is contrasted with the spectrum of perfused liver from a 24-hour fasted lean littermate (Fig. 89–1*a*). The wet weight of the ob/ob liver was 2.5 times that of the lean liver; much of this additional weight is made up of triacylglycerols, which had a concentration of about 250 μmol/g liver wt in the ob/ob liver compared with 30 to 40 μmol/g liver wt in the lean liver. Because triacyl-

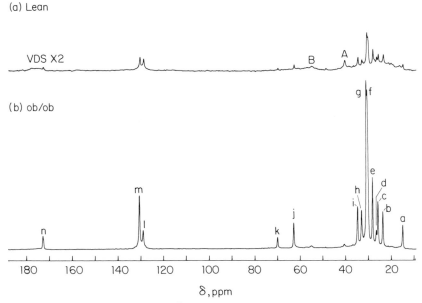

Figure 89–1. Natural abundance background ^{13}C NMR spectra at 90.5 MHz of isolated perfused liver, at 35°C, from (*b*) a genetically obese (ob/ob) mouse and (*a*) its lean littermate. Each spectrum represents 800 scans and required 10 min.[25] The notation VDS ×2 indicates that the gain on the vertical axis was increased twofold when spectrum (*a*) was read out.

glycerols are present in liver as neutral fat droplets[14] and therefore are reasonably mobile on the NMR time scale, carbon atoms in these compounds give rise to relatively sharp NMR peaks, as shown; in confirmation with this suggestion, it is noted that the spectrum of ob/ob liver shown in Figure 89–1b closely resembles that of adipose tissue.[16,17] However, beyond showing the increase in triacylglycerol content in ob/ob liver, an examination of the assignments of the labeled resonances in Figure 89–1, which are listed in Table 89–1, indicates another interesting difference; that is, the ratio of monounsaturated fatty acids to polyunsaturated fatty acids is manyfold greater in the ob/ob liver. Note that peak *l*, which arises only from polyunsaturated fatty acids, is relatively much less intense compared with peak *m*, which arises from *both* mono- and polyunsaturated fatty acids, in ob/ob liver (Fig. 89–1b) than in lean liver (Fig. 89–1a). Similarly, peak *d*, which can arise only from polyunsaturated fatty acids, is much less intense than peak *c*, to which all fatty acids may contribute, in ob/ob liver compared with the lean liver.

Using natural abundance ^{13}C NMR spectra of excised rat liver, Block[15] showed that ethionine-induced fatty liver was detectable by ^{13}C NMR and that the large increase in lipid resonances observable in ^1H and ^{13}C spectra of fatty liver as compared with control liver was attributable to triacylglycerides. We note, however, that in the ethionine-induced fatty livers the relative proportion of polyunsaturated fatty acids was not sharply reduced, as was observed in ob/ob liver.

Using the topical magnetic resonance (TMR) method in conjunction with radio-frequency (rf) surface coils, Canioni et al.[16] investigated the effects of chronic modification of dietary fat and carbohydrate on the natural abundance ^{13}C spectra of rat liver and adipose tissue in vivo. The TMR method was an early attempt by Gordon et al.[18] at spatial localization of resonances; in TMR the main magnetic field was profiled by the use of static field gradients so that only over a selected sample volume was the magnetic field homogeneous enough to permit the measurement of a high-resolution spectrum. Canioni et al.[16] found that, in general, the levels of carbohydrates and saturated and unsaturated lipids observed in ^{13}C TMR spectra of rat tissue were in accord with the relative amounts of these substances in the diet of the rat. In this study it was not possible to obtain TMR spectra of liver in vivo that were free of contributions from extrahepatic adipose tissue because the smallest attainable sensitive volume extended beyond the dimensions of liver in rat.[16]

Table 89–1. ASSIGNMENTS OF LIPID RESONANCES OBSERVABLE IN NATURAL ABUNDANCE ^{13}C NMR SPECTRA OF LIVER FROM OB/OB MOUSE

Resonance	Assignment	Chemical Shift (ppm)
a	$*CH_3$—CH_2—	14.73
b	CH_3—$*CH_2$—CH_2—	23.47
c	—$*CH_2$—CH_2—CO—	25.60
d	—CH=CH—$*CH_2$—CH=CH—	26.32
e	—CH_2—$*CH_2$—CH=CH	27.95
f	fatty acyl—$(*CH_2)$—	30.18
g	fatty acyl—$(*CH_2)$—	30.51
h	CH_3—CH_2—$*CH_2$—CH_2—	32.76
i	—CH_2—$*CH_2$—CO—	34.46
j	glycerol $*CH_2$	62.59
k	glycerol $*CH$	69.74
l	=$*CH$—CH_2—$*CH$=	128.73
m	—CH=$*CH$—CH_2—CH_2	130.35
n	—CH_2—CH_2—$*CO$—	172.43
A	unassigned	40.4
B	Choline$(CH_3)_3N$—	58.8

Difficulty had been encountered in maintaining liver glycogen levels in anesthesized fed rats during a ^{13}C TMR examination,[16] although signals from endogenous glycogen were observable by ^{13}C NMR in either excised liver or perfused liver from fed rats.[10] Alger et al.[11] were able to minimize the problem of hepatic glycogenolysis in vivo during NMR examination by pretreating the animal with alpha- and beta-adrenergic blockers; because respiratory motion reduces spectral resolution, paralysis was induced and respiration was assisted. Using this stratagem, Alger et al.[11] measured intense resonances for endogenous glycogen in ^{13}C NMR spectra of liver in vivo in a fed rabbit; spectra were acquired with a surface rf coil (no magnetic field profiling) with 10 min time resolution.

Adopting a modified approach to the measurement of natural abundance ^{13}C NMR spectra of rat liver in vivo, Stevens et al.[9] placed a small surface rf coil directly on the liver by means of an abdominal incision. Using an ordinary high-resolution NMR spectrometer that operated at 50 MHz for ^{13}C and had an extra wide-bore magnet, this group measured glycogen levels in the liver of fed gsd/gsd rats, which are phosphorylase kinase deficient and hence lack phosphorylase *a*, that were about 2.5 times greater than the glycogen levels observed in liver of fed normal control rats. Hepatic glycogen did not decrease after a 24-hour fast in this model of glycogen storage disease. Reo et al.[12,13] extended this approach by developing a surface-coil probe of improved design for acquiring proton decoupled ^{13}C NMR spectra using a standard wide-bore 8.4 tesla magnet. With this probe, ^{13}C spectra of surgically exposed rat liver in vivo were acquired in 3 to 10 min; thus it was possible to follow in rat liver in vivo the time course of glycogenolysis stimulated by the intravenous injection of glucagon.[13]

Metabolism of ^{13}C-labeled Substrates: Isolated Liver Cells from Euthyroid and Hyperthyroid Rats

To explore the potential of ^{13}C NMR in metabolic studies, comparison was made of gluconeogenesis from ^{13}C-labeled glycerols by hepatocytes from 24-hour fasted normal control rats and triiodothyronine (T3)-treated rats.[19] As expected for the major gluconeogenic pathway, with [1,3-^{13}C]glycerol as substrate, carbons 1,3,4, and 6 of glucose were strongly and approximately equally labeled; whereas with [2-^{13}C]glycerol as substrate, carbons 2 and 5 of glucose were strongly and about equally labeled. Time resolved ^{13}C NMR spectra showed that T3 treatment caused the rates of glycerol consumption and glucose production to increase twofold, while the levels of L-glycerol-3-P decreased to 40 percent of the control value. Beyond measurements of the major gluconeogenic pathway, the observed ^{13}C label distribution in glucose allowed the quantitative determination of flux through the pentose cycle directly in both rat liver cells and perfused mouse liver;[19,20] the pentose cycle is important in supplying nicotinamide-adenine dinucleotide phosphate (NADPH) for lipogenesis, for example. In the absence of pentose cycle activity, the directly labeled C-2 and C-5 sites in glucose synthesized from [2-^{13}C]glycerol are equally and exclusively labeled; the flux of hexose that cycles through the pentose phosphate pathway and back into the hexose pathway is measured directly by the ^{13}C enrichment at C-1 and C-3 of glucose (and by a concomitant decrease at glucose C-2). The distribution of ^{13}C label measured in the glucose produced by hepatocytes from [2-^{13}C]glycerol[19,20] agreed exactly with that predicted by the classic pentose cycle reaction scheme, but it did not agree with the predictions of an alternate mechanism that was proposed more recently. With the assumption of metabolic and isotopic steady state, it was possible to calculate pentose cycle activity (that is, the rate of glucose-6-P-dehydrogenase relative to the rate of glucose-6-phosphatase) from a straightforward expression that required only the relative ^{13}C specific enrichments at glucose C-1 and C-2. In experiments with [1,3-^{13}C]glycerol as substrate, the path through the nonoxidative pentose branch was examined as well by fitting the ^{13}C distributions measured in glucose, including the observed multiplet structure due to ^{13}C-^{13}C J coupling, to model pathways.[19] Because we make extensive use of the ^{13}C enrichments in key metabolites to estimate in-situ metabolic fluxes in liver, it is worth mentioning that in a study of gluconeogenesis from ^{13}C-labeled glycerols, each containing a tracer amount of the ^{14}C counterpart, it was demonstrated that the specific label distribution measured directly in the ^{13}C NMR spectra of the living cell agreed closely with the ^{14}C isotopic distributions determined by classic isolation and degradation procedures in extracts of the same double-labeled samples.[20]

The metabolism of [3-^{13}C]alanine was also followed in suspensions of hepatocytes from 24-hour fasted control and T3-treated rats by Cohen et al.[21] The competition between alanine and ethanol into the Krebs cycle was followed by the coadministration of either unlabeled ethanol or [2-^{13}C]ethanol with [3-^{13}C]alanine. The flux of label from [3-^{13}C]alanine was followed into the Krebs cycle and into glutamate, glutamine, β-hydroxybutyrate, and aspartate; gluconeogenesis was also followed and the ^{13}C distribution in glucose was measured. During gluconeogenesis from [3-^{13}C]alanine, the large stimulatory effect of this hormonal treatment on the flux from phosphoenolpyruvate (PEP) through pyruvate kinase as compared with the flux from PEP to glucose (see Fig. 89–2) was measured in situ by comparing the concentration of ^{13}C label at the randomized alanine C-2 position with that at the corresponding carbon, C-5, in glucose.[21] When ethanol was not coadministered with alanine, the relative flux through pyruvate kinase was about 3.5 times greater in hepatocytes from the T3-treated rats. The extension of the ^{13}C NMR method to the determination of the activity of the phosphoenolpyruvate futile cycle in perfused liver is described in more detail below.

Metabolism of ^{13}C-labeled Substrates: Effects of Insulin on Perfused Liver from Streptozotocin-Diabetic and Untreated Rats

We have recently used ^{13}C NMR to investigate the gluconeogenic pathway and to identify metabolites in perfused liver from streptozotocin-treated rats and their un-

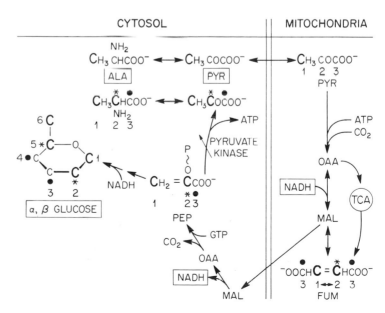

Figure 89–2. Simplified model gluconeogenic pathway. The original label at C-3 of alanine (boldface C) is followed into the Krebs (TCA) cycle where randomization by malate dehydrogenase and fumarase exchange occurs; thus, in fumarate (FUM) the label is found with equal probability at *either* of the two middle carbons (boldface Cs). (The *asterisk* follows the position of the randomized middle carbon). Further randomization in the Krebs cycle introduced a small amount of label into the terminal carbons of FUM (solid circle over C). The numbering of the carbons refers to their relationship with the carbons of glucose. MAL is malate and OAA is oxaloacetate.

treated littermates.[22] Both ^{13}C and ^{31}P NMR were useful in defining some of the changes in hepatic metabolism that occur in the streptozotocin model of Type 1, or insulin-dependent, diabetes. The activity of pyruvate kinase, which is known to be a target site for hormonal control of gluconeogenesis, was one of the changes monitored. To do so required the development of a ^{13}C NMR assay applicable to the time-sequential spectra of perfused liver under conditions of active gluconeogenesis from [3-^{13}C]alanine.[23] The importance of futile cycling, which causes ATP hydrolysis without a corresponding change in reactants, in metabolic regulation is generally accepted. Three futile cycles operate in hepatic glucose metabolism.[24] One of these is the PEP cycle (pyruvate → PEP → pyruvate), in which the path in the gluconeogenic direction from pyruvate to PEP is catalyzed by a complex sequence of enzymes; in the glycolytic direction only a single enzyme, pyruvate kinase, catalyzes the reaction PEP → pyruvate (Fig. 89–2). Our ^{13}C NMR assay hinges upon the observation that randomized label is introduced into PEP (C with * and C with ● in Fig. 89–2) prior to its appearance in pyruvate through action of pyruvate kinase. Subsequently, liver alanine aminotransferase activity converts this pyruvate to alanine. In the presence of a large trapping pool of alanine with the original unscrambled label at C-3, the relative ^{13}C enrichment at the randomized alanine carbons, compared to the enrichment at the corresponding carbons in glucose, provides a measure of the flux through pyruvate kinase as a fraction of the flux of PEP to glucose. (Measurement of the rate of gluconeogenesis then gives the absolute rate of flux.) Under our conditions of metabolic and isotopic steady state, this relative flux is given by the expression

$$\frac{\text{pyruvate kinase flux}}{\text{(gluconeogenic flux)}} = \frac{\text{Ala(C-2/C-3)}[1 + (1 - \phi)\text{Glc(C-6/C-5)} + (1 - \phi')\text{Glc(C-4/C-5)}]}{1 - [\text{Glc(C-6/C-5)}](\text{Ala(C-2)/C-3)})} \quad (2)$$

$$(1)$$

in which all components are readily measured in ^{13}C NMR spectra of perfused rat liver, such as Figure 89–3. That is, Ala(C-2/C-3) is the ratio of ^{13}C enrichment at C-2 to that at C-3 of alanine; Glc(C-6/C-5) is the corresponding ratio for glucose C-6 and C-5; and $\phi(\phi')$ is the fraction of the ^{13}C-labeled alanine pool in which *both C-2 and C-3* (*both C-1 and C-2*) are labeled in the same molecule.[23] The assay includes a check on the reuse of pyruvate with the randomized label, that is, on the adequacy of the trapping

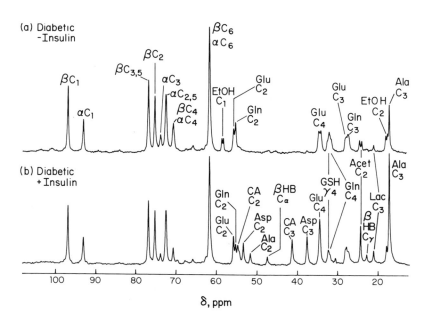

(a) Diabetic −Insulin

(b) Diabetic +Insulin

δ, ppm

Figure 89–3. 90.5 MHz ^{13}C NMR spectra of livers from streptozotocin-diabetic rats; livers were perfused in the absence (*a*) or presence (*b*) of insulin. Each spectrum is part of a time sequence of spectra and was accumulated during the interval 170–180 min after addition of 10 mM [3-^{13}C]alanine, 7.3 mM [2-^{13}C]ethanol; in (*b*) 7 nM insulin was also added. Each spectrum represents 800 scans, requiring 10 min data accumulation. The background ^{13}C spectrum, recorded under identical conditions before addition of labeled substrates, was subtracted. Abbreviations: α and β, α- and β-anomers of glucose; EtOH, ethanol; Gln, glutamine; Glu, glutamate; Asp, aspartate; Ala, alanine; βHB, β-hydroxybutyrate; CA, N-carbamoylaspartate; GSH, glutathione; Lac, lactate.[23]

pool; this check uses the ^{13}C enrichment measured at glutamate C-4 and C-5 to estimate the flux from recycled pyruvate into the mitochondrial acetyl-CoA pool.

Both an earlier ^{13}C NMR study[1] and the one under discussion[23] showed that the metabolic effect of insulin in vitro on perfused liver from fasted normal control rats was slight. In contrast, upon treatment of liver from streptozotocin-diabetic rats with 7 nM insulin in vitro, a partial reversal of many of the differences noted between diabetic and control liver was demonstrated by ^{13}C NMR (Fig. 89–3). The spectra in Figure 89–3 compare metabolism in diabetic liver perfused in the absence (Fig. 89–3a) or presence (Fig. 89–3b) of insulin; comparison is made at the same time post substrate and after addition of essentially the same total quantity of gluconeogenic substrate, [3-^{13}C]alanine. In both cases, as predicted by the main gluconeogenic pathway (Fig. 89–2), the newly synthesized glucose is strongly labeled at C-1, C-2, C-5, and C-6 and weakly labeled at C-3 and C-4. In the absence of insulin, the rate of ^{13}C-glucose synthesis was high (51.7 ± 7.7 μmol/g liver wet wt/h),[22] steady-state levels of certain amino acids were relatively low, and *no* ^{13}C enrichment was detectable at the randomized carbon of alanine, C-2, in diabetic liver ($n = 6$), as shown in Figure 89–3a. However, when perfused diabetic liver was incubated with insulin (Fig. 89–3b), the rate of ^{13}C-glucose synthesis fell off slightly to 44.0 ± 12 μmol/g liver wet wt/h, steady-state levels of ^{13}C-labeled aspartate and N-carbamoylaspartate[22] increased sharply, and, most significantly, the relative ^{13}C enrichment at the randomized alanine carbon (C-2) was brought into the range of enrichment observed in liver from 24-hour fasted control rats. Thus, the acute regulation of pyruvate kinase by insulin in vitro in diabetic liver was demonstrated by ^{13}C NMR. In addition to diabetic liver, two other types of liver preparations were studied so as to provide gradations of pyruvate kinase flux within the confines of our ^{13}C NMR assay's requirement of active gluconeogenesis; the other preparations were perfused liver from 24-hour and 12-hour fasted rats. By this NMR determination (Eq. 1), the rate of pyruvate kinase flux was 0.74 ± 0.04 of the gluconeogenic rate in 24-hour fasted controls; in liver from 12-hour fasted controls, the relative pyruvate kinase flux increased to 1.0 + 0.2. In diabetic liver, this flux was undetectable; as an upper limit, this flux was at least 7-fold lower than the flux measured in 24-hour–fasted controls. Treatment of diabetic liver with insulin in vitro produced the induction of a huge enhancement in the flux through pyruvate kinase, bringing the relative and absolute fluxes up to the level measured in 24-hour–fasted controls.[23] To complement these studies of experimental diabetes, we are currently using ^{13}C NMR to study hepatic metabolism in the genetically obese ob/ob mouse, a model of Type 2, or non–insulin dependent, diabetes.[25]

Metabolism of ^{13}C-labeled Substrates: Glycogenesis from ^{13}C-labeled Gluconeogenic Substrates in Perfused Liver from Fasted Rats

An investigation in which both ^{13}C and ^{31}P NMR spectra were acquired simultaneously through the use of a dual tuned rf probe[1] illustrates other kinds of information obtainable in ^{13}C NMR studies of hepatic metabolism. From the ^{13}C side of the study under consideration[1] it was possible in the *same* perfused liver to (1) follow gluconeogenesis and glycogenesis from [2-^{13}C]pyruvate ± insulin; (2) measure relative fluxes through the Krebs cycle and into glucose by a method based on the use of two different ^{13}C-labeled substrates; (3) estimate the intracellular level of free Mg^{2+} by a new ^{13}C NMR assay; and (4) observe the stimulation of glycogenolysis by glucagon. The three consecutive ^{13}C spectra shown in Figure 89–4 are from a sequence taken repetitively and show the time development of several metabolites over a period 17 to 67 min after

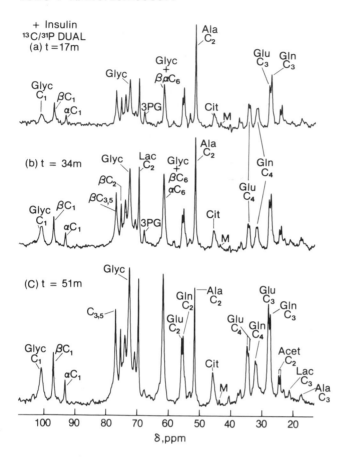

Figure 89–4. Shown are 90.5 MHz ^{13}C NMR spectra of an isolated perfused liver from a fasted normal rat. Time resolved ^{13}C spectra were accumulated concurrently with ^{31}P spectra over an interval 17–67 min after the addition of 9 mM [2-^{13}C]pyruvate, 7.3 mM [2-^{13}C]ethanol, 3.6 mM NH_4Cl, and 7 nM insulin. Each spectrum (800 scans) required 10.5 min data accumulation starting at the indicated time post substrate. The background ^{13}C spectrum was subtracted (see Fig. 89–3). Abbreviations are given in Figure 89–3, with the addition of: Glyc, glycogen; 3PG, 3-P-D-glycerate; Cit, citrate; M, malate; and Acet, acetate.[1]

the addition of [2-^{13}C]pyruvate, [2-^{13}C]ethanol, and NH_4Cl. Intense peaks are seen that arise from enrichment at alanine C-2 and lactate C-2, both of which are directly traceable to [2-^{13}C]pyruvate via alanine aminotransferase and lactate dehydrogenase, respectively. Note that ^{13}C enrichment at alanine C-2 is maintained at a high constant level, while that at lactate C-2 is seen to increase in time. Glutamate and glutamine are strongly labeled at C-2, C-3, and C-4 as well as C-5 (not shown). Krebs cycle activity is also visible in the distinct resonance arising from the methylene carbons of citrate, which grows more intense with time (Fig. 89–4c).

The most notable changes over time shown in Figure 89–4, however, are the synchronous increases in newly synthesized ^{13}C-labeled glucose (pathway similar to that shown in Fig. 89–2) and ^{13}C-labeled glycogen (spectral region from 60 to 105 ppm; note especially the unique glycogen C-1 peak at 100 ppm). In this study endogenous stores of glycogen were very low because (1) the donor rats were fasted for 16 hours in wire cages and (2) a 30 to 40 min period of nonrecirculation of perfusate, designed to wash out remaining endogenous substrates, took place before the addition of our labeled substrates. Thus, essentially the only glucose present was that synthesized from [2-^{13}C]pyruvate. Under these conditions, glycogenesis must be proceeding as a strictly gluconeogenic process. In this study the rates of glucose synthesis and glycogen synthesis were about equal and were unaffected by the presence of insulin in vitro; the *total* rate of gluconeogenesis (including glycogen synthesis) in perfused liver under these conditions was 34 μmol/g liver/h. ^{13}C NMR is probably unique in being able to monitor glycogenesis in perfused liver noninvasively.

Pyruvate is an important branch point in the gluconeogenic pathway, being able to enter the Krebs cycle in two different ways: by carboxylation to oxalacetate (OAA) via pyruvate carboxylase activity or by oxidative decarboxylation to acetyl-CoA via pyruvate dehydrogenase activity. By coadministering the substrates [2-¹³C]pyruvate and [1,2-¹³C]ethanol to perfused rat liver we were able to measure relative fluxes into the Krebs cycle by these two routes, as well as follow the competition between pyruvate and ethanol into acetyl-CoA.[1] Use of this substrate combination introduced well-defined multiplet structure, due to ¹³C-¹³C J coupling, into the NMR peaks of several important metabolites, including citrate, glutamate, β-hydroxybutyrate, and glucose. These spin-spin multiplets were used to unravel the pathways that the carbon backbones of these metabolites had followed in the Krebs cycle and to reveal each metabolite's labeled sources of OAA and acetyl-CoA and the extent of contributions from unlabeled endogenous sources. Because NMR peaks are broadened in spectra of perfused liver, intensities and splittings within the multiplets were measured in spectra of the perfusates and acid extracts of liver that had been freeze clamped at the end of the perfusion period (Fig. 89–5). This procedure gives representative results because of the maintenance of steady-state conditions during the perfusion.

As indicated in Figure 89–5, the main flux into the mitochondrial acetyl-CoA pool is via the oxidation of [1,2-¹³C]ethanol; the resultant labeled acetate can be converted to [1,2-¹³C]acetyl-CoA through the activity of the mitochondrial acetyl-CoA synthetase. ([2-¹³C]pyruvate would have produced [1-¹³C]acetyl CoA.) Acetyl-CoA carbons from ¹³C-labeled ethanol are denoted by boldfaced C with asterisk in Figure 89–5. As shown, the main flux of pyruvate into the Krebs cycle is via pyruvate carboxylase to OAA (the small O follows the original label at pyruvate C-2 into OAA). However, to the extent that randomization at the symmetrical molecule fumarate occurs (see Fig. 89–2), the ¹³C label in that portion of the OAA pool will be found with equal probability

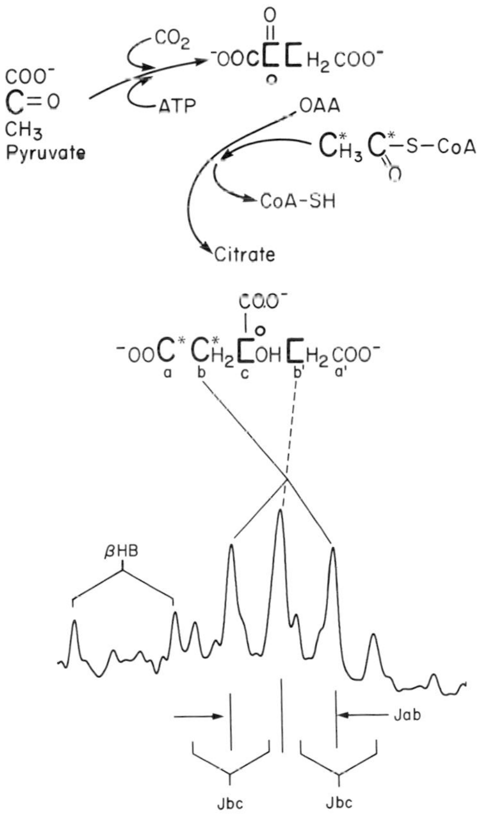

Figure 89–5. ¹³C NMR spectrum of perchloric acid extract of the liver shown in Figure 89–4, prepared after liver was freeze clamped at end of perfusion. The citrate methylene region is shown. *Top half* of figure gives a simplified model pathway.[1]

at *either* the methylene or the carbonyl carbon; this randomization is denoted by the boldface square C symbol in Figure 89–5. The assignments of the peaks and the corresponding J coupling constants are given in Figure 89–5. An analytical expression for the ratio of the total intensity of citrate C_b to that of C_b' can be written straightforwardly in terms of the frequency of appearance of all significant contributions to the mitochondrial OAA pool in combination with the two possible labeled forms in the acetyl-CoA pool. Similarly analytical expressions were written for the other metabolites; in this way a set of simultaneous equations was generated and solved in general form. When measured intensity ratios are substituted into these expressions, relative fluxes for a given experiment are estimated. Because the observation of multiplets for several metabolites overdefines the system, checks on self-consistency are built into the estimates.

Metabolism of ^{13}C-labeled Substrates: ^{13}C-Glucose/Glycogen Metabolism in Rat Liver in Vivo

Ackerman and co-workers have used the technique in which a rf surface coil is placed on surgically exposed liver to study the kinetics of glycogenesis from [1-^{13}C]glucose and subsequent stimulated glycogenolysis in vivo under a number of conditions.[13,26] Their most extensive set of experiments was carried out in the presence of a continuous infusion of somatostatin to suppress endogenous insulin and glucagon secretion; [1-^{13}C]glucose was given intravenously to fasted rats.[26] In this way the loss of hepatic [1-^{13}C]glucose and the incorporation of [1-^{13}C]glucose into glycogen was followed. Insulin under these conditions did not affect the incorporation of ^{13}C-glucose into glycogen when administered alone or with glucagon. As anticipated for these conditions, glucagon alone did not change serum glucose levels or hepatic ^{13}C-glucose levels, but it did cause loss of ^{13}C-glucose from glycogen and did inhibit the incorporation of ^{13}C-glucose into glycogen. It was also determined that with insulin administration, serum glucose levels fell below basal levels and hepatic ^{13}C-glucose levels declined more rapidly than in the absence of insulin.[26] Thus, the effects of hormonal treatment on hepatic glucose metabolism in vivo can be monitored by ^{13}C NMR methods.

Shulman et al.[27] used [1-^{13}C]glucose in a completely different ^{13}C NMR approach to study the mechanism of glycogen repletion in rat liver in vivo. In the Shulman study, [1-^{13}C]glucose at two dose levels was administered by gavage to awake fasted rats. At two times post dose, livers were freeze clamped and hepatic glycogen was extracted and hydrolyzed. Subsequent ^{13}C and ^{1}H NMR examinations of the specific ^{13}C enrichment of the carbons in the glucosyl units of the hydrolyzed glycogen and the ^{13}C enrichments of portal vein lactate and alanine were used to infer the pathways by which glycogen was repleted. Under these conditions, it was demonstrated that only one-third of liver glycogen repletion occurred by direct conversion of glucose to glycogen and that alanine and lactate account for a minimum of 7 and 20 percent of the repletion, depending upon the initial glucose dose. Futile cycling between fructose-6-P and fructose-1,6-bisphosphate was shown to be minimal. Most interestingly, these three pathways could account for only 50 percent of the total glycogen synthesized. While this information could be obtained, in principle, by ^{14}C isotopic methods, equally detailed radioactivity measurements would be too time consuming in a study as extensive as that of Shulman et al.[27] to be feasible. Thus, many valuable ^{13}C NMR studies of in-vivo metabolism, designed to parallel ^{14}C isotopic approaches, may require only a conventional high field, narrow bore high-resolution NMR spectrometer.

Metabolism ^{13}C-labeled Substrates: Ketogenesis in Rat Liver in Vivo

Seelig and co-workers[28] have used rf surface coils and judicious choice of ^{13}C-labeled substrate to achieve, in effect, the localization of signal from liver without surgery. That is, by following the flow of label from [1-^{13}C]butyrate into metabolites labeled only at the carbonyl carbon, many of the problems encountered in in-vivo ^{13}C NMR studies were avoided because the carbonyl spectral region (170 to 190 ppm) suffers relatively less from interferences from endogenous substances in liver and extrahepatic adipose tissue. In addition, only liver would metabolize ^{13}C-butyrate to acetoacetate and β-hydroxybutyrate. Glutamate and glutamine labeled at C-1 were also observed.

Metabolism of ^{13}C-labeled Substrates: Measurement of ^{13}C-labeled Metabolites in Urine Samples

A pioneering use of ^{13}C NMR in a clinical investigation was reported by Tanaka et al.[29] over a decade ago. On separate days, [α-^{13}C]- and [α,β-^{13}C]valine were administered to a 7-year-old boy with methylmalonic acidemia. Methylmalonic acid was isolated from multiple urine samples, purified, and analyzed by ^{13}C NMR. The labeling patterns measured in methylmalonic acid demonstrated unequivocally that, contrary to the prevailing view at that time, methylmalonic semialdehyde, formed from the metabolism of valine, was decarboxylated to propionate before conversion to methylmalonyl CoA. Despite the success of this first use of a ^{13}C-labeled compound as a nonradioactive tracer in a clinical investigation and despite the ease with which samples of urine or blood can be analyzed by conventional ^{13}C NMR techniques, few subsequent applications in this area have been reported.

^{13}C NMR SPECTROSCOPIC STUDIES OF HEART

Isolated Perfused Heart

Lavanchy et al.[30] were able to detect glycogen synthesis from [1-^{13}C]glucose in Langendorff perfused rat heart by ^{13}C NMR, but only when the rat had been pretreated in vivo with the beta-adrenergic agonist isoproterenol. Hearts from rats whose endogenous glycogen stores were not depleted by this pretreatment failed to show detectable incorporation of [1-^{13}C]glucose into glycogen. The pretreated rat model was used to show glycogenolysis during global ischemia; the appearance of label in lactate was also monitored under these conditions. Earlier Bailey et al.[31] followed the metabolism of [2-^{13}C]acetate in isolated heart perfused in the Langendorff mode. Time-resolved ^{13}C NMR spectra indicated that the incorporation of ^{13}C label into glutamate C-4, and subsequently C-2 and C-3, reached a steady-state level of enrichment after about 40 min of perfusion. Appearance of ^{13}C label in aspartate was promoted by decreasing the concentration of [2-^{13}C]acetate and increasing the level of unlabeled glucose, presumably by elevating oxalacetate levels and thereby shifting the equilibrium of aspartate aminotransferase towards the formation of aspartate. Chance et al.[32] used a more analytical approach in that they acquired ^{13}C NMR spectra only of perchloric acid extracts of Langendorff perfused hearts that had been freeze clamped at various times after the addition of either [2-^{13}C]acetate or [3-^{13}C]pyruvate to the perfusate. A mathematical model of the Krebs cycle and ancillary transamination reactions was constructed using the ^{13}C enrichments at specific carbons of glutamate and aspartate in ^{13}C spectra of the extracts; although the glutamate resonances were split into well-resolved multiplets, only the total ^{13}C enrichment at each carbon was used in this analysis.[32]

^{13}C NMR Studies of Guinea Pig Heart in Vivo

Cardiac metabolism in fed guinea pig in vivo has been studied by Neurohr et al.[33,34] by ^{13}C NMR at 20 MHz using a horizontal-bore magnet. A solenoidal rf receiver coil was placed around the heart in the open-chested guinea pig for these experiments.[35] In ^{13}C NMR spectra of guinea pig heart in vivo after the infusion of a total of 1.2 g of sodium [2-^{13}C]acetate, resonances arising from glutamate C-2, C-3, and C-4 and the methylene carbons of citrate were measured. Although endogenous glycogen was not detectable, it was possible to follow the incorporation of [1-^{13}C]glucose into glycogen during the infusion of 0.5 g of [1-^{13}C]glucose and 50 units of insulin. The specific enrichment at the C-1 carbons of the glucosyl units of glycogen was determined to be about 18 percent under these conditions. In other guinea pigs, after infusion of [1-^{13}C]glucose had labeled myocardial glycogen stores, various periods of anoxia were imposed and the degradation of the labeled glycogen was monitored by ^{13}C NMR. After only three minutes, about one-half of the ^{13}C enriched glycogen had been degraded; by seven minutes, glycogen was undetectable by ^{13}C NMR. ^{1}H NMR spectra of glycogen extracted from these hearts after an 8 min period of anoxia indicated that the remaining glycogen was not ^{13}C labeled and was only slightly diminished from the level of unlabeled glycogen extracted from other hearts before anoxia. These observations are consistent with the labeled glucose moieties being preferentially degraded during anoxia.[34]

^{13}C NMR SPECTROSCOPIC STUDIES OF BRAIN

Reports showing natural abundance ^{13}C NMR spectra acquired with rf surface coils placed over the brain of a rat in vivo have shown only lipid resonances, presumably arising from both brain and subcutaneous fat.[12,36] Only recently have preliminary studies been reported in which similar spectra were acquired of rat brain in vivo after the administration of [1-^{13}C]glucose.[37] Hammer et al.[38] have given a preliminary account of the first ^{13}C NMR studies of primate brain in vivo. In this investigation, 2 g of [1-^{13}C]glucose were administered intravenously to a rhesus monkey and ^{13}C NMR spectra of the brain were accumulated in a serial manner with 5 min time resolution. ^{1}H decoupled ^{13}C NMR spectra of monkey brain were acquired at 2.1 tesla using two orthogonal saddle shaped rf coils of $3\frac{1}{2}$ inches in diameter. Serial blood samples were taken from 10 to 90 min post glucose dose, concurrently with the ^{13}C NMR measurements. Hammer et al. reported that whereas the level of ^{13}C-glucose in blood had fallen by a factor of $\frac{1}{18}$ by 30 min post glucose, ^{13}C-glucose in the spectra of the brain peaked at 20 min post dose and showed a drop of less than 20 percent at 30 min post dose.[38] The hypothesis favored by these investigators as a possible explanation of these provocative observations involves the existence of a slowly metabolized pool of glucose in monkey brain, which suggests the need for a ^{13}C MRI technique so that the ^{13}C-glucose signals in brain can be localized in future studies.

^{13}C NMR SPECTROSCOPIC STUDIES OF ERYTHROCYTES AND MICRO-ORGANISMS

^{13}C NMR studies of micro-organisms are numerous and have received extensive review;[3,4,6,8,39,40] while this coverage will not be repeated here, we note that glucose catabolism in the parasitic protozoan *Trypanosoma brucei gambiense,* which is of considerable biomedical interest, has been investigated by ^{13}C NMR.[41]

Glycolysis in erythrocytes of mice infected with *Plasmodium berghei,* the malaria parasite of rodents, was studied by ^{13}C NMR by Deslauriers et al.[42] The effects of several antimalarial drugs, including chloroquine and primaquine, on the rate of conversion of [1-^{13}C]glucose to lactate was followed in both normal and infected erythrocytes.[42] MacKenzie et al.[43] reported a similar study of glycolysis in erythrocytes of mice infected with the protozoan parasite *Babesia microti;* the effect of a trypanocidal drug on the rate of conversion of [1-^{13}C]glucose to lactate was monitored in control and infected erythrocytes. In both of these studies,[42,43] lactate was the sole metabolite of ^{13}C-glucose that was detected.

The metabolism of [1-^{13}C]glucose by human erythrocytes was used to investigate the flux of ^{13}C label through the 2,3-bisphosphoglycerate bypass and to estimate the activity of the pentose phosphate shunt. Oxley et al.[44] measured resonances from ^{13}C, ^{31}P, and ^{1}H nuclei simultaneously in this study by using a rf probe tuned to all three frequencies.

With the exception of the report by Tanaka et al.,[29] in which a ^{13}C-labeled metabolite was measured in human urine, an absence of ^{13}C NMR clinical investigations will be noted. Natural abundance ^{13}C NMR spectra of human surgical muscle samples, before and after removal of neutral fat by extraction with isopentane, have been used by Bárány et al.[45] to differentiate between normal and diseased muscle. In an early feasibility test, Alger et al.[36] measured ^{1}H coupled natural abundance ^{13}C NMR spectra of muscle in vivo in the human arm. More recently, Starewicz et al.[37] acquired natural abundance ^{13}C spectra of a human subject using a whole body 1.4 tesla magnet; in this preliminary study, spectra were measured with a rf surface coil placed over the liver, the chest, or the head and, because no additional spatial localization technique was implemented, strong signals were also received from subcutaneous adipose tissue.

As the examples surveyed here may suggest, ^{13}C NMR can provide a wide range of detailed biochemical information on the regulation of metabolism in the whole cell, organ, or animal, in both physiological and pathophysiological contexts. The well-defined conditions that obtain for perfused organ preparations and cellular suspensions ensure that these applications will continue to be useful even after spectrometers suitable for whole body ^{13}C NMR spectroscopy become more available. Clearly, extensive application of whole-body ^{13}C NMR spectroscopy, without surgical exposure of tissue, is contingent upon the development of sensitive and practical techniques for the spatial localization of resonances.

References

1. Cohen SM: Simultaneous ^{13}C and ^{31}P NMR studies of perfused rat liver: Effects of insulin and glucagon and a ^{13}C assay of free Mg^{++}. J Biol Chem 14294, 1983.
2. Shaw D: Fourier Transform NMR Spectroscopy. New York, Elsevier, 1976.
3. Radda GK, Taylor DJ: Applications of nuclear magnetic resonance spectroscopy in pathology. Int Rev Exp Pathol *27*:1–58, 1985.
4. Scott AI, Baxter RI: Applications of ^{13}C NMR to metabolic studies. Ann Rev Biophys Bioeng *10*:151, 1981.
5. Cohen SM: Applications of nuclear magnetic resonance to the study of liver physiology and disease. Hepatology *3*:738, 1983.

6. Bock JL: Recent developments in biochemical nuclear magnetic resonance spectroscopy. *In* Glick D (ed): Methods of Biochemical Analysis. Vol. 31. New York, John Wiley & Sons, 1985, pp 259–315.

7. Foster MA: Magnetic Resonance in Medicine and Biology. New York, Pergamon Press, 1984.

8. Cohen SM: Applications of ^{13}C NMR to the study of metabolic regulation in the living cell. *In* Gupta RK (ed): NMR Spectroscopy of Cells and Organisms. Vol I Boca Raton, CRC Press, 1987, pp 31–49.

9. Stevens AN, Iles RA, Morris PG, Griffiths JR: Detection of glycogen in a glycogen storage disease by ^{13}C nuclear magnetic resonances. FEBS Letters *150*:489, 1982.

10. Sillerud LO, Shulman RG: Structure and metabolism of mammalian liver glycogen monitored by carbon-13 nuclear magnetic resonance. Biochemistry *22*:1087, 1983.

11. Alger JR, Behar KL, Rothman DL, Shulman RG: Natural-abundance ^{13}C NMR measurement of hepatic glycogen in the living rabbit. J Magn Reson *56*:334, 1984.

12. Reo NV, Ewy CS, Siegfried BA, Ackerman JJH: High-field ^{13}C NMR spectroscopy of tissue in vivo. A double-resonance surface-coil probe. J Magn Reson *56*:76, 1984.

13. Reo NV, Siegfried BA, Ackerman JJH: Direct observation of glycogenesis and glycogenolysis in the rat liver in vivo by high-field carbon-13 surface coil NMR. J Biol Chem *259*:13664, 1984.

14. Cohen SM, Shulman RG, McLaughlin AC: Effects of ethanol on alanine metabolism in perfused mouse liver studied by ^{13}C NMR. Proc Natl Acad Sci USA *76*:4808, 1979.

15. Block RE: Direct proton and natural abundance carbon-13 NMR observation of liver changes induced by ethionine. Biochem Biophys Res Commun *108*:940, 1982.

16. Canioni P, Alger JR, Shulman RG: Natural abundance carbon-13 nuclear magnetic resonance spectroscopy of liver and adipose tissue of the living rat. Biochemistry *22*:4974, 1983.

17. Williams E, Hamilton JA, Jain MK, Allerhand H, Cordes EH, Ochs S: Natural abundance carbon-13 nuclear magnetic resonance spectra of the canine sciatic nerve. Science *181*:869, 1973.

18. Gordon RE, Hanley PE, Shaw D, Gadian DG, Radda GK, Styles P, Bore PJ, Chan L: Localization of metabolites in animals using ^{31}P topical magnetic resonance. Nature *287*:736, 1980.

19. Cohen SM, Ogawa S, Shulman RG: ^{13}C NMR studies of gluconeogenesis in rat liver cells: Utilization of labeled glycerol by cells from euthyroid and hyperthyroid rats. Proc Natl Acad Sci USA *76*:1603, 1979.

20. Cohen SM, Rognstad R, Shulman RG, Katz J: A comparison of ^{13}C nuclear magnetic resonance and ^{14}C tracer studies of hepatic metabolism. J Biol Chem *256*:3428, 1981.

21. Cohen SM, Glynn P, Shulman RG: ^{13}C NMR study of gluconeogenesis from labeled alanine in hepatocytes from euthyroid and hyperthyroid rats. Proc Natl Acad Sci USA *78*:60, 1981.

22. Cohen SM: ^{13}C and ^{31}P study of gluconeogenesis: Utilization of ^{13}C-labeled substrates by perfused liver from streptozotocin-diabetic and untreated rats, Biochemistry *26*:563, 1987.

23. Cohen SM: ^{13}C NMR study of the effects of insulin on perfused liver from streptozotocin-diabetic and untreated rats: ^{13}C NMR assay of pyruvate kinase flux. Biochemistry *26*:573, 1987.

24. Katz J, Rognstad R: Futile cycles in the metabolism of glucose. Curr Top Cell Regul *10*:237, 1976.

25. Cohen SM: ^{13}C and ^{31}P NMR studies of hepatic metabolism in two experimental models of diabetes. Ann NY Acad Sci Nov 1987.

26. Siegfried BA, Reo NV, Ewy CS, Shalwitz RA, Ackerman JJH, McDonald JM: Effects of hormone and glucose administration on hepatic glucose and glycogen metabolism in vivo. J Biol Chem *260*:16137, 1985.

27. Shulman GI, Rothman DL, Smith D, Johnson CM, Blair JB, Shulman RG, DeFronzo RA: Mechanism of liver glycogen repletion in vivo by nuclear magnetic resonance spectroscopy. J Clin Invest *76*:1229, 1985.

28. Cross TA, Pahl C, Oberhansli R, Aue WP, Keller U, Seelig J: Ketogenesis in the living rat followed by ^{13}C NMR spectroscopy. Biochemistry *23*:6398, 1984.

29. Tanaka K, Armitage IM, Ramsdell HS, Hsia YE, Lipsky SR, Rosenberg LE: [^{13}C]Valine metabolism in methylmalonicacidemia using nuclear magnetic resonance: Propionate as an obligate intermediate. Proc Natl Acad Sci USA *72*:3692, 1975.

30. Lavanchy N, Martin J, Rossi A: Glycogen metabolism: A ^{13}C NMR study on the isolated perfused rat heart. FEBS Lett *178*:34, 1984.

31. Bailey IA, Gadian DG, Matthews PM, Radda GK, Seeley PJ: Studies of metabolism in the isolated, perfused rat heart using ^{13}C NMR. FEBS Lett *123*:313, 1981.

32. Chance EM, Seeholzer SH, Kobayashi K, Williamson JR: Mathematical analysis of isotope labeling in the citric acid cycle with applications to ^{13}C NMR studies in perfused rat hearts. J Biol Chem *258*:13785, 1983.

33. Neurohr KJ, Barrett EJ, Shulman RG: In vivo carbon-13 nuclear magnetic resonance studies of heart metabolism. Proc Natl Acad Sci USA *80*:1603, 1983.

34. Neurohr KJ, Gollin G, Neurohr JM, Rothman DL, Shulman RG: Carbon-13 nuclear magnetic resonance studies of myocardial glycogen metabolism in live guinea pigs. Biochemistry *23*:5029, 1984.

35. Neurohr KJ: An experimental setup for carbon-13 NMR studies of heart metabolism in live guinea pigs. J Magn Reson *59*:511, 1984.

36. Alger JR, Sillerud LO, Behan KL, Gillies RJ, Shulman RG, Gordon RE, Shaw D, Hanley PE: In vivo carbon-13 nuclear magnetic resonance studies of mammals. Science *214*:660, 1981.

37. Starewicz PM, Lund G, Johnson S: In vivo carbon-13 spectroscopy at 1.4T in a 1-m bore clinical MR imaging system. Radiology *157*(P):61, 1985.

38. Hammer BE, Sacks W, Hennessy MJ, Bigler RE, Sacks S, Fleischer A, Zanzonico PB: Investigations

of in vivo glucose metabolism in monkey brain by C-13 MR imaging [spectroscopy]. Radiology *157*(P):220, 1985.

39. Kuchel PW: Nuclear magnetic resonance of biological samples. *In* Campbell B, Meites L (eds): Critical Reviews in Analytical Chemistry. Boca Raton, Florida, CRC Press, 1981, p 155.

40. Shulman RG, Brown TR, Ugurbil K, Ogawa S, Cohen SM, den Hollander JA: Cellular applications of ^{31}P and ^{13}C nuclear magnetic resonance. Science *205*:160, 1979.

41. MacKenzie NE, Hall JE, Seed JR, Scott AI: Carbon-13 nuclear-magnetic-resonance studies of glucose catabolism by *Trypanosoma brucei gambiense*. Eur J Biochem *121*:657, 1982.

42. Deslauriers R, Ekiel I, Kraft T, Leveille L, Smith ICP: NMR studies of malaria. Tetrahedron *39*:3543, 1983.

43. MacKenzie NE, Johnson J, Barton G, Wagner GG, Scott AI: ^{13}C NMR studies of glycolysis in intra- and extra-erythrocytic *Babesia microti*. Mol Biochem Parasitol *13*:13, 1984.

44. Oxley ST, Porteous R, Brindle K, Boyd J, Campbell ID: A multinuclear NMR study of 2,3-bisphosphoglycerate metabolism in the human erythrocyte. Biochim Biophys Acta *805*:19, 1984.

45. Bárány M, Doyle DD, Graff G, Westler WM, Markley JL: Natural abundance ^{13}C NMR spectra of human muscle, normal and diseased. Magn Reson Med *1*:30, 1984.

90

The Biomedical Applications of Fluorine-19 NMR

STEPHEN R. THOMAS

The introduction of ^{19}F NMR techniques into medicine has created significant new approaches for highly sensitive investigations of the in-vivo properties and diagnostic capabilities of fluorine based compounds. The wide-ranging possibilities involving spectroscopy and/or imaging include research on metabolic processes using fluorine-labeled substrates; enzymatic activity, reaction mechanisms, and biomolecular binding; membrane and cell systems; perfluorocarbon compound utility; biodistribution and retention of fluorinated materials, including anesthetics; and gas phase applications. The characteristics of ^{19}F that make this nucleus uniquely suited for high contrast NMR studies in vivo are readily appreciated and include a high gyromagnetic ratio (40.05 MHz/tesla), spin 1/2, a sensitivity relative to protons of 0.83, 100 percent natural isotopic abundance, and an extremely low biological occurrence. The high gyromagnetic ratio represents a resonant frequency only approximately 6 percent lower than that for protons (42.58 MHz/tesla), which allows utilization of existing proton NMR instrumentation with a minimum of component adjustments and tuning procedural difficulties. The high sensitivity and 100 percent abundance provide the potential for achieving a signal-to-noise ratio comparable to that for protons on a nucleus-per-nucleus basis. The low endogenous total body levels provide the conditions required for high contrast ^{19}F tracer NMR imaging and spectroscopic analysis through utilization of suitable biocompatible fluorine compounds.

An evaluation of the intrinsic total body occurrence of fluorine in man relevant specifically to the possibility of ^{19}F tracer NMR imaging has been presented by Thomas et al.[1] Under the conservative assumption that the 2.6 g of fluorine per the standard kg man[2] is distributed uniformly throughout the body, the intrinsic concentration would be less than 2 mM. In fact, the actual soft tissue concentration would be much less because most of the ^{19}F is likely to be incorporated into bone minerals (fluoroapatite). Any resonance arising from such motionally hindered ^{19}F will be broadened and/or have so long a longitudinal relaxation time as to be unsuitable for standard imaging methods. (The development of solid-state imaging techniques, however, might hold some promise for visualizing nuclei confined within a rigid matrix.)

Estimates of 1 to 2 mM have been reported for the endogenous fluorine levels within canine myocardium.[3] Other investigators put the concentration of ^{19}F in biological tissue at much lower values, namely in the submicromolar range.[4] Nevertheless, even for the upper estimates, these levels of intrinsic concentration are too small to give any detectable ^{19}F signal under standard imaging protocols and would be impractical even for time averaged spectroscopic studies. Thus, these facts set the stage for high contrast ^{19}F tracer investigations if suitable biocompatible fluorine compounds can be developed for introduction into living systems. Through the applications to be discussed below, this chapter will review ongoing research and describe the potential applications of ^{19}F NMR in medicine.

METABOLISM

Various fluorine-labeled substrates are being utilized to investigate metabolic mechanisms in vivo. Through time sequenced NMR spectroscopy, chemical shift information may be analyzed to allow identification of different molecular species, thus enabling differentiation between various competing metabolic models. Such techniques hold forth the possibility for the development and verification of quantitative models of regional metabolism.

Fluorodeoxyglucose

Positron emission tomography (PET) procedures using the positron emitting nucleus ^{18}F are well documented and include extensive clinical research with ^{18}F-fluorodeoxyglucose (FDG) for investigations of brain and myocardial metabolism and infarct detection.[5-7] The potential for NMR imaging of stable ^{19}F-FDG has been considered.[1] It was estimated that the concentrations required for imaging would be at least several orders of magnitude greater than the intrinsic biological levels, or in the 0.1 to 1.0 M range. A 0.1 M solution of FDG represents a fluorine concentration approximately 1/1000 that of hydrogen in water, and since the time required to achieve a given signal-to-noise ratio is inversely proportional to the square of the concentration, severe sensitivity losses would be encountered, which must be overcome. Attempts to increase the quantity of this tracer introduced in vivo must analyze existing uptake and toxicity data.

As summarized in reference 1, two principal forms of FDG have been utilized: 2-deoxy-2-fluoro-D-glucose (2-FDG) and 3-deoxy-3-fluoro-D-glucose (3-FDG). These two compounds differ only in the position of the single fluorine atom within the molecule. Figure 90–1 shows the chemical structure of these two types of FDG along with a high resolution spectrum of 2-FDG taken at 2.1 tesla (84.7 MHz for fluorine). The spectrum exhibits a doublet of triplets due to spin-echo couplings. An image of a 2-FDG phantom taken at 0.66 tesla (26.5 MHz for fluorine) is shown in Figure 90–2. The complex spectrum evident in Figure 90–1b may have a direct effect on image quality (depending on factors such as gradient strength) in that it represents a broadened system response function (as opposed to a single sharp line), which degrades the spatial resolution. Deconvolution techniques may be applied to remove the effects of chemical shift and improve the resolution.[8,9]

The biokinetic characteristics involving trapping within the metabolic pathways of the brain have been studied through PET techniques more extensively for 2-FDG than for 3-FDG. However, work with rhesus monkeys has demonstrated that 3-FDG exhibits behavior identical to that of glucose in passing the blood-brain barrier[10] and thus also may be useful in the measurement of glucose metabolism in the brain (although the optimal time for imaging may be shorter than that for 2-FDG owing to the slightly different biokinetic properties observed). The toxicity data analysis would indicate that 2-FDG with a relatively high lethal dose in rats (LD_{50} = 600 mg/kg)[11] will be an unlikely candidate for a human in-vivo ^{19}F NMR imaging agent; whereas 3-FDG, which is considerably less toxic (nontoxic in rats at levels of 5 g/kg),[11] offers greater promise for NMR imaging applications in the study of glucose metabolism.

In-vivo rat brain studies by Nakada et al.[12-14] have demonstrated the presence of

A

2− deoxy−2− fluoro−D −glucose [2-FDG]

R_1=F
R_2=OH

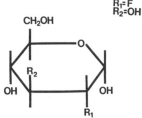

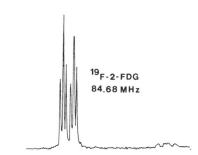

3− deoxy−3− fluoro−D −glucose [3-FDG]

R_1=OH
R_2=F

B

^{19}F-2-FDG
84.68 MHz

Figure 90–1. *A*, The inorganic chemical structure of 2-FDG and 3-FDG. The differing position of the single fluorine atom within each molecule is indicated. *B*, A high resolution fluorine spectrum of 2-FDG at 84.68 MHz (2.1 T). The doublet and triplet splittings are approximately 49 Hz and 13 Hz, respectively. The chemical shift is −33 ppm with respect to an external reference of C^6F^6.[1]

multiple metabolites of FDG. Table 90–1 provides a summary of the NMR characteristics of 2-FDG and a list of its known metabolites.[12] The early (3-hour) spectra were characterized by four resolvable resonant lines with discrete chemical shift positions (Fig. 90–3). Two were identified as 2-FDG (and/or FDG-6-PO$_4$) and FD-δ-PGL (and/or FD-6-PG) while the chemical identities of the other two could not be specified.[14] Later spectra indicated a relative dominance by one or more of the metabolites. The authors interpreted their results as evidence that the metabolism of FDG in vivo is more extensive than previously recognized and goes beyond the established hexokinase reaction. The possibilities of utilizing ^{19}F-FDG techniques to develop quantitative models of cerebral glucose metabolism were mentioned. Wyrwicz et al.[15] and Berkowitz et al.[16] (Fig. 90–4) have also applied time sequenced spectroscopic techniques to the study of 2-FDG metabolism in the rat brain and have demonstrated similar multiple metabolite formation. Babcock and Nunnally[17] have investigated the distribution of 2-FDG in the brain and myocardium of rabbits using NMR imaging and spectroscopy. In vivo, 3-FDG metabolism in the rat brain model has been studied by Kwee et al.,[80] with an indication that this fluorinated glucose analogue follows the aldose reductase sorbitol (ARS) pathway. These findings have a significant impact on the understanding

2-FDG, 0.7M

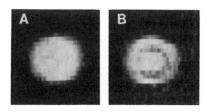

26.6 MHz

Figure 90–2. Images of phantoms containing approximately 0.7M 2-FDG: *A*, Cylindrical. *B*, Cylindrical with the addition of a central glass tube of wall thickness 1 mm and OD 6.8 mm. In each case, the 2-FDG sample height was 12 mm and the outer diameter 9 mm. The imaging technique involved 26.6 MHz (0.66 T for fluorine); TE 5 ms; TR 1000 ms; NSA 64; readout gradient 0.24 G/cm; acquisition matrix 64 × 128.

Table 90–1. 2-FLUORO-2-DEOXY-D-GLUCOSE (2-FDG): METABOLITES AND SPECTRAL ANALYSIS DATA*

A. Metabolites of 2-FDG
    (1) FDG-6-PO₄: 2-fluoro-2-deoxy-D-glucose-6-phosphate
    (2) FD-δ-PGL: 2-fluoro-2-deoxy-δ-phospho-glucose-lactose
    (3) FD-6-PG;   2-fluoro-2-deoxy-6-phosphogluconate
B. Spectral analysis data acquired at 188.2 MHz (4.69 tesla) at 23° C. Chemical shifts were measured with respect to an external standard of trifluoroacetic acid (10 mM TFA/D₂O). Proton decoupling techniques were utilized in the spectral data acquisition.

Compound	Anomeric Form	Chemical Shift (ppm)	Coupling constant (Hz)	
			F_2-H_2 Geminal	F_2-H_3 Vicinal
2-FDG	alpha	−123.79	49.1	13.6
	beta	−123.67	51.0	15.3
FDG-6-PO₄	alpha	−123.93	48.9	13.5
	beta	−123.76	50.9	15.2
FD-δ-PGL		−120.72	—	—
FD-6-PG		−120.82	49.3	25.3

* From Nakada T et al.: 19-Fluorine nuclear magnetic resonance spectra of 2-fluoro-2-deoxy-D-glucose and its metabolites. Biochem Arch *1*:163–166, 1985.

and modeling of glucose metabolism and the quantitative mapping of glucose utilization by tissue.

Fluorinated Antitumor Drugs

The fluoropyrimidines (5-fluorouracil, 5-fluorouridine, and 5-fluoro-2-deoxyuridine) have found extensive application in the treatment of disseminated human cancers. For chemotherapy regimens, using these agents alone or in combination with other drugs, the objective is to control the rate and fate of metabolism of the drugs and thus increase their therapeutic efficiency.[18] The noninvasive techniques available through ^{19}F NMR allow direct investigation of biological samples or of localized in-vivo regions, which provide simultaneous identification and quantitation of all the fluorinated metabolites without any requirement for differential labeling.[19]

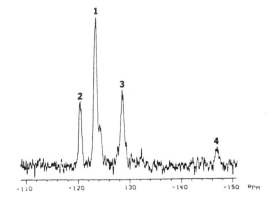

Rat Brain : 2-FDG
3Hour Data

Figure 90–3. The ^{19}F spectrum obtained in vivo at 188.2 MHz (4.7 T) from a rat brain 3 hours after 2-FDG infusion. Peak 1 has been associated with 2-FDG and/or FDG-6-PO₄, whereas peak 2 was attributed to FD-δ-PGL and/or FD-6-PG. The other peaks were unknown and not assigned. (From Nakada T et al.: Biochem Arch *1*:163, 1985. Used by permission.)

Rat Brain : 2-FDG (50 mg I. V.)

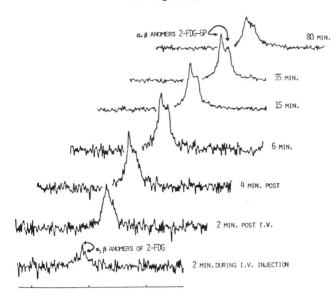

Figure 90–4. Proton decoupled time sequenced ^{19}F spectra from a rat brain obtained in vivo at 188.2 MHz (4.7 T) following intravenous administration of 50 mg of 2-FDG. This sequence demonstrates the time course for the rat brain metabolism from 2-FDG to 2FDG-6-P. (From Berkowitz BA, Ackerman JJH: Abstract. *In* Proceedings of the 4th Annual Meeting of The Society of Magnetic Resonance in Medicine, August 19–23, 1985, London, England. Used by permission.)

Stevens et al.[18] have studied the metabolism of intravenously injected 5-fluorouracil (5-FU) in situ for both implanted tumors and livers of C57 mice using surgically placed surface coils. Their investigation demonstrated the effectiveness of ^{19}F NMR techniques in the measurement of metabolism both at the site of drug action and at the sites of detoxification. The ability to monitor the adjuvant action of other drugs on the 5-FU metabolism was discussed also. Nunnally et al.[20] have reported observations on 5-fluorouracil metabolism in the liver of an intact rabbit. They mention extended studies designed to examine the metabolic effect in tumor and liver of combined radiation treatment or hyperthermia and 5-FU chemotherapy. Postulated also is the employment of double-tuned coils for the nearly simultaneous observation of ^{19}F and ^{31}P resonances for determination of the fluorine agent concentration, catabolic products, and bioenergetic status of the tumor or tissue. Other ^{19}F metabolic studies have been conducted on the drug 5'-deoxy-5-fluorouridine[21,22,81] (Fig. 90–5). All of this research indicates

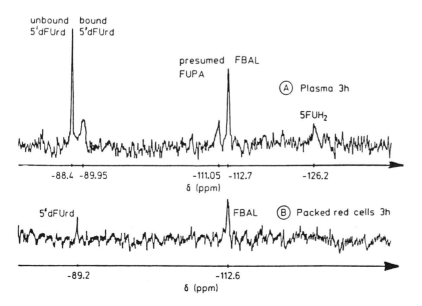

Figure 90–5. The three hour plasma (*A*) and packed red cell (*B*) ^{19}F NMR spectra for a patient who was undergoing an IV infusion of 5'-deoxy-5-fluorouridine (5'dFUrd) at a constant rate over six hours. The resonance at −89.95 ppm is assigned to 5'dFUrd bound to plasmatic proteins. Other notation: α-fluoro-β-ureidopropionic (FUPA); α-fluoro-β-alanine (FBAL); 5,6-dihydrofluorouracil (5FUH$_2$). The spectra were obtained at 250 MHz (6.2 percent) with the chemical shift related to an external standard of CF$_3$COOH (0.5 percent aqueous solution). (From Malet-Martino MC et al.: Cancer Chemother Pharmacol *13*:31, 1984. Used by permission.)

that ^{19}F NMR methods represent a potentially powerful methodology for evaluation of tumor therapy.

ENZYMATIC ACTIVITY AND BINDING MECHANISMS

A number of investigators have reported on the use of ^{19}F NMR for studying the energetics and catalytic action of various enzyme groups. Rigo et al.[23] have demonstrated that ^{19}F NMR techniques provide a means for obtaining a direct, specific assay of enzymes in biological materials free of interference by other molecules. The ^{19}F relaxation rates for bovine copper, zinc superoxide dismutase were found to depend on both the enzyme and F^- concentrations. The relaxation rate parameter furnished an effective probe of anion binding to the active site of the enzyme. Representative results indicated that the effect of copper, zinc, or manganese superoxide dismutase on this parameter was significantly greater than that of other copper and iron proteins.

Amshey et al.[24] have described ^{19}F magnetic resonance studies of fluorine-substituted benzoyl chymotrypsins in which they attempted to relate conditions of the active site environment to the kinetics of the deacylation step in the enzymatic reaction sequence through analysis of the fluorine chemical shift data (ranging from approximately 13 to 31 ppm for the specific derivatives investigated). However, the initial results did not succeed in establishing the sought-for correlation between active site polarity and solvent polarity. Other investigators have published on associated aspects within this field, including the binding of galactose to enzyme active sites (galactose oxidase-substrate binding);[25] determination of comparative molecular environment characteristics to establish the interactive links between fluorinated groups and an enzyme (fluorocinnamoylchymotrypsins);[26] and studies of enzyme activity during conditions of steady-state turnover (Cu, Zn super-oxide dismutase).[27] These reports have demonstrated the value of utilizing NMR techniques involving either relaxation or fluorine chemical shift analysis to effectively obtain information concerning the factors that influence enzymatic reactions.

Observation of various bound complexes by ^{19}F NMR has allowed characterization of the mechanism of specific catalytic reactions.[28] The versatility of this method is evident in the ability to monitor the free acid as well as the other fluorinated substrates

Riboflavin binding protein

Figure 90–6. The ^{19}F spectra at 23°C of 8-fluoro-8-dimethylriboflavin (FF) indicating its potential as a probe for the flavin-protein interaction. FF free in solution (*a*) 2 mH, pH 6.0, NSA 9000. FF bound to the hen egg white riboflavin binding protein apoRBP (*b*): 1.1 mM FF-apoRBP, pH 6.18, NSA 39,400. The spectra were obtained at 188 MHz (4.7 T) with the chemical shift expressed in ppm downfield from an external standard of 10 mM NaF in 0.1 M deuterated sodium phosphate buffer (pH 7.0). (From Miura PA et al.: Biochemistry *21*:615, 1982. Used by permission.)

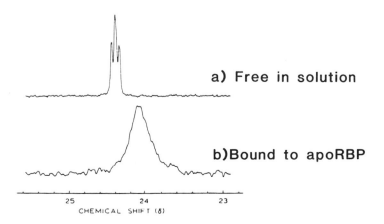

a) Free in solution

b) Bound to apoRBP

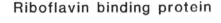

simultaneously. Additional research in associated areas includes development of specific fluorine-labeled reagents for the investigation of the energetics of the equilibrium between bound states (two nucleotide-free myosin subfragment 1 states with the chemical shift of the resonant line of the fluorine compound being sensitive to temperature, pH, ionic strength, and nucleotides bound in the active site);[29] the study of CO_2 binding to modified human hemoglobin;[30] and investigations of protein structure, interactions and binding (Fig. 90–6).[31-34]

MEMBRANE AND CELLULAR SYSTEMS

Molecular order and dynamics in model and biological membranes have been studied with considerable intensity using ^{19}F NMR techniques.[35] Investigations using specifically labeled phospholipids (e.g., fluorine-19 in the 8 position and deuterium in the 2, 7, and 9 positions of the 2-acyl chain) have demonstrated that ^{19}F provides a sensitive probe for the motional state of hydrocarbon chains in the liquid-crystalline phase of a lipid membrane.[36] Spectra obtained from both the macroscopically oriented bilayers and nonoriented liposomes of the phospholipids have been utilized in this analysis. The potential for examining the effect of incorporating various biomolecular complexes (such as cholesterol or proteins) into model bilayers containing a difluoromethylene group at various positions along the 2-acyl chain was mentioned.[35]

Fluorine-labeled phospholipid research has been extensive in many areas, including investigations of lipid-lipid and protein-lipid interactions;[37,38] differentiation between possible spectral line broadening mechanisms (e.g., the distribution of order parameters versus extra relaxation processes such as exchange or other slow motions);[39] preferential interaction of certain proteins with specific lipids;[40] the mobility of labeled amino acid residues in M13 coat protein;[41] and transmembrane channels and membrane structure.[42] Monofluorinated fatty acid probes have been utilized in the study of lipid fatty acyl chain order and dynamics in specific membrane models.[43,44]

Fluorinated molecules constrained to specific cellular compartments in complement with studies of other nuclei have been demonstrated to be useful in the investigation of cell systems such as human platelets;[45] while fluorine-labeled Ca^{2+} indicators have been used for direct identification of specific intracellular cation binding, internal calibration of $[Ca]_i$ and pH_i, and the simultaneous measurement of multiple indicators within the same cell suspension.[46] The chemical shifts of selected fluorinated compounds (e.g., trifluoroethylamine) are strongly pH dependent and provide a sensitive method for measuring pH gradients through the ability to observe discrete resonance lines within the intracellular and extracellular compartments[47] (Fig. 90–7). Intracellular pH has been determined in a perfused single frog skin model through combined ^{19}F

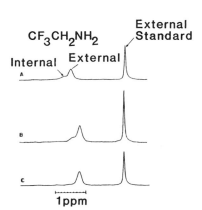

Figure 90–7. The proton decoupled ^{19}F NMR spectra of human erythrocytes plus trifluoroethylamine ($CF_3CH_2NH_2$). The data were taken at 4°C to reduce the rapid exchange process and allow resolution of the two separate resonances associated with the pH gradient across the cell membrane between the internal and external compartments. The spectra were obtained at 169.4 MHz (4.2 T) with the chemical shift relative to an external standard containing trifluoroacetate (with adjustments to a pH of 8.2). *A*, Whole erythrocytes, suspension pH 7.2. *B*, Whole erythrocytes, suspension pH 8.0. *C*, Lysed erythrocytes control, solution pH 8.1. With the suspension pH at 7.2 and 8.0, the internal pH was calculated to be 7.0 and 7.6, respectively. (From Taylor JS et al.: Anal Biochem *114*:415, 1981. Used by permission.)

and ^{31}P NMR analysis.[48] Because intracellular pH is a major determinant of cell function and biosynthesis, the evolving application of ^{19}F NMR investigative techniques holds important promise for efficient, noninvasive methods to measure intracellular pH continuously over an extended range of conditions within biological systems.[47]

PERFLUOROCARBON COMPOUNDS

Highly fluorinated organic compounds known as perfluorocarbons (PFCs) have shown increased utility as emulsions in biological and clinical applications.[49,50] The demonstration in 1966 by Clark et al.[51] that certain perfluorocarbon liquids could be breathed with survival initiated the use of PFCs for respiration and artificial blood (popularly referred to as "blood substitutes"). The suitability of the perfluorocarbons for these applications was based on their properties of chemical and biological inertness combined with the ability to dissolve up to 60 volume % of oxygen and 120 volume % of CO_2.[52] Initial research focused on the oxygen and carbon dioxide transport capability in an effort to identify fluorocarbons with the best molecular structure to form emulsions for intravascular use while confining body retention to the period of functional usefulness.[53]

The potential of ^{19}F NMR imaging[1,4,54–56] combined with spectroscopic techniques has now opened significant new avenues for highly sensitive investigations of the in vivo properties and diagnostic capabilities of the perfluorcarbon compounds. The feasibility of NMR imaging of PFC emulsions and neat liquids now has been demonstrated by a number of investigators.[4,57–62] The ^{19}F NMR spectra of some PFCs are shown in Figure 90–8. As evident in this figure, the PFCs have complex spectra, which result from the nonequivalent chemical environments for the individual fluorine atoms within the molecular configuration. Depending on the specific PFC spin-coupling characteristics and the NMR pulse protocols used (projection reconstruction versus two-di-

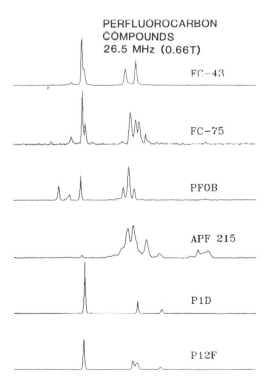

Figure 90–8. The chemical shift spectra for several perfluorocarbon compound neat liquids obtained in vitro at 26.5 MHz (0.66 T for fluorine). F-tributylamine (FC-43), F-butylfuran (FC-75), F-octylbromide (PFOB), F-phenathrene (APF 215), bis-isopropyl-ethyl ether (P1D), isopropyl-hexyl ether (P12F). The spectral width displayed is approximately 4.9 kHz, corresponding to 185 ppm.[64]

mensional Fourier transform echo techniques), these characteristics give rise to potential complications, including degradation of the signal-to-noise ratio, loss of spatial resolution, and introduction of chemical shift artifacts, which must be addressed in the NMR imaging phase.[8,9] On the positive side, exciting applications of chemical shift imaging[63] may be envisioned that exploit the profound chemical shift sensitivity to the molecular (and cellular) environment, including factors such as molecular-complex binding, pH, and local temperature.

Oxygenation State Indicator

One unique application for the PFCs in association with NMR is the potential for the in-vivo monitoring of the oxygen tension (P_{O_2}) in tissue and organs.[57,58,62,64] This possibility is based upon the intrinsic paramagnetism of O_2, which significantly affects the spin-lattice relaxation time $T1$ of the PFC. The relaxation rate $T1^{-1}$ has been found to increase linearly with P_{O_2}.[57,58,64-67] Examples of this linear relationship are shown in Figure 90–9. Regional differences in tissue oxygenation in organs concentrating the PFCs may be monitored qualitatively as well as quantitatively through the contrast enhancement provided in the image for those areas experiencing a higher P_{O_2} level. The enhancement is derived from the increased signal provided at moderate recycle delay times (TR) due to a reduced $T1$ value. Aspects of this application were demonstrated by Thomas et al.[62] for pulmonary NMR imaging following liquid breathing of PFC neat liquids. Figures 90–10 and 90–11 show some lung images obtained through

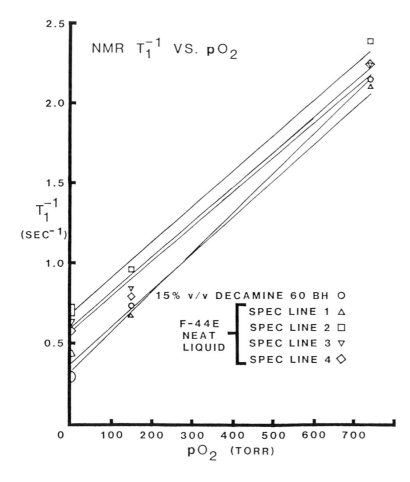

Figure 90–9. Data obtained at 84 MHz (2.1 T), which illustrate the linear relationship between the relaxation rate $(T1)^{-1}$ and the partial pressure of oxygen (pO_2) for several PFCs. The behavior of the four individual spectral lines of F-di-*n*-butyl dihydroethylene (F-44E) is shown, as well as that for the bridge head (BH) fluorine atoms in F-decalin.[58]

67% FC-75, 33% PFOB

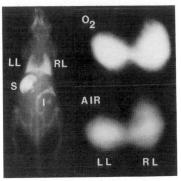

Figure 90–10. The posterior anterior radiograph (*A*) and transverse NMR lung images (*B*) of a mouse following liquid breathing of a 2-to-1 FC 75/PFOB mixture. The x-ray opacity is due to a single bromine atom incorporated at the end of the CF chain within PFOB. Some of the mixture had been swallowed during the liquid breathing procedure and is visualized in the stomach (S) and intestines (I), which illustrates the potential of using the PFCs as gastrointestinal NMR contrast agents. The transverse NMR images were obtained at 25.1 MHz (0.63 T) without slice selection and represent the signal from residual PFC trapped within the alveolar space following liquid breathing and partial draining. A signal enhancement of approximately 10 percent as the result of breathing pure oxygen during imaging was achieved.[62]

X-RAY TRANSVERSE NMR

A B

this research. General possible future uses of PFCs in the pulmonary system include diagnosis of a variety of lung diseases (ventilation defects, pulmonary carcinoma, etc.), monitoring neonatal lung mechanics, and possibly devising new treatments for cystic fibrosis and pulmonary emphysema. In addition, as evident in Figure 90–10, there are real possibilities for the use of PFCs as NMR gastrointestinal contrast agents. Investigations involving PFC accumulation in rat liver (Fig. 90–12) have demonstrated that, for certain PFCs, clinically significant Po_2 differentials may be determined in vivo with an eventual quantitative precision projected to be 10 torr over the physiologically important Po_2 range for the liver of 0 to 100 torr.[64]

Thermal Imaging

Another area of interest representing potential utility for NMR PFC investigations centers on the temperature dependent properties of some of these compounds.[68,69] The relative position, magnitude, and/or shape of various chemical shift spectral lines for a given PFC as a function of temperature may possibly be used to monitor temperature gradients in vivo. The nature of the different coupling mechanisms between non-equivalent fluorine atoms gives rise to intensity variations reflecting the relative rates of chemical exchange, which are directly related to the temperature. Figure 90–13 illustrates the relative spectral changes for perfluorodecalin as a function of temperature. The ratio of peak 1 to peak 2 increases significantly over the given temperature range.

PROTON APF-215

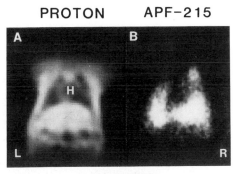

Figure 90–11. *A*, A 4 mm thick coronal proton NMR image through the thorax of a rat showing the lung field demarcated as a low signal area. (Even without cardiac gating, the heart wall [H] is visible). *B*, A non–slice selected coronal ¹⁹F image of APF-215 of the same rat lungs taken sequentially immediately following the proton image; although the scale is slightly different between the two images, the one-to-one anatomical correlation between the lung fields is evident. Both images were obtained at 0.14 T (6.0 MHz for protons and 5.7 MHz for fluorine).[62]

CORONAL

P1D, 26.5 MHz

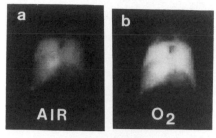

a

b

AIR

O₂

LIVER

Figure 90–12. Coronal, non–slice selected in vivo NMR images of a mouse liver containing P1D obtained at 26.5 MHz (0.66 T) under conditions of ambient air and pure oxygen breathing, demonstrating the enhanced signal resulting from the elevated pO_2 levels.[64]

Perfluorodecalin
26.5 MHz, NX 64, SW 3KHz, TE 22mS

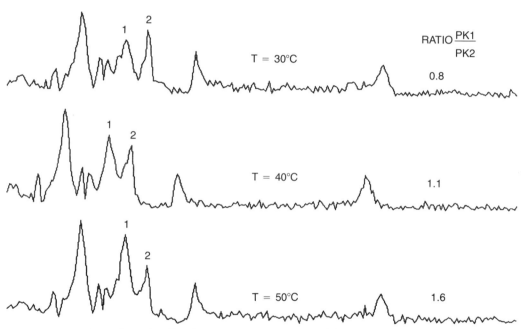

RATIO $\frac{PK1}{PK2}$

T = 30°C   0.8

T = 40°C   1.1

T = 50°C   1.6

Figure 90–13. Spectra for perfluorodecalin taken at 26.5 MHz (0.66 T) with 64 acquisitions and displayed at a spectral width of 3 kHz. The relative intensity ratio of the peaks labeled 1 and 2 is changing significantly over the temperature range 30°C to 50°C.[69]

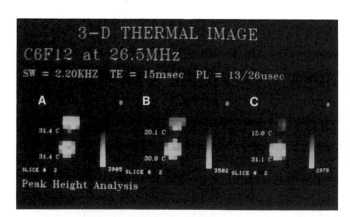

3–D THERMAL IMAGE
C6F12 at 26.5MHz
SW = 2.20KHZ   TE = 15msec   PL = 13/26usec

A   B   C

31.4 C   20.1 C   15.0 C

31.4 C   30.9 C   31.1 C

SLICE # 2   3905 SLICE # 2   3502 SLICE # 2   2978

Peak Height Analysis

Figure 90–14. An example of the potential for producing thermal images. The phantom consisted of two 8-mm tubes containing C_6F_{12}. The temperature of each tube was maintained independently of the other through individually controlled water jacket systems. The three-dimensional data acquisition involved two phase-encoded directions with the echo obtained with no readout gradient. A peak height analysis of the spectra obtained per matrix element (a single line for C_6F_{12}) provided the image intensity display. For panel *A* the two tubes were maintained at the same temperature (31.4°C), while for *B* and *C*, the temperature for the lower tube was held constant, with the upper tube cooled by successive amounts (to 20.1°C and 15.0°C). (Spectral width, SW; time to echo, TE; pulse length, PL for the 90 and 180 pulses.)[69]

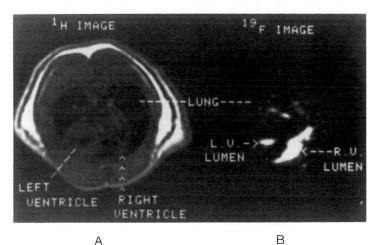

Figure 90–15. Axial images 2.5 mm thick through the thorax of a rat killed after perfluorotibutylamine infusion. *A*, Proton image exhibiting diminished signal intensity from the ventricular lumens. *B*, Fluorine-19 image showing the ventricular lumens as well as signals from the lungs and vessels around the heart. Magnetic field strength 1.4 T. (From Joseph PM et al.: J Comp Assist Tomogr 9:1012, 1985. Used by permission.)

A   B

An example of a three-dimensional thermal image involving a temperature controlled $C_6 F_{12}$ phantom is shown in Figure 90–14. The future objective is the development of thermal imaging over the narrower range of physiologically important temperatures using selected compounds.

Other NMR Fluorine-19 Studies Using PFCs

Additional areas of interest representing potential utility for NMR PFC investigations in vivo include (1) imaging of the vascular system, providing NMR equivalent cerebroangiography and cardioangiography (Fig. 90–15); (2) tumor marking through the imaging of macrophage based activity reflecting the natural affinity for macrophages to accumulate the PFCs; (3) quantitative studies on oxygen transport to increase tumor radiosensitivity; and (4) investigations to evaluate the extent to which the PFC reduces myocardial ischemic damage after coronary occlusion.

BIODISTRIBUTION, RETENTION, PERFUSION STUDIES

As a direct consequence of the negligible intrinsic biological concentrations of fluorine in tissue, any introduced fluorinated substrate, in principle, may be monitored by NMR techniques, including imaging as to its distribution and retention or perfusion in specific organ systems.

Anesthetics

The retention of fluorinated anesthetics has been studied spectroscopically in rabbit brains using surface coil ^{19}F-NMR methods by Wyrwicz et al.[70,71] The additional resonances observed as a function of time following administration for both 1 percent halothane and 1.5 percent isoflurane provide direct evidence of the kinetics associated with the formation of bound species or other molecular environment changes for these anesthetics (Fig. 90–16). Recent additional investigations have also reported on the research aspects of NMR techniques applied to the study of inhaled anesthetics.[72,73] Burt et al.[74] have published on the use of fluorinated anesthetics as probes of lipophilic environments in tumors. They also postulate the potential use of ^{19}F NMR spectroscopy

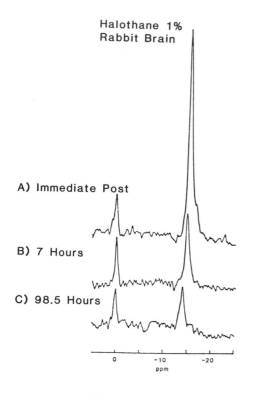

Halothane 1%
Rabbit Brain

A) Immediate Post

B) 7 Hours

C) 98.5 Hours

0   -10   -20
ppm

Figure 90–16. ^{19}F NMR spectra of a rabbit brain following a 30-minute administration of 1 percent halothane demonstrating the presence of significant levels of halothane or a halothane metabolite for long periods of time. The spectra were acquired at 75.5 MHz (1.89 T) with a surface coil centered on the head, over the calvarium. The chemical shifts were measured relative to an external 1,2-dibromotetrafluoro-ethane standard. (From Wyrwicz AM et al.: Science 222:429, 1983. Used by permission.)

to follow the degradation of the anesthetics by the liver, including identification of toxic derivative products. In addition, they indicate the possibility of monitoring drug and radiation response of tissue in a unique fashion through processes primarily involving the membrane.

Distribution Investigations

Bartels et al.[75] have utilized ^{19}F NMR for the quantitative determination of fluorinated neuroleptic levels following administration of psychopharmacological agents with the intent of correlating the administered neuroleptic dose with its clinical effect on the symptoms. The retention of the perfluorocarbon components within Fluosol 43 in whole blood has been investigated in mice using quantitative ^{19}F spectroscopic techniques.[76] Nunnally et al.[77] have evaluated the use of ^{19}F NMR imaging in the study of tissue perfusion. A water soluble ^{19}F-labeled compound (Mallinckrodt MP-312: a meglumine salt of trifluoromethyl sulfonic acid) was used to demonstrate a decrease in myocardial perfusion in a rabbit heart model involving coronary arterial ligation. It was proposed that these techniques would find future applications in diagnosis and evaluation of general perfusion defects, including clinical situations exhibiting enhanced as well as decreased perfusion characteristics.

FLUORINATED GAS RESEARCH

Gas phase ^{19}F NMR imaging has been reported by Heidelberger and Lauterbur,[78] who proposed that this technique could be used for ventilation imaging to visualize the distribution and exchange of gases within the lungs. Images of CF_4 were shown for various concentrations of the gas in phantom cylinders and within an excised pair of rabbit lungs. In other work, Bolas et al.[79] have demonstrated the potential for the noninvasive measurement of cerebral blood flow using a fluorinated gas such as Freon 22 ($CHClF_2$) and spectroscopic analysis.

APPLICATIONS SUMMARY

The biomedical applications of ^{19}F NMR are extending across the boundaries of various disciplinary research areas with dramatic effect. The investigations described in this review indicate wide ranging and consequential utilization of ^{19}F NMR techniques within medicine and varied biomedical fields. The extremely low endogenous concentrations of mobile fluorine within biological tissue coupled with the positive aspects of a high NMR sensitivity and 100 percent natural isotopic abundance contribute to make the ^{19}F nucleus uniquely suited for use in high contrast NMR studies in vivo involving the introduction of biocompatible fluorine-based tracer compounds. The in-vitro applications include multiple possibilities for utilizing specific fluorinated molecules as probes of the biomolecular environment and functional pathways. It would be expected that ^{19}F NMR techniques will continue to develop as powerful investigative tools with new methods evolving and contributing to these expanding areas of research.

ACKNOWLEDGMENTS

The author would like to acknowledge the other individuals who have been active in the ^{19}F-NMR research at the University of Cincinnati: Jerome L. Ackerman, Leland C. Clark, Jr., Lawrence J. Busse, Ronald G. Pratt, R. C. Samaratunga, Richard E. Hoffman, and Stephen L. Dieckman.

References

1. Thomas SR, Ackerman JL, Gobel JR, et al: Nuclear magnetic resonance imaging techniques as developed modestly within a University Medical Center Environment: What can the small system contribute at this point? Magn Reson Imag *1*:11–21, 1982.
2. Standard man–total body content for some elements. Radiological Health Handbook (Revised edition) p. 214. Washington, D.C., U.S. Government Printing Office, 1970.
3. Goldman MR, Fossel ET, Ingwall T, et al: Feasibility of ^{19}F as an agent for NMR imaging of myocardial infarction: An in vivo study (Abstract). J Nucl Med *20*:604, 1979.
4. McFarland E, Koutcher JA, Rosen BR, et al: In vivo ^{19}F NMR imaging. J Comput Assist Tomogr *9*:8–15, 1985.
5. Gallagher BM, Ansari A, Atkins H, et al: ^{18}F Labeled 2-FDG as a radiopharmaceutical for measuring regional myocardial glucose metabolism in vivo: Tissue distribution and imaging studies in animals. J Nucl Med *18*:990–996, 1977.
6. Phelps ME, Hoffman EJ, Selin C, et al: Investigation of ^{18}F 2-FDG for the measure of myocardial glucose metabolism. J Nucl Med *19*:1311–1319, 1978.
7. Phelps ME, Mazziotta JC: Positron emission tomography: Human brain function and biochemistry. Science *228*:799–809, 1985.
8. Harrison CG, Adams DF, Kramer PB: Imaging of complex NMR spectra. Invest Radiol *20*:180–185, 1985.
9. Busse LJ, Thomas SR, Pratt RG, et al: Deconvolution techniques for removing the effects of chemical shift in NMR imaging of perfluorocarbon compounds. Med Phys *13*:518, 1986.
10. Tewson TJ, Welsh MJ, Raichle JE, et al: ^{18}F labeled 3-FDG: Synthesis and preliminary biodistribution data. J Nucl Med *19*:1339–1345, 1978.
11. Bessel EM, Courtenay VD, Foster AB, et al: Some in vivo and in vitro effects of the FDGs. Europ J Cancer *9*:463–470, 1973.
12. Nakada T, Kwee IL, Rao GA, et al: 19-Fluorine nuclear magnetic resonance spectra of 2-fluoro-2-deoxy-D-glucose and its metabolites. Biochem Arch *1*:163–166, 1985.
13. Nakada T, Kwee IL: Non-invasive demonstration of in vivo 2-fluoro-2-deoxy-D-glucose metabolism in rat brain by ^{19}F NMR spectroscopy (abstract). Fourth Annual Meeting of the Society of Magnetic Resonance in Medicine, August 19–23, 1985, London, England, pp 806–807.
14. Nakada T, Kwee IL, Conboy CB: Noninvasive in vivo demonstration of 2-fluoro-2-deoxy-D-glucose metabolism beyond the hexokinase reaction in rat brain by ^{19}F nuclear magnetic resonance spectroscopy. J Neurochem *46*:198, 1986.

15. Wyrwicz AM, Murphy R, Prakash I, et al: 2-Fluoro-2-deoxy-D-glucose metabolism in the rat brain (abstract). Fourth Annual Meeting of the Society of Magnetic Resonance in Medicine, August 19–23, 1985, London, England, pp 827–828.

16. Berkowitz BA, Ackerman JJH: 2-Fluoro-2-deoxy-D-glucose (2FDG) metabolism in vivo: A ^{19}F-(^{1}H) NMR study (abstract). Fourth Annual Meeting of the Society of Magnetic Resonance in Medicine, August 19–23, 1985, London, England, pp 759–760.

17. Babcock EE, Nunnally RL: In vivo and in vivo determination of 2-fluoro-2-deoxyglucose by F-19 NMR imaging and spectroscopy (abstract). Fourth Annual Meeting of the Society of Magnetic Resonance in Medicine, August 19–23, 1985, London, England, pp 751–752.

18. Stevens AN, Morris PG, Iles RA, et al: 5-Fluorouracil metabolism monitored in vivo by ^{19}F NMR. Br J Cancer *50*:113–117, 1984.

19. Bernadou J, Armand JP, Lopez A, et al: Complete urinary excretion profile of 5-fluorouracil during a six-day chemotherapeutic schedule as resolved by ^{19}F nuclear magnetic resonance. Clin Chem *31*:846–848, 1985.

20. Nunnally RL, Babcock EE, Antich P: The direct observation of 5-fluorouracil metabolism by the liver in the intact rabbit: A 19-F NMR study (abstract): Fourth Annual Meeting of the Society of Magnetic Resonance in Medicine, August 19–23, 1985, London, England, pp 810–811.

21. Malet-Martino MC, Martino R, Lopez A, et al: Detection of fluoropyrimidines and their metabolites in biological samples by fluorine-19 NMR: Application to 5'-deoxy-5-fluorouridine. Biomed Pharmacother *37*:357–359, 1983.

22. Malet-Martino MC, Martino R, Lopez A, et al: New apporach to metabolism of 5'-deoxy-5-fluorouridine in humans with fluorine-19 NMR. Cancer Chemother Pharmacol *13*:31–35, 1984.

23. Rigo A, Viglino P, Argese E, et al: Nuclear magnetic relaxation of ^{19}F as a novel assay method of superoxide dismutase. J Biol Chem *254*:1759–1760, 1979.

24. Amshey JW, Bender ML: Fluorine magnetic resonance studies of fluorine-substituted benzoyl chymotrypsins. Arch Biochem Biophys *224*:378–381, 1983.

25. Marwedel RJ, Kurland RJ: Fluoride ion as an NMR relaxation probe of galactose oxidase-substrate binding. Biochem Biophys Acta *657*:495–506, 1981.

26. Gerig JT, Halley BA: Fluorine NMR studies of fluorocinnamoylchymotrypsins. Arch Biochem Biophys *209*:152–158, 1981.

27. Viglino P, Rigo A, Argese E, et al: ^{19}F relaxation as a probe of the oxidation state of Cu, Zn superoxide dismutase. Studies of the enzyme in steady-state turnover. Biochem Biophys Res Com *100*:125–130, 1981.

28. Anderson DC, Dahlquist FW: ^{19}F nuclear magnetic resonance observations of aldehyde dismutation catalyzed by horse liver alcohol dehydrogenase. Arch Biochem Biophys *217*:226–235, 1982.

29. Shriver JW, Sykes BD: Energetics of the equilibrium between two nucleotide-free myosin subfragment 1 states using fluorine-19 nuclear magnetic resonance imaging. Biochemistry *21*:3022–3028, 1982.

30. Knowles FC: Application of ^{19}F NMR spectroscopy to a study of carbon monoxide binding to human hemoglobin modified at Cys-β 93 with the S-trifluorethyl residue. Arch Biochem Biophys *230*:327–334, 1984.

31. Sakai TT, Dallas JL: Synthesis and properties of a fluorine-containing sulfhydryl reagent for ^{19}F NMR studies. FEBS Lett *93*:43–46, 1978.

32. Miura R, Kasai S, Horiike K, et al: 8-Fluoro-8-demethylriboflavin as a ^{19}F NMR study with egg white riboflavin binding protein. Biochem Biophys Res Com *110*:406–411, 1983.

33. Post JFM, Cottam PF, Simplaceanu V, et al: Fluorine-19 nuclear magnetic resonance study of 5-fluorotryptophan-labeled histidine-binding protein J of *Salmonella typhimurium*. J Mol Biol *179*:729–743, 1984.

34. Mirau PA, Shafer RH, James TL: Binding of 5-fluorotryptamine to polynucleotides as a model for protein-nucleic acid interactions: Fluorine-19 nuclear magnetic resonance, absorption, and fluorescence studies. Biochemistry *21*:615–620, 1982.

35. Ho C, Dowd SR, Post JFM: ^{19}F NMR investigations of membranes. Curr Top Bioenerg *14*:53–95, 1984.

36. Engelsberg M, Dowd SR, Simplaceanu V, et al: Nuclear magnetic resonance line-shape analysis of fluorine-19-labeled phospholipids. Biochemistry *27*:6983–6989, 1982.

37. Post JFM, Cook BW, Dowd SR, et al: Fluorine-19 nuclear magnetic resonance investigation of fluorine-19-labeled phospholipids. 1. A multiple-pulse study. Biochemistry *23*:6138–6141, 1984.

38. Dowd SR, Simplaceanu V, Ho C: Fluorine-19 nuclear magnetic resonance investigation of fluorine-19-labeled phospholipids. 2. A line-shape analysis. Biochemistry *23*:6142–6146, 1984.

39. Post JFM, DeRuiter EEJ, Berendsen HJC: A fluorine NMR study of model membranes containing ^{19}F-labeled phospholipids and an intrinsic membrane protein. FEBS Lett *132*:257–260, 1981.

40. Ong RL: ^{31}P and ^{19}F NMR studies of glycophorin-reconstituted membranes: Preferential interaction of glycophorin with phosphatidylserine. J Membrane Biol *78*:1–7, 1984.

41. Dettman HD, Weiner JH, Sykes BD: ^{19}F nuclear magnetic resonance studies of the coat protein of bacteriophage M13 in synthetic phospholipid vesicles and deoxycholate micelles. Biophy J *37*:243–251, 1982.

42. Weinstein S, Wallace BA, Blout ER, et al: Conformation of gramacidin A channel in phospholipid vesicles: A ^{13}C and ^{19}F nuclear magnetic resonance study. Proc Natl Acad Sci USA *76*:4230–4234, 1979.

43. MacDonald PM, McDonough B, Sykes BD, et al: Fluorine-19 nuclear magnetic resonance studies of lipid fatty acyl chain order and dynamics in *Acholeplasma laidlawii* B membranes. Effects of methyl-

branch substitution and of trans unsaturation upon membrane acyl-chain orientational order. Biochemistry 22:5103–5111, 1983.

44. McDonough B, MacDonald PM, Sykes BD, et al: Fluorine-19 nuclear magnetic resonance studies of lipid fatty acyl chain order and dynamics in *Acholesplasma laidlawii* B membranes. A physical, biochemical, and biological evaluation of monofluoropalmitic acids as membrane probes. Biochemistry 22:5097–5103, 1983.
45. Costa JL, Dobson CM, Kirk KL, et al: Studies of human platelets by ^{19}F and ^{31}P NMR. FEBS Lett 99:141–146, 1979.
46. Metcalfe JC, Hesketh TR, Smith GA: Free cytosolic Ca^{2+} measurements with fluorine labeled indicators using ^{19}F NMR. Cell Calcium 6:183–195, 1985.
47. Taylor JS, Deutsch C, McDonald GG, et al: Measurement of transmembrane pH gradients in human erythrocytes using ^{19}F NMR. Analy Biochem 114:415–418, 1981.
48. Civan MM, Lin-Er L, Peterson-Yantorno K, et al: Intracellular pH of perfused single frog skin: Combined ^{19}F- and ^{31}P-NMR analysis. Am J Physiol 247 (Cell Physiol 16):C506–C510, 1984.
49. Ohyanagi H, Toshima K, Sekita M, et al: Clinical studies of perfluorochemical whole blood substitutes: Safety of fluosol-DA (20%) in normal human volunteers. Clin Therap 2:306–312, 1979.
50. Perfluorochemical oxygen transport. Int Anesthesiol Clin 23(1). Boston, Little, Brown and Company, 1985.
51. Clark LC Jr, Gollan F: Survival of mammals breathing organic liquids equilibrated with oxygen at atmospheric pressure. Science 152:1755–1756, 1966.
52. Wessler EP, Iltis R, Clark LC Jr: The solubility of oxygen in highly fluoridated liquids. J Fluor Chem 9:137–146, 1977.
53. Clark LC Jr, Becattini F, Kaplan S, et al: Perfluorocarbons having a short dwell time in the liver. Science 181:680–682, 1973.
54. Holland GN, Bottomley PA, Hinshaw WS: [19]F magnetic resonance imaging. J Magn Reson 28:133–136, 1977.
55. Bottomley PA, Edelstein WA: NMR imaging applications in medicine and biology. Curr Prob Cancer 7:20–31, 1982.
56. Nelson RT, Newman FD, Schiffer LM, et al: Fluorine nuclear magnetic resonance: Calibration and system optimization. Magn Reson Imag 3:267–273, 1985.
57. Clark LC Jr, Ackerman JL, Thomas SR, et al: High contrast tissue and blood oxygen imaging based on fluorocarbon ^{19}F NMR relaxation times (abstract). J Magn Reson Med 1:135–136, 1984.
58. Clark LC Jr, Ackerman JL, Thomas SR, et al: Perfluorinated organic liquids and emulsions as biocompatible NMR imaging agents for ^{19}F and dissolved oxygen. In Bruley D, Bicher HI, Reneau D (eds): Advances in Experimental Medicine and Biology. Vol 180: Oxygen Transport to Tissue IV. New York, Plenum Publishing Corporation, 1985, pp 835–845.
59. Longmaid HE III, Adams DF, Neirinckx RD, et al: In vivo ^{19}F NMR imaging of liver, tumor, and abscess in rats. Preliminary Results. Invest Radiol 20:141–145, 1985.
60. Joseph PM, Yuasa Y, Kundel HL, et al: Magnetic resonance imaging of fluorine in rats infused with artificial blood. Invest Radiol 20:504–509, 1985.
61. Joseph PM, Fishman JE, Mukherji B, et al: In vivo ^{19}F NMR imaging of the cardiovascular system. J Comput Assist Tomogr 9:1012–1019, 1985.
62. Thomas SR, Clark LC Jr, Ackerman JL, et al: MR Imaging of the lung using liquid perfluorocarbons. J Comput Assist Tomogr 10:1–9, 1986.
63. Guilfoyle DN, Mansfield P: Chemical shift imaging. Magn Reson Med 2:479–489, 1985.
64. Clark LC Jr, Thomas SR, Pratt RG, et al: NMR determination of liver pO2 in vivo using perfluorocarbon emulsions (abstract). Fourth Annual Meeting of the Society of Magnetic Resonance in Medicine, London, England, August 19–23, 1985, pp 40–41.
65. Parhami P, Fung BM: Fluorine-19 relaxation study of perfluoro chemicals as oxygen carriers. J Phys Chem 87:1928–1931, 1983.
66. Lai CS, Stair SJ, Miziorko H, et al: Effect of oxygen and the lipid spin label TEMPO-laurate on fluorine-19 and proton relaxation rates of the perfluorochemical blood substitute, FC-43 Emulsion. J Magn Reson 57:447–452, 1984.
67. Reid RS, Koch CJ, Castro ME, et al: The influence of oxygenation in the ^{19}F spin-lattice relaxation rates of fluosol-DA. Phys Med Biol 30:677–686, 1985.
68. Ackerman JL, Clark LC Jr, Thomas SR, et al: NMR thermal imaging (abstract). Third Annual Meeting of the Society of Magnetic Resonance in Medicine, New York, New York, August 13–17, 1984, pp 1–2.
69. Dieckman SL, Kreishman GP, Pratt RG, et al: 19-F NMR thermal imaging utilizing perfluorocarbons (abstract). Sixth Annual Meeting, Soc. Magn. Res. Med. New York, August 17–21, 1987, p 815.
70. Wyrwicz AM, Pszenny MH, Schofield JC, et al: Noninvasive observation of fluorinated anesthetics in rabbit brain by fluorine-19 nuclear magnetic resonance. Science 222:429–430, 1983.
71. Wyrwicz AM, Ryback K, Pszenny MH: In vivo ^{19}F NMR study of fluorinated anesthetics elimination from a rabbit brain (abstract). Third Annual Meeting of the Society of Magnetic Resonance in Medicine, New York, New York, August 13–17, 1984, pp 763–764.
72. Conboy CB, Wyrwicz AM: Localization of halothane in a rat brain with 19-F NMR rotating frame zeugmatography (abstract). Fourth Annual Meeting of the Society of Magnetic Resonance in Medicine, London, England, August 19–23, 1985, pp 775–776.

73. Higuchi T, Naruse S, Horikawa Y, et al: In vivo 19-F NMR spectroscopic study of normal and pathological brains (abstract). Fourth Annual Meeting of the Society of Magnetic Resonance in Medicine, London, England, August 19–23, 1985, pp 795–796.

74. Burt CT, Moore RR, Roberts MF: Fluorinated anesthetics as probes of lipophilic environments in tumors. J Magn Reson 53:163–166, 1983.

75. Bartels M, Albert K, Kruppa G, et al: Fluorinated psychopharmacological agents: Noninvasive observation by fluorine-19 nuclear magnetic resonance (abstract). Fourth Annual Meeting of the Society of Magnetic Resonance in Medicine, London, England, August 19–23, 1985, p 755.

76. Malet-Martino MC, Betbeder D, Lattes A, et al: Fluosol 43 intravascular persistence in mice measured by ^{19}F NMR. J Pharm Pharmacol 36:556–559, 1984.

77. Nunnally RL, Babcock EE, Horner SD, et al: Fluorine-19 NMR spectroscopy and imaging investigations of myocardial perfusion and cardiac function. Magn Reson Imag 3:399–405, 1985.

78. Heidelberger E, Lauterbur PC: Gas phase ^{19}F-NMR zeugmatography: A new approach to lung ventilation imaging (abstract). First Annual Meeting of the Society of Magnetic Resonance in Medicine, Boston, August 16–18, 1982, pp 70–71.

79. Bolas NM, Petros AJ, Bergel D, et al: Use of ^{19}F magnetic resonance spectroscopy for measurement of cerebral blood flow (abstract). Fourth Annual Meeting of the Society of Magnetic Resonance in Medicine. London, England, August 19–23, 1985, pp 315–316.

80. Kwee IL, Nakada T, Card PJ: Noninvasive demonstration of in vivo 3-flouro-3-deoxy-D-glucose metabolism in rat brain by ^{19}F nuclear magnetic resonance spectroscopy: Suitable probe for monitoring cerebral aldose reductase activities. J Neurochem 49:428, 1987.

81. Malet-Martino MC, Armand JP, Lopez A, et al: Evidence for the importance of 5'-deoxy-5-fluorouridine catabolism in humans for 19-F nuclear magnetic resonance spectroscopy. Cancer Res 46:2105, 1986.

91

NMR of ^{23}Na in Biological Systems

P. A. NARAYANA
M. V. KULKARNI
S. D. MEHTA

The cellular composition of sodium and its concentration gradient across the plasma membrane play very important roles in various physiological processes. Excess accumulation of these ions inside the cell is implicated in various diseases, including cancer,[1,2] diabetes,[3] and hypertension.[4] The determination of sodium ion concentration and chemical state in cells is, therefore, of considerable importance. Most of the conventional methods used to determine the concentration of sodium ions in various tissues are invasive and require the destruction of the sample.[5-7] The noninvasive nature of nuclear magnetic resonance (NMR) is ideally suited for the determination of the properties of sodium ions in the cell and is a topic of numerous reviews.[8-11]

In order to appreciate the overall NMR sensitivity of ^{23}Na (100 percent natural abundance) in tissues, it is helpful to compare it with ^{1}H and ^{31}P, the two most commonly used nuclei for in vivo studies. The concentration of sodium in the human body is 44 mM, compared with 387 mM of phosphorus and 99.9 M of protons.[12] The overall NMR sensitivity of ^{23}Na in body is $4.1 \times 10^{(-5)}$ while it is $25.7 \times 10^{(-5)}$ for ^{31}P, assuming a unit sensitivity for ^{1}H.[11]

Even though the overall NMR sensitivity of ^{31}P in tissues appears to be better than ^{23}Na, in practice this is not the case. Firstly, owing to the multiple spectral nature of ^{31}P, the intensity is distributed in a number of spectral peaks. Secondly, in most of the NMR studies, signal averaging is an integral part of the experiment, and because ^{23}Na has a fairly short spin-lattice relaxation time ($T1$),[13] higher sensitivity per unit time can be achieved by decreasing the repetition time. Thus the overall sensitivity of ^{23}Na is higher than ^{31}P and is next only to ^{1}H.

The nature of information that can be obtained from the NMR studies of ^{23}Na differs somewhat from what is obtained from ^{1}H and ^{31}P studies. Because of its abundance in the tissues and its high NMR sensitivity and the dependence of the relaxation times on the type of tissues and the pathology, the ^{1}H nucleus is extensively used to generate images that exhibit exquisite anatomical details with excellent soft tissue contrast. The usefulness of ^{1}H and ^{31}P for in vivo spectroscopic studies stems from the fact that they exhibit a number of spectral peaks owing to the chemical shift. The chemical shift and the relative amplitudes of the various peaks reflect the tissue biochemistry and, therefore, tissue state. For instance, the chemical shift of inorganic phosphate peak relative to the phosphocreatine peak in the ^{31}P spectrum is related to the intracellular pH.[14] Similarly the amplitude of the phosphocreatine peak relative to the inorganic phosphate peak indicates the tissue state.

While ^{23}Na has been used for generating images,[15-17] owing to its relatively low sensitivity, the images do not provide anatomical details to the same extent as the proton images do. Owing to short relaxation times the contrast in the sodium images is fairly poor. Thus ^{23}Na is not a nucleus of choice for NMR imaging. It is also not a nucleus of choice for spectroscopy in the conventional sense. This is because the sodium ions exist generally in the form of aquo complexes both inside and outside the cell and, therefore, exhibit very small chemical shifts. In spite of these problems, great strides have been made in the last few years in applying ^{23}Na spectroscopy to the studies of tissues and relating them to various physiological processes.

Most of the ^{23}Na NMR spectroscopic studies on tissues have been carried out with the aims of (1) separating the nuclear resonant frequencies of intracellular and extracellular ions and (2) understanding the "NMR visibility." The sodium ions in cells are distributed between the intracellular and extracellular region. The intracellular sodium ion concentration is small compared with the extracellular concentration. Yet from a physiological point of view, the properties of the intracellular ions are much more interesting. Unfortunately it is difficult to distinguish between the ions associated with intracellular and extracellular regions based on the NMR spectrum because they resonate at the same frequency. With the development of paramagnetic shift reagents (SR)[18–21] it is now possible to induce frequency shifts between extracellular and the intracellular space.

It was observed by Cope[22–24] that the concentration of sodium ions as determined from the NMR measurements is smaller than the actual concentration, i.e., not all the sodium nuclei are NMR "visible." Similar observations were made by others in different biological samples. This is described in more detail below. It is now generally agreed that this is a consequence of the nuclear quadrupole interaction of ^{23}Na with the surrounding electric field gradients. A proper understanding of this effect will aid us in interpreting the chemical nature of the sodium ions in the cell. This review mainly deals with these two aspects. The imaging aspects of sodium will not be discussed because they are covered elsewhere in this book.

NUCLEAR QUADRUPOLE INTERACTION

^{23}Na differs from ^{1}H and ^{31}P in one important respect. It has a nuclear spin of I = 3/2 and, therefore, possesses a nuclear quadrupole moment. The quadrupole moment interacts with the electric field gradients set up by the asymmetric distribution of dipoles surrounding the nuclei.[25] If the surrounding dipoles are arranged such that they exhibit either a cubic or a spherical symmetry, no net electric field gradients exist at the site of the nucleus and, therefore, the quadrupole interaction is zero.

According to quantum mechanics, a nucleus with I = 3/2 has four energy levels in the presence of a magnetic field (Fig. 91–1a). Each one of these energy levels differs from the others only in the spin magnetic quantum number, which is denoted by m. According to quantum mechanics, transitions are allowed between two energy levels only if they differ in their m values by unity. Therefore, we expect to see only three transitions. In the absence of any other interactions besides the Zeeman interaction, the energy separation between the adjacent levels is the same and, therefore, all the three transitions occur at the same frequency, resulting in a single NMR line. The energy levels are, however, modified in the presence of quadrupole interaction. The quadrupole interaction depends on the symmetry of the dipoles around the sodium ions (loosely referred to as the molecular complex) and the orientation of the symmetry axis of the molecular complex relative to the external magnetic field. If we assume an axial symmetry for the molecular complex with its symmetry axis oriented at an angle θ

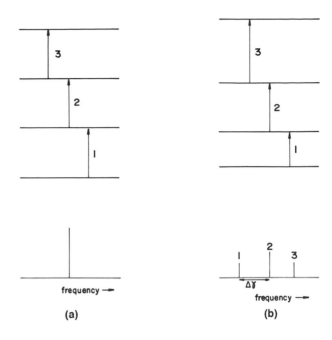

Figure 91–1. Energy level of an $I = 3/2$ nucleus in a magnetic field (a) with no quadrupole coupling and (b) with quadrupole coupling. In the absence of quadrupole coupling the three transitions denoted by 1, 2, and 3 occur at the same frequency, resulting in a single line. The quadrupole coupling separates these transition energies and gives rise to three lines shown at the bottom, at different frequencies. Transition 2 is independent of the quadrupole coupling to a first approximation.

relative to the external magnetic field, the energies of the four levels are given by

$$E(m) = E(m, 0) + (\tfrac{1}{16})e^2qQ(4m^2 - 5)(3\cos^2\theta - 1) \tag{1}$$

where $E(m, 0)$ is the Zeeman energy for the level m, eq is the electric field gradient, eQ is the quadrupole moment, and e is the charge. The energy level diagram in the presence of quadrupole interaction for the case where the molecular axis is parallel to the external magnetic field ($\theta = 0$) is shown in Figure 91–1b. It is clear from the above equation that in the presence of quadrupole interaction the three allowed transitions (denoted as 1, 2, and 3) occur at three different frequencies, i.e., three separate NMR peaks will be observed. It can also be seen from the above equation that the position of the center line (2), which originates from the transition $m = \tfrac{1}{2}$ to $m = -\tfrac{1}{2}$, is not affected by the quadrupole coupling. The transitions 1 and 3, whose energies are determined by the strength of the quadrupole interaction, lie on either side of the central line and are displaced by $\Delta\gamma = \pm(\tfrac{1}{2})e^2qQ$ from it. Quantum mechanical calculations show that the center line has 40 percent of the total intensity while each one of the outer lines contains 30 percent of the total intensity.[26] This is what was indeed observed from single crystal studies. The three expected transitions are shown at the bottom of Figure 91–1.

The transition energies due to quadrupole interaction depend on the orientation of the molecular symmetry axis relative to the external magnetic field. If σ is the angle between the magnetic field and the molecular symmetry axis, the positions of the outer lines with respect to the center line are given by

$$\Delta\gamma = (1/2)e^2qQ(3\cos^2\theta - 1) \tag{2}$$

The separation of the outer lines (1 and 3) relative to the central line varies with the orientation. For example, at $\theta = 55$, $3\cos^2\theta - 1 = 0$, and therefore the outer lines coalesce into the center line. The maximum splitting occurs when $\theta = 0$, and in this case, the outer lines are separated by e^2qQ from the center line. The NMR spectrum of Na in an oriented DNA recorded at $\theta = 0$ degrees, 55 degrees, and 90 degrees depicted in Figure 91–2 clearly shows this behavior.[27]

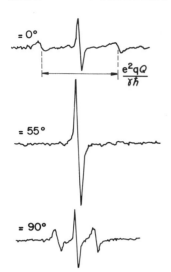

Figure 91–2. The ^{23}Na NMR spectrum of an oriented Na DNA complex at three orientations: $\theta = 0$ degrees, 55 degrees, and 90 degrees, where θ is the angle between the fiber axis and the magnetic field.[27] The separation between the outer lines is maximum at $\theta = 0$ degrees and is zero at $\theta = 55$ degrees. (From Gupta RJ et al: J Magn Reson *47*:344, 1982.)

In polycrystalline samples, the molecular complexes are randomly oriented. Since the position of the center line is independent of the orientation of the molecular complex, the random orientation does not affect the width of this line to a first approximation. However, the positions of the outer lines are distributed over a frequency range from 0 to $\pm e^2qQ$ from the center line. Since the area under these outer lines is constant, a frequency spread in their positions implies a reduction in the peak height. If, in addition, there is a heterogeneity in the molecular environment, the quadrupole interaction eq also varies. This in turn broadens the outer lines further. Under these circumstances the outer lines are broadened beyond detection. Therefore only 40 percent of the sodium ions contribute to the observed NMR spectrum. This is a static effect, and the resulting broadening of the outer lines is referred to as the heterogeneous broadening.

If there are molecular motions, they can cause fluctuations in the electric field gradients. These fluctuations reduce the average value of the quadrupole splitting and in the limit of fast fluctuations (small correlation time) the quadrupole splitting averages to zero, and therefore a single line is observed. However, these fluctuations can affect the relaxation times of the transitions 1 and 3. Thus, even though these transitions occur at the same frequency as the central transition because the average quadrupole coupling is zero, their relaxation times are so shortened as to broaden the lines beyond detection. Again 60 percent of total signal intensity is lost. This is a dynamic effect, and the line broadening of the outer lines is referred to as homogeneous broadening. The relaxation behavior of $I = 3/2$ system is discussed in greater detail by Hubbard[28] and Bull.[29]

NMR VISIBILITY

Using continuous wave NMR, Cope[22,23] observed that the sodium signals observed from muscle, kidney, and brain samples accounted only for about 30 to 40 percent of the total sodium content in these tissues. Similar observations were made in a number of different tissues by a number of other groups[29–42] and are summarized in Table 91–1. These observations were interpreted by postulating the existence of two populations of sodium ions, with approximately 60 percent of the sodium ions bound to the macromolecules and 40 percent of the ions assumed to be free.[22,23] The bound ions have long correlation times, and the NMR lines are broadened beyond detection. The observed NMR line was thought to originate from the free ions and, therefore, has only 40 percent of the total intensity. Cope's hypothesis was initially supported by similar results obtained by a number of investigators using more complex tissues (see Table 91–1). Further, the results of Czeisler et al.[31] based on the anomalous saturation behavior of the NMR spectrum also seemed to support the presence of a broad component arising from the bound ions. In addition, the pulsed NMR results have also established the presence of two transverse relaxation times.[13,32,43–45] The shorter relaxation time was interpreted as arising from the sodium ions bound to the macromolecule.

The tissues on which ^{23}Na NMR studies were reported are quite varied, with different concentrations of macromolecules. It is, therefore, surprising that they all should have approximately the same concentration of free sodium. It was Shporer and Civan[46] who first pointed out that these observations could be explained on the basis of a single population of sodium ions with a quadrupole coupling. Further evidence against the two-population interpretation was provided by the NMR studies on striated muscles by Berendsen and Edzes.[13] These authors observed a single spin-lattice relaxation time for ^{23}Na even though two spin-spin relaxation times were observed. If two populations with relative concentrations of 40 and 60 percent give rise to two distinct spin-spin relaxation times, there is no reason why two spin-lattice relaxation times should not be observed.

However, by invoking the quadrupole coupling, it is possible to explain why only 40 percent of the sodium was observed in the NMR spectrum. If the observed NMR line arises from the central transition ($m = \frac{1}{2} - m = -\frac{1}{2}$) of the quadrupole coupled ^{23}Na, we expect to observe only 40 percent of the intensity. The remaining 60 percent of intensity, which resides in the two outer lines, is broadened and cannot be detected. In biological samples the sodium complexes are randomly oriented and are in constant motion. Therefore, the broadening of the outer transition probably arises from both the homogeneous and the heterogeneous mechanisms described earlier. While this interpretation based on quadrupole coupling has gained wide acceptance, the precise nature of the quadrupole interaction is not clear (see, for instance, reference 8). It could arise either from a rapid exchange between a small fraction of bound ions with the bulk free sodium ions or from a homogeneous population of sodium ions with some sort of

Table 91–1. PERCENTAGE OF NMR VISIBLE ^{23}Na IN BIOLOGICAL SAMPLES

Tissue	NMR Visible ^{23}Na (%)	References
Frog muscle	28–37	23
	63	30
	37–45	31
Rat muscle	28–35	23
	38	32
Homogenized frog muscle	26–35	23
Rabbit muscle actomyosin	52	23
Frog skin	36–43	33
	56	34
Rat testicle	76	34
Rabbit kidney	30–42	23
Rat kidney	33	33
Rabbit brain	30–40	23
Rat brain	33	32
Rabbit myelinated nerve	44	35
Frog liver	34	30
Rat liver	39	36
Pseudomonas aeruginosa	40	37
Rat cardiac myocytes	100	38
Rabbit kidney tubules	59–73	39
Human erythrocytes	100	40
	100	41
Perfused rat heart	100	42

ordering of macromolecules within the cell. If the rapid exchange between two heterogeneous fractions of sodium ions is responsible for the observed quadrupole coupling, calculations indicate that the bound fraction should be fairly small, on the order of 1 percent.

Burnstein and Fossel[45] have recently made careful measurements of the relaxation times of the intracellular sodium using shift reagents (see below) in perfused hearts. In order to minimize the signal contamination from the large pool of extracellular sodium ions to the observed intracellular sodium signal, they have either presaturated the extracellular sodium signal or applied mathematical filtering. They have observed two $T2$ components and a single $T1$ component. The values of the two $T2$ components were 2 ms and 17 ms, with relative amplitudes of 0.47 and 0.53, respectively. However, based on the two mechanisms proposed for the quadrupole interaction, the short $T2$ component is expected to have 60 percent contribution while 40 percent of the total sodium ions should contribute to the longer $T2$ component. Based on these observations Burnstein and Fossel[45] postulate that probably a majority (over 80 percent) of intracellular sodium is in a homogeneous pool with $T2$ values of 2 ms and 15 ms and an average $T1$ value of 23 ms while a second pool of sodium ions has a fairly short correlation time, with $T1$ equal to approximately $T2$, which is between 20 ms and 25 ms.

PARAMAGNETIC SHIFT REAGENTS

In tissues, sodium exists in multicompartments. The NMR frequency of ^{23}Na is the same in all these compartments. It is not, therefore, possible to distinguish sodium ions in these various compartments based on their resonant frequencies. The problem is further aggravated by the fact that often one is more interested in the behavior of the intracellular ions whose concentration is small compared with the concentration of the relatively uninteresting extracellular ions. This hurdle has been overcome by using paramagnetic shift reagents (SR).[18–21] The SRs selectively induce a hyperfine frequency shift in the resonant frequency of the nuclei in the extracellular compartment. In the presence of the SR the NMR ^{23}Na consists of two separate peaks arising from the extracellular and intracellular ions. The ^{23}Na spectrum of a packed suspension of human erythrocytes at different concentrations of the SR [DY(PPP)$_2$]$^{7-}$ shown in Figure 91–3 clearly depicts this behavior.

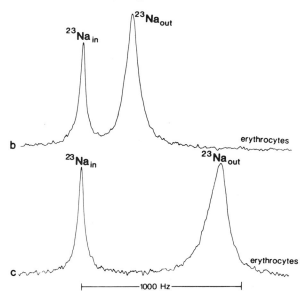

Figure 91–3. The ^{23}Na isotropic hyperfine shift induced by various paramagnetic complexes as a function of the stoichiometric molar ratio of shift reagent to Na$^+$. The concentration of NaCl was kept constant at 150 mM. The vertical scale is in ppm.[48] (From Springer CS et al: J Magn Reson 56:33, 1984.)

Studies indicate that SRs made of lanthanide ions chelated with anionic complexes possess desirable properties.[20,21,47,49] The anionic nature of the chelate minimizes the binding to the macromolecules and membrane surfaces, which have a net negative charge, and therefore reduces toxicity to the cells. Secondly, the rapid dynamic ion-pair equilibrium between the sodium ion and the shift reagent enables the magnitude of induced frequency shift to be controlled by varying the concentration of the paramagnetic complex. Because of the highly anionic nature of the SR, it does not enter the cell; therefore, the frequency of intracellular ^{23}Na remains unshifted. However, the extracellular ^{23}Na resonant frequency experiences a shift. The commonly used lanthanide ions are Dy^{3+}, Tm^{3+}, and Gd^{3+}. Some of the more popular chelates that have been used are PPP^{5-} (tripolyphosphate)[21] and $TTHA^{6-}$ (tetraethylene triaminehexacetic acid).[48]

The total observed hyperfine frequency shift induced by the SR is the sum of three terms, viz., (1) Fermi contact shift, (2) diamagnetic shift, and (3) pseudocontact or dipolar shift.[50] The Fermi contact shift is negligibly small because the sodium ion does not directly bind to the lanthanide ion. The other two contributions depend on both the electronic ground state of the lanthanide ion and the structure of the chelate. For ions like Gd^{3+} that have a spherically symmetric electron distribution in the ground state,[51] the pseudocontact term is very small. However, the chelate may modify the spherically symmetric ground state, and consequently it is possible to observe the pseudocontact induced shift. Chelates like EDTA (ethylenediaminetetraacetate) and DTPA (diethylenetriaminepentaacetate) do not significantly modify the ground state[52,53] of Gd^{3+}; therefore, in this case the observed hyperfine frequency shift originates mainly from the diamagnetic term due to complex formation. These complexes induce frequency shifts in ^{23}Na resonances that are fairly small, of the order of 2 ppm.[54] On the other hand Dy^{3+} has 6H5/2 ground state, and in this case the pseudocontact term is the most important source for the frequency shift. The structure of the chelate also plays an important role. Chu et al.[48] have measured the induced frequency shifts by Dy^{3+} and Tm^{3+} chelated to various complexes and observed that the complexes $[Dy(PPP)_2]^{7-}$ and $[Dy(TTHA)]^3$ induce the largest shifts. For this reason these two anion complexes seem to be very popular. Their results are shown in Figure 91 4. These authors have also observed that the larger the charge on the complex anion, the larger is the induced shift.

The shift reagents have been used mainly to determine the intracellular sodium ion concentrations and transmembrane transport in cell suspensions. These include yeast cells,[55,56] amphibian oocytes,[57] bacterial cells,[58] erythrocytes,[21,40,59-62] and rat myocytes.[38] For example, Gupta and Gupta[21] have studied packed human red cells using the shift reagent $[Dy(PPP)_2]^{7-}$. They estimated the intracellular sodium ion concentration to be 6 mM, which agrees well with the values reported using other techniques. These studies also indicate that all the sodium ions are NMR visible. Wittenberg and Gupta[39] have also used the same shift reagent to study cardiac myocytes at rest and to explore the magnitude and the reversibility of changes in the intracellular sodium concentration with and without the extracellular Ca^{2+}. They observed a significant change in the intracellular sodium concentration by removing the Ca^{2+} and its restoration to its normal value by adding Ca^{2+} to the medium. Thus these studies demonstrate that NMR could be used, without destroying the cells, to study sodium loading upon removal of the Ca^{2+} and its extrusion after restoring Ca^{2+}. Ogino et al.[40] have used the SR to measure the gramicidin induced ion transport in human erythrocytes.

The SR should not perturb the energy metabolism. Ogino et al.[40] have monitored the energy metabolism of human erythrocytes by measuring the ^{31}P NMR spectrum after introducing the SR $[Dy(P_3O_{10})_2]^{7-}$ into the medium. They have observed that the ^{31}P spectral features did not change before and after the addition of the shift reagents.

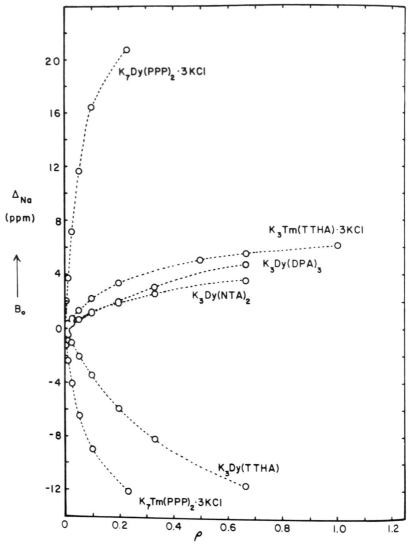

Figure 91–4. ^{23}Na NMR spectrum of ^{23}Na of a gently packed suspension of human erythrocytes in a medium containing 140 mM Na$^+$, 10 mM K$^+$, and the SR Dy(PPP)$_2$$^{7-}$. Spectrum (*a*) was recorded with an SR concentration of 2 mM, whereas spectrum (*b*) was recorded with 5 mM concentration. Na$_{in}$ and Na$_{out}$ represent the intracellular and extracellular sodium.[21] (From Edzes HT et al: Biochem Biophys Res Commun *46*:790, 1972.)

These studies seem to indicate that at least this shift reagent does not interfere with the energy metabolism. The limited number of studies on the toxicity of SRs seem to indicate that [Dy(PPP)$_2$]$^{7-}$ decomposes in the physiological medium, releasing toxic products.[11,63] Further, the divalent cations Ca^{2+} and Mg^{2+} were also found to compete with sodium for the shift reagents and also compete with the lanthanide ions for the chelate. Therefore, this SR may not be suitable for studying cells that are very sensitive to Ca^{2+} in the extracellular phase for prolonged periods of time.[49] The shift reagent [Dy(TTHA)]$^{3-}$ does not seem to suffer from these drawbacks to the same extent. It seems prudent to add Ca^{2+} to the physiological medium whenever SRs are used. Brown et al.[64] have recently suggested using the SR Gd-DPTA, which has been proved to be safe for in vivo applications. They have shown that a 20 mM of this complex induces a shift of 2.9 ppm. This is a small shift compared to the -21.6 ppm observed using

$[Dy(TPP)_2]^{7-}$. But the added advantage, besides being physiologically safe, is that it alters the relaxation times significantly and therefore may find application in sodium imaging.

Shift reagents have also been used to study intact tissues.[21,42,45,63-68] The situation involving tissues is clearly more complex than that encountered with cell suspension studies. The presence of more than one type of cell in tissues implies the presence of more than two compartments in which sodium ions can exist. In the absence of definite knowledge as to which compartment the SR enters, the interpretation of the ^{23}Na NMR results could be misleading. This is particularly true if the SR is introduced into the tissue by bathing the tissue in the solution containing the SR, as is done frequently.[21,63-66] In this case the SR enters the tissue through diffusion, which is a slow process. For instance, Gupta and Gupta[21] have observed with frog muscle that the unshifted resonance decreased in intensity over a period of time. This presumably represents the time required for the SR to diffuse through. Even after this time it is possible that the SR has not entered all the extracellular space. If all the unshifted resonance is attributed to the intracellular sodium, the value of the intracellular concentrations determined may be artificially higher than the actual value. For instance, it was pointed out by Springer[11] that for this reason the value of 44 mM for the intracellular sodium observed by Gullams et al.[66] for the rabbit renal cortical tubule cells may be high. This problem may be less severe if the tissue is perfused with the physiological medium containing the SR. Studies on perfused heart[67] indicate that more than 98 percent of the extracellular space is pervaded by the SR in a relatively short time.

The next logical extension of the application of SRs is in vivo animal and human studies. To the best of our knowledge only two abstracts have appeared on studies dealing with animals; none have appeared on studies dealing with humans. The animal studies were reported by Blum et al.[69] and Balschi et al.[70] Both of these studies deal with ischemic skeletal muscles in rats. Both these groups have correlated the accumulation of intracellular sodium with the deletion of high energy phosphate metabolites. The rate of sodium accumulation in the cell was shown to increase with the depletion of ATP.

Except for imaging,[15-17] no MR studies of ^{23}Na have been reported in humans. However, judging from the progress made in the last few years, it seems certain that in humans ^{23}Na NMR techniques will be applied to study various physiological processes in the very near future.

References

1. Cameron IL, Smith NKR, Pool TB, Sparks RL: Intracellular concentration of sodium and other elements as related to mitogens and oncogenesis *in vivo*. Cancer Res. *40*:1493–1500, 1980.
2. Boynton AL, McKeehan WL, Whitfield JF: Symposium on Ions, Cell Proliferation and Cancer. New York, Academic Press, 1982.
3. Moore RD, Munford JW, Pillsworth Jr TJ: Effects of streptozotocin diabetes and fasting on intracellular sodium and adenosine triphosphate in rat soleus muscle. J Physiol (Lond) *338*:277–294, 1983.
4. Blaustein MP: Sodium ions, calcium ions, blood pressure regulation, and hypertension: A reassessment and a hypothesis. Am J Physiol *232*:C165–C175, 1977.
5. Bosher SK, Warren RL: Measurement of element concentrations in small volumes of biological fluids. Tech Life Sci: Physiol *P1/2*:121–134, 1982.
6. Lechene CL: Electron probe microanalysis of biological soft tissues: Principle and technique. Fed Proc *39*:2876–2880, 1980.
7. Armstrong WM, Garcia-Diaz JF: Ion-selective microelectrodes: Theory and technique. Fed Proc *39*:2851–2859, 1980.
8. Civan MM, Shporer M: NMR of sodium-23 and potassium-39 in the biological systems. *In* Berlinear LJ, Reuben J (eds): Biological Magnetic Resonance. Vol I. New York, Plenum Press, 1978, pp 1–32.
9. Gupta RK, Gupta P, Moore RD: NMR studies of intracellular metal ions intact cells and tissues. Ann Rev Biophys Bioeng *13*:221, 1984.

10. Belton PS, Ratcliffe RG: NMR and compartmentation in biological tissues. Prog Nucl Magn Reson Spectrosc *17*:241–279, 1985.
11. Springer Jr C: Measurement of metal cation compartmentalization in tissue by high-resolution metal cation NMR. Ann Rev Biophys Chem *16*:375–399, 1987.
12. Zumdahl SS: Chemistry. Lexington, Massachusetts, Heath, 1986, p 943.
13. Berendsen HJ, Edzes HT: The observation and general interpretation of sodium magnetic resonance in biological material. Ann NY Acad Sci *204*:459–485, 1973.
14. Moon RB, Richards JH: Determination of intracellular pH by ^{31}P magnetic resonance. J Biol Chem *248*:7276–7278, 1973.
15. Hilal SK, Maudsley AA, Ra JB, et al.: In vivo NMR imaging of sodium-23 in the human head. J Comput Assist Tomogr *9*:1–7, 1985.
16. Ra JB, Hilal SK, Cho ZH: A method for *in vivo* MR imaging of the short T_2 component of sodium-23. Mag Reson Med *3*:296–302, 1986.
17. Turski PA, Houston LW, Perman WH, et al: Experimental and human brain neoplasms: Detection with *in vivo* sodium MR imaging. Radiology *163*:245–249, 1987.
18. Degani H, Baron Z: Nuclear magnetic resonance kinetic studies of diffusion and mediated transport across membranes. Period Biol *83*:61–68, 1981.
19. Bryden CC, Reilley CN, Desreaux JF: Multinuclear magnetic resonance study of three aqueous lanthanide shift reagents: Complexes with EDTA and axially symmetric macrocyctic polyamino polyacetate ligands. Anal Chem *53*:1418, 1981.
20. Pike MM, Springer CS: Aqueous shift reagents for high-resolution cationic nuclear magnetic resonance. J Magn Reson *46*:348–353, 1982.
21. Gupta RK, Gupta P: Direct observation of resolved resonances from intra- and extracellular sodium-23 ions in NMR studies of intact cells and tissues using dysprosium (III) tripolyphosphate as paramagnetic shift reagent. J Magn Reson *47*:344–350, 1982.
22. Cope FW: Nuclear magnetic resonance evidence for complexing of sodium ions in muscle. Proc Nat Acad Sci USA *54*:225–227, 1965.
23. Cope FW: NMR evidence for complexing of Na$^+$ in muscle, kidney, and brain and by actomyosis: The relation of cellular complexing of Na$^+$ to water structure and to transport kinetics. J Gen Physiol *50*:1353–1375, 1967.
24. Cope FW: A non-equilibrium thermodynamic theory of leakage of complexed Na$^+$ from muscle, with NMR evidence that the non-complexed fraction of muscle Na$^+$ is intravacuolar rather than extra-cellular. Bull Math Biophys *29*:691–704, 1967.
25. Das TP, Hahn EL: Nuclear quadrupole resonance spectroscopy. Solid State Physics Supplement I. New York, Academic Press, 1958.
26. Abragam A: The Principles of Nuclear Magnetism. London, Oxford University Press, 1961.
27. Edzes HT, Rupprecht A, Berendsen HJC: Observation of quadrupolar NMR signals of ^{7}Li and ^{23}Na in hydrated oriented DNA. Biochem Biophys Res Commun *46*:790–794, 1972.
28. Hubbard PS: Nonexponential nuclear magnetic relaxation by quadrupole interactions. J Chem Phys *53*:985–989, 1970.
29. Bull TE: Nuclear magnetic relaxation of spin-3/2 nuclei involved in chemical exchange. J Magn Reson *8*:344–353, 1972.
30. Martinez D, Silvidi AA, Stokes RM: Nuclear magnetic resonance studies of sodium ions in isolated frog muscle and liver. Biophys J *9*:1256–1260, 1969.
31. Czeisler JL, Fritz Jr OG, Swift TJ: Direct evidence from nuclear magnetic resonance studies for bound sodium in frog skeletal muscle. Biophys J *10*:260–268, 1970.
32. Cope FW: Spin-echo nuclear magnetic resonance evidence for complexing of sodium ions in muscle, brain and kidney. Biophys J *10*:843–858, 1970.
33. Rotunno CA, Kowalewski V, Cereijido M: Nuclear spin resonance evidence for complexing of sodium in frog skin. Biochem Biophys Acta *135*:170–172, 1967.
34. Reisin IL, Rotunno CA, Corchs L, Kowalewski V, Cereijido M: The state of sodium in epithelial tissue as studied by nuclear magnetic resonance. Physiol Chem Phys *2*:171–179, 1970.
35. Cope FW: Complexing of sodium ions in myelineated nerve by nuclear magnetic resonance. Physiol Chem Phys *2*:545–550, 1970.
36. Monoi H: Nuclear magnetic resonance of tissue ^{23}Na I. ^{23}Na signal and Na$^+$ activity in homogenate. Biophys J *14*:645–651, 1974.
37. Magnuson NS, Magnuson JA: ^{23}Na$^+$ interaction with bacterial surfaces: A comment on nuclear magnetic resonance invisible signals. Biophys J *13*:1117–1119, 1973.
38. Wittenberg BA, Gupta RK: NMR studies of intracellular sodium ions in mammalian cardiac myocytes. J Biol Chem *260*:2031–2034, 1985.
39. Boulanger Y, Vinay P, Pejedor A, Noel J: ^{23}Na NMR investigations of isolated kidney tubules (abstract). Fifth Annual Meeting of the Society for Magnetic Resonance in Medicine *3*:645–646, 1986.
40. Ogino T, Shulman GI, Avison MJ, Gullan SR, den Hollander JA, Shulman RG: ^{23}Na and ^{39}K NMR studies of ion transport in human erythrocytes. Proc Natl Acad Sci USA *82*:1099–1103, 1985.
41. Yeh HJC, Brinley FJ, Becker ED: Nuclear magnetic resonance studies on intracellular sodium in human erythrocytes and frog muscle. Biophys J *13*:56–71, 1973.
42. Fossel ET, Hoefeler H: Observation of intracellular potassium and sodium in the heart by NMR: A major fraction of potassium is "invisible." Magn Reson Med *3*:534–540, 1986.

43. Shporer M, Civan MM: Effects of temperature and field strength on the NMR relaxation times of ^{23}Na in frog striated muscle. Biochim Biophys ACTA *354*:291–304, 1974.

44. Chang DC, Woessner DE: Spin echo study of sodium-23 relaxation in skeletal muscle. Evidence of sodium ion binding inside a biological cell. J Magn Reson *30*:185–191, 1978.

45. Burnstein D, Fossel ET: Intracellular sodium and lithium NMR relaxation times in the perfused frog heart. Magn Reson Med *4*:261–273, 1987.

46. Shporer M, Civan MM: Nuclear magnetic resonance of sodium-23 linoleate-water: Basis for an alternative interpretation of sodium-23 within cells. Biophys J *12*:114–122, 1972.

47. Degani H, Elgavish GA: Ionic permeabilities of membranes. FEBS Lett *90*:357–360, 1978.

48. Chu SC, Pike MM, Fossel ET, Smith TW, Balschi JA, Springer Jr CS: Aqueous shift reagents for high resolution cationic nuclear magnetic resonance III Dy(TTHA)$^{3-}$, Tm(TTHA)$^{3-}$, and Tm(PPP)$_2$$^{7-}$. J Magn Reson *56*:33–47, 1984.

49. Pike MM, Yarmush DM, Balschi JA, Lenkinski RE, Springer Jr CS: Aqueous shift reagents for high-resolution cationic nuclear magnetic resonance. 2. ^{25}Mg, ^{39}K, and ^{23}Na resonances shifted by chelidan-mate complexes of dysprosium (III) and thulium (III). Inorg Chem *22*:2388–2392, 1983.

50. Soher P: Nuclear Magnetic Resonance Spectroscopy. Vol 2. Boca Raton, CRC Press, 1983, p 115.

51. Kuhn HG: Atomic Spectra. New York, Academic Press, 1962.

52. Huhuy JE: Inorganic Chemistry: Principles of Structure and Reactivity. New York, Harper and Row, 1972.

53. Elgavish G: The Rare Earths in Modern Science and Technology. Vol 3. New York, Plenum Press, 1982, p 193.

54. Brown MA, Stenzel TT, Ribeiro AA, Drayer BP, Spicer LD: NMR studies of combined lanthanide shift and relaxation agents for differential characterization of ^{23}Na in a two compartment model system. Magn Reson Med *3*:289–295, 1986.

55. Balschi JA, Cirillo V, Springer Jr CS: Direct high-resolution nuclear magnetic resonance studies of cation transport *in vivo*: Na$^+$ transport in yeast cells. Biophys J *38*:323–326, 1982.

56. Ogino T, den Hollander JA, Shulman RG: ^{39}K, ^{23}Na, and ^{31}P NMR studies of ion transport in *Saccharomyces cerevisiae*. Proc Natl Acad Sci USA *80*:5185–5189, 1983.

57. Morrill GA, Kostellow AB, Weinstein SP, Gupta RK: NMR and electrophysiological studies of insulin action on cation regulation and endocytosis in the amphibian oocyte: Possible role of membrane recycling in the meiotic divisions. Physiol Chem Phys Med NMR *15*:357–362, 1983.

58. Castle AM, Macnab RM, Shulman RG: Measurement of intracellular sodium concentration and sodium transport in *Escherichia coli* by ^{23}Na nuclear magnetic resonance. J Biol Chem *261*:3288–3294, 1986.

59. Pettegrew JW, Woessner DE, Minshew NJ, Glonek T: Sodium-23 NMR analysis of human whole blood, erythrocytes, and plasma: Chemical shift, spin relaxation and intracellular sodium concentration studies. J Magn Reson *57*:185–196, 1984.

60. Pike MM, Fossel ET, Smith TW, Springer Jr CS: High resolution ^{23}Na NMR studies of human erythrocytes: Use of aqueous shift reagents. Am J Physiol *246*:C528–C536, 1984.

61. Shinar H, Navon G: NMR relaxation studies of intracellular Na$^+$ in red blood cells. Biophys Chem *20*:275–283, 1984.

62. Boulanger Y, Vinay P, Desroches M: Measurement of a wide range of intracellular sodium concentrations in erythrocytes by ^{23}Na nuclear magnetic resonance. Biophys J *47*:553–556, 1985.

63. Matwiyoff NA, Gasparovic C, Wenk R, Wicks JD, Rath A: ^{31}P and ^{23}Na NMR studies of the structure and lability of the sodium shift reagent, B3(tripolyphosphate dysprosium (III) ([Dy(P$_3$O$_{10}$)]$^{7-}$) ion, and its decomposition in the presence of rat muscle. Magn Reson Med *3*:164–168, 1986.

64. Brown MA, Skenzel TT, Ribeiro AA, Drayer BP, Spicer LD: NMR studies of combined lanthanich shift and relaxation agents for differential characterization of ^{23}Na in a two-compartment model system. Magn Reson Med *3*:289–295, 1986.

65. Civan MM, Degani H, Margalit Y, Shporer M: Observations of ^{23}Na in frog skin by NMR. Am J Physiol *245*:C213–C219, 1983.

66. Gullans SR, Avison MJ, Ogino T, Giebisch G, Shulman RG: NMR measurements of intracellular sodium in the rabbit proximal tubule. Am J Physiol *249*:F160–F168, 1985.

67. Pike MM, Frazer JC, Dedrick D, et al.: ^{23}Na and ^{39}K nuclear magnetic resonance studies of perfused rat hearts. Biophys J *48*:159–173, 1985.

68. Springer Jr CS, Pike MM, Balschi JA, Chu SC, Frazier JC, Ingwall JS, Smith TW: Use of shift reagents for nuclear magnetic resonance studies of the kinetics of ion transfer in cells and perfused hearts. Circulation *72*:IV89–93, 1985.

69. Blum H, Schnall MD, Buzby GP, Chance B: Sodium flux and high energy phosphate content in ischemic skeletal muscle (abstract). Fifth Annual Meeting of the Society for Magnetic Resonance in Medicine *2*:339, 1986.

70. Balschi JA, Bittl JA, Ingwall JS: Ischemia in the intact rat leg by interleaved P-31 and Na-23 NMR wing: a shift reagent to discriminate intra and extracellular sodium (abstracts). Fifth Annual Meeting of the Society for Magnetic Resonance in Medicine *2*:343–344, 1986.

92

Chemical Shift Imaging

RICHARD B. BUXTON
THOMAS J. BRADY
GARY L. WISMER
BRUCE R. ROSEN

Soon after the demonstration of the phenomenon of nuclear magnetic resonance (NMR) in 1946,[9,48] it was shown that the resonant frequency of a nucleus depends in a small but measurable way on the surrounding chemical environment.[20,47] These small shifts in frequency—the chemical shift—are the basis of NMR spectroscopy. During the past three decades, the importance of the chemical shift effect was realized by many investigators studying biologically relevant nuclei, including ^{1}H, ^{13}C, and ^{31}P. Although early observations using NMR spectroscopy were limited to in-vitro measurements,[22] in recent years techniques have been developed for the acquisition of in-vivo metabolic data.[25,61] The central problem faced in such studies is how to localize the signal, so that only the tissue of interest contributes to the measured spectrum. Several schemes have been used, including (1) surface coil technology,[2,3,6,11,46] where a small receiving coil is used to acquire the resonance signal from tissue adjacent to the coil; (2) topical magnetic resonance (TMR), which uses specially designed magnets with time invariant high order gradient fields to define a small homogeneous B_0 region and acquire chemical shift data from volumes lying deep within subjects;[26] and, (3) sensitive point and line techniques,[7,10,59] which use linear magnetic field gradients to define a volume of interest. All three techniques are capable of providing spectral data; however, the sensitive volume for in-vivo spectroscopy with these methods is imperfectly determined and localized.

Concurrent with developments in in-vivo NMR spectroscopy, the last decade has witnessed the production of MR images. The first images were acquired by Lauterbur in 1973 using a modified spectrometer.[31] Soon afterward, data from this same laboratory demonstrated the feasibility of chemical shift imaging,[32] and the potential of combining the analytical power of NMR spectroscopy with the high resolution localization of signal that is possible with MR imaging was appreciated early.[19] However, the subsequent commercial development of MR imaging systems failed to take advantage (until recently) of this capability. In conventional imaging the field gradients that are applied to encode the spatial distribution of the signal dominate the chemical shifts, so that the only appearance of the chemical shift is as an artifact, the apparent displacement of fat and water images.

A number of investigators have outlined techniques for retaining chemical shift information. In this chapter we will try to provide some general bearings for understanding the different approaches to chemical shift imaging and some of the advantages and disadvantages of each. The field of chemical shift imaging is expanding rapidly, and it is not possible to discuss the many techniques in detail in the space of a few pages. For that reason we will concentrate on techniques that can be adapted with relative ease to conventional imaging systems and have been used for in-vivo imaging. Other methods, such as those requiring time-varying gradients,[37] while promising for the future, will not be discussed here.

THE CHEMICAL SHIFT

The phenomenon of magnetic resonance arises simply from the effects of a magnetic field acting on a magnetic moment. A nucleus that possesses angular momentum will also possess a magnetic moment, and when placed in a magnetic field $\bar{B}$ will precess with a frequency proportional to B:

$$\omega = \gamma B \tag{1}$$

where γ is a constant that depends on the nuclear species. However, when a sample of some material is put in a uniform external field B_0, the field felt by a particular nucleus in a particular molecule is not just B_0, but B_0 plus the local field produced by the rest of the sample:

$$B = B_0 + B_{local} \tag{2}$$

B_{local} has several sources, and the interaction of the nucleus with these sources leads to different effects. Unpaired electrons have a magnetic moment due to their spin and produce paramagnetic phenomena. Other nearby nuclei may also have magnetic moments, giving rise to the phenomenon of J-coupling. And finally, the motions of the electrons in the molecule produce magnetic fields, and these give rise to the chemical shifts of interest here.

In the absence of an external field, electron motions do not produce a net local magnetic field, but when a molecule is placed in a field B_0 the electron motions are perturbed, creating currents, which in turn create magnetic fields.[62] The field felt at a particular nucleus will depend on the detailed geometrical relationship between the currents and the nucleus. Currents far from the nucleus will have a small effect, while nearby currents can have a much larger effect. The perturbation in the electron motions is proportional to B_0, so the resulting local field is also proportional to B_0. The observed resonant frequency is then:

$$\omega = \gamma B_0 (1 + \sigma) \tag{3}$$

where σ is the chemical shift, usually expressed in parts per million (ppm). The value of σ is characteristic of the chemical environment of the nucleus and is independent of the applied field.

In biological tissues the ^1H NMR spectrum is composed of many lines but can be approximated accurately as two lines, arising primarily from fat $(-CH_2-)$ and water, with a separation of 3.7 ppm.[50,53,67] Since ^1H is by far the most abundant in-vivo NMR sensitive nucleus, most of the in-vivo applications of chemical shift imaging have focused on resolving the simple fat/water proton spectrum of tissue. In the following discussion we will emphasize proton chemical shift imaging, but many of the techniques are applicable to the spectra of other nuclei. In particular, ^{31}P has a rich spectrum that has been used frequently in studies of metabolism because of the important role played by phosphorus in cellular energy use.

CHEMICAL SHIFT IMAGING

In conventional MR imaging the spatial distribution of nuclear magnetization can be encoded in the measured signal in many ways, but the following are the most common:[38,49]

(1) Selective pulses. A radiofrequency (rf) pulse with a limited bandwidth applied in the presence of a z gradient excites only a limited slice perpendicular to z.

(2) Frequency encoding. The signal is measured in the presence of an x gradient, so that frequency reflects position in x.

(3) Phase encoding. Between excitation and data collection, a y gradient is turned on for a limited time. In subsequent pulses the gradient magnitude is incremented (or, equivalently, the duration is incremented) so that the signal magnitude on each pulse gives a different component of the Fourier transform in y.

With this type of imaging the chemical shift information is lost. Indeed, the chemical shift appears only as a hindrance, the "chemical shift artifact," which is an apparent displacement of the fat and water images due to the fact that frequency differences in the signal are interpreted as due to differences in x position.[63]

A useful way to understand the problem of retaining the chemical shift information in imaging is to think of the chemical shift dimension as a fourth spatial dimension, ω, that must be encoded in the measured signal. The distribution of spins in this dimension is then the distribution of spins among the different lines of the spectrum. But this fourth "spatial" dimension differs in an important way from the true spatial dimensions, x, y, and z: there is effectively a permanent, intrinsic gradient in this direction that cannot be altered. The problem of devising a method for chemical shift imaging is then the problem of doing normal spatial imaging in a situation in which there is an intrinsic gradient in one dimension.

The methods that have been developed for encoding the chemical shift dimension can be grouped into the same three categories described above for encoding spatial information in conventional imaging. The simplest method (in principle if not in practice) is to use selective pulses with no applied gradients to excite or saturate only one line in the spectrum.[12,24,27,30,55] This is equivalent to selecting a slice in the chemical shift dimension. The second approach is to "frequency encode" the chemical shift dimension.[13,28,40,50,57] That is, the data are collected with no applied gradients, so that differences in frequency directly reflect the distribution in the chemical shift dimension: the intrinsic gradient in the chemical shift dimension is used as a read gradient. And finally the chemical shift dimension can be phase encoded by allowing the spins to evolve for a time τ that changes incrementally with each pulse.[21,36,39,60] In other words, the intrinsic gradient in the chemical shift dimension is used as a constant phase encoding gradient, and the duration is changed on subsequent pulses to phase encode the chemical shift dimension.

Chemical shift imaging is not restricted to Fourier transform methods but can also be done by reconstruction from projections.[8,33] One may still view the chemical shift dimension as a new spatial dimension with a fixed gradient. The difference from normal projection imaging is that in addition to rotating the direction of the read gradient in the x-y plane, the magnitude of the gradient must also be varied. The reason for this is that in the three-dimensional space defined by the spatial x and y axes plus the chemical shift dimension (ω), the total gradient is the vector sum of the applied gradients in x and y plus the intrinsic gradient in the chemical shift dimension. If the magnitude of the applied gradient is zero, then the projection is simply along the chemical shift axis. When the applied gradient is increased, the resulting gradient will be in a direction between the chemical shift axis and the direction of the applied gradient. And if the applied gradient is much stronger than the intrinsic gradient, the total gradient will be close to the axis of the applied gradient. Note, however, that an applied x gradient would have to be infinite to get a projection truly along x, so that in practice some projections will be missing. Some correction for limited angle tomography is therefore necessary.[8,33]

SELECTIVE PULSE METHODS

The use of selective pulses in chemical shift imaging is an outgrowth of techniques developed by NMR spectroscopists.[18,65] If the effects of rf pulses can be limited to only one or a few lines of a simple spectrum, then conventional imaging techniques can be used to give an image of the excited line. Several groups of investigators[12,24] have used a selective saturation method to eliminate either the fat or the water signal from the in-vivo proton spectrum. In these methods the imaging sequence is preceded by a narrow bandwidth 90 degree pulse with no applied gradients, with the frequency band set so that only one of the spectral lines is affected. For example, if the saturating pulse is set to tip the water line, the magnetization of these spins is turned into the x-y plane, where it soon loses coherence and the signal dies away. It is then possible to image the fat line with a standard imaging sequence. A second image can then be made with the fat line saturated to give a water image.

An alternative use of selective pulses has been suggested by Joseph.[30] In this method no saturating pulse is used. Instead the 180 degree pulse selects only one spectral line, so that only one set of spins is refocused to produce a measurable signal. Except for the lengthened duration of the 180 degree pulse, the imaging sequence is a conventional one.

The advantage of these methods is that since the selectivity in the chemical shift dimension is done all at once at the beginning, a standard imaging sequence can then be used to encode the spatial dimensions. Thus the time required for separate fat and water images is just twice the time required to make a conventional image. The major disadvantage of these methods is that they put severe constraints on the B_0 inhomogeneity: over the entire slice being imaged the variation of the field (in ppm) must be much less than the separation of the lines. For fat and water imaging, the inhomogeneity must be less than ·1 ppm; a spectrum of the slice as a whole must show two distinct lines.

Selective saturation has another use that is important for imaging metabolites present in low concentration. As we have seen, in vivo the water resonance dominates in most soft tissues, with only aliphatic ($-CH_2-$) protons from lipids having a sufficiently high concentration to contribute to the measured proton chemical shift spectrum.[50] In addition to these two ^1H species, there are many important chemical moieties with well-defined proton resonances that are present in low concentration (<50 mM), including several amino acids and lactate. To acquire spectra of proton metabolites in millimolar concentrations, it is necessary to suppress the overwhelming water signal (solvent suppression), which causes dynamic range and digitization problems.[51,55]

Although saturation techniques can reduce the water signal by more than 90 percent,[55] it is unlikely that the water signal can be reduced below that of the metabolites of interest, such as lactate. Nevertheless, water suppression pulses may well be a prerequisite for imaging lactate with other chemical shift imaging techniques in order to avoid dynamic range problems. Work on lactate imaging will be discussed more fully in the next section.

THREE-DIMENSIONAL FOURIER TRANSFORM METHODS

The three-dimensional Fourier transform (3DFT) method[13,28,40,50,57] is the most robust chemical shift imaging technique, in the sense that it requires no prior knowledge of the spectrum and is relatively insensitive to inhomogeneities in the field. The first in-vivo proton chemical shift images were made with this technique by Pykett and

Rosen[50] using the pulse sequence shown in Figure 92–1. Slice selection is done with a narrow band pulse in the presence of a z gradient, both x and y are phase encoded, and the signal is collected with no applied gradients (the chemical shift dimension is "frequency encoded" using the "intrinsic gradient" in the chemical shift dimension). When properly Fourier transformed, the resulting data set is a separate image at each frequency, or, equivalently, an image in which each pixel is a full spectrum. This three-dimensional data set—x, y, and ω—is shown schematically in Figure 92–2. If the main field B_0 is perfectly homogeneous, a particular line (say, water) will always appear at the same value on the frequency axis. That is, in the three-dimensional space the water line would be a plane perpendicular to the frequency axis. In an inhomogeneous field the water resonant frequency will vary with position, and the water plane will then be warped, as shown in Figure 92–2. The effect of inhomogeneities is thus simply to shift the spectrum measured at each point. However, this should not interfere with identification of the lines of the spectrum, so the effects of inhomogeneities can easily be corrected. Indeed, as Maudsley et al.[40,42] have pointed out, this technique can equally well be used for field mapping, since the method simply measures the intensity at each frequency at each point in the field.

The major disadvantage of the 3DFT method is that the minimum time necessary to make an image with comparable resolution is much longer than with conventional methods. With a conventional method one spatial dimension (x) is frequency encoded—all the data are collected on each pulse—so the minimum imaging time is proportional to n_y, the number of pixels required in the y direction. With the 3DFT method, however, x must also be phase encoded, so the minimum imaging time is proportional to $n_x n_y$. A typical image size is 128×128, so a three-dimensional image of comparable resolution would require 128 times as much time as a conventional sequence. To limit imaging time it is therefore necessary to sacrifice resolution.

Three-dimensional In-Vivo Imaging Studies

While in-vivo chemical shift images in principle can be acquired from various NMR sensitive nuclei, to date in-vivo data have been limited to ^{1}H, ^{31}P and ^{19}F.[35] Because

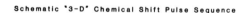

Schematic "3-D" Chemical Shift Pulse Sequence

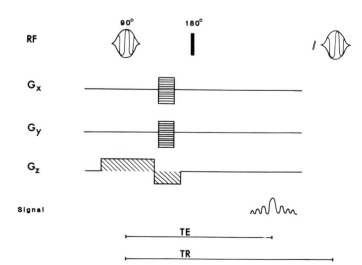

Figure 92–1. Schematic representation of generalized pulse sequence used to perform three-dimensional Fourier transformed chemical shift imaging. Note that both x and y are phase encoded and all gradients are off during data collection. (From Pykett IL, Rosen BR: Radiology *149*:197, 1983. Used by permission.)

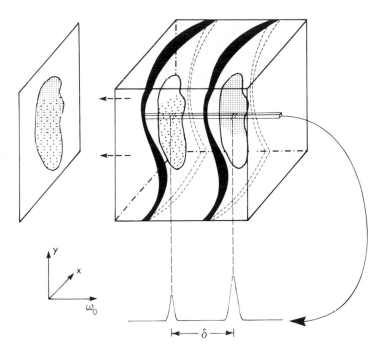

Figure 92–2. Three-dimensional image matrix formed by Fourier transform of the raw data (*top right*). An object with two chemical shift resonance peaks is represented; two spatial axes (x, y) and the frequency axis (ω_0) are displayed. A conventional MRI image is formed by summing all the data along ω_0 (*top left*). Regional spectral data can be extracted from any region and displayed (*bottom right*). Data contained in $-x$ and $-y$ planes are labeled "edge profiles" and provide chemical shift information along a single line in the (x, y) plane. (From Pykett IL, Rosen BR: Radiology *149*:197, 1983. Used by permission.)

of the large natural abundance and high NMR sensitivity of the ^1H nucleus, most work has focused on proton chemical shift imaging.

One of the first in-vivo chemical shift images, a proton chemical shift data set from a normal human forearm,[50] is shown in Figure 92–3. Chemical shift spectra have been extracted and displayed from muscle, subcutaneous fat, and bone marrow. Strong lipid signals are observed from regions of subcutaneous fat and bone marrow; the latter consists of fat in the long bones (nonhematopoietic) in adults. The prominent peak in muscle is from water protons, although lipid signal is present when fascial planes that contain lipid are volume averaged on these low resolution images.

Similar results have been obtained in normal cat heads (Fig. 92–4). From this chemical shift data set, no detectable lipid signal is observed in the brain despite the high concentrations of lipid in the white matter. In vivo spectroscopy of rat brain also failed to demonstrate a significant lipid signal, which supports the imaging data.[5] Unlike subcutaneous fat, brain lipids are incorporated into membrane (e.g., the myelin sheath

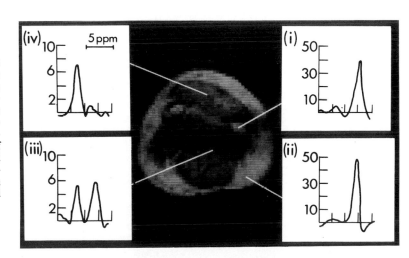

Figure 92–3. Data acquired from a human forearm using a spin echo 300/51 pulse sequence. Spectra are extracted from the central integrated (conventional) MR image and contain predominant mobile lipids from bone marrow (*i*) and subcutaneous fat (*ii*), admixture of water and lipid protons (*iii*), and predominant water signal from muscle (*iv*). (From Pykett IL, Rosen BR: Radiology *149*:197, 1983. Used by permission.)

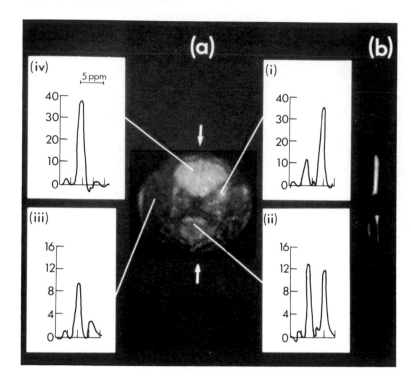

Figure 92–4. Data acquired from a coronal section through the head of a normal, anesthetized cat. The integrated image depicts normal anatomic structures. MR spectra from selected regions (*i–iv*) show clearly resolved peaks corresponding largely to water and to lipid resonances (*a*). An edge profile (*b*) taken through the head (location indicated by arrows in (*a*) clearly shows both lipid and water resonances in the tongue, but only the water line is visible in the brain. (From Pykett IL, Rosen BR: Radiology *149*:197, 1983. Used by permission.)

Spectral Intensity vs. τ

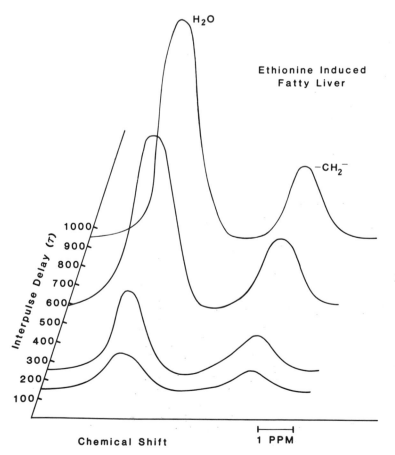

Figure 92–5. Four chemical shift spectra extracted using chemical shift imaging from a small volume (0.125 cc) within the liver of an L-ethionine-treated rat; TR values (τ) of 149, 245, 605, and 965 ms and TE of 30 ms were used. Lipid peak is to the right of the water peak. Integrated lipid and water peak intensities at each value of TR formed the basis of *T1* relaxation measurements. (From Rosen BR et al.: Radiology *154*:469, 1985. Used by permission.)

in white matter) rather than intracellular deposits. The difference in NMR signal between membrane and stored lipids is postulated to lie in the mobility of the protons. In membrane lipids, the highly ordered lattice leads to very short $T2$ relaxation time, resulting in broad spectral linewidth, while intracellular lipids are mobile with longer $T2$, resulting in narrow spectral linewidth. An important implication of this result is that discrimination between gray and white matter on conventional MR images of brain[17] is due to environmental modifications of water proton relaxation time rather than to direct observation of myelin lipid protons.

The 3DFT method has also been applied to an animal model of fatty liver infiltration.[53] Conventional MR imaging techniques may be insensitive to small amounts of fat deposition, since bulk relaxation times will only be changed slightly, as evidenced by a report in which conventional MR imaging failed to detect fatty liver changes when they were present without tissue necrosis.[64] Using similar models of chemically induced fatty liver infiltrate in rats treated with L-ethionine, Rosen et al.[53] demonstrated the appearance of a lipid (—CH$_2$—) peak from regions of fatty liver with three-dimensional chemical shift imaging. The spectra from a rat with chemically induced fatty liver change (Fig. 92–5) shows two spectral lines separated by 3.7 ppm in the region of the liver. This additional aliphatic line corresponds to an elevated triglyceride content in this animal. An excellent correlation ($r = 0.97$) was found to exist between the lipid image intensity and in-vitro measurements of triglyceride content in the liver of these animals (Fig. 92–6). These results suggest that three-dimensional chemical shift imaging may be clinically useful in the noninvasive detection and quantitation of fatty involvement in the liver and other tissues known to undergo fatty degeneration. In addition to the increased sensitivity and ability to quantitate fatty infiltration, proton chemical shift imaging may improve diagnostic specificity.

Using the same animal model, Rosen et al. acquired images at four TR values to

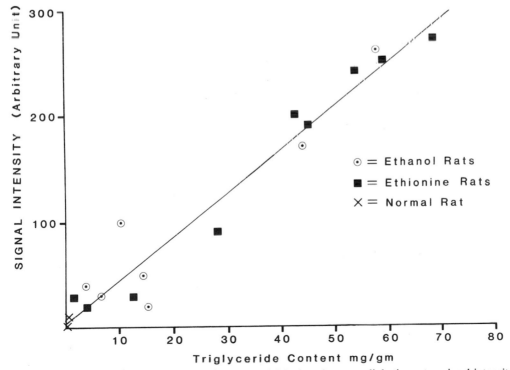

Figure 92–6. Liver triglyceride content (mg/gm wet weight) plotted versus aliphatic proton signal intensity from chemical shift imaging measurements within the liver. An overall correlation of $r = 0.97$ was determined. Lower right: 1 SD error bars. (From Rosen BR et al.: Radiology *154*:469, 1985. Used by permission.)

demonstrate the difference in relaxation times of the fat and water components. Chemical shift spectra were extracted from a small (2 × 2 voxel) area within the liver of these animals for each *TR* tested. From these data, *T1* relaxation times were calculated separately for the water and lipid protons, with corrections included for the effects of using a gaussian shaped selective pulse.[54] An average *T1* difference between aliphatic and water protons of 160 ms was measured, confirming the multiexponential relaxation behavior of tissues with nonexchanging proton populations. As expected, the relaxation times of the aliphatic protons were not strongly dependent on their proton concentrations (as reflected by triglyceride content) and were in fact quite similar in other drug models that produce fatty change without tissue necrosis. This is because fat appears as compartmentalized lipid droplets within fatty livers which are stable as triglyceride concentration increases.[58]

In-vivo chemical shift imaging of the phosphorus nucleus (^{31}P) with the 3DFT method has also been recently accomplished.[41] A number of factors make in-vivo ^{31}P studies technically challenging, and the production of even crude images is therefore impressive. First, the *T2* relaxation times of the α and β ATP phosphorus peaks are quite short (~1–20 ms), placing demands on the rapidity with which data are collected following initial excitation. Second and most important, the natural abundance of ^{31}P is quite small (<10 mM for PCr vs. ~80 M for water protons in tissue), and the intrinsic NMR sensitivity is reduced by greater than 10 times for a constant B_0 field strength in an imaging experiment. The overall signal obtained from naturally occurring ^{31}P is thus reduced by greater than 10,000 times compared to protons.

To combat this low sensitivity, relatively high field strength magnets (>1.5 tesla) are required. In addition, large voxels (coarse spatial resolution) must be used to increase the signal. Finally, the pulse sequence can be modified to include additional 180 degree refocusing pulses, which permit coherent addition of data from a train of spin echoes. Using these strategies, ^{31}P chemical shift images have been acquired from both normal and infarcted cat brains, and in human and cat legs with imaging times of approximately four hours.[41] These studies have imaged the large PCr peaks within normal muscle and brain and demonstrated changes under ischemic conditions, including elevation of Pi and decrease of PCr.

Although still quite primitive, these results represent a significant achievement. For studies of this kind to be clinically useful, imaging times will need to be reduced considerably. High field strength magnets and more efficient methods of data collection, including the use of surface coils, offer the hope that ^{31}P chemical shift imaging can be useful in at least a research setting.

Lactate Imaging

Protons in the CH_3 group of lactate are chemically shifted by about 3.4 ppm from water protons and can potentially be distinguished from water by using chemical shift imaging methods. In the brain, lactate is normally present at a low concentration, ~2 mM, but in ischemia it has been shown to increase 10- to 20-fold.[44,45,52] To image such a low concentration (<40 mM), the overwhelming water signal must be suppressed to avoid dynamic range problems. Although in-vivo imaging of lactate has not yet been reported, the feasibility of such measurements has been demonstrated by Rosen et al.[55] In this study, the water resonance was selectively saturated by applying a narrowband 90 degree selective pulse in the absence of any magnetic field gradient (Fig. 92–7). Following this preparatory pulse, plane selection and refocusing pulses were applied as in Figure 92–1 for 3DFT chemical shift imaging. Spoiler gradients were used to

SELECTIVE SATURATION PULSE SEQUENCE

For "3-D" Chemical Shift Imaging

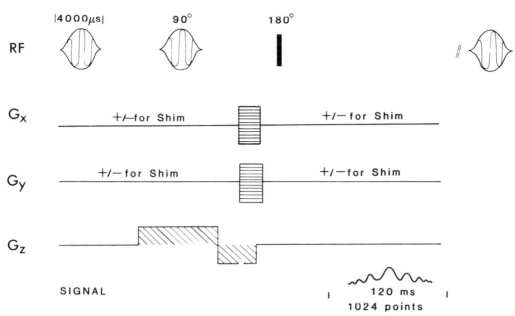

Figure 92–7. Adaptation of three-dimensional FT pulse sequence in Figure 92–1. Both saturating and plane selection pulses have a Gaussian profile. Slight G_x and G_y gradients are used to perform B_0 shimming from first-order variation. (From Rosen BR et al.: J Comput Assist Tomogr 8:813, 1984. Used by permission.)

dephase any residual transverse magnetization from the saturating pulse prior to plane selection.

In imaging experiments on dilute lactate phantoms, the water signal was reduced by more than 90 percent. With water suppression the methyl protons of lactate were visible at 40 mM, while without water suppression the lactate signal was not apparent even at 80 mM concentration (Fig. 92–8). The role of lactate in the etiology of irreversible CNS damage during ischemic insult makes imaging of this metabolite particularly important.[52] Although ^{31}P can provide information on cellular high energy metabolism, the ability to utilize proton NMR offers distinct advantages, including the intrinsically greater sensitivity of the hydrogen versus the phosphorus nucleus (greater than ten times for constant B_0) and more favorable relaxation times; the protons in lactate have a longer *T2* and shorter *T1* than several of the high energy ^{31}P nuclei, allowing for more efficient collection of imaging data. Thus, ^{1}H imaging times can be substantially less with better spatial resolution, ultimately making these examinations practical with field strengths of 1.5 tesla or above.

From this initial experience, imaging of lactate at ~20 mM concentration is feasible within imaging times of 30 minutes. This will require imaging systems with magnetic field homogeneity of <2 ppm or better over the entire imaged region. This level of homogeneity is certainly greater than that of most imagers currently in use. Newly designed systems with spectroscopic capabilities should meet this requirement. The presence of free lipid, with its dominant chemical shift resonance overlapping that of the terminal CH_3 of lactate, will necessitate more complex pulse sequences to image lactate in tissue that contains or is closely associated with fat, such as skeletal and cardiac muscle. In the brain, the lack of significant mobile lipids lessens this concern.[5,50]

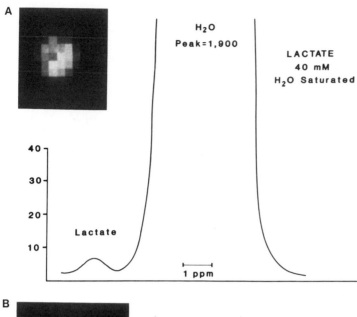

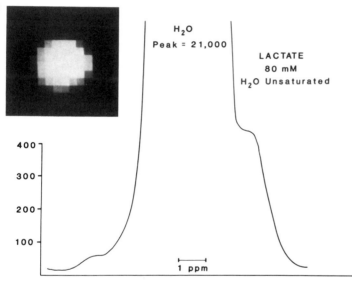

Figure 92–8. Total proton (lactate + water) images and chemical shift spectra extracted from a small region centered within 2-cm diameter aqueous lactate phantoms. *A*, Results from 40 mM lactate with water suppression. Note a clear lactate peak to the left of the central water remnant. *B*, Results obtained from 80 mM lactate, without water suppression. Note the relative water signal is increased 10×, and no clear lactate signal is visible. (From Rosen BR et al.: J Comput Assist Tomogr *8*:813, 1984. Used by permission.)

PHASE ENCODING METHODS

The essence of the phase encoding methods[21,36,39,60] is that the spins are allowed to evolve for a time τ at their natural frequencies so that a phase difference $\Delta\phi = \delta\tau$ develops between spins with a chemical shift δ. By repeating the pulse sequence with different τ values the entire spectrum can be reconstructed, just as the spatial distribution in y can be reconstructed by repeating a pulse sequence with different values of the phase encoding gradient.

Recently a method was described in which a standard spin-echo imaging sequence is modified by simply moving the time of the 180 degree pulse without changing the gradients,[21,60] as illustrated in Figure 92–9. There are two echo-forming processes at work in this pulse sequence. First, if no gradients were applied, a Hahn echo would occur at time *TE* when the dephasing effects of precession at different frequencies, due either to the intrinsic chemical shift or to inhomogeneities of the field, are refocused

SE Pulse Sequences

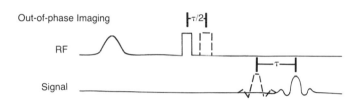

Figure 92–9. Schematic spin echo (SE) pulse sequences for standard in-phase imaging and for out-of-phase imaging with the Dixon method.[21] In the out-of-phase sequence the 180 degree pulse is shifted by a time $\tau/2$, with $\tau = \pi/\delta_0$, and δ_0 is the angular frequency difference of the fat and water lines. (From Buxton R et al.: J Magn Reson Med 3:881–900, 1986.)

by the 180 degree pulse. With the x gradients on, a gradient refocused echo will occur when the phase changes produced by the gradient G' are canceled by the phase changes produced by the gradient G. In a conventional in-phase imaging sequence these two echoes occur at the same time, so that all protons, regardless of their natural frequency, will be in phase with each other. For the fat/water system (with a frequency separation δ_0), the signal detected at a frequency ω is due to water protons at position x and fat protons at position $x + \Delta x$, where $\Delta x = \delta_0/G$ is the apparent displacement of the fat and water images (the chemical shift artifact). Since these fat and water protons are in phase, the image intensity will be proportional to the sum of the fat and water signals.

In the method of Dixon[21] and Sepponen et al.,[60] the time of the 180 degree pulse is shifted by a time $\tau/2$ so that the gradient echo and the Hahn echo are separated by a time τ. Since the applied gradients must be much larger than those due to static inhomogeneities for adequate spatial encoding, the gradient echo dominates so that the observed echo time does not change. The difference, however, is that now the phase changes due to chemical shift are no longer canceled by the 180 degree pulse. In effect, the spins will have been evolving at their natural frequencies for a time τ, so that the phase difference between fat and water is $\Delta\phi = \tau\delta_0$.

In the variation of this method proposed by Sepponen et al.,[60] images are made with many values of τ, and the values for each position in the image are then Fourier transformed to give the spectrum for that position. The phase in each pixel, as well as the magnitude, must be used in calculating this transform. Sepponen et al. used this method with 16 values of τ to detect pathological changes in the fat content of bone marrow.

The method proposed independently by Dixon[21] is a minimal form of this phase encoding method: only two images are made, one with fat and water in phase and one with them 180 degrees out-of-phase (the phase contrast image). The image intensities in these two sequences are then proportional to the sum and difference, respectively, of the fat and water signals:

$$S_{in} = S_W + S_F \tag{4}$$

$$S_{out} = S_W - S_F \tag{5}$$

This method has stirred much interest because of its ease of implementation, the modest time requirement (only one additional image), and the striking sensitivity of the method for detecting changes in the fat content of a tissue. This is illustrated by Figure 92–10, a plot of signal intensity vs. fat fraction (f) for a tissue with water $T1_w = .5$s and the fat $T1_f = .3$s. For a conventional pulse sequence the signal will change slightly as the fat content increases because the effective, bulk $T1$ of the tissue will approach the fat $T1$. However, because the signal intensity in the out-of-phase image is proportional to the *difference* between the fat and water signals, out-of-phase imaging is 3 to 7 times more sensitive[14] to changes in the fat content than in-phase imaging.

We have recently looked at questions related to the quantitative application of the Dixon method and found that the simple equations (4 and 5) for the in-phase and out-of-phase signal intensities describe measured data well when the effects of pulse shape are taken into account[54] and as long as field homogeneity within a voxel is reasonably good.[15,16] By imaging phantoms with a range of fat contents and relaxation times we found a good correlation ($r = .97$) between the $T1$'s calculated from image data and those calculated from "spectrometer mode" data (measuring FIDs with all gradients off), as shown in Figure 92–11. There was also a very tight correlation between the fat content calculated from the images and the fat content by weight ($r = .995$) as shown in Figure 92–12.

Although these quantitative tests are reassuring, the Dixon method is subject to systematic errors related to basic assumptions of the method. The method works with so minimal a data set because it is assumed that the spectrum is known before any data are taken. Specifically, it is assumed that the spectrum consists of two sharp lines with a known separation. The only unknown variables in the spectrum are then the two amplitudes, so that only two images are necessary to calculate them. The problem is that neither the assumption of known chemical shift nor narrow width may be true.

First, if the assumed chemical shift is incorrect, so that the τ value used is incorrect, then the out-of-phase image will not be completely out of phase. A similar systematic error can arise if the assumed chemical shift is correct but the in-phase sequence is

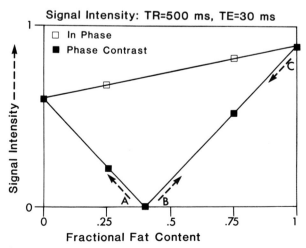

Figure 92–10. In-phase (open square) and phase contrast (solid square) signal intensities as functions of fat fraction for $TR = 500$ ms and $TE = 30$ ms. Relaxation parameters are $T1_W = 500$ ms, $T2_W = 40$ ms, $T1_F = 300$ ms, and $T2_F = 50$ ms. For normal tissues of mixed water and fat content, such as bone marrow (see Fig. 92–13B), phase contrast signal intensity is near the minimum value. Pathology affecting such tissues results in higher phase contrast signal intensity. For example, increased water will cause phase contrast signal to increase in the direction of arrow A, whereas increased fat results in phase contrast signal change in the direction of arrow B. Influx of water into predominantly fatty tissues will decrease phase contrast signal intensity in the direction of arrow C. In all cases, it is the steeper slope of the phase contrast plot relative to that of the in-phase signal intensity that accounts for the superior image contrast seen on out-of-phase images. Parenthetically, we note that magnitude data reconstruction accounts for the positive phase contrast signal intensity on both sides of the null point (i.e., value of F for which $S_{out} = 0$). Phase-corrected data display is possible, in which case the phase contrast curve becomes a straight line and S_{out} has negative values for lipid fraction short of the null point. (From Wismer GL et al.: *AJR* *145*:1031, 1985. Used by permission.)

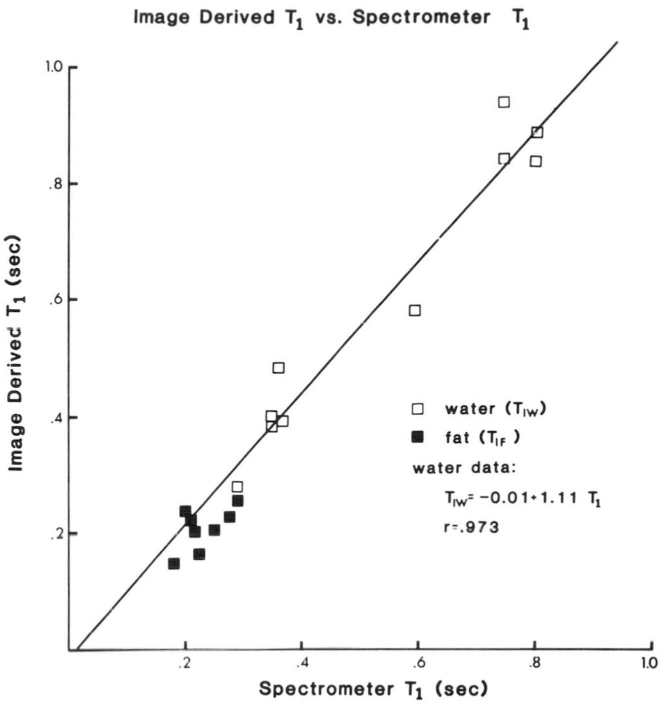

Image Derived T₁ vs. Spectrometer T₁

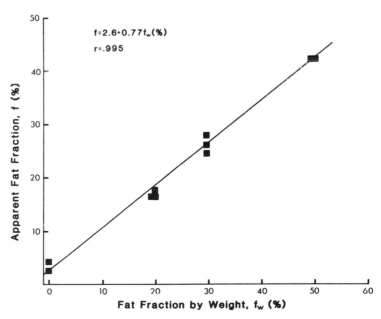

Figure 92–11. *T1* values, as calculated from image data for 10 phantoms, compared with the *T1* values measured with the same instrument in spectrometer mode (all gradients off). Phantoms were prepared from mayonnaise mixed in different proportions with agar gel and gadolinium $(DTPA)^{2-}$ to produce a range of water *T1* values and fat content. (From Buxton R et al.: J Magn Reson Med *3*:881–900, 1986.)

not properly set up. That is, if the pulse sequence timings are such that the Hahn echo and the gradient echo are slightly displaced for the in-phase image, then the fat and water signals will be slightly out of phase, and for the out-of-phase image the signals will not be fully out of phase. In either case, this problem will lead to systematic errors when the fat content or relaxation times are calculated from the images, but the magnitude of the error depends on the fat fraction of the tissue being imaged.[15,16] Calculations for a particular set of pulse sequences indicated that for an error of 5 percent

Apparent Fat Fraction vs. Fat Fraction by Weight

Figure 92–12. Apparent fat fraction, as calculated from image data for the same 10 phantoms as in Figure 92–11 compared with the fat fraction by weight, as calculated from the known fraction of mayonnaise in each phantom. (From Buxton R et al.: J Magn Reson Med *3*:881–900, 1986. Used by permission.)

in the τ value used or in the pulse timing, the resulting fractional errors in the calculated tissue parameters were less than 5 percent for tissues that are mostly water or mostly fat, but for tissues with $f \simeq .5$ the errors can be 7 to 10 percent.

A second source of error in the Dixon method is due to the finite width of the spectral lines due to inhomogeneities in the main field and the fact that each line is composed of several slightly displaced resonances. Since the Hahn echo and the gradient echo are displaced in the out-of-phase pulse sequence, the dephasing of the signal because of this spread in frequency is not canceled. The result is that the out-of-phase image intensity of even a single component sample (pure water or pure fat) will be reduced from the in-phase image intensity. If this systematic effect is not taken into account, it will lead to errors in the calculated relaxation times, but there tends to be some cancellation of this error, since the relaxation time calculations depend on ratios of image intensities; a 5 percent reduction in out-of-phase image intensity leads to comparable or much smaller errors in the relaxation times. The error in the fat content estimate is also small when $f \simeq .5$, but when f is small, the fractional error can be large. For accurately quantitating low fat content ($f < .1$) it will be necessary to correct for the effects of inhomogeneities by first measuring the signal reduction in the out-of-phase image with a single component phantom (pure water or pure fat) and scaling the out-of-phase image accordingly.

With careful attention to these potential systematic errors, the Dixon method is capable of yielding accurate quantitative data. And with the high sensitivity of out-of-phase imaging to differences in fat content,[14] this method should be very effective in studying pathology with associated changes in fat content.

The Dixon method is also of interest because it represents a different approach to extracting chemical shift information, by explicitly making use of prior knowledge of the spectrum. This is an approach that has been used in a few spectroscopic applications[4] and may in the future be adapted for imaging more complex spectra.[1]

In Vivo Applications

The first clinical application of the Dixon method was a study by Lee et al.[34] of fatty infiltration of the liver in three patients with evidence of fatty infiltration on computed tomography (CT) and two normal volunteers. As mentioned above, conventional MR imaging techniques have been reported to be sensitive to fatty infiltration of the liver.[64] Surprisingly, even non-uniform or focal fatty infiltration of liver, demonstrated by CT, appears normal on conventional spin-echo images. With the Dixon method, however, both diffuse and focal fatty infiltration can be readily detected. Lee et al.[34] showed normal livers to have a lipid signal constituting less than 10 percent of the water signal. In fatty livers this lipid signal fraction may be greater than 20 percent.

Clinical application of this technique has been shown for detection of liver cancer.[29] Fatty infiltration of the liver is a common problem in hospitalized patients; diffuse fatty infiltration can mask detection of metastases by CT, or alternatively focal fatty infiltration can mimic the CT appearance of liver cancer. On out-of-phase images lipid acts as an endogenous contrast material; fatty infiltration occurs only in functioning hepatocytes whereas tumor tissue has no NMR observable fat. Therefore, on out-of-phase images, fatty infiltrated liver tissue will show a reduced signal intensity, while the relative intensity (tissue contrast) of tumor tissue is increased. Similarly, areas of focal fat infiltration, suspicious for cancer by CT criteria, can be specifically identified as fatty liver tissue on the phase contrast image. Preliminary data suggest that phase contrast imaging can equal or better the performance of CT for the evaluation of suspected liver cancer.[29]

In addition to the assessment of tumor extension into fat and fatty infiltration into tissue, phase contrast imaging is also useful for the evaluation of hematopoietic marrow such as the sternum, ribs, and vertebrae. In adults, these tissues are composed of approximately 70 percent of cellular elements, containing mostly water protons, that are intimately admixed with fat (~30 percent). Wismer et al.[66] have recently demonstrated that a variety of lesions can be detected in marrow with out-of-phase images. The conspicuity of such lesions is enhanced over conventional (in-phase) MR images, making the phase contrast technique a sensitive indicator of pathologic involvement of marrow.

The distinctive features of conventional and out-of-phase images of bone marrow are illustrated in Figure 92–13, surface coil SE 500/30 images of the cervical spine and cord of a normal adult female. The in-phase image shows bright signal intensity from vertebral marrow due to the short *T1* of marrow fat. The low signal from vertebral marrow on the phase contrast image (*B*) is attributable to the high fractional volumes of both fat and water per image voxel in this tissue. In tissues that are composed of high proportions of either fat or water, the signal cancellation effect seen within vertebral marrow is not observed. Instead the signal intensities within such tissues are identical to those on conventional images, but a thin zone of low signal is observed at interfaces between tissues containing only fat or only water. This "edge effect" is clearly shown in Figure 92–14, which is an out-of-phase image from a patient with a large chondrosarcoma of the right ilium. Boundaries between the subcutaneous fat and the water in tumor or normal muscle are highlighted by a zone of low signal intensity at these interfaces. This effect may provide superior delineation of the extent of tumor or improved detection of involvement in adjacent fatty tissue, e.g., in assessing invasion of perirectal fat by cancer of the rectum. Although conventional MR imaging shows promise in evaluating lumbar disc disease,[23,43] out-of-phase images can further aid in the detection of herniated lumbar disc, especially at L5-S1 where there is usually ample epidural fat.[56]

In this chapter we have briefly reviewed the theory of chemical shift imaging using three basic approaches and have discussed their applications. All of these techniques

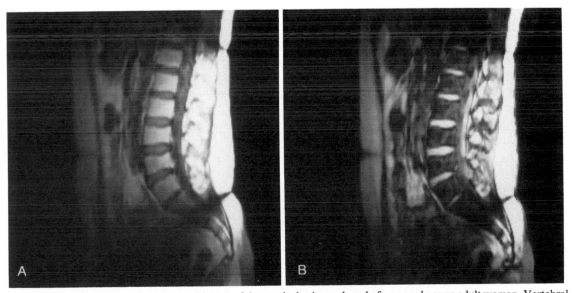

Figure 92–13. *A*, Conventional surface coil image of the cervical spine and cord of a normal young adult woman. Vertebral marrow contains approximately 30 percent aliphatic protons. The short *T1* of marrow fat accounts for the bright marrow signal in this image. *B*, Marrow signal cancels on the phase contrast image because of opposed contributions from aliphatic and water protons. Note the intensely bright signal from the purely water-containing intervertebral disks.

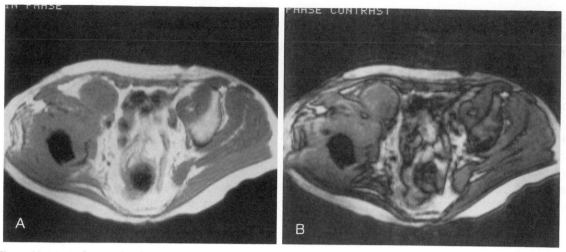

Figure 92–14. *A*, Conventional transverse image through the pelvis, showing a right iliac chondrosarcoma with poorly defined margins. *B*, Sharp definition of tumor extent caused by cancellation of signal at fat-water interfaces on the phase contrast image.

are capable of producing quantitative as well as qualitative information, and the choice of a technique will be determined by the clinical problem under investigation.

The 3DFT method is the most general and can be used for measuring spectra of any nucleus. Images of the spatial distribution of each spectral line can be formed using this technique with no prior knowledge of the spectrum, and the effects of B_0 inhomogeneity can be corrected. Since the minimum imaging time increases with the square of the linear resolution, images from three-dimensional data sets will in general have lower spatial resolution than conventional images. Therefore, this technique is suitable for the spectral assessment of large organs, e.g., liver, especially when involved with a diffuse disease. Complete three-dimensional chemical shift data sets can be obtained in as fast as six minutes with low (32 × 32) spatial resolution and a frequency resolution of 256 points providing both qualitative and quantitative information in vivo.

For proton imaging of fat and water, phase contrast and selective saturation methods can provide images with the same resolution as conventional images in just twice the imaging time. The phase contrast method has the additional advantage of immediate implementation on most magnet systems currently in use, and the requirement on B_0 inhomogeneity is only that the variation in B_0 across a voxel be less than the chemical shift. Selective saturation techniques as currently implemented require high homogeneity magnets for maximum efficiency; variation in B_0 across the entire slice must be less than the chemical shift.

For assessment of proton metabolites in millimolar concentration, the requirements for extensive signal averaging, along with large voxel size, mean that the trade-off between spatial and spectral resolution favors the use of three-dimensional techniques. Although quantitative applications are exciting, significant development will be required before these techniques can be implemented routinely.

It is evident that spatially localized metabolic data can be acquired noninvasively using both ^1H and ^{31}P nuclei. New techniques will no doubt emerge and may provide the investigator/clinician with additional alternatives. The ultimate clinical application of these techniques will depend upon several factors, including the refinement of equipment to facilitate data acquisition and analysis and improved understanding of the complex response of tissue in the NMR experiment.[68]

ACKNOWLEDGMENTS

This work was supported in part by the Technicare Corporation, Solon, Ohio, and by PHS grants 1 R01 CA40303-01 and 1 K04 CA00848-03, awarded by the National Cancer Institute, DHHS.

References

1. Ackerman JL, Koutcher J, Brady TJ: Minimal sampling of the free induction decay: applications to high speed chemical shift imaging and multidimensional spectroscopy. Presented at the Fourth Annual Meeting of the Society of Magnetic Resonance in Medicine, London, August 19–23, 1985.
2. Ackerman JJH, Grove TH, Wong GG, Gadian DG, Radda GK: Mapping of metabolites in whole animals by ^{31}P NMR using surface coils. Nature *283*:167–170, 1980.
3. Axel L: Surface coil magnetic resonance imaging. J Comput Assist Tomogr *8*:381–384, 1984.
4. Barkhuijsen H, DeBeer R, Bovee WMMJ, van Ormondt D: Retrieval of frequencies, amplitudes, damping factors, and phases from time-domain signals using a linear least-squares procedure. J Magn Reson *61*:465–481, 1985.
5. Behar KL, DenHollander JA, Stromski ME, Ogino T, Shulman RG, Petroff OHC, Prichard JW: High-resolution ^{1}H nuclear magnetic resonance study of cerebral hypoxia in vivo. Proc Nat Acad Sci USA *80*:4945–4948, 1983.
6. Bendall MR, Gordon RE: Depth and refocussing pulses designed from multipulse NMR with surface coils. J Magn Reson *53*:365–385, 1983.
7. Bendel P, Lai C-M, Lauterbur PC: ^{31}P spectroscopic zeugmatography of phosphorus metabolites. J Magn Reson *38*:343–356, 1980.
8. Bernardo ML, Lauterbur PC, Hedges LK: Experimental example of NMR spectroscopic imaging by projection reconstruction involving an intrinsic frequency dimension. J Magn Reson *61*:168–174, 1985.
9. Bloch F, Hansen WW, Packard M: Nuclear induction (letter to the editor). Phys Rev *69*:127, 1946.
10. Bottomley PA: Localized NMR spectroscopy by the sensitive-point method. J Magn Reson *50*:335–338, 1982.
11. Bottomley PA, Foster TB, Darrow RD: Depth-resolved surface coil spectroscopy (DRESS) for in-vivo ^{1}H, ^{31}P and ^{13}C NMR. J Magn Reson *59*:338–342, 1984.
12. Bottomley PA, Foster TH, Leve WM: In vivo nuclear magnetic resonance chemical shift imaging by selective irradiation. Proc Natl Acad Sci USA *81*:6856–6860, 1984.
13. Brown TR, Kincaid BM, Ugurbil K: NMR chemical shift imaging in three dimensions. Proc Natl Acad Sci USA *79*:3523–3526, 1982.
14. Buxton RB, Wismer GL, Brady TJ, Rosen BR: MR image contrast with out-of-phase proton chemical shift imaging. Presented at the Fourth Annual Meeting of the Society of Magnetic Resonance in Medicine, London, August 19–23, 1985.
15. Buxton RB, Wismer GL, Brady TJ, Rosen BR: Quantitative proton chemical shift imaging. Presented at the Fourth Annual Meeting of the Society of Magnetic Resonance in Medicine, London, August 19–23, 1985.
16. Buxton R, Wismer GL, Brady TJ, Rosen BR: Quantitative proton chemical shift imaging. J Magn Res Med *3*:831, 1986.
17. Bydder GM, Steiner RE, Young IR, Hall AS, Thomas DJ, Marshall J, Pallis CA, Legg NJ: Clinical NMR imaging of the brain: 140 cases. Am J Radiol *139*:215–226, 1982.
18. Clore GM, Kimber BJ, Gronenborn AM: The 1-1 hard pulse: A simple and effective method of water resonance suppression in FT ^{1}H NMR. J Magn Reson *54*:170–173, 1983.
19. Cox SJ, Styles P: Towards biochemical imaging. J Magn Reson *40*:209–212, 1980.
20. Dickinson WC: Dependence of the fluorine^{19} nuclear resonance position on a chemical compound. Phys Rev *77*:736, 1950.
21. Dixon WT: Simple proton spectroscopic imaging. Radiology *153*:189–194, 1984.
22. Dwek RA: Nuclear Magnetic Resonance in Biochemistry: Applications to Enzyme Systems. Oxford, Clarendon Press, 1973.
23. Edelman RR, Shoukimas GM, Stark DD, Davis KR, New PFJ, Saini S, Rosenthal DI, Wismer GL, Brady TJ: High resolution surface coil imaging of lumbar disc disease. AJR *144*:1123, 1985.
24. Frahm J, Haase A, Hanicke W, Matthaei D, Bomsdorf H, Helzel T: Chemical shift selective MR imaging using a whole-body magnet. Radiology *156*:441–444, 1985.
25. Gadian DG: Nuclear Magnetic Resonance and Its Application to Living Systems. London, Oxford University Press, 1982.
26. Gordon RE, Hanley PE, Shaw D: Topical magnetic resonance. Prog NMR Spect *15*:1–47, 1982.
27. Haase A, Frahm J, Hanicke W, Matthaei D: ^{1}H-NMR chemical shift selective (CHESS) imaging. Phys Med Biol *30*:341–344, 1985.
28. Hall LD, Rajanayagam V, Sukumar S: Chemical-shift-resolved tomography using four-dimensional FT imaging. J Magn Reson *61*:188–191, 1985.
29. Heiken JP, Lee JKT, Dixon WT, Ling D, Glazer HS: MR imaging of hepatic metastases. Presented at

the 70th Annual Meeting and Scientific Sessions of the Radiological Society of North America, Washington, D.C., 1984.

30. Joseph PM: A spin echo chemical shift MR imaging technique. J Comput Assist Tomogr 9:651–658, 1985.
31. Lauterbur PC: Image formation by induced local interactions: Examples employing NMR. Nature 242:190–191, 1973.
32. Lauterbur PC, Kramer DM, House WV, Chen C-N: Zeugmatographic high resolution nuclear magnetic resonance spectroscopy: Images of chemical inhomogeneity within macroscopic objects. J Am Chem Soc 97:6866–6868, 1975.
33. Lauterbur PC, Levin DN, Marr RB: Theory and simulation of NMR spectroscopic imaging and field plotting by projection reconstruction involving an intrinsic frequency dimension. J Magn Reson 1984; 59:536–541, 1984.
34. Lee JKT, Dixon WT, Ling D, Levitt RG, Murphy WA: Fatty infiltration of the liver: Demonstration by proton spectroscopic imaging. Radiology 153:195–201, 1984.
35. McFarland E, Koutcher JA, Rosen BR, Teicher B, Brady TJ: In vivo ^{19}F NMR imaging. J Comput Assist Tomogr 9:8–15, 1985.
36. Manassen Y, Navon G: A constant gradient experiment for chemical-shift imaging. J Magn Reson 61:363–370, 1985.
37. Mansfield P: Spatial mapping of the chemical shift in NMR. Magn Reson Med 1:370–386, 1984.
38. Mansfield P, Morris PG: NMR Imaging in Biomedicine. Washington, Academic Press, 1982.
39. Martin JF, Wade CG: Chemical shift encoding in NMR images. J Magn Reson 61:153–157, 1985.
40. Maudsley AA, Hilal SK, Perman WH, Simon HE: Spatially resolved high resolution spectroscopy by "four-dimensional" NMR. J Magn Reson 51:147–152, 1983.
41. Maudsley AA, Hilal SK, Simon HE: Multinuclear applications of chemical shift imaging. Magn Reson Med 1:202–203, 1984.
42. Maudsley AA, Simon HE, Hilal SK: Magnetic field measurements by NMR imaging. J Phys E 17:216, 1984.
43. Modic MT, Weinstein MA, Pavlicek W, Starnes DL, Duchesneau PM, Boumphrey F, Hardy RJ: Nuclear magnetic resonance imaging of the spine. Radiology 148:757–762, 1983.
44. Myers RE: Lactate measurements in cerebral ischemia. In Fahn S, Davis JN, Rowland LP (eds): Advances in Neurology. New York, Raven Press, 1979, pp 195–213.
45. Myers RE, Yamaguchi M: Effects of serum glucose concentration on brain response to circulatory arrest. J Neuropathol Exp Neurol 35:301, 1976.
46. Nunnally RL, Bottomley PA: Assessment of pharmacological treatment of myocardial infarction by phosphorus-31 NMR with surface coils. Science 211:177–180, 1981.
47. Proctor WG, Yu FC: The dependence of a nuclear magnetic resonance frequency upon a chemical compound. Phys Rev 77:717, 1950.
48. Purcell EM, Torrey HC, Pound RV: Resonance absorption by nuclear magnetic moments in a solid. Phys Rev 69:37–38, 1946.
49. Pykett IL, Newhouse JH, Buonanno FS, Brady TJ, Goldman MR, Kistler JP, Pohost GM: Principles of nuclear magnetic resonance imaging. Radiology 143:157–168, 1982.
50. Pykett IL, Rosen BR: Nuclear magnetic resonance: in-vivo proton chemical shift imaging. Radiology 149:197–201, 1983.
51. Redfield AG, Kunz SD, Ralph EK: Dynamic range in Fourier transform proton magnetic resonance. J Magn Reson 19:114–117, 1975.
52. Rehncrona S, Rosen I, Siesjo BK: Excessive cellular acidosis: an important mechanism of damage in the brain. Acta Physiol Scand 110:435–437, 1980.
53. Rosen BR, Carter EA, Pykett IL, et al: Proton chemical shift imaging: An evaluation of its clinical potential using an in vivo fatty liver model. Radiology 154:469–472, 1985.
54. Rosen BR, Pykett IL, Brady TJ: Spin lattice relaxation time measurements in two-dimensional magnetic resonance imaging: Corrections for plane selection and pulse sequence. J Comput Assist Tomogr 1984; 8:195–199, 1984.
55. Rosen BR, Wedeen VJ, Brady TJ: Selective saturation proton NMR imaging. J Comput Assist Tomogr 8:813–818, 1984.
56. Rosen BR, Wismer GL, McFarland EW, Brady TJ: Evaluation of intervertebral disk disease using MR proton chemical shift imaging and surface coils. Works in Progress, RSNA, 70th Scientific Assembly and Annual Meeting, Washington, D.C., 1984.
57. Satoh K, Kose K, Inouye T, Yasuoka H: Chemical shift imaging by spin-echo modified Fourier method. J Appl Phys 57:2174–2181, 1985.
58. Schlunk FF, Lombardi B: Isolation and chemical characterization. Lab Invest 17:30–38, 1967.
59. Scott KN, Brooker HR, Fitzimmons JR, Bennett HF, Mick RC: Spatial localization of ^{31}P nuclear magnetic resonance signal by the sensitive point method. J Magn Reson 50:339–344, 1982.
60. Sepponen RE, Sipponen JT, Tanttu JI: A method for chemical shift imaging: demonstration of bone marrow involvement with proton chemical shift imaging. J Comput Assist Tomogr 8:585–587, 1984.
61. Shulman RG: Biological Applications of Magnetic Resonance. New York, Academic Press, 1979.
62. Slichter S: Principles of Magnetic Resonance. New York, Springer-Verlag, 1980.
63. Soila KP, Viamonte M Jr, Starewicz PM: Chemical shift misregistration effect in magnetic resonance imaging. Radiology 153:819–820, 1984.

64. Stark DD, Bass NM, Moss AA, Bacon BR, McKerrow JH, Cann CE, Brito A, Goldberg HI: Nuclear magnetic resonance imaging of experimentally induced liver disease. Radiology *148*:743–751, 1983.
65. Turner DL: Binomial solvent suppression. J Magn Reson *54*:146–148, 1983.
66. Wismer GL, Rosen BR, Buxton R, Stark DD, Brady TJ: Chemical shift imaging of bone marrow: preliminary experience. AJR *145*:1031–1037, 1985.
67. Yoshizaki K, Seo Y, Nishikawa H: High-resolution proton magnetic resonance spectra of muscle. Biochim Biophys Acta *678*:283–291, 1981.
68. Twien DB, Katz J, Peshock RM: General treatment of NMR imaging with chemical shifts and motion. Magn Res Med *5*:32, 1987.

93

Technical Demands of Multiple Nuclei

A. A. MAUDSLEY

The predominant application of nuclear magnetic resonance (NMR) imaging has undoubtedly taken place using proton resonance for biomedical studies. The high NMR sensitivity of protons coupled with the high concentration of the NMR observable nucleus in tissue makes it the most favorable nucleus for study. Currently proton imaging is rapidly becoming a valuable tool for research and clinical diagnosis owing to its ability to observe remarkable detail within soft tissues. In the area of conventional NMR spectroscopy a wide range of other nuclei are more commonly observed for studies of, for example, molecular structure, dynamics, and rate constants. For spectroscopic studies of biological systems the most commonly observed nuclei include carbon-13, sodium-23, and phosphorus-31 as well as protons; and other nuclei such as nitrogen-15, oxygen-17, fluorine-19, and potassium-41 have been less frequently observed. It is of interest to investigate the potential of these nuclei for possible clinical applications and to develop appropriate data acquisition methods for observation using spatial localization techniques. Imaging may be performed using any observable nucleus, and techniques also exist that enable spectroscopic information to be obtained along with an image of the spatial distribution of that nucleus. However, imaging of other nuclei is not always a simple extension of existing methods, and frequently different experimental strategies and apparatus as well as methods of processing, displaying, and handling of the data are needed. It can also be said that the same limitations exist for observation of all nuclei and that the same compromises must be made to optimize data acquisition. Indeed the most demanding requirement for imaging of nuclei other than protons is to increase the sensitivity of observation, which is also a requirement for proton imaging in the quest to improve image quality. A discussion of the differences and similarities for multinuclear observation will be given, using the techniques and requirements of conventional proton imaging as a base for comparison.

Table 93–1 lists some parameters of those nuclei that are considered to have the most potential for imaging applications in biological systems. Proton observation of metabolites is included separately, being an application that is distinct from the more conventional proton spin density imaging. ^{19}F is potentially useful as a contrast agent which can be introduced in a variety of ways,[1,2] similar to ^{13}C where the fate of labeled substances may be monitored.[3] ^{23}Na has already found application in clinical studies[4] as has ^{31}P, which has been extensively studied using surface coil techniques[5,6] and has been investigated for imaging studies.[7]

Of significance in Table 93–1 is the typical concentration of the NMR observable compounds and the relative sensitivity of observation. Calculation of the relative sensitivity figures has included the NMR sensitivity of observation of that nucleus relative to protons for an equal number of nuclei at the same magnetic field strength, the con-

Table 93–1. PARAMETERS OF NUCLEI

Nucleus	Frequency at 2 tesla (MHz)	Chemical Shift Range (ppm)	Typical Observed Systems	Typical Concentration in Tissue (mM)	Approximate Relative Sensitivity*
^{1}H	85.1	10	water	110000	1
			metabolites	10	1×10^{-4}
^{13}C	21.4	200	natural	1–10	1×10^{-8}
			^{13}C enriched	5–50	5×10^{-7}
^{19}F	80.1	200	contrast agent	10–70	1×10^{-4}
^{23}Na	22.5	20†	CSF	160	5×10^{-4}
			tissue	40	1×10^{-5}
^{31}P	34.5	25	PI, PCr, ATP	1–10	4×10^{-6}

* Includes concentration, abundance of observable isotope, and NMR sensitivity of detection.
† Sodium chemical shifts as the result of shift reagents.

centration of the NMR observable nucleus in tissue, and an estimate of the effect of relaxation rate differences relative to protons. It can be seen that for all nuclei other than protons the sensitivity is several orders of magnitude smaller.

The low NMR sensitivity is the major consideration for observation of these nuclei. A variety of steps can be used to improve sensitivity or alternatively to reduce system noise. These include using higher field strengths, optimizing all receiver electronics for low noise, shielding the imaging apparatus from radio frequency (rf) interference, using more efficient rf receiver coils, optimizing the efficiency of data collection methods, and performing additional signal averaging. Associated with the last two points is the reduction of spatial resolution, which increases the volume of spins contributing to the signal at each point and generally reduces data acquisition times. Many variables are frequently related, for example, the data acquisition strategies may differ according to the choice of rf coil design and the type of information required. For some applications it is not necessary to obtain a two- or three-dimensional distribution of a particular nucleus, and a point measurement technique[8–11] may be applied. For these techniques surface coils are frequently used, as they can provide increased sensitivity of detection from a small region. While this advantage is particularly applicable for single point measurements, surface coils can also be applied for imaging limited regions with increased sensitivity. Other advantages of surface coils in clinical applications include the convenience of rapidly changing coils for multiple nuclei observation, lower rf transmitter power, and the ability to localize observation to a particular region.

Significant improvement in sensitivity can undoubtedly be obtained by using higher magnetic field strengths. Investigations of the dependence of the sensitivity on field strength indicate that an improvement as a linear function of field strength may be obtained rather than to the 7/4th power as theoretically predicted.[12,13] There is, however, an upper limit of the usable field strength, which is dependent upon a number of issues. For clinical studies, one limit of field strength occurs when rf absorption in tissue may produce an unacceptable heating effect. The heating effect is a function of the tissue type, object size, average rf powers used, and the frequency. Currently proton whole body imaging has been safely carried out at 85 MHz, which corresponds to a field strength of 2 tesla.[14] This would suggest that if rf absorption presented the limit of operating frequency, then for imaging of nuclei other than ^{1}H and ^{19}F field strengths of as high as 8 tesla could be used, and even higher if surface coil techniques are used. However, a much lower limit arises from concern of the biological effects of static magnetic fields, as well as the construction, cost, and siting of high field strength magnets. Current experience indicates that the existing 2 tesla magnets enable imaging of ^{23}Na with reasonable spatial resolution as well as surface coil observations of other nuclei. For imaging of ^{31}P distributions in vivo it is estimated that a field strength of at least 3 tesla is required,[7] which lies above the present guidelines for exposure to static magnetic fields.[15]

Observation of many of those nuclei listed in Table 93–1 allows considerable chemical information to be gained from their high resolution spectra. To observe these spectra it is necessary that the line broadening from the magnetic field variations be less than the frequency resolution required to observe the chemical shift. For this requirement, the field homogeneity specifications are again dependent upon the experiment technique used. For single point measurements it is relatively simple to obtain a small region within a large magnet that has the required homogeneity. One technique, that of topical magnetic resonance (TMR),[8] actually requires a very inhomogeneous field over the object except at a single point. With spectroscopic imaging techniques[16–18] the observed volume is the whole imaged plane over which considerable field variation may exist. The imaging procedure effectively divides the plane into an array of voxels, or resolved image points; and provided that field variations over each voxel are small, the high resolution spectrum can still be observed.[17] To obtain the distribution of a specific resonance the effects of field inhomogeneity must be corrected for. This may be as simple as taking the magnitude spectra for simple spectroscopic imaging[18] or may be performed by a more extensive field correction procedure for high resolution spectroscopic imaging.[17]

Many spectroscopic methods use a number of double irradiation techniques for such applications as simplification of spectra, to elucidate intermolecular couplings or for solvent suppression. These techniques place much greater demands on field inhomogeneity requirements. For water suppression using selective excitation or saturation pulses[19] it is necessary that the field variation over the whole of the observed plane be on the order of 2 ppm or less; otherwise the suppression of the water signal becomes less effective, and spectral information close to the water peak may be lost. For many double resonance studies using ^{13}C, where precise irradiation of narrow lines is required, homogeneity requirements must be better than 1 ppm. For volume imaging techniques these requirements become extremely difficult to satisfy, particularly in light of the fact that magnetic susceptibility variations within the object itself cause field variations of this order.[17] For these experiments, therefore, it is often necessary to use techniques that limit the observed volume to a small region, where high homogeneity can be achieved.

If spatial localization techniques are to be used for multinuclear observation, then the magnetic field gradient requirements must also be reviewed. For imaging methods, the observation gradient, which we assume to be G_x, is ideally set such that the line broadening caused by the gradient is equal to the inhomogeneity broadening, i.e.,

$$\Delta f = \frac{\gamma}{2\pi} \cdot \Delta B \cdot B_0 \tag{1}$$

$$= \frac{\gamma}{2\pi} \cdot \Delta x \cdot G_x \tag{2}$$

where Δf is the linewidth due to field inhomogeneity in Hz, γ is the gyromagnetic ratio, ΔB the inhomogeneity in ppm of the field strength B_0, Δx is the resolution dimension in meters and G_x is the gradient strength in gauss/m. Here it has been assumed that where necessary some suitable technique is used to resolve chemical shift information. From Equations 1 and 2 it can be seen that for a given magnetic field strength, homogeneity, and experimental technique the observation gradient strength is independent of the nucleus being studied. For observation of nuclei other than protons the resolution is typically reduced to improve sensitivity, and in practice lower gradient strengths may be used.

For slice selection using selective irradiation a different situation exists. Here the frequency spread of the selective pulse is set as:

$$\Delta f' = \frac{\gamma}{2\pi} \cdot \Delta z \cdot G_z \tag{3}$$

where Δz is the selected slice width and $\Delta f'$ is the frequency bandwidth of the selective pulse. Thus for the same selective pulse and slice thickness, for a nuclei of gyromagnetic ratio γ_n, the gradient strength must be changed by γ_h/γ_n, where γ_h is the gyromagnetic ratio of protons. Thus, for example, for ^{23}Na a four times stronger gradient would be required. However, for multinuclear studies the lower sensitivity generally means that thicker slices are observed than for protons with the result that similar selection gradient strengths are used.

For the phase encoding gradient in the commonly used Fourier methods of imaging, the $T2$ of the system under study must also be taken into account. The phase encoding gradients are set such that:

$$\pi = \gamma \cdot N \cdot \Delta y \cdot \int_{t=0}^{t=ty} G_y \cdot t \cdot dt \tag{4}$$

where N is the number of points of width, Δy is the resolution along the y direction, and ty is the time over which the maximum amplitude of the phase encoding gradient G_y is applied. For observation of systems having short $T2$ the time ty must be kept short in order to avoid unnecessary loss of signal during the phase encoding time period. This requires that gradient G_y be turned on as rapidly as possible, and to be of sufficient strength to satisfy Equation (4). Whereas switching times of 2 ms may be adequate for proton observation, times of 0.5 ms or less are desirable for observation of ^{23}Na or ^{31}P systems that have short $T2$ values.

The primary considerations in the design of the rf section of any NMR spectrometer system include the frequency range of interest and the rf transmitter and receiver amplifier specifications. The most immediate requirement of a multinuclear imaging system is that it must be able to observe nuclei having a range of gyromagnetic ratios. In most present-day systems, this is achieved by making the rf electronics broadband, rather than changing the magnetic field strength in order to operate at a fixed resonance frequency. Broadband rf power amplifiers are generally available at additional cost over narrowband units, while some reduction in cost at the expense of some flexibility may be achieved if a system is designed to operate at several spot frequencies.

Transmitter power requirements depend strongly on the experimental technique selected. The angle of rotation of the spins, θ, following a pulse of length t_p, and strength B_1, is given by:

$$\theta = \gamma \cdot B_1 \cdot t_p \tag{5}$$

For multinuclear studies, to achieve the same pulse lengths as for protons the rf field strength must be increased by a factor γ_h/γ_n, which corresponds to an increase in the rf power of $(\gamma_h/\gamma_n)^2$. Fortunately at a fixed field strength, this does not imply a corresponding increase in the rf power absorbed by the object, as the absorbed power is strongly dependent on the frequency,[20] which is lower by a factor γ_n/γ_h. For the receiver section, the gain selected at the preamplifier section should generally be larger for optimum sensitivity of nuclei other than protons, the exact gain figures depending on the field strength and object size. In all cases the noise figure of the first amplifier stage, which is the most critical, should always be low, i.e., less than 1 dB.

Relaxation rates must be considered with any NMR observation. Although $T1$ values will not alter apparatus, they affect the rate at which signal averaging can be performed and thereby influence the choice of data collection method and hence the effective sensitivity of observation. Observation of sodium, whose $T1$ is similar to $T2$

and lies in the range of 30 to 50 ms, can be done at a fast repetition rate. In this case a three-dimensional data acquisition is suitable as the large number of measurements required to obtain the full three-dimensional data may be rapidly acquired, and full advantage taken of the increased sensitivity of the volume acquisition method over two dimensional techniques.[21] On the other hand, phosphorus compounds may have $T1$'s of 2 to 3 seconds, and in addition chemical shift information is required. If a total volume imaging method were to be used in this case, a four-dimensional data set would result, and data collection times may become unreasonably long. Therefore it may be more appropriate to use multiple plane data acquisition methods that obtain information from a large volume over each $T1$ period while producing multiple three-dimensional data sets (two spatial and one frequency dimension). Short $T2$ values also influence the data acquisition method used. The phosphorus resonances of ATP have relatively short $T2$'s and when using a spin-echo sequence with Fourier imaging techniques the ATP signal is barely observable due to $T2$ relaxation.[7] Consequently to observe these resonances it is necessary to observe immediately after the excitation pulse. This can be achieved with either single point data acquisition methods, or a four-dimensional projection reconstruction method,[22] which would allow observation of chemical shifts and short $T2$ signals.

Present-day NMR spectroscopy uses a wide variety of computer software utilities for data processing, analysis, and storage, providing a sophisticated tool for spectral analysis. With the application of spectroscopic methods to imaging, many of these methods must also be used and frequently adapted to accommodate the additional spatial information that is available. The handling of the different data types must be carefully considered. For observation of multiple line, high resolution spectra where many narrow lines occur over a large range of chemical shifts, the acquisition of over one thousand points is typically required, and frequently as many as sixteen thousand. For proton spectroscopic imaging using only 512 points in the frequency domain and a 64×64 original spatial matrix size for a single plane, this can result in 136 Mbytes of data storage being used during the full data processing.[23] Processing of this amount of data may require several hours on a minicomputer unless consideration is paid to the computer hardware and software system design, including such items as array processors to rapidly perform the many Fourier transforms that are required.

At the present time, the application of NMR observation of nuclei other than protons for clinical studies has been limited to a few NMR research institutions. Should more extensive applications occur, then it would appear necessary for a wide range of suitable data processing and display utilities to be developed. For example, it may be of use to combine low resolution studies of phosphorus with high resolution proton images, which show the anatomy of the imaged section better. Many spectroscopic studies present the investigator with a wealth of spectral information, though some procedure that selects out one resonance of interest may be sufficient and enable easier analysis.

The application of multinuclear and spectroscopic studies for NMR imaging continues to expand the potential of the clinical application of NMR, providing a powerful tool for performing a non-invasive means of chemical analysis. Efforts continue to expand these NMR techniques and to investigate the clinical utility of these studies. With further improvements in the techniques and apparatus used we can expect to see increasing application of NMR observation of a wide range of nuclei.

References

1. Wyrwicz AM, Schofield JC, Tillman PC, Gordon RE, Martin PA: Noninvasive observation of fluorinated anesthetics in rabbit brain by fluorine-19 nuclear magnetic resonance. Science *222*:428, 1983.

2. McFarland E, Koutcher JA, Rosen BR, Teicher B, Brady T: In vivo ^{19}F NMR imaging. J Comput Assist Tomogr 9:8, 1985.
3. Alger JR, Shulman RG: Metabolic applications of high resolution ^{13}C nuclear magnetic resonance spectroscopy. Br Med Bull 40:160, 1984.
4. Hilal SK, Maudsley AA, Ra, JB et al: In vivo NMR imaging of sodium-23 in the human head. J Comput Asst Tomogr 9:1, 1985.
5. Radda GK, Bore PJ, Rajagopalan B: Clinical aspects of ^{31}P NMR spectroscopy. Br Med Bull 40:155, 1983.
6. Cresshull I, Dawson MJ, Edwards RHT et al: Human muscle analysed by ^{31}P nuclear magnetic resonance in intact subjects. Proc J Physiol 18P:317, 1981.
7. Maudsley AA, Hilal SK, Simon HE, Wittekoek S: In vivo MR spectroscopic imaging with P-31. Radiology 153:745, 1984.
8. Gordon RE, Hanley PE, Shaw D: Topical magnetic resonance. Prog NMR Spectr 15:1, 1982.
9. Hinshaw WS: Image formation by NMR: The sensitive point method. J Appl Phys 47:3709, 1976.
10. Damadian R, Minkoff L, Goldsmith M, Stanford M, Koutcher J: Field focussing nuclear magnetic resonance (Fonar): Visualization of a tumor in a live animal. Science 194:1430, 1976.
11. Aue WP, Mueller S, Cross TA, Seelig J: Volume-selective excitation: A novel approach to topical NMR. J Magn Reson 56:350, 1948.
12. Hoult DI, Lauterbur PC: The sensitivity of the zeugmatographic experiment including human samples. J Magn Reson 34:425, 1979.
13. Chen C-N, Sank VJ, Hoult DI: Probing image frequency dependence. Proceedings of the Society for Magnetic Resonance in Medicine, New York, 1984, p 148.
14. Bomsdorf H, Buikman D, Kuhn M et al: From Proceedings of the Society of Magnetic Resonance in Medicine, New York, 1984, p 61.
15. Alpen EL: Magnetic field exposure guidelines. Proceedings of the Biomagnetic Effects Workshop, Lawrence Berkeley Laboratory Report No. 7452, Berkeley, California, 1978, pp 19–26.
16. Maudsley AA: In-vivo spectroscopy by NMR imaging. In Gupta RK (ed): NMR Spectroscopy of Cells and Organisms. Boca Raton, CRC Press, 1987.
17. Maudsley AA, Hilal SK: Field inhomogeneity correction and data processing for spectroscopic imaging. J Magn Reson Med 2:218, 1985.
18. Dixon WT: Simple proton spectroscopic imaging. Radiology 153:189, 1984.
19. Hore PJ: Solvent suppression in Fourier transform nuclear magnetic resonance. J Magn Reson 55:283, 1983.
20. Bottomley PA, Andrew ER: RF magnetic field penetration phase shift and power dissipation in biological tissue: Implications for NMR imaging. Phys Med Biol 23:630, 1978.
21. Brunner P, Ernst RR: Sensitivity and performance time in NMR imaging. J Magn Reson 33:83, 1979.
22. Lauterbur PC, Levin DN, Marr RB: Theory and simulation of NMR spectroscopic imaging and field plotting by projection reconstruction involving an intrinsic frequency dimension. J Magn Reson 59:536, 1984.
23. Maudsley AA: Electronics and instrumentation for NMR imaging. IEEE Trans Nucl Sci NS-31:990, 1984.

94

NMR Evaluation of Tumor Metabolism

H. D. SOSTMAN
J. C. GORE
I. M. ARMITAGE
J. J. FISCHER

The detection and characterization of malignant tissue remain the most important problems in medical diagnosis. There are still significant limitations in our ability to detect cancer, to select optimal treatments, to evaluate the early response of tumors to therapy, and to distinguish between recurrent neoplasia and fibrotic or inflammatory sequelae of treatment.

Tumors can be diagnosed and classified with reasonable accuracy by biopsy and microscopic examination, but no noninvasive and generally applicable method is available that has acceptable specificity for cancer diagnosis, given the rigors of oncologic therapy and the grim outcome of untreated neoplasia. Modern imaging techniques have high sensitivity for detection of anatomic lesions or masses, although limitations exist in many clinical situations in which tumors are small or differ little in their physical properties from adjacent tissue.

Following diagnosis, selection and application of optimal therapy are hampered by numerous factors. Local or distant spread of tumor must be detected in order to determine if surgery is possible, to direct appropriate surgical intervention, or to outline radiation ports. This "staging" process suffers from many of the same deficiencies that affect the original diagnosis. If primary radiation or palliative or adjuvant radiotherapy or chemotherapy is contemplated to treat solid tumors, the presence of ischemic or hypoxic zones within the lesion constitutes a major obstacle to the success of most forms of such therapy. No clinically applicable method for detecting or quantifying the extent of such zones is now available. Once nonsurgical therapy is begun, it is typically difficult or impossible to individually optimize the sequence and schedule of treatment or to evaluate the response of the lesion at a stage before gross changes in its size begin to occur. Following completion of therapy, it is at times obscure whether anatomic changes at the site of the tumor represent recrudescence of neoplasia or a benign response to toxic therapy.

In addition to these pragmatic clinical problems, many aspects of tumor biology and metabolism in vivo are incompletely understood. This is the case with normal tissues as well, but the problem is magnified in neoplasms by the wide variety of their degrees of differentiation and by the complexity and importance of their interaction with the host.

This chapter reviews the applications of NMR spectroscopy to studies of tumors in light of some of the above problems and suggests some possible future applications of this technique in oncology.

METABOLISM OF TUMORS

The study of neoplasms has been linked with the study of metabolism for many years. The search for a unique biochemical feature of malignant cells has been extensive, but no convincing evidence has been found for a metabolic peculiarity present solely in malignant tissue. Recent authors have pointed out that this is an overly simplistic concept and should be abandoned. Conversely, when one searches for metabolic differences between most tumors and normal tissues, particularly the tissues from which the tumors originate, numerous metabolic disparities between normal and malignant cells can easily be found.

One of the central dogmas of tumor metabolism research is that genotypic aberrations lead to the phenotypic aberration of synthesis of novel enzymes or unusual isozyme patterns of common enzymes. Many of the metabolic consequences of malignancy are thought to follow from this. In particular, three phenotypic alterations already have been extensively studied by NMR spectroscopic techniques in tumors. These are glycolytic anomalies (particularly high aerobic glycolysis), abnormal pH and pH regulation, and abnormal properties of tumor cell membranes. In addition, of course, alterations in biochemical pathways may not be directly related to neoplastic transformation but may be secondary to the altered environment in which a neoplasm is situated.

The observation of high aerobic glycolysis in tumors was initially made by Warburg.[1] It is well known that when normal tissue is incubated in a nutrient medium containing glucose, but in the absence of oxygen, a rapid evolution of lactic acid takes place. When normal tissues are incubated in the presence of oxygen, however, glycolysis and lactic acid production virtually cease. The decrease in glycolysis brought about by oxygen exposure is termed the Pasteur effect. With tumor tissues anaerobic glycolysis is also high, and although a Pasteur effect is observed, it is far smaller. That is, the presence of oxygen does not lead to the elimination of glycolysis in tumor tissue. Aerobic glycolysis is present. Warburg thought the presence of high aerobic glycolysis was the result of a defect in oxidative respiration and was the key to neoplastic transformation. This hypothesis has subsequently been disproved.

Of particular interest in this regard have been studies done on the Morris hepatomas.[1] These are rat tumors of graded malignancy, which also have differing rates of aerobic glycolysis. In the better-differentiated versions of these hepatomas, there is low or negligible glycolysis. Respiration decreases with loss of differentiation, with a high level of aerobic glycolysis in the poorly differentiated lesions. The well-differentiated, slow growing, histologically minimally changed tumors, which do not utilize glucose, use fatty acids for metabolic fuel. In contrast, the poorly differentiated tumors are unable to utilize fatty acids for metabolism. The utilization of fatty acids by the well-differentiated hepatomas is linked to the retained capability of converting long and short chain fatty acids to acetoacetate (a characteristic function of normal liver), a capability that is lost in the poorly differentiated lesions expressing some genes (to increase their capability for glucose utilization) and suppressing other genes (those that code for the metabolic apparatus responsible for fatty acid oxidation).

Similar findings have been noted in clinically derived tumors. Metabolism in neuroectodermal tumors has been studied extensively. The respiration and oxygen consumption of even well-differentiated astrocytomas is low. On the other hand, oligodendrogliomas have shown much higher rates of oxygen consumption.[2] Interestingly, in this setting studies on the respiratory quotients of glial tumors have demonstrated that the values are much lower in malignant astrocytomas than in normal brain, suggesting that there is a considerable degree of oxidation of fatty acids. On the other hand, high respiratory quotients have been found in oligodendrogliomas, suggesting that they depend upon carbohydrate alone as an energy source. It has been pointed out that this higher glycolytic rate is not dissimilar to that found in embryonic cerebral tissue.

Many attempts have been made to find relationships between the uncontrolled proliferation of tumors, their metabolic activity patterns, and their enzyme activities.[3] Measurements of total enzyme activity have been unrevealing, and it is now believed that alterations of isozyme patterns are more likely to reflect the metabolism and growth of tumor cells.[1,2] Data collected to date indicate that it is likely that loss of regulatory enzymes that are determinants of metabolic processes is the key to both the unbridled proliferation and the metabolic anomalies found in cancer cells. Additionally, the similarity of these results to certain immunological properties of tumors is notable. In cancer, antigens that characterize differentiated tissues often disappear, while tumor specific neoantigens appear. In many instances, the neoantigens are identifiable as fetal proteins. An aberration of gene expression characterized by loss of both enzymatic and antigenic proteins normally present in adult, differentiated tissue and the acquisition of proteins (both enzymatically active and antigenically identifiable) present in fetal tissue are related to repression and expression of varying portions of the total cellular genome. Therefore, it is by no means surprising that characteristic metabolic changes can be found in various types of malignant tumors.

In addition to alterations in biochemical pathways directly related to molecular neoplastic transformation, there are also changes definable as a result of the altered environment in which the neoplasm is situated or which it creates for itself. For example, alterations in blood supply and metabolite availability may affect both the rate of growth and the viability of tumor cells. Mechanical factors, such as compression within fascial planes or orientation of fiber tracts in the nervous system, will also affect the direction and perhaps the rate of growth. Histologic examination of tumors often demonstrates differences in cell type and in degree of differentiation from one part of the tumor to another. This histologic variation may be associated with considerable variation in biochemical activity. In the case of human glial tumors,[2] it has been demonstrated that there are three main zones, each differing in their blood supply. In quite malignant tumors, there is a large area of central necrosis surrounded by a rim of living tumor. Vessels show a transition from capillaries to sinusoids, which are largest and fewest at the edge of the necrosis. The necrotic center contains only cell debris, extravasated blood, and thrombosed sinusoids. Marked endothelial cell proliferation is found in the actively growing superficial parts of the more malignant gliomas, and in the zone containing the largest sinusoids bordering the edge of the necrotic area marked adventitial proliferation may be found. This area has the greatest cellularity, the cells are better differentiated, and the rate of growth and mitosis is greatest. Cells in the mid zone are less well differentiated but show less evidence of mitotic activity than those in the outer zone. The description of oxygen availability in different parts of the tumor is therefore likely to be complex and dynamic throughout all stages of its growth.

Since the original description[3] of hypoxic but viable (Fig. 94–1) cell populations in solid tumors, a number of experimental neoplasms have been studied; most contain from 10 to 50 percent hypoxic cells,[4–8] which may be present in tumors as small as 1 mm.[7,8] Radiobiologic data suggest that hypoxic cell populations are also present in human tumors,[9–11] although rigorous experimental determinations are lacking.

Intermediary metabolism specifically in hypoxic tumor cells has in general been elucidated only indirectly. It was shown[12] in a DS-carcinosarcoma implanted into and replacing rat kidney (so that cannulation of the rat's renal artery and vein permitted measurement of tumor blood flow and effluent metabolites) that the critical radius[3] for O_2 diffusion was only 75 percent that for glucose. As tumor size increased, the lactate/

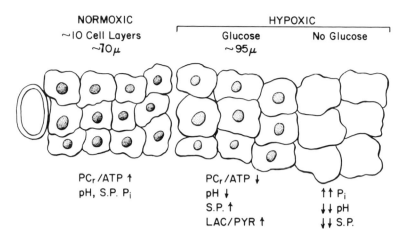

Figure 94–1. Pictorial representation of metabolic events in three hypothetical zones of a solid tumor: normoxic, hypoxic but viable and metabolizing, and hypoxic "doomed to die" cells are depicted.

pyruvate ratio in tumor venous blood increased and ($V_{O_2}/V_{Glucose}$) decreased. These findings support the contention that areas of anaerobic glycolysis occur in tumors,[13] related to the presence of hypoxic but metabolizing cells. Findings compatible with anaerobic glycolysis have been shown by ^{31}P NMR in five ischemic human kidneys containing hypernephromas, in which pH was lower and ATP higher in tumor tissue than in surrounding renal tissue.[14]

It is likely that specific enzyme levels, growth rates, or differentiation of different lines of tumor will have an effect on the specific responses of energy metabolism to hypoxia in tumor cells.[15] Interestingly, there is little evidence for the manner in which tumor cell metabolism adapts to chronic hypoxia. Activities of pyruvate kinase (PKI), phosphofructokinase (PFK), cytochrome oxidase (COX), and superoxide dismutase (SOD) in HeLa and HT 1080 fibrosarcoma cells do not change following exposure to hypoxia (PO_2 = 15 torr), while normal cells (rat lung fibroblasts and WI-38 human fibroblasts) show increases in PKI and PFK and decreases in COX and SOD[16] under these conditions. Adaptive alterations other than those in enzyme levels may occur in tumor cells, of course.

Another, more controversial metabolic alteration seen in neoplasms is aberrant pH values and presumably, therefore, abnormal pH regulation. It has even been proposed that a persistent change in the pH alters intracellular conditions in such a manner that control mechanisms of growth and regulation are disturbed.[17] Certainly, a lowering of pH can be caused by increased aerobic or anerobic glycolysis with concurrent production of lactic acid. For example, some tumor-inducing viruses have ATP-ase activity, which could contribute to the pool of available ADP and phosphate, thus inducing an increased glycolytic rate. However, increased acid production can take place entirely unrelated to glycolysis by an increased rate of lipolysis. Alternatively, increased glycolysis could be induced by increasing the flow of inorganic phosphate into the cell. Primary alterations in the cell membrane could affect the normally present sodium-proton antiporter. In this respect, it is interesting (although open to interpretation either as a cause or an effect) that sodium levels in malignant tumors appear typically to be very high.

As with energy metabolism, pH values expressed in tumors will be strongly dependent upon the tumor's environment. This is because the rate of delivery of acid-producing metabolic substrate, and the rate of removal of acid products of metabolism, will clearly be dependent upon the perfusion of the tissue and/or the level of oxygen available to the metabolic apparatus of the cell.

HIGH RESOLUTION NMR STUDIES OF TUMORS

Energy Metabolism in Cell Suspensions and Implanted Tumors

Studies of tumor cell suspensions, principally by ^{31}P NMR, have been carried out by several groups.

In 1977, Evans and Kaplan[18] and Navon et al.[19] studied ^{31}P spectra of HeLa and Ehrlich ascites tumor cells and their acid extracts. These and other investigators described prominent resonances from various phospholipid metabolites, which are discussed in a later section. In the acid extracts of HeLa cells, inorganic phosphate (P_i) was present in highest concentration (1.9 μmol), followed by ATP (1.3 μmol), phosphorylcholine (0.9 μmol), phosphocreatine (0.3 μmol, perhaps spuriously low due to acid lability), UTP (0.3 μmol), NAD pool (0.2 μmol), and sugar phosphates (glucose-6-P and fructose-1,6-diP, 0.03–0.17 μmol). Other resonances in the "sugar phosphate" region were not resolved or assigned. In contrast, Ehrlich ascites cells lacked UTP and phosphocreatine (PCr); glucose-6-P was not observed, while both fructose biphosphate anomers were present in larger amounts.[19] In a more recent study, however, PCr was observed in intact Ehrlich ascites cells by Gupta and Yushok.[20]

Navon et al.[4] estimated ATP/ADP ratios in HeLa, lymphoid, and Friend erythroleukemia cells; in the lymphoid cells, the ratio was high, while in the other lines it approached unity. In addition, the lymphoid cells showed less change than the other lines upon addition of glucose, and the authors speculated that this might reflect a slower rate of metabolism. Although changes in the "sugar phosphate" region were observed, they were generally not resolved owing to the inherent linewidths and multiple resonances in this region of the spectrum.

Treatment of HeLa cells with iodoacetate resulted in depletion of nucleoside triphosphates and phosphocreatine and accumulation of fructose-1,6-diP; dinitrophenol diminished ATP levels without accumulation of sugar phosphates.[18] These results are in accord with established theory, and similar findings were reported later by Yushok and Gupta.[22]

Several years later, Melner et al.[23] evaluated the effects of the mitogenic peptide epidermal growth factor (EGF) upon cultured A-431 human epidermoid carcinoma (EC) cells and SV-40 virus transformed mouse fibroblasts (MF). In neither of these cell lines is EGF mitogenic; rather, it inhibits their growth, an effect perhaps mediated by a protein kinase; morphologic changes are induced in EC cells, and uptake of deoxyglucose is stimulated in MF cells. In the EC cells, Melner et al. observed decreases in ATP levels and increases in P_i and "sugar phosphates" (or phosphomonoesters) between 80 and 160 minutes following exposure to EGF. Similar effects were observed from 20 to 40 minutes in MF cells. The NMR measurements were confirmed in EC cells by chemical determinations of ATP in perchloric acid extracts.

In 1981, Griffiths et al.[24] reported the first ^{31}P NMR investigation of a solid tumor in situ in a living animal. Walker 256 carcinosarcomas were implanted subcutaneously in rats. Spectra of tumors and normal muscle were obtained with surface coils in a topical magnetic resonance (TMR) spectrometer operating at 32.5 MHz. The tumors were found to lack observable phosphocreatine, and the ratios of sugar phosphates, P_i, and phosphodiesters to ATP were elevated. A later study by this group[25,26] evaluated human tumors implanted in mice: anaplastic MT tumors, fibrosarcomas, spindle cell sarcomas, Lewis lung carcinomas, and B16 melanomas. In all types of tumor, the ATP/P_i ratio (about 2.5 to 1) was lower than in contralateral, uninvolved skeletal muscle (about 8 to 1). These reports gave few details of the sizes of the tumors that were studied or of any variations of spectra with tumor growth.

In some tumor spectra PCr was relatively prominent, but controls were not done in this study to rule out the possibility that this resonance reflects spectral contamination by the high levels of PCr in muscle surrounding the tumor implants. An in vivo ^{31}P study by Griffiths et al.[27] of a primary rhabdomyosarcoma in situ on a human hand revealed a large PCr resonance. We have observed PCr both in acid extracts (Fig. 94–2) and in vivo studies (Fig. 94–3) of the BA1112 rhabdomyosarcoma in rats. In these studies, PCr levels varied with stage of development and therapy; changes in PCr resonances following antineoplastic therapy and stage of tumor development have been observed by others and will be discussed below. In addition, as Griffiths[26] has pointed out, the presence of PCr in tumors will vary according to the cell type of origin and degree of differentiation of the tumor.

A series of subcutaneously implanted tumors in mice were studied in vivo with ^{31}P NMR by Ng et al.[28,29] at rest, as a function of growth, and after therapy with alkylating agents, radiation, and hyperthermia.[30] Studies were performed at 80.9 MHz using surface coils. The tumors studied were MOPC 104E myeloma, Dunn osteosarcoma, Dunning M5076 ovarian, colon 26, mammary 16/C adenocarcinoma, and human colon, lung, and breast tumors.

In general, the human and murine tumors were considered to exhibit the same spectral features. No ^{31}P resonances unique to a given tumor type were observed in these experiments, although the amounts of different metabolites present in different tumors exhibited considerable variation. The authors suggested that the size and stage of growth of the tumors studied were responsible for the observed variations in levels of metabolites. All of the above tumors contained little ADP and pyridine nucleotide (NAD pool) relative to ATP. Some tumors exhibited a PCr resonance, particularly at early stages of growth, but most did not. Prominent peaks in the "sugar phosphate" (SP) region and high levels of P_i were a uniform feature, however.

In general, tumors appeared to become less metabolically active as they grew larger. Small tumors had high levels of ATP, PCr, P_i, and SP. Tumors of about 1 gram exhibited decreases in PCr and pH (assessed from P_i), little change in ATP, and elevations of P_i and SP. Large tumors (grossly necrotic, ulcerated lesions were not studied) usually had little or no observable PCr or ATP (although some tumor lines displayed ATP resonances even at very late stages of growth), more prominent SP and P_i res-

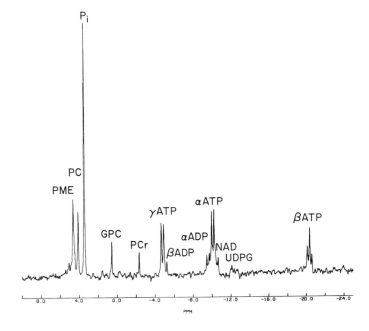

Figure 94–2. H-1 decoupled P-31 NMR spectrum at 80.9 MHz of a perchloric acid extract from a subcutaneously implanted BA1112 rhabdomyosarcoma in a rat. (From Sostman et al.: Magn Reson Imag 2:265–278, 1984. Used by permission of Pergamon Press, Ltd.)

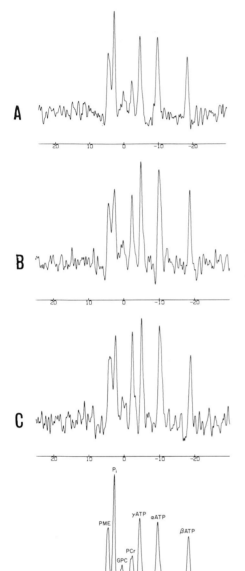

Figure 94–3. In vivo ^{31}P spectra of rat rhabdomyosarcoma before and at intervals after low-dose radiation therapy (3 Gy). *A*, Preirradiation. *B*, 17 minutes after irradiation. *C*, 6 hours after irradiation. *D*, 23 hours after irradiation. (From Sostman et al.: Magn Reson Imag 2:265–278, 1984. Used by permission of Pergamon Press, Ltd.)

onances, and further decreased pH.[29] These results are in general agreement with those of Carpinelli et al.,[31] and again one might implicate a relatively ischemic or hypoxic cell population in larger tumors.

Chemotherapy of MPOC 104E with BCNU or cyclophosphamide resulted in increases in PCr and decreased ATP/PCr ratios prior to changes in tumor mass (assessed by blood levels of tumor idiotypic IgM). Decreases in blood IgM lagged behind changes in phosphorus metabolites. These results suggest that in vivo metabolic studies can in at least some instances detect tumor response at an earlier stage than conventional methods. In the mammary 16/C tumor treated with adriamycin, there were smaller reductions in tumor mass that were associated with similar but far less dramatic metabolic changes.[28] Changes in tumor spectra following therapy have also been reported by others. In preliminary in vivo studies of rodents with subcutaneously implanted brain tumors,[32] administration of cyclophosphamide resulted in decreases in ATP and increases in P_i in tumor (but not in muscle) before histologic changes were seen in the tumor. A later study, by this group, of RIF-1 tumors treated with cyclophosphamide showed decreases in P_i to correlate with the initial decrease in cell proliferation and increases in pH to correlate with maximum regrowth delay.[33] A clinically apparent failure of response of a human rhabdomyosarcoma to adriamycin therapy was associated with a substantial decrease in PCr on a repeat examination.[27] As pointed out by Bore,[34] the problems of localization of the sources of signals inherent in surface coil technique and the numerous causes for changes in PCr levels render an unequivocal interpretation of the etiology of such changes difficult at this stage.

A study of 10 and 15 Gy irradiation of the mouse mammary carcinoma NU-82 demonstrated 30 percent decreases in ATP levels during the first 6 hours after treatment at 10 Gy, but 50 percent declines that lasted up to 48 hours for 15 Gy.[35] Mammary 16/ C carcinoma treated with radiation (14 Gy) showed complete disappearance of PCr within 15 minutes (Fig. 94–4). This was followed by changes similar to those induced by chemotherapy with subsequent increases in PCr associated with reduced tumor mass.[28,36] On the other hand, in the BA1112 rhabdomyosarcoma, we have observed significant early *increases* in PCr (Fig. 94–3) following a lower dose (3 Gy) of radiation and *decreases* in PCr following a higher dose (20 Gy).

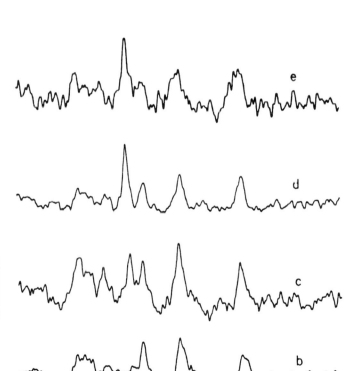

Figure 94–4. In vivo ^{31}P spectra of mouse carcinoma before (*a*) and at intervals of 15 min (*b*), 9 hr (*c*), 28 hr (*d*), and 40 hr (*e*) after radiation therapy (14 Gy). Peak assignments: ATP (I–III); Pcr (IV); P_i (VI); phosphomonoester (VII). V is not assigned. (From Evanochko et al.: PNAS *80*:334–338, 1983. Used by permission and the courtesy of Dr. William T. Evanochko.)

Hyperthermic exposure of Dunn osteosarcoma[30] and mammary 16/C adeno-carcinoma[36] resulted in decreases in ATP, PCr, and pH and a marked increase in P_i. The spectra were considered to approximate, to a first order, a weighted superposition of the spectra of dead cells and untreated cells. Changes in the ATP/P_i ratio were proportional to heat dose and cell kill,[30] as might be expected from the known effects of hyperthermia.[37]

The above studies comprise an extensive NMR survey of tumors and early descriptions of in vivo metabolic responses to therapy. Further work is needed to provide important correlative observations. For example, the radiation response could be interpreted in light of the phenomenon of "reoxygenation" (q.v.), but the fraction of hypoxic cells in the tumors at times coinciding with the spectra are not available. As another example, changes in PCr levels (in the absence of signal contamination by surrounding tissues) could reflect alterations in PCr formation, utilization, or both. Shifts in the creatine kinase equilibrium have been shown to occur with tissue growth.[38] Saturation transfer experiments could be of value in differentiating such processes and should be done in future studies in which artifactual changes are also excluded. The mechanisms of the changes described above are unproven and further research must be directed toward their elucidation, but the sensitivity and potential utility of NMR measurements are obvious from these results.

Studies of Tumor pH

From measurement of P_i chemical shift, it was shown in Ehrlich ascites cells that during both aerobic and anaerobic glycolysis, intra- and extracellular pH differed by less than the experimental accuracy of 0.2 pH unit.[19] This result agreed with pH measurements made using 5,5-dimethyl-2,4-oxazolidinedione (DMO). When the pH of the medium was decreased suddenly to demonstrate intracellular P_i, a pH gradient between intra- and extracellular compartments was measurable; it decayed with a time course in reasonable agreement with previous lactate transport measurements. Navon et al. also found no pH gradient in HeLa, Friend leukemia, and lymphoid cells.[21] A later study, however, showed the pH_i of Ehrlich ascites cells to be more alkaline (by 0.5 unit) than pH_e when oxygen was bubbled through the cells and pH_e was less than 7.1. When nitrogen was substituted or when pH_e was acidic, the pH gradient collapsed rapidly as ATP levels declined.[39] This study was performed at 37° C in an oxygenated medium, whereas the previous study was done at 20° C in a static suspension. This is a dramatic demonstration of the model dependence of results and indicates that Ehrlich cells do regulate pH and that this regulation depends upon energy metabolism.

In the in vivo studies of the Walker 256 carcinosarcoma performed by Griffiths et al.,[24] tumor pH (assessed by P_i chemical shift) was evaluated at rest and after infusions of glucose (0.6 g/kg) and deoxyglucose. There was a small (0.07 pH unit) but statistically significant difference between tumor and muscle pH, but no change in either tumor or muscle pH was observed after glucose infusion. However, when the tumor was rendered ischemic, a marked decrease in pH (0.78 pH unit) was produced. Deoxyglucose-6-phosphate (DG-6-P) caused transient acidification of tumors; interestingly, the P_i and DG-6-P chemical shifts gave different pH values in tumors but not in muscle. This finding was suggested to reflect either compartmentation effects or failure to adequately resolve DG-6-P from other "sugar phosphate" peaks, which are substantially more prominent in tumors than in normal tissues. In this group's study of human tumors implanted in mice, the pH_i was not significantly lower in tumors (7.15 ± 0.03) than in contralateral, uninvolved skeletal muscle.[25,26]

The relatively normal tumor pH and failure to acidify tumor with hyperglycemia as reported in the above studies[19,20,24-26] is in contrast to three more recent ^{31}P studies.

In studies of FLC cells in vitro and in vivo, Carpinelli et al.[31] observed a decrease in tumor pH_i by about 0.35 unit as tumor mass increased. This was associated with progressively increased signal from the "sugar phosphate" region, compared both with small tumors and with tumors grown in vitro.

Chan, Radda, and Ross[14] compared ^{31}P spectra from hypernephromas in situ in five ischemic human kidneys with spectra from the surrounding non-neoplastic renal tissue. They found higher ATP levels in the tumors (0.78 μmole/g) than in non-neoplastic tissue (0.23 μmole/g); this was confirmed by enzymatic assay. Tumor intracellular pH was 0.21 unit less than normal renal tissue.

Evelhoch et al.[40] administered glucose to female C_3H/Anf mice bearing subcutaneous murine RIF-1 tumors and observed a decrease in intracellular pH by about 0.45 pH unit coincident with elevation of serum glucose from 6 mM to 15–25 mM. Phosphocreatine decreased by about 50 percent during the same period. Normal muscle was unaffected by hyperglycemia. In four of nine tumors, two populations were observed; one was unaffected by hyperglycemia and the other showed a decrease in pH. The etiology of this effect is unknown, although it is tempting to speculate that a hypoxic, ischemic cell fraction is responsible in the latter group. The discrepancy between the findings of Griffiths et al.[24] and Evelhoch et al.[40] could reflect differences in metabolism or vascularization of the specific neoplasms studied, or in experimental conditions. Griffiths et al.[24] used a lower dose of glucose relative to the animal's body weight, and they did not measure blood glucose. Since it has been reported that substantial degrees of hyperglycemia (blood glucose, 25 to 50 mM) are required to depress tumor pH,[41] their results in this context must be regarded as inconclusive.

In evaluating the apparently conflicting results discussed above, one must consider that in addition to potential variation in pH response of different tumor types, the size and environment of the tumor may be of great importance. In both normo- and hyperglycemic rats, larger tumors may achieve lower pH values than smaller, presumably better vascularized tumors.[41] In vitro studies[42] indicate that at least some tumor cells may increase their glycolytic rate under hypoxic conditions, and the ability to rid both the cell and the interstitial fluid of resulting lactate would then be taxed severely under hypoxic conditions. In one report, tumors in an exponential phase of growth responded to hyperglycemia with a decrease in "extracellular" pH (measured by 1 mm electrode) by 0.54 pH unit but showed no change in intracellular pH (measured by DMO). This was associated with a threefold increase in both blood and tumor lactate levels;[43] tumor glucose was elevated for only two hours, but tumor lactate levels were elevated for 6 hours, and pH_e remained depressed for up to 12 hours. This suggests that impaired lactate clearance was partly (but not completely) responsible for the prolonged acidification of the tumors.

An important, recent in vivo study[44] of the murine RIF-1 tumor showed the aggregate tumor pH (determined from P_i) to correlate well ($r = .868$) with the mobile perfused fraction of the tumor (Fig. 94–5). An inverse correlation was also present with the P_i:ATP ratio. This is the first demonstration of an estimate of the hypoxic cell fraction by NMR in an in situ tumor.

Metabolism of Hypoxic Tumor Cells

The effects of hypoxia upon ATP levels and intracellular pH of suspensions of Ehrlich ascites tumor cells were studied with ^{31}P NMR by Navon et al.[19] They were

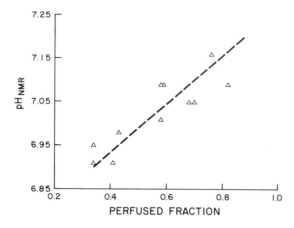

Figure 94–5. Correlation of tumor pH with perfused cell fraction. The pH was determined from P_i chemical shift. (Redrawn from Evelhoch et al.: Society of Magnetic Resonance in Medicine Third Annual Meeting Program, p. 223, 1984, through the courtesy of Dr. J. J. H. Ackerman.)

able to demonstrate preservation of ATP signal in hypoxic cells fed glucose and depletion of ATP in hypoxic cells fed deoxyglucose, which is not utilized beyond the hexokinase reaction. They also found that anaerobic glycolysis decreases the pH of the medium but observed no difference between intracellular and extracellular pH. One must, of course, distinguish between hypoxia and ischemia. Significant differences in the alterations in PCr and ATP levels attendant upon hypoxia[45] and ischemia[46] have also been shown in vivo by NMR in the gerbil brain. In general, in vivo, one would expect hypoxic tumor cells to be ischemic also.

A recent ^{31}P and ^{13}C NMR investigation of aerobic and anaerobic glycolysis in suspensions of Ehrlich ascites cells by Gillies[42] showed a 50 percent increase in glucose consumption and a 600 percent increase in lactate production under conditions of complete hypoxia (95 percent N_2:5 percent CO_2). This was accompanied by a drop in intracellular pH and rise in intracellular P_i beyond that elicited by addition of glucose (20 to 50 mM) under aerobic (95 percent O_2:5 percent CO_2) conditions. However, these experiments were also performed in static cell suspensions, which permitted accumulation of lactate and other metabolites; they thus include a significant component of "ischemia" as well as hypoxia.

The redox state of tumor cells and its measurement are obviously pertinent to the evaluation of hypoxia in tumors. Several attempts have been made to design chemotherapeutic agents active against hypoxic tumor cells.[4] This has resulted in evidence supporting the hypothesis[47] that hypoxic tumor cells exist in a reductive environment. This association of hypoxia and high reduction potential is predictable and had previously been demonstrated in anaerobic cultures of bacteria.[4] Two classes of drug have been developed that depend upon reductive activation for their toxicity: the quinone bioreductive alkylating agents (e.g., mitomycin C) and the nitroheterocyclic radiosensitizers (e.g., metronidazole). The former may require NADPH-dependent biotransformation in order to be activated to alkylating species.[48–51] The latter, in addition to sensitizing hypoxic cells to radiation effects, are directly and selectively toxic to hypoxic cells in vitro.[4] It appears that this toxicity depends upon reduction of the nitro group to *N*-hydroxy and amine metabolites,[4,52–54] which in turn depends upon the state of cellular oxygenation. The nitroreductive activity in hypoxic tumor cells has been suggested to be analogous to the NADH/NADPH-dependent nitro-reductive activity in liver microsomes. It is of interest in this context that liver hypoxia leads to increased levels of NADH and NADPH.[55] The latter would likely be a general phenomenon in all types of mammalian cells as a result of hypoxia[55–57] and might be detectable in neoplasms by ^{13}C NMR.[58,59]

Other findings have been reported that suggest differences between normoxic and hypoxic tumor cells that also might be demonstrable by NMR. Hypoxic cells are more sensitive to hyperthermia; this has been suggested to result from alterations in environmental pH,[60] nutritional status,[61] and the cell membrane.[62] The glucose analogs, 5-thio- and 2-deoxy-glucose, may be preferentially cytotoxic to hypoxic tumor cells.[63,64] This has been explained as reduction by nonmetabolizable substrate of catabolic capacity in hypoxic cells, although other mechanisms are not excluded. All of these alterations could be manifest in ^{31}P, ^{13}C, or ^{1}H NMR spectra.

Tumor Membranes and Phospholipid Metabolites in Tumors

Resonances from phosphodiester and phosphomonoester compounds involved in lipid metabolism have been detected in a variety of tumors[18,19,40,65,66] and other systems.[67-69] A potentially significant finding was that of Navon et al.,[69] who studied three mutant yeasts. Two strains (pgi—lacks phosphoglucose isomerase, and pfk—lacks phosphofructokinase) showed only a glycerophosphorylcholine (GPC) resonance, while the wild type exhibited GPC, glycerophosphorylethanolamine (GPE), and glycerophosphorylserine (GPS). Although these compounds as well as phosphorylcholine (PC) and phosphorylethanolamine (PE) had been detected in various tissues by classical methods, the work of Navon et al. directly related them to specific genome expression. This result is relevant to the studies of tumors described below, since tumor enzymes (both isozyme and protein contents) and phospholipid metabolites may both differ from those in analogous normal tissues. The former are known characteristically to reflect specific tumor genome expression,[3,70] which might suggest that the latter do also.[71]

Phospholipids are, of course, important components of biologic membranes. As GPC and GPE may be involved in phospholipid catabolism and PC and PE are involved in phospholipid synthesis, it is plausible that their proportions in cells may reflect membrane structure and that the flux through them may reflect rates of membrane synthesis and catabolism. This has been suggested by Agris and Campbell,[65] who observed a fourfold increase in cytoplasmic PC (and possibly GPC) during the DMSO-induced erythroid differentiation of Friend leukemia cells (FLC) using ^{31}P and ^{1}H NMR. At the same time, during differentiation, an increase of similar magnitude was found in resonances assigned to methylene protons of triglycerides. These observations would be consistent with an increase in phospholipid synthesis and perhaps also catabolism, which might reflect accelerated turnover of membrane components during differentiation. This might be consistent with the observation by Haran et al., using 0-17 NMR, of increased membrane permeability in DMSO-treated FLC.[72] A recent ^{31}P NMR study[31] of FLC includes a figure (I.b) that could be compatible with increased PC following DMSO exposure, associated with a decrease in GPC and GPE.

In addition to variation of phospholipid metabolites with differentiation of a particular cell line, marked differences in phospholipid metabolites have been noted between tumors of different lines. Evans and Kaplan[18] found little GPC or GPE in HeLa cells, although there was a large PC peak. Navon et al.[21] found that lymphoid cells, Friend leukemia cells, and HeLa S-3 cells had quite different levels of phospholipid metabolites; they also observed more GPC and less PC in HeLa cells than did Evans and Kaplan. The PC signal in the lymphoid cells increased upon addition of glucose in at least some instances, while GPC and GPE in the Friend and HeLa cells did not. Ehrlich ascites tumor cells exhibited PC, GPC, and GPE;[19] in this system, the concentration of PC in resting and glucose-fed cells was the same. Walker carcinosarcoma cells contain both GPC and PGE,[24] and PC has been tentatively identified in human hypernephroma.[14] In addition, it is likely that the alterations in the imperfectly resolved (in vivo) signals from the "sugar phosphate" region noted in a wide variety of resting and treated (chemotherapy, radiotherapy, and hyperthermia) human and animal tumor cells[28,30,36] may include alterations in PC or PE levels.[73]

Studies, using ^{31}P NMR, of FLC subcutaneously implanted in mice have shown significant increases in GPC and GPE with growth in tumor mass[31] temporally coincident with decreases in intracellular pH and increases in P_i. Although no mechanistic relationship is demonstrated, one might speculate that the elevation of GPC and GPE levels reflects membrane catabolism in cells undergoing ischemic injury.

Recent studies of two patients with metastatic neuroblastoma are of interest.[74] In both, elevated levels of phosphomonoester (PME), thought to be PE, were present in the tumors. As the metastases regressed following resection of the primaries, the PME levels decreased in one patient and normalized in the other.

Thus, although there is as yet no coherent explanation for the notable variations in phospholipid metabolites observed in tumors by NMR, it appears plausible that serial study of their concentrations in a particular cell line may yield information concerning membrane turnover or other metabolic events, and it might even be that patterns of phospholipid metabolites are a hallmark of different tumor types. Recent evidence suggests that resonances in the "sugar phosphate" region of ^{31}P spectra of several tumors that were previously considered to represent glycolytic intermediates are more likely PC and PE.[73] We have demonstrated the presence of PC in the BA1112 rhabdomyosarcoma. If confirmed in other systems, these findings would corroborate earlier work and suggest that alterations in phospholipid metabolites may be a useful tumor marker. Considering the alterations in these resonances with changes in the biologic status of tumors induced by growth, perhaps by hypoxia/ischemia, and by therapy, further study of the role of these metabolites seems to be warranted.

Studies of tumor cell membranes with NMR appear to be limited. A ^{31}P NMR study of isolated plasma membrane from normal hamster NIL 8 cells and cells transformed with hamster sarcoma virus revealed no differences, but ^{1}H spectroscopy of this preparation after incubation at 4° C for four days showed increased signal intensity from methylene groups and a prominent, narrow resonance from the phosphatidylcholine methyl protons.[75] This result is consistent with reduced lipid ordering in the transformed membrane, perhaps reflecting reduced interaction with membrane proteins[76] or changes in membrane composition.[77]

Block et al.[78] compared the ^{1}H spectra of intact EL-4 cells, membrane preparations and lipid extracts with those of mouse spleen cells and studied the effects of concanavalin-A (con-A) binding to cell membranes. Lipid resonances were observed in the intact cell spectra which corresponded to those in membrane preparations and lipid extracts. Those in the EL-4 spectra were sharper and better resolved than in the spleen cell spectra. This could reflect greater lipid mobility in the EL-4 membranes. Experimental conditions, such as sample inhomogeneity, could explain these differences, since spleen cells are somewhat prone to aggregation. However, other proton NMR experiments in a variety of normal, transformed, and malignant cells tend to confirm these results and the interpretation of greater lipid mobility.[79,80] Line broadening was produced when the EL-4 membranes were treated with con-A; control studies suggested that reduced lipid mobility was the cause of the broadening, an interpretation supported by the ^{1}H NMR studies of con-A binding to murine myeloma membranes reported by Tellier et al.[81]

Potential correlates of changes in lipid structure or lipid-protein interactions in tumor cell membranes could include alterations in contact inhibition, turnover of cell surface antigens (and thus tumor immunogenicity), and resistance to chemotherapy.[82,83] Studies of membrane lipid resonances in cell lines exhibiting variations in such properties might reveal findings of biologic interest and potential clinical usefulness.

Tumor Cell Differentiation

As described above, Agris and Campbell[65] have shown distinct changes in phospholipid metabolites upon differentiaton of FLC induced by DMSO.

Changes in the levels of phosphorus-containing metabolites were evaluated in two neuroblastoma clones by Pettegrew et al.[84] The N-18 line differentiates (forms neurites) when grown in presence of dibutyryl cyclic AMP (db-cAMP) or when observed in confluent culture, while the C-46 line shows no morphologic differentiation under either of these conditions. Both clonal lines were studied by ^{31}P NMR in the presence and absence of confluency and db-cAMP treatment. Irrespective of culture conditions, the N-18 cells showed much greater amounts of unidentified nucleoside monophosphate and phosphodiester compounds but less dipyrophosphodiester. The C-46 cells showed neither morphologic differentiation nor changes in ^{31}P spectra with culture conditions. The N-18 cells, which formed long (30 μ) neurites in confluent culture in the presence of db-cAMP, showed disappearance of another nucleoside monophosphate resonance, decrease in phosphodiester by 17.4 percent, and smaller decreases in PC, GPC, and GPE. These changes were accompanied by increases in dipyrophosphodiester, pyrophosphate, and "sugar phosphate" signals.

Navon et al.[85] studied the differentiation of neuroblastoma x glioma cells with ^{1}H spectroscopy. The cells were induced to differentiate with prostaglandin E_1 and theophylline. The differentiated cells were found to contain significantly higher levels of glutamine than did the undifferentiated precursors. Interestingly, fewer resolvable signals (including those from glutamine) were obtained with a spin-echo pulse sequence than with the use of solvent suppression with a repetitive low power selective pulse. It was suggested that the absence of sharp signals from glutamine on spin-echo sequences could reflect binding effects.

Differences between typical and variant small cell lung carcinoma lines grown from clinical specimens have recently been reported.[86] Phosphocreatine was present in large quantity in variant cells but absent in typical cells, despite equivalent levels of creatine kinase. Uridine diphosphoglucose was present in the tyypical cells but absent in the variant cells.

In studies of human breast carcinoma lines with and without estrogen receptors, several differences were observed,[87] including differences in PCr and phosphodiester levels and pH.

These studies indicate the potential of NMR studies for the metabolic characterization of tumors undergoing differentiation (or dedifferentiation) and distinguishing metabolic variants of tumors of the same class.

Summary

There are relatively few NMR studies of tumor metabolism, given the intense interest evoked by either subject individually. Certain common findings can be identified, while numerous areas of uncertainty and many incomplete and apparently contradictory results must be acknowledged.

The spectra of neoplasms are distinct from those of normal tissues. NMR studies of living cells confirm that the relative levels of ubiquitous metabolites, such as P_i and ATP, are regularly different in tumors from those in a variety of normal cells. Novel resonances have been found in the phosphodiester region, while unusually prominent signals regularly occur in the phosphomonoester region of ^{31}P spectra. Frequently, the assignments of these resonances are unknown or controversial, reflecting the difficulties in assigning the same ions of unknown and often imperfectly resolved compounds.

Whether different tumor lines present reproducible and distinct spectra is far less clear. Both positive and negative data relative to this question have been reported; whether this represents biologic or experimental variation or both is not yet clear. The acid-base status of tumors remains controversial after numerous NMR studies, which have not resolved the disputes engendered by microelectrode measurements. Given the multiplicity of factors that may influence tissue pH and its measurement, this is perhaps not too surprising.

Reported results make it clear that NMR experiments can monitor changes in the composition and metabolic status of tumors in real time, as they can in non-neoplastic tissues. Obvious alterations in spectra of neoplastic tissue obtained in vivo and in vitro have been observed consequent upon hypoxia, ischemia, growth, differentiation, nutritional status, and antineoplastic therapy. In general, however, the mechanisms of these changes and their significance are still unknown, and there is considerable descriptive and correlative work yet to be done in all of these settings.

As might be expected, studies of spontaneously arising neoplasms in situ in humans or animals are rare. Consistent differences between tumors grown in vitro and in animals, or between human and animal tumors in the same experimental setting, are not striking. However, comparisons in different laboratories and detailed studies are still lacking.

CLINICAL SIGNIFICANCE AND POTENTIAL APPLICATIONS

It is obvious that NMR studies can have great potential in the elucidation of the basic biology of tumors. The preceding considerations also indicate the potential for NMR spectroscopy to provide increased specificity in separating malignant neoplasms from normal tissue. This might be accomplished in the resting subject, but it is also possible that perturbations of the subject's physiology, such as induced hyperglycemia, may be required, or that isotopic enrichment (such as ^{13}C or ^{19}F glucose or glucose analogues, or ^{15}N amino acids) will prove useful. Certain biologically relevant nuclei, such as ^{15}N, have yet to be studied in much detail[88,89] in tumors, and high resolution proton spectroscopy of tumors has been explored only briefly.[75,85,90,91] If the considerable basic work still to be done continues to indicate that reproducible and quantifiable differences in metabolic processes between tumors and normal tissues are detectable by NMR, it will be necessary to achieve precise spatial localization of the volume of tissue from which spectra are received, and also to evaluate the metabolic processes of inflammatory lesions and benign neoplasms in greater breadth and depth than has yet been done. Differences in metabolism between tumors and benign neoplasms or abnormal but non-neoplastic tissues have been little studied so far. If these goals can be accomplished with results that continue to indicate usefulness, the effects upon the economics as well as the risks and discomforts of medical diagnosis could be enormous.

For example, in clinical radiation therapy tumors are typically treated with multiple small daily doses of radiation. If a relatively small dose of radiation were given to a tumor with a mixed cell population, one would normally expect that the population of well-oxygenated cells would be severely depleted while the population of hypoxic cells would be affected to a much lesser extent. If, shortly after this initial treatment, an experiment to measure the fraction of hypoxic cells were carried out, one would expect that the fraction of hypoxic cells among the survivors would have increased. This does occur if the "measurement" experiments are carried out immediately, but it is not always the case if there is some delay between the priming dose of radiation and measurement of the hypoxic fraction. In fact, the opposite may occur.[92] This observation has been explained by the concept of "reoxygenation." Surviving hypoxic cells may become well oxygenated owing to changes in vascular pattern and oxygen consumption within the tumor. Reoxygenation has been demonstrated in animal tumor systems, and it is felt to occur in at least some human tumors. It may, in fact, be one of the principal reasons for the empirically found success of prolonged radiation therapy treatment schedules. The possibility of reoxygenation makes the need for a method of directly measuring the proportion of hypoxic cells in tumors obvious, since it would then be possible to design treatment schedules to maximize this effect. For example, a single treatment could be given, the tumor observed for reoxygenation, and further treatment given at an optimal time. The necessity for use of radiation sensitizers or high LET radiation, both of which neutralize the relative advantage of hypoxic cells, could be more accurately assessed.

The influence of hypoxic cells on tumor cure is not limited to radiation therapy. Malignant solid tumors that are poorly vascularized or have a low growth fraction are the major cause of mortality from cancer and are typically resistant to cell cycle–active chemotherapy. Hypoxic tumor cells, in addition to their lack of proliferation, may be resistant to various antineoplastic agents for reasons that include achievable concentrations of drug in ischemic tissue, dependence upon aerobic metabolic activation, and participation of molecular oxygen in the drug's action. However, some agents are available that are preferentially toxic to hypoxic cells. Thus, the utility of knowledge of the existence and numbers of hypoxic cells in particular tumors to planning of chemotherapy is perfectly analogous to its importance for radiation therapy.

In addition, there is reason to believe that there must exist metabolic indicators of tumor response to therapy at an early stage. As described above, there is preliminary evidence that such changes may be observable by NMR. If detection of such changes could be accomplished, it would permit the minimization of the toxicity of radiation or chemotherapy to normal tissues while perhaps also improving therapeutic response by permitting not only more accurate design of treatment regimens as indicated above but potentially also improved accuracy in assessing which lesions require more aggressive therapy and which do not. Analysis of tumor differentiation or dedifferentiation resulting from therapy could also be of great value. Of course, the potential of NMR for the direct monitoring of toxic effects of therapy on normal tissues[93,94] is also important in this context, as is the ability to use certain nuclei such as ^{19}F to monitor metabolism of chemotherapeutic agents.[95]

Relaxation measurements and ^1H NMR imaging in tumors are potential sources of information complementary to high resolution spectroscopy. They may well prove to lack the intrinsic specificity of metabolic studies, although the spatial information provided may improve the predictive value of relaxation measurements in the characterization of lesions. Further, although relatively primitive analyses of imaging and proton relaxation data have shown poor specificity in cancer diagnosis, the evidence is hardly conclusive. If more sophisticated analytic techniques (which have yet to be applied to proton NMR tissue characterization) provide more encouraging results, improved accuracy of relaxation measurements in vivo would be a high priority. Such developments would no doubt have significant effects on oncologic practice as a result of the rapidly increasing availability of whole-body NMR imaging devices. The commercial development and medical use of NMR imaging may, as well, provide a critical impetus to the further developments necessary for in vivo spectroscopy to be performed with useful spatial localization.

ACKNOWLEDGMENT

The authors thank Mary Surowiecki for manuscript preparation.

References

1. Weinhouse S: Glycolysis, respiration and anomalous gene expression in experimental hepatomas: G.H.A. Clowes memorial lecture. Cancer Res. *32*:2007–1026, 1972.
2. Timperly WR: Glycolysis in neuroectodermal tumors. *In* Thomas DGT, Graham DI (eds.): Brain Tumours. London, Butterworths, 1980, pp 145–167.
3. Weber G: Enzymology of cancer cells. N Engl J Med *296*:486–493, 1977.
4. Kennedy KA, Teicher BA, Rockwell S, Sartorell AC: The hypoxic tumor cell: A target for selective cancer chemotherapy. Biochem Pharmacol *29*:1–8, 1980.
5. Kallman RF: The phenomenon of reoxygenation and its implications for fractionated radiotherapy. Radiology *105*:135–142, 1972.
6. Rockwell S, Kallman RF, Fajardo LF: Characteristics of a serially transplanted mouse mammary carcinoma and its tissue-culture-adapted derivative. JNCI *49*:735–749, 1972.
7. Rockwell S, Kallman RF: Cellular radiosensitivity and tumor radiation response in the EMT6 tumor cell system. Radiat Res *53*:281–294, 1973.
8. Suit HD, Shalek RJ: Response of anoxic C₃H mouse mammary carcinoma isotransplants (I-25 mm3) to X irradiation. JNCI *31*:479–509, 1963.
9. Bush RS, Jenkin RDT, Allt WEC, et al: Definitive evidence for hypoxic cells influencing cure in cancer therapy. Br J Cancer *37*(Suppl. 3):302–306, 1978.
10. Urtansun R, Band P, Chapman JD, et al: Radiation and high-dose metronidazole in supratentorial glioblastomas. N Engl J Med *294*:1364–1367, 1976.
11. Bush RS, Hill RP: Augmenting radiation effects and model systems. Laryngoscope *85*:1119–1133, 1975.
12. Vaupel P, Braunbeck W, Schultz V, Gunther H, Thews G: Critical O_2 and glucose supply and microcirculation in tumor tissue. Bibl Anat *12*:527–533, 1973.
13. Tannock IF: The relation between cell proliferation and the vascular system in a transplantable mouse mammary tumor. Br J Cancer *22*:258–273, 1968.
14. Chan I, Radda GK, Ross BD: P-31 NMR of renal cell carcinoma in intact ischemic human kidney. Magn Reson Med *1*:131, 1984.
15. Weber G, Stubbs M, Morris HP: Metabolism of hepatomas of different growth rates in situ and during ischemia. Cancer Res *31*:2177–2183, 1971.
16. Simon LM, Robin ED, Theodore J: Differences in oxygen-dependent regulation of enzymes between tumor and normal cell systems in culture. J Cell Physiol *108*:393–400, 1981.
17. Racker E: Bioenergetics and the problem of tumor growth. Am Scientist *60*:56–63, 1972.
18. Evans FE, Kaplan NO: P-31 nuclear magnetic resonance studies of HeLa cells. Proc Natl Acad Sci USA *74*:4909–4913, 1977.
19. Navon G, Ogawa S, Shulman RG, Yamane T: P-31 nuclear magnetic resonance studies of Ehrlich ascites tumor cells. Proc Natl Acad Sci USA *74*:87–91, 1977.
20. Gupta RK, Yushok WD: Noninvasive P-31 NMR probes of free Mg^{2+}, MgATP, and MgADP in intact Ehrlich ascites tumor cells. Proc Natl Acad Sci USA *77*:2487–2491, 1980.
21. Navon G, Navon R, Shulman RG, Yamane T: Phosphate metabolites in lymphoid, Friend erythroleukemia, and HeLa cells observed by high-resolution P-31 nuclear magnetic resonance. Proc Natl Acad Sci USA *75*:891–895, 1978.
22. Yushok WD, Gupta RK: Phosphocreatine in Ehrlich ascites tumor cells detected by noninvasive P-31 NMR spectroscopy. Biochem Biophys Res Comm *95*:73–81, 1980.
23. Melner MH, Sawyer ST, Evanchko WT, Ng TC, Glickson JD, Puett D: Phosphorus-31 nuclear magnetic resonance analysis of epidermal growth factor action in A-431 human epidermoid carcinoma cells and SV-40 virus transformed mouse fibroblasts. Biochemistry *22*:2039–2042, 1983.
24. Griffiths JR, Stevens AN, Iles RA, Gordon RE, Shaw D: P-31 NMR investigation of solid tumors in the living rat. Biosci Rep *1*:319–325, 1981.
25. Stevens AN, Adams GE, Gordon RE, Griffiths JR, Iles RA, Sheldon PW: P-31 nuclear magnetic resonance spectra of tumours and muscle in the anesthetized mouse. Biochem Soc Trans *10*:507–508, 1982.
26. Griffiths JR, Iles RA: NMR studies of tumours. Biosci Rep *2*:719–725, 1982.
27. Griffiths JR, Cady E, Edwards RHT, McCready VR, Wilkie DR, Wiltshaw E: P-31 NMR studies of a human tumour in situ. Lancet *1*:1435–1436, 1983.
28. Ng TC, Evanochko WT, Hiramoto RN, et al: P-31 NMR spectroscopy of in vivo tumors. J Magn Reson *49*:271–286, 1982.
29. Evanochko WT, Ng TC, Glickson JD, Durant JR, Corbett TH: Human tumors as examined by in vivo P-31 NMR in athymic mice. Biochem Biophys Res Comm *109*:1346–1352, 1982.
30. Lilly MB, Ng TC, Evanochko WT, et al: Loss of high-energy phosphate following hyperthermia demonstrated by in vivo P-31 nuclear magnetic resonance spectroscopy. Cancer Res *44*:633–638, 1984.
31. Carpinelli G, Maddaluno G, Podo F, Proietti E, Santurbano L, Bellardeli F: P-31 NMR studies on subcutaneous tumors in mice injected with Friend erythroleukemia cells. Magn Reson Med *1*:124, 1984.
32. Naruse S, Horikawa Y, Tanaka C, et al: P-31 in vivo NMR studies on experimental brain tumors using topical magnetic resonance. Magn Reson Med *1*:211, 1984.
33. Evanochko WT, Schiffer LM, Ng TC, Braunschweiger PG, Glickson JD: In vivo P-31 NMR as a noninvasive index for timing sequential doses of chemotherapeutic agents. Presented at the Third Annual Meeting of the Society of Magnetic Resonance in Medicine, New York, August, 1984.
34. Bore P: P-31 NMR studies of human tumours. Lancet *2*:458–459, 1983.
35. Sijens PE, Bovee WMMJ, Seijkens D: Dose-related radiation response of mammary tumors as inves-

tigated by in vivo P-31 spectroscopy. Presented at the Third Annual Meeting, Society of Magnetic Resonance in Medicine, New York, August, 1984.

36. Evanochko WT, Ng TC, Lilly MB, et al: In vivo P-31 NMR study of the metabolism of murine mammary 16/C adenocarcinoma and its response to chemotherapy, x-radiation, and hyperthermia. Proc Natl Acad Sci USA 80:334–338, 1983.

37. Vaupel P, Ostoheimer K, Muller-Kleiser W: Circulatory and metabolic responses of malignant tumors to localized hyperthermia. J Cancer Res Clin Oncol 98:15–29, 1980.

38. Victor TA, Shaer A, Kaye AM, Degani H: P-31 NMR studies of high-energy phosphate metabolism during estrogen-induced growth of rat uterus. Magn Reson Med 1:290, 1984.

39. Gillies RJ, Ogino T, Shulman RG, Ward DC: P-31 nuclear magnetic resonance evidence for the regulation of intracellular pH by Ehrlich ascites tumor cells. J Cell Biol 95:24–28, 1982.

40. Evelhoch JL, Sapareto SA, Jick DEL, Ackerman JJH: In vivo metabolic effects of hyperglycemia in murine RIF tumor: A P-31 NMR investigation. Magn Reson Med 1:209, 1984.

41. Jahde E, Rajewsky MF: Tumor-selective modification of cellular microenvironment in vivo: Effect of glucose infusion on the pH in normal and malignant rat tissues. Cancer Res 42:1505–1512, 1982.

42. Gillies RJ: P-31 and C-13 NMR analysis of glycolysis in Ehrlich ascites tumor cells. Biophys J 41:251a, 1983.

43. Dickson JA, Galderwood SK: Effects of hyperglycemia and hyperthemia on the pH, glycolysis and respiration of the Yoshida sarcoma in vivo. JNCI 63:1371–1381, 1979.

44. Evelhoch JL, Sapareto SA, Nussbaum GH, Purdy JA, Ackerman JJH: P-31 NMR spectroscopy of murine RIF-1 tumor in vivo: The effect of tumor composition on the observed spectrum. Presented at the Third Annual Meeting of the Society of Magnetic Resonance in Medicine, New York, August 1984.

45. Gyulai L, Chance B, Ligeti L, et al: Correlated in vivo P-31 NMR and NADH-fluorometric studies on gerbil brain in graded hypoxia. Magn Reson Med 1:160, 1984.

46. Thulborn FR, Boulay GH, Duchen LW, Radda G: A P-31 nuclear magnetic resonance in vivo study of cerebral ischemia in the gerbil. J Cereb Blood Flow Metabol 2:299–306, 1982.

47. Lin AJ, Cosby LA, Shansky CW, Sartorelli AC: Potential bioreductive alkylating agents. I. Benzoquinone derivatives. J Med Chem 15:1247–1252, 1972.

48. Schwartz HS: Pharmacology of mitomycin CC. III. In vitro metabolism by rat liver. J Pharmacol Exp Ther 136:250–258, 1962.

49. Iyer VN, Szybalski W: Mitomycin and porfiromycin: Chemical mechanism of activation and cross-linking of DNA. Science 145:55–58, 1964.

50. Kennedy KA, Sartorelli AC: Metabolic activation of mitomycin C by isolated liver nuclei and microsomes. Fed Proc 38:443, 1964.

51. Kennedy KA, Rockwell S, Satorelli AAC. Preferential activation of mitomycin C to cytotoxic metabolites by hypoxic tumor cells. Cancer Res 40:2356–2360, 1980.

52. Taylor YC, Rauth AM: Differences in the toxicity and metabolism of the 2-nitroimidazole (R$_o$-07-0582) in HeLa and Chinese hamster ovary cells. Cancer Res 38:2745–2752, 1978.

53. Wong TW, Whitmore GF, Gulyas S: Studies on the toxicity and radiosensitizing ability of misonidazole under conditions of prolonged incubation. Radiat Res 75:541–555, 1978.

54. LaRusso NF, Tomasz M, Muller M: In vitro interaction of metronidazole with nucleic acids. Gastroenterology 71:917, 1978.

55. Lemasters JJ, Ji S, Thurman RG: Centrilobular injury following hypoxia in isolated perfused rat liver. Science 213:661–663, 1981.

56. Barlow CH, Chance B: Ischemic areas in perfused rat hearts: Measurement by NADH fluorescent photography. Science 193:909–910, 1976.

57. Scholz R, Thurman RG, Williamson JR, Chance B, Bucher T: Flavin and pyridine nucleotide oxidation-reduction changes in perfused rat liver. J Biol Chem 244:2317–2324, 1969.

58. Unkefer CJ, Blazer RM, London RE: In vivo determination of the pyridine nucleotide reduction change by carbon-13 nuclear magnetic resonance spectroscopy. Science 222:62–65, 1983.

59. Hutson JY, Brainard JR, Unkefer CJ, London RE, Mastwiyoff NA: C-13 NMR studies on the effects of altered oxidation-reduction state on pyridine nucleotide ratios and gluconeogenic flux in the perfused hamster liver. Magn Reson Med 1:177, 1983.

60. Gerweck L, Rottinger E: Enhancement of mammalian cell sensitivity of hyperthermia by pH alteration. Radiat Res 67:508–511, 1976.

61. Hahn GM: Metabolic aspects of the role of hyperthermia in mammalian cell inactivation and their possible relevance to cancer treatment. Cancer Res 34:3117–3123, 1974.

62. Bass H, Moore JL, Coakley WT: Lethality in mammalian cells due to hyperthermia under oxic and hypoxic conditions. Int J Rad Biol 33:57–67, 1978.

63. Song CW, Clement JJ, Levitt SH: Preferential cytotoxicity of 5-thio-D-glucose against hypoxic tumor cells. JNCI 57:603–605, 1976.

64. Sridhar R, Kocj CJ, Stroude EC, Inch WR: Cell survival in V-79 multicell spheroids treated with de-hydroascorbate, 5-thio-D-glucose and 2-deoxy-D-glucose. Br J Cancer 37(Suppl. 3):141–144, 1978.

65. Agris PF, Campbell ID: Proton nuclear magnetic resonance of intact Friend leukemia cells: Phosphorylcholine increase during differentiation. Science 216:1325–1327, 1982.

66. Evans FE: P-31 nuclear magnetic resonance studies on relaxation parameters and line broadening of intracellular metabolites of HeLa cells. Arch Biochem Biophys 193:63–75, 1979.

67. Burt CT, Glonek T, Barany M: Phosphorus-31 nuclear magnetic resonance detection of unexpected phosphodiesters in muscle. Biochemistry 15:4850–4852, 1976.

68. Burt CT, Danon MJ, Millar EA, et al: Variation of phosphate metabolites in normal and Duchenne human muscle. Biophys J *21*:184a, 1978.
69. Navon G, Shulman RG, Yamage T, et al: Phosphorus-31 nuclear magnetic resonance studies of wild-type and glucolytic pathway mutants of Saccharomyces cerevisiae. Biochemistry *18*:4487–4499, 1979.
70. Weber G: Ordered and specific pattern of gene expression in neoplasia. Adv Eng Regul *11*:79–102, 1973.
71. Satouchi K, Mizuno T, Samejima Y, Kunihiko S: Molecular species of phospholipid in rat hepatomas and fetal, regenerating and adult rat livers. Cancer Res *44*:1460–1464, 1984.
72. Haran N, Malik Z, Lapidot A: Water permeability changes studied by O-17 nuclear magnetic resonance during differentiation of Friend leukemia cells. Proc Natl Acad Sci USA *76*:3363–3366, 1979.
73. Evanochko WT, Ng TC, Sakai TT, Krisna NR, Glickson JD: Development of improved techniques for in vivo NMR studies of tumors and other intact tissues. Magn Reson Med *1*:49, 1984.
74. Maris JM, Evans A, McLaughlin A, Bolinger L, Chance B: In vivo P-31 studies of human neuroblastoma. Presented at the Third Annual Meeting of the Society of Magnetic Resonance in Medicine, New York, August 1984.
75. McLaughlin AC, Cullis PR, Hemminga M, Brown FF, Brockelhurst J: Magnetic resonance studies of model and biological membranes. *In* Dwek RA, Campbell ID, Richards RE, Williams RJP (eds): NMR in Biology. New York, Academic Press, 1977, pp 231–246.
76. Davis DG, Inesi G: Phosphorus and proton nuclear magnetic resonance studies in sarcoplasmic reticulum membranes and lipids, a comparison of phosphate and proton group mobilities in membranes and lipid bilayers. Biochim Biophys Acta *282*:180–186, 1972.
77. Shinitzky M, Inbar M: Difference in microviscosity induced by different cholesterol levels in the surface membrane lipid layer of normal lymphocytes and malignant lymphoma cells. J Molec Biol *85*:603–615, 1974.
78. Block RE, Maxwell GP, Irvin GL, Hudson JL, Prudhomme DL: Nuclear magnetic resonance studies of membranes of normal and cancer cells. *In* Shultz J, Block RE (eds): Membrane Transformations in Neoplasia. New York, Academic Press, 1974.
79. Mountford CE, Grossman G, Reid G, Fox RM: Characterization of transformed cells and tumors by proton nuclear magnetic resonance spectroscopy. Cancer Res *42*:2270–2276, 1982.
80. Mountford CF, Grossman G, Gatenby PA, Fox RM: High resolution proton nuclear magnetic resonance: Application to the study of leukemic lymphocytes. Br J Cancer *41*:1000–1003, 1980.
81. Tellier C, Curtet C, Poignunant S, Godard A, Aubry J: Proton NMR study of the binding of concanavalin A on myeloma plasma membranes. Biochem Biophys Res Comm *104*:113–120, 1982.
82. Burns CP, Luttenegger DG, Dudley DT, Buettner GR, Spector AA: Effect of modification of plasma membrane fatty acid composition on fluidity and methotrexate transport in L1210 murine leukemia cells. Cancer Res *39*:1726–1732, 1979.
83. Glauniger D, Magrath IT, Joshi A: Membrane lipid structural order in doxorubicin-sensitive and resistant P388 cells. Cancer Res *43*:5533–5537, 1983.
84. Pettigrew JW, Glonek T, Baskin F, Rosenberg RN: Phosphorus-31 NMR of neuroblastoma clonal lines. Effect of cell confluency state and dibutyryl cyclic AMP. Neurochem Res *4*:795–802, 1979.
85. Navon G, Burrows H, Cohen JC: Differences in metabolite levels upon differentiation on intact neuroblastoma x glioma cells observed by proton NMR spectroscopy. FEBS Lett *162*:320–323, 1983.
86. Knop RH, Carney DN, Chen CW, Cohen JS: P-31 NMR differentiation of small cell lung cancer and non-small cell lung cancer human tumor cell lines. Presented at the Third Annual Meeting of the Society of Magnetic Resonance in Medicine, New York, August 1984.
87. Victor TA, Wiebolt RC, Shattuck N, et al: P-31 NMR studies of human breast carcinomas. Presented at the Third Annual Meeting of the Society of Magnetic Resonance in Medicine, New York, August 1984.
88. Lapidot A, Irving CS: Dynamic structure of whole cells probed by nuclear Overhauser enhanced nitrogen-15 nuclear magnetic resonance spectroscopy. Proc Natl Acad Sci USA *74*:1988–1992, 1977.
89. Schelstraete K, Simons M, Deman J, et al: Uptake of N-13-ammonia by human tumours as studied by positron emission tomography. Br J Radiol *55*:797–804, 1982.
90. Block RE, Maxwell GP, Prudhomme DP, Hudson JL: High resolution proton magnetic resonance spectral characteristics of water, lipid and protein signals from three mouse cell populations. JNCI *58*:151–156, 1977.
91. Tanaka C, Naruse S, Harakawawa K, Yoshizaki K, Nishikawa H: High resolution H-1-NMR spectra of tumors. Magr Reson Med *1*:264, 1984.
92. Howes A: An estimation of changes in the proportions and absolute numbers of hypoxic cells after irradiation of transplanted C_3H mouse mammary tumours. Br J Radiol *42*:441–447, 1969.
93. Ng TC, Daugherty JP, Evanochko WT, Digerness SB, Durant JR, Glickson JD: Detection of antineo-plastic agent induced cardiotoxicity by P-31 NMR of perfused rat hearts. Biochem Biophys Res Comm *110*:339–347, 1983.
94. Tamptsu H, Nakazawa M, Imai S, Watari H: P-31 Topical nuclear magnetic resonance studies of cardiotoxic effects of 5-fluorouracil and 5'-deoxy-5-fluorouridine. Jpn J Pharmacol *34*:375–379, 1984.
95. Stevens AN, Morris PG, Iles RA, Griffiths JR: 5-Fluorouracil metabolism monitored in vivo by F-19 NMR. Presented at the Third Annual Meeting of the Society of Magnetic Resonance in Medicine, New York, August, 1984.

95

Localization Methods in NMR

PONNADA A. NARAYANA
JOHN L. DELAYRE

One of the potentials of nuclear magnetic resonance (NMR) in medicine is its ability to yield highly specific biochemical information. The biochemical data include high resolution spectra and relaxation times. This information must be obtained from a small well-defined region if it is to be of practical use. In an imaging experiment, localization of the region of interest is achieved by applying field gradients.[1] However, these gradients broaden the NMR spectral lines and compromise the diagnostic potential. Also, under these conditions, the measured relaxation times represent a weighted average of different chemical species. In principle, it is possible to measure the NMR properties from a localized region of interest indirectly via chemical shift imaging[2-10] at a significantly reduced sensitivity and increased acquisition time. It is, therefore, necessary to employ more efficient and sensitive methods to achieve localization. A number of such methods have been reported in the last few years. The purpose of this review is to briefly summarize these methods and point out some of their salient features.

There are basically four methods to achieve localization. They involve (1) static magnetic field profiling, (2) radio frequency (rf) field profiling, (3) the use of surface coils, and (4) techniques based on imaging principles.

STATIC MAGNETIC FIELD PROFILING

In this method the main magnetic field is shaped so that it is homogeneous over a small volume and is very inhomogeneous everywhere else. The resonance condition is satisfied in this region, and the high resolution character of the spectrum is preserved. Outside this region, the sample experiences very strong magnetic field inhomogeneities, resulting in broadening of the spectral lines, and their contribution to the observed signal can be removed by standard deconvolution techniques.

Field Focused Nuclear Magnetic Resonance Technique

Localized NMR studies using static field profiling were reported by Damadian and his colleagues[11,12] using the field focused nuclear magnetic resonance (FONAR) technique. The static field is shaped like a saddle, as shown in Figure 95-1. The resonance condition is satisfied only at the saddle point. Damadian and his colleagues have observed the ^{31}P spectrum from skeletal muscle using this method. The sensitive volume is located at the center of the magnet system, and the different regions can be accessed by moving the sample physically.

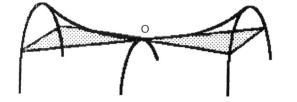

Figure 95–1. The saddle-shaped field pro-file used to define the resonance aperture at the saddle point.

Topical Magnetic Resonance

A second method for achieving localization, which is conceptually very similar to the FONAR method, is the topical magnetic resonance (TMR) technique.[13] The sensitive volume is defined by using the second and fourth order axial gradients generated by the room temperature profiling coils. These produce a roughly spherical sensitive volume of a diameter $2a = 3.1(B_2/2B_4)$ where B_2 and B_4 are the amplitudes of the second and fourth order gradients.[14] The field inhomogeneity across the sensitive volume increases as B_2/B_4. Thus the extent of useful central region can be varied by simultaneously adjusting the values of B_2 and B_4 within the tolerable value of the inhomogeneity across the sensitive volume. However, as with the FONAR method, the homogeneous region is restricted to the center of the magnet system. It is therefore necessary to move the object to access different regions.

The problem with both FONAR and TMR methods lies in determining the region from which the signals originate. For this reason both these methods, especially the FONAR method, are increasingly replaced by more elegant and efficient methods.

Sensitive Point

A method that involves dynamic profiling of the static field in order to move the sensitive volume electronically was proposed by Hinshaw.[15,16] This method, originally used for generating images, was more recently applied by Scott et al.[17] and Bottomley[18] for obtaining localized high resolution spectra. The basis for this method can be understood by referring to Figure 95–2. When a linear magnetic field gradient is reversed periodically, it produces a time dependent field everywhere except at the crossing point of the time dependent gradient. This position depends on the relative ratio of the currents in the pair of coils producing the gradient. The plane passing through this point and perpendicular to the gradient direction, referred to as the sensitive plane, does not experience any time dependent field. Everywhere else in the sample, the field and

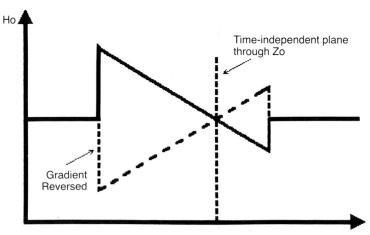

Figure 95–2. The effect of reversing a linear field gradient is to produce a time independent field in a plane where the gradients cross. This plane is perpendicular to the linear gradient. The position of the plane can be varied by changing the ratio of currents in the two coils producing the gradient.

hence the signal exhibit time dependence. This time dependent component of the rf signal can be eliminated with a low pass filter so that the NMR signal from the sensitive plane alone is detected. By applying three time dependent orthogonal gradients simultaneously, it is possible to localize the signal to a small volume. The three gradients should have different time dependences for this method to work. Hinshaw[16] originally applied three orthogonal gradients, two with the same frequency but with quadrature phases while the third gradient had a different frequency. The sensitive point method is generally used with a steady-state free precision (SSFP) technique[19,20] because it yields a relatively large and continuous signal. To avoid the frequency modulation of the time domain signal, the gradient frequency must be much lower than the pulse repetition rate.

It is possible to vary the size of the sensitive volume by varying the gradient amplitude and frequency. The center of the sensitive region can be translated along any axis by simply changing the ratios of the currents in the appropriate pair of coils. In this way different regions of the sample can be accessed.

The main problem with this method is that the localization is imperfectly defined. Part of the reason is the presence of spinning sideband type of artifacts produced by the time dependent gradients. In order to understand these sidebands let us assume a single gradient with an amplitude, G, and frequency, ω, which is much smaller than the homogeneous linewidth. With the additional assumption that the resonance offset is zero, it can be shown that the observed in phase component of the signal is given by:[16]

$$f = \gamma B_1 T_2 M_0 J_0^2 \left(\frac{\omega G x}{\omega} \right) \tag{1}$$

where γ is the gyromagnetic ratio, B_1 is the rf magnetic field, and M_0 is the equilibrium magnetization. The function $J_0(x)$ is the zeroth order Bessel function of the first kind. The thickness of the slice is given by the full width at half maximum of the above response function and is equal to 2.2 $\omega/\gamma G$. Besides the main peak, the response function exhibits side lobes, as shown in Figure 95–3. The first side lobe occurs at a distance

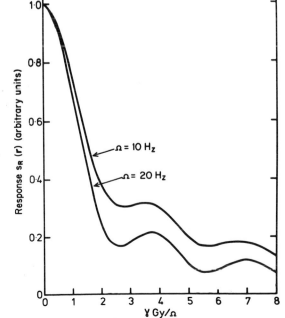

Figure 95–3. The response obtained in the presence of a time dependent gradient as a function of $\gamma G/\Omega$ for two gradient frequencies 10 and 20 Hz. Note the presence of strong side lobes.

of $x = 3.8\ \omega/\gamma G$ and has 16 percent amplitude of the center peak. Ljunggren[21] showed that a square wave modulation of the gradients reduces the amplitude of the side lobes and improves the localization. However, the improvement appears to be very marginal.

Scott et al.[17] have shown that if the echo, rather than the free induction decay (FID), is used for defining the sensitive volume, the problems associated with the side lobes and the line broadening can be minimized. In an SSFP method, rf pulses are applied rapidly and repetitively before the transverse magnetization decays. This leads to the spin-echo formation, which is separated in time from the FID due to inhomogeneous broadening. The presence of the time dependent fields destroys the echoes from outside the sensitive volume. Only the spins located in the sensitive volume contribute to the echo. Scott et al.[17] have demonstrated this by obtaining the high resolution spectra of ^{31}P from a localized region using a phantom. However, they found some phase anomalies in the signals with this technique. This method uses SSFP technique, which results in a poor signal to noise ratio (SNR). Further, the SSFP method can distort the amplitudes of spectral peaks such that the distortion depends on the relaxation times.[22]

RADIO FREQUENCY FIELD PROFILING

Another way to achieve localization is to employ switched rf field gradients. This method was proposed for imaging by Hoult,[23] who termed it rotating frame zeugmatography. It is based on the two-dimensional Fourier transformation (2DFT) introduced by Kumar et al.[24] for NMR imaging. The advantage of using rf gradients rather than static field gradients for localization is that the chemical shift information is preserved in the spectrum.

Rotating frame zeugmatography can be best understood by considering a one-dimensional sample lying along the x axis. If the sample is subjected to an rf field gradient, all the spins in the sample do not experience the same flip angle. Rather, the flip angle depends on the location of the spins in the sample. Spins located at position x are rotated by an angle $\theta = \gamma B_1 x t_1$ where B_1 is the amplitude of the rf gradient and t_1 is the rf pulse width (Fig. 95–4). The observed FID, following the application of the pulse sequence shown in Figure 95–4, is given by

$$S \propto -M_0(x)\ \sin(\gamma B_1 x t_1)\ e^{-t/T2} \tag{2}$$

where $T2$ is the spin-spin relaxation time and t is the data acquisition period. Equation (2) indicates that the signal intensity varies sinusoidally with the conjugate variables (x, t_1). Fourier transformation of Equation (2) with respect to t yields the high resolution spectrum. However, the contributions from various regions to the total signal intensity are scrambled. Thus a single FID does not give the spatial information. The spatial resolution can be obtained by collecting a number of FIDs as a function of t_1. Each of

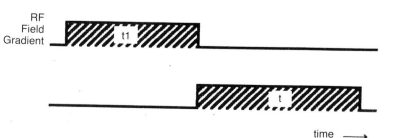

RF Field Gradient

t1

t

time ⟶

Figure 95–4. The pulse sequence used for one-dimensional rotating frame zeugmatography. Pulsed rf field gradient is applied to a time *T1* while the data is collected as a function of *t*. The Fourier transformation with respect to *t* gives the spectrum for a given pulsewidth t_1. Spectra are collected as a function of pulsewidth t_1. The Fourier transformation in the second dimension with respect to t_1 yields a one-dimensional image.

these FIDs is Fourier transformed with respect to t to obtain a series of high resolution spectra. A second Fourier transformation with respect to t_1 gives the spatial resolution; Cox and Styles[25] have shown that in a one-dimensional case, this technique preserves the high resolution character. It is possible to extend this technique to the second dimension by applying a second rf gradient orthogonal to the first gradient using a complicated probe arrangement. Extension of this technique to the third dimension requires the presence of a static field gradient during the data acquisition. The presence of this field gradient destroys the chemical shift information. This method, therefore, may not be very appropriate for volume localization studies.

SURFACE COILS

Perhaps the simplest and most popular way to achieve localization is by using special coils called "surface coils."[26,27] As the name implies, they are essentially useful for the study of tissues and organs lying close to the surface. Unlike an imaging probe that produces a very homogeneous rf field, surface coils exhibit a very inhomogeneous field distribution. For instance, a circular surface coil of radius a produces a field that falls off rapidly beyond a distance a from its center along its axis. A three-dimensional sensitivity profile of a circular surface coil is shown in Figure 95–5.[28] If such a coil is placed adjacent to the sample, it will excite approximately a bubble shaped region of radius a within the sample. By the same token, it also receives the signal from this small region within the sample. This is in contrast to the situation involving localization with imaging probes where the signal is received from a small region within the sample while the noise is received from the whole volume. Therefore, surface coils exhibit a higher SNR. Another advantage of the surface coils is that they can be made of any size and shape to conform to the shape of the organ to be studied.[29,31] Surface coils have been extensively used for high resolution spectroscopic studies to monitor metabolic activity. (For more recent work see references 32 to 35.) It has also been demonstrated that the relaxation times can be measured from a localized region with surface coils using inversion-recovery[36] and saturation-recovery techniques.[37] These coils are also increasingly being used as receiver coils to image superficial organs with high sensitivity and high spectral resolution.[38–44]

In spite of their many attractive features, surface coils suffer from poor localization properties due to their axial and radial field distributions. Thus in many instances it is difficult to identify the region from which the signals originate unless the tissue of

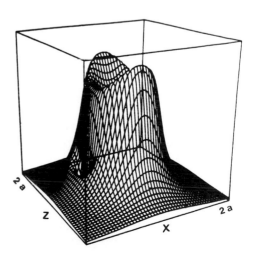

Figure 95–5. Calculated NMR signal intensity (vertical axis) as a function of position (horizontal axes) for a circular surface coil of radius a. The positions in the horizontal plane are given in a plane parallel to the surface coil and located at a distance of $0.5a$ from the coil. The total length of each of the horizontal axes is $2a$.

interest exhibits an identifiable indicator. This, for instance, is the case with kidneys, which can be identified by the absence of phosphocreatine signal.[45] Therefore, a number of methods have been proposed to improve the localization properties of surface coils. These methods can be basically divided into three categories, viz. (1) topical magnetic resonance, (2) rotating frame zeugmatography, and (3) multipulse sequences.

Topical Magnetic Resonance

This method[46] uses the surface coils in conjunction with the TMR method discussed earlier. If a surface coil is used to excite the spins in the sensitive volume defined by the field profile, a better defined localization can be obtained. One principal advantage of this method is its ability to remove the contaminating signals originating from the surface. This method is useful for studying superficial tissues only. One disadvantage of this method is that in a living organism it is difficult to define the size and the region from which the signal originates. Probably a more serious drawback of this technique is that different regions of the sample cannot be accessed without physically moving the sample.

Rotating Frame Zeugmatography

Another method aimed at improving the localization with surface coils is based on the rotating frame zeugmatography discussed earlier. This relies on the rf field gradient provided by the surface coils. A number of spectra are obtained as a function of the pulsewidth. Fourier transformation in the second dimension with respect to the pulsewidth yields a one-dimensional map of the sample while retaining the high resolution spectral information along this dimension. Haase, Malloy, and Radda[47] have demonstrated the effectiveness of this method by using phantoms containing glass bulbs filled with mixtures of sodium dihydrogen orthophosphate, adenosine triphosphate, or phosphocreatine in various combinations. The rf gradient produced by a circular surface coil is approximately linear in the range of $0.2a$ to $1.4a$ along the axis. Thus, the frequency in the second dimension is not linearly related to the axial distance outside this region. This results in a distorted spatial localization. Further, the SNR of this method is approximately half relative to that obtained in usual NMR experiments. A more serious problem arises due to the lateral extension of the rf field in the plane of the coil (see below), making it difficult to distinguish tissue lying directly on the coil axis from tissue far from the coil axis. The rotating frame zeugmatography involves the variation of pulsewidth for phase encoding. The dephasing of transverse magnetization, while negligible for shorter pulsewidths, could result in a smaller signal when larger pulsewidths are used. It is, therefore, hard to use this method for samples that exhibit short values of $T2$.

Rotating frame zeugmatography suffers from smearing artifacts induced by $T1$. These artifacts occur when short repetition times are used for obtaining optimal SNR. Under these conditions the longitudinal magnetization does not recover to its thermal equilibrium value. In order to understand the nature of this smearing artifact, we note that the FID obtained for a pulsewidth, t_1, is given by:[48]

$$S(t_1, t_2) \propto \mathrm{B_1^i} \sin(\Omega_1^i t_1) \exp\left(i\Omega_2 t_2 - \frac{t_1}{T2^{(1)}} - \frac{t_2}{T2^{(2)}} \right) \qquad (3)$$

where t_1 and t_2 are the evolution and detection periods, and Ω_1^i and Ω_2 are the frequencies during time periods t_1 and t_2 with the corresponding decays given by $T2^{(1)}$ and $T2^{(2)}$

The rf field B_1^i experienced by the element i is related to the pulse width as $\theta_i = \gamma B_1^i t_1 = \Omega_1^i t_1$. It is clear from Equation (3) that the signal amplitude is determined by B_1^i and oscillates as a function of t_1. For an efficient signal collection signal averaging is performed with a repetition time short compared to the time required for the magnetization to recover to its equilibrium value. In this case the FID is given by:

$$S(t_1, t_2) \propto B_1^i \sin(\Omega_1^i t_1) \frac{1 - \exp(-\tau/T1)}{1 - \cos(\Omega_1^i t_1) \exp(-\tau/T1)} \exp\left(i\Omega_2 t_2 - \frac{t_1}{T2^{(1)}} - \frac{t_2}{T2^{(2)}} \right) \qquad (4)$$

where τ is the total time ($t_1 + t_2$ + acquisition time) and $T1$ is the longitudinal relaxation time. Equation (4) clearly indicates that the signal does not oscillate in a purely sinusoidal fashion but depends in a complex way on t. Thus for $\tau/T1 < 1$, the data exhibit considerable distortion, leading to smearing artifacts in the imaging direction (ω_1 direction). Garwood et al.[49] have minimized these artifacts by using a preparation pulse to eliminate all the longitudinal magnetization followed by a delay τ^1 before the evolution pulse was applied. This delay allows for a partial recovery of the magnetization. The preparation pulse consisted of a phase cycled composite pulse sequence along each of the orthogonal axes in the rotating frame. Under these conditions, it can be shown that the signal in the frequency domain after double FT is given by:[49]

$$S(\omega_1, \omega_2) \propto B_1^i [1 - \exp(-\tau^1/T1)] \qquad (5)$$

and shows the absence of smearing artifacts.

From the above discussion, it is clear that only one-dimensional localization along the axis of the coil can be achieved with this method. Extension to other dimensions involves complex arrangements of more than one coil. However, no such experiments have been reported so far.

Multipulse Sequences

When a surface coil is excited by a single pulse that flips the magnetization at the position, x, by an angle θ, the signal intensity originating from this position is proportional to $\sin \theta$. Since θ varies with x, the NMR signal would have contributions from a large region within the sample. Thus a single pulse excitation exhibits a poor localization. It is, however, possible to achieve a better localization by exciting the surface coil with complex multipulse sequences. These include the depth pulses proposed by Bendall and Gordon,[50] the NOBLE (narrowband for localization of excitation) of Tycko and Pines,[51] and the sequence based on EXORCYCLE proposed by Shaka et al.[52] Such pulse sequences are commonly used in high resolution NMR studies to extract special spectral features (see, for example, reference 48). These are described below.

Depth Pulses

The depth pulse sequence proposed by Bendall and Gordon[50] is based on a phase cycling concept described by Bodenhausen et al.[53] to eliminate the ghost and phantom artifacts in two-dimensional NMR spectra. One of the simplest depth pulse sequences consists of four sequences with different phase combinations, with two pulses in each sequences. The sequence is shown in Table 95–1 and is designated as $\theta; 2\theta[\pm x, \pm y]$. Thus the sequence $2\theta[\pm x, \pm y]$ corresponds to four combinations of pulses applied along all the four axes in the transverse plane of the rotating coordinate system. The reference phase of the receiver is zero (+) whenever the rf pulse is applied along $+x$ or $-x$ axis and is inverted (−) whenever the rf pulse is applied along $+y$ or $-y$ axis.

Table 95–1. THE PHASES OF THE RADIO FREQUENCY PULSES AND THE CORRESPONDING RECEIVER PHASES EMPLOYED IN DEPTH PULSES

Radio Frequency Pulse		Receiver	
θ	2θ		
x	x	$+$	$+$
x	$-x$	$-$	$+$
x	y	$+$	$-$
x	$-y$	$-$	$-$

The θ pulse is always assumed to have zero phase, which is conveniently considered as applied along the the $+x$ axis. When the coil is excited by the depth pulse sequence, $\theta; 2\theta[\pm x, \pm y]$, the intensity of the signal is proportional to $\sin^3 \theta$. A plot of $\sin^3 \theta$ as a function of θ therefore represents the localization achieved. This plot is shown in Figure 95–6 (curve b) along with the localization obtained with a single θ pulse (curve a). It can be seen from this figure that for a significant deviation of θ from 90 degrees, the signal intensity is considerably reduced, i.e., this depth pulse sequence results in a better localization compared to a single θ pulse.

The localization can be futher improved by adding more $2\theta[\pm x, \pm y]$ pulses. For instance, a pulse sequence, $\theta; 2\theta[\pm x, \pm y]; 2\theta[\pm x, \pm y]$, which is represented as $\theta; 2\theta[\pm x, \pm y]_2$, yields a signal that is proportional to $\sin^5 \theta$. A plot of this function is shown in Figure 95–6 (curve c). A comparison of this curve with curve b clearly demonstrates an improved localization. In order to appreciate the rapid increase in the number of pulses with each addition of a $2\theta[\pm x, \pm y]$ sequence, let us take a closer look at the sequence $2\theta[\pm x, \pm y]_2$. For a proper functioning of this sequence, the phase

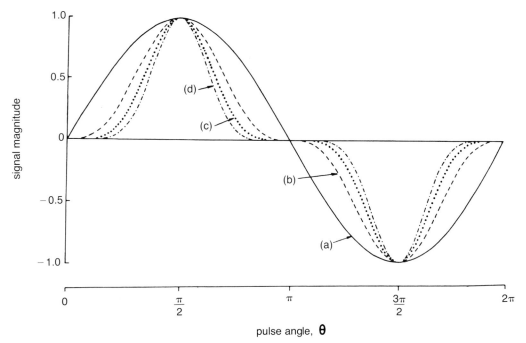

Figure 95–6. Signal amplitude as a function of the flip angle for a surface coil. The flip angle is a function of depth and therefore these plots represent the degree of localization obtained. The various curves represent (a) a single θ pulse with the signal proportional to $\theta \sin \theta$, (b) depth pulse sequence $\theta; 2\theta[\pm x, \pm y]$ with the signal proportional to $\sin^3 \theta$, (c) depth pulse sequence $\theta; (2\theta[\pm x, \pm y])_2$ with the signal intensity proportional to $\sin^5 \theta$, and (d) depth pulse sequence $\theta; (2\theta[\pm x, \pm y])_3$ with the signal proportional to $\sin^7 \theta$. Note the improvement in the localization from (a) through (d).

Table 95–2. RELATIVE PHASES OF RADIO FREQUENCY PULSES AND RECEIVER PHASES FOR THE DEPTH PULSE SEQUENCE $2\theta[\pm x, \pm y]_2$

Radio Frequency Phase		Receiver Phase
First 2θ Pulse	*Second 2θ Pulse*	
x	x	$+$
x	$-x$	$+$
x	y	$-$
x	$-y$	$-$
$-x$	x	$+$
$-x$	$-x$	$+$
$-x$	y	$-$
$-x$	$-y$	$-$
y	x	$-$
y	$-x$	$-$
y	y	$+$
y	$-y$	$+$
$-y$	x	$-$
$-y$	$-x$	$-$
$-y$	y	$+$
$-y$	$-y$	$+$

cycling of the first $2\theta[\pm x, \pm y]$ sequence should be independent of the phase cycling of the second $2\theta[\pm x, \pm y]$ sequence. Since each of these sequences contains four combinations, the $2\theta[\pm x, \pm y]_2$ sequence contains sixteen different combinations of the rf and the receiver phases. As before, we assume that the θ pulse has zero phase (i.e., applied along the $+x$ axis). All the sixteen combinations of the rf pulse and the receiver phases are shown in Table 95–2 for clarity.

The localization can be further improved by the successive addition of $2\theta[\pm x, \pm y]$ pulses, i.e., one can employ a sequence of the type $\theta; 2\theta[\pm x, \pm y]_n$, which results in a signal intensity proportional to $\sin^{2n+1}\theta$. At the same time, the number of pulses increases as 4^n. As an example the plot of $\sin^7 \theta$ is shown in curve d. In general, it is not worth increasing n beyond 2 because the marginal improvement in the localization does not justify the rapid increase in the number of pulses.

Another pulse sequence that was used for localization is $2\theta; \theta[\pm x]; 2\theta[\pm x, \pm y]$. As before, $2\theta[\pm x, \pm y]$ stands for four sequences with different rf and receiver phases (Table 95–1). The first 2θ pulse always has zero phase. Independent phase cycling of $\theta[\pm x]$ and $2\theta[\pm x, \pm y]$ requires the total number of combinations in this sequence be $2 \times 4 = 8$. These combinations are shown in Table 95–3. The signal intensity with this sequence is given by $\cos 2\theta \sin^3 \theta$. The variation of this function with θ is shown in Figure 95–7 (curve b). For comparison, the signal expected from a single θ pulse is shown in curve a. It can be seen from this figure that the depth pulse sequence improves

Table 95–3. THE RELATIVE PHASES OF THE RADIO FREQUENCY PULSES AND THE RECEIVER FOR THE SEQUENCE $2\theta; \theta[\pm x]; 2\theta[\pm x, \pm y]$. THE FIRST 2θ PULSE IS ALWAYS ASSUMED TO BE APPLIED ALONG THE $+x$ OF THE ROTATING FRAME (TAKEN AS ZERO PHASE)

2θ (First)	θ	2θ (Second)	Receiver
x	x	x	$+$
x	x	$-x$	$+$
x	x	y	$-$
x	x	$-y$	$-$
x	$-x$	x	$+$
x	$-x$	$-x$	$+$
x	$-x$	y	$-$
x	$-x$	$-y$	$-$

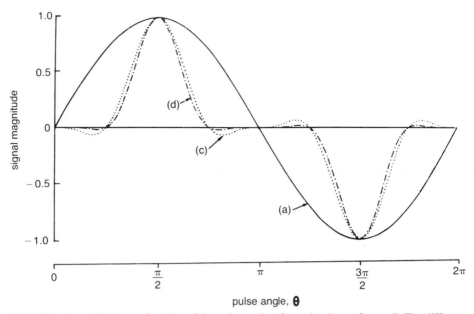

Figure 95–7. Signal amplitude as a function of the pulse angle θ for a circular surface coil. The different plots represent (*a*) a single pulse θ with the signal proportional to sin θ, (*c*) the depth pulse sequence 2θ; $\theta[\pm x]$; $2\theta[\pm x, \pm y]$ with the signal proportional to $-\cos 2\theta \sin^3 \theta$, (*d*) the depth pulse sequence 2θ; $\theta[\pm x]$, $(2\theta[\pm x, \pm y])_2$ with the signal amplitude proportional to $-\cos 2\theta \sin^5 \theta$. Note the improved localization from sequence (*a*) through (*c*).

the localization by reducing the contribution to the signal from the negative wings in the region 0 degrees < θ < 45 degrees and 135 degrees < θ < 180 degrees. As before, an improved localization can be obtained by adding more $2\theta[\pm x, \pm y]$ sequences. For instance, the depth pulse sequence 2θ; $\theta[\pm x]$; $2\theta[\pm x, \pm y]_2$ gives a signal proportional to $-\cos 2\theta \sin^5 \theta$. The shape of this function is shown in curve *c*. Successive addition of $2\theta[\pm x, \pm y]$ pulses would improve the localization somewhat, but the rapid increase in the number of pulses would offset the small improvement achieved in localization. These predictions were experimentally verified by Bendall and Aue.[54]

In order to reach larger depths in the sample, it is necessary to increase the pulse width. However, this increased pulsewidth results in large negative signals from regions close to the coil, where the condition $\theta = 270$ degrees is approximately satisfied. This problem can be greatly reduced by making the flip angle at the center of the coil approximately 225 degrees. In this case, signal is essentially obtained from the sample region lying between .7*a* to 1.3*a*.

As mentioned earlier, the contribution to the signal from the off axis regions of surface coil results in a poor localization. For depths less than 0.5*a* and an off axis distance of 0.7*a*, the signal arises from the same depth, i.e., the slice responsible for the observed signal is approximately planar. However, for off axis distances greater than 0.7*a*, there is a rapid decrease in the depth from which the signals originate. This effect arises owing to the curvature of the rf field lines, which must eventually loop around the surface coil wire. This region is loosely termed the "high flux" region. For example, if the flip angle is adjusted to be 90 degrees at a distance of *a* on the axis of the coil, the surface representing the distribution of this angle crosses the surface of the coil at a distance of 1.5*a* from the coil center. This is illustrated in Figure 95–8, which shows the regions from which signals arise for a circular surface coil excited by the depth pulse sequence 2θ; $\theta[\pm x]$; $(2\theta[\pm x, \pm y])_2$ as a function of the depth and off axis radius of the surface coil. One way to eliminate this problem is to use two surface coils of different sizes. The large coil is used for excitation while the smaller coil is

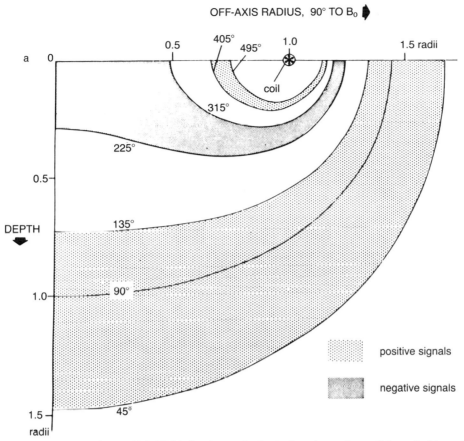

Figure 95–8. The regions from which NMR signals are obtained when the surface coil is excited by a depth pulse sequence 2θ; $\theta[\pm x]$; $(2\theta[\pm x, \pm y])_2$. The vertical axis represents the depth, i.e., distance from the center of the coil. The horizontal axis represents the off-axis distance. The positive and negative signals refer to the phase of the signal. Only the right half of the figure is shown. The left half is symmetric about the depth axis. Note the curving in of the signal region towards smaller depths for large off-axis distances.

used for detection. The shallow region excited by the large coil is not detected by the small coil. The two coils can be decoupled from each other using one of the schemes reported in the literature.[55-57] Results obtained by Bendall[58] indicate that the use of two coils improves the localization somewhat but is far from perfect. An overview of surface coil theory and technology is provided in Chapter 73 by Bendall.

Bendall[58] has also suggested using a slightly different pulse sequence to eliminate signals arising from the regions close to the surface of the sample. One such sequence is:

$$2\theta[\pm x]; \{(2/3)\theta + (4/3)\theta\}; (2\theta[\pm x, \pm y])_2$$

which is a shorthand notation for:

$$2\theta[\pm x]; (2/3)\theta; (2\theta[\pm x, \pm y])_2; \text{acquire}$$
$$+ 2\theta[\pm x]; (4/3)\theta; (2\theta[\pm x, \pm y])_2; \text{acquire}$$

In this case the signal intensity is proportional to

$$- \cos 2\theta \sin^4 \theta[\sin(2/3)\theta + \sin(4/3)\theta]/2$$

A plot of this function is shown in Figure 95–9 (broken line) along with the signal expected from the basic sequence 2θ; $\theta[\pm x]$; $2(\theta[\pm x, \pm y])_2$ (solid line). It can be seen

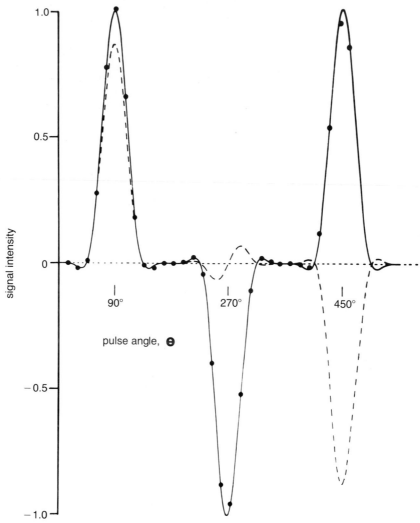

Figure 95–9. Signal amplitude as a function of the flip angle for a surface coil. The solid line represents the excitation pulse sequence 2θ, $\theta[\pm x]$, $2\theta[\pm x, \pm y]_2$ with the signal amplitude proportional to $-\cos 2\theta \sin^5 \theta$. The broken line represents the excitation pulse sequence $2\theta[\pm x]$; $[(2/3)\theta + (4/3)\theta]$; $(2\theta[\pm x, \pm y])_2$ with the signal amplitude proportional to $-\cos 2\theta \sin^4 \theta \, [\sin(2/3)\theta + \sin(4/3)\theta]/2$. Notice the significant reduction in the signal amplitude around $\theta = 270$ degrees (broken line).

from the above expression that signals from the 270 degree region are suppressed without reducing the 90 degree signal amplitude significantly. This helps in reducing the surface contribution.

NOBLE Sequence

Another special pulse sequence used in conjunction with the surface coil to obtain better localization is the NOBLE (narrowband for localization of excitation) sequence.[51] This relies on an rf pulse sequence that inverts the magnetization over a narrow range of rf amplitudes. The pulse sequence used is shown in Figure 95–10. The pulse, P, inverts the magnetization for a narrow range of rf amplitudes. For example, P represents a sequence of 27 pulses, each with a nominal flip angle of 180 degrees. The phases of these pulses are 0, 120, 240, 120, 240, 0, 240, 0, 120, 120, 240, 0, 240,

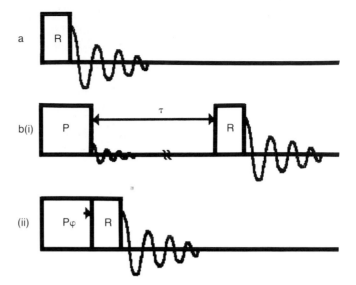

Figure 95–10. The NOBLE sequence used for localization. P denotes a narrowband inversion sequence, and R denotes the read pulse. In $b(ii)$, P_φ indicates a phase cycling through 0 degrees and 180 degrees.

0, 120, 0, 120, 240, 240, 0, 120, 0, 120, 240, 120, 240, 0. The read pulse, R, can be either a single pulse or a sequence of pulses. The FID is first obtained just with the read pulse alone, as shown in Figure 95–10a. Next, the FID is recorded with the pulse sequence shown in Figure 95–10b(i). The difference between the FIDs recorded with sequences in Figures 95–10a and 95–10b(i) gives the signal from the spins inverted by the sequence P alone. The delay, τ, between the pulses P and R in the sequence of Figure 95–10b(i) is needed to dephase the residual transverse magnetization. The decay of this residual transverse magnetization can be hastened by applying a static field gradient. Alternatively, the need for a static field gradient can be eliminated by using a sequence shown in Figure 95–10b(ii), where the phase of P is cycled between 0 and 180 degrees and the FIDs are added. This eliminates the contribution from the residual transverse magnetization. The FID recorded with R alone is then subtracted from the above sum. The resulting signal arises only from those spins inverted by P. The localization obtained with a surface coil using this method is shown in Figure 95–11a. Here B_1^0 is arbitrarily defined as rf amplitude, which corresponds to a 90 degree pulse. For comparison, the localization obtained by a single 180 degree pulse is shown in Figure 95–11b. An improved localization is apparent from this figure.

If we assume that B_1 is the amplitude of the rf field at the region of interest, there will be regions where the rf amplitudes are $3B_1$, $5B_1$, etc., which contribute to the

Figure 95–11. The spin inversion obtained as a function of the normalized rf field B_1/B_1^0 using a NOBLE sequence (solid line). The sequence consists of 27 rf pulses each with a nominal flip angle of 180 degrees. The phases of the pulses are 0,120,240,120,240,0,240, 0,120,120,240,0,240,0,120,0,120,240,240,0,120,0,120, 240,120,240,0. For comparison, the inversion obtained with a single 180 degree pulse is shown (broken line).

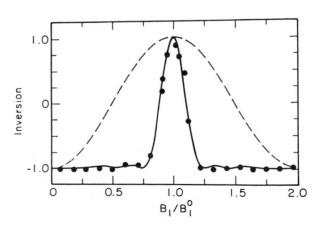

observed signal. If it is possible to increase the separation between the surface coil and the sample, the signal from the $5B_1$ region can be significantly reduced. The amplitude from the $3B_1$ region can be minimized by employing a 60 degree pulse for R. This, however, also reduces the signal from the 90 degree region to 87 percent of its maximum value while the signal from the $3B_1$ region is only about 7 percent of this value. It is possible to access different regions of the sample either by varying the rf power and keeping the pulse lengths constant or by proportionally varying the pulse lengths, keeping the rf power constant.

EXORCYCLE Sequence

Another method that improves the localization produced by a surface coil was proposed by Shaka et al.[52] Conceptually, it is very similar to the method proposed by Tycko and Pines.[51] The idea is to excite the transverse magnetization and invert it with one or more composite 180 degree pulses that are sensitive to the rf field strength. Signals from the sample region experiencing an rf field close to B_1 are obtained, while the signals from those regions that do not experience almost complete inversion are canceled by employing the EXORCYCLE scheme.[53] First, the NMR signal is excited by a nominal 60 degree pulse. A 60 degree pulse, instead of 90 degree pulse, eliminates the contributions from the region where the amplitudes of the rf field are $3B_1$, $5B_1$, etc. The transverse magnetization excited by the 60 degree pulse is then inverted twice by the cascade $Q^1 \tilde{Q}^1$ where

$$Q^1 = 2x \; \overline{2y} \; \overline{2x} \tag{6}$$

and

$$\tilde{Q}^1 = \overline{2x} \; \overline{2y} \; 2x \tag{7}$$

where $2x$ represents a nominal 180 degree pulse about the x axis; $2y$ a nominal 180 degree pulse about the y axis; and $\overline{2x}$ and $\overline{2y}$ represent 180 pulses along $-x$ and $-y$ axes, respectively.

It can be seen from the above definition that $\tilde{Q}^1$ is a time reversed Q^1 sequence. The cascade $Q^1 \tilde{Q}^1$ compensates for the sense of the resonance offset. All the component pulses are phase cycled according to the EXORCYCLE.[53] The receiver phase is inverted for each 90 degree rf phase shift in the component pulses of Q^1 or $\tilde{Q}^1$. All the rf and the receiver phase combinations are shown in Table 95–4. Different regions of the sample can be accessed by increasing the pulsewidths such that the correct proportion of the various flip angles is maintained while keeping the rf power constant. Shaka et al.[52] have verified this method by employing a phantom containing three bulbs filled with benzene, water, and cyclohexane and demonstrated a good localization along the axis of the surface coil.

The pulse sequences described above produce localization essentially along one direction of the coil and thus do not represent a true volume localization. In principle, the extension of localization to other dimensions can be achieved by using more than one coil.

Bendall and Pegg[59] have compared, theoretically, the performance of depth pulse and composite pulse sequences. Their analysis indicates that the off resonance performance of depth pulses is superior to that of the composite pulses. Solutions to remedy this problem with composite pulse sequences have been proposed by Shaka and Freeman.[60] However, one problem common to both depth and composite pulse sequences is the large number of pulses they employ for achieving only a moderate degree of localization. This large number of pulses might result in a large power deposition in

Table 95–4. PHASE COMBINATIONS OF THE RADIO FREQUENCY PULSES AND THE RECEIVER FOR EXORCYCLE SEQUENCE*

Radio Frequency Pulses						Receiver
2x	$\overline{2y}$	$\overline{2x}$	$\overline{2x}$	$\overline{2y}$	2x	+
$\overline{2y}$	$\overline{2x}$	2y	$\overline{2x}$	$\overline{2y}$	2x	−
$\overline{2x}$	2y	2x	$\overline{2x}$	$\overline{2y}$	2x	+
2y	2x	$\overline{2y}$	$\overline{2x}$	$\overline{2y}$	2x	−
2x	$\overline{2y}$	$\overline{2x}$	2y	2x	$\overline{2y}$	−
$\overline{2y}$	$\overline{2x}$	2y	2y	2x	$\overline{2y}$	+
$\overline{2x}$	2y	2x	2y	2x	$\overline{2y}$	−
2y	2x	$\overline{2y}$	2y	2x	$\overline{2y}$	+
2x	$\overline{2y}$	$\overline{2x}$	2x	$\overline{2y}$	$\overline{2x}$	+
$\overline{2y}$	$\overline{2x}$	2y	2x	$\overline{2y}$	$\overline{2x}$	−
$\overline{2x}$	2y	2x	2x	$\overline{2y}$	$\overline{2x}$	+
2y	2x	$\overline{2y}$	2x	$\overline{2y}$	$\overline{2x}$	−
2x	$\overline{2y}$	$\overline{2x}$	$\overline{2y}$	$\overline{2x}$	2y	−
$\overline{2y}$	$\overline{2x}$	2y	$\overline{2y}$	$\overline{2x}$	2y	+
$\overline{2x}$	2y	2x	$\overline{2y}$	$\overline{2x}$	2y	−
2y	2x	$\overline{2y}$	$\overline{2y}$	$\overline{2x}$	2y	+

* In this sequence $2x$ represents a nominal $\underline{180}$ degree pulse about the x axis and $\overline{2x}$ represents a nominal 180 degree pulse about the $-x$ axis. $2y$ and $\overline{2y}$ represent nominal 180 degree pulses applied along the $+y$ and $-y$ axes, respectively.

the sample and prove to be a serious problem for in-vivo studies in humans. In the case of depth sequence, Rothman et al.[61] have shown that, in many instances, it is possible to avoid the phase cycling by using spin echoes to acquire the data, thus reducing the total power deposition.

METHODS BASED ON IMAGING PRINCIPLES

A number of methods based upon imaging principles have been proposed to achieve good localization. They all use (a) a large transmitter coil to produce a homogeneous rf field over a reasonable volume and (b) switched field gradients for localizing the region of interest. Some of these methods use a second small coil as a receiver to improve the signal to noise ratio. The important point to note is that all the static field gradients are turned off during data acquisition so as to retain the high resolution character of the spectra.

The depth resolved surface coil spectroscopy (DRESS) proposed by Bottomley, Foster, and Darrow[62] is one such method. It eliminates the surface tissue contributions to the observed signal and provides an accurately controlled, depth resolved spectra for in-vivo applications. This method utilizes two rf coils. The transmitter coil can be either a large surface coil or a conventional coil to provide a uniform rf excitation over the sensitive volume. The receiver coil is a small surface coil. These two coils are decoupled from each other either by using a pair of crossed diodes[55] or by employing more elaborate detuning circuits.[56,57] Depth resolution is achieved by applying the selective excitation in the presence of a field gradient whose direction is parallel to the axis of the surface coil. Therefore, nuclei in a plane parallel to the plane of the coil alone are excited. The pulse sequence employed in these studies is shown in Figure

95–12. The thickness and the location of the selected plane are defined by the bandwidth of the excitation and the gradient field strength, while the extent of the sensitive volume within this plane is defined by the size of the surface coil. This sensitive volume can be approximated by a disk lying at the intersection of the selected plane and the three-dimensional field profile of the surface coil. This method was tested both with phantoms and live animals and seems to yield a good localization. This method is quite promising for studying superficial tissues.

A variation of the DRESS sequence, termed the SLIT DRESS (slice interleaved depth resolved surface coil spectroscopy) was proposed by Bottomley et al.[63] The advantage of this method is that localized spectra from a number of planes (typically 8) can be acquired in about the same time it takes to acquire data from a single plane. In NMR, generally, signal averaging is performed to improve the SNR by repeating the same pulse sequence. Typically, long repetition times (>1000 ms) are used to allow a substantial recovery of the magnetization. On the other hand, the data acquisition time is less than 100 ms. Thus a large amount of time is wasted inbetween the scans. In the DRESS sequence, spins are excited only in a selective plane. Therefore, except in this slice, spins in the rest of the sample are in thermal equilibrium. After collecting data from the plane that is selectively exited, it is possible to excite an adjacent plane by changing the center frequency of the selective pulse and record the data. This can be repeated by sequentially exciting a number of adjacent planes. By this time, the spins in the first plane would have sufficiently recovered. The first plane can therefore be excited again and the signal recorded for signal averaging. This procedure can be repeated for all the adjacent planes. Clearly this is a very efficient method. This strategy is similar to the one used in multislice imaging.[64]

Another method for achieving spatial localization was proposed by Mareci et al.[65] The same surface coil is used for both transmission and detection. This method can be understood by referring to the pulse sequence shown in Figure 95–13. A depth pulse sequence is applied to the surface coil in the presence of two gradients, G_x and G_z, where the y direction defines the axis of the surface coil. The depth pulse sequence θ; $2\theta[\pm x, \pm y]$, which was discussed earlier, provides the localization along the axis of the coil while the two gradients provide the localization in a plane perpendicular to this axis. The depth pulse sequence is repeated for different gradient amplitudes to provide the weighted acquisition necessary to define the localized region in the x and z direction.[66] The advantage of this method is that the exact location in the x and z directions can be selected after the data acquisition. The disadvantage is that a large amount of rf power is needed to implement the depth pulse sequence.

A third method for achieving localization was proposed by Gordon and Ordidge.[67]

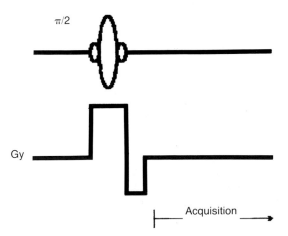

Figure 95–12. The DRESS sequence used for localization. The 90 degree selective pulse is applied in the presence of a gradient G_y where y is the axis of the coil. The negative G_y gradient is for refocusing the spins. The data is acquired in the absence of any gradient.

θ;2θ[±x, ±y]

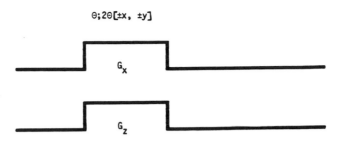

Figure 95–13. Timing sequence used by Mareci et al.[65] for achieving the localization with a surface coil. The depth pulse sequence θ; 2θ[±x, ±y] is applied in the presence of the gradients G_x and G_z. While localization along the y axis is obtained with the depth pulses, the localization in the other orthogonal direction is obtained by the application of the gradients G_x and G_z.

This uses three tailored rf pulses in the presence of field gradients as shown in Figure 95–14. The result of the application of the three selective pulses in the presence of the gradients is to generate transverse magnetization from a small volume within the sample. Signal from outside this selected volume is destroyed owing to the presence of residual field gradients. Generally the location of the sensitive volume is determined by the center frequency of the rf pulses while the size of volume is determined by the strength of the gradient and the bandwidth of the rf pulses. Nuclei that have short $T1$ values and that lie outside the sensitive region may contribute to the observed signal. This contribution, however, can be minimized by shortening the length of the whole sequence. This is truly a volume localization method that holds a great degree of promise.

Another method, called ISIS (which is an acronym for image selected in-vivo spectroscopy) was proposed by Ordidge.[68] This method is best understood by considering the pulse sequence (Fig. 95–15) appropriate for a one-dimensional sample lying along the z direction. Initially (experiment A) the FID from the whole sample is collected immediately following a nonselective 90 degree pulse. This FID is Fourier transformed and stored as spectrum S_1. (This signal is assumed to be positive.) Next (experiment B), spins from a selected region are inverted by applying a selective 180 degree pulse in the presence of a gradient G_z. After a brief waiting period for the gradient field to decay completely, the FID is recorded immediately following a nonselective 90 degree pulse, Fourier transformed and stored as spectrum S_2. The spins from the selected region are affected by both the selective 180 degree and the nonselective 90 degree pulse and therefore give a negative signal. Spins from the rest of the sample are effected by the nonelective 90 degree pulse only and therefore give a positive signal. The difference $S_1 - S_2$, therefore, contains signal from the selected region only. This method can be extended to volume localization easily by an appropriate combination of slice-selective gradients and receiver phase. It is easy to see that volume localization involves $2^3 = 8$ experiments. The sequences for volume localization are shown in Table 95–5. The position of the selective volume can be controlled by varying the frequency offset of the selected pulses while the volume of the localized region is determined by the bandwidth of the selective pulses and the strength of the gradients. One of the dis-

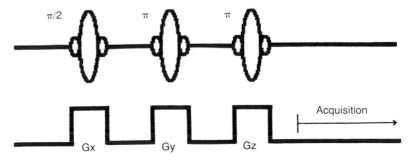

Figure 95–14. Timing sequence employed by Gordon and Ordidge[67] for localization studies. The three selective rf pulses applied in the presence of the three gradients result in a transverse magnetization only from small selected volume.

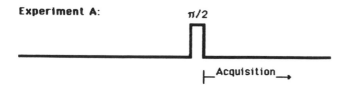

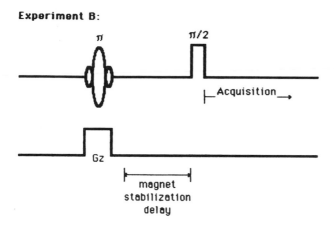

Figure 95–15. Timing sequence for one-dimensional image-selected in vivo spectroscopy (ISIS). The experiment consists of two parts, *A* and *B*. In part *A*, the spectrum S_1 is obtained from the entire sample using a hare 190 degree pulse. In part *B*, spins in the selected region are inverted by a selective 180 degree pulse in the presence of a gradient G_z and the spectrum S_2 is obtained using a 90 degree hard pulse. The difference $S_1 - S_2$ results in a spectrum from the selected region alone.

advantages of this method may be the large number of sequences needed to obtain one spectrum.

One of the most promising techniques for achieving localization is the volume selective excitation proposed by Aue et al.[69] This method can be best understood by referring to the pulse sequence shown in Figure 95–16. The "sandwich" pulse, which consists of two 45 degree selective pulses and a 90 degree nonselective pulse in the presence of gradient G_x, preserves the *z* magnetization in the *xy* plane of the sample and generates transverse magnetization everywhere. The successive application of the other two "sandwich" pulses in the presence of the other two orthogonal gradients results in a *z* magnetization in the sensitive volume. The magnetization everywhere else dephases under the influence of the gradients and does not contribute to the signal. The *z* magnetization can be detected using conventional NMR methods to obtain the high resolution spectrum or measure the relaxation times.

For an artifact-free localization, the nonselective 90 degree pulse of the sandwich pulse has to have a bandwidth that is large compared to the frequency spread introduced by the gradients. This necessitates the use of small pulsewidth and high rf power. Alternatively, the gradient needs to be switched off during the application of this pulse. This switching on and off of the gradients for a short time, however, poses considerable

Table 95–5. COMPLETE ISIS SEQUENCE FOR VOLUME LOCALIZATION

Experiment Number	Selective Pulses			Receiver Phase
	x	*y*	*z*	
1	off	off	off	+
2	on	off	off	−
3	off	on	off	−
4	on	on	off	+
5	off	off	on	−
6	on	off	on	+
7	off	on	on	+
8	on	on	on	−

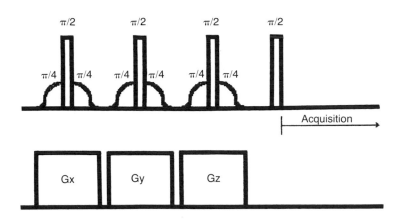

Figure 95–16. Timing sequence proposed by Aue[69] for volume localization. Each of the sandwich pulses consists of a hard 90 degree pulse sandwiched by two selective 45 degree pulses. Application of the three sandwich pulses in the presence of linear gradients results in a z magnetization only in a small selected volume. This magnetization can be recalled with a hard 90 degree pulse.

technical problems. In the absence of any gradients, the center of the sensitive volume is at the center of the magnet. The position of the sensitive volume can be changed by changing either the center frequency of the selective pulses or the offset of the magnetic field. The size of the sensitive volume can be adjusted by varying the gradient amplitudes and the width of the selective pulses. The success of this method was demonstrated with phantoms. The volume selective excitation has a number of advantages compared to other methods. (1) The method is not restricted to the superficial organs close to the surface. (2) The position and the size of the sensitive volume can be adjusted electronically. (3) The method is one dimensional and is therefore sensitive and simple. (4) The region of interest can be picked up from the proton images and (5) the magnetic field could be homogenized over the sensitive volume.

There are two problems associated with this method that need further investigation. (1) There is an ambiguity between the influence of the chemical shift and the gradients on the Larmor frequency. Presumably, the effect of chemical shift can be minimized by interrogating the selective magnetization using the spin-echo technique. In any case, this effect is relatively small. For example, for typical gradient values used for proton studies, the inaccuracy in the localization is <1 mm while for ^{31}P it is about 2 mm and so can be neglected. (2) The spins with short $T1$ and that lie outside the sensitive volume recover significantly before data acquisition and contribute to the final signal. This effect can be minimized by shortening the length of the whole sequence.

Mueller, Aue, and Seelig[70] have applied the VSE method using a surface coil for both transmission and detection. The inhomogeneous field distribution of the surface coil makes the determination of the sandwich pulse a little more difficult. Initially the plane of interest is determined by adjusting the gradient strength and the frequency of the selective pulses. The width and amplitude of the broadband pulses are determined as follows: The sample is excited by a broadband pulse and the magnetization is detected by the application of a second broadband pulse of the same amplitude and width as the excitation pulse. The data are collected in the presence of the same gradient used for slice selection. The acquired NMR signal represents the spin density profile. The first zero crossing occurs at the plane where both the excitation and the detection pulses are 90 degrees. The amplitude and duration of these pulses are adjusted so that this first-zero crossing occurs at the plane of interest. Unwanted signals arising from outside the selected plane due to pulse imperfection in the nonselective pulse can be eliminated to a significant degree by phase cycling the broadband pulse of the sandwich pulse. For instance, application of a sandwich pulse ($45^0_x - 90^0_x - 45^0_x$) in the presence of a y gradient results in magnetization along the $-z$ axis from the selected plane, which is detected and is denoted by S_1 (the subscripts x and $-x$ indicate the phase of the rf pulses). Application of a second sandwich pulse ($45^0_x - 90^0_{-x} - 45^0_x$) results in a magnetization from the selected plane along the z-axis, which is detected and is denoted as S_2. The difference of these two signals, therefore, contains the contribution from the selected plane alone, leaving very little unwanted signal. This method can be easily extended to volume localization by the application of three sandwich pulses in the presence of three orthogonal gradients. Since this method employs a single surface coil, it retains experimental simplicity and at the same time provides a good SNR. If, for instance, the distance between the surface coil and the imaging plane is greater than the coil radius, secondary signals originate close to the coil, leading to some ambiguity. Unambiguous information can, therefore, be obtained only from regions close to the surface coil. This method is, therefore, only suitable for investigating superficial tissues and organs.

A number of techniques proposed for localization have been reviewed. Some of these methods employ a large number of very complex pulses. This may result in an unacceptably large power deposition, particularly for the in-vivo studies involving human subjects. Even though many of these methods have been tested on phantoms, only a few of them were applied to animals and humans. This makes it very difficult to assess their performance. More work is needed to separate methods that are useful from those that are merely of academic interest.

References

1. Mansfield P, Morris PG: NMR Imaging. Advances in Magnetic Resonance, Supplement 2. New York, Academic Press, 1982.
2. Pykett JL, Rosen BR: Nuclear magnetic resonance: In vivo proton chemical shift imaging. Radiology *149*:197–201, 1983.
3. Maudsley AA, Hilal SK, Perman WH, Simon HE: Spatially resolved high resolution spectroscopy by "four dimensional" NMR. J Magn Reson *51*:147–152, 1983.
4. Sipponen RE, Sipponen JT, Tanttu JI: A method for chemical shift imaging: Demonstration of bone marrow involvement with proton chemical shift imaging. J Comput Asst Tomogr *8*:585–587, 1984.
5. McFarland E, Koutcher JA, Rosen BR, Teicher B, Brady TJ: In vivo 19F NMR imaging. J Comput Assist Tomogr *9*:8–15, 1985.
6. Haase A, Frahm J, Hanicke W, Matthaei D: 1H-NMR chemical shift selection (CHESS) imaging. Phys Med Biol *30*:341–344, 1985.
7. Hall LD, Sukumar S: Three dimensional Fourier transform NMR imaging: High resolution chemical shift resolved planar imaging. J Magn Reson *56*:314–317, 1984.
8. Mansfield P: Spatial mapping of the chemical shift in NMR. Magn Reson Med *1*:370–386, 1984.
9. Bernardo ML Jr, Lauterbur PC, Hedges LK: Experimental example of NMR spectroscopic imaging by projection reconstruction involving an intrinsic frequency dimension. J Magn Reson *61*:168–174, 1985.
10. Martin JF, Wade CG: Chemical shift encoding in NMR images. J Magn Reson *61*:153–157, 1985.
11. Damadian R, Minkoff L, Goldsmith M, Koutcher JA: Field-focusing nuclear magnetic resonance (FONAR): Formation of chemical scans in man. Naturwissenschaften *65*:250–252, 1978.
12. Damadian R: Field focusing NMR (FONAR) and the formation of chemical images in man. Philos Trans R Soc Lond B *289*:489–500, 1980.
13. Gordon RE, Hanley P, Shaw DG, Gadian DG, et al: Localization of metabolites in animals using ^{31}P topical magnetic resonance. Nature *287*:736–738, 1980.
14. Gordon RE, Hanley PE, Shaw D: Topical magnetic resonance. Progress in NMR spectroscopy. *15*:1–47, 1982.
15. Hinshaw WS: Spin mapping: The application of moving gradients to NMR. Phys Lett *A48*:87–88, 1974.
16. Hinshaw WS: Image formation by nuclear magnetic resonance: The sensitive-point method. J Appl Phys *47*:3709–3721, 1976.
17. Scott KN, Brooker HR, Fitzsimmons JR, Bennett HF, Mick RC: Spatial localization of ^{31}P nuclear magnetic resonance signal by the sensitive point-method. J Magn Reson *50*:339–344, 1982.
18. Bottomley PA: Localized NMR spectroscopy by the sensitive point-method. J Magn Reson *50*:335–338, 1982.
19. Carr HY: Steady-state free precession in nuclear magnetic resonance. Phys Rev *112*:1693–1701, 1958.
20. Schwenck A: NMR pulse technique with high sensitivity for slowly relaxing systems. J Magn Reson *5*:376–389, 1971.
21. Ljunggren S: The influence of the waveform of the time dependent magnetic field gradient on the spatial localization in the sensitive-point method of NMR imaging. J Magn Reson *54*:165–169, 1983.
22. Ernst RR, Anderson WA: Application of Fourier transform spectroscopy to magnetic resonance. Rev Sci Instrum *37*:93–102, 1966.

23. Hoult DI: Rotating frame zeugmatography. J Magn Reson *33*:183–197, 1979.

24. Kumar A, Welti D, Ernst RR: NMR Fourier zeugmatography. J Magn Reson *18*:69–83, 1975.

25. Cox SJ, Styles P: Towards biochemical imaging. J Magn Reson *40*:209–212, 1980.

26. Ackerman JJH, Grove TH, Wong GG, Gadian DG, Radda GK: Mapping of metabolites in whole animals by ^{31}P NMR using surface coils. Nature *283*:167–170, 1980.

27. Gadian DG: Nuclear Magnetic Resonance and Its Applications to Living Systems. Oxford, Clarendon Press, 1982.

28. Bottomley PA: NMR imaging techniques and applications: A review. Rev Sci Instrum *53*:1319–1337, 1982.

29. Clarke GD, Nunnaly RL: Investigation of NMR surface coil geometrics. Third Annual Meeting of the Society of Magnetic Resonance in Medicine, New York, 1984, abstracts 161–162.

30. Ross MS, Hasenfeld A, Bendall MR, Huesman RH, Budinger TF: Simulations of spatial sensitivity for multiple pulse sequences and selective excitation in inhomogenous B1 fields. Third Annual Meeting of the Society of Magnetic Resonance in Medicine, New York, 1984, abstracts 632–633.

31. Sauter R, Mueller E, Fritschy P: Design of special (surface) coils for MR imaging. Meeting of the Radiological Society of North America, Washington D.C., 1984, abstract 527.

32. Kantor HL, Briggs RW, Balaban RS: In vivo ^{31}P nuclear magnetic resonance measurements in canine heart using a catheter-coil. Circ Res *55*:261–266, 1984.

33. Evelhoch JL, Sapaareto SA, Jick DE, Ackerman JJ: In vivo metabolic effects of hyperglycemia in murine radiation-induced fibrosarcoma: A ^{31}P NMR investigation. Proc Natl Acad Sci USA *81*:6496–6500, 1984.

34. Reo NV, Siegfried BA, Ackerman JJ: Direct observation of glycogenesis and glucagon-stimulated glycogenolysis in the rat liver in vivo by high-field carbon-13 surface coil NMR. J Biol Chem *259*:13664–13667, 1984.

35. Younkin DP, Delivaria-Papadopousol M, Leonard JC, Subramanian VH, Eleff S, Leigh Jr JS, Chance B: Unique aspects of human newborn cerebral metabolism evaluated with phosphorus nuclear magnetic resonance spectroscopy. Ann Neurol *16*:581–586, 1984.

36. Evelhoch JL, Ackerman JJH: NMR T1 measurements in inhomogeneous B1 with surface coils. J Magn Reson *53*:52–64, 1983.

37. Matson GB, Schleich J, Serdahl C, Acosta G, Willis JA: Measurement of longitudinal relaxation times using surface coils. J Magn Reson *56*:200–206, 1984.

38. Axel L: Surface coil magnetic resonance imaging. J Comput Assist Tomogr *8*:381–384, 1984.

39. Bottomley PA, Edelstein WA, Hart HR, Schenck JF, Smith LS: Spatial localization in ^{31}P and ^{13}C NMR spectroscopy in vivo using surface coils. Magn Reson Med *1*:410–413, 1984.

40. Richards T, Budinger TF, Nunlist R: Phase encoded proton spectroscopy and imaging of the rat brain in vivo with the surface coil. Third Annual Meeting of the Society of Magnetic Resonance in Medicine, New York, 1984, abstracts 621–622.

41. Brandt G, Chang H, Leifer M: Multislice imaging with surface coils. Third Annual Meeting of the Society of Magnetic Resonance in Medicine, New York, 1984, abstracts 86–87.

42. Holcomb WG, Gore JC: Novel design for surface and intracavity coils for NMR imaging. Third Annual Meeting of the Society of Magnetic Resonance in Medicine, New York, 1984, abstract 333.

43. Sauter R, Fritschy P, Mueller E, Kaiser W, Reinhardt ER: Special coils and surface coils in magnetic resonance imaging. Third Annual Meeting of the Society of Magnetic Resonance in Medicine, New York, 1984, abstracts 656–657.

44. Stelling CB, Wang PC, Lieber A, Mattingly SS, Griffen WO, Powell DE: Prototype coil for magnetic resonance imaging of the female breast. Radiology *254*:457–462, 1985.

45. Radda GK, Ackerman JJH, Bore PJ, Sehr PA, et al: ^{31}P NMR studies on kidney intracellular pH in acute renal acidosis. Int J Biochem *12*:277–281, 1980.

46. Balaban RS, Gadian DG, Radda GK: Phosphorus nuclear magnetic resonance study of the rat kidney in vivo. Kid Int *20*:575–579, 1981.

47. Haase A, Malloy C, Radda GK: Spatial localization of high resolution ^{31}P spectra with a surface coil. J Magn Reson *55*:164–169, 1983.

48. Bax A: Two Dimensional Nuclear Magnetic Resonance in Liquids. Boston, D. Reidel Publishing Co., 1982, pp 22–30.

49. Garwood M, Schleich T, Matson GB, Acosta G: Spatial localization of tissue metabolites by phosphorus-31 NMR rotating-frame zeugmatography. J Magn Reson *60*:268–279, 1984.

50. Bendall MR, Gordon RE: Depth and refocusing pulses designed for multipulse NMR with surface coils. J Magn Reson *53*:365–385, 1983.

51. Tycko R, Pines A: Spatial localization of NMR signals by narrowband inversion. J Magn Reson *60*:156–160, 1984.

52. Shaka AJ, Keller J, Smith MB, Freeman R: Spatial localization of NMR signals in an inhomogeneous radiofrequency field. J Magn Reson *61*:175–180, 1985.

53. Bodenhausen G, Freeman R, Turner DL: Suppression of artifacts in two dimensional J spectroscopy. J Magn Reson *27*:511–514, 1977.

54. Bendall MR, Aue WP: Experimental verification of depth pulses applied with surface coils. J Mag Reson *54*:149–152, 1983.

55. Bendall MR: Portable NMR sample localization method using inhomogeneous RF irradiation coils. Chem Phys Lett *99*:310–315, 1983.

56. Bendall MR, McKendry JM, Cresshull ID, Ordidge RJ: Active detune switch for complete sensitive-

volume localization in in vivo spectroscopy using multiple RF coils and depth pulses. J Magn Reson *60*:473–478, 1984.

57. Haase A: A new method for the decoupling of multiple-coil NMR probes. J Magn Reson *61*:130–136, 1985.
58. Bendall MR: Elimination of high-flux signals near surface coils and field gradient sample localization using depth pulses. J Magn Reson *59*:406–429, 1984.
59. Bendall MR, Pegg DT: Comparison of depth pulse sequences with composite pulses for spatial selection in in vivo NMR. J Magn Reson *63*:494–503, 1985.
60. Shaka AJ, Freeman R: A composite 180 degree pulse for spatial localization. J Magn Reson *63*:596–600, 1985.
61. Rothman DL, Behar KL, DenHollander JA, Shulman RG: Surface coil spin-echo spectra without cycling the refocusing pulse through all four phases. J Magn Reson *59*:157–159, 1984.
62. Bottomley PA, Foster TB, Darrow RD: Depth-resolved surface-coil spectroscopy (DRESS) for in vivo ^{1}H, ^{31}P and ^{13}C NMR. J Magn Reson *59*:338–342, 1984.
63. Bottomley PA, Smith LS, Leue WM, Charles C: Slice-interleaved depth-resolved surface-coil spectroscopy (SLIT DRESS) for rapid ^{31}P NMR in vivo. J Magn Reson *64*:347–351, 1985.
64. Crooks LE, Ortendahl DA, Kaufman L, et al: Clinical efficiency of nuclear magnetic resonance imaging. Radiology *146*:123–128, 1983.
65. Mareci TH, Thomas RG, Scott KN, Brooker HR: Combination pulse gradient and surface coil localization of chemical shift resolved spectra. Third Annual Meeting of the Society of Magnetic Resonance in Medicine, New York, 1984, abstracts 493–494.
66. Mareci TH, Brooker HR: High-resolution magnetic resonance spectra from a sensitive region defined with pulsed field gradients. J Magn Reson *57*:157–163, 1984.
67. Gordon RE, Ordidge J: Volume selection for high resolution NMR studies. Third Annual Meeting of the Society of Magnetic Resonance in Medicine, New York, 1984, abstracts 272–273.
68. Ordidge RJ, Bendall MR, Gordon RE, Connelly A: Volume selection for in vivo biological spectroscopy. *In* Gorrl GV, Khetrafal CL, Saran A (eds): Magnetic Resonance in Biology and Medicine. New Delhi, Tata McGraw Hill, 1985, pp 387–397.
69. Aue WP, Muller TA, Cross TA, Sellig J: Volume-selective excitation: A novel approach to topical NMR. J Magn Reson *56*:350–354, 1984.
70. Miller S, Aue WP, Seelig J: NMR imaging and volume-selective spectroscopy with a single surface coil. J Magn Reson *63*:530–543, 1985.
71. Pekar J, Leigh JS Jr, Chance B: Harmonically analyzed sensitivity profile. A novel approach to depth pulses for surface coil. J Magn Reson *64*:115–119, 1985.
72. Ordidge RJ, Connally A, Lohman JAB: Image-selected *in vivo* spectroscopy (ISIS). A new technique for spatially selective NMR spectroscopy. J Magn Reson *66*:283–294, 1986.
73. Jensen DJ, Delayre JL, Narayana PA: Localized *T1* measurements using volume-selective excitation. J Magn Reson *69*:552–558, 1986.
74. Luyten PR, Marien AJH, Sijtsma B, den Hollander JA: Solvent-suppressed spatially resolved spectroscopy. An approach to high-resolution NMR on a whole-body MRI system. J Magn Reson *6*:148–155, 1986.
75. Luyten PR, Anderson CM, den Hollander JA: ^{1}H NMR relaxation measurements of human tissues *in situ* by spatially resolved spectroscopy. Magn Reson Med *4*:431–440, 1987.
76. Jensen DJ, Narayana PA, Delayre JL: Pulse sequence design for volume selective excitation in magnetic resonance. Med Phys *14*:38–42, 1987.
77. Bailes DR, Bryant DJ, Bydder GM, et al: Localized phosphorus-31 NMR spectroscopy of normal and pathological human organs *in vivo* using phase-encoding techniques. J Magn Reson *74*:158–170, 1987.
78. Frahm J, Merboldt K, Hanicke W: Localized proton spectroscopy using stimulated echoes. J Magn Reson *72*:502–508, 1987.

XVII

RESEARCH AREAS

96

Fast Scanning Methods in MRI

RONALD R. PRICE
DAVID R. PICKENS

Conventional magnetic resonance (MR) imaging methods are time consuming, requiring image acquisition times ranging from 2 to 10 minutes and longer. Long imaging times are not tolerated well by many patients, especially children, and are impossible for some critically ill patients. In addition, long imaging times amplify motion artifacts (particularly from respiration), leading to inferior image quality. The advantages of short imaging times, including better patient throughput for more efficient facility utilization and new dynamic imaging procedures, have added great impetus to the development of fast scanning techniques.

Most fast scan techniques employ a variation of the two-dimensional Fourier transform method (2DFT). In the 2DFT method, frequency encoding provides spatial localization along one axis of an image while phase encoding provides spatial location along a second orthogonal axis. This approach can be extended to three-dimensional Fourier transform (3DFT) imaging, where phase encoding provides spatial location along both of the other axes orthogonal to the frequency encoding axis. Phase encoding is accomplished by acquiring data N different times following independent applications of N different (systematically stepped) gradient strengths along the selected phase-encoded direction. The number of gradient applications (N) determines the number of pixels that will be present in the image in the phase-encoding direction, usually 128 or 256 gradient steps in typical 2DFT sequences. The magnitude of the gradient steps determines the field of view (FOV), so that the combination of the number of pixels and the FOV over which they are spread determines the spatial resolution.

The length of time between the acquisitions of each of the N gradient steps is the repetition time (TR). Frequently each gradient step will be repeated and the results averaged in order to improve the signal to noise ratio (S/N) of the image. The increase in S/N is proportional to the square root of the number of acquisitions (NA), which are averaged. Thus, the total time (T) needed to acquire an image is the product of the TR, the number of gradient steps (N), and the number of acquisitions (NA):

$$T = N \cdot TR \cdot NA. \tag{1}$$

Fast scanning techniques may be categorized with regard to which of the above variables (N or TR) is reduced for the purpose of minimizing the total acquisition time, T. Since the number of acquisitions, NA, is directly related to the signal sensitivity of the system as reflected by the S/N, a minimum number of acquisition averages to achieve a usable signal to noise ratio depends on the machine characteristics. The other quantities, however, have more interesting potentials for scan time shortening and likewise have more significant effects on the acquired image.

METHODS THAT REDUCE GRADIENT STEPS

Let us consider first those techniques that attempt to reduce the number of phase-encoding gradient steps (N) as the means of reducing T. Usually data are acquired once for each phase-encoding gradient step with each acquisition, providing an additional "view" in phase space. The number of "views" determines the number of pixels that will be created in the phase-encoding direction in the final image. For example, an image taken with 128 gradient steps will yield an image with 128 pixels in the phase-encoding direction. The number of pixels available in the frequency-encoded direction is determined by the number of samples taken by the analog-to-digital converter. The number of pixels in the phase-encoding and frequency-encoding directions do not have to be equal.

Half-Fourier Imaging

In the typical 2DFT technique described above, the phase-encoding gradient is usually stepped from some maximum negative value ($-G_y$) through zero ($G_y = 0$) to the maximum positive value ($+G_y$) in discrete steps. It has been recognized that the echo signal acquired following a negative value of G_y is mathematically related to the signal following the positive value of G_y at the same strength because of the property of symmetry of the Fourier transform. In this light, it is therefore possible to acquire data only from the negative gradient steps and then to "create" the positive signals. The obvious advantage of this method is to reduce the acquisition time by one-half. The disadvantage of the technique is a reduction of S/N because the redundant acquisitions provide additional signal averaging, which results in a reduced noise level in the images.

Echo-Planar Method

The echo-planar method, originally proposed by Mansfield,[1] and its variations use oscillating gradients. These methods tend to reduce the scan time by reducing the number of sequence repetitions required to create an image. In the full echo-planar method, data for an entire image can theoretically be acquired during a single sequence. As seen in Figure 96–1, the sequence is initiated by a slice-selecting pulse in the presence of a gradient field (G_z) in the desired slice-selection direction (logical Z). Following

Echo-Planar Method

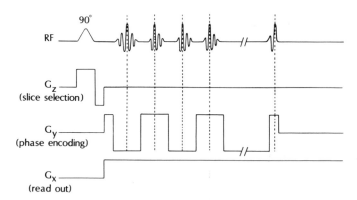

Figure 96–1. The echo-planar technique differs from the conventional two-dimensional Fourier transformation method in that the phase-encoding gradient is rapidly switched instead of being turned on in discrete steps with systematically increasing values for each acquisition. The echo-planar method acquires data adequate to reconstruct an entire image in a single sequence.

the 90 degree pulse, a series of phase encoded echoes are created by rapidly switching the gradient in the phase-encoding direction. Each digitized echo acquires a different phase as a result of the time intervals between each echo. Data from each echo then are used as a phase-encoded view in a conventional 2DFT image reconstruction. The limitations of the technique are primarily related to the capabilities of the gradient drivers to produce the required rate and magnitude of gradient field switching. If the switching rate is too slow, significant $T2$ decay will have occurred between each echo, resulting in an image in which each phase encoded view has a different $T2$ dependence. Similarly, the absolute magnitude of the signal would also be significantly different for each view and can vanish completely if the delay is too long. At the present time, gradient switching rates in the range of 1 KHz have allowed images to be made within about 40 ms with 32 phase encoded views (i.e., 32 × 32 images). Further improvements in gradient power drivers and signal averaging promise continued development of this technique.

Several variations on the basic method of echo-planar imaging have been investigated. These methods are generally referred to as "hybrid" imaging methods and incorporate aspects of both conventional 2DFT imaging and echo-planar imaging. Hybrid imaging sequences are generally less ambitious than the echo-planar sequences in that they attempt to acquire several phase-encoded views during each sequence rather than trying to record information for an entire image. For example, using a phase-encoding gradient that oscillates 8 times would reduce the total scan time by a factor of 8. Factors of 2 and 4 have already been demonstrated.[4] Several institutions are also investigating methods that utilize combinations of oscillating gradients in both axes of the two-dimensional image plane.

METHODS THAT REDUCE TR

The other category of fast scanning methods are those techniques that attempt to shorten the total imaging time, T, by shortening TR. The primary limitation on shorter TR's in the conventional spin-echo sequence is the $T1$ relaxation time of the tissue under study. The time interval between the last data acquisition and the start of the excitation pulse (90 degree pulse) of the next sequence is the time available for the recovery of the longitudinal magnetization (M_z). As the TR is shortened, there is less time for recovery of M_z, with the result that the spin system becomes saturated and the signal begins to vanish as TR progressively gets shorter than $T1$. The reduction in signal (S) follows the following relationship:

$$S = 1 - \exp(-TR/T1) \qquad (2)$$

Using partial flip angles, however, it is possible to reduce the TR while maintaining an adequate signal level.

Partial Flip Angles

The conventional spin-echo sequence utilizes a 90 degree excitation pulse and a 180 degree rephasing pulse. The 90 degree pulse is used because it yields the highest NMR signal, provided the spin system has fully recovered its longitudinal magnetization (M_z) at the start of each sequence. With short TR sequences this is not the case, and in fact, it can be shown that excitation angles of less than 90 degrees will produce a stronger signal by preserving the longitudinal magnetization.[2] As illustrated in Figure 96–2, a small flip angle (θ) will produce only a small change in the longitudinal mag-

Partial Flip Angles

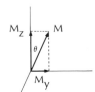

Figure 96–2. The transverse magnetization (M_y) is responsible for the magnitude of the NMR signal. Small flip angles (θ) are used to allow rapid recovery of the longitudinal magnetization (M_z). In relative terms, a small change in M_z results in a large change in M_y.

netization component while producing a very large change in the transverse component (M_y).[6] The large change in M_y occurs because $M_y = 0$ at equilibrium. With the magnetization largely remaining longitudinal, less time is needed for equilibrium to be established and consequently, a shorter *TR* may be used.

The conventional spin-echo sequence also uses a 180 degree radio frequency (rf) rephasing pulse to bring about an echo. Unfortunately, when *TR* becomes very short, the longitudinal magnetization will be inverted following each rephasing pulse with the eventual result being to create an equilibrium state in which the longitudinal magnetization goes to zero. For this reason fast scanning methods generally do not use slice selective 180 degree rephasing pulses but instead rely upon echo formation by gradient reversals, i.e., gradient echoes.[5]

Gradient Echo Methods

Most fast scanning methods now use imaging sequences that employ both partial flip angles and gradient echoes to achieve ultrashort *TR*'s, typically *TR*'s of 10 to 40 ms.[3] In gradient echo sequences, the 180 degree rf pulse is eliminated and the frequency-encoding gradient is modified to be bipolar in form (Fig. 96–3). By applying a negative gradient first, the spins will be dephased across the selected slice (with spins located at the center being the reference phase) such that spins in the higher gradient fields will accumulate a progressively larger phase difference as long as the gradient remains on. When the gradient is reversed, those spins that originally experienced fields that were larger than that of the reference spins will now experience fields that are correspondingly smaller than the reference, causing them to rephase at the same rate with which they originally dephased. The result is to create a rephased echo at the center of the positive lobe of the bipolar gradient. The echo is digitized and the image is created with the conventional 2DFT method. Figure 96–4 illustrates a more complete description of a full 2DFT imaging sequence with gradient echoes and partial spin flips. The

Gradient Echo

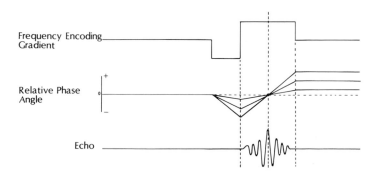

Frequency Encoding Gradient

Relative Phase Angle

Echo

Figure 96–3. Gradient echoes are formed by first applying a negative gradient, which causes spins to precess at different rates depending upon their location in the field and will accumulate a progressively larger negative phase (relative to stationary spins) until the gradient is reversed, i.e., areas originally experiencing negative gradient values will now experience positive gradients of equal magnitude. The result is to bring about rephasing (echo), since the spins will now reverse their rate of precession, i.e., rapidly precessing spins will slow down and slowly precessing spins will speed up.

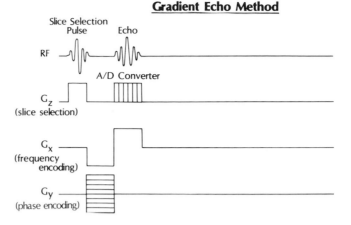

Gradient Echo Method

Figure 96–4. The gradient echo can be utilized as part of a two-dimensional Fourier transformation imaging sequence by eliminating the 180 degree rephasing pulse and replacing it with a bipolar gradient pulse in the read-out direction. The phase-encoding gradient and the slice selection gradient applications remain unchanged.

rf pulse consists of only a slice-selective pulse, which is usually a reduced flip angle of 10 to 45 degrees. It should be pointed out that another advantage of the gradient-echo method is reduction in rf power dissipation in the patient (as a result of the elimination of the 180 degree pulse). Power dissipation is an issue of great concern, especially in higher field systems when high duty factor multislice/multiecho imaging sequences are used. The disadvantage of the gradient-echo method is that the technique does not compensate for main field inhomogeneities as well as the spin-echo technique does and, therefore, places a premium on field uniformity.

Other than the elimination of the 180 degree rf pulse and the modification of the read-out gradient waveform, the rest of the sequence is identical to the 2DFT spin-echo sequence. In like manner, the total image acquisition time will be equal to the product of the number of phase-encoding gradient steps, the TR, and the number of acquisitions. A sequence that acquired 128 gradient steps with a TR of 40 ms and two acquisitions would require an imaging time of just over 10 seconds.

$$T = N \times TR \times NA$$
$$T = 128 \times 0.04 \text{ s} \times 2 \tag{3}$$
$$T = 10.2 \text{ s}$$

In general, the ultrafast scanning techniques will result in a loss of S/N. The image contrast, however, can be varied considerably by varying TR, flip angle, and TE.

Commercial vendors have implemented most of the above fast scan techniques and refer to them by various names. Most of the sequences are variations of the sequence that uses the combination of reduced flip angles and gradient echoes. In this category are included FAST (Fourier acquired steady-state technique), GRASS (gradient recalled acquisition of steady state), and FLASH (*Fast Low Angle SHot*), FISP (*Fast Imaging with Steady Precession*) both techniques involve reduced flip angle and gradient refocussing.

The FLASH and FISP techniques differ in that in the FISP method, the order of the phase encoding steps is reversed after each data collection. A comparison of a 40 degree flip angle FLASH image (TE/TR = 14 ms/30 ms) with a 90 degree flip angle FISP image (14 ms/30 ms) (Fig. 96–5) shows that the FLASH image provides better gray/white matter differentiation while the FISP image shows better contrast of edema and CSF.

In fast FISP techniques (50 s) with low flip angles, the cerebrospinal fluid (CSF) is visualized with high intensity much like a $T2$ weighted spin echo scan. Figure 96–6 is an axial C-spine scan with the scan techniques TE/TR/angle = 13 ms/100 ms/20

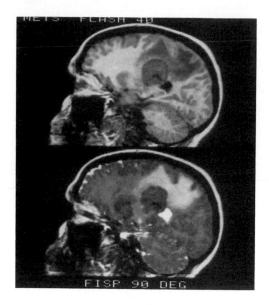

Figure 96–5. (Breast Mets) This is a direct comparison of FLASH 40 and FISP 90. Both images are from a set of 128 1.4 mm slices acquired in approximately 13 minutes. The FLASH image demonstrates excellent grey/white matter differentiation while the FISP images provide better contrast between tumor and edema. (Courtesy of Siemens Medical Systems.)

degrees. For very short $TR = 20$ ms, the CSF intensity is maximum at low flip angles (5 degrees) and diminishes with larger flip-angles (20 degrees). Comparisons of images $TE/TR = 12$ ms/20 ms for flip angles of 5, 10, 15, and 20 degrees are shown in Figure 96–7.

Fast imaging techniques can be utilized to make high spatial resolution images in reasonably short times. The extra time needed to form additional gradient steps for higher resolution is compensated for by the short TR values. In Figure 96–8 is a high resolution (512×512) image, which was acquired in 5.5 min. The in-plane resolution is 0.45 mm with a slice thickness of 5 mm. The technique was a 10 ms/20 ms/20 degree FLASH scan.

Fast scan techniques can also be used to produce high resolution three-dimensional image acquisitions. In Figure 96–9 is illustrated a FISP scan with a 40 degree flip angle (15 ms/30 ms) in which 64 contiguous slices were acquired in 7.6 minutes.

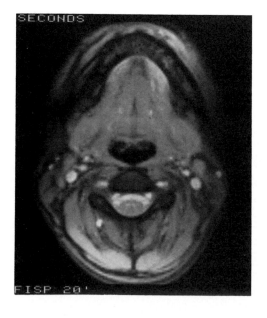

Figure 96–6. (50 sec) Axial C-Spine. Helmholtz coil. In this low angle FISP image (100/13/20 degrees) detail is visualized within the cord as in a *T1* weighted spin-echo scan, while CSF is visualized with high intensity as in a *T2* weighted scan. Dorsal and ventral nerve roots are seen. Transverse vessels can be distinguished as peripheral structures of high signal intensity. (Courtesy of Siemens Medical Systems.)

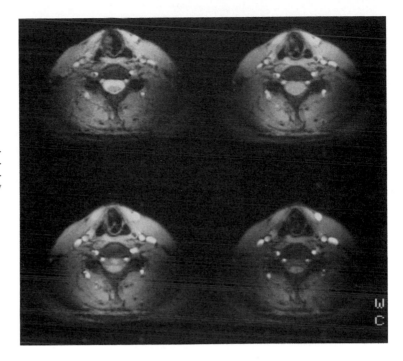

Figure 96–7. (0.33 min) Flip angle comparison. FISP 55, 10, 15, and 20. Increasing flip angle increases *T1* weighting and suppression of CSF. (Courtesy of Siemens Medical Systems.)

Fast imaging is also useful for producing cine-like presentations of the heart. A typical motion-corrected FISP image (22 ms/680 ms) of the heart is shown in Figure 96–10. This image is one of 30 images which were used to produce a "real-time" view of the beating heart.

Commercial vendors have also implemented a modified echo-planar method using oscillating gradients and have named the sequence HYBRID. Other fast scan techniques of interest are those that use a technique called "driven equilibrium," in which pulses are used to drive the magnetization to equilibrium without waiting. This technique has been called DEFT for driven equilibrium Fourier transform.

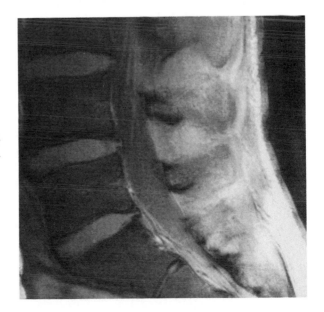

Figure 96–8. (Super-High Res) FLASH 20, 5.5 minutes. Nerve roots are visualized. In-plane resolution is 0.47 mm, 5 mm slice (1.1 mm cubed voxel). (Courtesy of Siemens Medical Systems.)

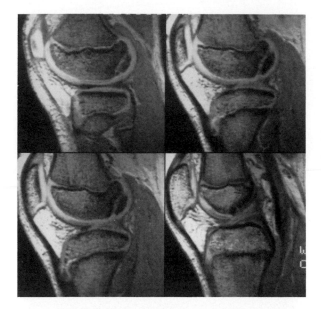

Figure 96–9. Example of three-dimensional imaging with FISP 40, in which 64 contiguous slices were acquired in 7.6 minutes. (Courtesy of Siemens Medical Systems.)

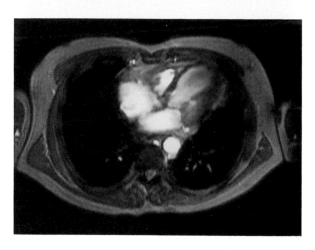

Figure 96–10. (Infarct, aneurysm) FISP can be combined with gradient motion rephasing to produce artifact-free images of the heart. This is one of 30 images that may be displayed in CINE fashion to provide a "real-time" view of the beating heart. (Courtesy of Siemens Medical Systems.)

Another technique for acquiring ultrafast scans reduces the number of phase encoding gradient steps while simultaneously reducing the field of view. In this manner scan time is reduced and spatial resolution is maintained at the expense of field of view. This method is generally referred to as "strip scanning."

At the present time much effort is being put into developing ultrafast scanning techniques, which allow MRI to enter into dynamic imaging protocols for the evaluation of the cardiovascular system, for the creation of noninvasive vascular images, and for rapid imaging of children and the critically ill. At the expense of S/N, high resolution scans on the order of 10's of seconds are now available. Further work and research will likely produce even shorter scan times with improved image quality.

References

1. Mansfield P, Morris PG: NMR imaging in biomedicine. In Waugh JS (ed): Advances in Magnetic Resonance. Supplement 2. New York, Academic Press, 1982.
2. Haase A, Frahm J, Matthaei D, et al: FLASH imaging: Rapid NMR imaging using low flip angle pulses. J Magn Reson 67:258–266, 1986.

3. Frahm J, Haase A, Matthaei D, et al: Three-dimensional NMR imaging using the FLASH technique. J Comput Asst Tomogr *10*:363–368, 1986.
4. Haacke EM, Bearden FH, Clayton JR, et al: Reduction of MR imaging time by the hybrid fast scan technique. Radiology *158*:521–529, 1986.
5. Wehrli FW, Shimakawa A, Gullberg GT: Time-of-flight MR flow imaging: Selective saturation recovery with gradient refocussing (SSRGR). Radiology *160*:781–785, 1986.
6. Wehrli FW: Introduction to Fast-Scan Magnetic Resonance. Milwaukee, Wisconsin, General Electric Company Publication, 1986.

97

Thin-Slice MRI

JOSEPH D. WEISSMAN
ALAN STEIN

In this chapter we will discuss the applications and limitations of various methods for the generation of thin-slice magnetic resonance images. We will arbitrarily define thin slices as 0.5 cm or less by full-width-half-maximum (FWHM), twice the distance between slice center and the point where the hydrogen nuclei produce a magnetic resonance signal that is half of the maximum signal amplitude. Each method presents a different tradeoff between imaging time, resolution, signal to noise ratio (SNR), and the ability to produce thin slices of high quality.

Slice thickness and positioning in MRI are under software control, are variable over a wide range, and can be optimized for particular diagnostic situations. This is in marked contrast to other tomographic imaging modalities in which slice thickness is fixed by hardware. In determining the optimal slice thickness for diagnostic applications of magnetic resonance imaging (MRI) the desire for anatomic resolution must be balanced against the unavoidable decreases in SNR from the smaller voxels that will be obtained.

Thin slices and fine in-plane resolution are essential for the imaging of detailed anatomy such as the sella, brainstem, orbit, temporal bone, and temporomandibular joint, where volume averaging would obscure detail. Here surface coils and signal averaging are used to maintain SNR. In other diagnostic situations thin slices are counterproductive.

For example, the recent work of Butch et al.[1] has demonstrated that relatively thick slices (1 to 1.5 cm) yield diagnostically superior transverse images of the liver when combined with short *TE* and *TR* acquisitions and extensive signal averaging. No respiratory gating is required, as the signal averaging reduces the ghost artifacts caused by motion.

Reduction of slice thickness has some unavoidable consequences for image quality. Regardless of the way thin slices are made, fewer hydrogen nuclei per voxel are producing the magnetic resonance signal. This reduces the maximum SNR and affects detectability. Slice thickness and resolution do not limit the detectability (the question of the absence or presence) of lesions or anatomy. An object smaller than the MRI voxel can be detected if its signal contribution changes the signal of the voxel to a significant degree. This occurs when a small high signal producing structure lies in a low signal environment. Conversely, a minimal contrast difference between a large object and its background can be masked by the decreased SNR associated with thin slices. Detection is determined by both contrast and resolution. Decreasing slice thickness increases the number of slices required for a given field of view and may increase the duration of acquisition, reconstruction, and archiving. Thinner and increased numbers of slices may also increase radio frequency (rf) energy deposition in the patient, depending on the pulse sequence, pulse rate, pulse width, and amplitude that are used.

Certain techniques can be used to improve signal strength and provide the ability to decrease slice thickness. With physiologic synchronization, even rapidly moving detailed anatomic structures such as the heart valves can be imaged with reduced motion effects (D. Feiglin, personal communication). Surface coils provide increased signal from a localized area and greatly increase the ability to collect adequate information for thin slice imaging. The falloff of sensitivity with distance that is common to all surface coil designs is a blessing in disguise, as it permits the use of increased gradient amplitude for zoomed acquisitions.

Two-dimensional multislice and three-dimensional volume techniques are the current alternatives for the production of thin slice magnetic resonance images. Each has its advantages with respect to slice definition, the production of thin slices, slice-slice interactions, the use of slice gaps, acquisition time, rf energy deposition in patient tissues, and motion artifact sensitivity. The relative merits and deficiencies of these techniques will be reviewed below.

TWO-DIMENSIONAL MR IMAGING

Selective Excitation

The basis of two-dimensional MRI techniques is selective excitation, a process that enables the hydrogen nuclei in a slice of tissue to be excited without affecting the state of the surrounding hydrogen nuclei. Ideally the slices should be well-defined (square or with very limited "tails"), and it should be possible to use two-dimensional multislice techniques without slice gaps or slice-slice interactions. In reality we do not achieve this perfection and must accept slice profiles that are not perfectly square and/ or have significant tails. The reasons for this are found in the physics of selective excitation.

To understand selective excitation we begin with the basic MR phenomenon: an MR-active nucleus or "spin" such as hydrogen-1 in a magnetic field of a given strength has a characteristic Larmor frequency at which it can absorb or emit energy. When linear magnetic field gradients are added, the Larmor frequency varies linearly with distance along the gradient direction.

A distance along a magnetic field gradient corresponds exactly with a range or "bandwidth" of Larmor frequencies. Selective excitation uses "selective" rf pulses (also known as narrow-band, soft, or shaped) with a controlled frequency range or bandwidth. Conversely, "nonselective" rf pulses have a broad frequency range and are variously known as wideband, hard, or square. When selective rf pulses are combined with magnetic field gradients, a slice of hydrogen nuclei is "flipped" selectively in the patient or experimental system (Fig. 97–1). The slice of tissue is oriented perpendicular to the magnetic field gradient. The thickness of the slice is proportional to the bandwidth of the exciting pulse and inversely proportional to the strength of the magnetic field gradient.

Selective excitation depends on the ability to create selective rf pulses. By controlling the shape or "envelope" of a rf pulse the frequency range of the pulse can be broadened from the carrier frequency to more or less uniformly cover a range of frequencies. A large number of rf pulse envelopes have been used in MR applications. In MRI some common pulse envelopes are square (nonselective), Gaussian ($\exp(-x^2)$), and $\sin(x)/x$, otherwise known as sinc. In the presence of a magnetic field gradient, a selective rf pulse, depending on its strength and the shape of its envelope, will selectively tip a different spatial distribution (otherwise called the excitation or slice profile)

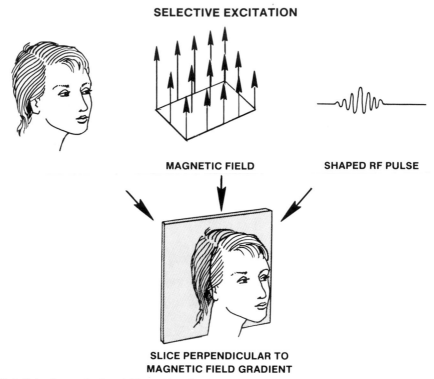

SELECTIVE EXCITATION

MAGNETIC FIELD   SHAPED RF PULSE

SLICE PERPENDICULAR TO
MAGNETIC FIELD GRADIENT

Figure 97–1. Selective excitation. *i*, The subject lies in a uniform magnetic field. *ii*, Simultaneously, magnetic field gradients and shaped rf pulses are applied. *iii*, Hydrogen nuclei are "flipped" within a slice with thickness proportional to the length of the rf pulse and the reciprocal of the strength of the gradient.

of nuclear magnetization along the direction through the slice. At each point along the excitation profile the nuclear magnetization has a direction in space and a magnitude.

The Bloch equations (for a useful discussion of the Bloch equations, see reference 2) are a set of differential equations that define the relationship between the nuclear magnetization and applied static and rf magnetic fields. Using a computer simulation of the Bloch equations, the excitation profile of a given rf pulse envelope can be calculated exactly. The slice profile resulting from an entire multislice imaging pulse sequence may be simulated with a slightly more elaborate computer program. Given these slice profiles, the optimal spacing of multislice acquisitions can be determined.

A prevalent but overused approximation is the Fourier transform relationship between slice profiles and pulse envelopes. Although valid for low (<30 degrees) tip angles, and a very rough approximation of 90 degree slice profiles, it is completely incorrect for 180 degree slice profiles. It is not sufficiently accurate to predict the relative merit of different rf pulse envelopes and slice profiles, the magnitude of slice-slice interactions, or the slice profiles of complete MRI pulse sequences. For all of these reasons Bloch equation simulations are preferred to the Fourier transform relationship.

Each rf pulse envelope has its characteristic excitation and slice profiles. These may be calculated or directly measured. In Figure 97–2, sinc (*B* and *D*) and Gaussian (*A* and *C*) envelopes are shown together with the excitation and slice profiles calculated by the Fourier transform relationship and by Bloch equation simulations of 90 degree pulses and 90 to 180 degree pulse combinations.

The slice profiles show the relationship between the transverse and longitudinal components of magnetization of hydrogen nuclei along a line running through the slice. In this and subsequent discussions the magnetization is displayed as the magnitude of

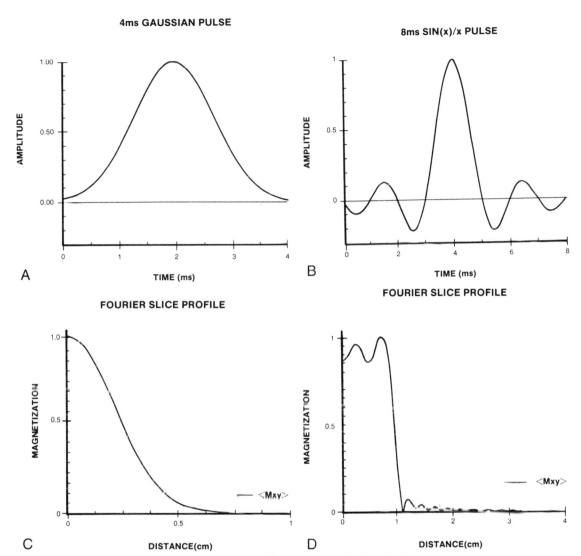

4ms GAUSSIAN PULSE

8ms SIN(x)/x PULSE

A

B

FOURIER SLICE PROFILE

FOURIER SLICE PROFILE

C

D

Figure 97–2. Slice and excitation profiles—sinc and Gaussian. *A* and *B,* The rf pulse envelopes are used to amplitude modulate the transmitter output as in AM radio broadcasting. The Gaussian envelope (*A*) is a smooth positive peak which rapidly decreases to the baseline. The sinc envelope (*B*) is a more complex damped oscillation with positive and negative lobes which do not rapidly reach baseline. For this reason the sinc envelope must be truncated in actual use. The time scale in these plots is the same for both pulses. *C* and *D,* Fourier transform slice profiles. These represent what the slice profile would look like if the selective excitation process followed the simple Fourier transform relationship. The Gaussian rf pulse has a Gaussian profile, and the sinc pulse has a square profile with some "ringing." *Illustration continued on following page*

E and *F,* Bloch equation simulations of isolated rf and magnetic field gradient pulses. The combination of the shaped rf pulses and magnetic field gradients produces the excitation profiles shown. The excitation profiles show the transverse and longitudinal components of magnetization as a function of distance off slice center. In this constant gradient strength simulation the gradient strength was 0.25 g/cm. No relaxation effects are included in these simulations of 4 ms Gaussian and an 8 ms sinc pulses. *G* and *H,* Bloch equation simulations of entire imaging pulse sequences. A real MRI pulse sequence contains gradient and RF pulses for slice selection, frequency encoding, and phase encoding. The sinc and Gaussian slice profiles both show trailing slice profiles and surrounding extensive areas of saturation due to the use of "wide" 180 degree slice profiles to obtain central regions of uniform refocusing ability. These effects define a requirement for slice gaps which are typically 10 to 30 degrees of the full-slice thickness.

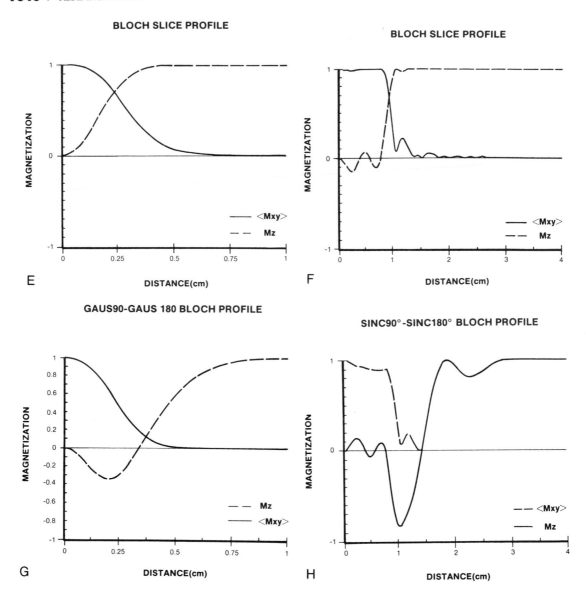

BLOCH SLICE PROFILE

E DISTANCE(cm)

BLOCH SLICE PROFILE

F DISTANCE(cm)

GAUS90-GAUS 180 BLOCH PROFILE

G DISTANCE(cm)

SINC90°-SINC180° BLOCH PROFILE

H DISTANCE(cm)

the component within the transverse plane, (M_{xy}), and as the longitudinal component, M_z. In an imaging pulse sequence it is (M_{xy}) that produces the magnetic resonance signal, but M_z is also important, as discussed below.

The Fourier transform calculations (Fig. 97–2C and D) show only (M_{xy}) and suggest, as expected, that the Gaussian envelope has a Gaussian slice profile and that the truncated sinc envelope has a roughly square slice profile.

A more exact calculation is shown in the Bloch equation simulations of the selective excitation from isolated 90 degree sinc and Gaussian rf pulses (Fig. 97–2E and F). (M_{xy}) and M_z are shown. The (M_{xy}) slice profiles corresponding to the Gaussian rf pulses are Gaussian-like and blunted at the slice center compared to Figure 97–2C. The (M_{xy}) slice profiles corresponding to the sinc rf pulse envelope have a large hump outside an otherwise square profile. The changes in M_z for both sinc and Gaussian pulse envelopes extend outside the profile as defined by (M_{xy}). This means that the selective excitation defines a signal producing slice that is surrounded by a region of saturation.

A practical discussion of slice profiles must include the effects of complete imaging pulse sequences using selective 180 degree and 90 degree pulses. In two-dimensional multislice-multiecho (20-MS/ME) sequences both types of pulses are used. Figure 97–2G and H shows the (M_{xy}) and M_z slice profiles from a Bloch simulation using selective 90 and 180 degree sinc and Gaussian pulses. The (M_{xy}) profiles are more distorted than in Figure 97–2E and F, particularly the sinc pulse. For both sinc and Gaussian pulses the M_z effects extend far outside the slice as defined by (M_{xy}). In this region no signal is produced, but the state of the hydrogen nuclei is perturbed so that it would cause signal intensity changes in adjacent slices. In other words, the imperfections in real slice profiles require that slice gaps be used. Typically these must be 10 to 30 percent of the full slice thickness to prevent reduction in SNR and alterations in tissue contrast by slice-slice saturation interactions.

Several useful generalizations can be made about rf pulses and slice profiles. First, for a given envelope shape, the wider the rf pulse envelope (in time), the proportionately narrower its bandwidth (in frequency) and, in the example shown, the narrower the slice profile (in space) that it creates (Fig. 97–3a to d).

Second, more complicated rf pulse envelopes, such as sinc (for 90 degree and lower tip angles), are used to create slices with squarer profiles. They generally do so at the cost of increased pulse duration. When the length of the rf pulse interval is fixed, a Gaussian or similar pulse will produce a thinner slice as defined by FWHM. Conceptually, the central lobe of a sinc pulse does the major portion of spin flipping in the slice and the side lobes of the sinc pulse rf envelope "square up" the slice profile, which would result if the center lobe was used alone. The side lobes contribute to rf deposition and make the sinc pulse less efficient in terms of patient heating. Thus, under conditions of constant gradient strength, rf pulse duration and *TE*, one can always produce a thinner slice (by FWHM) with Gaussian than with sinc or other complex pulses. More complex rf pulses must be longer in duration than Gaussian pulses to

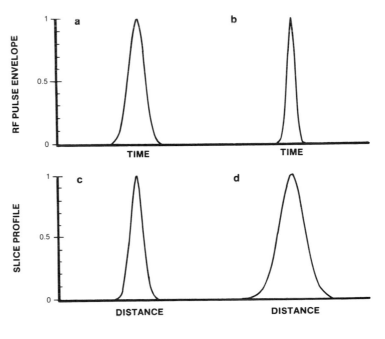

THE EFFECT OF RF PULSE DURATION ON SLICE PROFILE

Figure 97–3. Slice profiles as a function of pulse duration. Here the Gaussian rf pulse envelope is varied in duration by a factor of two. Plots (*a*) and (*b*) show the two RF pulse envelopes using the same time scale. Plots (*c*) and (*d*) show the corresponding slice profiles using the same distance scale. The pulse with the shorter duration has a profile that is twice as thick.

achieve the desired FWHM and squarer slice profiles with the same gradient strengths[3] (Fig. 97–4).

Third, saturation affects signal intensity and is determined by pulse sequence repetition rate (*TR*), *T1*, and the tip angle of the rf pulses. Since the slice profile measures both tip angle and phase, the slice profile will vary with saturation and slice profile overlap when relaxation is considered.[4]

Fourth, the slice profiles for 180 degree pulses differ markedly from those of 90 degree pulses. The slice profiles of isolated 180 degree pulses may be calculated with Bloch equation simulation programs. A 180 degree Gaussian rf pulse has a central 180 degree region surrounded by tails, where there is essentially 90 degree tipping. The 90 degree areas can give rise to free-induction decay signals, which can result in artifacts on MR images. The sinc-180 slice profile shows an irregular profile, again with extensive effectively 90 degree tipping side lobes. Similar undesirable effects are found with most commonly used rf pulse envelopes.

There are several ways to cope with the effects of nonselective inversion pulses. Since the central portion of a sinc or Gaussian 180 degree pulse slice profile is an effective inverter, using imaging sequences with 180 degree profiles that are twice as thick as the 90 degree profiles (and using appropriate signal averaging with phase shift-

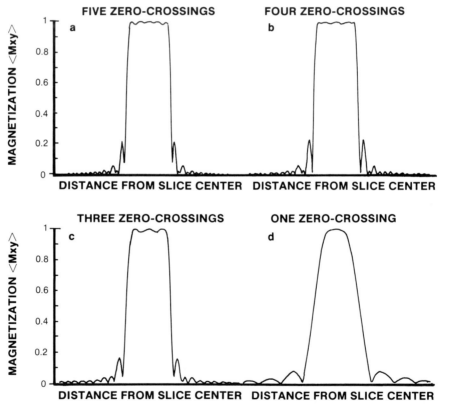

Figure 97–4. The effect of pulse envelope truncation. The sinc envelope, unlike the Gaussian, does not rapidly approach zero amplitude. As a result it is necessary to use truncated sinc pulses. The shape factor of a given sinc envelope is the number of zero-crossings in a given waveform. For example, a sinc pulse with a shape factor of five will have five zero-crossings on either side; it is truncated after five zero-crossings. Truncation reduces the quality of the slice profile. Here slice profiles have been simulated for imaging pulse sequences with 90 degree sinc pulses with five, four, three, and one zero-crossings. The envelopes were consecutive truncations of the same sinc function. The Bloch equation calculations assumed a single slice with a nonselective 180 degree pulse. For multislice operation the effects of nonideal refocusing pulses and slice-slice interaction cause further degradation in the slice profile. Parts *a* through *d* show the slice profiles of sequences with sinc pulses with five, four, three, and one zero-crossings. The progressive degradation is obvious.

ing) will produce slices with profiles that do not neglect the irregularities of the selective 180 degree pulse. The slice profiles in Figure 97–2*G* and *H* were produced using 180 degree pulses with slice profiles that were twice as wide as those of the 90 degree pulses.

Another approach is to design selective 180 degree pulse envelopes using Bloch equation simulations and modeling algorithms. The WOW-180 pulse[5] produces localized inversion with minimal tails or other side effects (Fig. 97–5*a* and *b*).

In multiecho imaging the effects of nonideal inversion pulses are cumulative. "Nonharmonic" sequences that allow short and long *TE* multiecho data acquisition without intervening 180 degree pulses reduce the nonideal effects directly by reducing the number of 180 degree pulses.

Most of the above that is important in daily use can be summarized in a simple relationship:

$$\text{FWHM} = \frac{(\text{gradient pulse amplitude}) \times (\text{rf pulse shape factor})}{(\text{rf pulse width})} \qquad (1)$$

The rf pulse shape factor is specific for a given rf pulse envelope. The effects of gradient strength and pulse duration are complementary: increasing either will result in reduced slice thickness.

Two-Dimensional Single Slice, Two-Dimensional Multiecho and Two-Dimensional Multislice-Multiecho

A simple two-dimensional MRI pulse sequence requires slice selection, spatial encoding in the in-plane directions, and the production of a spin echo (Fig. 97–6). Note that the *x*, *y*, and *z* axes as shown on the pulse sequence diagram are symbolic and can be related to any real coordinate axis by software operations. The multiecho version of this sequence is shown in Figure 97–7.

Two-dimensional multiecho (2D-ME) is also multislice compatible (Fig. 97–8). In 2D-MS/ME a number of slices are performed *nearly* simultaneously by the use of se-

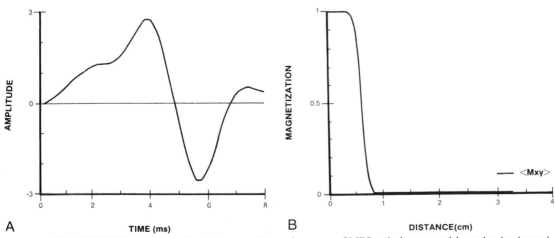

Figure 97–5. The WOW-180 pulse. In order to improve the performance of MRI techniques requiring selective inversion computer optimization methods were used by Lent and Kritzer to custom-design a rf pulse envelope. The result is the strikingly nonintuitive time-asymmetric envelope shown here. Interestingly, the envelope works just as well reversed in time (personal communication.)

2D SINGLE SLICE PULSE SEQUENCE

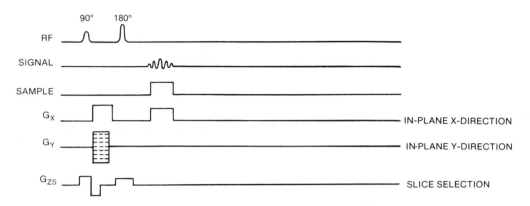

Figure 97–6. Two-dimensional single-slice pulse sequence. The simultaneous application of a 90 degree rf pulse and gradient (Gzs) defines the slice to be imaged. The subsequent 180 degree pulse recalls a spin-echo which is sampled by an A/D converter N_x times during the application of the read gradient (G_x). The number of sampling intervals determines the x resolution. The y direction of spatial information is obtained via spatial encoding from the y gradient pulse. The above sequence is repeated N_y times, each time with an increment of the y gradient. Each such sequence is known as a y line. A number of y lines may be averaged to remove artifact and improve signal-to-noise. The data from the above acquisition does not directly yield the image information but must first be processed by a two-dimensional Fourier transform reconstruction to give a N_x by N_y resolution image.

2D MULTI-ECHO PULSE SEQUENCE

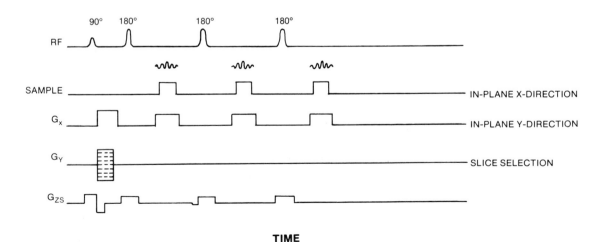

Figure 97–7. Two-dimensional multislice pulse sequence. The two-dimensional multiecho pulse sequence is similar to the two-dimensional single-slice pulse sequence in that the 180 degree pulses may be either selective or nonselective. Here they are shown as selective pulses. Slice selection, x encoding, and y encoding are performed using the z, x, and y gradients. A series of 180 degree pulses recalls successive "harmonic" echoes. At each echo the data collection is repeated for a separate reconstruction and image. A separate two-dimensional Fourier transform is required for reconstruction of each slice.

2D MULTI-SLICE MULTI-ECHO PULSE SEQUENCE

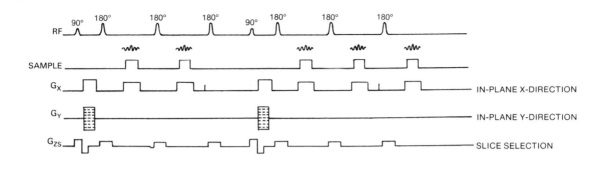

TIME

Figure 97–8. Two-dimensional multislice multiecho pulse sequence. Two-dimensional multislice multiecho pulse sequence. Selective 180 and 90 degree pulses allow the acquisition of multislice and multiecho data. The different slices are acquired in a time-staggered fashion instead of simultaneously. The length of the TR interval determines the number of slices and the number of echoes per slice. A separate two-dimensional Fourier transform is required for reconstruction of each echo image from every slice.

lective 90 and 180 degree rf pulses. Slice selection, phase encoding, and frequency encoding are done separately and consecutively for each slice. In this way rf pulse operations on one slice do not affect other slices. As noted, slice profiles are not perfectly square, and slices tend to interact with each other. Thus two-dimensional multislice (2D-MS) operation requires the use of 10 to 30 percent gaps between slices to minimize slice profile overlap and maintain image quality. Alternatively one can use the inefficient procedure of separate staggered acquisitions with a slice gap equal to the slice thickness.

In 2D-MS/ME MRI the number of slices that can be acquired in a single acquisition is determined by the time per slice (last echo time + a constant) and the length of the TR interval:

$$N = \frac{TR}{(TE_{\text{last}} + T_{\text{delay}})} \qquad (2)$$

T_{delay} is determined by instrumental factors such as gradient rise and fall times and the length and center point of the data collection window. The important thing to remember about 2D-MS/ME is that the number of slices and echoes is limited by the TR. If slice thickness is reduced, it may not be possible to acquire enough slices to cover the field of view without increasing the TR (with its attendant effects on image contrast and scan times).

Implications for Thin-Slice Imaging with Two-Dimensional MRI

SLICE-SLICE INTERACTIONS

Given that two-dimensional slice profiles are imperfect, the spatial overlap of slice profiles reduces the effective TR and signal and can markedly alter image contrast. When thin two-dimensional slices are made, these effects are more significant because the thinner voxels produce less signal and usually contain finer detail. T2 weighted (long TE and long TR) spin-echo images of tissues with long T1 and T2 such as the cerebrospinal fluid (CSF) are particularly sensitive to image contrast alterations arising from slice-slice interactions. The signal intensity from CSF from a multislice acquisition suffering from excessive slice overlap effects will be less than from a comparable single-slice image (Fig. 97–9A). As expected, slice-slice interactions increase as slice gaps (expressed as a fraction of slice thickness) are reduced. The question is: How does one balance the negative aspects of slice-slice interactions with the need to have full tissue coverage?

The solution is twofold. First, space the slices as far apart as possible in time by using a two pass interleaved slice order within a given acquisition (Fig. 97–10). Second, use slice gaps of 10 to 30 percent to provide a good balance between image quality and tissue coverage (Fig. 97–9B and C).

CHEMICAL SHIFT

All two-dimensional MRI applications involve chemical shift effects along the read-out and slice selection directions. The chemical shift artifact is due to the difference between the Larmor frequencies of fat and water protons. The frequency difference is proportional to magnetic field strength. As a result there is an offset between the fat and water components of the MR image along the gradient axis. This causes separate fat and water images to be misregistered in the image plane along the direction of the read-out gradient (the x direction chemical shift artifact). Chemical shift artifacts along the x direction affect all MR images as a function of the strength of the read-out gradient and are independent of slice thickness. The chemical shift artifact from the slice selection gradient also causes the components to arise from slices that are offset from each other (the z direction chemical shift artifact). The offset is proportional to the

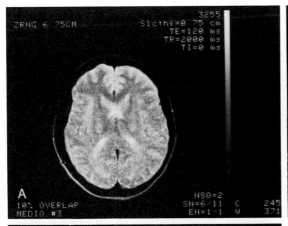

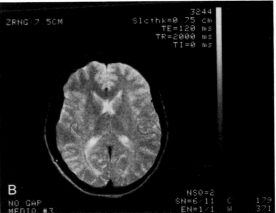

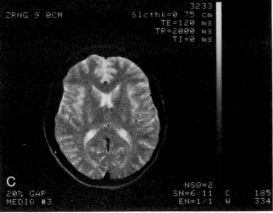

Figure 97–9. Effect of slice profile overlap (SPO) on image contrast. SPO causes reductions in image contrast and overall SNR. The loss of image quality is clearly demonstrated on these axial multislice images of the brain made with and without SPO. In *A* a 10 percent slice overlap causes a marked reduction in grey-white distinction and in overall image quality. Contiguous (*B*) and 20 percent gap (*C*) acquisitions show progressive improvements in image quality.

TWO-PASS INTERLEAVED SLICE ORDER

Figure 97–10. Dual interleaved slice order for two-dimensional multislice. The slices are numbered according to their position in space. In order to minimize slice-slice interactions each slice must be "spaced" as far as possible from its adjacent slices in two-dimensional multislice or two-dimensional multislice/multiecho acquisitions. This is most easily accomplished if a two-pass interleaved order of slice acquisition is used. In this example the odd-numbered slices are acquired first, followed by the even-numbered slices.

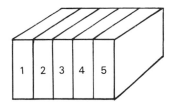

ORDER OF SLICES
IN SPACE

1   3   5   2   4

ORDER OF SLICES
IN TIME

strength of the slice selecting gradient pulse but not to its duration. The z direction chemical shift artifact can be very significant with thinner two-dimensional slices. It can cause the fat and water components to arise from totally nonoverlapping slices.

Chemical shift effects are prominent in Figure 97–11. Figure 97–11*A* shows a *T1* weighted sagittal image of the lumbar spine made at 0.15 telsa. Note the even spacing between the vertebrae marrow and the intravertebrae discs. The corresponding image made at 0.5 telsa shows the marrow fat demonstrated relative to discs. Techniques to

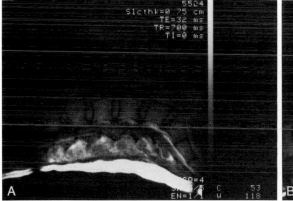

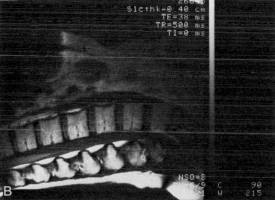

Figure 97–11. Chemical shift effects. The fat and water components are displaced along the read-out gradient direction as a result of the chemical shifts of their respective protons. These *T1* weighted midsagittal images of the lumbar spine were made with similar gradient and timing parameters and surface coils of nearly identical shape. The 0.15 T (*A*) image shows little chemical shift effect. The chemical shift is visible in the 0.6 T (*B*) and 1.5 T (*C*) images as a proportionately greater shift of the fat component to the left of the viewer. (Courtesy of Drs. Messina and Leibeskind of New York City, Drs. Brady and New of Massachusetts General Hospital, and Dr. Weinstein of the Cleveland Clinic Foundation.)

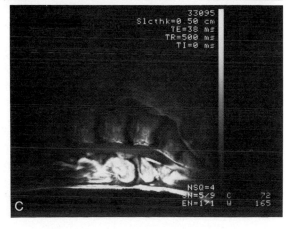

separate fat and water components are well known but their application to 2D-MS/ME is complicated by the side effects of selective excitation.

CONCLUSION

Two-dimensional MRI methods are often effective when short acquisition times, long *TR T2* weighted images, and the benefits of signal averaging (for increasing SNR and for motion artifact reduction) are desirable. Unfortunately, chemical shift artifacts, gradient generated acoustic noise, the requirement for slice gaps, time lag between slices, and limitations on the number of slices for a given *TR* interval are inherent features of two-dimensional MRI. Experience has also shown that slice gaps (expressed as a percent of FWHM) must increase somewhat as two-dimensional slice thickness is reduced in order to maintain image quality. When these limitations interfere with the diagnostic goal the various three-dimensional magnetic resonance imaging methods are possible solutions and are discussed in the following section.

THREE-DIMENSIONAL FULL VOLUME AND LIMITED VOLUME MRI

Overview of Three-Dimensional MRI Methods

In three-dimensional MRI the same techniques that are used for in-plane phase encoding of the *y* axis in two-dimensional MRI are used for encoding of the (slice) *z* axis. The resulting acquisition has variable resolution in *x, y,* and *z* and requires a three-dimensional Fourier transform for reconstruction. The resolution can be equal in all directions (isotropic three-dimensional full volume [3D-FV] MRI) or it can be fine in-plane (*x* and *y* dimensions) and coarse in the slice thickness (*z*) dimension (anisotropic 3D-FV MRI). Anisotropic 3D-FV acquisitions are often referred to as three-dimension multislice. Here, for clarity, we will refer to the *z* voxel dimension as the slice thickness.

A typical 3D-FV pulse sequence is shown in Figure 97–12. The conventions regarding the *x, y,* and *z* dimensions and pulse repetition parameters are retained from the two-dimension discussion. There is an additional line representing the *z* phase encoding gradient step, which is incremented throughout the acquisition. Because selective excitation methods are not used there is no slice selection gradient on during rf pulses. As a result, 3D-FV acquisitions image the full active volume of the rf coil and every MR-active hydrogen nucleus in this volume is affected by every rf pulse.

There are a number of consequences of using phase encoding to resolve slices. As in the phase encoding that produces in-plane resolution,

1. The number of *z* phase encoding steps is equal to the number of slices along the *z* axis, *N*.

2. The imaging time is directly proportional to the number of phase encoding steps.

3. The dimension of the voxel in the slice direction is determined by the area under the *z* axis phase encoding gradient pulse.

4. There can be "aliasing" or "rollover" of the image if the subject occupies a larger distance along *z* than the image volume $= N_z x$ (slice thickness).

5. The slices along *z* are contiguous, just as the pixels are in the in-plane dimension.

6. There is no chemical shift artifact along the *z* axis.

Three-dimensional methods rely on phase encoding by *z* gradient pulses. Because it is the area under the gradient pulse and not the amplitude that determines the slice thickness, gradients are used more efficiently. For the same reasons, three-dimensional methods can produce thinner and more contiguous slices than two-dimensional methods

3D FULL-VOLUME PULSE SEQUENCES

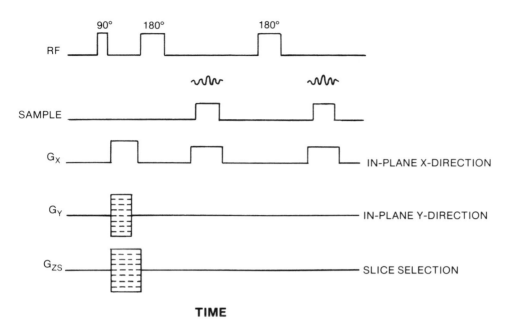

TIME

Figure 97–12. Three-dimensional full volume pulse sequence. A nonselective 90 degree pulse tips all of the hydrogen nuclei within the rf coil. The read-out gradient is used to encode the information along the x axis. The y and z spatial information are both obtained by phase encoding techniques. This means that the entire subject must be imaged with the same resolution even if only a small part is of interest. The reconstruction of the data for a three-dimensional acquisition involves a three-dimensional Fourier transform.

for a given *TE*. Acoustic noise and eddy currents are reduced accordingly. The reduction in the number of gradient pulses per *TR* interval implies improved multiecho performance.

Image contrast in 3D-FV acquisitions is determined by the same factors as in two-dimensional MRI (*T1, T2, N(H), TE,* and *TR*). Because there is no issue of overlapping slice profiles as in two-dimensional MRI, in 3D-FV MRI the effective *TR* is *the TR* and image contrast may be improved. In other words, slice-slice interactions are reduced. There is no need to increase the *TR* of *T1* weighted 3D-FV acquisitions so that an adequate number of slices can be imaged in a single acquisition. Thus image contrast and tissue parameter determination with 3D-FV are potentially more optimal, reproducible, and/or accurate. The analysis of eightfold multiecho 3D-FV images of the head with multiplanar reformatting capability has also provided insight into the basis of tissue contrast changes in pathologic states.[6]

A typical 3D-FV anisotropic image data set might contain $128 \times 128 \times 32$ pixels and take 20 minutes (for $TR = 300$) to collect. Among the current applications for such contiguous three-dimensional pixel "blocks" produced by 3D-FV MRI are the generation of three-dimensional contour surface displays (Fig. 97–13). 3D-FV image data also allow reformatting along the sagittal, coronal, and transverse planes. This flexibility partially offsets the increased acquisition time in some cases.

The combination of two-dimensional selective excitation and three-dimensional phase encoding slice methods yields 3D-LV MRI, which combines the advantages of both. The concept of a slice used in two-dimensional methods is extended to a slab, a thick slice of the subject that can be resolved into thinner slices with phase encoding methods (Fig. 97–14).

The basic rationale behind 3D-LV is the use of three-dimensional methods over a

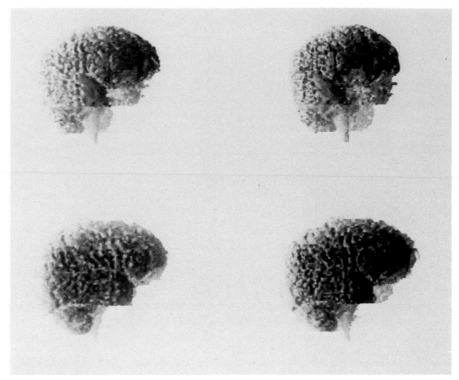

Figure 97–13. Multiplanar and contour display of full-volume 30 data. Transverse, sagittal, and coronal reconstructions from a 0.6T TR 250 TE 27 128 × 96 × 96 30 FV data set. (Courtesy of CEMAX Corporation.)

limited region of space. When the anatomic region of interest can be contained within a slab that is smaller than the active volume of the rf coil, the imaging time is proportionately reduced compared to 3D-FV because the number of slices is reduced. 3D-LV is particularly effective in the imaging of small structures with high resolution.

Figure 97–15 shows a 3D-LV pulse sequence. It contains both three-dimensional and two-dimensional components. Selective 90 degree rf and z gradient pulses are used

THREE-DIMENSIONAL LIMITED-VOLUME MRI

SELECTIVE EXCITATION DEFINES THE SLAB

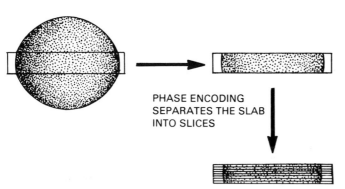

Figure 97–14. Three-dimensional limited volume MRI.

PHASE ENCODING
SEPARATES THE SLAB
INTO SLICES

3D LIMITED VOLUME PULSE SEQUENCE

Figure 97–15. Three-dimensional limited volume pulse sequence. The three-dimensional limited volume sequence contains elements of both two-dimensional single slice and three-dimensional full volume sequences. Instead of using a nonselective 90 degree pulse to begin the sequence a selective pulse defines a thick slice or slab. Phase encoding methods are used to break the slab up into thin slices in a fashion exactly analogous to three-dimensional full volume. X and Y encoding are done as with two-dimensional and three-dimensional full volume sequences. Please see the text for further explanation.

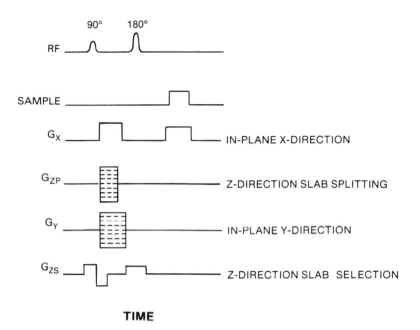

for slab selection via selective excitation. The splitting of the slab into thinner slices is accomplished by *z* gradient phase encoding methods. These are performed on the same physical gradient, but the functions are shown separately on the figure for clarity. As in 3D-FV, the number of *z* axis phase encoding steps determines the number of slices that the slab is split into. However, unlike 3D-FV, only part of the active volume of the rf coil is imaged.

The phase encoding process defines a "stack" of slices that must be positioned within the slab defined by selective excitation. Proper operation of a 3D-LV acquisition requires that the slab excitation volume be contained within the phase-encoded volume.

3D-LV reduces the imaging time compared to 3D-FV without loss of *z* resolution or aliasing. At constant slice thickness (*z* axis resolution) imaging time for 3D-LV versus 3D-FV is reduced proportionately to the reduction in the number of slices. As a result, 3D-LV imaging times become more comparable to those of 2D-MS/ME with the same *TR*, etc. The reduction in imaging time facilitates the use of greater in-plane resolution, signal averaging, etc. Single excitation imaging in a head coil with 3D-LV can provide high-quality contiguous slices with under 2 mm thickness (Fig. 97–16).

Imaging Time, SNR, and Radio Frequency Deposition Compared for Three Dimensions and Two Dimensions

Two-dimensional multislice-multiecho imaging is the most frequently used modality in clinical MRI today. This is because of the efficiency of data collection in many current diagnostic applications as compared with earlier sensitive point, two-dimensional single-slice and three-dimensional full volume methods. For both two-dimensional and three-dimensional MRI, acquisition time is given by:

$$t = TR \times N_y \times N_z \times NSQ \tag{3}$$

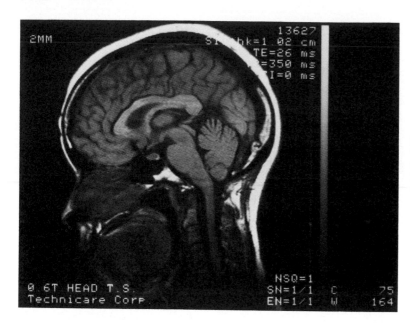

Figure 97–16. Shown here is a 0.6 T TR300/TE26 2 mm NSQ:1 midsagittal image of the head from a 16 slice 17 minute three-dimensional limited volume acquisition.

where TR = sequence repetition rate; N_y = number of y lines = number of y phase encoding steps; NSQ = number of data acquisition sequences averaged per phase-encoded steps; and N_z = number of slices = number of z phase encoding steps = 1 for two-dimensional methods.

This calculation does not reflect acquisition time per two-dimensional slice, which is determined by the number of slices per TR interval. It applies equally to two-dimensional, 3D-FV, and 3D-LV acquisitions. Inspection reveals that imaging time for three-dimensional acquisitions is longer than for two-dimensional acquisitions by a factor of N_z (the number of slices) if repetition rates and signal averages are held constant. This is significant in the case of a isotropic 3D-FV acquisition with N_z = 128. If N_z is reduced by using either fewer voxels (anisotropic 3D-FV) or only part of the active volume of the rf coil (3D-LV), then imaging time is reduced by the same proportion. The majority of 3D-LV clinical applications use anisotropic voxels and NSQ = 1 so that the total imaging times are usually only 1 to 4 times that for two-dimensional methods with constant TR.

Surface coils provide an increased SNR, which may be used to overcome the signal losses associated with reduction of TR. This is a useful means to provide $T1$ weighted three-dimensional images in times comparable to two-dimensional acquisition, particularly when limited volume techniques are used (Figs. 97–17 and 97–18). Radio frequency energy deposition (see below) and other factors place limitations on the number of two-dimensional slices that can be done in a short TR interval.

Since the acquisition time is shorter for two-dimensional acquisition, signal averaging is used to increase the signal-to-noise ratio and to reduce certain artifacts of the imaging process that arise from selective excitation.

A disadvantage of 3D-FV methods is that $T2$ weighted acquisitions (long TE and long TR) are very long, and motion artifacts are more prominent compared to two-dimensional operation. On the other hand, multiecho operation is enhanced, with eight or more high-quality echoes easily available without limitations on slice number.

The signal to noise ratio per pixel in two-dimensional and in three-dimensional acquisitions is determined by the same factors: slice or z resolution, in-plane resolution, bandwidth, signal averaging, and, of course, tissue properties and TE and TR. However, every excitation in a 3D-FV or 3D-LV acquisition contributes to the signal of every

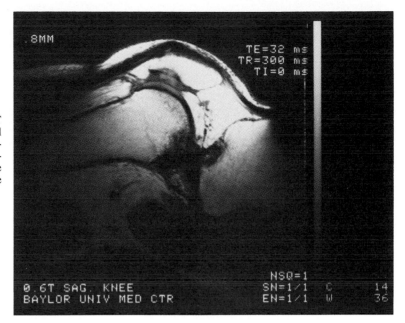

Figure 97–17. Shown here is a 0.6 T TR300/TE32 0.8 mm NSQ:1 sagittal image of the knee through the intercondylar notch from a 16 slice 17 minute three-dimensional limited volume acquisition. (Courtesy of Dr. Steve Harms, Baylor University.)

pixel in every slice. In 2D-MS/ME each rf pulse affects and contributes to the signal of only one slice. The following equation gives the relative SNR for both two-dimensional and three-dimensional acquisitions for spin-echo sequences:

$$SNR = K\,N(H)\,V_{vox}\,f(v)\,C(T1,T2,TE,TI,TR)\,[NSQ\,N_y\,N_z]^{1/2}$$
$$= [exp\text{-}[TE/T2]\,[1 - exp\text{-}[(TR - TE)/T1]$$

(4)

where K = constant factor; $N(H)$ = spin density; $f(v)$ = velocity effect term; $C(T1 \ldots TR)$ = tissue contrast term; TR = sequence repetition rate; N_y = number of y lines = number of y phase encoding steps; NSQ = number of data acquisition se

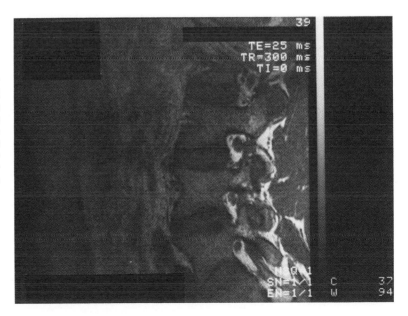

Figure 97–18. Shown here is a 0.6 T TR300/TE25 0.8 mm NSQ:1 sagittal image of the lumbar spine through the intervertebral foramina showing the nerve roots in their dural sheath surrounded by epidural fat. This was from a 16 slice 17 minute three-dimensional limited volume acquisition. (Courtesy of Dr. Steve Harms, Baylor University.)

quences averaged per phase-encoded line; N_z = number of slices = number of z phase encoding steps = 1 for two-dimensional method; and V_{vox} = volume of the voxel.

Equation (4) enables the computation of relative SNR for different acquisitions as a function of tissue properties, timing parameters, and voxel dimensions but does not address bandwidth or slice profile overlap effects, which are assumed constant in any comparison.

A quick look at Equation (4) shows that the SNR is proportional to the volume of the voxels. Both voxel volume and the number of voxels along each dimension are usually changed simultaneously, as in going from a 128 × 256 to a 256 × 256 matrix. In this case the area under the y gradient phase encoding pulse is doubled and the number of y gradient phase encoding steps is doubled. The resulting voxel volume is halved, the number of pixels along the y axis is doubled, the acquisition time is doubled (due to the increased number of y lines), and the SNR decreases by a factor equal to the square root of two.

Further inspection shows that N_z, N_y, and NSQ all contribute to SNR by a factor of the square root. As mentioned above, the three-dimensional acquisition will also be longer in duration by a factor of N_z. In this way the effect of z phase encoding on imaging time and SNR is similar to signal averaging; thus the time efficiency with respect to SNR is the same for two-dimensional or three-dimensional acquisition if all of the slices in the desired region can be imaged in one scan. The SNR of a 3D-FV acquisition is greater than that of a comparable 2D-MS/ME acquisition (same *TE*, *TR*, in-plane resolution, and NSQ) by a factor of the square root of N_z. In actual application, the increased SNR of three-dimensional acquisitions (see below) allows single excitation (no signal averaging) operation and reductions in *TR*, which reduce acquisition times accordingly.

Signal averaging increases SNR and is feasible with the comparatively short acquisition time of two-dimensional MRI sequences. It also tends to diminish image artifacts arising from the side effects of selective excitation, tip angle misadjustment, and motion.

Radio frequency pulses, whether selective or not, deposit rf energy as heat in all tissues within the active region of the rf coil. The rate of energy deposition is a function of the amplitude of the rf pulse squared. Since, for a given pulse envelope, the area under the envelope is proportional to the tip angle, shorter rf pulses deposit proportionately more energy than long ones. For similar reasons 180 degree selective pulses deposit much more energy than their 90 degree counterparts. The pulse amplitude is greater not only because of the increased tip angle but also because the 180 degree pulse width is sometimes reduced to allow for a wider excitation profile, as discussed above. This results in greater rf deposition. Nonselective 180 degree pulses have the greatest rf deposition effects.[7,8] Radio frequency deposition increases in 2D-MS/ME operation in proportion to the increased rate of application of selective 180 degree pulses. The use of thinner slices tends to increase rf deposition in actual use because there is a motivation to cover the same field of view in the same acquisition time. The result is a proportionately higher duty cycle if rf pulse width is held constant. This effect is offset somewhat if the selection of thinner slices is accomplished by increasing rf pulse width (with attendant rf pulse attenuation) instead of increasing slice selection gradient strength.

Radio frequency energy deposition increases at a rate close to the second power with increasing field strength.[9] At higher field strengths, such as 1.5 tesla, rf deposition becomes a limitation with 2D-MS/ME operation (where selective 180 degree pulse repetition rates are the highest). In 3D-FV multiecho operation the nonselective 180 degree pulses contribute the greater part of the total rf deposition. This is usually not a limitation with respect to the safety guidelines at commonly used repetition rates.

Most manufacturers have developed software and hardware functions that prevent unauthorized operation with any pulse sequence above the current NEMA guidelines for rf energy deposition.

Technical Challenges in Three-Dimensional Full Volume and Limited Volume MRI

3D-FV MRI has a more stringent requirement than two-dimensional MRI for uniform sensitivity and phase response of the rf coil system. This may require design compromises with other desirable coil properties, such as sensitivity. The present limited clinical use of 3D-FV methods may not justify these compromises.

For 3D-LV the requirements on coil design are less critical than for 3D-FV, but it desirable to have good control of the slab profile, particularly to minimize trailing edges that can cause aliasing. Sinc 90 pulses can produce thick, square slab profiles and are useful in this regard. Gaussian slab selection will result in marked falloff in signal intensity on the off-center slices or aliasing of signals.

Periodic and erratic subject motions are associated with image artifacts of the ghost variety on three-dimensional techniques. These are similar to those on two-dimensional MRI, except that ghosts propogate along the y and z axes of the image block. The absence of signal averaging (with phase alternation, as is conventionally done in two-dimensional acquisitions) makes the ghosts more prominent than on two-dimensional images. This has restricted 3D-FV to applications where there is little physiologic motion.

Chemical shift artifacts occur along the read out gradient direction on MRI images and also in the direction of slice selection in two-dimensional MRI images. Phase encoded directions are essentially unaffected by chemical shift. In the case of 3D-LV the selective excitation phase excites separate "fat" and "water" slabs, which are offset by the chemical shift between fat and water. The z phase encoding treats the fat and water components according to their true position and there is no chemical shift artifact. It is important to ensure that the chemical shift caused by slice selection does not cause aliasing: the offset fat and water excitations must be contained within the phase encoded volume. It is sufficient that the outer phase encoded slice on either side of the slab has no or only minimal signal.

Future Directions: Multislab and Contrast Agents

3D-LV methods can be extended from single- to multi-slab where many slabs can be imaged in the same time as one,[10] (see Figs. 97–17 and 97–18). This is analogous to the progression from two-dimensional single slice to two-dimensional multislice methods. The slabs can be contiguous or they may be widely separated in space.

The multislab pulse sequence (Fig. 97–19) shows features common to both 3D-LV and two-dimensional multislice. A technical challenge is posed by the need for 180 degree pulses that have very broad and square excitation profiles. Conventional Gaussian and sinc envelopes perform poorly in this regard, as their excitation profiles show a gradual transition between 180 degree tip angles at the slice center plane and 0 degrees in the area outside the slice. WOW-180 pulses perform this function well. An example multislab study of the cervical spine and segments of the carotid vessels is shown in Figure 97–20.

A shortcoming of 3D-LV MRI is that acquisition times for $T2$ weighted images will be longer than for a comparable two-dimensional multislice study with the same

MULTI-SLAB PULSE SEQUENCE

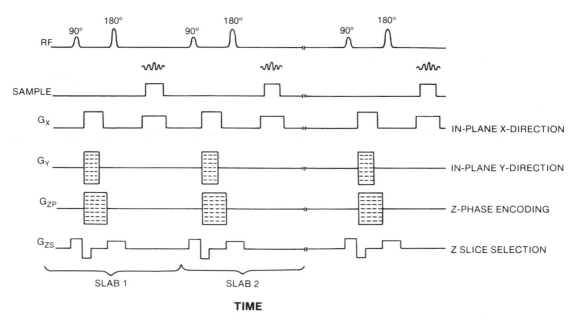

Figure 97–19. Two-dimensional multislab pulse sequence. The multislab pulse sequence combines three-dimensional limited volume and two-dimensional multislice techniques. The use of selective 90 degree and 180 degree pulses in combination with z-phase encoding enables the nearly simultaneous acquisition of multiple slabs, each with a number of phase encoded slices. In-plane phase encoding is done as before. Multislab imaging requires a separate three-dimensional reconstruction for each slab of slices.

TE, *TR*, and in-plane resolution by a factor of $N_z/2$ (assuming that a single signal average is used on the two-dimensional study and not on the 3D-LV study). Although the acquisition time is still long, the 3D-LV approach represents a relative improvement over the 3D-FV. Acquisition times for 3D-LV can be reduced somewhat by decreasing resolution and repetition times.

Despite the decreased SNR, *T2* weighted images are more sensitive to pathologic change and are essential in many diagnostic situations. The pathologic sensitivity provided by *T2* weighted acquisitions may also be provided by the use of strongly *T1* weighted acquisitions with paramagnetic contrast agents such as Gd-DTPA. The preliminary clinical and pharmacological experience suggests that various types of tissue injury cause accumulation of the agent in the extracellular extravascular space.[11] The proton relaxation effect of the Gd-DTPA causes the local *T1* and *T2* to decrease. (The *T1* effect predominates unless the concentration of the relaxation agent becomes very high, as in the urinary bladder.) A 3D-LV study of a dog with a 2 mm tumor implant in the left cerebellar hemisphere 5 min following the intravenous administration of .1 mmole/Kg Gd-DTPA is shown in Figure 97–21. The tumor is visualized well on the post contrast study as a bright signal from the left cerebellar hemisphere. It is poorly seen, if at all, on the precontrast study made with the same acquisition parameters.

We have discussed two-dimensional and three-dimensional methods for the acquisition of magnetic resonance images. Each method has its characteristic advantages and disadvantages; no method is good for all situations. The proper use of these alternative imaging methods requires an understanding of the tradeoffs between image contrast, resolution, signal to noise ratio, motion artifact sensitivity, slice number, slice definition, and throughput.

Two-dimensional MRI has the advantages of throughput (in many but not all sit-

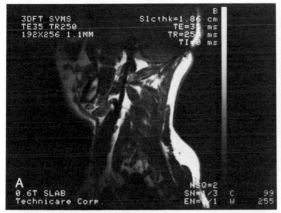

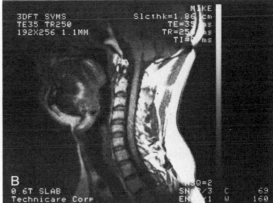

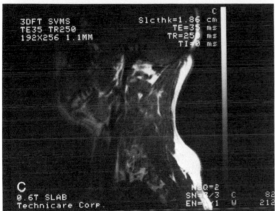

Figure 97–20. Three-dimensional multislab C-spine and carotid segments. In a multislab acquisition two-dimensional and three-dimensional techniques are combined to allow multiple three-dimensional limited volume studies to be performed at the same time. *A* and *C* show slices through the carotid vessels taken from the ouside slabs in a three-slab sagittal multislab acquisition. *B* shows the midsagittal slice from the center slab.

uations), relative immunity to motion artifacts, and the ability to easily produce *T2* weighted images. The disadvantages include the requirement for slice gaps and limitations on slice number in a given *TR* interval.

Three-dimensional MRI can produce thinner and more contiguous slices than two-dimensional methods. The principal disadvantage is increased acquisition time and a relative sensitivity to motion artifacts compared to two-dimensional acquisitions. The

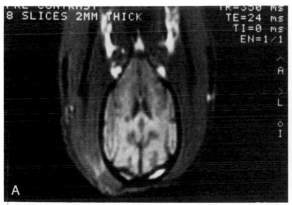

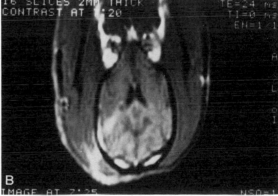

Figure 97–21. Three-dimensional limited volume image of dog brain with infarct and Gd-DTPA. The dog had a surgically implanted brain tumor that was less than 5 mm in diameter. Prior to the administration of contrast a three-dimensional limited volume image showed only the surgical entry scar (*A*). The area of the tumor was well visualized following the administration of a gadolinium-containing contrast agent (*B*). These agents may enable short-TR three-dimensional limited volume imaging techniques to provide the tissue contrast associated with *T2* weighted acquisitions.

absence of slice-slice interactions allows the production of high-quality thin-slice magnetic resonance images with reduced reliance on gradient strength.

At present two-dimensional methods dominate in clinical MRI because they are generally more efficient at data collection. Three-dimensional limited volume techniques are less widely used owing to the relatively recent introduction of the necessary software to the clinical environment. In diagnostic situations where high-quality contiguous thin multislice and four- or eight-fold multiecho data are of value 3D-LV techniques will be recognized as powerful tools.

ACKNOWLEDGMENTS

We would like to express our thanks to Drs. David Kramer, Waldo Hinshaw, Arnold Lent, and James Murdoch for their invaluable technical advice and comments, which contributed greatly to the discussion in this chapter.

References

1. Butch RJ, Stark DD, Wittenberg J, Brady TJ, Ferrucci JT: MRI of the abdomen and pelvis. Fourth Annual Meeting of the Society of Magnetic Resonance in Medicine, 1985, pp 216–217.
2. Hinshaw WS, Lent AH: An introduction of NMR imaging: From the Bloch equation to the imaging equation. Proc IEEE *71*:338–350, 1983.
3. Silver MS, Joseph RI, Chen C-N, Sank VJ, Hoult DI: Selective population inversion in NMR. Nature *310*:681–683, 1984.
4. Edelstein WA, Bottomley PA, Hart HR, Smith LS: Signal, noise and contrast in nuclear magnetic resonance (NMR) imaging. J Comput Assist Tomogr *7*:391–401, 1983.
5. Lent AH, Kritzer MR: A new RF pulse shape for narrow-band inversion: The WOW-180. Fourth Annual Meeting of the Society of Magnetic Resonance in Medicine, 1985, p 1015.
6. Harms SE, Brown MB: Multiple-echo magnetic resonance imaging. Unpublished ms.
7. Brandt G, Wilfley B: Tissue heating by radiofrequency magnetic fields during magnetic resonance imaging. Diasonics Corporation (preprint).
8. Hill BC: Considerations of RF power deposition with the 1.5 tesla teslacon. Technicare Corporation (preprint).
9. Chen C-N, Sank VJ, Hoult DI: A study of RF power deposition in imaging. Abstracts Society of Magnetic Resonance in Medicine, 4th Annual Meeting, 1985, pp 918–919.
10. Dramer DM, Compton RA, Yeung HN: A volume (3D) analogue of 2D multislice or "multislab" MR imaging. Fourth Annual Meeting of the Society of Magnetic Resonance in Medicine, 1985, pp 162–163.
11. Carr DH, Brown J, Bydder GM, Steiner R, Weinmann HJ, Speck V, Hall AS, Young IR: Gd-DPTA as a contrast agent in clinical MRI: Initial clinical experience in 20 patients. Am J Roentgenol *143*:215–224, 1984.

98

MRI of Blood Flow

LEON AXEL

Effects of fluid flow or motion were observed early in studies of magnetic resonance.[1–3] They were explained as being due either to the effects of washout of saturated or excited spins from the region being studied or to phase shifts acquired due to motion of excited spins along magnetic field gradients. It was soon proposed to use these effects to measure flow.[4,5] The introduction of magnetic resonance imaging revealed a variety of effects of flow on images[6–12] and opened up the possibility of using these effects to make localized measurements of flow within particular vessels or to make images that would selectively display vessels owing to their containing moving blood. We will briefly review some aspects of the circulation relevant to flow imaging. Then we will describe the basic flow effects in magnetic resonance and how they arise in conventional imaging techniques.[13] Finally, we will consider how these effects may be applied in techniques specifically designed for flow imaging.

ASPECTS OF BLOOD FLOW

We will review some basics of the physical aspects of blood flow to provide a background on what will be measured with magnetic resonance imaging (MRI).[14] The velocity of blood is a vector quantity whose direction and speed vary both with position within the vessel and with time. The frictional drag of the walls results in a velocity profile within the vessel, with slow flow at the periphery and more rapid flow in the middle. Alterations of the flow by curves or bifurcations of vessels result in asymmetry of the velocity distribution within the vessel. Although the flow within the normal circulation is smooth (laminar), vessel stenosis commonly results in turbulence. Finally, both the speed and the distribution of velocities within the vessel may depend on the phase of the cardiac and respiratory cycles. Thus, to fully define the patterns of flow within a vessel will require many measurements. Even if only knowledge of the average net flow through a given vessel is desired, it may be necessary to measure velocities at many points in the vessel at different phases of the cardiac cycle and appropriately average them together in order to accurately compute the net flow.

Flow in the heart and large vessels differs significantly from that in the tissue capillaries. In the heart, the velocities are high during systole but low during diastole; the average cardiac output is on the order of 5.5 liters/min. The flow is turbulent in the ventricles and probably also in the atria (which makes sense teleologically as providing good mixing of the blood).

The larger vessels (arteries and veins) serve to distribute the blood to the tissues. Their diameters range from around 2.5 cm down to millimeters. In the aorta, the mean velocity is on the order of 30 cm/s, but the peak velocity may be on the order of 100 cm/s. Although there may be great variations in the blood flow, especially on the arterial side (the velocity may actually reverse in the aorta during diastole), the flow is generally not turbulent.

The capillaries, which allow for exchange of water and solutes between the blood and the tissues, are different in many respects from the larger vessels. Their diameters are approximately 7 μ, well below the likely resolution of any conventional MR image. Their lengths are on the order of a millimeter and the velocity less than a millimeter a second, implying a transit time of a second or more. However, as diffusional exchange across the capillary walls can be of the order of ten times the flow through the capillary, spins entering one end of the capillary are likely not to exit promptly at the other end. Whereas the flow of blood within a large vessel has a well-defined direction, the capillaries usually make up an isotropic network with no net direction of flow. The capillaries typically make up only a few percent of the tissue volume, resulting in a large background of "stationary" water. Thus, capillary flow may be difficult to distinguish from diffusion of water within tissues. Finally, flow within tissues is typically patchy and phasic, with significant local time-dependent variations. The net result of all this is that tissue perfusion is likely to be difficult to measure.

The kinds of flow changes likely to be of interest to study with MRI are local obstructions or stenoses, such as could be due to plaque, clot, tumor, trauma, etc., or altered flow due to more distant obstructions or shunts. The clinical questions most likely to be addressed by MRI are those concerning vessel patency and geometry. The direction of flow is also likely to be readily determined. Measurement of volume of flow in a given vessel is more difficult, as it may require integrating measurements of velocity across the vessel lumen and over different phases of the cardiac cycle, but it is in principle straightforward. As an intermediate step in this calculation, we would also obtain a velocity waveform, although this is less often likely to be clinically useful. As discussed above, measurement of tissue perfusion will be difficult, although probably of the greatest clinical interest.

BASIC MR FLOW EFFECTS

Magnetic resonance provides three basic means of noninvasively "tagging" the blood in order to detect its motion: local changes in the longitudinal magnetization, limited to times on the order of $T1$, local changes in the transverse magnetization, limited to times on the order of $T2$, and local changes in the phase of the transverse magnetization, again limited to times on the order of $T2$. In addition, we can use the injection of tracer substances in order to monitor their distribution as a measure of blood flow. Such tracer substances could contain paramagnetic components to alter the $T1$ or $T2$ of spins in their environment or they could contain nuclei, such as fluorine, not normally found in the body in significant quantities. We will not consider the use of such tracer substances further in this chapter.

The simplest flow effect to understand is that of washout or time of flight. When the longitudinal or transverse magnetization of the spins in a particular region have been altered by selective saturation or excitation, flow may partially or completely remove them from this region before a subsequent excitation or detection of the spins (Fig. 98–1). When flow results in the replacement of saturated spins by less saturated spins, the signal will increase; it will decrease when the reverse takes place. If excited spins move between the time of their excitation and their detection, an apparent displacement of their position may be seen. With a spatially selective detection process, motion of the spins between excitation and detection may result in a loss of signal.

A somewhat subtler effect is the phase shifts that excited spins may experience owing to motion along magnetic field gradients. Compared with a spin that remains

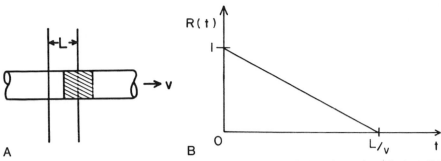

Figure 98–1. Plug flow (single velocity). Washout from rectangular profile imaging region (slice). *A*, Schematic representation of previously tagged (e.g., saturated or excited) fluid (shaded region) being washed out of slice of thickness L by flow of velocity, v. *B*, Fraction of spins remaining in slice, $R(t)$, after tagging at time $t = 0$. (From Axel L: AJR *143*:1157, 1984. Used by permission.)

stationary, a moving spin will experience a range of different local fields (and thus different precession rates) in the presence of a magnetic field gradient along the direction of motion. Thus a refocusing radiofrequency (rf) pulse or reversal of the magnetic field gradient that will resynchronize the phases of the stationary spins to form a spin echo may not refocus the moving spins to the same phase as the stationary spins.

CONVENTIONAL MRI AND FLOW

Magnetic field gradients are used (typically as pulses) for two main purposes in conventional MRI: selective excitation and position encoding. The signal is detected as a "free induction decay" (FID) (in practice generally formed as a gradient echo), or as a spin echo, produced by a refocusing rf pulse (generally 180 degrees) that may be spatially selective or nonselective. Currently, most conventional MRI systems use some form of two-dimensional Fourier transform (2DFT) MRI.[15,16] A simplified timing diagram of a representative 2DFT imaging sequence is shown in Figure 98–2. The 180 degree refocusing rf pulse is frequently made selective in order to permit interleaved imaging of multiple planes.

Flow effects can arise in multiple ways in such an imaging technique. Replacement of partially saturated spins within the slice by spins from upstream will result in a change in signal intensity. If the spins from upstream are more fully magnetized, this will tend to result in an increase in signal intensity, appearing as an effective decrease in *T1* (Fig. 98–3). However, if the spins from upstream are even less magnetized than those being washed out of the slice, then the signal intensity may actually decrease owing to the washing in of the spins from upstream. This may result when the slice being imaged is in the interior of a stack of slices being "simultaneously" imaged or when the 180 degree refocusing rf pulse is not spatially selective, so that it acts as an inverting pulse outside the slice being imaged.

A different effect of washout that can result from the use of selective 180 degree refocusing rf pulses is that the spins excited by the initial selective 90 degree pulse may be partially washed out of the slice by the time the selective 180 degree refocusing pulse is applied. As only those spins that experience both pulses will contribute to the signal detected as the resulting spin echo, the signal will decrease owing to this effect, with an apparent decrease in the effective *T2*. As the time to echo formation (*TE*) is shorter than the pulse sequence repetition time (*TR*), this effect will be seen for higher flow velocities than the effect of saturated spins washout for a given slice thickness (Fig. 98–4).

TIMING DIAGRAM

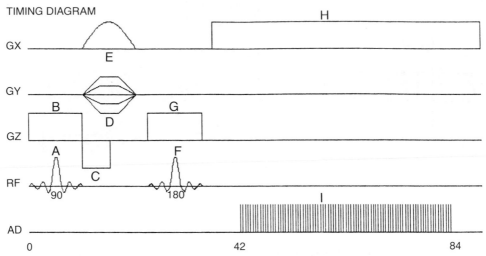

Figure 98–2. Pulse sequence timing diagram for conventional two-dimensional Fourier transform MR imaging. The five lines represent the timing of pulses of frequency-encoding magnetic field gradient (G_X), phase-encoding magnetic field gradient (G_Y), slice-selective magnetic field gradient (G_Z), radio frequency excitation (*rf*), and signal acquisition (*AD*). Initial excitation by an rf pulse A in the presence of pulse B for spatial selectivity is followed by pulse C to synchronize the phases of stationary spins. Variable pulse D provides phase encoding of position. Pulse E provides a preliminary dephasing so that the spins will rephase during the frequency-encoding pulse H. Pulse F is used to produce a spin echo; it may be made spatially selective with the optional pulse G.

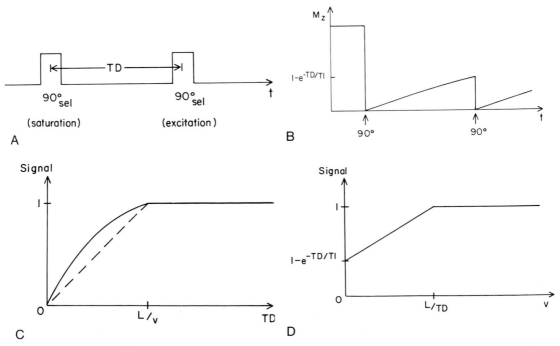

Figure 98–3. Effect of washout as in Figure 98–1, with tagging by saturation. *A*, Schematic rf pulse sequence: selective saturation pulse followed after delay of TD by selective excitation pulse at same location. *B*, Longitudinal magnetization, M_z, as function of time, *t*, with this pulse sequence, for spins remaining in slice for both pulses. *C*, Effect of varying TD (for fixed velocity) on signal produced by excitation pulse for replacement of "saturated" spins by fully magnetized spins. Solid line shows result for $T1 = L/v$; broken line shows limit for very long $T1$. *D*, Effect of increasing velocity (for fixed TD) on signal strength. (From Axel L: AJR *143*:1157, 1984. Used by permission.)

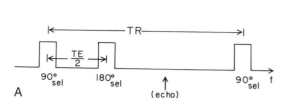

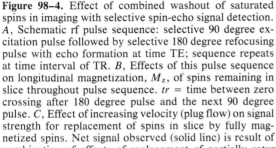

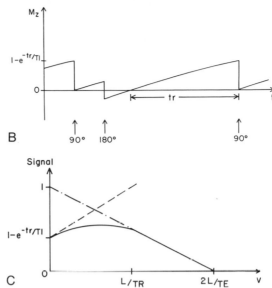

Figure 98–4. Effect of combined washout of saturated spins in imaging with selective spin-echo signal detection. *A*, Schematic rf pulse sequence: selective 90 degree excitation pulse followed by selective 180 degree refocusing pulse with echo formation at time TE; sequence repeats at time interval of TR. *B*, Effects of this pulse sequence on longitudinal magnetization, M_z, of spins remaining in slice throughout pulse sequence. *tr* = time between zero crossing after 180 degree pulse and the next 90 degree pulse. *C*, Effect of increasing velocity (plug flow) on signal strength for replacement of spins in slice by fully magnetized spins. Net signal observed (solid line) is result of combination of effects of replacement of partially saturated spins (broken line) and loss of excited spins from refocusing region (dot-dash line). (Axel L: AJR *143*:1157, 1984. Used by permission.)

If there is a component of the flow velocity within the plane of the image, a different flow effect may be seen owing to displacement of the blood between the time it is excited and the time its position is encoded by magnetic field gradient pulses. In the case of 2DFT imaging, there will be an asymmetry in the amount of apparent displacement of the blood for a given velocity, depending on the components of the velocity within the image, as the phase-encoding gradient pulses are applied prior to the frequency encoding gradient.

The use of different magnetic field gradients in imaging leads to different phase shift effects. In the presence of a constant gradient such as might result from a magnetic field inhomogeneity, a constant velocity will result in the phase shift of a first spin echo that is proportional to the velocity of the spin (and proportional to the square of the echo time)[3] (Fig. 98–5). For a multiple spin-echo train, the phase shift will cancel out and will be zero for the even-numbered echoes. In imaging, magnetic field gradients are usually applied as pulses, resulting in somewhat different effects.[13] For the bipolar magnetic field gradient pulse typically used for selective excitation, there will be a phase shift proportional to the component of velocity perpendicular to the slice (Fig. 98–6). Similarly, for a selective 180 degree rf refocusing pulse, moving spins will acquire a phase shift proportional to velocity; for a train of spin echoes the even-numbered selective 180 degree pulses will cancel out the phase shift effects of the odd-numbered selective pulses, similar to the effect of multiple spin echoes in constant magnetic field gradients (Fig. 98–7). The use of paired defocusing/refocusing magnetic field gradient pulses for frequency encoding of position will also result in phase shifts proportional to the component of velocity along this direction; the relatively long "baseline" in time between the paired pulses can result in these phase shifts being relatively great. Finally, the magnetic field gradient pulses of varying strength used for phase encoding of position will also result in phase shifts for blood moving along the direction of this gradient.

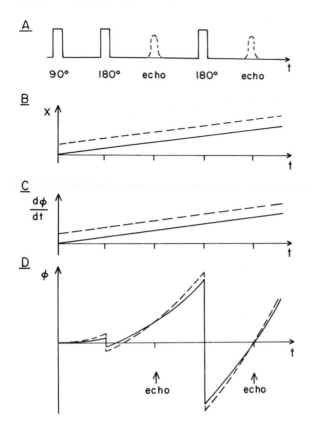

Figure 98–5. Effect of constant velocity motion along constant magnetic field gradient on phase of excited spins. *A*, Schematic rf pulse sequence with formation of pair of spin echos (broken lines). *B*, Position of spins along direction of gradient, *x*, as function time, *t*, for two different initial positions (broken and solid lines). *C*, Corresponding rate of change of phase, *dφ/dt*, due to changing local value of magnetic field. *D*, Net phase accumulated by moving spins. Effect of 180 degree pulses is to reverse value of phase. Note that at time of echo formation, phase is independent of initial position, but is nonzero (proportional to velocity) for first echo; phase is zero for second echo independent of velocity. (From Axel L: AJR *143*:1157, 1984. Used by permission.)

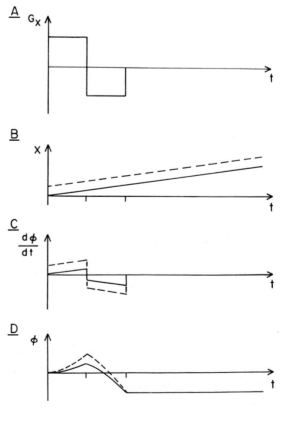

Figure 98–6. Effect of constant velocity motion along bipolar pulsed magnetic field gradient on phase of excited spins. *A*, Schematic gradient pulse sequence. *B*, Position of spins with two different initial positions, as in Figure 98–5*B*. *C*, Corresponding rate of change, as in Figure 98–5*C*. Note reversal of sign of rate of change corresponding to reversal of gradient. *D*, Net phase accumulated by moving spins. Note that although phase can be adjusted to be independent of initial position ("gradient reversal echo"), it is nonzero (proportional to velocity). (Axel L: AJR *143*:1157, 1984. Used by permission.)

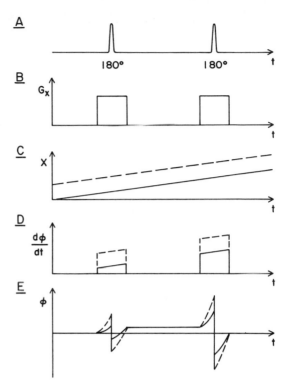

Figure 98–7. Effect of constant velocity motion with selective refocusing pulses on phase of excited spins. *A*, Schematic rf pulse sequence. *B*, Corresponding magnetic field gradient pulse sequence. *C*, Position of spins with two different initial positions, as in Figure 98–5B. *D*, Corresponding rate of change of phase, as in Figure 98–5C. *E*, Net phase accumulated by moving spins. Note that phase is proportional to velocity after first refocusing pulse but zero after second pulse. (From Axel L: AJR *143*:1157, 1984. Used by permission.)

However, in this case, the phase shift is proportional to the strength of the gradient and can result in an apparent displacement in the position along this direction.

Most images are displayed as the magnitude of the signal, so that phase shifts due to motion are not directly apparent. However, as there is generally a range of velocities (and thus phase shifts) within a picture element of a vessel lumen, particularly toward the vessel wall, the corresponding range of phases will result in partial cancellation and a reduction in the net signal.

As the final result of most of the effects described above is an alteration in signal intensity dependent on the velocity, the variations in velocity due to pulsatile flow will result in corresponding variations in intensity. This, in turn, can result in artifacts, such as "ghost" images of arteries analogous to those produced by respiratory or other regular motions.

The flow effects arising in conventional MRI can be used to extract some flow information from the images. The presence of the effects described above can help determine the presence or absence of flow. For example, the relative increase in signal that may be observed on the second of a pair of spin echoes due to compensation of phase shifts can help identify regions of flow. By noting whether there is increased signal within the vessel lumen due to washing in of fresh spins at the top or bottom of a stack of simultaneously acquired slices, the direction of the flow within the vessel can be determined. Determining the echo time at which the signal will be lost due to washout of excited spins from the slice will provide a rough measure of velocity (given the slice thickness). Using cardiac gating to acquire a pair of images, one in diastole and one in systole, and then subtracting the images will create a difference image that brings out arterial structures.[17] Displaying the phase information in the image, rather than just the conventional magnitude, will help bring out moving structures and flowing blood.[18]

MODIFIED MRI TECHNIQUES TO STUDY FLOW

The flow effect of washing out saturated spins can be exploited to measure the component of velocity at right angles to the slice by adding a preliminary pulse to produce saturation of the spins in the slice prior to the actual imaging excitation pulse. Measuring the effect on the signal of varying the time delay between the preliminary saturating pulse and the imaging excitation pulse makes it possible to calculate the velocity.[19]

The time of flight effect of motion of excited spins between initial excitation and the detection of a spin echo can also be used to study flow. If the selective 180 degree refocusing pulse is adjusted to affect a region in space displaced from the originally excited slice, only those excited spins that are carried into the region affected by the refocusing pulse will contribute to the signal;[20] varying the separation of the excitation and refocusing regions or the delay between the pulses will permit an assessment of velocity. Using a selective excitation pulse with a frequency encoding magnetic field gradient ("read-out gradient") oriented at right angles to the plane of excitation permits directly imaging the amount of displacement of the spins between excitation and signal detection.[21]

The phase shifts acquired by excited spins moving along magnetic field gradients can be used to study flow. Applying additional balanced magnetic field gradient pulse pairs designed to affect the phase of only the moving spins can enable separation of moving from stationary spins in several different ways. Stepping through a series of such balanced gradient pulse pairs and performing a Fourier transform of the resulting series of signals will enable calculation of the corresponding velocities along the corresponding direction.[22] By keeping the motion-induced phase shift less than 180 degrees, the velocity can be computed directly from the phase shift.[23]

As discussed above, tissue perfusion is similar in many respects to diffusion. Thus, techniques similar to those used to study diffusion, such as measuring the change in signal after the addition of balanced pulses of magnetic field gradients, may be useful in studying perfusion. The greater degree of order of the motion of the spins in perfusion than in diffusion may still permit some separation of these two processes.

Although the basic mechanisms of flow effects in MRI seem well understood and a wide variety of techniques to exploit them have been proposed, practical implementations for routine clinical applications have not yet come into general use. In part, this is due to the complex nature of blood flow, which may necessitate multiple measurements and thus be time consuming. The clinical importance of disorders of blood flow ensures that this will remain an active area for investigation.

ACKNOWLEDGMENT

Leon Axel is an Established Investigator of the American Heart Association and is supported in part by the Pennsylvania Chapter.

References

1. Hahn HL: Spin echoes. Phys Rev *80*:580–594, 1950.
2. Suryan G: Nuclear resonance in flowing liquids. Proc Indian Acad Sci [A] *33*:107–111, 1951.
3. Carr HY, Purcell EM: Effects of diffusion on free precession in nuclear magnetic resonance experiments. Phys Rev *94*:630–638, 1954.
4. Singer JR: Blood flow rates by nuclear magnetic resonance measurements. Science *130*:1652–1653, 1959.
5. Hahn EL: Detection of sea-water motion by nuclear precession. J Geophys Res *65*:776–777, 1960.
6. Hinshaw WS, Bottomley PA, Holland GN: Radiographic thin section image of the human wrist by nuclear magnetic resonance. Nature (Lond) *270*:722–723, 1977.

7. Young IR, Burl M, Clark GJ, et al: Magnetic resonance properties of hydrogen: Imaging the posterior fossa. AJR *137*:895–901, 1981.
8. Crooks L, Sheldon P, Kaufman L, Rowan W, Miller T: Quantification of obstructions in vessels by nuclear magnetic resonance (NMR). IEEE Trans Nuc Sci NS *29*:1181–1185, 1982.
9. Kaufman L, Crooks LE, Sheldon RE, Rowan W, Miller T: Evaluation of NMR imaging for detection and quantification of obstruction in vessels. Invest Radiol *17*:554–560, 1982.
10. Crooks LE, Hoenninger JC, Arakawa M: *In* Partain CL (ed): Pulse sequences for NMR imaging using multidimensional reconstruction techniques. Nuclear Magnetic Resonance and Correlative Imaging Modalities, New York, Society of Nuclear Medicine, 1984, p. 69.
11. Grant JP, Bank C: NMR rheotomography feasibility and clinical potential. Med Phys *9*:188–193, 1982.
12. Wehrli FW, MacFall JR, Axel L, Glover GH, Herfkens JR: Approaches to in-plane and out-of-plane flow imaging. Noninvasive Med Imag *1*:127–136, 1984.
13. Axel L: Blood flow effects in magnetic resonance imaging. AJR *143*:1157–1166, 1984.
14. Caro CG, Pedley TJ, Schroter RC, Seed WA: The Mechanics of the Circulation. New York, Oxford University Press, 1978.
15. Kumar A, Welti D, Ernst R: NMR Fourier zeugmatography. J Magn Reson *18*:69–85, 1975.
16. Edelstein WA, Hutchinson JMS, Johnson G, Redpath T: Spin warp NMR imaging and applications to whole body imaging. Phys Med Biol *25*:751–756, 1980.
17. Wedeen VJ, Meuli RA, Edelman RR, et al: Projective imaging of pulsatile flow with magnetic resonance. Science *230*:946–948, 1985.
18. van Dijk P: Direct cardiac NMR imaging of the heart wall and blood flow velocity. J Comput Assist Tomogr *8*:429–436, 1984.
19. Singer JR, Crooks LE: NMR blood flow measurements in the human brain. Science *221*:654–656, 1983.
20. Feinberg DA, Crooks LE, Hoenninger J, Arakawa M, Watts J: Visualization of pulsatile blood flow velocity in human arteries by magnetic resonance imaging. Radiology *153*:177–180, 1984.
21. Axel L, Shimakawa A, MacFall J: A time-of-flight method of measuring flow velocity by MRI. Magn Reson Imag *4*:199–206, 1986.
22. Moran PR: A flow velocity zeugmatographic interlace for NMR imaging in humans. Magn Reson Imag *1*:197–203, 1982.
23. O'Donnell J: NMR blood flow imaging using multi-echo phase contrast sequences. Med Phys *12*:59–64, 1985.

99

High Field MRI

ROBERT J. HERFKENS

In 1946, two separate groups, one led by Bloch and the other by Purcell, described the nuclear magnetic resonance (NMR) phenomenon for hydrogen protons. They subsequently won the Nobel Prize for their description, demonstrating absorption of energy by atoms with odd-numbered protons in a magnetic field.[1,2] Further development led to instrumentation capable of detecting the weak signals produced by this resonant phenomenon, leading to a tool that allowed nondestructive characterization of chemical compounds. It was in the early 1950s that the biomedical potential of this phenomenon generated worldwide enthusiasm. As the NMR technology improved in the 1950s and 1960s, the potential utility for biomedical applications became increasingly obvious. The development of these technologies resulted from improved electronics and increasing magnetic field strengths. In-vitro data in the 1970s suggested that NMR signal changes may have a use in diagnosing diseases in vivo. Parallel with this, larger magnets and specialized coils were built to examine the potential of human imaging. The development of human imaging technology paralleled the development of NMR spectroscopic capabilities. Initial experimentation and developments were made at relatively low field strengths utilizing resistive magnets. The development of large bore superconducting magnets quickly changed the emphasis to intermediate field strengths in the range of 0.3 tesla.[3,4] Throughout this period there was continued skepticism about problems encountered at moving to higher field strength imaging. There was significant concern over the ability to build a radio frequency (rf) coil that would work efficiently at higher field strengths. Additionally, questions about rf absorption and potential phase shifts associated with these higher frequencies led many observers to believe NMR imaging at 1.5 tesla to be impossible.[5]

With the development of large bore superconducting magnets operating in the range of 1.0 to 2.0 tesla, imaging and spectroscopy on the same system became a reality[6] (Fig. 99–1). The advent of high field systems generates a significant increase in engineering complexity and system cost. It becomes important for the user to understand some of the potential benefits and limitations dependent upon magnetic field strength.

EFFECTS OF MAGNETIC FIELD STRENGTHS

The intrinsic signal that comes from tissue on NMR imaging is dependent upon a number of factors, including the hydrogen density, *T1* (longitudinal relaxation time or spin-lattice relaxation time) and *T2* (transverse relaxation time or spin-spin relaxation time). The overall diagnostic quality of an image is based on the ability to discriminate between two different tissue types. This is image contrast; however, the real factor that determines the ability to discriminate changes in the clinical arena is contrast to noise. One of the significant drives from increasing field strength has been the increase

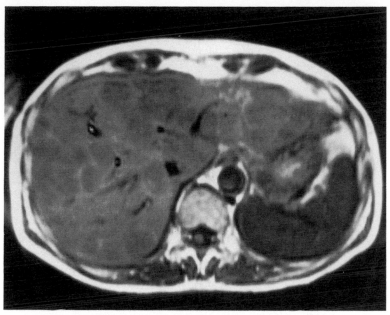

Figure 99–1. A transaxial image through the upper abdomen obtained at 1.5 tesla with a repetition time (*TR*) of 500 ms and an echo delay time (*TE*) of 25 ms. This image was obtained with two excitations and respiratory compensation. Note that there is no evidence of significant focal reduction in signal secondary to phase shifts or rf inhomogeneities as was suspect at higher field strengths. Multiple metastases are present as low intensity areas throughout the liver.

in signal to noise, and ultimately contrast to noise, achieved with higher field strength magnets. The number of hydrogen nuclei that participate in the resonant process is relatively small, in the range of a few parts per million: as the field strength increases, the total number of nuclei available for magnetic resonance increases. At relatively low field strength, noise is dominated by the rf receiver coil and its surroundings. At higher frequencies, the noise is dominated by the human body. The increase in relative signal with field strength is ultimately compromised by noise dominated within the imaging object, the patient. This improvement in signal to noise translates into the ability to obtain thin slices, thus reducing the potential partial volume effects.[7] Improvement in spatial resolution can be obtained when signal to noise increases, allowing finer spatial resolution (Fig. 99–2).

The ultimate test of a diagnostic procedure is its ability to discriminate two tissues. This again is contrast resolution. There are other changes associated with increasing field strength that have an affect on contrast. Specifically, the *T1* relaxation times increase with field strength. The relative increase in these tissues is a moderately complex relationship affecting different tissues to different degrees. The increase in *T1* of water-containing soft tissue structures is approximately 400 to 500 ms/tesla. The increase in fat-containing structures is significantly less, in the range of 200 ms/tesla.[8] The *T2* of tissues is not significantly affected by field strength on the whole; however, certain tissues that contain iron may have a reduction in *T2*. This complex relationship affects image contrast and in certain cases may increase or decrease the relative difference between two tissues. However, with the significant reduction in noise there is an overall increase in contrast to noise as field strength increases.[9–11]

There are a number of ways to improve signal to noise. These include increasing the overall imaging time by signal averaging. This can allow comparable signal to noise to be obtained at lower field strength magnets. A specific potential advantage at higher field strengths is the ability to reduce the scan time. The contrast to noise and signal to noise per unit time is increased, reducing the acquisition time. One of the more recent advances has been the introduction of gradient refocused, limited flip angle images that utilize very short repetition times and echo delay times, allowing for rapid imaging. The high homogeneity and improvement in signal to noise at higher field

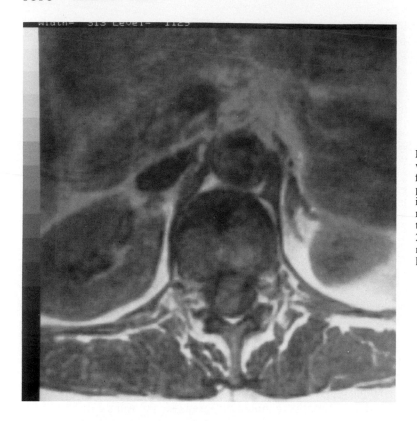

Figure 99–2. Surface coils combined with the high signal to noise of higher field strength systems allow an improvement in spatial resolution. This image through the region of the adrenal was obtained with a repetition time of 500 ms, an echo delay time of 25 ms, and four excitations for this 5 mm thick slice. Note the excellent delineation of the left adrenal gland.

strengths allow excellent image quality to be obtained in two seconds (Fig. 99–3). Although rapid imaging techniques are possible at virtually any field strength, the intrinsic improvement of signal to noise available at higher field strengths adds a significant potential advantage for these methods to decrease overall imaging time.

The improvement in image quality related to signal to noise with higher field strength is not without some disadvantages. There is a 3.5 ppm chemical shift separation between water protons and fat (CH_2) protons at all field strengths. With linear magnetic field gradients applied, there is a slight displacement or separation of these two chemical moieties in the frequency direction. This leads to a relative void at junctions of fat- and water-containing tissues. This void is proportional to the ratio of field strength to gradient amplitude. If gradients are kept constant and field strength increases, the chemical shift would be field dependent. The effect is reasonably subtle but can be increased if gradients are kept constant.[12] The high homogeneity of high field strength magnets and improvement in signal to noise make the chemical shift phenomenon more obvious. In the general clinical realm, the improvement in signal to noise and crispness of the chemical shift phenomenon do not make it a significant problem in routine clinical practice. Another potential difficulty with increasing field strength is the presence of eddy currents. Since tissues are electrically conductive, the changing magnetic fields potentially set up small currents within the tissue, inducing small magnetic fields and inhomogeneities. This is potentially a problem that causes significant shading in the image. The advent of circular polarized rf fields and homogeneous rf fields has essentially eliminated this effect. Although these are theoretical limitations, they appear to have little effect on the overall diagnostic quality of the images provided at 1.5 tesla.

Motion affects the overall signal intensity in an NMR image. This effect does not appear to be significantly field dependent; however, with the improvement of signal to noise at higher field strengths, the specific motion-induced ghosts in the phase direction

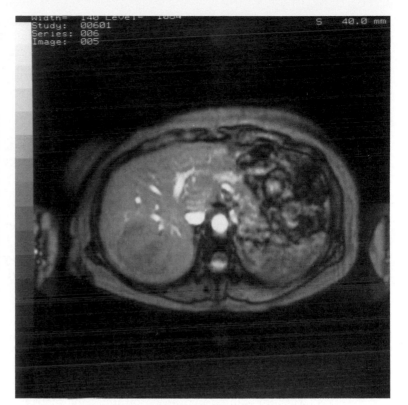

Figure 99–3. A 1 cm thick transaxial slice obtained with a limited flip angle (25 degrees) and gradient refocused echo with a *TE* time of 12 ms was obtained with a total scan time of 2.2 s. Note the excellent delineation of vascular structures and sufficient content to resolve the intrahepatic metastasis. The advantages of limited flip angle gradient refocused acquisition, coupled with the high homogeneity and signal to noise of higher field strength magnets, may prove to be a routine clinical tool.

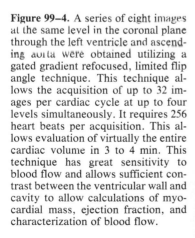

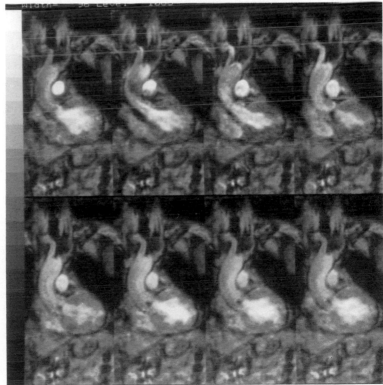

Figure 99–4. A series of eight images at the same level in the coronal plane through the left ventricle and ascending aorta were obtained utilizing a gated gradient refocused, limited flip angle technique. This technique allows the acquisition of up to 32 images per cardiac cycle at up to four levels simultaneously. It requires 256 heart beats per acquisition. This allows evaluation of virtually the entire cardiac volume in 3 to 4 min. This technique has great sensitivity to blood flow and allows sufficient contrast between the ventricular wall and cavity to allow calculations of myocardial mass, ejection fraction, and characterization of blood flow.

can be seen at times to be more distinct. The application of motion compensation techniques such as cardiac gating or respiration compensation techniques improves image quality significantly without affecting the overall image acquisition time, providing excellent diagnostic utility in the abdomen and chest (Fig. 99–4).

SPECTROSCOPY

Spectroscopy was the initial utilization of NMR techniques that spurred the development of imaging systems. It is in many respects simpler than imaging in the basic acquisition. The performance of spectroscopy depends upon the chemical shift or slight difference in resonant frequency associated with slightly different molecular environments of atoms. This is essentially the same effect as previously noted related to the differences between fat and water. These slight differences in resonant frequency are the basis for spectroscopy. A number of compounds have been proposed for which spectroscopy may be potentially useful. These include phosphorus-31, sodium-23, fluorine-23, carbon-13, and several others. The potential specificity provided by direct chemical measurements may ultimately enhance our ability to characterize disease processes.[13,14]

The performance of in-vivo spectroscopy is dependent upon a number of factors. Magnetic field homogeneity is a principal determinant of quality of the spectra obtained. High homogeneity is necessary. There is a significant improvement in chemical dispersion at higher field strengths, allowing the separation of chemically shifted peaks (Fig. 99–5). It is clear that with today's 1.5 tesla systems, chemical shift imaging and spectroscopy can be performed on the same instrument utilized for imaging. The ultimate utility of spectroscopy is yet to be determined.

SITING

The installation of an NMR device poses many difficulties that are not encountered in a routine radiology department. The effects of high magnetic fields on the immediate environment dictate specific siting requirements. Many of these requirements are made more difficult as field strength increases. The fringe fields of a magnet increase with the field strength. This requires an increase in the space required to site a high field magnet in order to physically separate the magnetic field from its environment. This

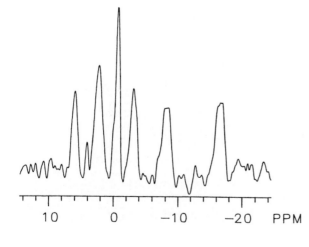

Figure 99–5. A spatially localized phosphorus spectrum obtained through the region of the temporal lobe of a normal volunteer. The spectra was obtained with an acquisition time of approximately 10 min. Note the excellent resolution of phosphocreatine at 0 ppm, and the three ATP peaks to the right.

can be accomplished by shielding the magnetic field by placement of a steel environment surrounding the magnet. This solution, however, requires significant amounts of iron to be present, increasing the weight required of the structure and its overall expense. Additionally, in order to take advantage of the high signal to noise, radio frequency shielding is required in order to eliminate extraneous sources of radio frequencies that are common in hospitals and urban environments.

Another concern associated with high field strength is an increased potential for ferromagnetic objects to act as projectiles and fly directly into the magnet. The environment must be severely restricted to eliminate the potential of anyone carrying ferromagnetic materials into the area. Routine screening for intracranial aneurysm clips, pacemakers, and prosthetic heart valves is accomplished by strict clinical screening.

The increased costs associated with the purchase and siting of higher field strength magnets need to be taken into account in relation to the overall benefits gained. The increase in signal to noise, contrast to noise, and the potential for spectroscopic studies must be related to the overall specific needs of the individual hospital. The increased diagnostic utility obtained by reducing slice thickness and improving spatial resolution are factors that need to be placed in the context of the individual institution.

NMR imaging technology has rapidly developed over the last ten years. This improvement can quickly be related to increasing field strength. The other "hardware" advances can only further improve on basic gains made at higher field strengths. The ability to perform proton imaging and spectroscopy on the same device allows the unique opportunity to improve diagnostic care of patients. The improvement of signal to noise, contrast to noise, and ultimate image resolution associated with higher field strength magnets had led to a significant advantage in localizing and defining normal and pathologic anatomy without prolonging imaging time. The development of rapid imaging techniques may significantly improve our ability to reduce scan time and enhance overall patient care in the future.

References

1. Bloch F, Hansen WW, Parkard ME: Nuclear induction. Phys Rev 127:23–27, 1946.
2. Purcell EM, Torrey HC, Pond RV: Resonance absorption by nuclear magnetic moments in a solid. Phys Rev 37:41–45, 1946.
3. Kaufman L et al: The potential impact of nuclear magnetic resonance imaging on cardiovascular diagnosis. Circulation 67:251–257, 1983.
4. Crooks LE, et al: NMR whole body images operating at 3.5 Kgauss. Radiology 143:159–174, 1982.
5. Bottomley PA, Andrews ER: RF magnetic field penetration, phase-shift and power dissipation in biological tissue: implications for NMR imaging. Phys Med Biol 23:630–643, 1978.
6. Bottomley PA, Hart HR, Edelstein WA, Schenck JF, Smith LS, et al: Anatomy and metabolism of the normal human brain studies by magnetic resonance at 1.5 Tesla. Radiology 150:441–446, 1984.
7. Daniels DL, Herfkens RJ, Gager WE, et al: Magnetic resonance imaging of the optic nerve and chiasm. Radiology 152:79–83, 1984.
8. Johnson GA, Herfkens, RJ, Brown MA: Tissue relaxation time: In vivo field dependence. Radiology 156:805–810, 1985.
9. Edelstein WA, Bottomley PA, Hart HR, et al: Signal, noise, and contrast in nuclear magnetic resonance (NMR). J Comput Assist Tomogr 7:391–401, 1983.
10. Wehrli FW, MacFall JR, Shutts D, et al: Mechanisms of contrast in NMR imaging. J Comput Assist Tomogr 8:369–380, 1984.
11. Hart HR, Bottomley PA, Edelstein WA, et al: NMR imaging as a function of magnetic field: The contrast to noise ratio. AJR 141:1195–1201, 1983.
12. Babcock EE, Brateman L, Weinreb JC, et al: Edge artifacts in MR images: Chemical shift effect. J Comput Assist Tomogr 9:252–257, 1985.
13. Bottomley PA, Hart HR, Edelstein WA, et al: Anatomy and metabolism of the normal human brain studied by magnetic resonance at 1.5 Tesla. Radiology 150:441–446, 1984.
14. Bottomley P: Noninvasive study of high energy phosphate metabolism in the human heart by depth resolved ^{31}P NMR spectroscopy. Science 229:769–772, 1985.

100

Advanced Methods for Spin Density, T1, and T2 Calculations in MRI

THOMAS E. CONTURO
RONALD R. PRICE
ALBERT H. BETH
MARK R. MITCHELL

Determination of the values and standard errors of the three principal nuclear magnetic resonance (NMR) tissue parameters, $T1$, $T2$, and relative hydrogen spin density (N_r), is important for several reasons. These reasons include characterization of pathologic and normal tissues,[2] selection of pulse sequences for optimal image contrast,[17,44] assessment of the time course of pathologic changes and therapeutic responses,[30,48] evaluation of paramagnetic contrast enhancement,[8,34] production of synthetic signal intensity images[47,50] and parametric N_r, $T1$, and $T2$ images[53,54] and extraction of biophysical information on the states of water in tissues.[33]

These measurements should possess six basic features to be appropriate for these applications. First, all three parameters must be measured. This is of particular importance for characterization of pathological and normal tissues, for pulse sequence optimization, and for production of synthetic images. Although the importance of N_r has generally been de-emphasized as a contributor to contrast in MR imaging, N_r measurement is required for all of these applications.

Second, these measurements should be as precise and reproducible as possible. This is important for confident clinical decision making and for characterization of tissues having subtle differences in tissue parameters. More precise measurements would also provide the basis for computation of less noisy parametric and synthetic images, which might provide anatomic detail otherwise masked by image noise.

Third, these measurements should be as accurate as possible. They should reflect intrinsic tissue parameters and should be minimally dependent on instrumental factors. This would best allow standardization of values obtained from different installations and should minimize the dependence of those values on day to day instrumental variations and on particular pulse sequence techniques.

Fourth, some assessment of the confidence limits of the measurement should be provided. This may be a useful parameter for statistical tissue characterization[6] and for determination of the significance of pathological changes and therapeutic responses.

Fifth, the measurement should allow, in a single experiment, accurate and precise determination of the full range of tissue parameter values that are present in all possible biologic fluids, soft tissues, and pathologic and contrast enhanced tissues. Accuracy and precision should also be somewhat uniform throughout that range. This would enable characterization of all tissues in a given image without repeat scanning and without an a priori knowledge of the pertinent tissues, the occurring pathologic processes, or their respective parameter values. These features should also enable computation of N_r, $T1$, and $T2$ images and synthetic images in which all anatomic regions have good signal to noise and should allow better imaging of the effects of paramagnetic contrast agents, which can drastically and unpredictably alter tissue relaxation times.

Sixth, the measurement must be clinically efficient. The data acquisition time should be as short as possible to avoid errors due to patient motion and to provide a patient throughput that is competitive with routine NMR imaging. In particular, measurements that require sequences having repetition times (TR) much greater than $T1$ should be avoided. Also, although the greatest limitation on clinical efficiency is scan time, the method should be computationally efficient.

In contrast to these desired features, routine measurements generally provide an N_r that is $T1$ or $T2$ dependent and is accurate only over a narrow range of $T1$ or $T2$ values. Secondly, routine methods produce parameter values that are imprecise and parametric images that are substantially noisier than routine signal intensity images. This is particularly true for substances having short $T2$ values and long $T1$ values. Thirdly, routine methods often require long scanning times because separate data acquisitions and calculations are used to determine $T1$ and $T2$; because acquisitions must often be signal averaged to reduce the noise of the calculated values; and because sequences with $TR > 5\ T1$ must often be collected. Such a sequence is particularly time consuming in MR imaging where $T1$ values can be greater than 3 seconds, requiring more than 30 minutes of acquisition time for unaveraged two-dimensional Fourier transform (2DFT) imaging with 128 phase encoding steps. Two-point measurements and linear regression $T1$ measurements also require the collection of sequences with $TR \gg T1$, as will be discussed.

The purpose of this chapter is to describe new techniques developed in an attempt to include all of the above six features without having the preceding three limitations. Compared to routine methods, the presented multiple-delay multiple-echo (MDME) pulse sequence strategy and three-parameter data analysis[15] enable measurement of a wide range of $T1$ and $T2$ values,[11] enable accurate measurement of N_r over a wider range of relaxation times,[14] provide precise measurement of all three parameters with standard errors as low as about 0.4 percent,[13] particularly provide precise $T2$ values, which are much shorter than the shortest available echo time,[14] require a maximum timing interval that is only about half the longest $T1$ value, and do not require that acquired intensities be signal averaged. Because of the latter two features, the measurement requires a scanning time that is nearly the same as for routine imaging of signal intensity.

The rationale for parameter measurement general to both NMR spectroscopy and MR imaging will first be discussed, followed by a discussion of the limitations of imaging approaches compared to spectroscopic approaches to parameter measurement.

BACKGROUND

For image intensity or spectroscopic signal intensity to be a basis for N_r, $T1$, and $T2$ measurement, it is essential that the intensity be sensitive to the desired parameter value. For example, if $T1$ is to be measured, image intensity must change with changing $T1$ so that the actual $T1$ value will be "registered" in the value of the intensity. The larger this sensitivity, given mathematically by $\partial I/\partial T1$,[44] the more useful the intensity will be for $T1$ determination. Similarly, N_r and $T2$ measurements require collection of intensities possessing N_r sensitivity and $T2$ sensitivity, given by $\partial I/\partial N_r$ and $\partial I/\partial T2$, respectively.

Spectroscopic Measurements

The simplest pulse sequence for *T1* measurement in NMR spectroscopy is the saturation-recovery (SR) sequence, diagrammed by [90° – FID – *TR*]$_n$ (Table 100–1, Fig. 100–1*A*), where *n* indicates that the sequence is repeated *n* times ($n \geq 2$) with the same repetition time, *TR*. At steady state, the signal intensity of the Fourier transform of the free induction decay (FID) is given by

$$I = N_r(1 - e^{-TR/T1}) \tag{1}$$

The absolute *T1* sensitivity of this sequence is graphed versus *T1* for a particular *TR* in Figure 100–2. As seen, a given pulse sequence with a given *TR* timing interval is sensitive to a narrow range of *T1* values. Specifically, sensitivity is maximal when *TR* = *T1*, but is less than half maximal when *T1* is less than about one third or greater than about four times the selected *TR* interval. For *T1* values for which sensitivity is low, different *T1* values would only produce subtle differences in intensity, which would be masked by image noise and would produce a very imprecise or noisy measurement. A given SR sequence will thus provide information for measurement of only a narrow range of *T1* values, and an a priori knowledge of the approximate parameter value

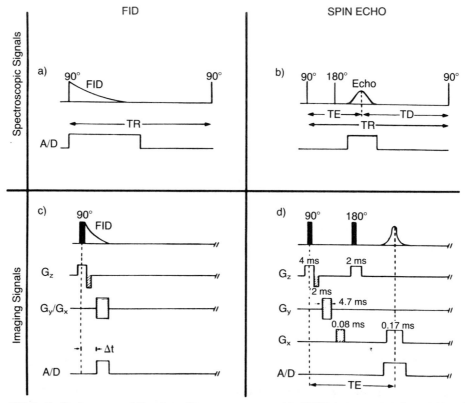

Figure 100–1. Radio frequency (rf) and gradient sequences used in NMR spectroscopy (*a* and *b*) and MR imaging (*c* and *d*). Spin-echo (SE) and free induction decay (FID) acquisition are both available in MR imaging and NMR spectroscopy. While FID acquisition delays (Δt) and echo times (TE) can be made very short in NMR spectroscopy, these times are finite in MR imaging, being limited by the time required for operation of slice selective (G_z) and phase-compensating (hatched) gradients, frequency-encoding gradients (G_x/G_y in the FID acquisition and G_y in the SE acquisition), and phase-encoding gradients (G_x in the SE acquisition). Typical gradient durations used in our multislice imaging SE sequence with 1.0 cm slice selection are labeled. These finite limitations on Δt and TE cause the imaging FID and SE signals to be significantly *T2** and *T2* weighted, respectively.

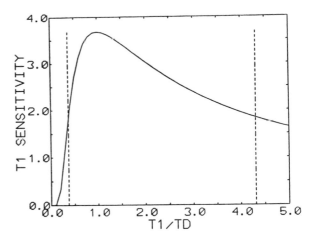

Figure 100–2. *T1* sensitivity (S_{T1}) of the signal intensity of a given spectroscopic saturation recovery (SR) sequence, where $S_{T1} = \partial I/\partial T1$. S_{T1} is maximal when *T1* = *TD* (S_{T1} is calculated for a fixed TD of 100 ms). Half maximal sensitivity is obtained for *T1* values of 0.37 and 4.3 TR (dashed lines). Thus, a given pulse sequence with a fixed timing interval will provide information for precise measurement of only a narrow range of *T1* values.

would be required for selection of the *TR* timing interval appropriate for the measurement.

Even if an intensity having sensitivity to the *T1* of interest is collected, the *T1* value cannot be directly calculated from this intensity. Absolute spin density, sampling volume, and internal electronic scaling can all affect intensity so that there is not a 1:1 correspondence between intensity and *T1*. If the scale factor is linear, all three of these contributions are combined to give relative spin density, N_r. To determine *T1* from a single intensity, one could assume a spin density of H_2O and calibrate the maximal signal for a given sampling volume. More commonly, the intensity is "normalized" by dividing it by a measured N_r. Normalization can be achieved by directly measuring N_t from the first FID of a double FID experiment (Table 100–1). If the sequence must be acquired at steady state for signal averaging or other reasons, the normalized SR sequence is used (Table 100–1), and a sequence having a *TR* > 5*T1* must be collected (Table 100–1) so that full *T1* relaxation will have occurred.

Alternatively, the long *TR* can be reduced to shorten scan times while still providing information for N_r and *T1* measurement (Table 100–1). The two *TR* intervals have been optimized theoretically to give maximal precision in a minimal amount of spectrometer time[1,23] and imager time,[37] predicting optimal *TR* intervals that are <5*T1*, and in which calculated noise per unit time is decreased. For example, the long *TR* of the theoretically optimized imaging sequence (Table 100–1) is only about 2.5 *T1*,[37] but this measurement has poor precision if *T1* is outside of the range from 0.6 to 1.3 times the anticipated *T1* value.[37,58] Moreover, this two-point measurement uses a combined sequence having an overall *TR* > 5*T1*, which causes long acquisition times for measurement of samples having long *T1* values.

As with two-point *T1* measurements, *T2* can be determined from the normalized intensity of a spin echo[22] acquired with a single SE sequence diagrammed by 90° – τ – 180° – τ – echo (Fig. 100–1*B*, Table 100–1), which has an echo time (*TE*) of 2 τ. The sensitivity profile of this sequence is identical to that of the SR sequence (Fig. 100–2), with a maximum at *TE* = *T2*. If a single repetition is acceptable, the signal can be normalized by an additional FID acquisition at little cost in scanning time to give both N_r and *T2*. However, if the sequence must be acquired at steady state, only *T2* will be provided from the normalized SE sequence (Table 100–1), and selection of a *TR* > 5*T1* will be required for N_r measurement (Table 100–1). Alternatively, spectral line widths obtained from the Fourier transform of the FID can be used for one-point *T2* measurement without intensity normalization, but this is valid only if *T2* ≪ *T1* (often not the case in proton NMR) and *T2** ≈ *T2*, where *T2** is the time constant of the FID (which is usually significantly shorter than *T2*).

Table 100–1. TYPICAL PULSE SEQUENCES USED IN NMR SPECTROSCOPY AND NMR IMAGING FOR PARAMETER MEASUREMENT*

Sequence†	Diagram^a	N_r^b	T1	T2	TR,TD >5T1?	Range^c
Spectroscopic Sequences **One Point or Normalized One Point**						
Single FID	90·FID	y	n	n^d	n	–
Double FID	90·FID·TR·90·FID	y	y	n	n	N
Steady-state FID (SR)	[90·FID·TR]$_n$	T1-w^e	n	n^d	y^f	–
Normalized SR	[90·FID·TR1·90·FID·TR2]$_n$	y	y	n^d	y^g	N
Single SE	90·τ180·τ·echo	T2-w^h	n	n	n	–
Steady-state SE	[90·τ·180·τ·echo·TD]$_n$	T1, T2-w	n	n	n	–
Normalized SE	[90·FID·TR·90·τ·180·τ·echo·TD]$_n$, TR = TD	T1-w^e	n	y	y^f	N
Multipoint						
Repeated SR	[90·FID·TR$_i$. . .]$_n$	y	y	n^d	n	W
Repeated IR	[180·T1$_i$·90·FID·TD. . .]$_n$	T1-w^{e,l}	y	n	y^f	W
Single ME	90·(τ·180·τ·echo)$_m$	y	n	y	n	W
Steady state ME	[90·(τ·180·τ·echo)$_m$·TD]$_n$	T1-w^e	n	y	y^f	W
Imaging Measurements **Two Point and Normalized One Point**						
FID	[90·Δt·FID − TD]$_n$	T1, T2*-w^e	n	n	n	–
Normalized FID	[90·Δt·FID·TD1·90·Δt·FID·TD2]$_n$	T2*-w	y	n	y^g	N
Optimized 2-point T1‡	[180·T1·90·τ·180·τ·echo·TD·90·τ·180·τ·echo·TD]$_n$	T2-w	y	n	y^i	N
Double SE	[90·(τ·180·τ·echo)$_2$·TD]$_n$	T1-w^e	n	y	y^f	N

Multipoint

Repeated FID	$[90 \cdot \Delta\tau \cdot FID \cdot TD_i \ldots]_n$	$T2^*\text{-w}$	y	n	n	W
Repeated SE	$[90 \cdot \tau \cdot 180 \cdot \tau \cdot echo \cdot TD_i \ldots]_n$	$T2\text{-w}$	y	n	n	W
Repeated ISE	$[180 \cdot TI_i \cdot 90 \cdot \tau \cdot 180 \cdot \tau \cdot echo \cdot TD \ldots]_n$	$T1, T2\text{-w}^{e,l}$	y	n	n	W
Repeated IME^j	$[180 \cdot TI_i \cdot 90 \cdot (\tau \cdot 180 \cdot \tau \cdot echo)_m \cdot TD \ldots]_n$	$T1\text{-w}^{e,l}$	y	n^k	n	W
ME	$[90 \cdot (\tau \cdot 180 \cdot \tau \cdot echo)_{ri} \cdot TD]_n$	$T1\text{-w}^{e,f}$	n	y	y^b	W
Repeated ME (MDME)	$[90 \cdot (\tau_i \cdot 180 \cdot \tau_i \cdot echo)_{mi} \cdot TD_i \ldots]_n$	y	y	y	n	W

* Steady-state sequences acquired for signal averaging or spatial encoding are diagrammed with closed brackets and subscripts representing that the sequence is repeated n times with the same timings ($n \geq 2$). Parameters that can be measured from fit to the acquired signals are listed for each sequence, as well as the range of parameters that can be measured by a given sequence and whether or not sequences with long TD or TR are required.

† Abbreviations: FID = free induction decay, SE = spin echo, IR = inversion recovery, ME = multiple spin echo, ISE = inversion spin echo, IME = inversion with multiple echo, MDME = multiple-delay multiple-echo, SR = saturation recovery.

‡ The optimized timings are predicted to be $TI = 0.8T1$ and $TD = 2.5T1$.[37,58]

^{a} Sequences that are repeated with varying timings are labeled as "repeated" and the timing that is varied is subscripted with i (timings that are not varied are not subscripted). For normalized sequences, parameter values are obtained from the ratio of the two signals. Echo trains of multiple echo sequences are subscripted by m, the number of echoes in the train.

^{b} $T1\text{-w} = T1$-weighted, $T2\text{-w} = T2$-weighted, etc; y = yes, the pure parameter can be measured; n = no.

^{c} W = wide range, N = narrow range.

^{d} $T2$ can be measured from line widths, but only if $T2 \approx T2^* \ll T1$.

^{e} $T1$-weighting can be eliminated by choosing $TD > 5T1$.

^{f} Only required for N_r correction.

^{g} For optimal $T1$ measurement, but timings can be shorter.

^{h} $T2$-weighting can be reduced in spectroscopy by using a very short TE.

^{i} Optimal $T1$ measurement is with both TD intervals set to $2.5T1$.

^{j} N_r and $T1$ determined by two-parameter fit to echo intensities extrapolated to $TE = 0$ (reference 53).

^{k} $T2$ could be obtained from the extrapolation procedure.

^{l} $T1$-weighting can potentially be corrected since $T1$ is measured.

These spectroscopic two-point and normalized one-point methods have two severe limitations. First, measurements are only appropriate for a narrow range of $T1$ or $T2$ values, as other values are either poorly measured or inaccessible. Second, if the sequence must be acquired at steady state, an intensity with $TR \gg T1$ must be collected for normalization, N_r determination, or optimized two-point $T1$ measurements. As discussed, this can be impractical in MR imaging.

These limitations can be avoided by using intensities collected with a variety of timing intervals for $T1$ or $T2$ measurement. For example, if intensities are collected using repeated SR sequences having several different TR intervals (the repeated FID sequence in Table 100–1), $T1$ sensitivity will be provided over a wider range than would be provided by a single sequence. This is illustrated in Figure 100–3, where selection of five different TR intervals provides intensities that have at least 90 percent of the maximal $T1$ sensitivity over a range of $T1$ values from 40 ms to 3 s (sensitivity to percent change in $T1$ as graphed, as will be discussed later). $T1$ can then be determined from a nonlinear regression fit of N_r and $T1$ to these intensities, which is preferred over a linear regression fit of $\ln[(N_r - I)/N_r]$ versus TR because N_r need not be separately measured, and calculations are less noisy.[60] For a given $T1$ value this multiple measurement may not provide as much precision per scan time as will the optimized two-point methods in which the target $T1$ is accurately set,[1] but such accurate estimations are difficult in NMR spectroscopy and are meaningless if different $T1$ values are to be measured by the same sequence, as desired in MR imaging.

Similarly, a single-repetition multiple spin-echo (ME) sequence (either the Carr-Purcell[10] sequence or the Meiboom-Gill variation[41]), given by $90° - (\tau - 180° - \tau - \text{echo})_m$, can be used to collect multiple echoes at different echo times (Table 100–1). By virtue of the single repetition of this sequence, N_r and $T2$ can be directly determined from fit to these echoes (Table 100–1). If this sequence must be repeated for signal averaging or for other reasons, the steady-state ME sequence results, given by $[90° - \tau - (180° - \tau - \text{echo} - \tau)_m - TD]_n$ (Table 100–1), where TD is the delay time.[12] In this case, a $T1$ weighted N_r is obtained with $T2$, and a "pure" spin density can be directly measured by this sequence only if $TD > 5T1$.

Thus, in NMR spectroscopy one can directly determine N_r and $T1$ using SR sequences repeated at different TR intervals, avoiding acquisition of a sequence having $TR > 5T1$ and presumably providing sensitivity to and measurement of a wider range of $T1$ values than is provided by a normalized single-point or two-point measurement. A multipoint $T2$ can be determined but, unlike the multipoint $T1$ measurement, this provides direct N_r determination only if a single-repetition ME sequence is used or if a $TD > 5T1$ is chosen for the steady-state ME sequence.

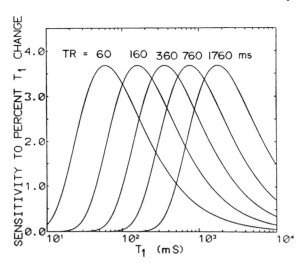

Figure 100–3. Sensitivity to percent change in $T1$, $\partial I/\partial(\ln T1)$, provided by five different SR sequences having five different TD intervals. With the geometric progression of fixed TD intervals, the sensitivity profiles are uniformly distributed across a range of $T1$ values. Approximately uniform net sensitivity to percent change in $T1$ will thus be provided for a range of $T1$ values so that the random error in the calculated values will be approximately uniform throughout the calculated range (see text).

Imaging Measurements

While these multipoint methods provide adequate parameter measurement in NMR spectroscopy, they are non-ideal for MR imaging because of inherent technical restrictions and because of practical limitations on scanning times.

The first of these technical restrictions is that, while NMR spectra (particularly proton water spectra) can sometimes be collected with a single repetition of a pulse sequence, spatial encoding of NMR images requires several steady-state repetitions of a given pulse sequence. This imposes a $T1$ dependence on all NMR image intensities, preventing the use of sequences such as the single-repetition FID or single-repetition ME sequence, which allow direct measurement of N_r without $TD > 5T1$ (Table 100–1).

Secondly and more importantly, spectroscopic NMR intensities can be measured immediately after the 90 degree pulse and thus can be derived from the entire time course of the FID, which is well characterized because of the high field homogeneity and long $T2^*$ time constant in NMR spectroscopy (Fig. 100–1A). In MR imaging, on the other hand, the FID cannot be collected immediately after the 90 degree pulse. Time is required for the operation of gradients for selective excitation,[57] phase compensation,[57] and frequency encoding[36] (Fig. 100–1C). These extra imaging operations delay the acquisition of the FID by a time Δt in Figure 100–1C, which may be on the order of milliseconds after the 90 degree pulse. With the poorer field homogeneity in imaging systems, the actual Fourier transformed image intensity is thus significantly attenuated by $T2^*$ at the time of data collection.[49,63]

Alternatively, image intensities can be collected by formation of steady-state spin echoes with the imaging SE sequence $[90 - \tau - 180 - \tau - echo - TD]_n$. This is used in the more conventional two-dimensional Fourier transform (2DFT) method[36] because the signal can be phase encoded during the τ interval. However, TE intervals are then limited by the operation of the gradients for selective excitation, gradient compensation, phase encoding, and signal read-out. Thus, while echo times can be made very short in NMR spectroscopy (Fig. 100–1B), these times are limited to several milliseconds in MR imaging (Fig. 100–1D), causing the imaging spin echo acquisition to have significant $T2$ dependence. All NMR image intensities are thus dependent on N_r, $T1$, and either $T2$ or $T2^*$.

Owing to the mixed dependence of the steady-state spin-echo signal intensity on all three tissue parameters, separate measurement of $T1$ in MR imaging requires that $T2$ dependence be fixed, while separate measurement of $T2$ requires that $T1$ dependence be fixed. This is true for both the two-point and the multipoint methods. For example, to determine $T1$, either two-point[37,49] or multipoint spin-echo methods can be used (Table 100–1). In both cases, the TE intervals of the SE sequences must be held constant while $T1$ dependence (e.g., TD) is varied.

Likewise, $T2$ can also be separately measured by two-point methods[43] or multipoint methods[3,53] using the double SE or (ME) sequences, respectively (Table 100–1). Conveniently all echoes in this sequence have the same $T1$ dependence and TD interval.[12,27] (In comparison, separate SE sequences having different TE intervals do not have the same TD interval or $T1$ dependence.)

Limitations of Imaging Measurements

Three limitations particular to separate imaging $T1$ and $T2$ measurements are to be discussed: (1) accurate N_r cannot be easily measured; (2) measurements are noisy; and (3) measurements are time inefficient. First, since separate single-point or multipoint $T1$ or $T2$ measurements require that $T2$ or $T1$ dependence, respectively, be fixed, accurate N_r cannot easily be obtained. In particular, acquisition of intensities by spin echo causes the N_r calculated with *T1* to be underestimated by the *T2* relaxation that occurs during the fixed *TE* interval, while acquisition of steady-state intensities causes the N_r calculated with *T2* to be underestimated by incomplete *T1* relaxation during the fixed *TD* interval.[3,53]

These N_r errors are demonstrated by collecting intensities from a phantom containing fifty-five different $CrCl_3$ solutions (Fig. 100–4), with ion concentrations ranging from 0 to 10 mM. Data for these and all other experimental studies in this chapter were collected using a Technicare 0.5 tesla clinical superconducting system with 2DFT data acquisition, 10 mm slice thickness, and 128 phase encoding steps without signal averaging. Mean intensities were collected from a 27-pixel ROI (1.2 mm by 1.2 mm pixel size interpolated from 1.2 mm by 2.4 mm voxels) and, unless otherwise stated, were corrected by subtracting the average background intensity of air measured from the corresponding image. N_r was obtained from a separate *T1* measurement by a nonlinear least squares fit to the mean ROI intensities of unaveraged SE sequences with *TE* = 30 ms and *TR* values of 0.3, 0.4, 0.6, 1.0, and 2.0 s (Fig. 100–5A) as in the repeated SE sequence (Table 100–1). Although these solutions should have equivalent N_r, the calculated N_r is underestimated at high ion concentrations (short *T2*) while it is stable at low ion concentrations (long *T2*). The underestimation is due to the significant *T2* decay at the time of echo collection, which cannot be completely eliminated due to instrumental limitations on how short *TE* can be (Fig. 100–1D). Unlike the *T2** weighting that would occur with FID acquisitions,[38] this *T2* weighting is theoretically independent of instrumental factors and so might easily be corrected. This demonstrated N_r error is clinically significant because normal muscle[5] and tendon,[21] and certain paramagnetic enhanced[18,34] and pathologic tissues have *T2* values corresponding to the range of concentrations for which N_r is underestimated in Figure 100–5A.

Similarly, N_r and *T2* can be calculated from the same phantom using an unaveraged eight-echo ME sequence (Table 100–1) having a *TD* of 1.76 ms (Fig. 100–5B) and *TE* = 30, 60, 90, . . . , 240 ms. In this case, N_r is underestimated at low ion concentrations (long *T1*) owing to incomplete *T1* relaxation during the *TD* interval. Unlike the *T2*

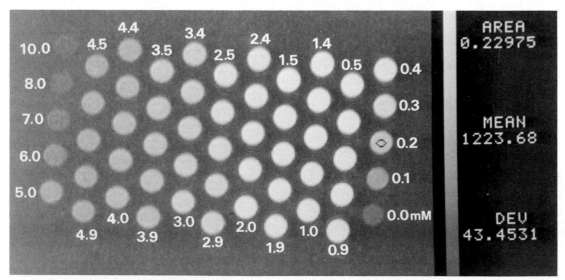

Figure 100–4. Sample two-dimensional FT image of the test phantom. The image was generated from the first echo (*TE* = 30 ms) of the ME sequence having a *TR* of 600 ms and a *TD* of 60 ms. The phantom contained aqueous solutions of $CrCl_3$ which ranged in concentration from 0 to 5 mM, in steps of 0.1 mM, and with extra solutions of 6, 7, 8, and 10 mM as labeled. The image had a slice thickness of 1 cm in the transverse plane and was not signal averaged. The 27-pixel region of interest (ROI) used for data collection is indicated.

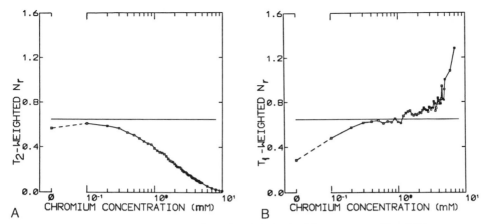

Figure 100–5. *T2* weighted N_r (*A*) and *T1* weighted N_r (*B*) obtained from separate *T1* and *T2* measurements, respectively. The *T2* weighted N_r (*A*) was obtained in the two-parameter nonlinear least squares fit to the unaveraged intensities in the open row of Figure 100–6, and *T1* weight N_r (*B*) was obtained from a two-parameter nonlinear least squares fit to the unaveraged intensities in the shaded column of Figure 100–6. The solid line of constant N_r is drawn to fit the N_r values at low ion concentration in *A*. At concentrations above 0.2 mM (*T2* < 180 ms), the N_r calculated with *T1* (*A*) is significantly below this line due to failure of the separate *T1* measurement to correct for the finite *T2* relaxation occuring during the first TE interval of 30 ms. Similarly, at ion concentrations below 0.4 mM (*T1* > 475 ms), the N_r calculated with *T2* (*B*) is significantly below this line owing to failure of the separate *T2* measurement to correct for the incomplete *T1* relaxation during the 1.76 s TD interval.

weighted N_r obtained with *T1* measurements, this error in Figure 100–5*B* can be eliminated by choosing *TD* > 5*T1*, but, as discussed, this demands prohibitive scanning times if accurate N_r is to be obtained for all biologic tissues and fluids. Values of N_r determined from separate multipoint *T1* or *T2* measurements are thus either *T1* or *T2* weighted by these effects.

As a modification, inversion spin-echo (ISE) sequences, [180° – *TI* – 90° – τ – 180° – τ – echo – *TD*]$_n$, with varying inversion times (*TI*) have been proposed for both two-point[37,49] and multipoint[3] imaging *T1* measurements in the hope of increasing *T1* sensitivity and *T1* precision (Table 100–1). However, these sequences also have mixed N_r, *T1*, and *T2* dependence and provide N_r measurements that possess both *T1* and *T2* weighting. Secondly, the ISE sequence, or the spectroscopic inversion-recovery (IR) sequence (Table 100–1) is very inefficient for measurement of long *T1* values.[19]

Three methods have previously been attempted to eliminate *T1* or *T2* weighting from N_r measurements. First, as mentioned, *T1* weighting can be virtually eliminated from N_r by performing multipoint *T2* measurements using SE or ME sequences with *TD* intervals on the order of five times the longest *T1* of biologic tissues,[3] but this is clinically impractical. Two other methods are directed at correcting N_r by making estimates of signal loss due to *T2* relaxation or incomplete *T1* relaxation. The first of these is to use the *T1* calculated from a separate data acquisition to correct the *T1* weighted N_r obtained in a *T2* measurement,[25,32] or using a separately measured *T2* to correct a *T2* weighted N_r obtained in a *T1* measurement. This approach, however, might be expected to result in unnecessary propagation of random and systematic *T1* and *T2* errors into N_r errors, as will be shown. The second correction method is to extrapolate multiple echo signal intensities to a zero *TE*, from which N_r and *T1* can be determined. However, extrapolation would be expected to be imprecise for samples with short *T2* values. (Similarly, extrapolation of the FID to the time of the 90 degree pulse would theoretically eliminate the *T2** weighting of the N_r obtained from an imaging SR sequence, but this would also be imprecise.) Moreover, the particular extrapolation study[53] used an inversion with multiple echo (IME) sequence, [180° – *TI*

$- 90° - (\tau - 180° - \tau - \text{echo})_M - TD]_n$ (Table 100–1) with varying TI intervals, causing N_r to be TI weighted by the incomplete TI relaxation during the TD interval.

The second major limitation of imaging measurements is sensitivity to image noise. This is particularly the case for measurement of short $T2$ values, as will be shown later, since the low signal to noise and sensitivity of the late echoes produces noisy $T2$ measurements[40] and $T2$ images. Attempts have been made to improve $T2$ precision by signal averaging the input intensities[3] or by averaging groups of rapidly produced multiple echoes.[53]

The third major limitation of imaging measurements is that long scan times are required. This is because, as mentioned, a $TD \gg TI$ is usually chosen for accurate N_r measurements and for two-point TI measurements. Long scan times are also caused by the need to signal average acquisitions to obtain improved noise levels in the calculated values, especially for short $T2$. Finally, most methods use separate data acquisitions and calculations to determine TI and $T2$, from which N_r can be determined. While attempts have been made to optimize selection of pulse sequences and timing intervals to provide the maximum measurement precision in the minimum scan time,[37,60] these studies assumed that only TI or $T2$ was to be measured. Thus separate acquisitions, although optimized for separate TI or $T2$ measurement, may not necessarily be the optimal use of scanning time for determination of all three principal parameters.

MULTIPLE-DELAY MULTIPLE-ECHO METHOD

Rather than signal average an ME sequence to obtain acceptable $T2$ precision (e.g., averaging the intensities in the row in Fig. 100–6), which only provides a "pure" N_r if $TD > 5TI$, one can instead collect unaveraged ME intensities using different ME subsequences with different TD intervals. The resulting multiple-delay multiple-echo (MDME) data set collected with five different TD intervals (Fig. 100–6) should, in principle, provide nearly the same potential for reducing the calculated $T2$ noise as is provided by an ME sequence signal averaged using the same TD interval. Since the MDME data set possesses information for measurement of TI as well as $T2$, the data should provide the potential for correction of N_r without separate measurement of TI or $T2$ and without use of sequences with $TD > 5TI$. The latter, combined with the ability to use unaveraged data, might also be expected to enable the MDME data set

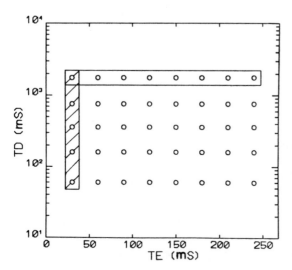

Figure 100–6. Array of TE and TD timing intervals used for multiple delay–multiple echo (MDME) data collection. Each circle locates a single collected image by its corresponding pair of timing intervals. The collected images are used as input to the three-parameter Gauss-Newton nonlinear least squares computation of N_r, TI, and $T2$ (see Figs. 100–7 and 100–8). Separate TI calculation requires fixing $T2$ dependence by using data with a fixed TE interval (preferably with the shortest TE, as indicated by the shaded column). Separate $T2$ calculation requires fixing TI dependence by using data with a fixed TD interval (preferably with the longest TD, as indicated by the blocked row). The results of a two-parameter fit of N_r and TI to the shaded column of intensities is given in Figures 100–5A and 100–14B for comparison. The results of a two-parameter fit of N_r and $T2$ to the blocked row of intensities is given in Figures 100–5B, 100–13A, 100–13C, and 100–14 for comparison. The MDME data set, which provides information for measurement of all three NMR parameters, is collected with virtually the same scanning time as is required for collection of the shaded column of intensities required for separate calculation of TI and a $T2$ weighted N_r.

to be collected in a reasonable scan time. The MDME data set can be collected in virtually the same time as the data set required for separate $T1$ calculation (i.e., the column of intensities in Fig. 100–6), since collection of ME intensities merely postpones the beginning of net $T1$ relaxation to the longest TE.[12,16]

In processing the MDME data set, particular attention should be paid to correction of N_r, minimization of the noise in all three calculated NMR parameters, and provision of parameters whose values are maximally independent of the other two parameter values. For example, one could separately determine $T1$ from different columns of the data set as suggested by Riederer et al.,[51] but this may cause high correlation between parameters, as will be shown. Alternatively, one could extrapolate each row of intensities to a zero TE, as discussed, but this may be a source of noise. We have instead chosen to use the entire MDME data set to simultaneously determine all three parameters. The performance of three-parameter Gauss-Newton least squares was investigated for this purpose. As will be shown, this provides an inherent N_r correction, utilizes the signal averaging potential of the MDME data set, and reduces interdependence between the three parameters.

Theory

The theory for the Gauss-Newton nonlinear least squares procedure is given elsewhere,[61] but certain formulae will be reiterated here for reference throughout the discussion.

The signal intensity (I) of a pixel or ROI in the MDME data set can be mathematically modeled as:

$$I_{C_{ij}} = f(N_r, T1, T2, TE_{ij}, TD_j) \tag{2}$$

where N_r is the relative hydrogen spin density, which is a combination of absolute spin density, electronic scale factors, and voxel volume; TD_j is the delay time of the j-th ME pulse subsequence; TE_{ij} is the echo time of the i-th echo in the j-th multiple-echo train; and $I_{C_{ij}}$ is the intensity calculated for the i-th echo in the j-th subsequence according to the model (where the MDME array in Fig. 100–6 is indexed by i and j). The least squares criterion for best fit is minimization of the expression

$$D = \sum_{ij} \omega_{ij}(I_{O_{ij}} - I_{C_{ij}})^2 \tag{3}$$

by selection of appropriate tissue parameter values $\hat{p} = (\hat{N}_r, \hat{T1}, \hat{T2})$, where $I_{O_{ij}}$ is the observed intensity collected with timings TE_{ij} and TD_j, $I_{C_{ij}}$ is the intensity calculated from equation (2), ω_{ij} is a relative weight assigned to each intensity, and the sum is over all combinations of TE and TD in the MDME array.

For minimization of Equation (3), the calculated intensity is linearized with respect to N_r, $T1$, and $T2$ using a truncated Taylor series expansion about initial estimated parameters $p_0 = (N_0, T1_0, T2_0)$. Using the linear approximation that all partial derivatives evaluated at $\hat{p}$ can be substituted by derivatives evaluated at p_0, the approximate parameters $\hat{p}$ can be obtained by solving the matrix equation:

$$\begin{bmatrix} \sum_{ij} \omega_{ij}(S_{Nr_{ij}})^2 & \sum_{ij} \omega_{ij}S_{Nr_{ij}}S_{T1_{ij}} & \sum_{ij} \omega_{ij}S_{Nr_{ij}}S_{T2_{ij}} \\ \sum_{ij} \omega_{ij}S_{T1_{ij}}S_{Nr_{ij}} & \sum_{ij} \omega_{ij}(S_{T1_{ij}})^2 & \sum_{ij} \omega_{ij}S_{T1_{ij}}S_{T2_{ij}} \\ \sum_{ij} \omega_{ij}S_{T2_{ij}}S_{Nr_{ij}} & \sum_{ij} \omega_{ij}S_{T2_{ij}}S_{T1_{ij}} & \sum_{ij} \omega_{ij}(S_{T2_{ij}})^2 \end{bmatrix} \begin{bmatrix} \hat{N}_r - N_{r0} \\ \hat{T1} - T1_0 \\ \hat{T2} - T2_0 \end{bmatrix} = \begin{bmatrix} \sum_{ij} \omega_{ij}\Delta I_{ij}S_{Nr_{ij}} \\ \sum_{ij} \omega_{ij}\Delta I_{ij}S_{T1_{ij}} \\ \sum_{ij} \omega_{ij}\Delta I_{ij}S_{T2_{ij}} \end{bmatrix} \tag{4}$$

or

$$\mathbf{Ax} = \mathbf{v} \tag{5}$$

where $\Delta I_{ij} = I_{O_{ij}} - I_{C_{ij}}$ and $S_{Nr_{ij}} = \partial I_{C_{ij}}/\partial N_r$, $S_{T1_{ij}} = \partial I_{C_{ij}}/\partial T1$, and $S_{T2_{ij}} = \partial I_{C_{ij}}/\partial T2$

represent the N_r, $T1$, and $T2$ sensitivities for a particular intensity collected with timing intervals TE_{ij} and TD_j, with all derivatives evaluated at the initial estimated values p_0.

The parameters $\hat{p}$ are obtained by multiplication of Equation (5) by A^{-1}:

$$x = A^{-1}v. \tag{6}$$

Because of the above linear approximation, $\hat{N}_r$, $\hat{T1}$, and $\hat{T2}$ calculated from x in Equation (6) will be only approximately correct. However, if the p_0 estimates are good, the new values will be better approximations than are the original p_0 values. These new parameters can be used as new estimates for a second calculation of x, and the calculation is then iterated until x converges to the zero vector.

The accuracy and precision of the nonlinear least squares method can be inferred from further theory. There are four causes of inaccuracy in this numerical method: (1) convergence to local minima, (2) fit to incorrect mathematical models, (3) inappropriate weighting of intensities, and (4) interdependence among the measured parameters. First, if relative minima in D in Equation (3) are present (as is often the case when observations are noisy or when complicated mathematical expressions are fit), the computation may yield incorrect parameters by converging to these local minima, from certain starting values. Next, if incorrect mathematical models are used, calculated values will have systematic error even though the computation may still converge to absolute minima and yield unique values. Such is the case when the SR signal intensity Equation (1) is often assumed for the ME sequence,[43] where fit gives well-converged but inaccurate $T1$ values.[12] As both convergence to local minima and improper mathematical models lead to poor fit to the MDME data set, the presence of these two situations can be detected by a large minimized value of D. Alternatively, we have defined agreement factors modified from Rollet[52] (pages 245 and 407) as follows:

$$R = \sqrt{\frac{|\sum_{ij} \omega_{ij}(I_{O_{ij}} - I_{C_{ij}})|}{\sum_{ij} \omega_{ij}(I_{O_{ij}})}} \tag{7}$$

$$R' = \sqrt{\frac{\sum_{ij} \omega_{ij}|(I_{O_{ij}} - I_{C_{ij}})|}{\sum_{ij} \omega_{ij}(I_{O_{ij}})}} \tag{8}$$

The R agreement factor is calculated from the sum of the difference in I_O and I_C, while R' is calculated from the sum of the absolute differences. Thus, random errors (i.e., image noise) would contribute to R' but not to R, since I_O would be randomly distributed about I_C and the sign of their difference is only preserved in the definition of R. On the other hand, systematic error (i.e., use of inappropriate mathematical models) would most likely result in a consistent displacement of I_C from I_O and would contribute equally to R and R'. Thus, for a situation in which the error in the fit is due to purely random error (i.e., fit of noisy data to a perfectly accurate mathematical model), $R \approx 0$ and $R' > 0$. For a situation in which the error is due to purely systematic error (i.e., fit of noiseless data to inappropriate models) or a situation in which mixed random and systematic errors occur, $0 < R \leq R'$ with greater deviation of R from R' for greater random errors. The agreement factors are normalized in Equations (7) and (8) so that their values are independent of both the size of the data set and the scaling of the intensities.

Thirdly, converged $\hat{p}$ values are dependent on the weighting of the observations. Often, the weights of all observations are set to unity. However, if the standard deviations of the observations are known, the most appropriate weights are given by:[42]

$$\omega_{ij} = \frac{1}{\sigma_{ij}^2} \tag{9}$$

where σ_{ij} is the standard deviation of the observed intensity collected with a given pair of timings TE_{ij} and TD_j. The single-pixel standard deviation (σ_{pixel}) was obtained from the ROI using system software:

$$\sigma_{pixel} = \sqrt{\frac{\sum_{l=1}^{L} (I_l - I_{ave})^2}{L - 1}} \tag{10}$$

where I_l is the intensity of a single pixel in the ROI, I_{ave} is the average ROI intensity, and L is the number of pixels in the ROI. As 27-pixel ROI was used to collect all intensities, the standard deviations of all mean intensities are proportional to the single pixel standard deviations given in Equation (10) so that relative weights could be assigned as $\omega = \sigma_{pixel}^{-2}$.

Finally, the interdependence among the measured parameters can be assessed in this analysis. Coefficients that describe this correlation between all pairs of parameters, ranging from 0.0 (no correlation) and 1.0 (full correlation), can be calculated from the elements of the inverse matrix by the equation from Rollett[52] (pages 99–106):

$$\rho_{kl} = \frac{b_{kl}}{\sqrt{b_{kk}b_{ll}}} \tag{11}$$

where ρ_{kl} is the coefficient describing the correlation between the k-th and l-th parameters, and $k, l = 1, 2, 3$ correspond to N_r, $T1$, and $T2$. High correlation coefficients indicate that the values of the k-th parameter will be significantly dependent on the value of the l-th parameter and vice versa. High correlations also indicate that the parameters may not be uniquely determined and that the full matrix **A** should be used rather than the more efficient block-diagonal forms.[56]

The precision of the calculation can also be assessed directly from theory. If the statistical weighting in Equation (9) is used, the standard errors of the resulting parameters are approximated by Rollett[52] (pages 112 to 114):

$$SE_k = \sqrt{\frac{b_{kk}D}{n - 3}} \tag{12}$$

where b_{kk} is the k-th diagonal element of the inverse matrix in Equation (6), n is the number of intensities in the MDME data set, D is given by Equation (3), and k is as in Equation (11). This error analysis assumes that there is no correlation between parameters and that image noise is the only contribution to D. In reality, systematic differences in I_O and I_C caused by improper convergence or use of inappropriate mathematical models will also contribute to D and will cause the errors calculated by Equation (12) to overestimate the precision.

Mathematical Model

As multiple-echo intensities are to be used to calculate $T1$ as well as $T2$, the $T1$ dependence of the ME subsequence must be mathematically defined. The signal intensity Equation (2) for the ME subsequence can be derived from the Bloch equations[4,28] in a manner similar to that done for the spin-echo sequence.[29] Using the timings defined in Table 100–2, this equation was derived for an eight-echo ME subsequence with equally spaced echoes (i.e., $TE_{ij} = 2i\tau$) as follows:[12]

$$I_{C_{ij}} = N_r e^{-TE_{ij}/T2}[1 - e^{-TR_j/T1}(1 - 2e^{\tau/T1} + 2e^{3\tau/T1} - 2e^{5\tau/T1} \tag{13}$$
$$+ 2e^{7\tau/T1} - 2e^{9\tau/T1} + 2e^{11\tau/T1} - 2e^{13\tau/T1} + 2e^{15\tau/T1})]$$

Table 100–2. TIMING INTERVALS FOR THE SIX MULTIPLE SPIN-ECHO (ME) SEQUENCES USED TO COLLECT MULTIPLE DELAY-MULTIPLE ECHO (MDME) INTENSITIES*

Sequence Number	τ (ms)	TE (ms)	TD (ms)	TR (ms)	Scan Time[a] (minutes)
1	15	30, 60, . . . , 240	60	300	0.64
2	15	30, 60, . . . , 240	160	400	0.85
3	15	30, 60, . . . , 240	360	600	1.28
4	15	30, 60, . . . , 240	760	1000	2.13
5[b]	15	30, 60, . . . , 240	1760	2000	4.27

* Each sequence has 8 echoes spaced 30 ms apart, and no sequences were signal averaged.
[a] Total scanning time is 9.7 minutes.
[b] Used to calculate the N_r values, $T2$ values, and errors graphed in Figures 100–5B, 100–13A, and 100–13C.

where τ is the interval from the 90 degree pulse to the 180 degree pulse. This equation, as well as other equations derived for multiple echoes,[3,53] becomes very complicated when many echoes are generated. As fit to complicated mathematical expressions can affect the accuracy and efficiency of the convergence of this algorithm, this expression was derived for an arbitrary number of echoes and was mathematically simplified to:[16]

$$I_{C_{ij}} = N_r e^{-TE_{ij}/T2}\left\{1 - \frac{e^{-TD_j/TI}}{\cosh(\tau_j/TI)}\{1 + (-1)^{M_j}e^{-2\tau_j M_j/TI}[\cosh(\tau_j/TI) - 1]\}\right\} \quad (14)$$

where τ_j is the τ interval of the j-th ME subsequence, and M_j is the total number of echoes in the j-th ME sequence. All ME subsequences were chosen to have the same τ (15 ms) and M (8 echoes), but this is not essential, since TI dependence need not be fixed as it must in separate $T2$ measurements. Equations (13) and (14) assume that (1) $TD \gg T2^*$ so that magnetizations are at steady state, (2) longitudinal and transverse relaxations are monoexponential, (3) the radio frequency (rf) pulses have tip angles that are uniform throughout the slice thickness, (4) phase is coherent throughout the slice thickness, (5) TI and $T2$ do not change with the variation in resonance frequency through the slice thickness, (6) the rf pulse is of negligible duration, and (7) translational self-diffusion, flow, and convection are absent. Unlike some signal intensity equation,[43,58] this equation accounts for TI relaxation during the generation of echoes and does not assume that $TI \gg \tau$.[12,16] If $TI \gg \tau$, Equations (13) and (14) approximate an equation similar to that of the SR sequence in Equation (1):[12,16]

$$I_{C_{ij}} = N_r e^{-TE_{ij}/T2}(1 - e^{-TD_j/TI}) \quad (15)$$

From this equation it is obvious that TI relaxation effectively begins approximately after the last echo and effectively occurs during the TD interval.

The partial derivatives used for calculation of the matrix elements in Equation (4) can be derived from the signal intensity Equation (14) and the resulting equations written into the algorithm:

$$\frac{\partial I_{C_{ij}}}{\partial N_r} = e^{-TE_{ij}/T2}\left\{1 - \frac{e^{-TD_j/TI}}{\cosh(\tau_j/TI)}\{1 + (-1)^{M_j}e^{-2\tau_j M_j/TI}[\cosh(\tau_j/TI) - 1]\}\right\} \quad (16a)$$

$$\frac{\partial I_{C_{ij}}}{\partial TI} = \frac{N_r}{TI^2} e^{-TE_{ij}/T2} e^{-TD_j/TI}\{\tau_j[(-1)^{M_j}e^{-2\tau_j M_j/TI} - 1]\tanh(\tau_j/TI)\text{sech}(\tau_j/TI)$$
$$- TD_j\text{sech}(\tau_j/TI) + (-1)^{M_j}TR_je^{-2\tau_j M_j/TI}[\text{sech}(\tau_j/TI) - 1]\} \quad (16b)$$

$$\frac{\partial I_{C_{ij}}}{\partial T2} = \frac{TE_{ij}N_r}{T2^2} e^{-TE_{ij}/T2}\left\{1 - \frac{e^{-TD_j/TI}}{\cosh(\tau_j/TI)}\{1 + (-1)^{M_j}e^{-2\tau_j M_j/TI}[\cosh(\tau_j/TI) - 1]\}\right\}, \quad (16c)$$

where TR is the pulse sequence repetition time and $TR_j = TD_j + 2\tau_j M_j$. Use of these analytical expressions improves the efficiency and accuracy of the computation compared to numerical determination of these derivatives.

Timing Interval Selection for MDME Data Set

As discussed, measurement of parameters requires intensities that are sensitive to those parameter values. Thus, the unaveraged MDME data are to be collected at TD and TE intervals chosen to provide sensitivity[44] to a full range of N_r, $T1$, and $T2$ values. Secondly, the timing intervals should also be chosen so that the percent calculated noise will be approximately uniform across the calculated range. This will enable all tissue values to be precisely measured from a single data set without repeat scanning and without an a priori knowledge of those values often required for timing interval selection. From Equation (15) and its resemblance to Equation (1), the $T1$ sensitivity (S_{T1}) of the ME sequence is maximal when $TD \approx T1$ (reference 32), and $T2$ sensitivity (S_{T2}) is maximal when $TE = T2$ (reference 44). Thus, the range of TE and TD timings in the MDME data set (Fig. 100–6) is chosen to approximate the desired range of $T1$ and $T2$ values, respectively. In selecting timing intervals to provide uniform percent precision, it is then noted by manipulation of Equations (4) and (12) that the standard errors are approximately proportional to the inverse of the sum of sensitivities over the entire MDME data set (assuming no correlation of data). To obtain percent precision that is uniform throughout the calculated range, timing intervals should thus be chosen so that the summed sensitivity to *percent* change in $T1$ (given by $(\partial I/\partial T1)/T1 = \partial I/\partial(\ln T1)$ in Tsui et al.[59]) is uniformly provided for the full range of $T1$ values. To accomplish this, a geometric progression of timings should be selected, as shown in Figure 100–3. Note here that the profiles of sensitivity to percent $T1$ change are the same shape across the range of $T1$ values and that a choice of a logarithmic (i.e., geometric) progression of TD intervals uniformly distributes these profiles. Sensitivity to $T1$ would then be within 90 percent of maximal sensitivity for all $T1$ values, rather than from 0 to 100 percent maximal for two-point measurements (Fig. 100–2). Thus net sensitivity would be approximately uniform throughout the range of $T1$ values.

For these reasons, the longest TD was chosen to be only 1.76 s to avoid long scanning time while providing some sensitivity to the pure water $T1$ value of about 3.6 s,[26,35,55] assumed to be the longest possible biologic hydrogen $T1$ value. Then, a geometric progression of TD values given by $TD_{j-1} = 0.5\, TD_j$ was chosen so that the five ME subsequences had TD intervals of 60, 160, 360, 760, and 1760 ms as in Figure 100–6. On the other hand, an arithmetic progression of TE values ($TE = 30, 60, 90, 120, \ldots, 240$ ms) was chosen because, with a minimum allowed intraecho time of 30 ms ($\tau = 15$ ms) set by the gradient durations, an arithmetic TE progression would provide the greatest number of signal reads per scan time, whereby a geometric progression ($TE = 30, 60, 120, 240$ ms) would provide less signal reads in the same scan time. The resulting 40 intensities of the MDME data set (Table 100–2, Fig. 100–6) are collected from five separate ME subsequences in a total acquisition time of 9.7 minutes with 128-step phase encoding. An MDME pulse sequence with interleaved collection of these five ME subsequences has a net TR of 4.3 s, which is on the order of the longest desired $T1$.

RESULTS AND DISCUSSION

Convergence of the Algorithm

Convergence to maxima or relative minima in D in Equation (3) would be expected to yield incorrect parameters for particular sets of starting parameters p_0. To evaluate this possibility, MDME intensities having timings listed in Table 100–2 were collected from a 0.6 mM solution of $CrCl_3$, which exhibits $T1$ and $T2$ values characteristic of biologic soft tissues. An array of starting p_0 values, varying independently from 0.02

to 50 times their converged value in 25 geometrically progressing steps, was used as input. For all above 15,625 independent triplets of starting values, the calculation either converged to unique $\hat{p}$ values within at least the sixteenth significant figure or failed to converge to the zero vector x. In the case of failure, the algorithm generated either (a) a negative parameter value, (b) a parameter value greater than 10^9, or (c) a singular matrix A. This indicates that the MDME data set has sufficient signal to noise and that Equation (14) adequately parameterizes the image intensity so that convergence is always to an absolute minimum in D.

The calculation was then performed on ME intensity data collected from all other $CrCl_3$ solutions in Figure 100–4 using the same set of timings (Table 100–2) and requiring three separate sets of starting values. Resulting longitudinal and transverse relaxation rates are graphed in Figure 100–7 versus $CrCl_3$ concentration. The computation did not converge for the 10 mM solution regardless of starting value. These relaxation rates are linear with respect to ion concentration (Fig. 100–7), without erratic deviation from the regression line that might result from convergence to maxima or relative minima. The calculated N_r graphed in Figure 100–8 also does not demonstrate grossly anomalous values, although there are systematic trends, which will be discussed. Similarly, although there are trends in the R and R' agreement factors calculated according to Equations (7) and (8) and graphed in Figure 100–9, there are no anomalously high factors that might result from sporadic convergence to a maximum or a relative minimum in D.

While the computation appears to converge to an absolute minimum, the method may still be practically limited by restrictions on the accuracy of the starting values. Specifically, the range of p_0 values from which the calculation can converge will be restricted by the linear approximations implicit in the truncation of the Taylor series and in substitution of derivatives evaluated at p_0 for derivatives evaluated at $\hat{p}$. These approximations often cause fit of strongly nonlinear functions to converge from only a very narrow range of starting values. To investigate this behavior, all combinations of p_0 that resulted in a converged calculation for the 0.6 mM solution are graphed in Figures 100–10A and 100–10B. The height of the surface in Figure 100–10A represents the maximum starting $T2_0$ value, relative to the converged $\hat{T2}$ value, which resulted in convergence for the given $N_{r0}/\hat{N}_r$ and $T1_0/\hat{T1}$ values. The surface is graphed such that all intermediate $T2_0/\hat{T2}$ values also resulted in convergence for the same starting $N_{r0}/\hat{N}_r - T1_0/\hat{T1}$ pair. The height of the surface in Figure 100–10B is as in Figure 100–

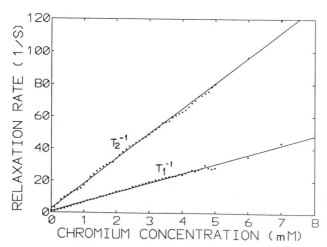

Figure 100–7. Relaxation rates obtained from three-parameter fit to MDME intensity data. Data were collected from the fifty-five $CrCl_3$ solutions in the test phantom (Fig. 100–4) using a 27-pixel ROI. Three separate sets of starting values were used to calculate these values. Starting N_{r0}, $T1_0$, and $T2_0$ values of 650, 200 ms and 80 ms were used to obtain values for solutions up to 2.2 mM. From 2.3 to 7.0 mM, N_{r0}, $T1_0$, and $T2_0$ were 650, 45 ms, and 20 ms, respectively. For the 8.0 mM solution, N_{r0}, $T1_0$, and $T2_0$ values of 650, 20 ms, and 15 ms were used. Computation failed for the 10 mM solution regardless of starting values. This was presumably because the MDME data set lacked sensitivity to the short $T1$ and $T2$ values of this solution, causing generation of a zero diagonal element. $T1$ and $T2$ relaxivities calculated from the drawn regression lines were 5.91 and 15.6 mM^{-1}s^{-1}, respectively, with respective correlation coefficients of 0.9976 and 0.9983. The values of the 8 mM solution were not included in the graph or regression analysis since their standard errors were in excess of 50 percent (see Fig. 100–12).

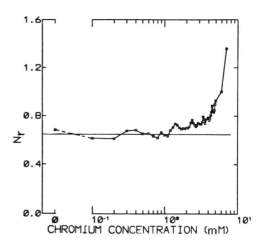

Figure 100–8. Relative spin density (N_r) calculated by the three-parameter fit to MDME data. The horizontal line is a theoretical line of constant N_r drawn from Figure 100–5. Compared to separate $T1$ (Fig. 100–5A) and $T2$ (Fig. 100–5B) measurements, the above N_r has automatically been corrected for $T2$ relaxation during the first TE interval and for incomplete $T1$ relaxation during the TD intervals. The drift in N_r at higher ion concentrations is present despite removal of the above $T1$ and $T2$ effects, and reflects minor residual $T1$ and/or $T2$ dependence in the calculated N_r. Local N_r fluctuations are also present, but random error is low.

Figure 100–9. Agreement factors R and R'. These factors were determined as in Equations (7) and (8). Consistent trends in R' suggest that convergence was to an absolute minimum in D for all ion concentrations. High R was obtained from low ion concentrations, indicating the presence of unmodelled systematic effects on image intensities collected from samples possessing long $T1$ and $T2$ values.

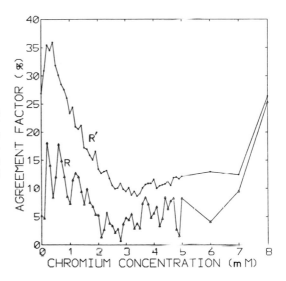

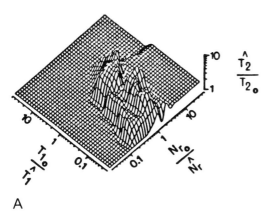

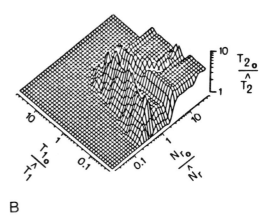

A

B

Figure 100–10. Graph of all combinations of starting N_{r0}, $T1_0$, and $T2_0$ values from which the computation converged. The axes are the starting parameter values relative to the final converged values (i.e., $N_0/\widehat{N_r}$, $T1_0/\widehat{T1}$, and $T2_0/\widehat{T2}$, using notation defined in the text). The height of the surface in A represents the maximum $T2_0/T2$ from which convergence was achieved for the given $N_0/\widehat{N_r}$ and $T1_0/\widehat{T1}$ pair. The height in figure B is as in A, but with the height representing the minimum $T2_0/\widehat{T2}$ which resulted in convergence. For a given $N_0/\widehat{N_r}$ and $T1_0/\widehat{T1}$ pair, convergence also resulted from all intermediate $T2_0/\widehat{T2}$ in A and B. In flat regions where $T2_0/\widehat{T2} = 1$, the computation failed to converge when $T2_0 = \widehat{T2}$ as described in the text.

10A, but represents the minimum $T2_0/\hat{T2}$, which resulted in convergence. Flat regions with a $T2_0/\hat{T2}$ of 1.0 represent starting $N_{r0}/\hat{N}_r$ and $T1_0/\hat{T1}$ values in which there were no starting $T2_0/\hat{T2}$ values that resulted in convergence. Taken together, then, Figures 100–10A and 100–10B represent the volume of p_0 starting vectors from which convergence could be assured, although convergence also occurred sporadically outside of this region. As demonstrated in these figures, the starting N_{r0} can be overestimated by at least 50 times and the starting $T1_0$ can be underestimated by as much as 50 times with convergence still achieved when the starting $T2_0$ is between 0.5 to 3.7 times its converged value. The dramatic asymmetry of the region of convergence in Figure 100–10 is due to the distorted distribution of parameter values for which the fitted function approaches linearity.[40]

Calculated Range of T1 and T2

The range of measured $T1$ and $T2$ values approximates the range of TE and TD timings in the MDME data set (Fig. 100–6) as anticipated. Three parameter fit to the MDME data set provides measurement of $T1$ values from 21 ms to at least 3.4 s, and $T2$ values from 6 ms to at least 714 ms. This range of $T1$ extends from 0.4 times the shortest TD interval to 2 times the longest TD interval in the MDME data set (Table 100–2), and this range of $T2$ values extends from 0.2 times the shortest TE interval to 3 times the longest TE interval. Successful calculation of all intermediate values indicates that the MDME timings in Table 100–2 are spaced closely enough to give adequate net sensitivity to a continuous range of $T1$ and $T2$ values so that calculation of intermediate values does not fail. Attainment of shorter $T1$ and $T2$ values is limited by the shortest TE interval rather than the shortest TD interval, since the $T2$ sensitivity available when $T2 = 0.2TE$ is less than the $T1$ sensitivity available when $T1 = 0.4TD$. This is supported by the addition of intensities collected with a 20 ms TD to the MDME data set, which did not extend the range of measured values (data not shown). With a minimum TE of 30 ms, there is very little net N_r and $T2$ sensitivity provided for samples having $T2$ values shorter than the measured range. Accordingly, as elements of **A** in Equation (5) are obtained from these net sensitivities, calculation of parameters for the 10 mM solution failed for all attempted starting values because low net N_r sensitivity caused generation of a zero first diagonal element in **A** and failure of the matrix inversion in Equation (6).

By comparison, a two-point $T1$ measurement using the optimized two-point method in Table 100–1[37,58] allowed precise assessment of $T1$ values only as short as 119 ms (data not shown), presumably because of short $T2$ values and concomitant poor signal to noise. While this limit appears to be shorter than the $T1$ values of most normal soft tissues, the presence of disease states[9] and use of paramagnetic contrast agents[18,34] may yield tissue $T1$ values significantly shorter than this. Determination of $T2$ by a nonlinear regression fit of the eight echo intensities collected with the 1.76 s TD interval enabled reliable measurement of $T2$ values only down to about 25 ms (Fig. 100–13A). Shorter linear regression $T2$ values were imprecise and based on fit to a linear regression line, as will be discussed. Normal soft tissues such as muscle,[5] tendon,[21] and possibly some contrast enhanced[18] and pathologic soft tissues can have $T2$ values in this range.

Improved Precision

As well as having an extended range, the method also has good precision throughout that range. The high precision is qualitatively demonstrated by the excellent fit of relaxation rates to the lines in Figure 100–7. However, these relaxation rate graphs are not optimal indicators of the precision or accuracy of the parameters. For example, relaxation rates that are inaccurately calculated by fitting the data with inappropriate signal intensity equations may also appear to be linear with respect to ion concentration.[12] Furthermore, systematic effects on signal intensity may affect the accuracy of long $T1$ and $T2$ values,[19] which would not be easily detected in a graph of relaxation rate versus ion concentration. In such a graph, errors in long $T1$ and $T2$ values would cause a negligible displacement of the relaxation rates from the line in Figure 100–7, compared to the displacement caused by errors in short $T1$ and $T2$ values. Similarly, as we have chosen the timings with the goal of obtaining uniform percent random error, the rate graph is deficient, since, for a constant percent random $T1$ or $T2$ error, more noise would be demonstrated in the graph at high concentrations than at low concentrations. For this reason, the log relaxation time versus the log of ion concentration was graphed. In such a graph the $T1$ and $T2$ values should fit a line with negative unit slope[19] if $T1 \ll T1_{H_2O}$ and if $T2 \ll T2_{H_2O}$, respectively, where $T1 \ll T1_{H_2O}$ and $T2 \ll T2_{H_2O}$ are the respective $T1$ and $T2$ values of pure water. This type of graph would be expected to give a better indication of the error in a wide range of $T1$ and $T2$ values, since the displacement of these values from the log-log negative unit slope line would always be directly proportional to the percent random or systematic error in those values.

To determine how well the actual data would be expected to fit the negative unit slope line, the relaxivities calculated in Figure 100–7 and pure water $T1$ and $T2$ values of 3.6 s[26,35,55] were used to generate the theoretical $T1$ and $T2$ values graphed in Figure 100–11A. Values for solutions having an 0.5 mM or higher ion concentration fall on the line of negative unit slope. At lower concentrations the data deviate from this line as $T1 \approx T1_{H_2O}$ and $T2 \approx T2_{H_2O}$, with a greater deviation present in $T1$ values than in $T2$ values. Thus, fit of data to the line at concentrations above 0.5 mM, and fit to the theoretical deviation of data in Figure 100–11A at concentrations less than 0.5 mM, can be used as an estimate of percent random or systematic error.

The actual calculated relaxation times are graphed logarithmically in Figure 100–11B with the negative unit slope line of Figure 100–11A superimposed. The log-log fit to the negative unit slope line appears to be good throughout the full range of measured $T1$ and $T2$ values, with the exception of the deviation of long $T1$ values expected from Figure 100–11A and systematic underestimation of long $T2$ values as will be described. This indicates that the percent noise in the $T1$ or $T2$ measurement is approximately uniform for the full measured range, as anticipated based on selection of timing intervals. The actual percent noise in the calculated values is estimated by calculating the standard errors according to Equation (12), graphed as percent standard error in Figure 100–12. Percent standard errors are as low as 0.45 percent, which compares favorably with the measured precision of other methods,[31] and are highest for $T1$ and lowest for $T2$. Despite the apparent uniformity in percent random error demonstrated by the log-log graphs, the calculated percent standard errors in Figure 100–12 are paradoxically increased at the extremes of the measured range. This trend in standard errors can be partly explained by a lower net sensitivity to the $T1$ and $T2$ values, which extend beyond the limits of TE and TD in the MDME data set. However, part of the increase in calculated standard errors at low ion concentrations is artifactually contributed to by unmodeled systematic effects on intensity, to be discussed, which are present at these low ion concentrations and affect $T2$, as apparent from the log-log graphs. The increase in R' at these low ion concentrations is accompanied by an increase in R (Fig. 100–9), indicating that the increase in these agreement factors (and in the standard errors) is probably due mostly to systematic error in the fit to the intensities of these solutions. (On the other hand, if the increased standard errors were principally due to decreased

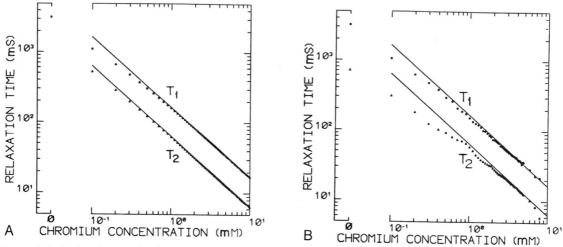

Figure 100–11. Log-log graph of theoretical (*A*) and experimental (*B*) relaxation times. The theoretical values were calculated using pure water *T1* and *T2* values of 3.6 s and using the *T1* and *T2* relaxivities obtained from the data in Figure 100–7. The theoretical *T1* and *T2* values are expected to form a line of negative unit slope if *T1* ≪ 3.6 s and if *T2* ≪ 3.6 s, respectively. The solid lines of negative unit slope are drawn tangent to the theoretical values at high ion concentrations, where values are expected to best obey the above conditions. Theoretical *T1* values greater than 300 ms, present at ion concentrations less than 0.5 mM, progressively deviate from the negative unit slope line. All other *T1* values and nearly all *T2* values obey the above conditions and fit the negative unit slope line. Fit of the experimental *T1* and *T2* values (*B*) to these negative unit slope lines can be used as a criterion for percent error, with exception made for the slight theoretical deviation of long *T1* values. The full range of experimental *T1* values (*B*) fit the theoretical negative unit slope line well, with the minor deviations in long *T1* values expected at ion concentrations below 0.5 mM. Short experimental *T2* values fit the theoretical line well, but longer *T2* values are progressively underestimated. The displacement of these *T2* values from the theoretical line is proportional to the percent systematic error in these values. As random displacement from the negative unit slope line is minimal, the percent random error in *T1* and *T2* appears to be low and approximately uniform throughout the range of values.

precision, R' would be increased with no increase in R). Thus, the log-log graph (Fig. 100–11*B*) demonstrates good precision for values obtained from low ion concentrations despite the calculation of high standard errors. If the systematic effects present at low ion concentration could be modeled or minimized by better imaging techniques, smaller and more accurate standard errors would probably be obtained for long *T1* and *T2* values.

The high precision of the presented method is also indicated by comparison of the *T2* derived from the two parameter fit to ME data (Fig. 100–13*A*) with the *T2* derived

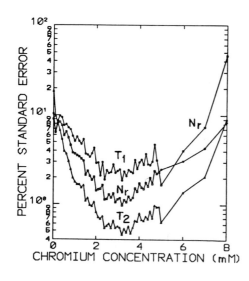

Figure 100–12. Percent standard errors in N_r, *T1*, and *T2* calculated from the three-parameter fit to MDME data. These errors are obtained from the diagonal elements of the matrix A as in Equation (12). Errors are higher at low and high ion concentrations than at intermediate ion concentrations because corresponding *T1* and *T2* values extend beyond the limits of the array of TD and TE timings, respectively (Fig. 100–6). Errors may also be artifactually high at low ion concentrations because of systematic effects on image intensity which are not modeled in the analysis (see text).

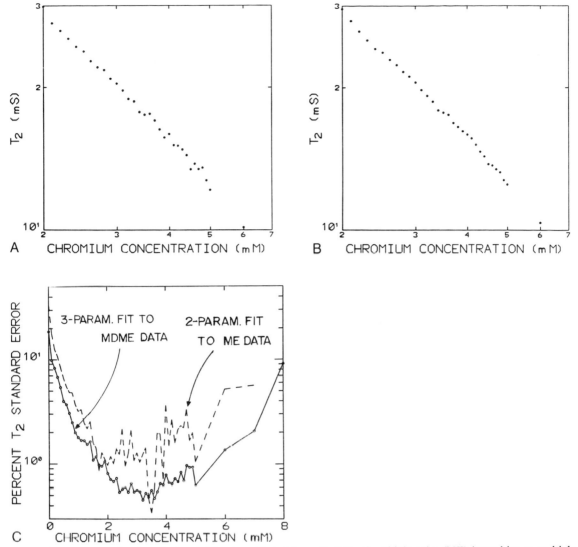

Figure 100–13. Reduction in calculated *T2* noise effected by collection of multiple echo (ME) intensities at multiple delays. From fit to the negative unit slope line, it can be seen that the *T2* obtained from two-parameter fit to a single unaveraged ME sequence (the open row of intensities in Figure 100–6, with *TD* = 1.76 s) has increased percent random error (*A*) for *T2* values less than the shortest TE of 30 ms. Rather than signal average this acquisition at a cost in scanning time, precision of the *T2* values is instead improved by collecting four other unaveraged ME subsequences with shorter TD intervals of 0.76, 0.36, 0.16, and 0.06 s, followed by three-parameter fit to the resulting MDME data set. This gives high precision for all short *T2* values (*B*). The standard errors (*C*) for the calculations in *A* (dashed line) and *B* (solid line), obtained from Equation (12), indicate as much as a two-fold improvement in the *T2* precision as a result of collecting multiple delays and fitting all three parameters to the MDME data set.

from the three parameter fit to MDME data (Fig. 100–13*B*). Relative to the *T2* obtained from the single unaveraged ME sequence, the *T2* obtained from the unaveraged MDME data demonstrates substantial signal averaging of the noise in the short *T2* values. The calculated standard errors (Fig. 100–13*C*) obtained from fit to the MDME data are as small as half the percent standard errors derived from single-delay multiple-echo data. Since both *T2* calculations were performed using intensity data that were not signal averaged, pooling of multiple-echo data from five different ME subsequences having different delay times, accompanied by a three parameter fit, thus provides an effective means of averaging the signal of each echo and improving *T2* precision.

Inherent Correction of N_r for T1 and T2 Weighting

As anticipated, the presented method also measures a more accurate N_r. Relative to the N_r obtained in a separate *T1* measurement (Fig. 100–5A), the N_r obtained with the three parameter fit to MDME data (Fig. 100–8) is more accurate for samples having short *T2* values. Similarly, in contrast to the N_r obtained in a separate *T2* measurement (Fig. 100–5B), the N_r obtained by the three parameter fit to MDME data is accurate for samples with long *T1*. Therefore, as anticipated, the three parameter fit to MDME data appears to provide an inherent correction for the *T2* relaxation occurring during the first echo time and for the incomplete *T1* relaxation during the *TD* interval.

Reduced Parameter Interdependence

Besides providing a reduced *T1* and *T2* weighting of N_r, the three parameter fit to MDME data also decreases the correlation between N_r and the two relaxation times. For example, fit of N_r and *T1* to intensities collected with a fixed *TE* and varying *TD* (i.e., the shaded column in Fig. 100–6), not only provides a *T2* weighted N_r but also gives high correlation between N_r and *T1* (Fig. 100–14). In this case, random and systematic errors in *T1* might be propagated into N_r errors, and nonunique solutions might be produced. This correlation could be reduced by choosing $TD > 5T1$, but only at the expense of scanning time. Worse N_r–*T1* correlations are found for samples having long *T1* values as there is greater uncertainty in the asymptote of the relaxation curve.

Similarly, a two-parameter fit of N_r and *T2* to the ME intensities of the row in Figure 100–6 contributes a high N_r–*T2* correlation for samples having short *T2* values, since there is some uncertainty in the intercept of the *T2* relaxation curve. Reduction of this correlation would require shorter *TE* intervals.

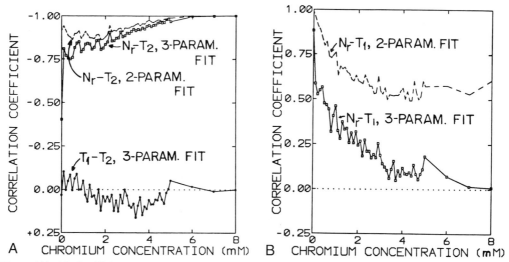

Figure 100–14. Coefficients of correlation between the three parameters. The dotted line represents no correlation, where correlation coefficients are determined by Equation (11). Coefficients obtained from the three-parameter fit to MDME data (solid lines) are graphed with coefficients obtained from separate *T1* and *T2* measurements using a two-parameter fit to the column and row of intensities in Figure 100–6, respectively (dashed lines). At high concentrations, N_r and *T2* are highly negatively correlated (*A*), while at low ion concentrations N_r and *T1* are highly positively correlated (*B*). The former indicates that slight underestimation of *T2* at high concentrations (as in Fig. 100–11B) would be expected to cause large overestimation of N_r (as in Fig. 100–8). Compared to the separate *T1* and *T2* measurements, the three-parameter fit to MDME data results in reduced N_r–*T2* correlation (*A*) and substantially reduced N_r–*T1* correlation (*B*). On the other hand, the three-parameter fit introduces only minimal correlation between *T1* and *T2* at all concentrations (*A*).

On the other hand, relative to the separate $T1$ and $T2$ measurements, the three parameter fit to MDME data reduces the N_r–$T2$ correlation and substantially reduces the N_r–$T1$ correlation (Fig. 100–14), while contributing negligible $T1$–$T2$ correlation. Thus, inclusion of both $T1$ and $T2$ in the fit serves to constrain the fit of N_r. As a result, N_r values obtained from the three parameter fit to MDME data would be expected to be less sensitive to the random and systematic errors in $T1$ and $T2$, and the computation may be less likely to converge to a nonunique solution.

Measurement Efficiency

In the same time that is required for collection of data for a multipoint measurement of $T1$ and a $T2$ weighted N_r (diagrammed by the shaded column of intensities in Fig. 100–6), the data can be collected with multiple echoes to provide an MDME data set that enables measurement of $T1$, $T2$, and an N_r that is minimally $T1$ or $T2$ dependent. This reduces the calculated $T2$ noise relative to a two-parameter fit of a single unaveraged ME sequence (diagrammed by the row of intensities in Fig. 100–6), which would otherwise require signal averaging for noise reduction, and also reduces the correlation between parameters. Thus, although the input intensities may be noisy, signal averaging is not required to obtain high precision in the calculated parameters. This, combined with collection of a maximal TD of only half the longest desired $T1$, enables the MDME data set to be collected in only 9.7 minutes for 128-step 2DFT imaging. This is considerably shorter than the acquisition times of other measurements and is similar to the times required for obtaining SE images having good signal to noise. The method could also be used in conjunction with fast imaging techniques such as echo-planar imaging[39] to further improve imaging times.

The efficiency of MDME data collection relative to data collection for separate $T1$ and $T2$ measurements is demonstrated by considering the number of intensities used for these measurements. In particular, determination of $T1$ and a $T2$ weighted N_r from the intensities in the shaded column in Figure 100–6 would use five intensities to determine two parameters, a 2.5:1 data-to-parameter ratio, while determination of all three parameters from the entire data set uses forty intensities, a 13.3:1 ratio. By a similar argument, separate $T2$ calculation by linear regression fit of the open row of intensities in Figure 100–6 has a 4:1 ratio. However, the time for signal averaging that might be needed to reduce the noise in this calculation (Fig. 100–13A) would undoubtedly be better spent obtaining four other sets of unaveraged multiple-echo intensities with geometrically decreasing delays, which only doubles the scanning time. This would yield a 13.3:1 ratio, allow accurate and precise measurement of very short $T2$ values, and also enable measurement of $T1$ and a minimally $T1$ dependent N_r. The improved ratios result in high precision in all three parameters and are achieved by simultaneously determining all three parameters from the entire MDME data set.

Parameter Accuracy

Despite removal of the above $T1$ and $T2$ effects on N_r and reduction in the parameter interdependence, there is a residual N_r error. This is seen as a trend of increasing N_r for increasing ion concentrations, as well as fluctuations in N_r, which are localized to the peripheral regions of the phantom in Figure 100–4. The former trend of increasing N_r is reproducible using different phantom orientations and using sagittal and transverse slices (data not presented), indicating that it is not due to position-dependent errors, such as external field inhomogeneity, but is rather due to the influences of *T1* and *T2* on the calculated N_r. The large negative correlation coefficient between *T2* and N_r at these high ion concentrations (Fig. 100–14) suggests that the systematic increase in N_r at higher concentrations may be a result of small systematic underestimation of short *T2* values. Systematic underestimation of *T2* does in fact appear to occur in the calculation of values for the 5 mM, 6 mM, and 8 mM solutions, based on fit to the negative unit slope line (Fig. 100–11*B*). One possible source of this error could be the assignment of the beginning of the *TE* interval to the center of the rf pulse. With a 4 ms pulse duration, *T2* relaxation might effectively begin at a time significantly later than the center of this pulse. This would be expected to cause a significant overestimation of N_r and a slight underestimation of *T2* at high ion concentrations, as is observed. Change in slice thickness due to the dependence of rf pulse shape on *T1* could also contribute to this trend in N_r.

This residual dependence of N_r on *T1* and *T2* is probably accentuated in this study by the measurement of such a wide range of *T1* and *T2* values. In contrast, verification of N_r measurements by using aqueous solutions that varied only in D_2O/H_2O concentrations[3,38,54] may not have demonstrated this effect because of the presence of only small variations in *T1* and *T2*. Regardless of the specific causes, the N_r errors and the underestimation of long *T2* values are probably not caused by computational errors but rather by inherent unmodeled systematic effects on intensity.

Furthermore, unmodeled systematic effects on intensity seem to be present for samples having long *T1* and *T2* values, since the *R* agreement factors are high for solutions having low ion concentration (Fig. 100–9). To investigate the accuracy of these long relaxation times, fit to the negative unit slope line in the log-log graphs (Fig. 100–11*B*) is considered. This demonstrates little systematic error in *T1* values but does show some systematic shortening of long *T2* values. This systematic error is not manifest in the relaxation rate graph (Fig. 100–7) as anticipated, although these graphs have been used by others as a criterion for accuracy.[3]

The systematic error revealed by log-log graphs is supported by comparison with literature values. The *T2* of pure water was measured to be about five times as short as the frequency independent literature value of about 3.6 s, while there is good agreement between measured and literature *T1* values for pure water (Table 100–3). Modeling th effect of dissolved oxygen and scalar coupling to ^{17}O reduced the theoretical water *T2* to be closer to the calculated value.[15] Shorter literature *T1* and *T2* values, determined for Cr^{3+} solutions by NMR spectroscopy,[7,24,45] compare favorably with the values obtained by the method of this paper (Table 100–3). Unlike some other methods,[43,58]

Table 100–3. COMPARISON OF LITERATURE VALUES WITH VALUES OBTAINED FROM THREE-PARAMETER GAUSS–NEWTON FIT TO MDME DATA*

Source	[CrCl$_3$] (mM)	*T1* (ms)	S.E.	*T2* (ms)	S.E.
Hindman et al 1973[a]	0.0	3518	—	3518[b]	—
MDME method[c]	0.0	3180[d]	330	714[d]	133
Hausser and Noack 1964	1.41	97	—	37.2	—
MDME method	1.4	111	6	38.4	0.6
Brown et al 1960	4.98	31.0	—	17.1	—
MDME method	5.0	35.5	0.8	12.5	0.1

* The literature values were determined spectroscopically at different frequencies and have been interpolated to 20.9 MHz using the graphs produced by the authors.
[a] At 24.45°C and at 60 MHz—these values can be compared with the values measured at 20.9 MHz by the presented method since pure water *T1* and *T2* values are approximately equal and are frequency independent.[20,24]
[b] Assuming *T1* = *T2* for pure water.
[c] Simultaneously calculated by three-parameter least squares fit to MDME data, as presented in this paper.
[d] At 24 ± 2°C—Over this range, literature values vary from 3.2 to 3.6 s.[26]

the presented method accurately measures short $T1$ values, since Equation (14) accounts for $T1$ relaxation during the production of echoes and does not assume that $T1 \gg TE$.[12]

Thus, because of the trends in agreement factors and the progressive underestimation of longer $T2$ values, which are manifest in the log-log graphs and confirmed by comparison with spectroscopic literature values, there appear to be systematic effects on the intensity of samples with long $T2$ values that are not adequately modeled by Equation (14).

Effect of Background Subtraction and Statistical Weighting

The choice of weighting schemes and the need for background subtraction can similarly be evaluated by log-log graphs. At ion concentrations greater than 2 mM, $T2$ values that are calculated without background subtraction (Fig. 100–15A) do not fit the negative unit slope line as well as $T2$ values calculated with background subtraction (Fig. 100–15C). Specifically, short $T2$ values are overestimated relative to those obtained with background subtraction. Since the background signal was constant for all echoes in a single ME sequence (data not shown), this can be explained by the presence of late echo background intensity despite complete decay of transverse magnetization. Fit to this late echo background would be expected to result in overestimation of short $T2$ values, as is observed.

Similarly, both $T1$ and $T2$ values calculated by assigning unit weights to the intensities (Fig. 100–15B) fit the theoretical negative unit slope line less well than the values in Figure 100–15C, which are calculated using the statistical weights defined in Equation (9). These results support the need for background subtraction and statistical assignment of relative weights to obtain maximal accuracy.

The presented method utilizes background-subtracted and statistically weighted spin echo intensities collected at multiple echo and delay intervals chosen to give sensitivity to a wide range of $T1$ and $T2$ values and to approximately provide uniform precision in the calculated parameters. A simple mathematical expression is then fit to the full set of MDME intensities by simultaneously varying N_r, $T1$, and $T2$. This enables measurement of N_r with minimal $T1$ and $T2$ weighting without using sequences with $TD > 5T1$, and results in reduced interdependence among parameters. $T1$ values from 21 ms to 3.4 s and $T2$ values from 6 ms to 714 ms were measured in only 9.7 minutes of scanning time for 128-step 2DFT imaging. Measurements are particularly extended to short $T1$ and $T2$ values, the former achieved by accurate parameterization of the mathematical model, and the latter achieved by the signal averaging potential of the MDME data set. Precision is roughly uniform throughout the measured range and is as low as 0.4 percent for certain $T2$ values.

These features, combined with the assurance of convergence to an absolute minimum and the generous and predictable limits on starting values, should eliminate the need for an a priori knowledge of the parameter of interest and its expected value. The set of ME sequences, or a single integrated MDME sequence with interleaved collection of the ME data sets, could thus be performed routinely to generate images or ROI values of the three principal tissue parameters for any set of normal, pathologic or contrast enhanced soft tissues or biologic fluids.

The presented methodology could also conceivably be used to give the same benefits in NMR spectroscopy, where separate $T1$ and $T2$ measurements are currently used and where $T1$ values and acquisition times are long owing to high fields and inherent properties of nuclei such as ^{13}C. For example, spin-echo signals obtained in an MDME sequence could be Fourier transformed, which, in the absence of homonuclear coupling,

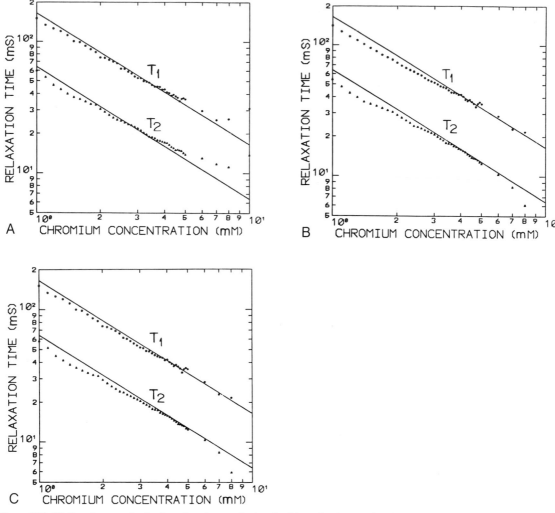

Figure 100–15. Log-log graph of relaxation times calculated without background subtraction (*A*) and with unit weighting (*B*). In the absence of background subtraction, the fit of short *T2* values to the negative unit slope line drawn from Figure 100–11*A* is not as good as the fit of those values following background subtraction (see *C*). Without background subtraction, the persistence of intensity at later echoes causes a biased overestimation of short *T2* values. Similarly, unit weighting of all observed intensities causes the fit of *T1* and *T2* values to the negative unit slope line (*B*) to be worse than when the statistical weights defined in Equation (9) are used (see *C*).

would accurately produce an array of spectra having multiple delays and multiple echoes. Spectral intensities could then be processed by the presented mathematical and computational method to obtain the three parameters for all spectral components.

Further research is needed to include the rationale of MDME data collection in the framework of the previous theoretical optimizations of measured precision per scanning time. For this purpose it will be necessary to use the criterion of minimizing the noise of all three parameters. In particular, the chosen distribution of *TE* and *TD* intervals may need to be better optimized, and alternate schemes for processing the MDME data set need to be considered. These predictions would then need to be verified by actual measurements of calculated noise, which should be best obtained from processed images rather than from matrix calculations of standard errors since the latter are affected by both random and systematic errors. Thirdly, the systematic effects responsible for the underestimation of long *T2* values and overestimation of N_r values associated with short *T2* values need to be characterized. Both instrumental factors (e.g., rf) and inherent physical properties (e.g., diffusion) should be considered, and the mathematical model should be adjusted appropriately. Finally, the effect of other factors that influence the signals from tissues (e.g., multiexponential relaxation and flow) need to be considered and modeled.

ACKNOWLEDGMENTS

We wish to thank Drs. R. Arenstorf and I. Lowe for their helpful discussions, Drs. S. J. Gibbs and P. G. Lenhert for providing software, Dr. A. D. Eisenberg for help with data collections, Dr. D. Pickens, III and E. Lagan for assistance with equipment, C. Miles for tuning the head coil, Dr. J. Erickson for editorial assistance, and B. Norman for artwork. This work was supported in part by a predoctoral fellowship from the Middle Tennessee Chapter of the American Heart Association, by NIH grant Nos. HL30372 and HL34737, and NIH MSTP grant GM07347.

References

1. Atkinson AC, Hunter WG: The design of experiments for parameter estimation. Technometrics *10*:271, 1968.
2. Bachus R, Konig H, Lenz G, Deimling M, Reinhardt, ER: Differentiation in MRI by means of pattern recognition. Proceedings of the Society of Magnetic Resonance in Medicine, London, England, 1985, p 18.
3. Bakker CJG, de Graaf CN, van Dijk P: Derivation of quantitative information in NMR imaging: A phantom study. Phys Med Biol *29*:1511–1525, 1984.
4. Bloch F: Nuclear induction. Phys Rev *70*:460–474, 1946.
5. Bottomley PA, Foster TH, Argersinger RE, Pfeifer LM: A review of normal tissue NMR relaxation times and relaxation mechanisms from 1–100 MHz. Med Phys *11*:425–448, 1984.
6. Bottomley PA, Hardy CJ, Argersinger RE, Allen GR: Relaxation in pathology: Are $T1$'s and $T2$'s diagnostic? Proceedings of the Society of Magnetic Resonance in Medicine, London, England, 1985, p 28.
7. Brown TH, Bernheim RA, Gutowsky HS: Temperature dependence of proton relaxation times in aqueous solutions of paramagnetic ions. II. $CrCl_3$. J Chem Phys *33*:1593–1594, 1960.
8. Bryant RG, Polnaszek C, Kennedy S, Hetzler J, Hickerson D: The magnetic field dependence of water proton $T1$ in aqueous solutions: Implications for magnetic imaging contrast media. Med Phys *11*:712–713, 1984.
9. Burnett KR, Wolf GR, Goldstein EJ, Joseph PM: The contribution of liver ferritin to $T1$ and $T2$ relaxation in iron storage diseases: A laboratory model. Proceedings of the Society of Magnetic Resonance in Medicine, New York, 1984, p 120.
10. Carr HY, Purcell EM: Effects of diffusion on free precession in nuclear magnetic resonance experiments. Phys Rev *94*:630–638, 1954.
11. Conturo TE, Mitchell MR, Price RR, Partain CL, James AE Jr: Simultaneous calculation of spin density, $T1$ and $T2$ from multiple echo MRI data. Invest Radiol *20*:S7, 1985.
12. Conturo TE, Mitchell MR, Partain CL, James AE Jr: Dependence of signal intensity on $T1$ and $T2$ in the multiple echo MRI pulse sequence. Invest Radiol *20*:S13, 1985.
13. Conturo TE, Mitchell MR, Price RR, Partain CL, James AE Jr: Simultaneous full-matrix non-linear least squares calulation of N, $T1$ and $T2$ and their standard errors from multiple echo MRI data. Proceedings of the Society of Magnetic Resonance in Medicine, London, England, 1985, pp 42–43.
14. Conturo TE, Mitchell MR, Price RR, Beth AH, Partain CL, James AE Jr: Improved accuracy of N(H) and $T2$ by simultaneous calculation of N(H), $T1$ and $T2$ from MR image data. Radiology *157*:238, 1985.
15. Conturo TE, Mitchell MR, Price RR, Beth AH, Partain CL, James AE Jr: Improved determination of spin density, $T1$ and $T2$ from three-parameter fit to multiple delay-multiple echo (MDME) NMR images. Phys Med Biol *31*:1361–1380, 1986.
16. Conturo TE, Beth AH, Arenstorf R, Price RR: Simplified mathematical description of longitudinal recovery in multiple echo sequences. Magn Res Med *4*:282–288, 1987.
17. Edelstein WA, Bottomley PA, Hart HR, Smith LS: Signal, noise, and contrast in nuclear magnetic resonance (NMR) imaging. J Comput Assist Tomogr *7*:391–401, 1983.
18. Eisenberg AD, Conturo TE, Mitchell MR, Schwartzberg MS, Price RR, Rich MF, Partain CL, James AE Jr: Enhancement of red blood cell proton relaxation with chromium labeling. Invest Radiol *21*:137–143, 1986.
19. Farrar TC, Becker ED: Pulse and Fourier Transform NMR. New York, Academic Press, 1971, p 22.
20. Franks F: Water: A Comprehensive Treatise. Vol. 5. New York, Plenum Press, 1973, p 320.
21. Fullerton GD, Cameron IL, Ord VA: Orientation of tendons in the magnetic field and its effect on $T2$ relaxation times. Radiology *155*:433–435, 1985.
22. Hahn EL: Spin echoes. Phys Rev *80*:580–594, 1950.
23. Harris RK, Newman RH: Choice of pulse spacings for accurate $T1$ and NOE measurements in NMR spectroscopy. J Magn Reson *24*:449, 1976.

24. Hausser R, Noack F: Kernmagnetische relaxation und korrelation in Zwei-Spin-Systemen. Z fur Physik *182*:93–110, 1964.
25. Hickey DS, Naughton A, Zhu XP, Checkley D, Jenkins JPR: Structure dependent spatial variation in 2DFT MR images and clinical relaxation times estimated from several tau values. Proceedings of the Society of Magnetic Resonance in Medicine, New York, 1984, p 319.
26. Hindman JC, Svirmickas A, Wood M: Relaxation processes in water: A study of the proton spin-lattice relaxation time. J Chem Phys *59*:1517–1522, 1973.
27. Hinshaw WS, Kramer DM, Young H-N, Hill BC: The Fundamentals of Magnetic Resonance Imaging. Solon, Ohio, Technicare Corp, 1985, p 47.
28. Hinshaw WS, Lent AH: An introduction to NMR imaging: From the Bloch equations to the imaging equation. Proc IEEE *71*:338–350, 1983.
29. Jones JP, Partain CL, Mitchell MR, Patton JA, Stephens WH, Price RR, Kulkarni MV, James AR Jr: Principles of magnetic resonance. *In* Kressel HY (ed): Magnetic Resonance Annual. New York, Raven Press, pp 71–111.
30. Karlik SJ, Gilbert JJ, Noseworthy JH: Proton relaxation time changes in myelin basic proteins—Induced acute experimental allergic encephalomyelitis (EAE). Proceedings of the Society of Magnetic Resonance in Medicine, London, England, 1985, p 68.
31. Kjos BO, Ehman RL, Brant-Zawadzki M: Reproducibility of *T1* and *T2* relaxation times calculated from routine MR imaging sequences: Phantom study. Am J Roentgenol *144*:1157–1163, 1985.
32. Kjos BO, Ehman RL, Brant-Zawadzki M: Reproducibility of relaxation times and spin density calculated from routine MR imaging sequences: Clinical study of the CNS. Am J Roentgenol *144*:1165–1170, 1985.
33. Koenig SH, Brown RD: The importance of the motion of water for magnetic resonance imaging. Invest Radiol *20*:297–305, 1985.
34. Koenig SH, Brown RD, Goldstein EJ, Burnett KR, Wolf GR: Magnetic field dependence of proton relaxation rates in tissue with added Mn^{2+}: Rabbit liver and kidney. Magn Reson Med *2*:159–168, 1985.
35. Krynicki K: Proton spin-lattice relaxation in pure water between 0°C and 100°C. Physica *32*:167–178, 1966.
36. Kumar A, Welti D, Ernst RR: NMR Fourier zeugmatography. J Magn Reson *18*:69, 1975.
37. Kurland RJ: Strategies and tactics in NMR imaging relaxation time measurements. I. Minimizing relaxation time errors due to image noise–The ideal case. Magn Reson Med *2*:136–158, 1985.
38. Lerski RA, Straughan K, Orr JS: Calibration of proton density measurements in nuclear magnetic resonance imaging. Phys Med Biol *29*:271–276, 1984.
39. Mansfield P: Multiplanar image formation using NMR spin echoes. J Phys C: Solid State Phys *10*:L55, 1977.
40. Marquardt DW: An algorithm for least squares estimation of non-linear parameters. J Soc Ind Appl Math *11*:431–441, 1963.
41. Meiboom S, Gill D: Modified spin echo method of measuring nuclear relaxation times. Rev Sci Instrum *29*:688–691, 1958.
42. Mellor JW: Higher Mathematics for Students of Chemistry and Physics. New York, Dover, 1955, pp 548–555.
43. Mills CM, Crooks LE, Kaufman L, Brant-Zawadzki M: Cerebral abnormalities: Use of calculated *T1* and *T2* magnetic resonance images for diagnosis. Radiology *150*:87–94, 1984.
44. Mitchell MR, Conturo TE, Gruber TJ, Jones JP: Two computer models for selection of optimal magnetic resonance imaging (MRI) pulse sequence timing. Invest Radiol *19*:350–360, 1984.
45. Morgan LO, Nolle AW: Proton spin relaxation in aqueous solutions of paramagnetic ions. II. Cr^{+++}, Mn^{++}, Ni^{++}, and Gd^{+++}. J Chem Phys *31*:365–368, 1959.
46. Nolle AW, Morgan LO: Frequency dependence of proton spin lattice relaxation in aqueous solutions of paramagnetic ions. J Chem Phys *26*:642–648, 1957.
47. Ortendahl DA, Hylton NM, Kaufman L, Crooks LE: Signal to noise in derived NMR images. Magn Reson Med *1*:316–338, 1984.
48. Palubinskas FS, Davis PL, Brito A, Dolkas CB: In-vivo measurement of rat skeletal muscle parameters *T1*, *T2*, and *N*(H) following various exercise regimens. Proceedings of the Society of Magnetic Resonance in Medicine, London, England, 1985, p 94.
49. Pykett IL, Rosen BR, Buonanno FS, Brady TJ: Measurement of spin-lattice relaxation times in nuclear magnetic resonance imaging. Phys Med Biol *28*:723–729, 1983.
50. Riederer SJ, Suddarth SA, Bobman SA, Lee NJ, Wang HZ, MacFall JR: Automated MR image synthesis: Feasibility studies. Radiology *153*:203–206, 1984.
51. Riederer SJ, Bobman SA, Wang BZ, Lee JN, Farzeneh F, MacFall JR: Improved precision in calculated *T* images using multiple spin-echo data. Invest Radiol *20*:S44, 1985.
52. Rollett D: Computing Methods in Crystallography. Oxford, Permagon Press, 1965.
53. Schneiders NJ, Post H, Brunner P, Ford J, Bryan RN, Willcott MR: Accurate *T2* NMR images. Med Phys *10*:642–645, 1983.
54. Schneiders NJ, Ford JJ, Bryan RN: Accurate *T1* and spin density images. Med Phys *12*:71–76, 1985.
55. Smith DWG, Powles JG: Proton spin lattice relaxation in liquid water and liquid ammonia. Mol Phys *10*:451–463, 1966.
56. Stout GH, Jensen LH: X-ray Structure Determination. New York, Macmillan Publishing Co., Inc., 1968, pp 389–393.
57. Sutherland RJ, Hutchison JMS: Three-dimensional NMR imaging using selective excitation. J Phys E *11*:79–83, 1978.

58. Teslacon Operator's Manual. Technicare Inc., 29100 Aurora Road, Solon, OH 44139, USA, 1984.
59. Tsui BMW, Turner TE, DiBianca FA, McCartney WH, Staab FV: Effects of pulse sequence on magnetic resonance images. Radiology *153*:369, 1984.
60. Weiss GH, Gupta RK, Ferretti JA, Becker ED: The choice of optimal parameters for measurement of spin lattice relaxation times. I. Mathematical formulation. J Magn Reson *37*:369–379, 1980.
61. Whittaker ET, Robinson G: The Calculus of Observations. New York, Dover Publications, 1967, pp 209–259.
62. Young IR, Bailes DR, Burt M: Initial clinical evaluation of a whole body nuclear magnetic resonance (NMR) tomograph. J Comput Assist Tomogr *6*:1–18, 1982.
63. Young IR, Dickinson RD, Hall AS: Demonstration of changes of temperature in vivo during hyperthermia using MR imaging. Radiology *157*:280, 1985.

101

Distinction of the Normal, Preneoplastic, and Neoplastic States by Water Proton NMR Relaxation Times

P. T. BEALL
C. F. HAZLEWOOD

The utilization of the behavior of cellular water as a probe of the physiologic state of tissues and cells has a long history, going back to the ancient Greeks. The idea that water may play a role in the cancerous process is based on early experimental evidence. Cramer, perhaps, was the first to present evidence that the percentage of water in tumors is related to their rate of growth, with faster growing tumors often having a higher water content.[26] McEwen et al. later reported that at least part of the elevated levels of water in the tissues could be due to an actual uptake of water by the transformed cells.[56] An elevated water content of tissues distant from the organ containing a tumor, termed the *systemic effect* of tumors, was observed by Schlottman and Rubenow.[80] Using multiple beam interference microscopy, Mellors et al. showed that individual sarcoma cells contained more water than normal fibroblasts.[66] Downing et al.[33] also used interferometry and reported that the increased hydration of tumors was probably intracellular. These early studies implied a relationship between water content and the growth of cells. Unfortunately, even with these remarkable correlations between water content and the transformation process, no general theory was developed to describe an active role for water in the cancerous process. Further pursuit of these observations seems to have been impeded by both lack of technology and theory.

With the development of nuclear magnetic resonance (NMR) spectroscopy, the interests of biologists were revived and the interests of physicists awakened to the study of water in biologic systems and in particular to water in cancer. With this technique, the characteristics of hydrogen nuclei of tissue water could be examined in a nondestructive manner in living cells.

Damadian[27] first reported that the NMR relaxation times of water protons in Walker sarcoma and Novikoff hepatomas were significantly higher than those of the normal tissues of origin. Damadian's findings were confirmed[44,45] and extended to preneoplastic and neoplastic mammary tissue. Rapidly, other reports confirmed this finding.[27,45–59,78] A sampling of these reports, which noted a difference in the spin-spin and spin-lattice relaxation times for water protons in normal and neoplastic tissues, is presented in Table 101–1. In general, although not in all cases, tumors have longer *T1* and *T2* values than the tissues of origin. The potential of NMR as a screening or diagnostic procedure for cancers is just beginning to be explored. The use of nuclear magnetic resonance spectroscopy to study in a nondestructive manner the water content

Table 101-1. NMR RELAXATION TIMES OF WATER PROTONS IN TISSUES

Tissue	Spin-Lattice Relaxation Time $T1$ (ms) Normal	Neoplastic	Reference
Rat (24 MHz)			
Liver	293	826	27
Muscle	538	736	"
Mouse (30 MHz)			
Mammary	380	920 D_2	44
		887 C3H	"
		906 C3Hf	"
		721 CD_3	"
(Preneoplastic Nodules)		(350) CD_3	"
		(709) D_2	"
		(451) D_2	"
		(657) D_1	"
Mouse (24 MHz)			
Liver	350	670	25
Human (24 MHz)			
Lung	788	1110	28
Breast	367	1080	"
Skin	616	1047	"
Stomach	765	1238	"
Intestine	641	1122	"
Muscle	1023	1413	"
Bladder	891	1245	"
Bone	554	1027	"
Liver	570	832	"
Spleen	701	1113	"
Ovary	989	1282	"
Thyroid	882	1072	"
Mouse (100 MHz)			
Muscle	850	880	48
Liver	420	480	"
Brain	840	930	"
Mouse (24 MHz)			
Muscle	471	662	46
Liver	263	798	"
Human (24 MHz)			
Kidney	459	638	46
Colon	475	553	"
Lung	404	420	"
Rat (24 MHz)			
Liver	467	652	21
Muscle	850	1150	"
Rat (25 MHz)			
Liver	273	749	23
Human (32 MHz)			
Thyroid	700	700	79
Chicken (32 MHz)			
Bone marrow	408	717	71
Liver	208	370	"
Spleen	596	641	"
Human (24 MHz)			
Breast	191	575	35
Colon	552	595	"
Thyroid	410	679	"
Lung	270	555	"
Rat (60 MHz)			
Liver	527	1150	52
		1093	"
		1025	"
Human (30 MHz)			
Breast	682	874	62
Human (25 MHz)			
Breast	415	819	51
Stomach	841	997	"
Cervix	825	1089	"
Skin	360	1037	"
Human (30 MHz)			
Breast	682	874	14
Human (25 MHz)			
Esophagus	797	959	75

and the physical properties of water in tissues has added a powerful tool to the investigation of the process of neoplastic transformation. Changes in water content and water mobility can be examined throughout the spectrum of cancers in all kinds of animals. Commonalities and differences can be sought from the normal state and the development of the preneoplastic and neoplastic states can be followed. Bottomley has recently catalogued and modeled changes in proton NMR relaxation times in various malignancies.[87]

DISTINCTION OF PRENEOPLASTIC AND NEOPLASTIC TISSUES OF THE BREAST

Mammary cancer, comprising 23 percent of all cancers in women, is the most prevalent cancer and a primary cause of death among females in the United States. Incidence is approximately 100,000 new cases per year, with the mortality rate reaching 40,000. The age-adjusted mortality index for women in their most productive years (ages 30 to 45) is 105 per 100,000 (NIH, 1973). Despite advances in diagnosis and treatment, the mortality rate for mammary cancer has remained fairly constant over the past 30 years, indicating that the cure rate has managed to just keep up with the increased incidence rate of approximately 10 percent over this time period.[1] These facts clearly demonstrate the need for innovative approaches to early detection, diagnosis, treatment, and management of human mammary cancer. We will indicate one such approach to diagnosis by reviewing some fundamental aspects of experimental mouse and human mammary cancer and draw on information learned in other cancer systems to aid in the interpretation of NMR results.

Mouse Mammary Cancer

The murine mammary tumor system is one of the most extensively studied model systems available and offers many advantages for experimental investigation. Mammary tumors are easily induced in mice by a variety of agents. Induction in inbred strains of mice allows easy transplantation of the tumor and extensive manipulation of the syngeneic hosts. The majority of murine mammary tumors are adenocarcinomas, which are influenced by a variety of factors, including viruses, chemical carcinogens, hormones, genetic backgrounds, diet, and the immune status of the host. A major effort has been directed over the past 30 years at unraveling the interactions among the many different factors that influence the induction and progression of mammary tumors.

One of the most important factors influencing mammary tumorigenesis is the presence of mammary tumor viruses (MMTV).[17,68] MMTV is transmitted through milk and germ cells.

The MMTVs have several well-documented effects on the host in addition to inducing preneoplastic mammary nodules and mammary tumors. It is well established that the presence of MMTV can alter tissue responsiveness and systemic functions. MMTV increases the responsiveness of the mammary gland to growth hormone and prolactin,[67] alters the hormonal sensitivity of DNA synthesis and mitosis in nodules,[6] shortens the life span of male and female mice in certain strains,[82] and depresses the immune response and alters NMR relaxation times in various organs.

The mouse mammary tumor system is characterized by the presence of *preneoplastic* lesions, termed hyperplastic alveolar nodules (HAN), which are altered from normal mammary alveoli in a number of properties.[60] The ability to transplant HANs into the gland-free mammary fat pads of syngeneic mice has established the preneoplastic nature of these lesions.[31] HANs are considered preneoplastic since mammary tumors arise more frequently from HANs than from normal cells.[31] HANs are visualized histologically in nonpregnant, nonlactating mice as foci of compact alveolar hyperplasia and are morphologically similar to the mammary lobuloalveolar development seen in mid-to-late pregnant mice.

It is known that HANs arise in mice treated with chemical carcinogens, in MMTV-infected mice, and in old, retired BALB/c female breeder mice free of MMTV. HAN outgrowth lines can be established by serially transplanting the tissue into the cleared fat pads of young mice and, therefore, may be considered analogous to established tumor lines or in-vitro cell lines. HANs are characterized by a set of criteria that distinguish them from normal and neoplastic cells:

1. Nodule lines, like tumors, can be serially propagated indefinitely.[30] This property is not virus or neoplastic dependent but appears to be acquired by the nodule state.

2. HANs do not require estrogens for maintenance, although estrogen is necessary for induction and proliferation in some strains such as C3H.[18] Normal mammary gland requires ovarian steroids for growth and maintenance, whereas mammary tumors are independent of ovarian steroids for growth.

3. Nodules, like normal mammary gland, are mammary fat pad dependent, do not grow in subcutaneous tissue[37] or beyond the limits of the mammary fat pad,[38] and are subject to local growth-regulatory factors exerted by normal duct cells.[19] Mammary tumors are not limited by any of these factors.

4. HANs are antigenic; however, these antigens so far have been associated with MMTV virions. Unique nodule-specific antigens analogous to mammary tumor-specific antigens have not been reported.

Several other intermediate cell populations occur in the mammary gland, particularly in chemical carcinogen treated mice.[57,58,63] These include ductal hyperplasias, fibrous nodules characterized by predominant connective tissue proliferation, alveolar adenosis, and nodules exhibiting epidermoid metaplasia. These lesions have not been well characterized biologically.

The scheme for mammary tumorigenesis suggests the presence of at least two sequential transformations, i.e., the nodule and the neoplastic transformations. Both types of transformed cells are remarkably stable; also, they can be separated from each other and from normal cells by relatively simple criteria. Understanding the pathogenesis of mammary tumors depends on understanding these intermediate lesions.

The concept of mammary tumorigenesis as developed in the mouse has direct applicability to mammary tumor pathogenesis in the chemical carcinogen-induced rat model and in human breast cancer.[76,85] The cellular type involved in the preoplastic lesions in the three species varies with the etiologic agent and the species, but the model is applicable to all.

The first NMR study on cancer was made on transplanted tumor lines.[27] To determine whether these results could be related to early spontaneously arising neoplastic tissue from the preneoplastic state, we concentrated experiments in our laboratory on primary mammary adenocarcinomas of the mouse.[44]

Normal mammary tissues were taken from the inguinal mammary glands of 17- to 19-day-old pregnant BALB/c and C3Hf mice. Preneoplastic nodule tissues were taken from Balb/c mice bearing nodule outgrowth lines D1 and D2 and from C3Hf mice bearing a C3Hf nodule outgrowth line. The tumor producing capabilities have been well defined under various experimental conditions. Outgrowth line D1 produced 2 percent mammary tumors after 360 days, whereas line D2 produced 45 percent mammary tumors after 360 days. The nodule outgrowth lines are morphologically similar to normal mammary tissues found in mid-to-late pregnant mice. Mammary tumors were taken as primary tumors arising in these nodule outgrowth lines.

For some of these experiments, samples of the nodule outgrowth lines were transplanted into the inguinal mammary gland–free fat pads of 3-week-old BALB/c female mice by the standard method of DeOme et al.[31] and analyzed 12 to 16 weeks later by NMR spectroscopy.[44]

For other experiments[13,44] mammary tumors from C3H and C3Hf mice were transplanted subcutaneously into 4-month-old syngeneic female mice near the right axilla. The C3H neoplasms were second-generation transplants from tumors that arose in breeding C3H stock mice. The C3Hf tumors were second- and third-generation transplants from tumors that arose from nodule outgrowth line F_2 in C3Hf mice. All tumors were analyzed within 1 month after transplantation. When the tumors reached 10 mm in diameter, they were surgically excised. Necrotic, nonviable areas of the tumor were carefully avoided in the preparation of the samples for NMR and tissue hydration analysis. All NMR measurements were made at 30 MHz and 25°C.

Early results of measurements of $T1$, $T2$, and D (self-diffusion coefficient for water) of water protons in normal mammary glands, preneoplastic nodules, and neoplastic tissue are summarized in Table 101–2. The relaxation times and the diffusion coefficient of water protons in these tissues are shorter than those for pure water. This agrees with the notion that the water molecules within living cells are strongly influenced by water-ion-macromolecular interactions. Table 101–2 also shows that the three morphologic states (normal, preneoplastic, and neoplastic) of mammary tissue can be distinguished by the average values of the physical parameters $T1$, $T2$, and D.

More extensive studies on several types of preneoplastic breast nodules in mice are summarized in Table 101–3.[13] The relaxation times of water protons in tumors are almost doubled relative to mammary gland tissue from pregnant animals and to preneoplastic nodule tissue. The relaxation times for the nodule (preneoplastic) tissues also appear to be slightly longer than those for mammary gland tissue from pregnant animals.[44]

These results indicate that it is possible with the use of NMR parameters to distinguish between preneoplastic nodule tissue (a population at high risk for developing tumors) and normal tissue in pregnant mice. Previous results demonstrated that mammary tumors could be distinguished from nodule tissues and normal tissues (Table 101–2).[44] Table 101–3 demonstrates that all NMR parameters increase monotonically and distinguishably from normal cells to nodule cells to tumor cells in the development of mammary tumors in mice. These data support the hypothesis that the preneoplastic HAN cells represent an altered population with properties intermediate between normal

Table 101–2. RELAXATION TIMES AND DIFFUSION COEFFICIENT OF WATER PROTONS IN WATER AND MOUSE MAMMARY TISSUE

Tissue	$T1$ (ms)	$T2$ (ms)	D ($cm^2/s \times 10^{-5}$)
Pure water	3100	1430 ± 270	2.38 ± 0.02
Tumor (5)	920 ± 47	91 ± 8	0.7 ± 0.05
Preneoplastic Nodules			
Series 1 (5)	450 ± 21	53 ± 1	0.44 ± 0.03
Series 2 (9)	681 ± 40	54 ± 1	0.67 ± 0.06
Normal			
Series 1 (5)	380 ± 41	39 ± 2	0.34 ± 0.04
Series 2 (8)	357 ± 47	47 ± 1	0.35 ± 0.03
High Tumor Potential			
D2 (4)	709 ± 29	54.1 ± 1.2	0.623 ± 0.057
Low Tumor Potential			
D1 (5)	657 ± 68	54.7 ± 1.8	0.708 ± 0.090

Data (obtained at 30 MHz) are given as mean value ± SEM. These data show a lack of correlation of the NMR parameters with the tumor potential of the nodule. Number of tissue samples is shown in parentheses. All values are given as the average ± SE. Normal tissue was 15- to 17-day pregnant mammary gland.[44,45]

Table 101–3. NMR RELAXATION TIMES OF WATER IN MOUSE MAMMARY TISSUE[13]

Tissue	(n)	T1 (ms)	T2 (ms)	%H$_2$O
Virgin Controls	(22)	275 ± 46	84 ± 8	26.8 ± 8.4
Pregnant Controls	(5)	380 ± 41		
	(8)	357 ± 47	47.1 ± .9	34.0 ± 1.9
Preneoplastic				
Hyperplastic Alveolar Nodules				
D$_1$	(5)	657 ± 68	54.7 ± 1.8	58.5 ± .1
(HAN)D$_2$	(4)	709 ± 29	54.1 ± 1.2	
CD-3	(17)	350 ± 75	85 ± 18	31.10 ± 13.1
Mammary Adenocarcinomas				
D$_2$	(5)	920 ± 47	91 ± 8	
C3H	(7)	887 ± 40	78.8 ± 8.2	83.1 ± 1.0
C3Hf	(12)	906 ± 43	80.3 ± 5.9	84.0 ± 0.3
CD-3	(19)	721 ± 98	98 ± 20	74.6 ± 11.7

From Danadian R: NMR Basic Principles and Progress. Berlin, Springer Verlag, 1981.

cells and neoplastic cells. In addition, they provide a theoretical basis for the possible use of NMR spectroscopy in the detection of suspected preneoplastic cell populations in the human breast.

The water proton *T1* and *T2* appear to be characteristic of the particular developmental state of the mammary gland. This is true for most biologic and hormonal parameters associated with preneoplastic and neoplastic mammary tissue. Thus, alterations in growth rate and hormonal responsiveness are not quantitatively correlated with the exact tumor potential of a nodule line (Table 101–2) but are associated with the developmental state of a high-risk population, i.e., the preneoplastic HAN. Similarly, changes in water proton *T1* and *T2* are associated with the preneoplastic HAN but are not quantitatively correlated with the actual tumor potential.

Human Mammary Cancer

Neoplasms of the human breast arise principally from the ductal epithelium in the terminal ducts of the mammary lobule. These neoplasms can be noninfiltrating ductal and lobular carcinomas (i.e., in situ carcinomas) or infiltrating carcinomas subdivided into a variety of classes (i.e., papillary, colloid, medullary, lobular, and comedocarcinoma). The cytologic and behavioral characteristics of these malignant neoplasms have been well defined and the course of treatment well established.[36,55] Of at least equal importance, however, are the benign proliferative breast lesions, including proliferations of epithelial and stromal elements, that present so worrisome a problem to the pathologist and physician; these include fibrocystic disease, which can be a very complex lesion. In its simplest form it shows alterations only in the ductal epithelium, but in complex forms it can also include hyperplasias of myoepithelial cells, metaplasia, sclerosis, and intraluminal proliferation of duct cells. This lesion is quite common in both cancerous and noncancerous breast.

Nevertheless, the significant patterns associated with fibrocystic disease remain largely unknown. Potter reported a 480 percent increased risk of mammary cancer for women with benign lesions.[69] Lobular and ductal carcinoma have been reported to arise out of foci of fibrocystic disease and fibroadenomas.[55] Little is known, however, about the neoplastic potential of the various cell populations that comprise fibrocystic disease. For example, this disease, as defined by Foote and Stewart,[41] can include among its atypia duct papillomatosis (atypical intraductal hyperplasia), an instance of lesions that are cytologically borderline. Their prognosis is not understood, although they manifest a few features of early intraductal carcinoma, notably, some cribriform pattern.[41]

The problem of preneoplastic lesions in the human breast is formidably complex, yet essentially the significant unanswered question concerns the long-term biologic fate of the various dysplasias. Here one does not have the advantage of an experimental model system of isotopic transplantation sites yielding indications of the neoplastic potential of suspect lesions. This difficulty may, in part, be overcome by using naturally or experimentally induced immunosuppressed hosts; however, the experiments so far have not shown promise. The need for better procedures to detect breast disease at both the precancerous and cancerous levels is attested by the relatively constant morbidity and mortality rates in breast cancer.

Advances in mammography and thermography in the past decade have contributed significantly to detection of breast malignancy at early stages. Such approaches, while beneficial, however, present fresh problems. On the one hand, the suspected neoplasm is caught early enough to offer a better prognosis for the patient; on the other, the early lesion may be more dificult to diagnose histopathologically. Thus, atypical intraductal hyperplasias, which are cytologically borderline lesions, are more frequently identified. It is an impossible task to study microscopically every duct and stroma, let alone the entire course of each lesion, within a patient's breast. Hence, many early lesions go undetected by routine microscopic analysis. Again, the situation requires new tools and procedures for enabling the pathologist to assess high-risk lesions. The need has become all the more pressing with the recognition that noninfiltrating breast cancer—*in situ* lobular and *in situ* ductal carcinomas—are being diagnosed more frequently today. Such contributions as the hypothesis of Jensen et al. concerning the origin and the progression of duct carcinomas from terminal duct lobular units[50] makes all the more obvious the importance of these lesions and their early diagnosis, as well as the compelling need for more accurate prognosis.

It is for these reasons that new approaches are so imperative in every aspect of the progression and treatment of breast cancer. It is hoped that one such approach, the utilization of NMR spectroscopy, will provide a powerful, routinely available tool equipping the pathologist with the means to determine which lesions have high risk of progressing to malignant neoplasia. Some of our continuing efforts in that direction are detailed here.

The studies by Damadian and associates[29] indicated that the $T1$ and $T2$ of water protons in neoplasic tissues could be distinguished from those in normal tissues. Damadian et al.[28,29] reported observations on 106 human tumors, representing the gastrointestinal tract, urinary bladder, lung, endocrine glands, lymph nodes, bone, melanomas, muscle, liver, breast, and skin. The neoplastic tissues could always be distinguished from normal by NMR. This group reported $T1$ routinely and $T2$ on some neoplasms; however, diseased nonneoplastic tissues were not studied.

We concentrated on the capability of NMR spectroscopy to distinguish between normal, diseased, and neoplastic human breast tissue.[62] The aims of this study were to demonstrate whether the mean $T1$ and $T2$ of the different cell populations were significantly different, and if so, to determine whether individual samples could be distinguished by NMR techniques.

Samples of human breast tissue were obtained as fresh, unfixed biopsy specimens. Diagnosis was confirmed by frozen sections and histologic examination. Samples for NMR were trimmed of observable fat and analyzed within 1 to 4 hours of the biopsy. After NMR analysis, the samples were fixed in formalin and stained in hematoxylin or Masson's trichome. Histologic examination was done on the tissue from which the NMR sample originated.

Fibroadenomas are recognized readily, but fibrocystic disease is sometimes loosely defined. In our study, fibrocystic disease included fibrosis, apocrine metaplasia, duct dilation, or cysts, with varied degrees and severity of ductal epithelial hyperplasia. This hyperplasia was the most important feature and the one required for fibrocystic disease to be present.

Most carcinomas examined were infiltrating ductal carcinomas. The data were evaluated by a variety of statistical tests, which included the Mann-Whitney U test (nonparametric statistics), Student's t-test (difference between two means), and Bartlett's χ^2 test for equality of variance.

The results of these studies on human breast tissues are summarized in Table 101–4. The mean values of the proton relaxation times ($T1$ and $T2$) of human mammary adenocarcinomas can be distinguished from those of normal breast tissue and fibrocystic disease but not from fibroadenomas. The mean values ($\pm$ SE) of $T1$ (in ms) for normal breast tissue, fibrocystic disease, fibroadenomas, and adenocarcinomas were 682 ± 32, 655 ± 21, 980 ± 51, and 874 ± 28 ms, respectively. The mean $T1$ values for the adenocarcinomas were significantly different from those for both normal breast tissue ($P < 0.001$) and fibrocystic disease ($P < 0.001$), but not significantly different from those for fibroadenoma ($0.5 < P < 0.10$). Bartlett's χ^2 test suggests the variance in $T1$ for fibrocystic disease was not significantly different from that for adenocarcinoma.

Values of $T2$ for normal breast tissue, fibrocystic disease, fibroadenomas, and adenocarcinomas were 35.5 ± 3.5, 37.0 ± 3.0, 62.5 ± 7.3, and 68 ± 2.3 ms, respectively. The mean $T2$ values for the adenocarcinomas were significantly different from those of both normal breast ($P < 0.001$) and fibrocystic disease ($P < 0.001$) but not significantly different from those for fibroadenoma ($P < 0.3$). The data were evaluated

Table 101–4. WATER PROTON RELAXATION TIMES OF HUMAN BREAST DISEASE BIOPSIES

Normal (7)*		Fibrocystic (21)		Fibroadenoma (8)		Adenocarcinoma (17)	
T1	T2	T1	T2	T1	T2	T1	T2
701	26.3	601	27.9			961	75.4
810	41.4	681	36.6			804	63.4
614	29.0	690	34.4	963	47.0	999	56.3
736	42.0	756	27.3	725	47.8	822	81.8
719	50.6	697	49.3	1,194	36.8	1,120	83.7
643	32.6	576	36.6	1,008	56.1	816	71.2
550	26.5	457	30.2	1,080	90.1	939	60.3
		630	38.5	1,080	94.7	881	85.6
		792	40.9	899	66.1	849	65.6
		610	27.3	891	61.0	666	62.5
		546	26.3			809	62.1
		648	24.7			748	61.3
		697	60.0			805	77.6
		728	45.0			930	62.0
		613	46.0			987	63.2
		696	29.4			753	60.0
		625	38.9			964	74.8
		677	35.6				
		576	15.3				
		598	24.3				
		936	82.7				
Mean	682	35.5	655	37.0	980	62.5	874	68.6
$\pm$ SE	$\pm$ 32	$\pm$ 3.5	$\pm$ 21	$\pm$ 3.0	$\pm$ 51	$\pm$ 7.3	$\pm$ 28	$\pm$ 2.3

* The number of tissue samples in each of the four groups is given in parentheses. Pairs of value of $T1$ and $T2$ are listed individually for each sample.[62]

by both the Student's t-test and the Mann-Whitney U test, a nonparametric statistical test. Both demonstrated that the *T1* and *T2* were stochastically smaller for the fibrocystic population than for the adenocarcinoma population. The variance in *T2* was significantly less for adenocarcinoma than for fibrocystic disease. Similar results were seen by Goldsmith et al.[43] for human mammary cancers. In addition, Goldsmith has combined *T1* and *T2* into a "malignancy index," which was claimed to distinguish human cancers with greater accuracy than either relaxation time variant alone.

Water proton relaxation times (*T1* and *T2*) can be utilized to distinguish normal, preneoplastic, and neoplastic tissues in animals and humans. In most reported cases *T1* is longer in cancer biopsies than in comparable normal tissues. This phenomenon is not solely dependent on tissue hydration,[13,14,73,84] and the mechanism for this difference is not totally understood. In animal model studies the *T1* and *T2* values for particular types of cancers and preneoplastic lesions are very reproducible. In the mouse mammary cancer model, distinction between the normal, pregnant, preneoplastic, and neoplastic states[13] is clear. In the more diverse human population, it is possible to distinguish normal tissues and some dysplasias from carcinomas. It is more difficult to separate metastatic carcinomas from the relatively benign fibroadenomas. The identification of preneoplastic states among a population of human breast dysplasias has not thus far been demonstrated by NMR techniques. A combination of NMR parameters or analysis of other nuclei (e.g., sodium) or both may yield a better definition. Certainly, careful consideration of the preneoplastic state should be given to interpretations of NMR scanning data and the search for parameters to identify this state in whole organs should be sought. One way to approach the problem is to seek those factors that distinguish the preneoplastic cell from the cancer cell in tissue culture.

DISTINCTION OF PRENEOPLASTIC AND CANCEROUS CELLS IN VITRO BY NMR

Numerous cancer cells from human and animal models have now been established as tissue culture cell lines and utilized in seeking a better understanding of the transformation process. Some of these cell lines have been examined for water proton relaxation times and their values are summarized in Table 101–5. Most of the established cell lines have *T1* and *T2* values similar to or higher than their tissue of origin (usually tumors or cells from metastatic sites). Differences between cell cannot be explained totally by hydration values.[7,8,11,73,84] In two cases, we have completed in-depth investigations of particular series of human breast cancer and human colon cancer cell lines to attempt to correlate NMR relaxation times with some functional or structural properties of these cells.

Human Breast Cancer Cells

Table 101–6 shows the results of a study of a diverse series of human breast cancer cell lines. In 10 established human mammary carcinoma cell lines, the range of visually estimated population doubling times ranged from 24 hours to several weeks. The cells were grown as monolayers in Leibovitz (Gibco-L15) medium supplemented with 15 percent fetal calf serum, glutathione, antibiotics, and insulin. Spin-lattice and spin-spin relaxation times, *T1* and *T2*, respectively, of the cellular water hydrogen protons were determined by the nondestructive nuclear magnetic resonance technique. In pure liquid water, the *T1* value is approximately 3000 ms, whereas in these living cells, the *T1* varies between 500 and 1000 ms, indicating restricted mobility and a more complex

Table 101—5. NMR RELAXATION TIMES OF WATER IN ESTABLISHED CANCER CELL LINES AND SINGLE CELL TYPES

Cell Type	*T1* (ms)	*T2* (ms)	%H_2O	Reference
Rat cancer cells (60 MHz)				
Ehrlich ascites	1150			52
Walker 256	1093			
Ehrlich solid	1025 ± 7	38.2 ± 6		
Established lines of mouse mammary cancer (30 MHz)				
ESD/BALB CL3	632 ± 8	113 ± 8	85.1 ± 0.7	11
MTV-L/BALB CL2	762 ± 26	105 ± 5	83.9 ± 0.7	
DMBA/BALB CL2	739 ± 33	109 ± 8	83.8 ± 0.2	
Mouse lung fibroblasts (30 MHz):				
BALB 3T3	1250	160		12
SV3T3	757 ± 58	84 ± 5		
Cultured cells				
Hela (Human cervical Ca)	1038 ± 975			84
HLS-2 (Human liposarcoma)	1093 ± 914			
VTC-4 (Human amnion)	749			
VERO (Monkey kidney)	724			
CEC (Chick embryo)	784 ± 733			
Ehrlich Ascites Cells	815 ± 7	61 ± 2	80.8 ± 0.34	54
Human cervical carcinoma (30 MHz)				
M_0 (0 min)	1020	130	88.2	7
M_{30} (30 min)	817	127	87.5	
G_1 (4 hrs)	638	110	85.8	
S (12 hrs)	534	117	84.4	
G_2 (18 hrs)	621	100	84.5	
G_2 (19 hrs)	690	96	84.3	
G_2 (20 hrs)	739	116	84.3	
Random (25 MHz)	990			72
Human leukemic cells				
Active	1031			72
After treatment of patient	612			
Human breast cancer (30 MHz)				
MDA-MB 231	934 ± 78	123 ± 31	86.5 ± 1.3	16
157	907 ± 10	135 ± 4	87.4 ± 0.1	
361	849 ± 25		88.4 ± 0.2	
134	717 ± 64	145 ± 39	88.9 ± 0.4	
453	770 ± 15	113 ± 18	87.4 ± 2.1	
330	752 ± 39		88.5 ± 1.4	
435	607 ± 9	112 ± 13	87.3 ± 0.9	
331	549 ± 136	75 ± 20	88.5 ± 0.1	
431	521	126		
436	499 ± 49	100 ± 20	84.3 ± 0.4	
231 (slow)	622 ± 70	104 ± 18		
157 (slow)	669 ± 52	102 ± 18	85.2 ± 1.0	
Human Leukocytes				
Normal	715 ± 23			36
Leukemic (active)	855 ± 42			
Leukemic (remission)	739 ± 54			
Human colon cancer (30 MHz)				
LS 180	643 ± 60	119 ± 12	85.5 ± 2.4	15
LS 174 T	744 ± 16	121 ± 3	86.6 ± 0.5	
LS 174 T 3-5 clone	663 ± 65	127 ± 11	89.7 ± 1.9	
LS 174 T 6-6 clone	716 ± 39	114 ± 16	86.4 ± 1.2	
HT 29	686 ± 21	108 ± 7		
SW 480	982 ± 9	176 ± 6	90.1 ± 1.4	
SW 1345	460 ± 45	83 ± 6	83.6 + 1.8	

Table 101–6. NMR RELAXATION TIME OF HUMAN BREAST CANCER CELLS[16]

Cell Line MDA-MB	T1 (ms)	T2 (ms)	%H2O	PDT (days)
231	934 ± 78	123 ± 31	86.5	1
157	907 ± 10	135 ± 4	87.4	1–1.5
361	849	—	88.4	1.5
134	717 ± 64	145 ± 39	88.9	1.5–2
453	770 ± 15	113 ± 18	87.4	1.5–2
330	752 ± 39	—	88.5	1.5–3
435	607 ± 9	112 ± 13	87.3	6–7
331	549 ± 136	75 ± 20	88.5	5–7
431	521	126	—	12–14
436	499 ± 49	100 ± 20	84.3	16–18
213 (slow)	662 ± 70	104 ± 18	—	2
157 (slow)	669 ± 52	102 ± 18	85.2	2.5

PDT = Population Doubling Time

environment for water molecules in some of the cells. The fastest growing cells had the longest $T1$ values (or the most mobile water), and the slower the cells grew, the shorter the $T1$ values (or the more restricted the water molecules). The differences in $T1$ values were not due solely to differences in hydration. One explanation for the exponential relationship between doubling time and $T1$ values is that a more complex or a different type of macromolecular lattice exists in the slower growing cells and has a greater influence on the motion of water. This study suggests the possibility of defining the differences among a series of individual cell lines of the same type of diagnosed cancer. A fundamental relationship between the physical state of cellular water and the factors that control cells in division is suggested by these studies.[9,13]

Human Colon Cancer Cells

Investigations of rat and human gastrointestinal cancers usually show normal intestine to have lower $T1$ and $T2$ relaxation times for water protons than does cancerous intestine.[25,28,34,43,46,53,73,81] The causes of differences in NMR relaxation times are difficult to interpret in whole tissue samples of the gastrointestinal tract, which may be covered with mucus and consist of several layers of epithelial and smooth muscle cells as well as blood, lymph, and extracellular spaces.

NMR measurements on pure populations of cells derived from tumors and established in cell culture may be more easily interpreted.[7–9,54,72,84] Such studies of cultured cells can eliminate some of the variables in the examination of cancer by NMR.

Human tumor biopsies are very heterogeneous samples. Koutcher et al.,[53] in an NMR study of human colon cancer, reported biopsies to contain between 1 and 60 percent cancer cells as determined by serial sectioning. $T1$ values for the biopsies varied from 455 to 756 ms, with a mean $T1$ value of 260 ± 58 ms for the series of 20 biopsies.[53] Normal colon from individuals without cancer gave $T1$ values with a mean of 330 ± 129 ms. Distinction between normal and cancerous biopsies required a formula involving the $T1$ from normal and cancer groups or the combined malignancy index.[53] These types of studies cannot determine whether NMR relaxation time differences are a function of a sample heterogeneity, variable extracellular spaces, hydration changes, or true differences between the relaxation times of intracellular water in normal and cancer cells.

In our study[15] advantage was taken of the existence of a number of established cell populations of human colon cancer. Established lines from several patients (LS180,

Table 101–7. WATER PROTON RELAXATION TIMES IN LINES AND CLONES OF HUMAN CANCER OF THE COLON[15]

Cell Line	(n)	Passage Number	PDT (hr)	T1 (ms)	T2 (ms)	%H$_2$O
LS 180	(5)	41	24.5	643 ± 60	119 ± 12	85.6 ± 2.4
LS 174T	(6)	37	20.3	744 ± 16	121 ± 3	86.6 ± 0.5
Clone 3-5	(6)	93	19.1	663 ± 65	127 ± 11	89.7 ± 1.9
Clone 6-6	(7)	60	20.5	716 ± 39	114 ± 10	86.4 ± 1.2
HT 29	(7)	140	12.2	686 ± 21	108 ± 7	—
SW 480	(4)	614	39.4	982 ± 9	176 ± 6	90.1 ± 1.4
SW 1345	(6)	55	51.1	460 ± 45	83 ± 6	83.6 ± 1.8

PDT = Population Doubling Time

LS174T, HT29, SW1345) had water proton NMR spin-lattice relaxation times of 460 ± 45 ms to 982 ± 9 msec and spin-spin relaxation times of 83 ± 6 msec to 176 ± 6 ms (Table 101–7). Two single cell clones derived from line LS174T were similar in T1 and T2 times to the parent line. Differences among the cell lines were not solely a function of cellular hydration. These cell lines of human colon cancer maintained water proton relaxation times similar to the original colon cancer biopsy values. Along with other morphologic and biochemical criteria, the consistency of relaxation times suggests that the established cell lines may serve as a good experimental model for the study of human colon cancer. The most intensively studied lines (LS and HT lines) had T1 values near the mean of 620 ms seen for tumor tissues in the Koutcher et al.[53] study. Cell lines with proven epithelial morphology and the capability to produce tumors in nude mice may serve as a good experimental models to examine the role of water in the neoplastic process.

Studies in rat and human gastrointestinal cancer have indicated that in the whole tissue, lower T1 values are found for normal tissue than for tumors. We wanted to test this hypothesis in the cultured cell system. Adult cell populations were cultured from nonmalignant tissue located away from tumor in two patients with colon cancer. Two populations of fetal intestinal cells were provided. All normal cells were wetter and had higher T1 and T2 values than all but one of the established cancer cell lines (Table 101–8).

Examination of the evidence suggests a possible reason for this apparent contradiction. Owing to current limitations in tissue culture technology and the possibility of genetic limits to the number of cellular divisions, normal human cell populations have short lifetimes in culture with a limited range of possible passages or cell divisions. Since all the normal cells in this study are early passage cell populations (<27 passages), they may not be appropriate controls. The established tumor cell lines have been passaged many times and have reproducible characteristics. In a study of parallel primary cultures of mouse mammary normal, preneoplastic, and neoplastic cells, Beall et al.[11] have shown that normal cells have lower T1 values than cancer cells, just as they do

Table 101–8. WATER PROTON RELAXATION TIMES IN HUMAN NORMAL COLON CELLS[15]

Cells	(n)	Passage Number	T1 (ms)	T2 (ms)	%H$_2$O
Adult Non-involved:					
NBV	(2)	12	1214 ± 46	207 ± 7	92.3 ± 0.4
NBM	(3)	13	1009 ± 7	191 ± 3	91.4 ± 0.4
Fetal:					
Hs 0677	(2)	20	1058 ± 13	221 ± 3	90.6 ± 0.4
Hs 0074	(2)	27	1106 ± 24	163 ± 23	—

in whole tissue biopsies.[44] However, all three primary cell types had higher *T1* and hydration values than three established lines of mouse mammary cancer. Ling and Tucker[54] suggest that normal tissue slices may be used as controls for ascites cancer cells in the mouse and rat. Established cell lines in our study had *T1* values similar to cancer biopsies and were higher than normal tissues in the Koutcher et al.[53] study.

Distinction of Normal, Preoplastic, and Neoplastic Mouse Mammary Cells in Primary Cell Culture

The basis for differences in the relaxation times of water in normal and cancerous whole tissues is complicated by contributions from connective tissue, vascular fluids, tissue hydration levels, and lipid hydrogen signals from fat. Since we had shown earlier that the normal, preoplastic, and neoplastic mouse mammary *glands* could be distinguished on the basis of *T1* and *T2*,[44] we chose to prepare primary cell cultures of these tissues to determine whether NMR properties could distinguish the individual cell types as well. Enriched populations of epithelial cells without the extraneous materials of the tumor, rather than whole tissues, were compared. With cultures of epithelial cells, it was possible to distinguish normal, preoplastic, and neoplastic cells with a high degree of accuracy ($P < .001$) on the basis of water proton NMR relaxation times.

Mammary tissues from BALB/cCrgl female mice were aseptically removed and washed three to four times in HEPES-buffered Dulbecco's balance salt solution (DBSS), pH 7.3, and minced into 1 to 2 mm^3 pieces. The pieces were incubated in collagenase solution as described[4] to prepare isolated cells. The cells were washed and plated into flasks and incubated at 37°C in 92.5 percent air–7.5 percent CO_2 in Dulbecco's modified Eagle's medium (DMEM) with 13 percent fetal bovine serum and 5 μg per ml insulin. Cells were grown for 5 days and harvested for NMR measurements. Each type of primary culture was reinoculated into the mammary fat pads of 3-week-old syngeneic female mice and examined histologically after 8 weeks to demonstrate their morphogenic potential of either normal, preoplastic, or neoplastic growth.

Established mouse mammary tumor lines. ESD/BALB CL3, MTV-L/BALB DL2, and DMBA/BALB CL2[22] were grown in DMEM with 10 percent fetal bovine serum, 15 mM HEPES buffer and 10 gm per ml and 100 units per ml of streptomycin and penicillin at 37°C in 90 percent air–10 percent CO_2 for comparison studies.

Primary cell cultures and established cancer cell lines were coded and identified only after the *T1* and *T2* measurements were complete. After NMR measurements, the cell pellets were dried to a constant weight at 105°C to determine the grams of water per gram of dry solids (or percentage of H_2O). The experimental results in Table 101–9 show that after removal of fat, connective tissue, vascular elements, and necrotic regions through the use of primary cell culture, it still remains possible to distinguish among normal, preoplastic, and neoplastic mammary epithelial cells by NMR with a high degree of accuracy ($P < .001$). *T1* and *T2* values of preoplastic cells in primary cultures were consistently found to be intermediate between those of normal and neoplastic cells. The *T1* values of primary cultures initiated from 13- to 14-week-old preoplastic nodule outgrowths were similar to those of primary cultures derived from 16- to 17-week-old nodule transplants, even though tumors start to appear around 19 weeks of age. This may indicate that nodules (HANs) do not progress continuously toward the neoplastic state but may undergo abrupt spontaneous changes toward neoplasia at some critical age or size.

The results of this study with primary cell cultures were compared with *T1* and *T2* values of three established cell lines of mouse mammary tumors that had been

Table 101–9. NMR RELAXATION TIMES OF WATER IN NORMAL, PRENEOPLASTIC, AND NEOPLASTIC MOUSE MAMMARY TISSUES AND PRIMARY CELL CULTURES[11]

	Whole Tissue		Primary Cell Cultures*		
Cell Type	T1 (ms)	T2 (ms)	T1 (ms)	T2 (ms)	%H2O
Normal Pregnant	380 ± 41	39 ± 2	916 ± 24	158 ± 6	90.8 ± 0.4
Hyperplastic Alveolar Nodules (D2-HAN)	451 ± 21	53 ± 1	1029 ± 24 ($P < .005$)†	187 ± 7 ($P < .01$)	90.0 ± 0.5 ($P > .7$)
Mammary Adenocarcinoma (D2)	920 ± 47	91 ± 8	1155 ± 42 ($P < .001$)	206 ± 8 ($P < .001$)	91.4 ± 0.2 ($P > .3$)

* n = 15 samples of each type or a total of 45 samples
† P calculated between test group and normal group by a Student-t test

serially passaged in culture for more than 3 years[22] (see Table 101–5). All three lines displayed lower $T1$, $T2$, and water percentage values than the primary cell cultures. Two important points can be made from these data: (1) even in the established cell lines, $1/T1$ versus grams of water per gram of dry solids does not show a monotonic relationship (which would be expected if the NMR differences were due solely to hydration differences), and (2) the three established cell lines are different from one another, although they were all derived from mouse mammary adenocarcinomas. It is, therefore, invalid to compare directly established neoplastic cell lines with normal primary cultures used as controls. In the case of these experiments, established neoplastic cell lines would have shown lower $T1$ and $T2$ values than "normal" cells.

Several authors[34,39,46,49] have suggested that the mechanism of increased $T1$ and $T2$ values for water in cancer is a result of an increased hydration of the tumor tissue (relative to normal tissue). Although there now exist a number of papers that show that $1/T1$ does not always vary in a direct relationship with grams of water per gram of dry solids in animal tissues and human tissues[23,24,51,73] and cultured cells,[7,8] this interpretation is still often used as an explanation for the increases observed in $T1$ and $T2$ between normal, preneoplastic, and neoplastic cells. Moreover, the differences in $T1$ and $T2$ remain, even when there is no difference in hydration between the groups.

Identification of the preneoplastic or transformed state by other than histologic staining has proved difficult. Transformed fibroblasts, when present in a mixed culture with normal cells, can be detected and isolated from their untransformed neighbors by a number of criteria, including changes in size or shape, differential staining characteristics, and altered growth properties. In contrast, the quest for markers that will identify or select preneoplastic or malignant mammary epithelial cells from their normal counterparts has proved a long, arduous, and frequently frustrating task.[64] It is especially complicated because mammary tissues are composed of heterogeneous populations of epithelial cells. Differentiated mammary gland contains, in addition to stromal and vascular cells such as fibroblasts, lipocytes, and endothelial cells, three types of epithelial cells: ductal, alveolar, and myoepithelial. Markers that would permit identification of the three types of normal mammary epithelial cells under various in-vivo and in-vitro conditions would be invaluable for following the roles and fates of these cells during mammary dysplasias and tumorigenesis. The questions and points raised here are pertinent to interpretation of the NMR studies. The molecular basis for the differences in cultures of normal, HAN, and tumor cells obtained by NMR has not been established.

Despite this limitation, NMR studies provide revealing information in several areas and lay the foundation for future investigations. First, the data indicate that the degree of hydration is similar in the cells grown from normal, preneoplastic, and neoplastic tissues and that this parameter therefore is not responsible for the observed dissimilarities in NMR values. Second, the use of the primary cultures enabled us to establish that the differences found in the tissues are probably due to actual properties of the cells rather than to changes in stroma or fat content of the tissues. Third, as the growth rates and number of dividing cells in the three types of cultures are similar,[11] it is unlikely that the observed NMR differences can be explained by these factors.

It has been underscored repeatedly in investigations on cancer markers that striking differences exist between the properties of normal, preneoplastic, and neoplastic mammary cells in primary cultures and established mammary tumor culture lines. An example of this is found in the NMR studies in which the *T1* and *T2* water proton values for cultures of three tumor lines were shorter than those of all three types of primary cultures (Table 101–5). Cells of the established tumor lines also differ from primary culture cells, regardless of neoplastic state, in morphology. Their surface topographies, visualized by scanning electron microscopy,[63] agglutinability by lectins,[4] association with fibronectin,[5] response to cytochalasin B–induced multinucleation,[64] and intermediate filament composition,[3] are all different. Whether these phenotypic differences are due to adaptation to prolonged cultivation in an artificial environment, selection of a subpopulation, or a malignant progression of the cells is unclear. When the properties of mammary cells in vivo have been compared with those cells cultured in vitro, however, as in the NMR and fibronectin studies,[5] the results indicate a strong correlation between the characteristics of cells in the tissues and properties of cells in the primary cultures. Thus, for now, mammary cells in primary cultures are the in vitro system of choice for investigating markers and identifying features at the cellular level that reflect as closely as possible the phenotype of the cells in mammary tissues.

The mechanism for the increased relaxation times of water protons in neoplastic cells is presently unknown. One current explanation for the reduction of *T1* and *T2* values for water protons in living cells (i.e., compared with pure water, which has a *T1* of 3000 ms), involves the interaction of water molecules with macromolecular surfaces inside cells. Such intracellular components as membranes, chromatin, microtubules, intermediate filaments, and microfilaments may interact with water to reduce the average motional freedom of cellular water. Antibody immunofluorescence and electron microscopic analysis of microfilaments and microtubules in normal, preneoplastic, and neoplastic mouse mammary cells revealed no differences in these components among the three cell types.[3] In contrast, studies of the protein constituents of intermediate filaments in the three types of mammary cells by two-dimensional gel electrophoresis revealed that the tumor cells were missing about three to five protein bands that were present in preparations from normal and preneoplastic cells.[3] Interlaced filamentous protein lattices such as the microtrabeculae described by Wolosewick and Porter[86] may interact with water and reduce its mobility by increasing macromolecular surface interactions.

THE SYSTEMIC EFFECT OF PRENEOPLASTIC, BENIGN, AND CANCEROUS DISEASE ON UNINVOLVED TISSUES AND SERA

The Systemic Effect in Tissues

ANIMAL MODELS

The utilization of NMR to study the transformed state has resulted in an interesting by-product. Since the presence of a tumor may result in physiologic changes throughout the body of an animal, it is not surprising that changes in the NMR properties of water in distant organs and the sera are found in tumor bearing animals. Investigators utilizing NMR scanning devices should be aware that these changes may be reflected in their data.

The discovery by Schlottman and Rubenow[80] that uninvolved tissues in animals bearing tumors could have higher than normal water contents was followed by the discovery of Frey et al.[42] that some uninvolved organs in an animal bearing a tumor could demonstrate elevated spin-lattice relaxation times (*T1*) for water protons when compared with the same organs in animals without tumors. This phenomenon was termed the *systemic effect*. In Frey's study, MCI tumors were transplanted to the hind leg muscles of C3H/HeJ mice and allowed to grow for 6 to 10 days to palpable size. The results of the study, shown in Table 101–10, demonstrate the type of conclusions typical of a study of the systemic effect of transplanted tumors. Usually one finds that (1) the *T1* of water protons in the tumor is longer than in the comparable normal tissue from a nontumor-bearing animal, (2) other tissues in the tumor-bearing animal may also have slightly elevated *T1* values compared with control nontumor-bearing animals, and (3) infectious diseases and bodily stress do not cause such changes.

Frey et al. concluded that the elevated *T1* values in distant organs ". . . may imply that some chemical or biological intermediate is introduced into the bloodstream during growth of the neoplasm, acting directly or indirectly to bring about changes in water structure in non-malignant tissues. Isolation of this intermediate, the effect of which we observe through *T1*, may turn out to be a useful diagnostic tool."[42]

Frey's results were followed by a series of investigations supporting these findings of elevated water relaxation times in tissues of tumor-bearing animals[42] (Table 101–11).

Table 101–10. ELEVATION OF WATER PROTON SPIN-LATTICE RELAXATION TIME (*T1*) IN THE SERA OF ANIMALS WITH VARIOUS CANCERS

Animal	Serum-Normal	Serum-Cancerous	Reference
Mouse	*T1* (ms) (Blood Plasma)	*T1* (ms)	
(Ehrlich Ascites)			
Day 1	1370	1580	40
Day 2	1370	1380	
Day 3	1370	1580	
Day 4	1370	1580	
Day 5	1370	1610	
Rat			
(Morris Hepatoma)	*T1* = (*T1* can − *T1* norm)		
Day 5	+45 ms		47
Day 8	+0 ms		
Day 12	+55 ms		
Day 15	+60 ms		
Day 20	+55 ms		
Day 21	+75 ms		
Day 28	+100 ms		
Day 40	+160 ms		
Day 46	+210 ms		
Rat	*Control*	*Carcinogen Treated*	
1 week (A)	750 ms	770 ms	40
2 weeks (A)	740 ms	780 ms	
4 weeks (A)	700 ms	810 ms	
4 weeks (A)	770 ms	780 ms	
Human			
Leukemia (active)			
Serum	1230 ± 170 (n = 7)	—	36
Plasma	1260 ± 60 (n = 7)	1105 ± 100 (n = 10)	
Leukemia (remission)	1230 ± 170 (n = 7)	1170 ± 100	
Carcinoma of cervix	1230 ± 170	1230 ± 90 (n = 15)	
Carcinoma of breast	1230 ± 170	1260 ± 80	

Table 101–11. SPIN-LATTICE RELAXATION TIME ($T1$) IN NONINVOLVED TISSUES OF ANIMALS WITH CANCERS

Animal & Type of Cancer	Tissue	$T1$ (ms) of Nontumor Bearing Animal	$T1$ (ms) of Tumor Bearing Animal	Reference
Mouse (MCI-tumor) $T1 = 853 \pm 19$ ms	Heart	650 ± 6	705 ± 5	42
	Brain	646 ± 4	618 ± 41	
	Lung	641 ± 9	665 ± 47	
	Muscle	615 ± 10	643 ± 10	
	Spleen	571 ± 8	731 ± 8	
	Kidney	470 ± 6	601 ± 19	
	Liver	386 ± 13	461 ± 9	
	Skin	390 ± 39	442 ± 37	
	Intestine	366 ± 19	399 ± 29	
	Stomach	294 ± 23	317 ± 29	
Mouse (MH134-tumor)	Muscle	850	880	48
	Liver	420	480	
Mouse (Fibrosarcoma) $T1 = 1000$ ms	Brain	840	930	34
	Liver	243–262	293–357	
	Kidney	272–307	337–422	
	Liver Mitochondria	354	701	
Rat (Rhabdomyosarcoma R)	Liver	467 ± 26	556	21
	Muscle	850 ± 29	882	
	Kidney	668 ± 31	811	
	Spleen	582 ± 18	686	
Rat (Adenocarcinoma 4658) $T1 = 1138$ ms	Liver	467 ± 26	628	21
	Muscle	850 ± 29	894	
Rat (Reticulum sarcoma 2880) $T1 = 1138$ ms	Liver	467 ± 26	652	21
	Muscle	850 ± 29	921	
Rat (Adenocarcinoma 3207) $T1 = 1279$ ms	Liver	467 ± 26	528	21
	Muscle	850 ± 29	903	
Mouse (Mammary carcinoma C3H)	Liver	341 ± 5	335 ± 28	49
	Spleen	523 ± 7	492 ± 27	
	Kidney	452 ± 5	463 ± 19	
	Muscle	590 ± 8	599 ± 25	
		ΔT1 between normal and tumor bearing after 46 days		
Rat (Morris hepatoma— leg 3924A)	Liver	up 120 ms		47
	Kidney	up 75 ms		
	Spleen	up 140 ms		
	Heart	no change		
	Skeletal muscle	no change		
Mouse (C3H) $T1 = 887 \pm 4$ ms	Liver	438 ± 36	468 ± 35	45
	Spleen	737 ± 6	734 ± 12	
	Kidney	503 ± 11	577 ± 14	
Mouse (C3Hf) $T1 = 906 \pm 43$ ms	Liver	412 ± 12	374 ± 25	
	Spleen	671 ± 9	716 ± 7	
	Kidney	551 ± 9	537 ± 17	
Human Esophageal adenocarcinoma $T1 = 959 \pm 39$	Noninvolved esophagus	797 ± 39		75
	Tissue near tumor		1042, 1018	
Human Colon cancer $T1 = 620 \pm 58$	Colon	330 ± 129	elevated	53
Human Gastrointestinal tumors $T1 = 644 \pm 136$	GI tract	416 ± 103	612 ± 123	43

Table 101–11. SPIN-LATTICE RELAXATION TIME (*T1*) IN NONINVOLVED TISSUES
OF ANIMALS WITH CANCERS (*continued*)

Animal & Type of Cancer	Tissue	*T1* (ms) of Nontumor Bearing Animal	*T1* (ms) of Tumor Bearing Animal	Reference
Mouse	Liver	341 ± 5	347 ± 7	49
(Isoimplants of C3H)	Spleen	523 ± 7	551 ± 24	
	Kidney	452 ± 5	448 ± 10	
	Muscle	590 ± 8	586 ± 7	
Mouse	Liver	(Normal)	(Treated)	40
(Injected	Day 1	700	820	
ascites-	Day 2	800	830	
Ehrlich)	Day 3	750	790	
	Day 4			
	Day 5	500	720	
	Blood			
	Day 1	1380	1580	
	Day 2	1380	1380	
	Day 3	1380	1580	
	Day 4	1380	1580	
	Day 5	1380	1610	
Mouse	Liver	225 ± 5	283 ± 8	47
(Lymphosarcoma	Kidney	322 ± 11	365 ± 23	
6C3HED)	Muscle	465 ± 49	458 ± 51	
T1 = 674 ± 10 ms				

Hollis et al.[47] conducted a study to follow the time-dependent changes in *T1* after the injection of a Morris hepatoma in the hind leg of a rat. Liver, spleen, and kidney tissues demonstrated elevated *T1* values during the course of tumor growth, while heart and skeletal muscle did not. The same paper reported elevated *T1* times in the liver and kidneys of mice with lymphosarcoma.

Floyd et al.[39] reported on two groups of rats fed a fast-acting carcinogen or a slow-acting carcinogen for 4 weeks. Only the fast-acting carcinogen produced elevated liver *T1* values after 4 weeks of treatment, when preneoplastic nodules were apparent in the liver. *T1* values for spleen displayed an unusual behavior that could be correlated with detectable iron levels in that organ.[20,32,39]

Human Tissues

The systemic effect has also been detected in humans having various types of tumors. Goldsmith et al.[43] found, in a survey of various types of human gastrointestinal tumors, that the *T1* value for tumors (644 ± 136 ms) was distinguishable from the *T1* of normal colon tissue removed from bodies not bearing tumors (416 ± 103 ms). However, pathologically normal tissues taken from the sites adjacent to or far from the tumor had *T1* values of 612 ± 123 ms, apparently demonstrating the systemic effect. In a followup to this study, Koutcher et al.[53] showed specifically that for tumors of the colon *T1* times were 620 ± 58 ms and for normal human colon *T1* was 330 ± 129 ms. However, all apparently normal colon samples taken from cancer patients had elevated *T1* values.

In a study of squamous cell carcinoma and adenocarcinomas of the esophagus, Ranade et al. detected elevated *T1* values for grossly uninvolved tissues (*T1* = 1042, 1018 ms), while tissues away from the tumor had *T1* times of 797 ± 39 ms.[75]

The evidence in this study suggests that the systemic effect of elevated *T1* and *T2* relaxation times, owing to cancer in the host, also exists in humans; but it is impossible to draw conclusions concerning the mechanisms of the systemic effect from such investigations. The following generalizations, however, may be made: (1) In all types of cancers studied in a number of animal models, at least one uninvolved organ and sometimes a number of organs demonstrate elevated $T1$ values; (2) $T2$ values have only occasionally shown an elevation in animals with cancer; and (3) the magnitude of the effect differs with the type of cancer and animal species.

The Systemic Effect in Sera

While investigators were exploring the phenomenon of elevated $T1$ values of uninvolved organs of cancer-bearing organisms, Floyd et al.[40] found that this phenomenon extended to the serum as well. It has been suggested by Frey et al.[42] that cancer cells might secrete some substance into the blood that would travel to distant organs and cause the elevated $T1$ values seen in the systemic effect. Economou et al.[34] had also stated that preliminary evidence in their laboratory suggested that $T1$ might be elevated for the sera of human cancer victims.

In a careful study, Floyd et al.[40] inoculated mice intraperitoneally with living and dead Ehrlich-Lettre ascites cells. Mouse plasma $T1$ values in response to live tumor cells were elevated 14 to 19 percent on the first day after injection, fell to approximately normal on day 2, and then rose steadily to a level of 6 to 8 percent above normal by the fifth day (see Table 101–11). Hollis et al.[47] studied the time course of changes in the serum $T1$ in rats with Morris hepatoma implanted in their hind legs. Serum $T1$ values above the control were detected from day 1 through the 46 days of the experiment. The final $T1$ values were 210 msec above the original control $T1$ values. The $T1$ values increased proportionally with the size of the tumor after day 8 of the experiment (see Table 101–12). Floyd et al.[39] returned to this interesting problem in rats fed fast and slow acting liver carcinogens for up to 4 weeks. The $T1$ of sera in animals fed the fast acting carcinogen was significantly elevated after 4 weeks but was not elevated in the slow acting carcinogen fed animals (see Table 101–11).

Additional experiments were undertaken in our laboratory on an animal model to determine if the systemic effect could be useful in cancer detection by NMR. A detailed examination of these studies may elucidate some of the problems and potentials of this phenomenon. Our study was designed to follow the effect of benign and malignant tumors on serum $T1$ values. Since Hazlewood et al.[44] had already been able to distinguish between normal, preneoplastic, and malignant mouse mammary cancer tissue by NMR techniques (Table 101–2), we thought the mammary cancer system would be

Table 101–12. SPIN-LATTICE RELAXATION TIME ($T1$) OF WATER IN SERA OF NORMAL, DISEASED, AND CANCER-BEARING MICE[10]

Group	$T1$ (Mean ± SD ± SE)† (n)*	(ms)	Total Serum Iron (µg%)	Total Serum Protein (mg%)	P Value‡ Vs. Normal for $T1$
Normal virgins	(24)	1554 ± 93 ± 19	229	4.95	
Mammary duct hyperplasia (CDH-1)	(4)	1575 ± 44 ± 22	—	—	<.5
Ductal papilloma (benign)	(4)	1719 ± 44 ± 22	—	—	<.005
Preneoplastic alveolar nodules (C4)	(14)	1564 ± 48 ± 13	210	5.60	<.5
Mammary carcinoma	(17)	1801 ± 189 ± 46	229	5.60	<.001
Protein malnourished	(5)	1565 ± 13 ± 6	214	3.80	<.5

* n = Number of animals in pooled and individual samples
† Mean ± SD ± SE = mean ± standard deviation ± standard error of the mean
‡ P = calculated according to Students-t test with P tables

excellent for determination of the effect of the malignant and preneoplastic states on serum $T1$ values. A benign ductal papilloma arising from mammary ductal hyperplasia was also studied. The effects of whole body stress from low protein diets, serum iron levels, and serum protein concentrations were included in the study. This experiment showed a significant early elevation of serum $T1$ values in malignant and benign tumor bearing animals. No detectable difference from normal controls was seen for ductal hyperplasia or the preneoplastic state of mammary cancer in the early stages of tumorigenesis (Table 101–12). Sera collected from 24 normal virgin mice had a mean water proton spin-lattice relaxation time ($T1$) of 1554 ± 93 ms. The low standard deviation indicates that normal mouse serum has a reproducible spin-lattice relaxation time. The sera of animals with transplanted papillary ductal hyperplasias and preneoplastic alveolar nodules showed no significant difference from normal mouse serum (see Table 101–12). The sera of mice with developed benign mammary ductal papilloma ($T1$ = 1719 ± 44 ms) and malignant mammary adenocarcinoma ($T1$ = 1801 ± 189 ms) were clearly distinct from sera or normal control mice. Serum iron values between the groups showed no significant difference.

Total serum protein determinations on pooled normal and preneoplastic nodule sera were compared with the mean of four determinations of malignant mammary cancer sera. No significant difference was seen that could account for the elevation of $T1$. In fact, the slightly higher protein concentration would, according to Hollis,[47] tend to lower the $T1$. Nearly the same serum protein concentration was found in groups of mice bearing two types of preneoplastic nodules and two types of malignant tumors. In order to lower serum protein concentration in living animals, a protein-deficient diet was provided. Sera from mice on a protein-free, all glucose diet for 5 days did have a lower serum protein concentration (3.8 gm per dl compared with 4.95 gm per dl for normal mice), but their serum $T1$ values were indistinguishable from normal. Certainly, these data do not support the idea that serum $T1$ values are *only* a function of protein and water concentration. Recent work in Italy[65] suggests a difference in electrophoretic patterns of serum proteins between normal and cancer patients. Thus, relative amounts of different proteins may control $T1$ more than the total amount of protein does.

The conclusions of this study and others in our laboratory were that both benign and malignant mammary carcinomas could produce elevated $T1$ values in serum and uninvolved organs. The malignant state produced the highest elevation of serum $T1$ and there was no elevation in the preneoplastic state or studied disease states (Table 101–12).

THE SYSTEMIC EFFECT IN THE SERA OF HUMANS WITH CANCER

Ekstrand et al.[36] investigated a small number of sera and white blood cells of humans with active leukemia, leukemia in remission, carcinoma of the cervix, and carcinoma of the breast. They found no difference in the sera or plasma $T1$ values between normal and cancer patients (Table 101–11). Leukocyte $T1$ values were elevated only in patients in the active phase of leukemia. This study, however, suffers from several problems common to research in humans. Normal sera taken from only seven individuals had a greater range of values and standard deviation than those of the cancer patients. This may be an indication that serum $T1$ values vary as a function of age, sex, and other human variables. Control groups must be matched to the patient group before one can say there are no significant differences. In addition, when dealing with human populations, sample size should be increased to fully explore trends in the data.

A study in our laboratory sought to determine whether the systemic effect of an elevation of $T1$ in the serum also occurs in humans with cancer and to determine whether this effect is of enough significance to be useful in the detection of cancer in human beings. Samples of human sera were collected from several sources, including fresh serum samples drawn from female volunteers, a group of frozen human sera from normal males and females, sera from breast cancer patients, preoperative blood bank sera from breast cancer patients, and a sampling of preoperative sera from many human cancers. Serum protein concentrations were determined with a refractometer calibrated against solutions of bovine serum albumin. The results are summarized in Table 101–13.

Both normal groups of males and females showed an unusually reproducible mean value, although the samples were taken from men and women of all ages, races, and weights, were measured fresh or from frozen samples of up to 3 years, and were taken at all times of the day. Normal females had a mean serum $T1$ value of 1534 ± 178 ms. The large variance may reflect the differences in the samples. Preoperative sera of females entering the hospital for the primary removal of a palpable breast nodule showed $T1$ values of 1612 ± 45 ms compared with a matched control sample of women with a serum $T1$ of 1535 ± 59 ms. Such preliminary results can only be indicative, but it appears that very small tumors (<1 cm in diameter) may be detectable by an elevated serum $T1$ value if proper control groups are available. In a large group of female breast cancer patients who had complete removal of the involved breast, months to years before recurrence of cancer, serum $T1$ values reflected the state of the disease as follows. Patients known to have cancer, but being treated with chemotherapy and radiation (and classified as being in remission) showed a mean serum $T1$ value of 1460 ± 91 ms, somewhat below that of the normal group. Since cell division is often retarded by such management, it is possible to speculate about an interesting mechanism for the lower $T1$ values related to products of rapidly dividing cells. Serum protein concentrations in all groups were similar, except for those patients with active metastases. Patients with active cancer recurrence responding somewhat to drugs and radiation (but not in remission) demonstrate an elevated mean serum $T1$ value of 1618 ± 112 ms. Patients who are not responding to treatment and have active metastases to various organs such as lung, liver, and brain display a definitely elevated mean serum $T1$ value of 1734 ± 71 ms. These patients also have a lowered serum protein value compared with normals.

The preliminary results in human mammary cancer suggest that whatever mechanism is operating in the mouse mammary cancer system may also be operative in humans. Table 101–14 provides additional information concerning the systemic effect in humans by showing that serum $T1$ values of 1688 ± 105 ms may be found in a sampling of humans with cancer of many different organs.

Table 101–13. ELEVATION OF $T1$ IN SERA OF HUMANS WITH BREAST CANCER[13]

Sample Groups	Number of Samples (n)	Mean $T1$* (ms)	Mean $T1$ (ms)	Serum Protein (mg/ml)
Normal females (fresh)	(10)	1,535 ± 59	—	—
Normal males (frozen)	(30)	1,503 ± 146	488 ± 63	7.8 ± 1.0
Normal females (frozen)	(30)	1,534 ± 178	475 ± 68	7.8 ± 1.5
Biopsy females (small tumors, preoperative)	(10)	1,612 ± 45	—	—
Patients in remission (chemotherapy + radiation)	(20)	1,460 ± 91	474 ± 46	7.7 ± 0.9
Patients with cancer (but on drugs, not in remission)	(22)	1,618 ± 112	491 ± 61	7.1 ± 1.3
Patients with metastases (at time serum was taken)	(5)	1,734 ± 71	551 ± 46	6.5 ± 0.6

* Mean ± SD

Table 101—14. SERUM SPIN-LATTICE RELAXATION TIME (*T1*) OF HUMANS WITH VARIOUS CANCERS[13]

Type of Cancer		Serum *T1* (ms)
Normal sera		(1,535 ± 59)
Meningioma of the brain		1,615
Carcinoma of the lung	(A)	1,648
	(B)	1,642
	(C)	1,658
Carcinoma of the chest wall		1,513
Carcinoma of the kidney	(A)	1,669
	(B)	1,656
Carcinoma of the lymph node	(A)	1,583
	(B) metastatic	1,690
	(C)	1,852
Squamous carcinoma of the lymph node		1,632
Carcinoma of the omentum		1,906
Carcinoma of the prostate		1,798
Ovarian adenocarcinoma		1,743
Carcinoma of the colon		1,802
Adenocarcinoma of the small bowel		1,605
	Mean	1,688
	SD	105
	SE	21

This study has shown preliminary results that indicate that the systemic effect of elevated serum *T1* values may occur in humans with cancer, as in animal model systems. Disagreement with the study of Ekstrand et al.[36] may be a function of type of cancer, sample size, and lack of matched control groups. The question remains as to whether results in humans are significant enough to be useful in the early detection of cancer. At present, it appears that serum *T1* values are only definitely elevated during active metastases. In order to fully answer this question, it will be necessary to design much more careful studies in humans, where the members of a group are matched by sex, age, weight, race, state of health, and time of day the serum was drawn. Once proper normal control values are established for these groups, it will be possible to determine whether cancer patients have *T1* values for serum above those for their specific control group. The potential of this phenomenon as an inexpensive, low-risk, and quick, preliminary screening method for cancer detection in humans makes it important that additional research be done.

The additional possibility of utilizing easily obtained serum samples to monitor the state of remission and onset of recurrence in cancer patients encourages continued research in this area. Recent results with ^{31}P NMR spectroscopy in serum from cancer patients suggest the possibility of an inexpensive screening tool for occult malignancy.[88]

References

1. American Cancer Society. Cancer Facts and Figures 1980.
2. Asch BB, Leonardi C, Burstein NA, Rubin RW: Analysis of cytoskeletal models from normal and neoplastically transformed cells. J Cell Biol *83*:470a, 1970.
3. Asch B, Medina D, Brinkley BR: Microtubule and actin containing filaments of normal, preneoplastic, and neoplastic mouse mammary gland. Cancer Res *39*:893, 1979.
4. Asch B, Medina D: Concanavalin A—induced agglutinability of normal, preneoplastic, and neoplastic mouse mammary cells. J Natl Cancer Inst *61*:1423, 1978.
5. Asch BB, Kamat B, Burstein NA: Deposition of fibronectin in normal, dysplastic, and malignant mammary tissues and cell cultures. Cancer Res *41*:2115, 1981.
6. Banerjee M: Hormonal control of DNA synthesis: Altered responsiveness of hyperplastic alveolar nodules of mouse mammary gland. J Natl Cancer Inst *42*:227, 1969.

7. Beall PT, Hazlewood CF, Rao PN: Nuclear magnetic resonance patterns of intracellular water as a function of HeLa cell cycle. Science *192*:904, 1976.
8. Beall PT, Hazlewood CF, Rao PN: Non-linearity of relaxation times versus water content. Science *194*:213, 1976.
9. Beall PT, Cailleau RM, Hazlewood CF: The relaxation times of water protons and division rates in human breast cancer cells: A possible relationship to survival. Physiol Chem Phys *8*:281, 1976.
10. Beall PT, Medina D, Chang DC, Seitz PK, Hazlewood CF: A systemic effect of benign and malignant mammary cancer on the spin-lattice relaxation time, $T1$, of water protons in mouse serum. J Natl Cancer Inst *59*:1431, 1977.
11. Beall PT, Asch BB, Chang DC, Medina D, Hazlewood CF: Distinction of normal, preneoplastic, and neoplastic mouse mammary primary cell cultures by water nuclear magnetic relaxation times. J Natl Cancer Inst *64*:335, 1980.
12. Beall PT, Chang DC, Hazlewood CF: Proton NMR relaxation times of water in contact and noncontact inhibited cells. Fed Proc *39*:1758, 1980.
13. Beall PT, Asch BB, Medina D, Hazlewood CF: Distinction of normal, preneoplastic and neoplastic mouse mammary cells and tissues by nuclear magnetic resonance techniques. *In* Cameron I, Pool T (eds): The Transformed Cell. New York, Academic Press, 1981, pp 293–325.
14. Beall PT, Medina D, Hazlewood CF: The systemic effect of elevated tissue and serum relaxation times for water in animals and humans with cancer. *In* Diehl P, Fluck E, Kosfeld R (eds): NMR Basic Principles and Progress. Vol. 19. Heidelberg, Springer Verlag, 1981, pp 39–57.
15. Beall PT, Hazlewood CF, Rutzky LP: NMR relaxation times of water protons in human colon cell lines and clones. Cancer Biochem Biophys *6*:7, 1982.
16. Beall PT, Brinkley BR, Chang DC, Hazlewood CF: Microtubule complexes correlated with growth rate and water proton relaxation times in human breast cancer cells. Cancer Res *42*:4124, 1982.
17. Bentvedzen P, Brinkhof J, Westenbrink F: Expression of endogenous mammary tumor virus in mice. *In* Essex H, Todaso T (eds): Viruses in Naturally Occurring Cancers. Cold Spring Harbor Laboratory, NY 1980.
18. Bern HA, Nandi S: Recent studies of the hormonal influence in mouse mammary tumorigenesis. Prog Exp Tumor Res *2*:90, 1961.
19. Blair PB: The mammary tumor virus (MTV). Curr Top Microbiol Immunol *45*:1, 1968.
20. Block RE: Factors affecting proton magnetic resonable linewidths of water in several rat tissues. FEBS Letters *34*:109, 1973.
21. Bovee W, Huisman P, Smidt J: Tumor detection and nuclear magnetic resonance. J Natl Cancer Inst *52*:595, 1974.
22. Butel JS, Dudley JP, Medina D, et al.: Comparison of the growth properties *in vitro* and transplantability of continuous mouse mammary tumor cell lines and clonal derivatives. Cancer Res *37*:1892, 1977.
23. Chaughule RS, Kasturi SR, Vijayaraghavan R, Ranade SS: Normal and malignant tissues—an investigation by pulsed nuclear magnetic resonance. Indian J Biochem Biophys *11*:256, 1974.
24. Chaughule RS, Kasturi SR, Ranade SS: Proton spin-lattice relaxation times and water content in human tissues. Proc Nucl Phys Solid State Phys Sym *17c*:1974.
25. Cottam G, Vasek A, Lusted D: Water proton relaxation rates in various tissues. Res Comm Chem Pathol Pharmacol *4*:495, 1972.
26. Cramer W: On the biochemical mechanism of growth. J Physiol *50*:322, 1916.
27. Damadian R: Tumor detection by nuclear magnetic resonance. Science *171*:1151, 1971.
28. Damadian R, Zaner K, Hor D: Human tumors by NMR. Physiol Chem Phys *5*:381, 1973.
29. Damadian R, Zaner K, Hor D: Human tumors detected by nuclear magnetic resonance. Proc Natl Acad Sci USA *71*:1471, 1974.
30. Daniel CW, DeOme KB, Young LJT, Blair PB, Faulkin LJ: The *in vivo* lifespan of normal and preneoplastic mouse mammary glands. A serial transplantation study. Proc Natl Acad Sci *61*:52, 1968.
31. DeOme KB, Faulkin LJ Jr, Bern HA, Blair PB: Development of mammary tumors from hyperplastic alveolar nodules transplanted into gland-free mammary fat pads of female C3H mice. Cancer Res *19*:515, 1959.
32. Dodd HJF: Electron spin resonance study of changes during the development of a mouse myeloid leukemia. I. Paramagnetic metal ions. Br J Cancer *32*:108, 1975.
33. Downing JE, Christopherson WM, Broghamer WL: Nuclear content during carcinogenesis. Cancer *15*:1176, 1962.
34. Economou JS, Parks LC, Saryan LA, Hollis DP, Czeisler JL, Eggleston JC: Detection of malignancy by nuclear magnetic resonance. Surg Forum *24*:127, 1973.
35. Eggleston JC, Saryan LA, Hollis DP: Nuclear magnetic resonance investigations of human neoplastic and abnormal non-neoplastic tissues. Cancer Res *35*:1326, 1975.
36. Ekstrand KE, Dixon RL, Raker M, Ferree CF: Proton NMR relaxation in the peripheral blood of cancer patients. Phys Med Biol *22*:925, 1977.
37. Faulkin LJ Jr, DeOme KB: The effect of estradiol and cortisol on the transplantability and subsequent fate of normal, hyperplastic, and tumorous mammary tissue of C3H mice. Cancer Res *18*:51, 1958.
38. Faulkin LJ Jr, DeOme KB: Regulation of growth and spacing of gland elements in the mammary fat pads of the C3H mouse. J Natl Cancer Inst *24*:953, 1960.
39. Floyd RA, Yoshida T, Leigh JS: Changes in tissue water proton relaxation rates during early phases of chemical carcinogenesis. Proc Natl Acad Sci *72*:56, 1975.

40. Floyd RA, Leigh JS, Chance B, Miko M: Time course of tissue water proton spin-lattice relaxation in mice developing ascites tumor. Cancer Res *34*:89, 1974.

41. Foote FW, Stewart FW: Comparative study of cancerous versus non-cancerous breasts. Ann Surg *121*:6, 1945.

42. Frey HW, Knispel RR, Kruvv J, et al.: Proton spin-lattice relaxation studies of non-malignant tissues of tumorous mice. J Natl Cancer Inst *49*:903, 1972.

43. Goldsmith M, Koutcher J, Damadian R: NMR in cancer. XI. Application of NMR malignancy index to human gastro-intestinal tumors. Cancer *41*:183, 1978.

44. Hazlewood CF, Chang DC, Medina D, Cleveland G, Nichols BL: Distinction between the preneoplastic and neoplastic state of murine mammary glands. Proc Natl Acad Sci *69*:1478, 1972.

45. Hazlewood CF, Cleveland G, Medina D: Relationship between hydration and proton nuclear magnetic resonance relaxation times in tissues of tumor bearing and non-tumor bearing mice: Implications for cancer detection. J Natl Cancer Inst *52*:1849, 1974.

46. Hollis DP, Economou J, Parks L, Eggleston JC, Saryan LA, Czeisler JL: Nuclear magnetic resonance studies of several experimental and human malignant tumors. Cancer Res *33*:2156, 1973.

47. Hollis DP, Saryan LA, Economou JS: Nuclear magnetic resonance studies of cancer. V. Appearance and development of a tumor systemic effect in serum and tissues. J Natl Cancer Inst *53*:807, 1974.

48. Iijima N, Saitoo S, Yoshida Y, et al.: Spin-echo nuclear magnetic resonance in cancerous tissue. Physiol Chem Phys *5*:431, 1973.

49. Inch WR, McCredie A, Knispel RR: Water content and proton spin relaxation time for neoplastic and non-neoplastic tissues from mice and humans. J Natl Cancer Inst *52*:353, 1974.

50. Jensen HM, Rice JR, Wellings SR: Preneoplastic lesions in the human breast. Science *191*:295, 1976.

51. Kasturi SR, Ranade S, Shah S: Tissue hydration of malignant and uninvolved human tissues and its relevance to proton spin-lattice mechanism. Proc Indian Acad Sci *84*:60, 1976.

52. Kiricuta IC, Simplanceanu V: Tissue water content and nuclear magnetic resonance in normal and tumor tissue. Cancer Res *35*:1167, 1975.

53. Koutcher JA, Goldsmith M, Damadian R: NMR in Cancer X. A malignancy index to discriminate normal and cancerous tissue. Cancer *41*:174, 1978.

54. Ling GN, Tucker M: Nuclear magnetic resonance and water contents in normal mouse and rat tissues and in cancer cells. J Natl Cancer Inst *64*:1199, 1980.

55. McDivitt RW, Stewart FW, Berg JW: Tumors of the breast. *In* Atlas of Tumor Pathology. Armed Forces Institute of Pathology, Second Series, Fascicle 2, 1968.

56. McEwen IID, Haven FL: Effect of carcinosarcoma 256 on the water content of liver. Cancer Res *1*:148, 1974.

57. Medina D: Mammary tumorigenesis in chemical carcinogen-treated mice. I. Incidence in Balb/c and C57BL mice. J Natl Cancer Inst *53*:213, 1974.

58. Medina D: Mammary tumorigenesis in chemical carcinogen-treated mice. II. Dependence on hormone stimulation for tumorigenesis. J Natl Cancer Inst *53*:223, 1974.

59. Medina D, DeOme KB: Effects of various oncogenic agents on the tumor-producing capabilities of the D series of Balb/c mammary nodule outgrowth lines. J Natl Cancer Inst *45*:353, 1970.

60. Medina D, Young L, DeOme KB: The tumor-producing capabilities of hyperplastic alveolar nodules occurring in virgin and pituitary-stimulated Balb/cfC3H and C3Hf mice. J Natl Cancer Inst *44*:167, 1970.

61. Medina D, Stockman G, Griswold D: Significance of chemical carcinogen-induced immuno-suppression in mammary tumorigenesis in Balb/c mice. Cancer Res *34*:2663, 1974.

62. Medina D, Hazlewood CF, Cleveland GG, Chang DC, Spjut HJ, Moyers R: Nuclear magnetic resonance studies on human breast dysplasias and neoplasms. J Natl Cancer Inst *54*:813, 1975.

63. Medina D, Asch BB, Brinkley BR, Mace ML Jr: *In vivo* and *in vitro* models for transformation of breast cells. *In* Brennan MI, Rich M, McGrath C (eds): Breast Cancer: New Concepts in Etiology and Control. New York, Academic Press, 1979, pp 53–66.

64. Medina D, Oborn CJ, Asch BB: Distinction between preneoplastic and neoplastic mammary cell populations in vitro by cytochalasin B-induced multinucleation. Cancer Res *40*:329, 1980.

65. Mela GS, Bianco B, Drago GP, Marchesi M, Martini C, Reghitto MR, Ridella S, Sacchetti C: Differences in the hydration of blood serum proteins between normal and untreated cancer human subjects. IRCS Medical Science *7*:537, 1979.

66. Mellors RC, Kupfer A, Hollender A: Quantitative cytology and cytopathology. Cancer *6*:372, 1953.

67. Nandi S: Interactions among hormonal, viral, and genetic factors in mouse mammary tumorigenesis. Proc Can Cancer Res Conf *6*:69, 1966.

68. Nandi S, McGrath CM: Mammary neoplasia in mice. Adv Cancer Res *17*:353, 1973.

69. Potter KF, Slimbaugh WP, Woodward SC: Can breast cancer be anticipated? A followup of benign breast biopsies. Ann Surg *167*:839, 1968.

70. Prehn RT: Function of depressed immunologic reactivity during carcinogenesis. J Natl Cancer Inst *31*:791, 1963.

71. Ratkovic S, Rusov C: Magnetic relaxation of water protons in the detection of tissue changes induced by erythroleukosis. Period Biol *76*:19, 1974.

72. Ranade SS, Chaughule S, Kasturi SR: Pulsed nuclear magnetic resonance studies on human malignant tissues and cells *in vitro*. Indian J Biochem Biophys *12*:229, 1975.

73. Ranade SS, Shah S, Korgaonkar KS, Kasturi SR, Chaughule RS, Vijayaraghavan R: Absence of cor-

relation between spin-lattice relaxation times and water content in human tumor tissue. Physiol Chem Phys 8:131, 1976.

75. Ranade SS, Shah S, Advani SH, Kasturi SR: Pulsed nuclear magnetic resonance studies of human bone marrow. Physiol Chem 9:297, 1977.

75. Ranade SS, Shah S, Talwalkar GV: Histopathological evidence in support of the association of elevated proton spin-lattice relaxation times with the malignant state. Tumori 65:157, 1979.

76. Russo J, Saby, I, Isenberg WM, Russo IH: Pathogenesis of mammary carcinomas induced in rats by 7, 12-dimethylbenzanthracene. J Natl Cancer Inst 59:435, 1977.

77. Saprin AN, Nagler LG, Koperina YV, Kriglyakova KY, Emanuel NM: Kinetics of change in the content of free radicals in both blood organs of mice with experimental leukemia. II. Biofizika 11:706, 1976.

78. Sarayan LA, Hollis DP, Economou JS, Eggleston JC: Nuclear magnetic resonance studies of cancer: IV. Correlation of water content with tissue relaxation times. J Natl Cancer Inst 52:599, 1974.

79. Schara M, Sentjuro M, Auersperg M, Golouh R: Characterization of malignant thyroid gland tissue by magnetic resonance methods. Br J Cancer 29:483, 1974.

80. Schlottman H, Rubenow W: Uber der wassergehalt der gewebe normaler und krebskranker ratten. Z Krebsforsch 36:120, 1932.

81. Schmidt K, Breitmaier E, Aeikens B: Spingitter relaxationzeit der protonen des zellwassers in normalen und tumorosen geweben des menschen. Z Krebsforch 80:209, 1973.

82. Storer JB: Non-specific life shortening in male mice exposed to the mammary tumor agent. J Natl Cancer Inst 37:211, 1966.

83. National Cancer Program: The Strategic Plan. U.S. Department of Health, Education and Welfare, Publication No. (NIH) 74-569, Washington, 1973, pp 1–6.

84. Wagh UV, Kasturi SR, Chaughule RS, Shah SS, Ranade SS: Studies on proton spin-lattice relaxation time (T1) in experimental cell cultures. Physiol Chem Phys 9:167, 1977.

85. Wellings SR, Jensen HM, Marcum RG: An atlas of subgross pathology of the human breast with special reference to possible precancerous lesions. J Natl Cancer Inst 55:231, 1975.

86. Wolosewick JJ, Porter KR: Stereo high-voltage electron microscopy of whole cells of the human diploid line, WI-38. Am J Anat 147:303, 1976.

87. Bottomley PA, Hardy CJ, Argersinger RE, Allen-Moore G: A review of ^{1}H NMR relaxation in pathology: Are T1 and T2 diagnostic? Med. Phys. 14:1, 1987.

88. Fossel ET, Carr JM, McDonagh J: Detection of malignant tumors: Water-suppressed proton nuclear magnetic resonance spectroscopy of plasma. N Engl J Med 315:1369, 1986.

102

Hydrodynamic Blood Flow Analysis with Low-Temperature NMR Spin-Echo Detection

WILFRIED H. BERGMANN

Early in 1946, Bloch[1,2] and Purcell[3] published independently the invention of nuclear magnetic resonance (NMR), a discovery that won the 1952 Nobel Prize in Physics. NMR is a method for the excitation of nuclei with spin into temporary coherent resonance motion. As this resonance depends not only on the nuclear species under observation but also on its intra- as well as extra-molecular linkage, NMR experiments yield not only information on abundance and structure, as in NMR tomography (imaging) and phosphorus NMR metabolite spectroscopy, but also dynamic information. The latter includes statistical measures of molecular motion in terms of diffusion and turbulence as well as the coherent molecular motion of flow.[4,5]

As of 1959, attempts to determine the flow rate of blood were among the first NMR flow measurements. These yielded completely noninvasive techniques (without any mechanical and electrical contacts), in which the sensitivity to fluid properties such as conductivity, temperature, viscosity, density, entrainment, or opacity may be controlled. The flow rate is determined generally from the transit time of some bolus of fluid labeled by some NMR technique. Effects of the flow type, such as laminar, turbulent, or non-Newtonian flow, or of the self-diffusion and the relaxation times on this magnetic labeling were compensated for by appropriate calibration. This development is well documented by Zhernovoi and Latyshev[6] and Jones and Child.[7]

Similiar methods for the in-vivo determination of the flow rate in biological objects, e.g. plants, animals, and human beings, have been developed. Hemminga et al.[8,9] published some pulse methods for the determination of flow rates in the range from 0.5 to 25 mm/s of a very small amount (down to 2 percent) of flowing fluid in the presence of a large amount of a stationary one. Other techniques were developed with the aim of observing at least qualitatively the flow of blood and atherosclerotic lesions in major blood vessels, e.g., the aorta and the iliac and femoral arteries, with presently available NMR imaging equipment.[10] Another approach to blood flow measurements in the human brain, e.g., in the internal jugular vein, was demonstrated by Singer and Crooks.[11] The rate of flow is obtained in this technique from the observation of the average cross-sectional area of the blood vessel and of the time required to refill that vessel after a depolarization pulse with fully magnetized (polarized) fresh blood. A determination with an accuracy of about 10 percent was obtained within approximately 20 minutes of imaging time.

NMR experiments may be conducted directly in the frequency domain by continous wave (cw) techniques or in the time domain by pulse methods or free precession techniques. A Fourier transform links the results of both experiments. Pulse and spin-echo methods were developed by Hahn[12] in 1950. In the latter technique the excitation of NMR is well separated in time from the observation of its signal, the spin echo. These two items opened up the approach to the development of an absolute (requiring no calibration) and quantitative hydrodynamic analysis of flow.

Its first step was the development of the multi-pulse spin-echo technique of the $\pi/2 - \tau - (\pi - \tau -)_n$ sequence by Carr and Purcell[13] in 1954 and their observation of first evidence of diffusion and flow (convective motion). In 1956, Torrey[14] extended Bloch's equations to include diffusion. Unangst[15] allowed in 1961 for the magnetization achieved by a stationary laminar flow through a constant magnetic field. In 1965, Arnold and Burkhart[16] determined the average nuclear magnetization of such a flowing sample, having not achieved equilibrium magnetization for spin-echo techniques. In the same year Stejskal[17] published generalized Bloch equations, including anisotropic diffusion and flow to be determined by spin-echo techniques in pulsed magnetic field gradients.[18] He observed that diffusion causes an additional attenuation while flow will shift the phase of the signal. In 1969, de Gennes[19] derived a theory of spin echoes in a turbulent fluid, and Packer[20] published a study of slow coherent molecular motion (of the order of 10^{-3} cm/s) moving with uniform velocity (plug flow) by pulsed nuclear magnetic resonance in time-constant uniform magnetic field gradients.

This work was extended into laminar flow with an average velocity of up to 3 cm/s and also with pulsed field gradients by Packer et al.[21,22] In 1971, Deville and Landesman[23] tested de Gennes' predictions experimentally, suggesting approaches to check the velocity correlation laws. Grover and Singer[24] determined, by the Hahn multiple exposure two-pulse single spin-echo technique of the $n(\pi/2 - \tau - \pi - \tau)$ sequence, the echo amplitude as a function of time in the direction of an applied time constant linear field gradient of a stationary laminar flowing fluid at equilibrium magnetization and of the average blood flow in a human finger. This information in the time domain is transformed by a Fourier cosine transform into the frequency domain. The resulting frequency distribution can be correlated with the relative velocity distribution as the fluid is Larmor phase labeled in the applied field gradient. Flow calibration measurements are required to obtain the absolute number of spins flowing in a given velocity range. Garroway[25] determined analogously the spatial profile of the velocity distribution as well as the relative velocity distribution using a $\pi/2_{x'} - (\tau - \pi/2_{y'} -)_n$ pulse sequence and a steady linear magnetic field gradient in the direction of some laminar flow as well as perpendicular to it to produce a spatial dependent Larmor frequency.

The preceding discussion demonstrates that spin-echo techniques have enabled diffusion, relative laminar velocity distributions, and some turbulence to be observed one at a time on stationary flows at equilibrium magnetization. These present important prerequisites for the development of a hydrodynamic analysis for the diagnosis of benign and malignant blood flows. This flow of blood is transient and in particular pulsatile in all arteries and in veins near the heart. It changes from laminar to turbulent during pulsation in arteries. It is lacking the necessary transition length for the flow to fully develop its equilibrium flow pattern, even where stationary flow is established. Furthermore, the walls of blood vessels are elastic and participate in the transport of blood by pulse wave propagation. Finally blood is under certain circumstances a non-newtonian fluid. It would be most desirable therefore that such a method should encompass the following capabilities:

1. Reduction of localized NMR imaging towards an angiogram without the use of contrast agents.

2. Real-time analysis of the pulse cycle (no averaging by trigger to the heart beat required). Such "instantaneous" spin-echo measurements demand pulse sequences of a duration no longer than 0.1 s for the analysis of the transient pulsating blood flow.

3. All flow quantities to be determined absolute (requiring no calibration measurements). This necessitates the complete mathematical treatment of the involved magnetic and electromagnetic fields.

4. Absolute and quantitative determination of the local pulsating flow cross-section and pressure and their variation with time.

5. Absolute and quantitative determination of the translatory and turbulent velocity spectra and their correlation for an analysis of laminar, turbulent, and non-newtonian flows.

6. Measurements to be performed also at nonequilibrium magnetization of the blood.

The above surveyed developments offer some important elements for the achievement of some of our goals. In these experiments the motion of the resultant nuclear magnetization $\overline{M}$ of a definite spin population is observed as function of time. It is defined by a particular labeling procedure, e.g., a $\pi/2$ – pulse, bringing all the spins under observation into coherent Larmor precession. The Bloch equation, in the generalized form of Torrey[14] and Stejskal[17] describes phenomenologically the motion and the magnitude of that resultant vector of magnetization $\overline{M}$ of that labeled spin system (fluid) as a function of time under the influence of statistical (rotatory) and coherent (translatory) motion in reference to the detection coil encompassing it.

$$\frac{\partial \overline{M}}{\partial t} = \gamma(\overline{M} \times \overline{H}) - \frac{M_x \cdot \overline{i} + M_y \cdot \overline{j}}{T2} - \frac{M_z - M_z(\infty)}{T1} \overline{k} - \nabla \bar{\bar{D}}_s \nabla [\overline{M}_z(\infty) - \overline{M}] - \nabla \overline{v} \overline{M} \quad (1)$$

In this equation $\overline{H}$ designates the local Larmor (Zeeman) field, $T1$ and $T2$ the spin-lattice or longitudinal and the spin-spin or transversal relaxation times, $\bar{\bar{D}}$ the diffusion tensor, and $\overline{v}$ the fluid velocity. Usually one attempts to solve that equation for the spin-echo amplitudes as a function of time in the presence of some boundary conditions, e.g., some time-dependent inhomogeneous magnetic fields. Stejskal[17] points out, in a general analysis of the effects of diffusion and flow on spin-echo amplitudes, that flow causes a shifting of the phase of the nuclear transverse magnetization in contrast to diffusion, which produces an attenuation, i.e., a dephasing effect. de Gennes[19] derives some particular effects of turbulence on the spin-echo amplitudes of a Carr-Purcell-Meiboom-Gill (CPMG) pulse sequence.[26] Packer[20] modifies this pulse sequence, taking into account both random (self-diffusion) and coherent (flow) motion. Using the original Hahn spin-echo technique,[12] Grover and Singer[24] demonstrate for a stationary laminar stream in truncated magnetic fields the same (sin x)/x spin-echo amplitude time dependence as Packer and collaborators.[21,22] The application of a Fourier cosine transform to the envelope of the spin-echo amplitudes yields the relative velocity distribution $f(v)$, the relative velocity spectrum of the laminar flow under observation. Garroway[25] shows that a $\pi/2_{x'} - (\tau - \pi/2_{y'} -)_n$ pulse sequence also produces spin-labeling along the direction of an applied magnetic field gradient like a CPMG pulse sequence.[26]

One goal of our development is to devise an experimental layout that is accessible in every regard to a quantitative mathematical treatment, without any truncations. We want a complete hydrodynamic analysis for an in vivo blood flow investigation not only of slow laminar flows, but even more so of fast transient (pulsatile) laminar as well as turbulent flows, their instantaneous mass or volume flow rates, cross-section, and pressure drop.

Today's magnet technology and mathematical computer methods offer every prerequisite for the achievement of the first requirement. That starts with a precise description of the induced transverse and rf magnetizations within the fluid traversing the Zeeman and Larmor fields by convolution. It is not necessary to achieve equilibrium magnetization. A twofold labeling in regard to some bandwidth in Larmor frequency and initial phase coherence is introduced. Each spin contributes conservatively to the integral phase of the fluid under observation owing to its translatory component of motion and contributes dissipatively to the dephasing of the initially phase coherent labeled sample owing to its rotatory (turbulent) component of motion. The mathematical analysis of this time domain function requires some particular two-dimensional Fourier (integral) transform in regard to frequency and attenuation, yielding a translatory and a turbulency velocity distribution function (spectrum) and their correlation.

We illustrate this with an oszillogram (Fig. 102–1) of a spin-echo experiment performed according to the preceding on a stationary turbulent flow with a Reynolds number of about 6250. The flow had achieved only about 10 percent of its equilibrium magnetization at the entrance into the coaxial the flow encompassing rf coil. The excitation was performed by a CPMG pulse sequence.[26] The field gradient in the direction of flow was about 2.10^{-6} tesla/m. The two-envelope structure of the "even" and "odd" echoes predicted by de Gennes[19] is evident. The "even" echoes are large and slowly decreasing, while the "odd" echoes are small and slowly increasing.

In the analysis of such an experiment the signal amplitude is computed quantitatively initially as function of time from the mathematical descriptions of the interacting magnetic and rf fields by convolution and the experimental parameters. Independent determinations of the volume flow rate and the fluid temperature and pressure as well as of both of the relaxation times and the coefficient of self-diffusion are made. Agreement within the accuracy of observation has to result between both of the time functions. Later integral transforms are being applied to these time functions for a determination of the velocity spectra and their correlation.[29]

Hinshaw's sensitive-point method[27] is to be applied to this hydrodynamic analysis for localized blood flow measurements. This technique confines the resonance volume by detuning the Larmor field. Furthermore, the unwanted signal contribution of the surrounding tissue can be eliminated by an appropriate delay time between an initial $\pi - \pi/2$ pulse sequence. That provides a method for the generation of NMR angiograms without the application of any contrast medium to the blood flow.

The mass, m, of fluid within the resonance volume is quantitatively determined by integration over the translatory velocity distribution function:

$$\int_{v_{\min}}^{v_{\max}} F(v) \cdot dv = m \tag{3}$$

This method becomes an absolute one by validation of this equation, requiring no calibration. In addition, the instantaneous mass flow rate, $\dot{m}$, can be determined according to:

$$\int_{v_{\min}}^{v_{\max}} F(v) \cdot v \cdot dv = \dot{m} \tag{4}$$

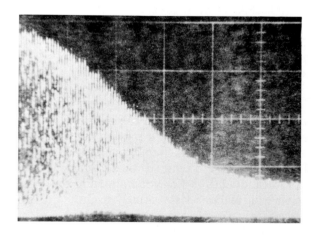

Figure 102–1. Spin-echo sequence of stationary turbulent flow with Reynolds number of about 6250.

The instantaneous flow cross-section F_w follows accordingly:

$$F_w = \frac{\dot{m}}{\rho \cdot \bar{v}} \tag{5}$$

with ρ the density of the blood and $\bar{v}$ its mean velocity, to be determined from the translatory velocity distribution function.

The hydrodynamics of pulsatile blood flow may be analyzed by application of physics of the propagation of pulse waves in elastic walled tubes. A rapid sequence of the previously described $T2$-type relaxation measurements is taken for observation of these pulse waves. The sequence of instantaneous translatory velocity distribution functions as a function of the pulsation yield the wave volume flow rate $\dot{m}/\rho = i_w$ of the circulating blood in the vessel under observation. Its pulsating cross section F_w may be derived from these data as function of time. These again yield the pulse wave rate c_w and the volume modulus of elasticity η.

$$\eta = \frac{dp}{dV} \cdot V = \rho \cdot c_w^2 \tag{6}$$

The wave resistance or impedance,

$$z = \frac{p_w}{i_w} = \frac{\rho \cdot c_w}{F_w} \tag{7}$$

establishes the instantaneous absolute pressure

$$p_w = \frac{i_w \cdot \rho \cdot c_w}{F_w} \tag{8}$$

The wave volume flow rate, i_w, yields the cardiac systolic discharge volume (ejection fraction) by appropriate integration. Analogously, the entire pressure-volume-time characteristic of the heart or any particular blood vessel, e.g., the aorta, may be determined in vivo completely noninvasively from such a sequence of instantaneous integral state of flow measurements.

We have also observed successive frequency bifurcations (period doubling) and band splitting in the power spectra of flows with Reynolds numbers in the vicinity of the transition from the laminar to the turbulent flow regime, as theoretically derived from a renormalization group treatment by Feigenbaum[30,31] and experimentally observed by Libchaber and Maurer.[32] Other transitions to turbulence (onset of chaos) should be observable too by this unique experimental technique, like the intermittency described by Ahlers and Behringer[33] and by Manneville and Pomeau.[34] Similar intermittent transitions were investigated experimentally also by Meseth,[35] Walden and Donelly,[36] Fenstermacher, Swinney and Gollub,[37] and Gollub and Benson.[38] Such investigations will be of great interest not only to hydrodynamics and chaos research but also to medical differential diagnostics. For example, in arteriosclerosis, our method is not only completely noninvasive but also nonlocal (integral), since it is able to analyze the hydrodynamic state of an entire flow field integral from one single spin-echo series and not only differential (one single discrete point) as for instance by laser Doppler anemometry.

The preceding discussion should furnish evidence of a quantitative and absolute hydrodynamic analysis of the transient blood flow by spin-echo techniques, provided these NMR methods attain sufficient sensitivity. We have devised also for the latter a novel approach.[28,39] We presented in the preceding the principle of our hydrodynamic analysis of transient flows, which can be extended into the observation of multiphase flows even during phase transition and the reconstruction of three-dimensional images of inhomogeneous distributions of phases. Further details of the hydrodynamics of pulsatile blood flow may be studied with improving quality of the observed spin-echo series.

The major prerequisite for the utilization of increased detection sensitivity is noise reduction. Noise emanating from exterior sources must be shielded by conventional means and by compensating with appropriate superconducting shielding. Compensation is also effected by differentiating the sensitivity of the detection coil with regard to exterior and interior sources by using a gradiometer design.[40] The latter is also used to protect against microphonics and perturbations originating from relative movements between different coil systems, as well as from vibrations and natural oscillations. Special attention is given to the elimination of possible motion of the probe relative to the detection coil system.

The internal, or Johnson, noise is due to the thermal fluctuations of charge carriers in thermal equilibrium with their lattice. These create statistically fluctuating voltages within the detection circuit, limiting its minimum detectable signal. Reduction of the Johnson noise implies operation of the detection system at very low temperatures, preferably in the superconducting state.

One possible experimental approach is the use of the NMR spin-echo technique. This is characterized by the spin echoes being received in an appropriate fashion by the gradiometer coil as transient electromagnetic wave trains of the pertinent Larmor frequency modulated in amplitude. These are coupled inductively by a flux-transformer into a *s*uperconducting *qu*antum *i*nterference *d*evice (SQUID) and are detected with an appropriately fast phase-sensitive detector[41] in quadrature. Preferably a bias frequency in the range above 1 GHz[42] is chosen, as the amplitude of the output signal and the signal to noise ratio increase proportional to the pump frequency. The SQUID is operated reflectively, to guarantee the necessary band width,[43] and preferably in the nonhysteretic mode tuned off resonance, to achieve the maximum flux sensitivity.[44–46]

The layout of this NMR system (Fig. 102–2) shows the arrangement of the different coils for the production of the individual fields in relation to the patient. The electromagnet, expediently laid out as a superconducting system for generation of the homogeneous magnetic field H_0 in the z direction, is extremely constant in time. The coil systems for the generation of the slowly variable field gradients in the x direction and for the fast field gradient pulses in the x direction are also indicated. The analogous coil systems for the production of the corresponding field gradients in the y and z directions are not shown.

H_1 is produced by means of an rf transmission coil. The slowly variable field gradients and the fast field gradient pulses in the x direction are also seen. The control volume, the region of observation and measurement, happens to be at the origin of the coordinate system, owing to the disposition of the slowly variable field gradient (see Fig. 102–2).

A gradiometer coil, in this particular case of the second order, comprises four windings (Fig. 102–3). This arrangement acts like switching in series two gradiometers of the first order in opposition. An array of fast switching ($\approx 10^{-7}$ s) thin film cryotrons follows further on. It prevents any pickup current from reaching into the SQUID during transmission times of H_1 and field gradient pulses. Simultaneously, it terminates the gradiometer dissipatively. Supercurrents within the gradiometer system induced by spin echoes during its receiving period (data acquisition) are coupled, preferably inductively, by a flux transformer into the SQUID detector by the field transfer coil, which toroidally surrounds the weak link (Josephson junction). Maximum amplification is achieved within the flux transfer circuit. Superconducting shielding is applied appropriately. Further the detection circuit comprises essentially a microwave generator supplying microwave power in the range of 10^{-9} W via an attenuator, an isolator, a directional coupler, and an appropriate impedance transformer, preferably designed as a near

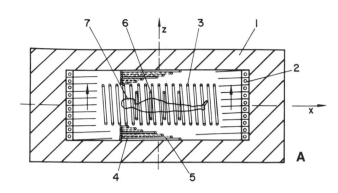

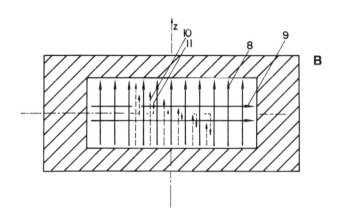

Figure 102–2. *A*, Layout of the NMR system. (1) Superconducting electromagnet, (2) superconducting excitation windings, (3) rf transmission coil, (4) slowly varying gradient coils, (5) fast pulsed gradient coils, (6) gradiometer coil, and (7) patient. *B*, Magnetic field directions. (8) Homogeneous magnetic field H_0 in the *z* direction, (9) the rf field H_1, (10) fast field gradient pulses, and (11) slowly variable field gradient pulses.

optimum taper[41] to the SQUID. The microwaves reflected from the SQUID are amplified by tunnel-diode amplifiers, then rectified by a Schottky diode and detected by a phase sensitive detector, preferably in quadrature. All microwave components are plated on the inside with appropriate superconductors or are made of such superconducting metals as niobium. With the exception of the generator, these parts are operated at temperatures within the range of their superconductivity, in particular at temperatures below 1.85 K, in order to reduce noise and thermal radiation effects to a minimum.

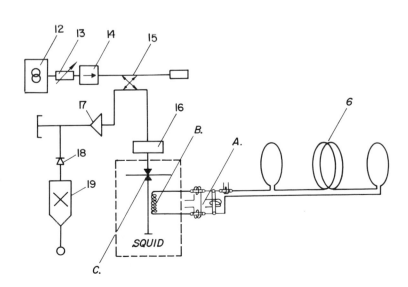

Figure 102–3. NMR signal detection circuit. (12) Microwave generator, (13) attenuator, (14) isolator, (15) directional coupler, (16) impedance transformer, (17) tunnel-diode amplifier, (18) Schottky diode, (19) phase sensitive detector, (A) an array of thin film cryotrons, (B) field transfer coil, and (C) Josephson junction.

Significant improvements on sensitivity have been achieved by cooling a detection circuit to liquid helium temperatures.[47]

References

1. Bloch F, Hansen WW, Packard M: Nuclear induction. Phys Rev 69:127, 1946.
2. Bloch F: Nuclear induction. Phys Rev 70:460–474, 1946.
3. Purcell EM, Torrey HC, Pound RV: Resonance absorption by nuclear magnetic moments in a solid. Phys Rev 69:37–38, 1946.
4. Bergmann WH: On fluid dynamic observations with nuclear magnetic resonance. Proc SENSOR '83 2/3:20, 1983.
5. Bergmann WH: Possibilities in flow imaging and analysis. J Comp Assist Tomogr 5:300, 1981.
6. Zhernovoi AI, Latyshev GD: Nuclear magnetic resonance in a flowing liquid. New York, Consultants Bureau, 1965.
7. Jones DW, Child TF: NMR in flowing systems. Advances in Magnetic Resonance. 8:123, 1976.
8. Hemminga MA, de Jager PA, Sonneveld A: The study of flow by pulsed nuclear magnetic resonance. I. Measurement of flow rates in the presence of a stationary phase using a difference method. J Magn Reson 27:359–370, 1977.
9. Hemminga MA, de Jager PA: The study of flow by pulsed nuclear magnetic resonance. II. Measurement of flow velocities using a repetitive pulse method. J Mag Reson 37:1–16, 1980.
10. Herfkens RJ, Higgins CB, Hricak H, Lipton MJ, Crooks LE, Sheldon PE, Kaufman L: Nuclear magnetic resonance imaging of arteriosclerotic disease. Radiology 148:161, 1983.
11. Singer JR, Crooks LE: Nuclear magnetic resonance blood flow measurements in the human brain. Science 221:654, 1983.
12. Hahn EL: Spin echoes. Phys Rev 80:580–594, 1950.
13. Carr HY, Purcell EM: Effects of diffusion on free precession in nuclear magnetic resonance experiments. Phys Rev 94:630–638, 1954.
14. Torrey HC: Bloch equation with diffusion terms. Phys Rev 104:563–565, 1956.
15. Herms W: Kerninduktionsuntersuchungen an stroemenden Proben. Ann Physik VII 8:280–286, 1961.
16. Arnold DW, Burkhart LE: Spin-echo NMR response from a flowing sample. J Appl Phys 36:870–871, 1965.
17. Stejskal EO: Use of spin echoes in a pulsed magnetic field gradient to study anisotropic, restricted diffusion and flow. J Chem Phys 43:3597–3603, 1965.
18. Stejskal EO, Tanner JE: Spin diffusion measurements: Spin echoes in the presence of a time-dependent field gradient. J Chem Phys 42:288–291, 1965.
19. de Gennes PG: Theory of spin echoes in a turbulent fluid. Phys Lett 29A:20–21, 1969.
20. Packer KJ: The study of slow coherent molecular motion by pulsed nuclear magnetic resonance. Mol Phys 17:355, 1969.
21. Packer KJ, Tomlinson DJ, Rees C: Spin-echo amplitude time dependence. Adv Mol Relax Proc 3:119, 1972.
22. Hayward RJ, Packer KJ, Tomlinson DJ: Pulsed field-gradient spin echo NMR studies of flow in fluids. Mol Phys 23:1083, 1972.
23. Deville G, Landesman A: Expériences d'echos de spins dans un liquide en écoulement. Le Journal de Physique (Paris) 32:67–72, 1971.
24. Grover T, Singer JR: NMR spin-echo flow measurements. J Appl Phys 42:938–940, 1971.
25. Garroway AN: Velocity measurements in flowing fluids by NMR. J Phys D 7:L159, 1974.
26. Meiboom S, Gill D: Modified spin-echo method for measuring nuclear relaxation times. Rev Sci Instr 29:688, 1958.
27. Hinshaw WS: Image formation by nuclear magnetic resonance: The sensitive point method. J Appl Phys 47:3709, 1976.
28. Bergmann WH: In Erne SN et al (eds): Biomagnetism. Proceedings-3rd Int'l Workshop on Biomagnetism. Berlin-New York, W. de Gruyter, 1981, pp 535–548.
29. Bergmann WH: On a hydrodynamic analysis of stationary and transient single and multi-phase flows by spin-echo methods Nucl Magn Reson (in press).
30. Feigenbaum MJ: Quantitative universality for a class of nonlinear transformations. J Stat Phys 19:25–31, 1978.
31. Feigenbaum MJ: The universal metric properties of nonlinear transformations. J Stat Phys 21:669–706, 1979.
32. Libchaber A, Maurer J: Une expírience de Rayleigh-Benard de geometric reduite; multiplication, accrochage et demultiplication de frequences. J Phys Paris 41/C3:51, 1980.
33. Ahlers G, Behringer RP: The Rayleigh-Bénard instability and the evolution of turbulence. Prog Theor Phys (Suppl) 64:186, 1978.
34. Manneville P, Pomeau Y: Intermittency and the Lorenz model. Phys Lett 75A:1, 1979.
35. Meseth J: Dissertation University of Gottingen (July, 1973).
36. Walden R, Donnelly R: Reemergent order of chaotic circular Couette flow. Phys Rev Lett 42:301–302, 1979.

37. Fenstermacher PR, Swinney HL, Gollub J, et al: Dynamical instabilities and the transition to chaotic Taylor vortex flow. J Fluid Mech 94:103–128, 1979.
38. Gollub J, Benson S: Many routes to turbulent convection. J Fluid Mech 100:449–469, 1980.
39. Bergmann WH: Method for improvement of the sensitivity of NMR measurements on samples which have to remain at their own characteristic temperature and which have a non-negligible electrical conductivity. (to be published). U.S. Pat. 4, 442, 404 (April 10, 1984).
40. Wikswo JP Jr.: Optimization of SQUID differential magnetometers. In Deaver BS et al (eds): Proceedings of the Conference on Future Trends in Superconducting Electronics. New York, AIP, 1978, p 146.
41. Rogall H, Heiden C: A SQUID system for low-drift magnetization measurements. Appl Phys 14:161, 1977.
42. Hollenhorst JN, Giffard RP: High sensitivity microwave SQUID. IEEE Trans Mag 15:474, 1979.
43. Kamper RA, Simmonds MB: Broadband superconducting quantum magnetometer. Appl Phys Lett 20:270, 1972.
44. Hansma PK: Superconducting single junction interferometers with small critical currents. J Appl Phys 44:4191, 1973.
45. Erne SN, Hahlboom H-D, Lübbig H: Theory of rf-based super conducting quantum interference devices for nonhysteretic regime. J Appl Phys 47:5440, 1976.
46. Lübbig H: Analytic study on the influence of the weak link parameters on the resonance circuit of the nonhysteretic RF SQUID. In Deaver BS et al (eds): Proceedings of the Conference on Future Trends in Superconducting Electronics. New York, AIP, p 140.
47. Styles P, Soffe NF, Scott CA, Cragg DA, Row F, White DJ, White PCJ: A high-resolution NMR probe in which the coil and preamplifier are cooled with liquid helium. J Magn Reson 60:397–404, 1984.

103

The Physiological Chemistry of Creatine Kinase in the Heart: Phosphorus-31 Magnetization Transfer Studies

JOANNE S. INGWALL

[31]P nuclear magnetic resonance (NMR) spectroscopy is now widely used to study the metabolism of phosphate-containing compounds in cells, organs, and intact animals.[1-3] Information contained in the ^{31}P NMR spectrum of heart includes (1) identification and concentration of phosphorus-containing metabolites present in concentrations greater than 0.6 mM in the cytoplasm, (2) intracellular pH, and (3) the fractions of metabolites that are Mg bound. ^{31}P NMR spectra of isolated buffer-perfused rat and rabbit hearts (Fig. 103–1A, B, and D) show that the metabolites readily observable by this technique are ATP, creatine phosphate (CrP), the nicotinamide adenine nucleotides (NAD(H)), and inorganic phosphate (Pi). Note that in the rabbit heart an additional resonance, attributed to glycerolphosphorylcholine (GPC), is also observable (Fig. 103–1D). For the rat heart in situ, diphosphoglycerate (2,3-DPG) is also observable. The relative concentrations of ATP, CrP, and Pi differ with the carbon substrate used to support ATP synthesis. In the rat heart the ratio of [CrP] to [ATP] is ~1.4 for glucose-perfused (11 mM) hearts, ~1.8 for pyruvate-perfused (10 mM) hearts, and ~1.8 for the blood perfused heart in situ. In all cases the intracellular pH is ~7.1 (Fig. 103–1A–C).

The in vivo NMR experiment provides the opportunity to obtain biochemical information repetitively while simultaneously monitoring cardiac performance. Consequently, ^{31}P NMR of heart has been used to measure time-dependent changes in metabolism and performance in experimental protocols designed to mimic various pathophysiological states. For example, changes in the tissue contents of ATP, CrP, and Pi and in cardiac performance can be followed during periods of ischemia and reperfusion with and without interventions designed to salvage myocardial tissue.

Perhaps the most important application of ^{31}P NMR to studies of myocardial energetics is the use of magnetization transfer techniques to study the whole organ enzymology of phosphate exchange reactions. The technique can be used to study reactions under steady-state conditions whose rate constants are on the order of 1 s^{-1}. Reactions amenable to study in heart include ATP synthesis and hydrolysis, creatine kinase, and adenylate kinase. A unique feature of the use of magnetization transfer NMR to study biological systems is that this information can be obtained while simultaneously respecting the physiological integrity of the system. In our studies of the physiologic chemistry of phosphate exchange reactions in the heart, we have used isolated heart preparations that mimic the in vivo situation as closely as possible while simultaneously permitting careful manipulation of the experimental conditions. In ad-

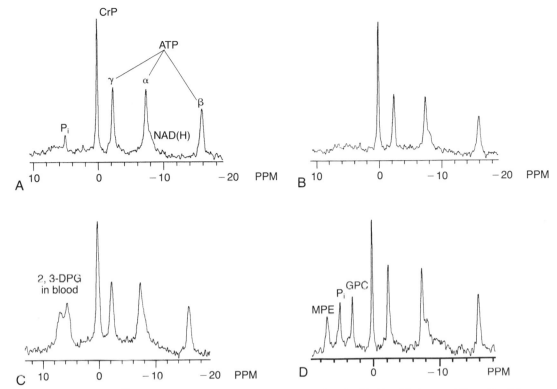

Figure 103–1. One-pulse ^{31}P NMR spectra of isolated rat heart perfused with 11 mM glucose (*A*) or 10 mM pyruvate (*B*), the blood perfused rat heart in situ (*C*) and the isolated perfused rabbit heart (*D*). Isolated hearts were perfused isovolumically. Spectra were obtained at 8.4 tesla as described in the text. (Abbreviations: adenosine triphosphate, ATP; creatine phosphate, CrP; diphosphoglycerate, 2,3-DPG; inorganic phosphate, Pi; glycerolphosphorylcholine, GPC; mon-ophosphate esters, MPE; nicotinamide adenine dinucleotide, NAD.)

dition, we have compared results obtained using in vitro preparations to those obtained in situ. In this chapter, we discuss our results using magnetization transfer NMR to study the physiological chemistry of creatine kinase in heart. The importance of optimizing the physiological aspects of the biological NMR experiment for proper interpretation of the results is emphasized.

Creatine kinase (creatine-N-phosphotransferase, EC 2.7.3.2.) is a dimeric enzyme (80 kdal) that catalyzes the transfer of high energy phosphate between ADP and creatine:

$$H^+ + MgADP + CrP \rightleftharpoons MgATP + creatine$$

In enzyme solutions mimicking physiological conditions of ionic strength, pH and temperature, the reaction has an equilibrium constant of ~170.[4] Four electrophoretically distinct isozymes have been characterized: BB, MB, MM, and mitochondrial creatine kinase. Creatine kinase is present in high activity in heart (~7 International Units/mg noncollagen protein in the rat heart). Thus, as ATP is utilized during contraction, creatine kinase catalyzes the transfer of a high-energy phosphate group from CrP to ADP to insure a constant supply of ATP. Early studies that sought direct evidence of ATP utilization by the myocardium observed only creatine phosphate hydrolysis.[5,6] Creatine kinase resynthesizes ATP so rapidly that direct measurement of the reaction rates in muscle has not been possible using conventional techniques. Using magnetization transfer techniques to investigate the kinetics of the creatine kinase reaction and ATP synthesis in the rat and rabbit heart, we found that flux through the creatine kinase reaction is an order of magnitude higher than ATP synthesis rates. We have also found that flux through the creatine kinase reaction increases as cardiac performance and oxygen consumption (and ATP synthesis) increase; that is, energy transfer via the creatine kinase reaction is coupled to energy demand.

PHYSIOLOGICAL HEART PREPARATIONS

The size ($\sim$1.5 g) and shape (slightly oval) of the adult rat heart permit the use of commercial 20 mm NMR probes, making the isolated rat heart the most widely studied organ in NMR spectroscopy. Young rabbit hearts can also be easily accommodated in commercial probes. There are three types of isolated perfused heart preparations: the Langendorff heart preparation, the working heart preparation of Neely and Morgan,[7] and the isovolumic heart preparation. Each can be readily adapted to interface with the NMR experiment,[1,8] and each permits analysis of phosphate metabolism in a viable, beating heart. Each preparation has advantages and limitations.

The Langendorff-perfused heart is useful for studies requiring viable myocardial cells but is seriously limited in studies of phenomena related to cardiac performance. Since these hearts perform no external work, Langendorff-perfused hearts consume only low levels of oxygen; i.e., ATP synthesis and hydrolysis rates are low. In terms of cardiac performance, this preparation is intermediate between the viable, nonbeating (produced for example by KCl-arrest) heart and a heart functioning in the normal physiological range. Thus, extrapolation of results obtained using this preparation to those obtained in hearts functioning in the normal range of cardiac performance is limited.

The full range of cardiac performance can be achieved in both the working and isovolumic heart preparations. In the Neeley-Morgan working heart preparation, the movement of fluid is the same as in the heart in situ: buffer enters the left atrium, passes into the left ventricle via the mitral valve, and is ejected through the aortic valve. Afterload (the resistance to aortic flow) and preload (atrial perfusion pressure) can be readily altered and monitored with pressure transducers. The advantage of this left heart model is fidelity to the in vivo setting. A disadvantage is that it is difficult to assess diastolic properties of the heart. The isovolumic heart preparation is well suited to measurement of diastolic as well as systolic performance. In this preparation, a fluid-filled latex balloon is inserted into the left ventricle via the mitral valve. The volume in the balloon can be altered via a catheter. Thus, diastolic pressure can be varied, and cardiac performance can be carefully monitored. In this preparation, flow is retrograde down the aorta; in this respect, the model does not mimic the heart in situ.

Both the ejecting and the isovolumic heart preparations can be blood perfused. Blood perfusion requires priming the perfusion system with blood donated from additional animals. Care must be taken to minimize foaming and to eliminate clotting. The major advantage of blood perfusion is that cardiac performance closely approximates normal physiology. For example, in buffer-perfused hearts, coronary flow is $\sim$20 ml/g, but in blood-perfused hearts, flow is nearly physiologic at $\sim$2 to 3 ml/g.

Open[9] and closed[10] chest rat heart preparations have been adapted for use in high-field spectrometers in spite of their relatively narrow bores (89 mm). Use of surface and implanted coils permits measurement of biochemistry in an ideal physiological setting.

The contractile state of the heart is best quantitated by oxygen consumption measurements. For buffer-perfused hearts, oxygen tension is measured in the perfusion medium and in the coronary effluent with a Clark-type electrode, and oxygen consumption is calculated according to the formula: (aortic-effluent pO_2 difference) $\times$ (solubility of O_2 in H_2O/mmHg) $\times$ (coronary flow)/dry weight.[11] For blood-perfused hearts, oxygen content is measured. Mechanical performance is defined as the rate-pressure product (mmHg/min), i.e., the product of heart rate and developed pressure (the difference between systolic and diastolic pressures). Since most of the oxygen consumed by a working rat heart under normal physiological conditions supports mechanical performance, these two parameters are closely related, and measuring either parameter is generally adequate. For the rat, the slope of the relationship between cardiac performance and myocardial oxygen consumption is 1.05. It should be noted, however, that in some settings this relationship is poor (except during postischemia), while in other settings it is not possible to measure oxygen consumption (except the rat heart in situ). In these cases, cardiac performance must be used to assess contractility.

Hearts must be continuously assessed throughout a protocol for physiologic and metabolic criteria of stability. In our studies, during the initial 10 to 30 min equilibration period, hearts are required to maintain a heart rate > 250 beats per min, be in normal sinus rhythm, and have flow (aortic plus coronary) > 20 ml/(min·g wet weight). In addition to physiological stability, the chemical concentration of NMR-observable substrates must not change during normoxia. If the metabolite concentrations were to change during the course of a magnetization transfer NMR experiment, changes in the resonance areas would no longer be due solely to changes in magnetic lifetime, making the results difficult to interpret. Characteristics of the ^{31}P NMR spectrum used to assess stability include the constancy of the $[\gamma\text{-P}]ATP$ resonance, the stability of the CrP resonance and negligible accumulation of Pi.

NMR EXPERIMENTS

The NMR experiments were carried out in a Nicolet wide-bore NT 360 pulsed Fourier transform NMR spectrometer, equipped with broad-banded electronics, a dedicated 128K 1280 minicomputer, a CDC dual moving head disc system, and 89 mm bore 82.5 kG superconducting magnet. Experiments on perfused hearts were carried out in 20 mm sample tubes in either fixed frequency or tunable probes. Experiments on open-chest rat hearts were carried out using surface coil tunable to either ^{31}P or ^{23}Na. To homogenize the magnetic field, we used an 18-channel Oxford Instruments Shim Supply and maximized the signal intensity from sodium in the heart and perfusate.

Observation of the steady-state content of the phosphate-containing substances CrP, ATP, and Pi was accomplished by obtaining conventional one-pulse NMR spectra of the isolated heart. Spectra were obtained under conditions where all resonances are fully relaxed so that equal resonance areas represent equal concentrations of metabolites. This permits analysis of relative concentrations of different metabolites and of time-dependent changes in relative concentrations in the same heart. With appropriate calibration, calculation of absolute concentrations can also be made. Figure 103–1A–D shows one-pulse spectra obtained for beating rat and rabbit hearts.

One-pulse ^{31}P NMR spectroscopy yields the tissue concentrations of CrP and ATP. Magnetization transfer provides measurement of the pseudo–first order unidirectional rate constants, k_{for} and k_{rev}, of the creatine kinase reaction:

$$CrP \underset{k_{rev}}{\overset{k_{for}}{\rightleftharpoons}} [\gamma\text{-P}]ATP$$

Fluxes through the forward and reverse creatine kinase reaction are calculated as the products of rate constant and appropriate metabolite concentrations, k_{for} [CrP] and k_{rev} [ATP], respectively. In a magnetization transfer experiment a magnetic label is applied at one or more resonances. The transfer of the magnetic label between chemical sites reflects both the chemical reaction rate, k, and the intrinsic relaxation time, $T1$.

In our experiments, we use the simplest form of magnetization transfer, namely saturation transfer.

Figure 103–2A illustrates the saturation transfer method. We irradiate either CrP or [γ-P]ATP with a long pulse of low-power radio frequency. The irradiation stacks the Boltzmann energy levels equally and thus nullifies or "saturates" the NMR signal (the shaded area represents the saturated moiety). As the time of saturation is prolonged, exchange via the creatine kinase reaction begins to alter the ^{31}P NMR spectrum as the phosphorus signal at CrP is transferred to the irradiated [γ-P]ATP site. In a reciprocal manner, the irradiated phosphorus from [γ-P]ATP moves to the CrP site. The stack of ^{31}P NMR spectra obtained for an isolated rat heart displayed in Figure 103–2B shows that the magnitude of the CrP signal diminishes exponentially with time of saturation. This is true as long as the chemical exchange rate, k, exceeds the rate of magnetic relaxation, $1/T1$, of CrP. The time dependence of the magnetization of CrP, M(CrP), is governed by[12]

$$\frac{dM\,(\text{CrP})}{dt} = \frac{M_0\,(\text{CrP})}{T1\,(\text{CrP})} - \frac{M\,(\text{CrP})}{\tau_1(\text{CrP})} \tag{1}$$

where

$$\frac{1}{\tau_1(\text{CrP})} = \frac{1}{T1\,(\text{CrP})} + k_{\text{for}} \tag{2}$$

The solution of Equation (1) is:

$$M\,(\text{CrP}) = M_0\,(\text{CrP}) \left[\frac{\tau_1(\text{CrP})}{\tau(\text{CrP})} \bullet \text{Exp}\left(\frac{-t}{\tau_1(\text{CrP})}\right) + \frac{\tau_1(\text{CrP})}{T1\,(\text{CrP})} \right] \tag{3}$$

where $1/\tau(\text{CrP}) = k_{\text{for}}$. As the saturating pulse becomes infinitely long, the exponential term approaches zero, yielding:

$$\frac{M_\infty(\text{CrP})}{M_0(\text{CrP})} = \frac{\tau_1(\text{CrP})}{T1\,(\text{CrP})} \tag{4}$$

Thus, the slope of the exponential function yields the value for $-1/\tau_1(\text{CrP})$. The ratio

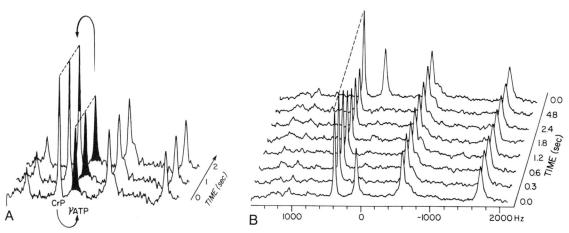

Figure 103–2. A, Schematic illustrating the measurement of the creatine kinase reaction using the saturation transfer technique. A low power pulse at the [γ-P]ATP resonance completely saturating the resonance area. The shaded areas represent saturated phosphate exchanging between CrP and [γ-P]ATP. See text for further description. B, Stack of ^{31}P NMR spectra obtained from a saturation transfer experiment of an isolated KCl arrested rat heart. The first and last spectra are one-pulse spectra showing metabolic stability of the preparation, and the intervening spectra were obtained for saturating times varying from 0.3 to 4.8 s. (From Ingwall JS, Balschi JA: In Pohost GM et al.: New Concepts in Cardiac Imaging, Vol. 2. Chicago, Year Book Medical Publishers, 1986, pp. 251–269. Used by permission.)

of the initial and infinity values of M defines the quotient, $T1$ (CrP)/τ_1(CrP). The absolute values of k_{for} and $T1$ (CrP) emerge from substitution into Equation (2).

Formally, the same approach can be used to probe the creatine kinase reaction in reverse. When the CrP resonance is selectively saturated, creatine kinase transfers magnetization from [γ-P]ATP to CrP. By substituting [γ-P]ATP for CrP in Equations (1) to (4), k_{rev} and $T1$ ([γ-P]ATP) can be calculated. As will be discussed below, however, this approach may underestimate the creatine kinase reaction in reverse.

Figure 103–3 shows magnetization transfer data for the forward creatine kinase reaction obtained for two perfused hearts, one working at a high level of cardiac performance and another in full KCl arrest. As the time of saturation increased, the magnetization approached an asymptote, M_∞. The asymptote can be measured experimentally after a sufficiently long saturating pulse or estimated from computer fits of data obtained at shorter times of saturation. If M_∞ is estimated by a single long period of saturation, $T1$ must be obtained from a separate experiment. We prefer to estimate M_∞ and $T1$ using computer fits of data obtained using multiple times of saturation ranging from 0 to 4.8 s, since both parameters are then obtained for the same heart during the same time interval. We use variance-weighted nonlinear regression as the method of analyzing the data because of its reproducibility, documentation of goodness-of-fit, and freedom from bias. Ideally, the greater the number of points, the more precise the fit. In practice, the length of each experiment is limited by the stability of the heart preparation (60 to 90 min for buffer-perfused hearts) and the number of experiments to be done per heart.

As shown in Figure 103–3, the shape of the relationship between resonance area and time of saturation, as well as the value of M_∞, varies with physiological performance. Depending on the number of points used for the computer fits, values for $T1$ differ despite excellent regression coefficients ($r^2 > 0.98$) and goodness of fit parameters (F and p values). Data given in Table 103–1 for hearts operating at high and low levels of cardiac performance show that results obtained using shorter times of saturation (to 1.2 s) yield values for $T1$ that are consistently 20 to 40 percent lower than results obtained from data sets, including longer times of saturation (to 2.4 and 4.8 s). On the

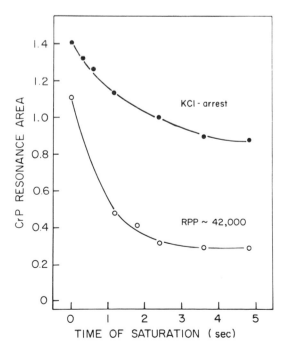

Figure 103–3. Relationship between CrP resonance area (where 1 represents CrP resonance area equal to β-ATP resonance area) and time of saturation for a KCl-arrested heart (filled circles) and a beating heart operating at a rate-pressure product of 42,000 mmHg/min. For the KCl-arrested heart, τ was 1.10 s^{-1}, $T1$ was 1.8 s and k_{for} was 0.34 s^{-1}; for the beating heart, τ was 0.53 s^{-1}, $T1$ was 2.0 s and k_{for} was 1.4 s^{-1}. (From Ingwall JS et al.: *In* Gupta RK (ed): NMR Spectroscopy of Cells and Organisms. Boca Raton, CRC Press, 1987, pp. 51–68. Used by permission.)

Table 103–1. CHARACTERISTICS OF COMPUTER FITS OF SATURATION TRANSFER DATA FOR THE FORWARD CREATINE KINASE REACTION: EFFECTS OF VARYING TIME OF SATURATION†

	High Workload ($n = 4$)			Low Workload ($n = 3$)		
	to 1.2 s	to 2.4 s	to 4.8 s	to 1.2 s	to 2.4 s	to 4.8 s
Parameters of Fit for Equation:						
Magnetization = $A + B\ exp(-C * time\ in\ s)$						
A	398 ± 18	333 ± 26	317 ± 18	679 ± 34	627 ± 15	629 ± 9
B	856 ± 50	856 ± 85	854 ± 75	733 ± 33	782 ± 17	781 ± 11
C	2.52 ± 0.33	1.80 ± 0.26	1.67 ± 0.15	1.56 ± 0.16	1.37 ± 0.08	13.7 ± 0.06
Goodness of Fit Parameters						
F	160	60	97	1,069	1,418	2,588
r^2	>.99	>.98	>.98	>.99	>.99	>.99
p	0.056	0.017	0.002	0.022	0.001	0.001
Results						
$T1$ (s)	1.25	1.98	2.21	1.33	1.64	1.64
k (s^{-1})	1.72	1.30	1.22	0.75	0.76	0.76
Flux (μmol/(gdw·s))	54	38	36	29	27	27

† Saturation transfer data for isolated isovolumic rat hearts at high (oxygen consumption 33 μmol/(g dry weight·s)) and low (oxygen consumption 18 μmol/(g dry weight·s)) workloads were obtained for 0, 0.3, 0.6, 1.2, 2.4, and 4.8 s of saturation at [γ-P]ATP. Shown here are the results of fitting the data to an exponential function, using 4, 5, or 6 points, i.e., to 1.2 s, 2.4 sec or 4.8 s.

other hand, values for k and hence flux did not vary for low-workload hearts and varied for only one test case for high-workload hearts. In these experiments, the total time required to obtain each saturation transfer spectrum differed, with the shortest delays between applying the unsaturated pulse used for spectra with 0, 0.3, and 0.6 s of selective saturation at the [γ-P]ATP resonance and the longest delays between unsaturated pulses used for spectra with 4.8 s of selective saturation. This is one practical way to reduce the total time of the saturation transfer experiment and thus ensure physiological stability throughout the measurement. In these examples, the time differential is considerable, from ~90 to ~35 mins. However, the degree of saturation of the CrP resonance with respect to saturation processes varied during the measurement. This may explain the consistent differences obtained for estimates of $T1$ (CrP). The results suggest that variations in k estimated in these experiments are relatively small. The reason for this is that the value for k depends primarily on the initial slope of the relationship between M and time of saturation; at these times, extent of CrP saturation from relaxation processes is nearly constant.

THE CREATINE KINASE REACTION IN SOLUTION

In order to validate the saturation transfer method, the forward and reverse fluxes for the creatine kinase reaction in solution have been measured using magnetization

Table 103–2. PHYSIOLOGIC PREPARATIONS DEMONSTRATING COUPLING BETWEEN CREATINE KINASE FLUX AND ATP SYNTHESIS RATES

Isolated Heart Preparations
Neely-Morgan working rat heart
  with glucose as substrate
  with pyruvate as substrate
Isovolumic (ballon-in-LV) rat heart
Isovolumic rabbit heart
In Vivo **Preparation**
The open-chest rat heart

transfer NMR. As expected, unidirectional flux or reaction velocity depends on enzyme concentration, on pH, and on temperature. Also as expected, the forward and reverse fluxes were indistinguishable. Furthermore, over the range of CrP/creatine ratios varying from 0.1 to 5, flux did not change.[13] These results show that the saturation transfer technique is valid and can be used to quantitate the dependence of flux on a variety of parameters.

This observation has been made by several groups. Kuprianov et al.[14] demonstrated not only that the method correctly shows that the enzyme in solution is in equilibrium but that the method measures the off-rate of the reaction products. Degani et al.[15] demonstrated equality of creatine kinase fluxes in solution using both saturation and inversion transfer methods. Mayer et al.[16] found a small difference between the forward and reverse fluxes in solution, but this difference is probably not significant.

THE CREATINE KINASE REACTION IN THE HEART

We have defined the relationships between creatine kinase flux and cardiac performance (and thus ATP synthesis rates) in well-oxygenated isolated perfused hearts in five different settings and in the open-chest rat heart (Table 103–2).[8,13,17–19] In each case, creatine kinase flux increased with cardiac performance and hence ATP synthesis. In isolated hearts, creatine kinase flux increased with cardiac performance (1) in isovolumic rat and rabbit hearts,[19,20] (2) in both the isovolumic and Neely-Morgan working heart preparations,[8] (3) in hearts with either glucose or pyruvate as substrate,[13,15] and (4) in both beating and nonbeating isovolumic rat hearts.[19,21] In the open-chest rat heart, cardiac performance was varied by using various levels of halothane anesthesia or norepinephrine. Here, too, creatine kinase flux increased with performance.[9]

Figure 103–4 shows results defining the relationship between creatine kinase flux and ATP synthesis, measured as oxygen consumption, for the isolated isovolumic rat heart operating at five levels of cardiac performance ranging from full KCl arrest to rate-pressure products (i.e., heart rate × developed pressure) as high as 45,000 mmHg/min. The shape of this relationship may be helpful for understanding regulation of the creatine kinase reaction. The data suggest that the coupling of creatine kinase flux and ATP synthesis is a saturable process that follows Michaelis-Menten kinetics, i.e., that the same metabolites regulate both reactions. Maximum flux (V_{max}) of the forward

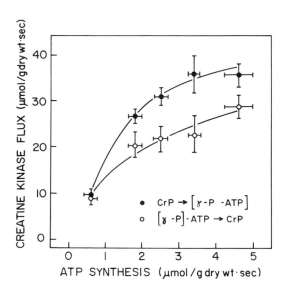

Figure 103–4. Relationship between creatine kinase flux and ATP synthesis for isovolumic rat hearts over the range of cardiac performance varying from 0 to 45,000 mmHg/min. The filled and open circles are data for the forward and reverse creatine kinase reactions, respectively. Values for $T1$ of CrP and [γ-P]ATP did not change with workload and averaged 2.06 +/− 0.13 sec and 0.75 +/− 0.08 s, respectively. The rate constant for the forward creatine kinase reaction increased from 0.27 to 1.30 s^{-1} and the rate constant for the reverse reaction increased from 0.31 to 1.14 s^{-1}. The tissue level of CrP decreased by 21 percent with increased workload; ATP content was unchanged. ATP synthesis was calculated from oxygen consumption measurements assuming a P:O ratio of 3.0. For further details, see reference 19. (From Ingwall JS et al.: *In* Gupta RK [eds]: NMR Spectroscopy of Cells and Organisms. Boca Raton, CRC Press, 1987, pp. 51–68. Used by permission.)

reaction is ~56 μmol/(g dry weight · sec). The reaction operates at half-maximum when the ATP synthesis rate is ~2.6 μmol/(g dry weight · s).[19]

These results show that over the entire range of cardiac performance possible to achieve in a buffer-perfused heart, flux through the creatine kinase reaction and ATP synthesis are coupled with a gain of ~0.5. If one considers only hearts operating at low levels of performance or only beating hearts operating at normal physiologic range, different conclusions could be drawn. For example, creatine kinase flux is 2.8 times greater in beating hearts operating at low levels of cardiac performance than in KCl arrested hearts. Over this range of performance, both ATP synthesis and creatine kinase flux increase ~2.8-fold; i.e., the coupling gain is ~1.0. In contrast, in the beating heart, creatine kinase flux increases 1.4-fold while oxygen consumption increases 2.6 times; i.e., the coupling is 0.5. Based on these results, one would predict that the coupling factor for creatine kinase flux and oxygen consumption would be highest in arrested hearts for which performance was altered by altering wall stress. This was indeed observed. In arrested hearts with varying extents of wall stress creatine kinase flux increased twofold while oxygen consumption increased by only 20 percent; i.e., creatine kinase flux and ATP synthesis were coupled with a gain of 1.7.[21] These results suggest that flux through the creatine kinase reaction is highly responsive to the demand on the heart. They also suggest that creatine kinase plays a relatively more important role in maintaining normal ATP levels in hearts operating at low levels of cardiac performance than at high levels of performance.

Our observations that creatine kinase flux measured by ^{31}P NMR magnetization transfer techniques increases with cardiac performance have now been confirmed by several groups. Miceli et al.[22] observed a linear increase in creatine kinase flux and cardiac performance in perfused isovolumic rabbit hearts in which cardiac performance was altered by pacing. Using the same protocol as ours, Kuprianov et al.,[14] studying the isolated perfused rat hearts, have also observed this coupling. Although the point was not made, Nunnally and Hollis[23] also observed a large increase in creatine kinase flux in normal compared with KCl arrested isovolumic rabbit hearts. Studying hearts operating at different but high levels of performance, Ugurbil et al.[24] observed a small increase in flux through the creatine kinase reaction. In contrast, Matthews et al.[25] using isolated Langendorff-perfused rat hearts, observed a decrease in k_{for} in hearts in KCl arrest compared with hearts perfused at high pressure. The inconsistencies between this study and the work of others, both in methods and results, make comparison difficult.

APPARENT DISCREPANCY BETWEEN FORWARD AND REVERSE CREATINE KINASE FLUXES

The results displayed in Figure 103–4 also show that, at each level of cardiac performance, there is an apparent discrepancy between the forward and reverse fluxes. Since the creatine kinase reaction operates at steady state, maintaining constant CrP and ATP concentrations at each level of cardiac performance, the discrepancy in the fluxes must be an apparent one. Otherwise, high energy phosphate content would change. It is assumed that the two-site exchange model reliably predicts k_{for} because CrP participates in no reaction other than creatine kinase. However, the two-site exchange model could underestimate k_{rev} by ignoring ATP synthesis and the possibility of metabolite compartmentation.

The two-site exchange model underestimates k and flux through the reverse creatine kinase reaction by ignoring other ATP reactions.[17] The results given in Figure 103–4 show that flux through the forward creatine kinase reaction is an order of magnitude greater than ATP synthesis rates calculated from oxygen consumption. This might suggest that ATP synthesis could be ignored. Nonetheless, since the Pi resonance area also changes when [γ-P]ATP is saturated, ATP synthesis can be detected by this technique and should be taken into account.[19] Since ATP synthesis rates increase with cardiac performance, the discrepancy between the forward and reverse creatine kinase fluxes should be greatest in high performance hearts and lowest in KCl arrested hearts. The results are consistent with this prediction. In the example shown in Figure 103–4, the ratio between the forward and reverse fluxes is smallest for KCl arrested hearts (1.1) but averaged ~1.4 for all beating hearts. We observed a similar discrepancy in the Neely-Morgan working heart.[17] Nunnally and Hollis[23] also observed equality of fluxes for KCl-arrested hearts. Degani et al.[15] observed no discrepancy for Langendorff-perfused hearts operating at low levels of performance.

In order to quantitate creatine kinase flux in the presence of multiple exchanges, experiments in which the magnetic lifetimes of ATP, CrP, and Pi are measured when resonance areas are saturated singly or in combination are currently under way in several laboratories. Ugurbil et al.[26] developed a technique whereby the saturation transfer experiment is made while the "interfering" resonance is continuously saturated. For example, to study the reverse creatine kinase reaction, the Pi resonance is continuously saturated while saturation transfer from [γ-P]ATP to CrP is measured. Ugurbil et al.[24] found that when this technique is applied to beating hearts, ATP synthesis accounts for most of the observed discrepancy between the forward and reverse fluxes through the creatine kinase reaction. We have developed a technique whereby two resonances can be saturated simultaneously. This technique yields rate constants and fluxes for ATP synthesis and hydrolysis, which incorporate rate constants for the forward and reverse creatine kinase reaction.[27] In hearts performing at a high level of cardiac performance, this approach yields the expected equivalence in creatine kinase fluxes and in ATP synthesis and hydrolysis.

As pointed out by Nunnally and Hollis,[23] the apparent difference between fluxes could also be due to compartmentation of substrate pools. If a fraction of [γ-P]ATP is sequestered in a very slowly exchanging, magnetically visible compartment, Equations (1) to (4) must be modified.[19] ATP compartmentation increases k_{rev} by decreasing the ratio of exchangable M_∞[γ-P]ATP to exchangeable M[γ-P]ATP in the appropriate forms of Equations (2) and (4). However, the value of F_{rev}, calculated in the presence of a compartmentalized pool of ATP, will be proportionately decreased because the sequestered ATP does not participate in the reaction. This analysis shows that compartmentation of the fraction of ATP in a slowly exchanging pool does not alter calculations of the forward and reverse fluxes. Other types of compartmentation may alter the calculation. We have developed a mathematical model that accounts for the presence of two ATP compartments, one that is NMR visible and saturable and another that is NMR invisible and nonsaturable. Assuming that the two compartments represent the cytosol and mitochondria, modeling of the saturation transfer data for the forward creatine kinase reaction predicts rates of the cytosolic and mitochonrial creatine kinase reactions and net ATP-ATP exchange between the mitochondrial and cytosol.[28]

REGULATION OF CREATINE KINASE FLUX IN HEART

The results summarized in this chapter show that flux through the creatine kinase reaction increases with cardiac performance and, thus, with ATP synthesis rates. Since it has been assumed that creatine kinase is at or near equilibrium in vivo, this result is unexpected and merits comment. Generally, enzyme reaction rates are altered by changes in enzyme content, pH, substrate content, and allosteric modulation such as phosphorylation. The changes observed for creatine kinase flux in heart described here are not due to changes in total enzyme content or intracellular pH. Since the rate constants measured by magnetization transfer techniques, k_{for} and k_{rev}, are pseudo first order rate constants (where $k_{for} = k[ADP]$ and $k_{rev} = k'[Cr]$ for the reaction $CrP + ADP \overset{k}{\rightleftharpoons} ATP + Cr$), it is possible that the observed increase in flux is due to changes in substrate ADP and creatine) concentrations, the true rate constant or both. The free creatine pool can be experimentally determined. However, since the free ADP concentration in the cytoplasm is on the order of 20 to 50 μM, even large changes in ADP concentrations could have occurred and not have been detected as either an increase in ADP or a decrease in the large ATP pool. It seems unlikely, however, that changes in ADP or creatine concentrations totally account for the changes in flux observed here for two reasons.

First, the assumption that creatine kinase is at or near equilibrium in vivo does not fit the data. Let us consider the consequences of assuming that the changes in flux are due to changes in metabolite concentration. The physiological condition in which the reaction should be closest to equilibrium is the nonbeating KCl arrested heart. Using the equilibrium constant at 166[4] and the experimentally determined CrP/creatine ratio of 2, the calculated concentration of ADP for the arrested heart is ~30 μM, a reasonable value. If we assume that the reaction is still at equilibrium at high workload, the concentration of ADP is calculated to be 60 μM. Over this wide range of cardiac performance, ADP content increased twofold and the free creatine concentration increased by ~50 percent. Yet, creatine kinase flux increased fourfold. A more striking example of the failure for substrate regulation to account fully for changes in flux is the comparison of hearts working at low workload and the arrested heart: creatine kinase flux increased nearly threefold but the tissue contents of CrP, creatine, or ATP—and therefore ADP—did not change. These observations and the assumption of equilibrium can be reconciled, for example, by postulating compartmentation of creatine and ADP, or by changes in the tissue content of other effectors, such as nitrate, known to influence the creatine kinase reaction. There is, however, no evidence supporting such postulates.

Second, we have measured creatine kinase flux and metabolite levels under conditions in which ADP was expected to accumulate and found that creatine kinase flux decreased instead of increased. During mild ischemia in the rat heart, the changes in metabolite levels are similar to those observed during increased work; i.e., CrP decreases slightly while ATP remains essentially unchanged. Surprisingly, in this setting, flux through the creatine kinase reaction decreased, not increased.[29] This change cannot be accounted for by changes in enzyme content or intracellular pH. Rather, it seems likely that creatine kinase flux is regulated by another unknown mechanism.

Compartmentation of creatine kinase isozymes may play a role in coupling creatine kinase flux and ATP production. The mitochondrial isozyme of creatine kinase is localized on the inner mitochondrial membrane[30,31] and, in rat heart, constitutes ~25 percent of total creatine kinase activity. As respiratory ATP production increases to meet demand due to increased cardiac performance, flux through mitochondrial creatine kinase activity should increase. Magnetization transfer results for hearts with varying amounts of mitochondrial creatine kinase activity suggest that this isozyme reaction is NMR observable. In hypertrophied spontaneously hypertensive rat hearts in the transition to failure, total creatine kinase activity was decreased by ~20 percent, mitochondrial creatine kinase activity was reduced by ~50 percent, and creatine kinase flux was threefold lower compared both with age-matched normotensive rats and with younger rat hearts with compensated hypertrophy operating at the same level of cardiac performance.[32,33] These results suggest that creatine kinase isozyme distribution and content influence creatine kinase flux in the beating heart.

^{31}P NMR: CLINICAL APPLICATIONS

^{31}P NMR spectroscopy of organs, both perfused and in situ, permits measurement not only of the concentrations of phosphorus-containing metabolites but also of their lifetimes. Magnetization transfer techniques allow direct measurement of reaction rates and chemical fluxes of certain phosphate exchange reactions in physiologically intact organs. The feasibility of applying these techniques to the clinical situation is high. Part of this optimism is based on improved technology. Excellent ^{31}P NMR spectra of large animal organs at relatively low field can now be obtained using surface coils and depth resolution techniques.[34] Chemical shift images of ATP, CrP, and Pi in the cat brain[35] demonstrate that phosphorus images are feasible. Part of the optimism is also based on the enormous clinical value of obtaining information about the metabolic status of diseased organs. Metabolic imaging will provide unique information to the clinician. The impetus to develop techniques to apply the kinds of studies described here for the isolated organ to the clinical setting clearly exists.

References

1. Ingwall JS: P-31 spectroscopy of cardiac and skeletal muscles. Am J Physiol *242*:H729, 1982.
2. Shulman RG, Brown TR, Ugurbil K, Ogawa S, Cohen SM, den Hollander JA: Cellular applications of ^{31}P and ^{13}C NMR. Science *205*:160, 1979.
3. Radda GK, Seeley PJ: Recent studies on cellular metabolism by NMR. Ann Rev Physiol *41*:46, 1979.
4. Lawson JWR, Veech RL: Effects of pH and free Mg^{2+} on the K_{eq} of the creatine kinase reaction and other phosphate hydrolyses and phosphate transfer reactions. J Biol Chem *254*:6528–6537, 1979.
5. Hohorst HJ, Reim M, Bartels H: Studies on the creatine kinase equilibrium in muscle and the significance of ATP and ADP levels. Biochem Biophys Res Commun *7*:142–146, 1962.
6. Mommaerts WFHM: Energetics of muscular contraction. Physiol Rev *49*:427–508, 1969.
7. Neely JR, Rovetto MMJ: Technique for perfusing isolated rat heart. *In* Harmand JG, O'Malley BW (eds): Methods in Enzymology, XXXIX. New York, Academic Press, 1975, p 289.
8. Ingwall JS, Kobayashi K, Bittl JA: Creatine kinase reaction rates in the isolated perfused rat heart: P-31 NMR magnetization transfer studies. *In* Gupta RK (ed): NMR spectroscopy of Cells and Organisms. Boca Raton, CRC Press, 1987, pp 51–68.
9. Bittl JA, Balschi JA, Ingwall JS: The effects of norepinephrine infusion on myocardial high-energy phosphate content and turnover in the living cat. J Clin Invest *79*:1852, 1987.
10. Koretsky AP, Wang S, Murphy-Boesch J, Klein MP, Janis TJ, Weiner MW: ^{31}P NMR spectroscopy of rat organs in situ using chronically implanted rf coils. PNAS *80*:7491, 1983.
11. Neely JR, Liebermeister H, Battersby EJ, Morgan HE. Effect of pressure development on oxygen consumption by isolated rat heart. Am J Physiol *212*:804–814, 1967.
12. Forsen S, Hoffman RA: Transfer of magnetization. J Chem Phys *39*:2892, 1963.
13. Ingwall JS, Kobayashi K, Bittl JA: In vivo enzymology of the creatine kinase reaction in the isolated rat heart: ^{31}P magnetization transfer. *In* Smirnoff VN, Katz A (ed): Proceedings of the Sixth Joint USA-USSR Symposium on Myocardial Metabolism. New York, Gordon and Breach, 1987, pp 30–48.
14. Kuprianov VV, Steinschneider EK, Ruuge EK, Kapelko VI, Zueva MY, Lalomkin VL, Mirnov VN, Saks VA: Regulation of energy flux through the creatine kinase reaction in vitro and in perfused hearts: ^{31}P NMR studies. Biochim Biophys Acta *805*:319–331, 1984.
15. Degani H, Laughlin M, Campbell S, Shulman RG: Kinetics of creatine kinase in heart: A ^{31}P NMR saturation and inversion transfer study. Biochemistry *24*:5510–5516, 1985.
16. Mayer RA, Kushmerick MJ, Brown RT: Application of ^{31}P NMR spectroscopy to the study of striated muscle metabolism. Am J Physiol *242*:C1, 1982.
17. Kobayashi K, Fossel ET, Ingwall JS: Analysis of the creatine kinase reaction in the isolated perfused rat hearts using ^{31}P NMR saturation transfer. Biochem J *37*:123a, 1982.
18. Ingwall JS, Kobayashi K, Bittl JA: Measurement of flux through the creatine kinase reaction in the intact rat heart: ^{31}P NMR studies. Biophys J *41*:1a, 1983.
19. Bittl JA, Ingwall JS: Reaction rates of creatine kinase and ATP synthesis in the isolated rat heart: A ^{31}P NMR magnetization transfer study. J Biol Chem *260*:3512–3517, 1985.
20. Ingwall JS, Dygert MK, Perry, SB: Localization of creatine kinase on heart mitochondria increases the rate of creatine phosphate synthesis from oxidation ATP. Biophys J (abstract) *51*:245a, 1987.
21. Bittl JA, Ingwall JS: The energetics of myocardial stretch: Creatine kinase flux and oxygen consumption in the non-contracting rat heart. Circ Res *58*:378, 1986.
22. Miceli MV, Hoerter JA, Jacobus WE: Evidence supporting the phosphocreatine-ATP energy transport shuttle in perfused rabbit hearts: A ^{31}P NMR saturation transfer study. Circulation *68*:III-65, 1983.

23. Nunnally RM, Hollis D: ATP compartmentation in living hearts: A ^{31}P NMR saturation transfer study. Biochemistry *18*:3642, 1979.

24. Ugurbil K, Petein M, Maidan R, et al: Measurement of an individual rate constant in the presence of multiple exchanges. Application to myocardial creatine kinase reactions. Biochemistry *25*:100, 1986.

25. Matthews PM, Bland JL, Gadien EG, Radda GK: A ^{31}P NMR saturation transfer study of the regulation of creatine kinase in the rat heart. Biochim Biophys Acta *721*:312, 1982.

26. Ugurbil K: Magnetization transfer measurements of individual rate constants in the presence of multiple reactions. J Magn Reson *64*:207–219, 1985.

27. Spencer RS, Leigh JS, Balschi JA, Ingwall JS: Double saturation transfer measurements of ATP synthesis and degradation in the perfused rat heart at high workload. Biophys J (abstract), *49*:101a, 1986.

28. Zahler R, Bittl JA, Ingwall JS: Analysis of compartmentation of ATP in skeletal and cardiac muscle using ^{31}P NMR saturation transfer. Biophys J *51*:883, 1987.

29. Kobayashi K, Ingwall JS. In preparation.

30. Saks VA, Kuprianov VV: Intracellular energy transport and control of cardiac contraction. *In* Chazav, Smirnov, Dhalla (eds): Advances in Myocardiology, 3. New York, Plenum Press, 1982, p 475.

31. Moreadith RW, Jacobus WE: Creatine kinase of heart mitochondria. J Biol Chem *257*:899, 1982.

32. Ingwall JS: The hypertrophied myocardium accumulates the MB-creatine kinase isozyme. Eur Heart J *5*(Suppl 7):129–139, 1984.

33. Bittl JA, Ingwall JS: Intracellular high-energy phosphate transfer in normal and hypertrophied myocardium. Circulation *75* (I):96, 1987.

34. Bottomley PA: Noninvasive study of high-energy phosphate metabolism in human heart by depth resolved ^{31}P NMR spectroscopy. Science *229*:769–771, 1985.

35. Maudsley AA, et al: In vivo MR spectroscopic imaging with ^{31}P: Work in progress. Radiology *153*:745–750, 1984.

36. Ingwall JS, Balschi JA: NMR spectroscopy of the heart. *In* Pohost GM, Higgins CB, Morganroth J, Ritchie JL, Schelbert HR (eds): New Concepts in Cardiac Imaging, Vol. 2. Chicago, Year Book Medical Publishers, 1986, pp 251–269.

104

MRI Synthesis

STEPHEN J. RIEDERER

Several years ago, when magnetic resonance (MR) imaging was being transferred from the research laboratory to the clinical setting, a number of investigators studied the mechanisms of contrast in MR imaging.[1-4] This work showed in a quantitative way how the MR signals from different materials depend both on intrinsic tissue properties (proton density, relaxation times, chemical shift, etc.) as well as operator-selected variables (the specific pulse sequence used as well as the interpulse time delays). Although this work was valuable in predicting which timing parameters would provide optimum contrast for given materials of interest, it also demonstrated the myriad of available acquisition techniques and the potential ambiguity in the decision concerning which to use for routine clinical work. Additional efforts were devoted to determining which pulse sequences might be "near optimum" for a large percentage of potential pathologies. Despite these important efforts the question still remained: Is there an "optimum" pulse sequence for clinical scanning, and if so, what is it? The attempt to answer this question is what motivated our group's investigation into the technique of MR image synthesis.

In the intervening years as clinicians have gained familiarity with MRI and confidence in their ability to interpret the results, determination of the "optimum" sequence may no longer be the most relevant question. Rather, the issue of patient throughput becomes important. That is, is it possible to scan a patient and acquire effective diagnostic images that are sensitive to alterations in both $T1$ and $T2$ and do this in a limited amount of time? Equivalently, can a standardized acquisition protocol be devised that provides effective MR images but still allows high patient throughput? Although these latter questions are somewhat different from the one raised earlier about the existence of an "optimum" pulse sequence, we believe that the technique of image synthesis addresses all of them.

The technique of MR image synthesis consists of three steps. First, images are acquired in the normal fashion at several repetition (TR) and echo (TE) times. Second, from this acquired data estimates are made for the proton density $N(H)$ and $T1$ and $T2$ relaxation times, and computed images of these quantities are generated. Third, the actual synthesis step consists of taking the computed images and inserting them into the mathematical equations that describe a particular pulse sequence of interest. At this stage the operator also selects arbitrary timing parameter values for insertion into the equation. The equation is then evaluated for every pixel, which results in a "synthetic" image corresponding to the timing parameters selected. It should be emphasized that the timing parameters used in the synthesis step need not match those used for the acquisition, and, in fact, images can be synthesized for a pulse sequence that is different from that of the acquisition. Thus, the technique of image synthesis is a retrospective one: After the original data is acquired, the operator can manipulate it and generate an image for an arbitrary pulse sequence.

The concept of MR image synthesis was proposed independently by three different groups, one at the University of California at San Francisco,[5,6] the second at the Deutsche Klinik für Diagnostik in Wiesbaden, West Germany,[7] and the third at Duke University.[8-10] This chapter is a discussion of the investigations of this last group. In the next two sections we briefly describe our initial feasibility studies and present analysis of the precision of image synthesis. We then describe how we have attempted to optimize each of the three steps—acquisition, fitting, and synthesis—that constitute image synthesis. Finally, we describe what we see as the major specific applications of this technique.

FEASIBILITY STUDIES

Perhaps the first question one has about the feasibility of the image synthesis technique is whether the results correspond to actual acquired images. Equivalently, are synthetic images credible representations of what one would have actually obtained if the synthetic timing parameters had been used in a direct acquisition? We attempted to answer this question in some of the earliest studies of this technique.[10,11] Before discussing these initial studies, however, it is useful to consider Figure 104–1, a schematic diagram of the detected MR signal M at some arbitrary pixel. This signal is plotted as a function of the repetition time, TR, and echo time, TE. The time constant or curvature in the TR direction is simply the longitudinal relaxation time, $T1$, while that in the TE direction is $T2$. The asymptotic limit of the curve for very long TR times and a TE of zero is a signal proportional to the proton density, $N(H)$. The concept of image synthesis can be viewed simply as attempting to determine such a curve or surface for every pixel in the image. Although this may seem at first to be a mammoth task, it is greatly simplified by noting that an entire surface for one arbitrary pixel can be reproduced by knowing the three "basis" quantities, $T1$, $T2$, and $N(H)$, for that pixel. These in turn can be estimated from measurements made at several TR and TE times. In the example of this figure, a total of eight measurements are assumed, four echoes at each of the two TR times. As will be seen later in this chapter, such sampling requirements can be relaxed depending upon the desired accuracy, scan time, and noise level.

Our initial studies consisted of acquiring multiple spin-echo (MSE) images consistent with the sampling of Figure 104–1, synthesizing spin-echo images at various TR and TE combinations, and comparing the synthetic results with images directly acquired at the same times. This was done in an increasingly stringent fashion. First, at a given

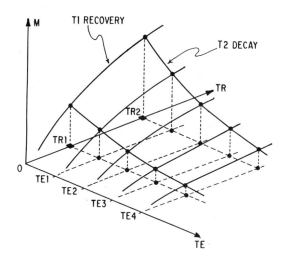

Figure 104–1. Schematic representation of the magnetization M measured at an arbitrary pixel in a spin-echo MR acquisition. As the repetition time TR increases, the signal recovers with a characteristic time constant of $T1$. As the echo time TE increases, the signal is diminished due to $T2$ related decay. The goal of MR image synthesis can be viewed as attempting to determine such a surface for every pixel in the image. Data is acquired at the TE and TR combinations corresponding to the closed circles.

TR time, four spin echoes were acquired and used to determine *T2* and pseudodensity (*PD*) images. *PD* is defined as the MR signal measured in the limit of a TE of zero and corresponds to measurements made at the squares of Figure 104–1. Synthetic results were formed from *PD* and *T2* at the same four echo times as the acquisition. These were then compared with the original acquired images. A sequence of synthetic versus acquired images at several echo times is shown in Figure 104–2. Qualitatively the match appears very close in both the average signals within each pair (accuracy) as well as the degree of graininess or ''noise'' in the synthetic image (precision).

In a more quantitative comparison, pixel values from the same 25-pixel region of interest (ROI) were tabulated in both synthetic and acquired images and plotted side by side versus the echo time, TE. Such a plot is shown in Figure 104–3 for the glioblastoma of Figure 104–2. For each of the four echo times the values from the acquired image are displaced slightly to the left and those from the synthetic image slightly to the right. For each time note that the average synthetic signal (the midpoint of the range of signal values) in general falls within the range of acquired signals (i.e., the method is accurate). Likewise, note that the range of synthetic signals is not appreciably

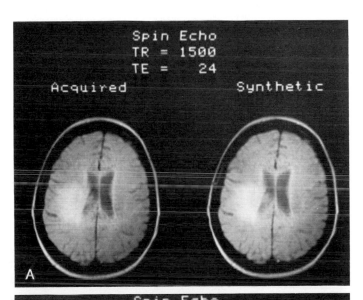

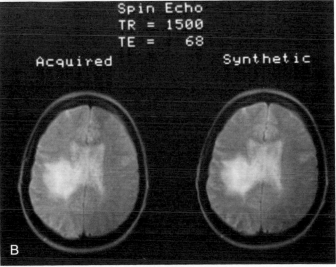

Figure 104–2. Feasibility studies of MR image synthesis comparing acquired and synthetic spin-echo images at TR/TE combinations of 1500/24 ms (*A*) and 1500/68 ms (*B*). Each synthetic image was generated from acquired images at the same TR and echo times of 24, 48, 68, and 92 ms. In each case the synthetic result compares favorably with the acquired image in both accuracy and precision.

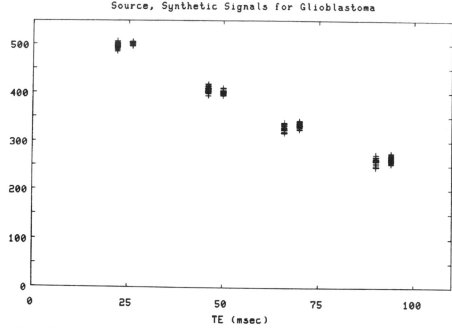

Figure 104–3. Plot versus the echo time of signal values measured in a 25 pixel region of interest of the glioblastoma visualized in the results of Figure 104–2. For each echo time the measurements from the acquired image are shown slightly displaced to the left and those from the corresponding synthetic image slightly to the right. The spread of the values is a measure of the noise magnitude in the image.

larger than the range of acquired signals. This means in this example that statistical noise in the measurements is not amplified appreciably by the synthesis process (i.e., the method has good precision). Similar comparisons for other materials of the brain yielded equivalent results. This implies for the echo times, the materials considered, and signal-to-noise ratios (SNRs) encountered in such imaging that the use of a single exponential model of *T2* relaxation is adequate.

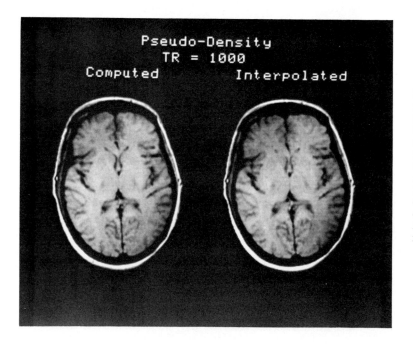

Figure 104–4. Comparison of directly computed (*left*) and synthetic (*right*) pseudodensity images generated for a TR of 1000 ms. These images correspond to the squares of Figure 104–1. The left image was computed from multiple spin echo measurements made at the same repetition time, 1000 ms. The right image was generated by interpolation of pseudodensity images formed at TR times of 500 and 2000 ms. Visually, the two results appear comparable.

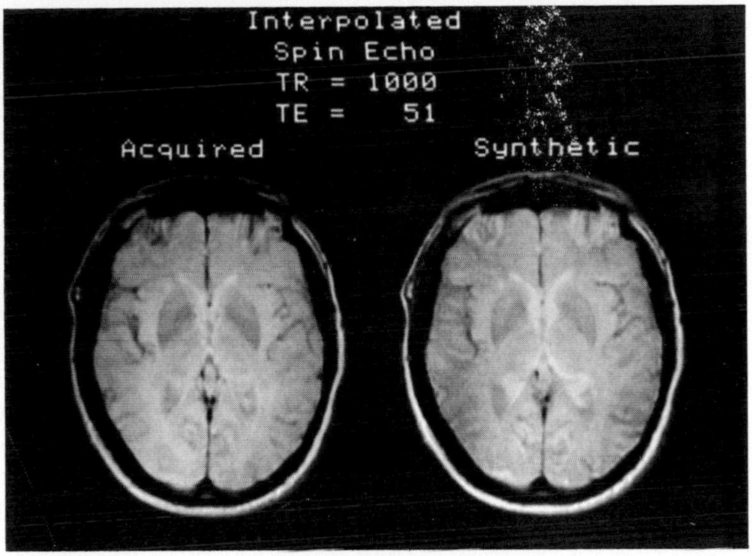

Figure 104–5. Plot versus the repetition time of signals measured in 25 pixel regions of interest from an area of the gray matter. As in Figure 104–3 the signals on the left of each pair correspond to the directly generated results while those on the right are for the synthetic image. Values plotted at TR of 1000 ms are from the images of Figure 104–4.

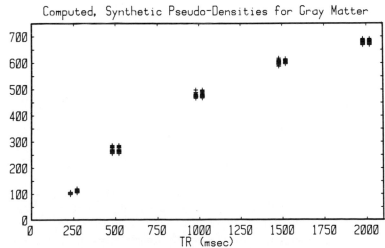

Similar comparisons were also performed to study the behavior in the TR direction. In this case acquisitions were made at TR times of 500 and 2000 ms; $T1$ and $N(H)$ were estimated via a two-point fit; and results were synthesized at various other TR times. Sample results are shown in Figure 104–4, a comparison of directly obtained and synthetic pseudodensity images for a TR of 1000 ms. Again, there is close correspondence between the two. Quantitative analysis of several ROIs was also performed similar to that discussed above for Figure 104–3. Results are shown in Figure 104–5 for the directly obtained and synthetic signals plotted versus the repetition time. The plotted points correspond to samples of the smooth surface of Figure 104–1 along the TR axis. As before, note the high degree of both accuracy and precision.

The results thus far have shown that it is possible to reproduce the original measurements synthetically (Figure 104–2) or to interpolate or extrapolate along the TR direction (Figure 104–4). Ideally one would like to perform such extrapolation or interpolation simultaneously in both TR and TE. Such a comparison was also performed, and results are shown in Figure 104–6. The synthetic image for TR of 1000 ms was generated from data acquired at TRs of 500 and 2000 ms. Likewise, interpolation

Figure 104–6. Comparison of a directly acquired image at TR/TE of 1000/51 ms with an image synthesized for the same scan parameters. The synthetic result has been simultaneously interpolated in TR and TE from the times at which the original data were acquired.

in TE was also performed. As before, acquired and synthetic results correspond closely in both accuracy and precision.

These results suggest that it is possible to acquire images at several TR and TE times in accordance with the sampling suggested in Figure 104–1 and synthesize spin-echo images at arbitrary TR and TE times with a high degree of fidelity. Having determined this, the next task was to optimize each stage of the synthesis process, to generate effective acquired images, and to transform them expeditiously into synthetic ones.

ANALYSIS OF MR IMAGE SYNTHESIS

In MR imaging in general, the SNR of an image increases as the scan time increases. The same concept applies to MR image synthesis as well. As one uses more and more scan time to obtain either a greater number of acquired images or images that have improved SNR, then the quality of the synthetic images improves as well. The possible drawback is that any improved capability offered by the synthesis method may be offset by a potentially unacceptable scan time. The feasibility studies of the previous section showed that reasonable synthetic images could be generated from acquisitions consisting of four spin echoes at repetition times of 500 and 2000 ms. Two broad questions subsequently arise. First, given the same number of images and the same expenditure of time (a total TR of 500 + 2000 ms, or 2500 ms), is it possible to improve the quality of the synthetic results over that of the feasibility studies? Second, what is the degradation in quality of synthetic images if the total scanning time and/or number of acquired images is decreased? In this section we describe how we attempted to answer these two broad questions. In doing this we concentrated our attention on the use of multiple spin-echo pulse sequences at several TR times. That is, we excluded consideration of alternative sequences such as inversion recovery (IR). We next describe our analysis of synthesis first along the *T1* or TR direction of Figure 104–1, and second along the *T2* or TE direction.

T1 Related Analysis

If one assumes that a single exponential model of longitudinal relaxation is accurate, then acquisition at only two different TR times is sufficient for estimating *T1*. The main issue then becomes one of precision, as illustrated in Figure 104–7. Shown in the figure are measured signals with error bars that are assumed to have been acquired at the two TR times, *TR1* and *TR2*. As stated earlier, image synthesis can be considered as an interpolation or extrapolation from acquired data to estimated signals at alternative TR times. That is, from the two measured signals we wish to estimate or synthesize a signal at a different TR time. As shown in the figure, given the uncertainty in the original measurements, the uncertainty or noise in a synthetic signal at a longer TR time can be appreciably greater. Thus, in this example the synthesis process would have poor precision in estimating the signal at the long TR time. We wished to study analytically what these noise propagation characteristics were of synthesis and determine how any propagation could be minimized by judicious selection of the TR times at which data were acquired. Much of the analysis next presented is taken from the work of Lee et al.[12]

The propagation of noise in image synthesis consists of two stages. First, any uncertainties in the acquired signals can be propagated into uncertainties or noise in the calculated *T1* values. Second, noise in these estimated *T1* times is in turn transformed into noise in the synthetic signals. Noise analysis of the first of these stages

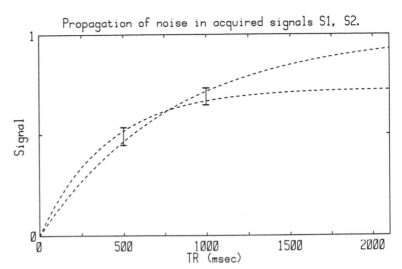

Propagation of noise in acquired signals S1, S2.

Figure 104–7. Schematic illustration of how noise amplification can occur in synthetic saturation recovery imaging. *S1* and *S2* correspond to original measurements, each with a statistical uncertainty (error bars). When extrapolation is performed from these measurements out to longer TR times, the resultant error bars at such times can be appreciably larger. This is equivalent to extensive noise amplification due to the synthesis process. By judicious selection of *TR1* and *TR2* such noise propagation can be minimized.

has been studied in detail in NMR spectroscopy[13–16] and more recently in the MR imaging context by Kurland.[17] Using such work as a starting point, Lee[12] has also accounted for the second stage. In this presentation we omit noise derivations for the sake of brevity and instead describe the results.

In the following discussion we assume that synthesis is done at the same echo time as the acquisition. Thus, it is possible to ignore any dependence on the echo time, TE, and the *T2* relaxation time. In this case, as discussed by Lee,[12,18] the equations that describe spin-echo signal behavior revert to those describing a saturation recovery (SR). Additionally, rather than a calculation of the true spin density, $N(H)$, the density actually determined is proportional to $N(H)$, with the proportionality factor equal to the *T2* exponential term.

Assume then that SR measurements are acquired at time *TR1* and *TR2*; they are then used to estimate *T1* and a density, *D*, and these in turn are used to synthesize a signal at time *TR*. We pose the question: how does the noise level in the synthetic signal compare with that in the acquired signals? It should be clear that it depends upon *TR1*, *TR2*, *T1*, and *TR* as well as the noise level of the acquisition. Lee has derived general formulas for this behavior, and a representative result is shown in Figure 104–8. Plotted there as the solid curve is the standard deviation in the synthetic signal at

Figure 104–8. A plot of the relative noise level (standard deviation) in direct acquisition (dashed curve) and in synthetic saturation recovery signals generated at the TR times shown (solid curve). Note that the noise level in synthetic signals need not match that in the acquisition. The latter signals are assumed to have been synthesized from data acquired at *TR1* and *TR2* times of 400 and 1500 ms. Additionally, the material under study is assumed to have a *T1* relaxation time of 770 ms. The squares correspond to direct measurements made under the same conditions as the curves. Note the close match of theory and experiment.

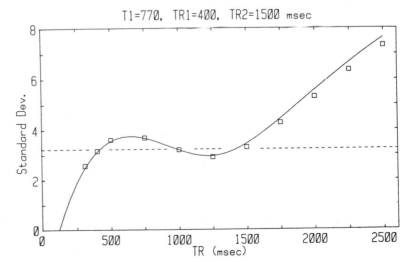

T1=770, TR1=400, TR2=1500 msec

time *TR* versus *TR*. This result assumed $TR1 = 400$, $TR2 = 1500$, and $T1 = 770$ ms. Also shown as a reference is the noise level in the acquired images. For TR times at which the smooth curve is higher than the dashed curve, the synthetic results appear noisier; while if lower than the dashed curve, the synthetic signal can actually be less noisy. This analysis was tested experimentally as well. A phantom was scanned at two TR times and images of the phantom synthesized at a variety of TR values. Noise levels were determined in the synthetic images and compared with that in the acquired images. Experimental results are also shown in Figure 104–8 as squares and demonstrate a close match with the theoretical prediction.

Having derived and experimentally verified the noise propagation formula, the next step was to apply it. Specifically, we wished to answer the two questions posed at the outset of this section. For a scan time equivalent to a total TR of, for example 2000 ms, what *TR1* and *TR2* would yield the best possible synthetic results and how would the results compare with acquired signals? Selection of these optimum times can be appreciated from Figure 104–9, which shows the noise in a synthetic SR signal versus the synthetic time TR for three different combinations of acquisition times. In all three cases *TR1* and *TR2* add to 2000 ms. As shown, the (300, 1700) combination provides the smallest maximum noise amplification over the 2000 ms range. This plot is for a specific *T1*, 800 ms. Fortuitously, for *T1* relaxation times in the range 400 to 1500 ms (the physiologic range at 1.5 tesla) the (300, 1700) choice for *TR1* and *TR2* is either at or near optimum as well. Thus, for acquisition of signals to be subsequently used for image synthesis, the optimum TR times used should be approximately 300 and 1700 ms, assuming that the total scan time is to be equivalent to a TR of 2000 ms. With this acquisition the noise in any signal synthesized for a TR in the 200 to 2000 ms range will be at most 20 percent higher than the noise in a signal directly acquired at the same TR. If the total TR were to be 2500 ms, then *TR1* and *TR2* should be approximately 370 and 2130 ms. Similar analysis can be done for any desired total TR.

A logical question that arises is to what extent image synthesis can be used to potentially reduce the scanning time. That is, is it possible to acquire signals at two "short" TR times and synthesize at a "long" TR and thereby decrease the total scan time. Using analysis similar to the preceding we investigated this question. Suppose that scans are done at *TR1* and *TR2*, and the sum $TR1 + TR2$ equals 1600 ms. Next, suppose that this acquired data is used to synthesize a signal at a *TR* of 2000 ms. In this case the scan time requirements would have been reduced by 20 percent, from a

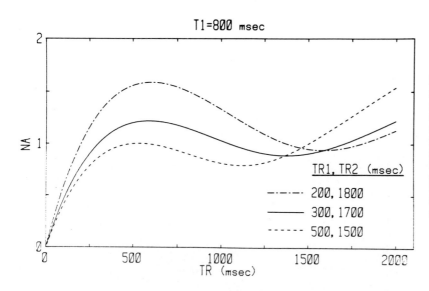

Figure 104–9. Plot of the relative noise level in synthetic saturation recovery signals as a function of the synthetic TR time. A *T1* value of 800 ms is assumed. Three different acquisition strategies are shown, all of which are equivalent in total scan time to a single acquisition at a *TR* of 2000 ms. The *TR1/TR2* combination of 300/1700 ms (solid curve) provides the lowest overall noise level.

TR of 2000 to 1600 ms. Analysis shows in this example that the noise in the synthetic signal at 2000 ms would be double that in the acquired signal. A 20 percent time reduction resulted in a 50 percent loss of SNR. For greater time reduction the penalty is more severe: 50 percent reduction in time would cost a 90 percent reduction in SNR. For this reason, the use of MR image synthesis to reduce scan time requirements in this fashion is not expected to be viable.

T2 Related Analysis

The analysis and results of the preceding section showed how proper selection of *TR1* and *TR2* is important in optimizing the precision of image synthesis along the TR direction. The same considerations apply for synthesis at various echo times as well. Although scan time is not substantially affected by selection of the echo times used for acquisition, the quality of synthetic spin-echo images is heavily dependent on these times. In this section we present our results for this *T2* related behavior.

Just as for the *T1* analysis described previously, the analysis of precision of synthetic spin-echo images consists of two stages. First, uncertainties in the measurements are propagated into uncertainties in the computed *T2* and pseudodensity values, and second, these are transformed into noise in the synthetic signals. In his work Kurland[17] considered the first of these, and recently MacFall et al.[19] have accounted for the second stage as well. In this case a set of spin-echo measurements are assumed to have been acquired at some given repetition time, *TR*. These measured signals are then used to estimate *T2* and the pseudodensity (*PD*). *PD* and *T2* are then used to synthesize a spin-echo signal at an arbitrary echo time, *TE*, for the same repetition time *TR*. As expected, the noise level in the synthetic signal depends on the echo times of the acquisition, the SNR of the measurements, the *T2* of the material under study, and the synthetic echo time *TE*. Again, for brevity the mathematical derivations are not presented here but rather the results.

Figure 104–10 shows the SNRs in an acquired (solid curve) and synthetic (dashed curve) spin-echo signal plotted as a function of the echo time *TE*. Because the noise level in the acquisition is the same for all echo times the SNR of the acquisition is simply proportional to the signal, the characteristic exponential decay. On the other

Figure 104–10. Plot of the signal-to-noise ratio (SNR) in acquired (solid curve) and synthetic (dashed curve) spin-echo signals. In each case the material under study is assumed to have a *T2* relaxation time of 100 ms. The synthetic result is assumed to have been generated from spin echoes acquired at 25, 50, 75, and 100 ms. Because the noise level is the same for all acquired echoes, the SNR of the acquired signal matches the signal behavior, the characteristic exponential decay. However, because the noise level in synthesis is dependent upon the synthetic echo time, improved SNR is possible. As shown, for four-echo acquisitions the resultant synthetic signal has superior SNR for echo times exceeding the first echo.

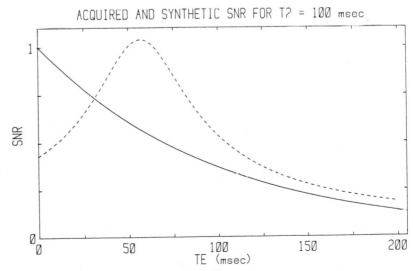

ACQUIRED AND SYNTHETIC SNR FOR T2 = 100 msec

hand, the result of MacFall's analysis shows that the noise in spin-echo synthesis can vary markedly with *TE*, yielding the dashed curve shown. It is noteworthy that the SNR of the synthetic signal essentially matches that of the acquired signal at approximately the first echo time and exceeds it thereafter. Although the plot shown is for a specific case of acquired echoes at 25, 50, 75, and 100 ms and a *T2* of 100 ms, this general behavior is similar for most four-echo acquisitions.

These theoretical predictions were tested experimentally with measurements made on phantoms. Spin-echo images were acquired, the *T2* and *PD* regressions were performed, and synthetic images generated at a variety of echo times. Sample results are shown in Figure 104–11, which is a plot versus *TE* of the standard deviation or noise (as opposed to Figure 104–10, which showed the SNR). The horizontal dashed curve is a plot of the noise level of the acquired images. The smooth curve is the theoretically predicted noise level, assuming acquired echoes at 20, 40, 60, and 80 ms and a *T2* of 93.8 ms. Finally, the circles with error bars are the measured standard deviations in the experimental synthetic spin-echo images. Note the close agreement between theory and experiment.

A clinical example of the improvement in SNR provided by image synthesis is shown in Figure 104–12. The left image is a directly acquired spin-echo result at an echo time of 120 ms of a patient having a hematoma. From this image and additional ones acquired at 30, 60, and 90 ms the synthetic result at the right was generated. It clearly has superior SNR. Note, for example, the interhemispheric fissure, which is not visualized at all in the acquired image.

Figures 104–10 to 104–12 all assumed that four echoes were used in the acquisition. One might ask whether these many echoes are required in general for effective synthetic results. In general, as the number of echoes is decreased, the quality of synthesis also diminishes. However, by judicious selection of the echo times themselves high precision can be maintained. In fact, it can be shown that if only two echoes are used for acquisition, that optimum precision in synthetic spin-echo images is obtained if an interecho time equal to the *T2* under study is chosen.[20] This means that for brain imaging, for example, in which case the *T2* values of interest are in the 50 to 70 ms range, then the two echoes used should be separated by about 60 ms. For example, acquisitions at times of 10 and 70 ms would be effective. It can also be shown in this case that the SNR of the synthetic signal always matches or exceeds the SNR of a direct spin-echo signal for echo times exceeding that of the first acquired signal. This result is important

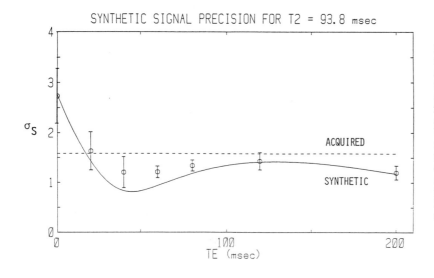

Figure 104–11. Plot of the relative noise level (standard deviation) in acquired (dashed curve) and synthetic (solid curve) spin-echo imaging for a *T2* time of 93.8 ms and four-echo acquisition at 20, 40, 60, and 80 ms. The circles with error bars correspond to measurements made under conditions identical to those for the solid theoretical curve. Note that the noise in the synthetic signal is less than that in the acquired signal, as shown in Figure 104–10. Also note the close match of theory with experiment.

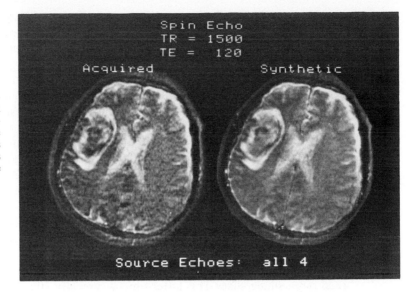

Figure 104–12. Experimental demonstration of the SNR improvement provided by spin-echo image synthesis. The synthetic image at the 120 ms echo, generated from echoes at 30, 60, 90, and 120 ms, clearly has superior SNR in comparison to the directly acquired result.

in that it shows that the SNR improvement of spin-echo images discussed earlier can be obtained with MR image synthesis even with the acquisition of only two spin echoes.

The results of these last two sections can now be used in formulating the ideal acquisition protocol for MR image synthesis.

ACQUISITION OF SOURCE IMAGES

We now specify the desired acquisition protocol for image synthesis. We assume first that scanning is to be performed at a field strength of 1.5 tesla, and thus the physiologic *T1* and *T2* relaxation times are in the 400 to 1500 ms and 50 to 90 ms range, respectively. Then, if scanning is to be done in a time equivalent to a TR of 2000 ms, the *TR1* and *TR2* values to be used in acquisition are 300 and 1700 ms. If the equivalent total *TR* is extended to 2500 ms for somewhat improved SNR, then the *TR1* and *TR2* values should be 370 and 2130 ms. In either case effective synthetic results can be obtained if two echoes are acquired at the long TR and one echo at the short TR. The first echo at the long TR and the echo at the short TR should be at the same echo time and as early as possible, such as 10 to 20 ms. Such early times yield source images that have high intrinsic SNR, which is important for determination of the computed *T1*, *T2*, and *N(H)* quantities. The late echo at the long TR time should be separated from the early echo by a time approximately equal to the average *T2* relaxation of interest. For example, if this average *T2* time is 60 ms and the early echo is at a *TE1* of 20 ms, then the late echo should occur at a *TE2* of 80 ms. Thus, this protocol consists of three acquired images: one early spin echo at a short *TR* and an early and late spin echo at a long *TR*. With this protocol synthetic images can be generated at any *TR* time not exceeding the total reference TR and for any echo time exceeding *TE1* with at most a 20 percent penalty in SNR. In many cases, such as at echo times exceeding *TE2*, the SNR in the synthetic images exceeds that in an image directly acquired using the same synthetic timing parameters.

As stated earlier, as more images are acquired and used in the image synthesis process, the quality of the synthetic results can improve. For example, if four rather than two spin echoes were acquired at the long TR, the SNR improvement would be even more pronounced than for the two-echo case. However, the protocol discussed above is roughly equivalent, if not less, in time consumption to that used for routine scanning. Additionally, it provides synthetic results essentially equivalent (within 20 percent) or even superior to direct acquisition. For this reason this is our targeted acquisition strategy.

Ideally this acquisition would be performed on a multislice basis. That is, in one scan equivalent to the reference TR of 2000 or 2500 ms, data would be acquired for two TRs, one or two echo times, and multiple slices. At this time we are developing such a sequence.

It is worthwhile to point out that such a pulse sequence could potentially be valuable for routine scanning irrespective of subsequent image synthesis. Common protocols now require images at both a long and a short TR from multiple slices. A pulse sequence such as that described here could be used for such protocols and eliminate the time overhead of resetting parameters between the long and short TR scans.

A second point to make is that the image synthesis acquisition protocol can potentially increase the number of slices that are imaged in one scan sequence. The reason for this is as follows. The number of slices imaged is proportional to the TR time used and inversely proportional to the time required to apply 90 and 180 degree pulses and read out a single slice. This latter time is typically 10 ms in excess of the last echo time used. For example, if the *TR* used were 1500 ms and the last echo were at 120 ms, then 1500/130 or approximately 11 slices could be scanned. On the other hand, if scanning were done at the same TR and echoes acquired at 20 and 80 msec, and synthesis performed to yield images at the desired 120 ms, then the number of slices in this case would be 1500/90 or 16, a considerable improvement.

COMPUTATION OF T1, T2 AND N(H) IMAGES

The second step of the image synthesis process is the computation of images of $T1$, $T2$, and $N(H)$ from the acquired image. These are now done using standard algorithms. In fact, such algorithms can be expedited using real-time digital video techniques, which enable computed images to be on the order of several seconds.[21] We next briefly outline the specific algorithms used.

If MR measurements $S1$ and $S2$ are made at the same echo time at each of two different repetition times $TR1$ and $TR2$, and if the ratio R of these measurements is taken, then R is equal to a function of $T1$ and known scanning parameters. For example, for the case of a simple saturation recovery pulse sequence, R is given by:

$$R = \frac{S1}{S2} = \frac{1 - e^{-TR1/T1}}{1 - e^{-TR2/T1}} \tag{1}$$

Note that the dependence on the $T2$ relaxation time is eliminated by taking the ratio. Even if other pulse sequences were used or more accurate mathematical models employed, in general a similar expression would result and the only unknown quantity appearing on the right side of the equation would be $T1$, the quantity of interest. Inspection of this equation shows that R is monotonically decreasing with respect to increasing $T1$. Although it is not possible to analytically invert Equation (1) and directly solve for $T1$, this monotonic behavior means that $T1$ can be determined via a lookup table. This is illustrated in Figure 104–13, which is a plot of R versus $T1$ for acquisitions done at $TR1$ of 500 ms and $TR2$ of 1500 ms and the same echo time for each. Any value of R, a quantity determined explicitly from the measurements, can be uniquely mapped to a $T1$ value, the $T1$ for that pixel at which $S1$ and $S2$ were measured. This is the essence of a two-point fit for $T1$. With the protocol discussed in the previous section

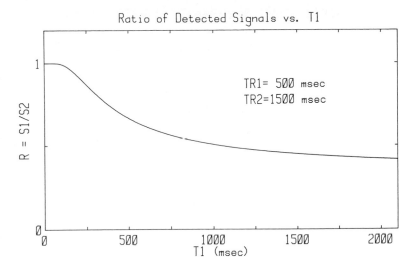

Figure 104–13. Plot of the ratio R of saturation recovery signals *S1* and *S2* measured at repetition times *TR1/TR2* of 500/1500 ms. Note that *R* decreases monotonically with increasing *T1*, thereby enabling estimation of *T1* from *R* values via a simple table lookup.

the two measurements used would correspond to the early echo at the long TR and the only echo at the short TR.

T2 fitting is performed by first modeling the signals (S_i) measured at echo time (TE_i) as a simple exponential related to the *T2* relaxation time of interest and the pseudodensity, *PD*.

$$S_i \simeq PD\ e^{-TE_i/T2} \tag{2}$$

Determination of *T2* is facilitated by taking the logarithm of both sides of Equation (2). When $ln(S_i)$ is plotted versus the echo times, then *T2* is recognized as the negative inverse slope of the line of regression.[19]

For the case in which only two echoes are acquired, this reverts to:

$$\frac{1}{T2} = \frac{ln\ S1 - ln\ S2}{TE2 - TE1} \tag{3}$$

If more than two echoes are acquired, then performing a least squares minimization yields *T2* as a function of various summations of the measured signals weighted by the echo times used. For the acquisition protocol discussed in the previous section, Equation (3) is used in conjunction with the two spin echoes acquired at the long repetition time.

Both of the algorithms outlined in Equations (1) and (3) can be performed using high-speed digital video techniques, as has been recently been discussed by Wright.[21] The two main requirements are adequate frame memory for image storage and enough capability in high speed hardware for performing the necessary mathematical manipulations. Such requirements are similar to those for performing the actual image synthesis at high speed. As an example, if Equation (3) is to be performed, then one starts by loading the acquired images *S1* and *S2* into frame memory. These are then separately transformed into logarithms via a lookup table, requiring a 1/30 s video frame interval for each. The *lnS1* and *lnS2* images can be written over the original *S1* and *S2* images or stored in additional frame memory if available. In the third frame interval the difference of the logged signals is generated, yielding the numerator of the right side of Equation (3). Finally this result is multiplied by the constant *1/(TE2-TE1)* to yield an image of *1/T2*. Thus, computation time for a *1/T2* image from two measurements is four video frame intervals, about 130 ms. This increases somewhat due to software overhead. If desired, the *1/T2* result can be inverted to provide the *T2* image. A similar approach can be used to generate images of *T1* and *N(H)*.

REAL–TIME MR IMAGE SYNTHESIS

The third and final step of the image synthesis process is the actual synthesis. From the outset of this project our aim has been to perform the synthesis at high speed. This enables the viewer to interactively optimize contrast through manipulation of TE and TR times in much the same way as window and level adjustments are made on a CT display. Indeed, our earliest feasibility studies demonstrated this in a crude manner.[8] Lee and coworkers[22] have shown how the synthesis computations can be done at high speed and with high numerical precision using generic digital video imaging device. Here we discuss these methods but omit the details for brevity.

The targeted configuration for the real time synthesis device is shown in Figure 104–14. For a specific slice, the computed $T1$, $T2$, and $N(H)$ images are contained in three video frame memories. These are fed in parallel to a digital video processor (DVP), where high speed mathematical manipulations are performed. Simultaneously with this, the operator is in putting the desired pulse sequence (SE, IR, SR, etc.) as well as specific values for the timing parameters such as TR and TE. A microprocessor acts as a controlling device and loads these timing parameters into the DVP. Then in a pipeline fashion the synthetic signal for the first pixel in the image is computed according to the appropriate mathematical equation. The signal for the second pixel is next computed using the same equation but with its own specific values for $T1$, $T2$, and $N(H)$. This is repeated for all pixels, and the resulting pixel stream is converted into an analog video signal and directed to a TV monitor. In response to visualizing the display the operator can readjust the scan parameters.

Some of the requirements of the DVP can be determined by consideration of a simple saturation-recovery pulse sequence, in which case the synthetic signal S is computed according to:

$$S = N(H) \cdot (1 - e^{-TR/T1}) \tag{4}$$

Inspection of Equation (4) shows that multiplication of one quantity by another must be allowed (e.g., TR by $1/T1$), addition or substraction (the exponential subtracted from 1), and exponentiation (the exponential of $-TR/T1$). High speed multiplication can be performed using hardware multipliers, while addition and subtraction are permitted with arithmetic logic units (ALUs). The exponentiation, and in fact arbitrary transformations, can be performed in a high-speed random access memory used as a lookup table (LUT). These devices can all operate at the 10 MHz pixel rates required for 512 × 512 real time digital video imaging. A pipelined digital video processor that can perform these necessary operations is shown in Figure 104–15. Although not designed

NMR IMAGE PROCESSOR

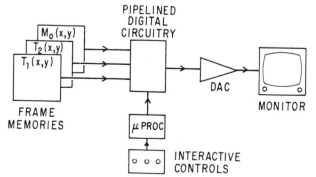

Figure 104–14. Basic schematic diagram of the desired instrumentation for high speed interactive MR image synthesis.

PIPELINED DIGITAL CIRCUITRY

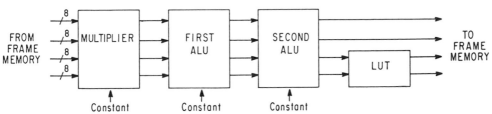

Figure 104–15. Schematic of the pipelined digital video processor (DVP) used for high speed synthesis.

so that the synthetic signal S of Equation (4) can be generated for each pixel in only one pass through the DVP, all necessary operations can be performed at some stage in the DVP.

Perhaps the fastest time in which an image could be synthesized according to the general schematic of Figure 104–14 is one video frame interval. That is, once the operator makes some alteration in one of the scan parameters, the corresponding synthetic image is generated and appears 1/30 s later on the monitor. As mentioned above, because the DVP is not configured to perform all of the required manipulations for a specific pulse sequence in a strict pipeline fashion, such a fast computation time is not possible. As an alternative our group has devised a method in which the synthetic signal (S of Equation 4) is constructed one term at a time, with one video frame interval required per term. As an example we again consider the saturation recovery pulse sequence of Equation (4).

Operation commences with the $N(H)$, $T1$, and $T2$ images (or reciprocal images of these latter two quantities) stored in video frame memory. Next, suppose the operator specifies some repetition time, TR, at which an image is to be synthesized. Then, during the first video frame interval, the $1/T1$ image is read from frame memory and multiplied in the multiplier stage of the DVP of Figure 104–15 by the constant TR. The product is passed through the subsequent arithmetic logic unit (ALU) and LUT stages without alteration and stored back into a scratch frame memory. During the second frame interval this newly formed $TR/T1$ image is read from the scratch memory and passed through the LUT where it is transformed into the $(1 - \exp[-TR/T1])$ term of Equation (4). That is, each $TR/T1$ input to the LUT can be uniquely assigned to the appropriate exponential. The resultant image is again stored in scratch frame memory. During the final frame interval of computation the exponential image is read from scratch memory simultaneously with the $N(H)$ image being read out from its memory. They are both presented to the multiplier of the DVP, where the images are multiplied together on a pixel by pixel basis in pipeline fashion. During this frame interval the result can be directly converted into analog video signal for display. In practice it may be directed to a buffer frame memory used to continuously refresh the video monitor. In either case, the total computation time in this example is three video frame intervals, 1/10 s. In actual practice the software overhead required to reconfigure the DVP pathways between the various passes may increase this time somewhat. Additionally, for more mathematically complicated pulse sequences additional passes would be required. However, we have been able to successfully generate images for all the standard pulse sequences (IR, SE, SR) in times of 600 ms or less.

One of the technical issues concerning the generation of synthetic images in this fashion is that of numerical precision. Equivalently, how many bits should be maintained at each stage of the computations? This topic has been studied in detail by Lee.[22] He has shown that with 16 bit arithmetic it is possible to generate images for all of the standard pulse sequences using standard timing parameters with errors no greater than 0.4 percent of $N(H)$, the maximum MR signal. This is generally comparable or less than the intrinsic noise level in the acquired images themselves.

APPLICATIONS

We expect that the technique of real time MR image synthesis has a number of potential applications, ranging from a learning tool to a routinely used clinical technique. Regardless of how the acquired images are generated, the ability to sit at a console, interactively adjust timing parameters, and dynamically see how the contrast in MR images varies in response to these changes is a very graphic demonstration of the contrast dependence in MR imaging. For clinical sites that are still in the process of formulating acquisition protocols the method of image synthesis can be used to retrospectively optimize contrast for a particular pathology. The sequences so determined can then be used on patients who subsequently present with the same suspected diagnosis.

For more routine clinical work it is uncertain whether radiologists will interactively use synthesis on all slices to retrospectively optimize contrast. This is particularly true for those who are confident in the inherent sensitivity of the pulse sequences used. On the other hand, the technique of image synthesis is seen as a useful technique for standardizing acquisition protocols and improving patient throughput. After a short sequence is used to verify proper patient position, a compound multi-TR multiecho multislice sequence can be performed using the protocol outlined above. After this temporally efficient pulse sequence is done for the desired slice orientations (axial, coronal, sagittal), the acquisition is over and the patient can be removed from the scanner.

At this point the acquired images are transferred to the high speed circuitry that performs first the computation of the $N(H)$, $T1$, and $T2$ images, and second, the actual image synthesis. Synthetic results would be computed for desired timing parameters in addition to and different from those used in the acquisition. For example, these could include intermediate echo (40 to 50 ms) results, late echo times (120 ms or longer), or inversion recovery images.

The two specific applications of this method are the formation of late-echo highly $T2$ sensitive spin-echo images and synthetic inversion recovery images. The importance of the former has been discussed with respect to the sensitivity for detecting many lesions.[23] Previously we discussed the fact that the price of acquiring such late echoes directly is a decreased number of slices, a price diminished by the synthesis process.

The second major application is pulse sequence extrapolation.[24] With this method images are acquired with one pulse sequence (e.g., spin-echo) and used to synthesize images for a different pulse sequence (e.g., inversion recovery). Validation studies of this method have been discussed recently by Bobman et al.[25] Examples are shown in Figure 104–16. The left of each figure is an inversion-recovery image acquired directly at the timing parameters shown. The subject was a normal adult male. The right image of each figure is an IR image synthesized at the same timing parameters. Each IR image was formed from multiple spin-echo images acquired at repetition times of 450 and 1600 ms, equivalent to a total TR of 2150 ms. Although there are perceptible differences between the acquired and synthetic images that comprise each pair, the relative trend of signal behavior with TI is consistent. For example, the white matter has slightly decreased signal intensity at the shorter TI time (50 ms, Figure 104–16A), while its contrast has reversed with respect to the surrounding brain at the longer TI time (600

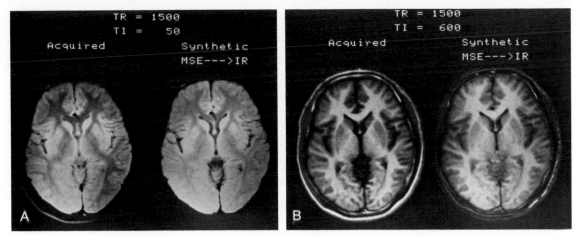

Figure 104–16. Demonstration of pulse sequence extrapolation using MR image synthesis. The left of each pair is a directly acquired inversion recovery (IR) image. The right of each is an IR image synthesized from multiple spin-echo acquisitions at 450 and 1600 ms. Results are shown for a *TR* time of 1500 ms and *TI* times of 50 (*A*) and 600 (*B*) ms.

msec, Figure 104–16*B*). This technique is expected to enhance the sensitivity to *TI* related pathology.

We have presented the method of magnetic resonance image synthesis and discussed its principles. Feasibility studies showed a high correlation between acquired and synthetic images in both accuracy and precision. We have performed detailed analyses of the precision of image synthesis and determined the acquisition protocol optimum for maximizing the precision. This protocol can be performed using a multi-TR multiecho multislice acquisition with a scanning time equivalent to a total TR of 2000 ms. Even if not used for synthesis, such a sequence is of potential value for routine clinical scanning. Once the scanning is completed, the two remaining stages of image synthesis, formation of computed images and the actual synthesis, can be performed at high speed using realtime digital video circuitry. Most of the required components for such hardware are found on commercial MR systems. Computed images of $N(H)$, *T1*, and *T2* can be generated in times of about two seconds apiece. Synthesis of images for arbitrary timing parameters for the standard pulse sequences can be done in times of about 600 msec or less. The method is seen as a means of standardizing and facilitating the acquisition of MR images and thus improving patient throughput. Expected applications are the synthesis of late echo spin-echo images and synthetic inversion recovery imaging.

ACKNOWLEDGMENTS

This investigation was supported by PHS grant number I RO1 CA37993, awarded by the National Cancer Institute, the Department of Health and Human Services, General Electric Medical Systems, and the Whitaker Foundation.

References

1. Wehrli FW, MacFall JR, Glover GH: The dependence of nuclear magnetic resonance (NMR) image contrast on intrinsic and operator-selectable parameters. Proc SPIE *419*:256–264, 1983.
2. Wehrli FW, MacFall JR, Newton TH: Parameters determining the appearance of NMR images. *In* Newton TH, Potts HG (eds): Modern neuroradiology advanced imaging techniques. Vol. 2. San Anselmo, Clavadel, 1983, pp 81–117.

3. Young IR, Bryan DTR, Payne JA, et al: Contrast in NMR imaging. Paper presented at the Society of Magnetic Resonance in Medicine, San Francisco, 1983.
4. Perman WH, Hilal SK, Simon HE, Maudsley AA: Contrast manipulation in NMR imaging. Magn Reson Imaging 2:23–32, 1984.
5. Ortendahl DA, Hylton NM, Kaufman L, Crooks LE: Signal to noise in derived NMR images. Magn Reson Med 1:316–338, 1984.
6. Ortendahl DA, Hylton NM, Kaufman L, Watts JC, Crooks LE, Mills CN, Stark DN: Analytical tools for magnetic resonance imaging. Radiology 153:479–488, 1984.
7. Bielke G, Meves M, Meindl S, et al: A systematic approach to optimization of pulse sequences. In Esser PD, Johnston RE (eds): Technology of nuclear magnetic resonance. New York, Society Nuclear Medicine, 1984, pp 109–117.
8. Riederer SJ, Suddarth SA, Bobman SA, Lee JN, Wang HZ, MacFall JR: Automated MR image synthesis: feasibility studies. Radiology 153:203–206, 1984.
9. Riederer SJ, Bobman SA, Suddarth SA, Lee JN, Wang HZ, MacFall JR: NMR image synthesis in realtime. In Esser PD, Johnston RE (eds): Technology of nuclear magnetic resonance. New York, Society Nuclear Medicine, 1984, pp 97–107.
10. Bobman SA, Riederer SJ, Lee JN, Suddarth SA, Wang HZ, MacFall JR: Synthesized MR images: comparison with acquired images. Radiology 155:731–738, 1985.
11. Bobman SA, Riederer SJ, Lee JN, Suddarth SA, Wang HZ, Drayer BP, MacFall JR: Cerebral MR image synthesis. Am J Neuroradiol 6:265–269, 1985.
12. Lee JN, Bobman SA, Johnson JP, Farzaneh F, Riederer SJ: The precision of TR extrapolation in MR image synthesis. Med Phys 13:170–177, 1986.
13. DeFontaine DL, Ross DK, Ternai B: A fast nonlinear least squares method for the calculation of relaxation times. J Magn Reson 18:276–281, 1975.
14. Liepert TK, Marquardt DW: Statistical analysis of NMR spin-lattice relaxation times. J Magn Reson 24:181–199, 1976.
15. Crouch R, Hurlbert S, Ragouzeos A: An iterative linear method for calculation of spin-lattice relaxation times. J Magn Reson 49:371–382, 1982.
16. Granot J: Optimization of spin-lattice relaxation time measurements: statistical analysis by stochastic simulation of inversion-recovery experiments. J Magn Reson 53:3386–397, 1983.
17. Kurland RJ: Strategies and tactics in NMR imaging relaxation time measurements. I. Minimizing relaxation time errors due to image noise—the ideal case. Magn Reson Med 2:136–158, 1985.
18. Lee JN, Riederer SJ: A modified saturation-recovery approximation for multiple spin-echo pulse sequences. Magn Reson Med 3:132–134, 1986.
19. MacFall JR, Riederer SJ, Wang HZ: An analysis of noise propagation in computed T2 and pseudo-density and synthetic spin-echo images. Med Phys 13:285–292, 1986.
20. Lee JN, Riederer SJ: Optimum acquisition times of two spin-echoes for MR image synthesis. Magn Reson Med 3:634–638, 1986.
21. Wright RC, Riederer SJ, Lee JN, Farzaneh F, DeCastro JB: High-speed techniques for estimating T1 and T2 images. Proc SPIE 626:196–199, 1986.
22. Lee JN, Riederer SJ, Bobman SA, Farzaneh F, Wang HZ: Instrumentation for rapid MR image synthesis. Magn Reson Med 3:33–43, 1986.
23. Brant-Zawadzki M: Nuclear magnetic resonance imaging: the abnormal brain and spinal cord. In Newton TH, Potts DG (eds): Modern neuroradiology: advanced imaging techniques, San Anselmo, Clavadel Press, 1983, pp 159–186.
24. Bobman SA, Lee JN, Suddarth SA, Wang HZ, Riederer SJ, MacFall JR: Comparison of synthesized NMR images with their source images. Association of University Radiologists, Newport Beach, May 1984.
25. Bobman SA, Riederer SJ, Lee JN, Farzaneh F, Wang HZ: Pulse-sequence extrapolation using MR image synthesis. Radiology 159:253–258, 1986.

105

MRI Parameter Selection Techniques

DOUGLAS A. ORTENDAHL
NOLA M. HYLTON

The enthusiasm with which magnetic resonance imaging (MRI) has been accepted by clinicians is due in large part to the technique's dependence on multiple tissue parameters: the hydrogen density $N(H)$, the relaxation times, $T1$ and $T2$, and the state of motion of the hydrogen. This multiparametric dependence offers high sensitivity to disease and the hope of higher specificity by tailoring the acquisition technique to the potential pathology. Therein lies the opportunity of MRI as well as what can be perceived as the frustration of having to deal with what could be a never-ending stream of data acquisition modes, each with a particular advantage or rationale. Since it is clearly impractical to try every technique in each patient, research in MRI is devoted to finding optimal protocols for various disease states and developing screening techniques.

What would need to be done if we desired to assess experimentally the clinical utility of MR techniques? Consider just one imaging technique, spin echo (SE). The parameter TR ($T1$ sensitive imager parameter) can be easily varied from 20 ms to as much as three times the $T1$ of CSF ($TR = 10$ s). This means that for a complete evaluation, some 30 points should be sampled in TR space. TE (the $T2$ sensitive parameter) could be varied between 20 and 300 ms in another 30 steps or so, so that to sample the SE technique response about 900 points would need to be considered. Inversion recovery (IR) adds a third parameter, TI, which can vary between zero and TR, so that the possible sampled space would easily be 7 to 8 times larger than for SE, or 7000 points. But, there exists in addition an infinite set of other imaging techniques, each with its own set of sampling parameters. It is clear that clinical efficacy studies cannot be done in an exhaustive manner, i.e., by sampling all possible techniques. In practice, we have used data on the behavior of normal and abnormal tissues in rats and later in humans to obtain what appear to be very sensitive imaging techniques.[1-4] For examination of the head, our routine screening technique has $TR = 2$ s and $TE = 30$ and 60 ms. Long TR times are also valuable for studying the pelvis and vascular disease, but elsewhere in the body shorter TR values find utility. In the case of liver lesions, the most effective technique we have found is an IR with $TR = 1.8$ s, TI $= 0.28$ s, and $TE = 28$ ms. New techniques are typically checked against the best prior technique. We have examined the same patient with up to four techniques at a time, but this reaches the limit of practicality, since a one-hour study is the longest that even a well-motivated patient will stand for.

An alternative approach is to try to understand how the images respond to changes in imaging parameters and to predict the effectiveness of various imaging procedures. This approach has been taken by several investigators. Droege[5] has used a computational technique to sample the space of all possible brain lesions to find which sequences provide optimal performance. Not surprisingly he finds that good sensitivity would be predicted from a $TE = 80$ ms, $TR = 2.7$ s SE sequence. The parameter sensitivity technique proposed by Mitchell et al.[6] has a similar goal: to find protocols that will give high confidence for detecting deviation from a given set of parameter values. Both of these methods attempt to find a protocol that will best detect lesions in a particular background tissue and as such primarily suggest screening techniques.

The emphasis of the work described here is different.[4,7,8] We start with a knowledge of the parameters of the tissues that are to be visualized. These parameters could be postulated, but usually they will have been determined from measurements within a particular patient, which is valuable, since results in normal patients will often not be indicative of success in the clinic. A methodology of this kind can serve various purposes:

1. It is a teaching tool to understand the effect of changes of imaging technique on object contrast.

2. Within the bounds of the noise introduced by the calculational process we can retrospectively obtain images better suited to the highlighting of particular processes.

3. Rather than implement every possible technique in an imager and use it on patients, this method can be used to select those techniques worthy of experimental study. This can be done with actual patient data rather than on the basis of phantoms or other computer models.

METHODOLOGY

The need for such a methodology follows from the fact that the relationships between the parameters are complex and the results of particular combinations of imaging parameters are not intuitive. In particular, great care must be taken with conclusions drawn solely on the acquired intensity images without the benefit of calculations. The tendency to use the terms $T1$ weighted and $T2$ weighted images is especially dangerous here. These terms are not in the ACR glossary, but are used because of the sense of simplification that they provide. The pitfall is that it is possible to draw completely wrong conclusions with such simplifications. In Figure 105–1, in the $TR = 0.5$ s, $TE = 28$ ms image the tumor has a mean intensity of 1659 while the white matter is 1462. The conventional wisdom for this "$T1$ weighted image" would be to conclude that the tumor has a shorter $T1$ than the white matter. In fact, by doing the necessary calculations we find $T1$, $T2$ and $N(H)$ for both tumor and white matter to be respectively 637 ms, 83 ms, 4649 and 415 ms, 56 ms, 3550. $T1$ is significantly longer for the tumor. The tumor is more intense in the $TR = 0.5$ s image because of the longer $T2$ value and increased $N(H)$ relative to the white matter.

A proper understanding of the process must start with the fundamental parameters $T1$, $T2$, and $N(H)$, which are calculated from the acquired images. With these parameters we may make predictions about the effectiveness of various imaging techniques. The MR intensity for spin echo (SE) and inversion recovery (IR) can be modeled as:

$$I(SE) = N(H)f(v)\exp(-TE/T2)[1 + g(T1)] \tag{1}$$

$$I(IR) = N(H)f(v)\exp(-TE/T2)[1 - 2\exp(-TI/T1) - g(T1)] \tag{2}$$

$$g(T1) = -\exp(-TR/T1) + 2\exp[-(TR - .5TE)/T1] - 2\exp[-(TR - 1.5TE)/T1] \tag{3}$$

where $f(v)$ is a function of the flow and will be assumed to be 1 for this analysis. This model includes corrections for the two additional 180 degree radio frequency (rf) pulses that are required to collect two spin echoes. The spin echo corrections are important,

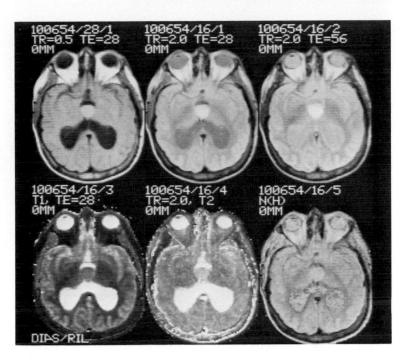

Figure 105–1. For a patient with a tumor of the third ventricle, we show acquired intensity images and images of *T1*, *T2*, and *N(H)*. The *TR* = 0.5 s, *TE* = 28 ms image shows higher intensity for the tumor as compared to white matter even though it has a longer *T1* than the white matter.

since errors of up to 20 percent in calculated *T1* may occur if they are neglected.[9] A similar result can be found from the Bloch equations for any number of spin echoes. The calculation of *T1*, *T2*, and *N(H)* is done by inversion of Equation (1). *T2* requires images at two different TEs while *T1* requires two different TRs. A basic assumption is made that the relaxation times are monoexponential, which has been shown to be true for the range over which we sample through extensive work in our laboratory.[4,10]

Calculated Images

Once the relaxation times have been determined, the intensity equations may be used to predict images at any desired values of the acquisition parameters. These calculated intensity images (some authors use the term synthesized images[11]) have been shown to be predictive of acquired images.[11-13] In Figure 105–2 we show examples of images calculated throughout the parameter space. In the SE images we see that contrast between the tumor and the brain can be reversed and made to disappear. With inversion recovery we can obtain more dramatic shifts in contrast. One particular application is the calculation of late echo (long TE) images, which are desirable for enhancing long *T2* valued tissue. As seen in the example of Figure 105–3, the calculated late-echo images are just as diagnostic as the acquired images. This allows us to avoid the necessity of acquiring these images, an advantage since late-echo imaging can impact on the ability to accumulate multisection images. Time is better spent acquiring additional sections rather than waiting for long TE images, which can just as well be calculated.

Signal Difference Maps

The calculated images themselves do not solve the problem of proliferation of imaging protocols, but this capability can provide a framework for evaluating the rela-

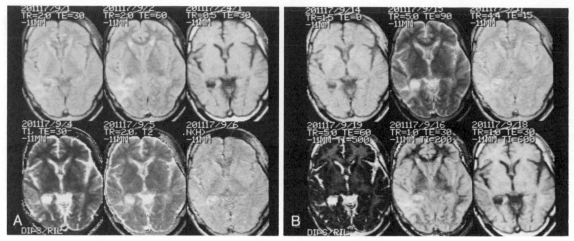

Figure 105–2. *A,* Acquired and relaxation time images of a patient with a brain tumor. The tumor is seen to have both a long *T1* and *T2*. *B,* Various calculated SE and IR images show that contrast may be varied over a wide range.

tive merit of various protocols. The goal of any diagnostic procedure is to separate the area of the pathology from the normal background tissues, and it is on this basis that they should be evaluated using a criterion of acceptable differentiation. In conventional imaging techniques, we search for contrast, i.e., C = (lesion − background)/background, in the terms defined by Rose.[14,15] In evaluating how well an object is visualized we must in addition to the contrast know something about the noise, an independent quantity. The output contrast in an image is dependent on the tissue parameters, the imager parameters, and if the feature is small, the spatial resolution. But noise does influence how well that contrast may be perceived, namely the confidence with which the presence of a lesion may be called. It is common to hear the comment that a noisy image shows "poor contrast." What is really meant is that the noise makes it impossible to confidently appreciate the contrast in the image. Our confidence depends on how much the perceived contrast will change if the experiment is repeated; this is the contrast noise. The significant parameter is contrast/(contrast noise), which is essentially

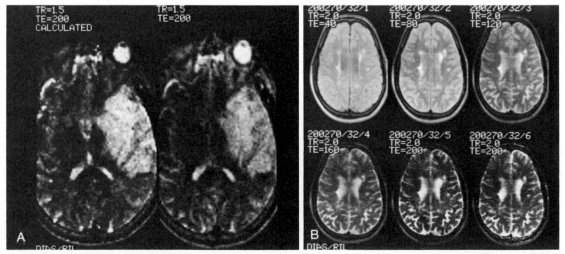

Figure 105–3. *A,* Acquired (*right*) and calculated *TE* = 200 ms images of a patient with an infarct. *B,* Five acquired images at different TE times and one calculated *TE* = 200 ms image (*lower right*) for a patient with multiple sclerosis. In both cases the late echo images were calculated using *TE* = 40 and 80 ms images and are diagnostically equivalent to the acquired images.

the confidence factor, k, which Rose suggests needs a value of 4 or so. For our purposes we need only be concerned with relative values of k, since we are comparing techniques. An alternative parameter that may be used is signal difference, D = lesion − background. This parameter must also be normalized by the noise so that the significant factor is difference/noise (D/N). This is a logical measure of confidence, since the larger the signal difference is relative to the noise in the image, the better we will be able to detect the lesion. We have found this to be completely equivalent to using contrast/contrast noise, and throughout the rest of this chapter we will use D/N in our evaluations.

In a well-tuned MR system the noise is almost totally introduced by random thermal currents within the patient.[12] As such, the noise will be independent of the choice of TE and TR, assuming that the number of acquisitions or redundant data sets remains the same. Since we are interested in relative values, we may neglect the noise entirely and consider only the signal difference. This simplification is one of the motivations for using difference rather than contrast, since contrast noise is always a function of TE and TR, as can be verified by standard techniques of error propagation. To efficiently evaluate a number of acquisition parameter pairs, we developed a tool called the difference map.[4] A two-dimensional space was used, with TE along the vertical axis and TR along the horizontal axis. The absolute signal difference (ASD) is plotted as a function of the TE and TR and is encoded in either a pseudocolor scale or in a black and white gray scale. This is one case where color has a significant advantage over black and white. The absolute value of the difference is used, since from a formal point of view it does not matter what sign the parameter has; the investigator may reverse the gray scale as he/she wishes. An example of an ASD map for lesion and white matter is shown in Figure 105–4 with the corresponding calculated images in Figure 104–5. The color scale we use is a rainbow, with red representing low intensity or in this case low signal difference while violet and then white indicate high intensity. The map shows two areas of high intensity separated by a dark valley. The valley shows the area of the TE, TR space, where very poor differentiation between lesion and white matter will be obtained. Crossing this dark area in TE, TR space will result in a contrast reversal. At short TR values the white matter is more intense while at long TRs it is less intense. Maximum absolute signal difference is obtained at the long TR values. The color scale shows that we should expect less absolute signal difference from images within the short TR region, as is verified by the $TR = 0.5$ s, $TE = 0$ ms image.

Figure 105–4. ASD map is shown for the patient of Figure 105–5. (See also Plate I, Figure *A*.)

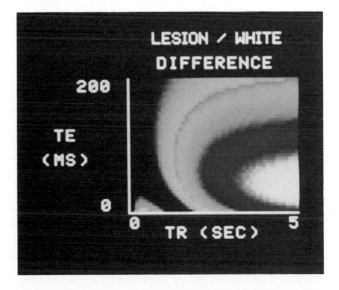

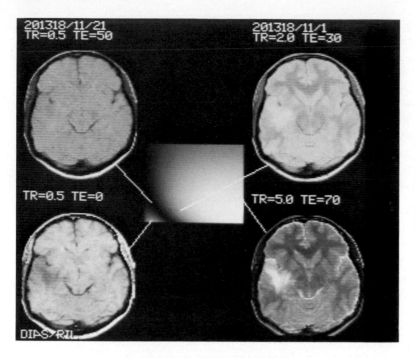

Figure 105–5. For a patient with metastasis to the brain from breast carcinoma we show an ASD map (see in color in Figure *A* of Plate I) for lesion/white matter difference. Note the contrast reversal as the dark band is crossed. An image obtained within the band shows no signal difference.

The ASD map provides information on the relative signal difference/noise, which can be obtained with various values of the acquisition parameters. It explicitly assumes that we are predicting the expected value of D/N for an *acquisition* at those particular parameter values. On the other hand, as shown previously, we may easily calculate images at any desired value of the acquisition parameters, but it is then no longer true that the noise is constant throughout the parameter space. The calculations involved in this process propagate the noise. *T1*, *T2* and *N*(*H*) are required for the calculations, and these parameters themselves have an error associated with them due to the noise in the original intensity images. The uncertainty will also depend on what acquisition points were sampled, since improper sampling of the decay curve could lead to additional error in the relaxation time. To account for these problems we use an additional map, the difference/noise or noise-corrected ASD plot. The signal difference is calculated at each point in the TE, TR space using the values of *T1*, *T2* and *N*(*H*) for the lesion and background. The intensity error is assumed to be independent of TE and TR, as previously stated. Using standard techniques of propagation of errors we can determine the noise in the calculated differences relative to the noise in the intensity images. This propagated difference noise is calculated at every point to normalize the difference values. This gives an indication of what quality of image we will be able to calculate at points other than the acquisition points.

An example of the noise corrected difference map is shown in Figure 105–6. The difference map shows a large area where maximum signal difference could be obtained by acquiring the image. But in the noise corrected image the area of maximum intensity has shifted toward shorter TR values and is now smaller. It is characteristic of these maps that the difference/noise peaks very close to the location of the acquired data upon which we base the calculations. It should not be surprising that the confidence with which we can predict goes down as we move away from the area where we have firm data points. In Figure 105–7 we see that the acquired image at *TR* = 2.0 s, *TE* = 30 ms shows maximum signal/noise. The short TR image where we have a contrast reversal is reduced in quality as predicted by the lower intensity seen in the noise corrected ASD map. The images calculated at *TR* = 5.0 s show high signal difference

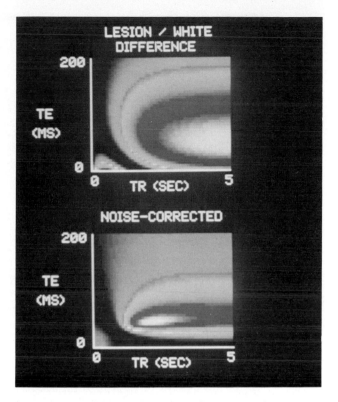

Figure 105–6. ASD and noise-corrected ASD maps for lesion/white contrast for the patient of Figure 105–7. (See also Plate I, Figure *B*.)

over a wide range of TE values as expected from the ASD plot. The noise-corrected map shows increased noise as *TE* is increased, which is seen in the *TE* = 120 ms image. Even though the relative confidence does go down, we can produce excellent quality calculated images far from the area of the original acquisition.

We can take a more detailed look at the problem of signal/noise in calculated images, with the plot of Figure 105–8. There are several points to make. First, the

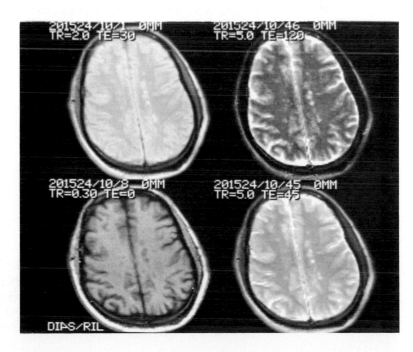

Figure 105–7. For a patient with multiple sclerosis we show calculated images corresponding to various points within the ASD maps of Figure 105–6. Maximum signal/noise is found at *TR* = 2.0 sec, *TE* = 30 ms, which is one of the acquired images and is near the maximum of the noise-corrected ASD plot.

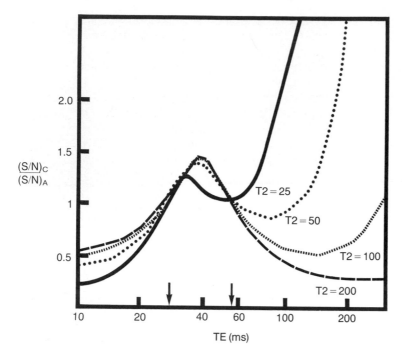

Figure 105–8. Ratio of S/N for calculated to S/N for acquired images for echoes calculated at different TE values (horizontal axis). The acquired echoes (arrows) are assumed to be at 28 and 56 ms. Results are shown for four *T2* values that cover the range of interest.

increase in signal/noise when we choose a TE value between the two acquisition points shows the benefit of interpolation between two known points, as has been observed by other investigators.[11] Unfortunately, this is not the region where we typically need to calculate images. For the short TE regime, we lose in relative signal/noise because we are extrapolating, and it gets worse the longer our lever arm is from the anchors provided by the acquired data points. The behavior here shows a weak dependence on the value of *T2*. For longer calculated TE values, the situation is much different. For the longer *T2* tissues, the signal/noise degrades, since the acquisition points poorly sample the decay curve. But the short *T2* values show an improvement in signal/noise even for an extrapolation. This surprising result can be understood by realizing that these short *T2*'s will produce close to zero signal in this region, and in the calculation we can say this with great certainty. On the other hand, the acquired image will also measure close to zero signal, but this will be modulated by the same amount of noise that is seen at the other TE points. This effect helps to contribute to the excellent diagnostic quality that is obtained in the calculated late echo images. The normal brain shows an increase in signal/noise for the calculated images relative to the acquired ones that more than compensates for the reduced signal/noise that may be present in the long *T2* structures.

APPLICATIONS

Inversion Recovery

The examples presented so far have shown parameter selection for the case of spin echo imaging where only two parameters, TE and TR, are of interest. The same tools may be used to examine the contribution of other parameters. For inversion recovery, of the three parameters available, TE, TR, and TI, it is natural to plot TR and TI, since the motivation for using inversion recovery is to enhance the contrast due to *T1* differences. We of course remain cognizant of the importance of possible *T2* contributions, and in fact the usual practice at our institution is to thoroughly investigate the use of spin-echo sequences prior to turning to inversion recovery. For the inversion recovery ASD map in Figure 105–9, it is only necessary to plot half of the TI, TR space, since by definition TI can never be larger than TR. This IR map was calculated at a *TE* of 45 ms. In Figure 105–10C the map is made at *TE* = 30 ms. This map shows two dark bands through the image compared to the single band seen in the SE difference maps. The contrast mechanism for inversion recovery allows for a disappearance of contrast when the magnetizations are equal and also when they are equal in magnitude and opposite in sign. For this reason we see a contrast reversal between the images at *TR* = 2.0 s, *TE* = 30 ms, *TI* = 200 ms and at *TR* = 3.0 s, *TE* = 45 ms, *TI* = 500 ms. This change in the map due to a change in TE shows how important it is to be cognizant of all the parameters that may be affecting the image. Inversion-recovery contrast can be more sensitive to changes in parameters than SE: a change in TI of only a few hundred milliseconds can dramatically change the contrast.

Multiple Tissues

The discussion so far has centered on the problem of distinguishing a pair of tissues. Often the problem is one in which we desire to be able to separate several tissues in the same image. For this we need to find an area where the difference map for each

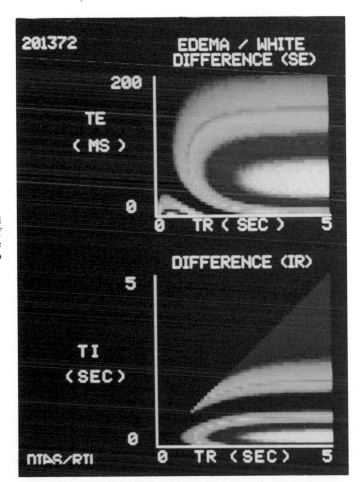

Figure 105–9. ASD maps for both spin echo and inversion recovery are shown for the patient of Figure 105–10 for edema vs white matter. The IR map is calculated at *TE* = 45 ms. (See also Plate I, Figure *C*.)

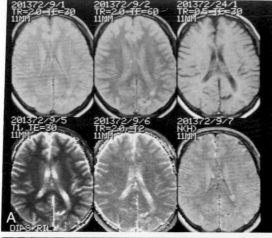

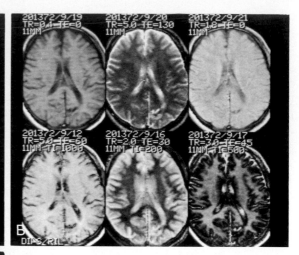

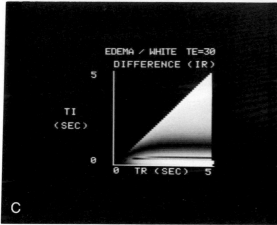

Figure 105–10. *A*, Acquired intensity images and relaxation time images are shown for a patient with an area of edema near the base of the brain on the left side. This is seen just below the area of low signal in the $TR = 0.5$ s, $TE = 30$ ms image. *B*, Calculated SE and IR images are shown corresponding to points in the ASD maps of Figure 105–9. *C*, An IR ASD map that was calculated at $TE = 30$ ms is shown. This map contains an additional dark band at short TI, which can cause additional contrast reversal not seen in the map in Figure 105–9.

of the pairs of tissues shows a relatively high intensity. This usually means a compromise in image contrast. Displaying this information is more of a problem, but one possible way is shown in Figure 105–11. This requires a threshold of acceptable discrimination. For this example we have used 50 percent of the maximum signal difference in each of the three difference plots. The multiple tissue map with this definition has four colors: white means that all three pairs are differentiated, medium gray where two pairs of tissue would be above threshold, dark gray for one pair and black where none of the differences would be above this limit. We can do a similar analysis using inversion recovery. In Figure 105–12 we show a patient with a metastasis with hemorrhage. By looking at each of the acquired intensity images it is determined that the area of the lesion is composed of two parts, an area of bleeding and an area of tumor. In order to obtain this separation in the same image along with the contrast against normal brain, inversion-recovery difference maps were studied. The calculated inversion-recovery image shows good contrast for all three tissues.

Magnetic Field

There are other parameters and topics that may be studied with tools of this kind. One of these is the strength of the static magnetic field used. Field-dependent relaxation time changes can also be modeled and used to predict the effects of field strength

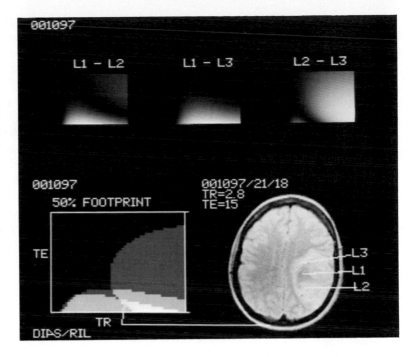

Figure 105–11. For a patient with a left parietal tumor we identify three separate components within the lesion. The three ASD maps between these tissues show substantial differences between them, indicating that the best image for differentiating between one pair will not necessarily be good for the other tissue. In the footprint, the small area in white shows the area of the TE, TR space where all three may be distinguished.

changes on image contrast and lesion detectability. The question of static magnetic field often relates to the topic of image signal/noise.[16] Increasing the operating field strength is often suggested as a means of improving the S/N. However, in addition to S/N, lesion conspicuousness is also affected by contrast, which is a function of the relaxation time differences between tissues. $T1$ values in particular have been found to increase with increases in field strength.[17,18]

Using data obtained in our laboratory at several field points between 1.4 and 7.0 kgauss we have fit the relaxation times as a function of field for tissues including gray and white matter, fat, muscle, and CSF.[19,20] For $T1$ we found a square root of field

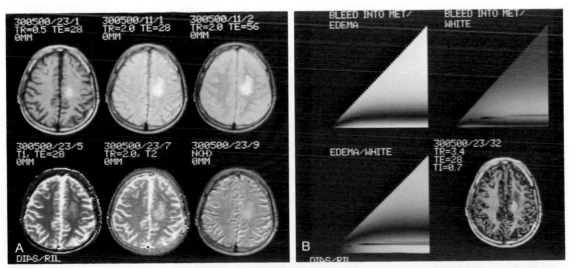

Figure 105–12. This patient was diagnosed as having metastatic disease with associated hemorrhage. *A*, Intensity and relaxation time images show structure within the lesion but do not allow normal white matter, the tumor and the hemorrhage to be clearly shown all in the same image. *B*, Using IR difference maps for all three pairs of tissues, we are able to find an IR image with TR = 3.4 s, TE = 28 ms, TI = 0.7 s, which allows all three tissues to be clearly appreciated.

strength dependence as a function of tissue group. The exception was CSF, which behaved similarly to pure water and exhibited no measurable changes in *T1* with field. *T2* appeared to be largely independent of field. The models of *T1* vs. the static field for the five tissue categories were used to extrapolate *T1* values for each pixel within the image from 3.5 kgauss, the operating field strength of the imager at the time of data acquisition, to any new value of field strength with the important assumption that the models remain valid outside of the range of field strengths used to establish them. These models are based on very limited data and are not purported to be precise. Rather, it is the method of evaluation that is of significance. As more experimental data become available, the models can be easily updated. Nevertheless, the trends established in the models have been supported by the published work of other investigators.[17,21]

T1 images calculated from data at 3.5 kgauss were extrapolated, creating *T1* images at new field strengths. The extrapolated *T1* images, along with *T2* and *N(H)* images, were used to calculate intensity images at new field strength values with any value of the acquisition parameters. Such images reflect the effects of field-dependent *T1* changes only and not of changes in S/N that would be expected if the new field image were actually acquired. ASD plots can similarly be extrapolated to new fields to show the effects of field strength on contrast for given values of the imaging parameters. Figures 105–13 and 105–14 show results for an extrapolation to 20 kgauss for a patient with an infarct in the brain. The color difference maps show very clearly that in order to obtain the same signal difference at the two field strengths, a longer TR and hence lengthened imaging time will be required at higher fields. Images at the same value of TE and TR show reduced contrast between the lesion and white matter at 20 kgauss. Note also the loss of contrast between the white and gray matter in the higher field image.

Lesion Size and Conspicuousness

It is obvious at this point that choice of acquisition parameters will affect lesion detectability. It should be equally clear that acquisition choice should affect the perceived size of the pathology. These tools were used to study this question retrospectively using data acquired for routine purposes.[22] Images were calculated at various MRI parameters for both SE and IR sequences. For each image, lesion size was estimated. An example from a patient with multiple sclerosis is shown in Figure 105–15.

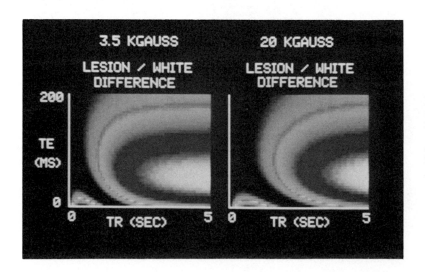

Figure 105–13. ASD maps are shown for field strengths of 3.5 and 20 kgauss for the patient of Figure 105–14. Equivalent signal difference requires longer TR values at higher field. (See also Plate I, Figure *D*.)

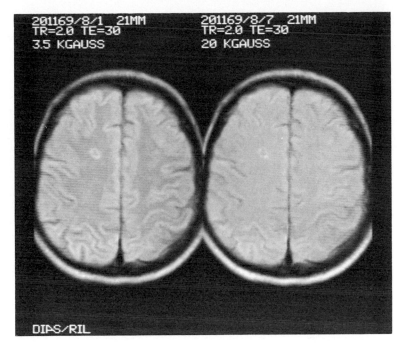

Figure 105–14. Calculated images at $TR = 2.0$ s, $TE = 30$ ms for a patient with an infarct show reduce image contrast at a field of 20 kgauss compared to 3.5 kgauss.

Lesion size is shown in Figure 105–16 as a function of TR with the TE fixed at 28 ms. There is significant variation in size and conspicuity for TR less than 2 to 3 seconds. In particular, some of the plaques were inapparent at $TR = 0.1$ to 0.5 s. For a fixed $TR = 2.0$ s and a variable TE, lesion size tended to stabilize at $TE = 28$ to 56 ms and remained relatively constant for longer TE times. Lesions were generally smaller and less conspicuous, with very short TE intervals, including $TE = 0$, which is essentially a free induction decay image (FID). For inversion recovery, size was quite variable. The dip in the curves occurs as the null point is crossed where intensity drops drastically and contrast with the brain disappears. The model of magnetic field described earlier can be used to predict the effect of changing the static field on lesion visibility. For short TR's there is significant variation in size for various field strengths. At some

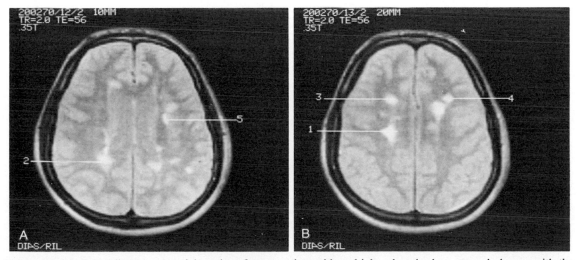

Figure 105–15. Two adjacent transaxial sections from a patient with multiple sclerosis show several plaques with the numbered lesions corresponding to the data of Figure 105–16.

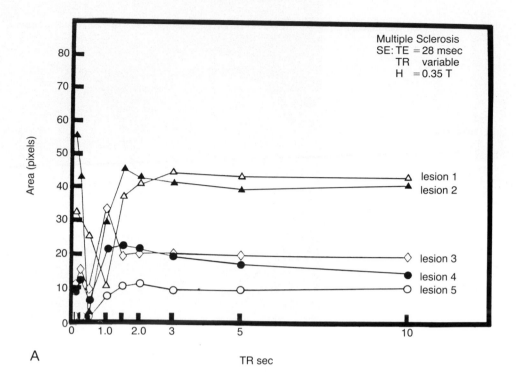

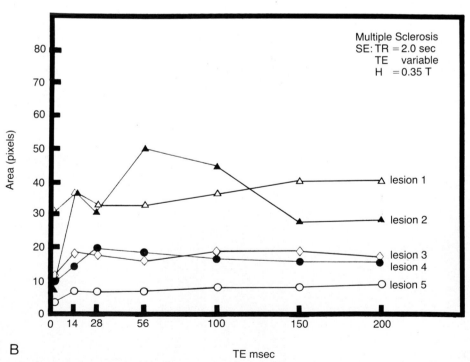

Figure 105–16. *A*, Lesion size is plotted as a function of TR for SE images for the patient of Figure 105–15. *B*, Lesion size is shown as a function of TE.

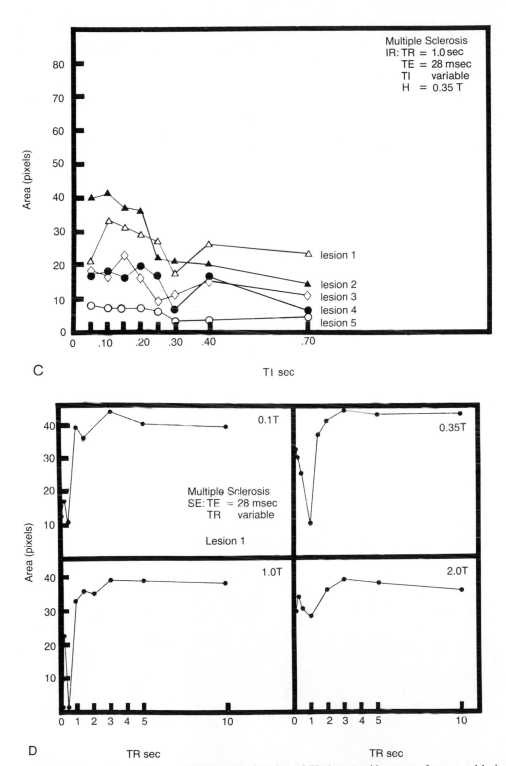

C

D

Figure 105–16 *Continued C*, IR images plotted as a function of TI show a wide range of measured lesion size. *D*, Using calculated images at four different field values. For short TR intervals (*TR* < 2–3 sec) every field shows significant variability in lesion size.

fields and techniques ($H = 1$T, $TR = 0.5$ s, $TE = 28$ ms) the lesion is not apparent. This is important to know, since it not unlikely that some patients may have images performed at different institutions using substantially different magnetic field strengths and different techniques. This method provides a way of reconciling the different images.

Variable Flip Angles

In spin-echo imaging it is customary to use a 90 degree pulse for the initial excitation to rotate the magnetization into the transverse plane. But it is possible to use other values for this "flip angle." The Bloch equations can be solved for this case and give an intensity:

$$I(SE) = \frac{N(H)f(v)\sin(\theta)\exp(-TE/T2)[1 + g(T1)]}{1 - \cos(\theta)\exp(-TR/T1)} \tag{4}$$

where θ is the flip angle. The sin term in the numerator gives an overall scale factor, but the cos term in the denominator includes both $T1$ and TR, suggesting that changes in the flip angle might produce changes in $T1$ contrast and might allow contrast to be improved at shorter TR values. The ASD map allows this question to be explored retrospectively.[23] The natural variables are TR and flip angle since we would like to trade flip angle for reductions in TR. Figure 105–17 shows an example for a patient with a frontal lobe mass. The lesion is well seen in the $TR = 2.0$ s image, but would be missed in the $TR = 0.5$ s image. The ASD map shows that there are isocontours, which allow equal signal difference to be obtained at a flip angle of 90 degrees and using a shorter TR with a flip angle less than 90 degrees. This can be verified with a calculated image; the $TR = 0.5$ s image with the flip angle of 35 degrees shows excellent contrast between lesion and the normal brain. The results of this retrospective study suggest that implementation of a reduced flip angle imaging sequence could prove useful in providing improved contrast along with a reduction in TR and hence imaging time. This particular study is designed solely to evaluate a new technique for future appli-

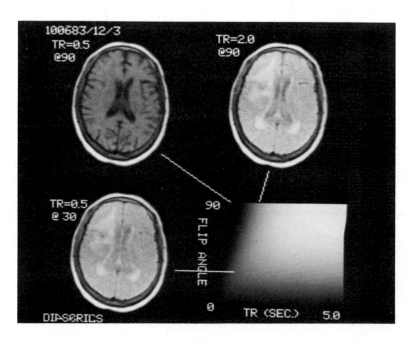

Figure 105–17. For a patient with a frontal lobe mass we show a difference map (TR vs. flip angle) for lesion − white matter difference. The lesion, which is well seen in the $TR = 2.0$ s image but not in the $TR = 0.5$ s image using a 90 degree flip angle, can be differentiated using the short TR sequence by reducing the flip angle to 30 degrees.

cation in the imager. In this case as in the magnetic field study there is no reason to use changes in flip angle to retrospectively improve image contrast, since the same effect can be obtained with changes in TR or TE. For this reason, noise-corrected maps are of little interest and we do not take the trouble to produce them.

Only a fixed amount of experimental work can be done in a given amount of time. Difference maps permit assessment of a large parameter set at a glance, and calculated images allow us to study the overall impact of different imaging techniques. All this is done with actual patient data and images, so we are not misled by using stylized or preconceptualized phantoms. This capability suggests that an effective imaging strategy is to obtain sufficient data to permit the calculation of accurate relaxation time and $N(H)$ images with other images calculated only as desired.[24]

ACKNOWLEDGMENTS

This work is supported in part by Diasonics (MRI), Inc.; by USPHS Grant CA 32850 from the NCI; and by USPHS Research Career Development Award GM00493 from the NIGMS(DHHS).

References

1. Davis PL, Sheldon PE, Kaufman L, et al: Nuclear magnetic resonance imaging of mammary adenocarcinomas in the rat. Cancer *51*:433, 1983.
2. Lukes SA, Crooks LE, Aminoff MJ, et al: Nuclear Magnetic Resonance Imaging in Multiple Sclerosis. Ann Neurol *13*:592, 1983.
3. Hricak H, Crooks LE, Sheldon P, Kaufman L: Nuclear magnetic resonance imaging of the kidney. Radiology *146*:425, 1983.
4. Ortendahl DA, Hylton NM, Kaufman L, et al: Analytical tools for MRI. Radiology *153*:479, 1984.
5. Droege RT, Weiner SN, Rzeszotarski MS: A strategy for magnetic resonance imaging of the head: Results of a semi-empirical model. Part II Radiology *153*:425, 1984.
6. Mitchell MR, Conturo TE, Gruber TJ, et al: Prosepctive selection of optimal magnetic resonance imaging (MRI) pulse sequence timing intervals. Abstract. Third Annual Meeting of the Society of Magnetic Resonance in Medicine, New York, 1984.
7. Hylton, NM: Computational techniques for the simulation and evaluation of hydrogen NMR imaging methods. Doctoral Thesis, Department of Applied Physics, Stanford University, 1985.
8. Hylton NM, Ortendahl DA: Simulation techniques for evaluating magnetic resonance imaging. *In* Bacharach SL (ed): Proceedings of the 9th International Conference on Information Processing in Medical Imaging. Martinus Nijhoff Publishers, The Hague, 78, 1986.
9. Ehman RL et al: Spin echo imaging: Method for correction of systematic errors in calculated *T1* and spin density. Third Annual Meeting of the Society of Magnetic Resonance in Medicine, New York, 1984.
10. Brant-Zawadski M, Bartokowski HM, Ortendahl DA, et al: NMR in experimental cerebral edema: Value of *T1* and *T2* calculations. Am J Neuroradiology *5*:125, 1984.
11. Bobman SA, Riederer SJ, Lee JN, et al: Synthesized MR images: Comparison with acquired images. Radiology *155*:731–738, 1985.
12. Ortendahl DA, Hylton NM, Kaufman L, Crooks LE: Signal to noise in derived NMR images. Magn Reson Med *1*:316, 1984.
13. Feinberg DA, Mills CM, Posin JP, et al: Multiple spin-echo magnetic resonance imaging. Radiology *155*:437, 1985.
14. Rose AA: Vision: Human and Electronic. New York, Plenum Press, 1973.
15. Shosa DW, Kaufman L: Methods for evaluation of diagnostic imaging instrumentation. Phys Med Biol *26*:101–112, 1981.
16. Hoult DI, Richards RE: The signal-to-noise ratio of the nuclear magnetic resonance experiment. J Magn Reson *24*:71–85, 1976.
17. Hart HR, Bottomley PA, et al: Nuclear magnetic resonance imaging: Contrast-to-noise ratio as a function of strength of magnetic field. AJR *141*:1195–1201, 1983.
18. Kaufman L, Crooks LE: Technical advances in magnetic resonance imaging. Presented at the Annual Postgraduate Course in MRI, CT and Interventional Radiology, San Francisco, 1985.
19. Crooks LE, Arakawa M, Hoenninger J et al: Magnetic resonance imaging: Effects of field strength. Radiology *151*:127, 1984.
20. Posin JP, Arakawa M, Crooks LE et al: Hydrogen MR imaging of the head at 0.35 T and 0.7 T: Effect of magnetic field strength. Radiology *157*:679, 1985.
21. Bottomley PA, Foster TH, et al: A review of normal tissue hydrogen NMR relaxation times and relaxation mechanisms from 1-100 MHz: Dependence on tissue type, NMR frequency, temperature, species excision, and age. Med Phys *11*:425–488, 1984.

22. Posin JP, Ortendahl DA, Hylton NM, et al: Variable magnetic resonance imaging parameters: Effect on detection and characterization of lesion. Radiology *155*:719–725, 1985.
23. Mills TC, Ortendahl DA, Hylton NM: Investigation of partial flip angle magnetic resonance imaging. IEEE Trans Nucl Sci *NS-33*:496, 1986.
24. Ortendahl DA, Hylton NM, Kaufman L, Crooks LE: Optimal strategies for obtaining the minimal NMR data set. IEEE Trans Nucl Sci *NS-32*:880, 1985.

106

Advanced Statistical Methods for Tissue Characteristics

EDWARD J. DUDEWICZ
GEORGE C. LEVY
MRUTYUNJAYA J. RAO
FELIX W. WEHRLI

Clinical utilization of MRI data in diagnostic medicine will require reliable controls over experimental procedures; optimum utilization of such data will also require effective statistical and other data handling methods. Furthermore, in this early but active stage of MRI methods development, powerful statistical techniques can give initial insight into the relationships between experiments, magnetic resonance imaging (MRI) parameters ($T1$, $T2$, and ^{1}H density), and tissue characterization (type and health).

The main goal of an interdisciplinary research program under way at Syracuse University is to design and conduct an experimental and computer aided data analysis protocol that will evaluate significant factors affecting experimental data obtained from normal human subjects as well as from a set of clinical cases, using a combined statistical/heuristic (logic programming) approach. Another goal is the development of an adaptive computer software methodology that eventually will lead to MRI expert systems that will have clinical utility in diagnosis of human disease. A unique feature of this project is the utilization of a large and well-defined training set to evaluate the applicability of advanced statistical and heuristic methods.

The potential of MRI in diagnostic medicine is currently unfolding in dramatic fashion.[6,17,21,23] Along with significant anatomical imaging capability, MRI observables can uniquely give information related to cellular processes. Unfortunately, most of those relationships are not yet fully understood and consequently, the full potential of MRI techniques in medicine is not yet close to realization. There are recent reviews of interesting applications to cardiac studies,[22] the urological/pelvic region,[37] chest,[33] and the central nervous system.[3] MRI studies of the brain (that avoid loss of detail/contrast from the surrounding skull) and clinical MRI modalities are advancing rapidly for evaluation of vascular disease, white matter disease, tumors of the brain, trauma, etc.[3,4,14,18]

The role $T1$ and $T2$ play in determining tissue contrast in various MRI pulse sequences is generally understood, although little is currently known as to why these parameters vary in healthy and diseased tissues, even where such variation is well established experimentally.[4,7,8,12,15] Full statistical use of $T1$, $T2$ and ^{1}H density, later possibly supplemented by separated values for fat and water components of tissues, offers a powerful route to differentiation of tissues.

Tests for validity of univariate statistical assumptions are widely performed and material on how to conduct them is accessible in "how-to" form.[30] However, powerful techniques have not yet been brought to bear on many multivariate problems due to a lack of software. In addition to making this methodology available for the first time on medical data, we will be in a position to transform the model as needed to meet model assumptions,[2,32,38] as an example of a tool for the community of researchers who have a need to test model assumptions—with an even greater need to know how to modify their procedures if those assumptions are violated.

The sophisticated statistical methods to be used in this project can be expected to elucidate all factors varying observables across the data to be examined, including physiological and experimental factors as well as environmental, primary data work-up, ROI homogeneity, and random factors.

This project has just begun. Nevertheless, we have obtained significant results from a first study of 40 MRI scans on normal volunteers. In each case a single transaxial brain slice was observed, at the level of the lateral ventricles. The brain was chosen for a first study, since it and other experimental parameters could be better controlled over this relatively small volume.

DATA

We were provided, by General Electric Medical Systems, with data on 40 magnetic resonance imaging scans labeled "Study #" 1 through 25 and 34 through 48. The data provided on the original data sheets consisted of the following:

1. Age, sex, weight, height, race, alcohol consumption, smoking habits, how long ago person had last eaten before scan, occupation, and medications of the person.
2. Scan date.
3. $T2$, $\sum T2$, ROI Size; $T1$, $\sum T1$, DEN, ROI Size, QDEN, $\sum$ QDEN for each of the 11 brain regions: left and right cortical white matter, left and right caudate nucleus, left and right thalamus, left and right internal capsule, left and right putamen, and corpus callosum. (Note that not all of the data described was available for each scan; in particular, full demographic data were not available for the first 22 scans, Study #'s 1 to 22, and other missing values were scattered about the data set.)

A RAW data set was assembled from tables of $T1$, $T2$, and ^{1}H density provided for the 11 regions of interest (ROIs) as identified by a consulting radiologist (Dr. Robert Breger).

The data set RAW was then subjected to a screening stage of statistical analysis for the purposes of detecting "outliers," i.e., egregious numbers as well as numbers that (while not so blatant) are detected as being "different" from the others (which is often a sign of incorrect recording, problems in execution of the scans, failure to follow the protocol, or sometimes of an unexpected but perhaps important phenomenon). One of the key tools used in this analysis was an interactive program prepared in our NMR Group that allows us to explore crossplots of variables in the data set. (For a description of crossplots and their power, see Section 4 of reference 20. For details of some possible problems in interpretation of crossplots, see "Crossplots and Their Hazards" in reference 11.)

Unfortunately, in our initial study, no internal ^{1}H density phantom was present, and thus, we were restricted in our utilization of reported ^{1}H densities.[17]

Some of the most important facts about Data Set RAW emerging from the cross-plots analysis are, in summary form, the following:

1. There are time trends of variables with SCANDATE. For example, there is a time trend for $T1$ of cortical white matter to increase, and there is a time trend for $T2$ of cortical white matter to decrease. Similarly there are trends in "corrected" ^{1}H density QDEN (increasing) and the new average density, AD, calculated as the percentage QDEN is of the average QDEN in brain tissues scanned in each subject (de-

creasing) of cortical white matter. (The above are all cortical white rightside.) Similar trends of *T1* increasing, *T2* decreasing, and AD decreasing with Scandate are (while not universal; e.g., *T1* of corpus callosum vs. scandate) widespread throughout the data set. While some of the indication of trend may be the result of outliers (discussed further below), we *determined that these time trends indicate the need for an independent standard for (T1, T2, QDEN) calibration (e.g., via phantom) in each scan.* (The need for such a phantom in terms of ^{1}H density values was first noted by Levy et al.[17]

2. There are outliers in Data Set RAW.

3. The time trends of *T1*, *T2*, and QDEN are even more marked if scan within day of scan is accounted for.

4. Almost all replication scans of an individual are in the later part of the data set.

5. There are linear relationships between each of QDEN CWRT, ICRT, CRT, TRT, and CC. The intercepts and slopes of the lines have not been analyzed, but may differ from line to line (which could be used as a possible tissue discriminator if it were not for the RF gain factor as a cause).

6. The transformation to average density comparison within a scan (AD values) eliminates most of this dependency, without "tagging" a region (such as cortical white right matter).

The data set after screening, with additions of variables noted above, and several data point deletions, is called dataset SCREENED.

REDUCTION

Dataset SCREENED includes a number of scans for several persons in the study, and one scan each for many others. In the population of persons, there is variability in brain tissue. To avoid a situation in which we give more weight to the values represented by one person, we have reduced dataset SCREENED by averaging over cases where the same person is represented more than once (represented by multiple occurrences of the same SUBJECT NUMBER); while such multiple occurrences are of value for, e.g., analysis of experimental error, they are not directly (by direct retention in the data set) for (e.g.) discriminant and other analyses (where their value is via averaging, which yields a more precise determination of the true values of a person who has been scanned more than once: such values have less variability than those for a person who has had only one scan, assuming that true values have not changed from scan to scan of the same person).

The data set resulting from this reduction is called Data Set REDUCED.

NORMALITY EVALUATION/TRANSFORMATION

Many statistical procedures have been developed under assumptions of an underlying normal probability density for the data. If the data follow the normal probability density (approximately), then these statistical procedures are optimal (approximately). Hence, if the data are (or can be transformed to be) normal, it will often be desirable to use these procedures. Therefore, a stage of data analysis entered into after screening and reduction is that of evaluation of, and (if the evaluation states "non-normal") transformation to, normality.

There are many tests of normality (e.g., see reference 30). One of the most powerful is that of Shapiro and Wilk, which uses what is generally called the W statistic (small values of which indicate lack of normality). If a set of data values $X_1, X_2, \ldots, X_n$

(e.g., these might be the values of *T1* in Data Set REDUCED, where $n = 24$ for cortical white right matter) fails to be normal, then often some function of them will be normally distributed. Most frequently in practice, one finds that that function is $\log(X_1)$, $\log(X_2)$, ..., $\log(X_n)$ or X_1^L, X_2^L, ..., X_n^L for some power L. (The latter, powers of the variable, are today called Box-Cox transformations.)

We have constructed a computer program that (1) sorts the data; (2) prints the sorted data; and (3) calculates the W statistic and its significance probability (SP) for the data as given, the data raised to powers ($-10 \leq L \leq 15$), the logarithm of the data, and the data exponentiated. A normal probability plot (different plotting positions can be chosen as options), with a least squares line (a Kolmogorov-Smirnov line is available as an option) and 95 percent confidence bands, is plotted for the original data and the best-looking (highest W statistic value) transformation of the data. Note that modern statistical practice stresses that one should not rely on any one or several statistics but should also "look at the data;" in the context of normality testing, it is usually recommended that this be (in the univariate case) by a normal probability plot, which may reveal deviations that while real were not caught by the test statistic. Different test statistics are sensitive to different types of deviations from normality, and while the Shapiro-Wilk test statistic is one of the most powerful, it is not a panacea.

Detailed results of applying this program to *T1*'s of corpus callosum (CC) are as follows. There are $n = 19$ such values in Data Set REDUCED. We find the W statistic values for the powers, log, and exp transformation noted above in this section. The W values are evaluated by their Significance Probability (SP) values: at the $100p\%$ level of significance, one rejects the normality of any transformation for which SP $\leq p$. While different values of p may be used by different experimenters, rarely would anyone consider a p of .50 or higher. Thus, transformations with an SP of .50 or more are considered normal; in this data set, we see that for *T1* of CC these transformations are X^L for L between -1 and 4.5, and $\log(X)$.

Commonly, level of significance $p = .05$ is employed (with this choice, we will reject normality, when it is true, 5 percent of the time that we run such a test). With that choice, we are interested in all transformations that yield an SP of .05 or higher. For *T1*'s of CC, this was X^L for L between -3.25 and 6.75, and $\log(X)$.

In evaluating values, bear in mind that when applying tests at level of significance .05 multiple times, some rejections are expected even if all the hypotheses are true. (For example, in 20 independent applications of tests at level of significance .05, one expects to find 1 rejection even if the hypotheses are all true [and as many as 3 would not be surprising statistically].) From this point of view, since nearly all *T1*'s and *T2*'s evaluated have some transformation that is normal by this test, we conclude that we can transform to normality. For use in discriminant analysis, we would like to use the *same* transform for *T1* in all tissues (since without knowing the tissue type we would not otherwise know what transform to use if the transforms were different). Seeking common transforms for *T1* across brain regions, we conclude that *T1* itself is sufficiently normal across tissues in the brain. Similarly, we conclude that *T2* is normal in probability distribution. We also conclude that AD and DEN are *not* normal, but that AD^{-2} and DEN^{-2} are each normal in probability distribution.

SUMMARY STATISTICS

There are a number of what are called "summary statistics" (measures for summarizing a data set) that are commonly employed in statistical analyses, and are also studied for their own sake (i.e., for the information they provide about the data set). These include the sample mean, sample variance, sample correlation coefficient (of 2 variables), minimum, maximum, and Q-contour value (of 2 variables). Of these, the least-known is the Q-contour value. Briefly, if variables X_1 and X_2 have a bivariate normal probability distribution, then they can be characterized by their means, variances, and correlation coefficient (respectively). It is then the case that the probability that the random pair (X_1, X_2) observed falls inside the ellipse

$$\left(\frac{x_1 - \mu_1}{\sigma_1}\right)^2 - 2\rho\left(\frac{x_1 - \mu_1}{\sigma_1}\right)\left(\frac{x_2 - \mu_2}{\sigma_2}\right) + \left(\frac{x_2 - \mu_2}{\sigma_2}\right)^2 = -2(1 - \rho^2)ln(1 - P) \equiv Q^*$$

is P. Q^* is called the Q-contour value; it is different for every P $(0 < P < 1)$ and changes as ρ changes (from variable pair to variable pair).

BIVARIATE NORMAL CONTOURS ANALYSIS

Bivariate normal probability distributions were fitted to a number of pairs of variables involving $T1$ and $T2$ (which were concentrated on owing to the difficulties with ^{1}H density described earlier). Using the methods discussed in the preceding discussion, contours were plotted for these situations.

T1 × T2 Tissue Plots

The first type of plot constructed is typified by Figure 106–1. Here, we have cortical white left matter, with $T1$ on the x axis and $T2$ on the y axis. The points plotted are the $(T1, T2)$ pairs for cortical white left matter in Data Set REDUCED.

There are 24 such pairs. The mean of $T1$ is 694.57, with standard deviation 53.61; the mean of $T2$ is 74.99, with standard deviation 5.07; the correlation coefficient of the $(T1, T2)$ pairs is $-.36$. Using the methods of the preceding section, we fit a bivariate normal probability distribution to this data, and in the plot of Figure 106–1, the inner (——) contour has probability .25 of containing a point. The next (——————) contour has probability .50 of containing any observation point, while the third (–··–··) contour from the center has a 75 percent chance of containing an observation pair. The outer (— —) contour has a 95 percent chance of containing an observation. The plot indicates a visually good fit of the bivariate normal to the data (recall that we saw in the preceding section on Normality Evaluation/Transformation that each of $T1$, $T2$ was individually normal in this setting; we now have evidence from the plot that in fact $T1$ and $T2$ are bivariate normal for cortical white left matter).

A similar plot for cortical white right matter yields the same conclusion of bivariate normality of the pair $(T1, T2)$. Similar plots, with similar conclusions (of bivariate normality) have been obtained for: thalamus, left and right; internal capsule, left and right; caudate, left and right; putamen, left and right; corpus callosum.

Right vs. Left Tissue (T1, T2) Distribution

A question of interest is: Do the $(T1, T2)$ pairs have the same chances of falling in the same regions, within a specific tissue type, irrespective of the side (right or left) of the brain? To approach this question, we can overplot the right side and left side $T1 \times T2$ tissue plots just discussed. For example, below we have, for cortical white matter, an overplot of the right side (solid) contours and the left side (dashed) contours (and the data points). From this we conclude that $(T1, T2)$ has the same distribution in cortical white right matter as in cortical white left matter (since the contours are, except for random variability, the same ellipses Fig. 106–2).

PLOT OF T2CWL VS T1CWL

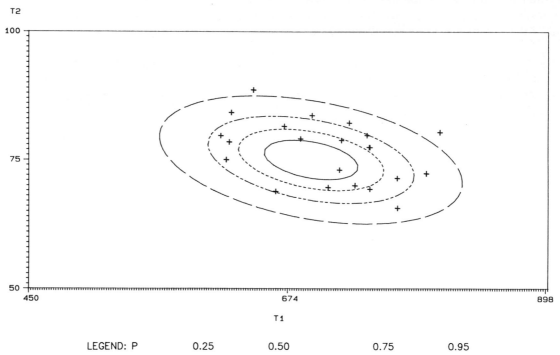

LEGEND: P   0.25   0.50   0.75   0.95

Figure 106–1. Data and bivariate normal probability contours for *T1* and *T2* of cortical white matter, left.

PLOT OF T2CW VS T1CW

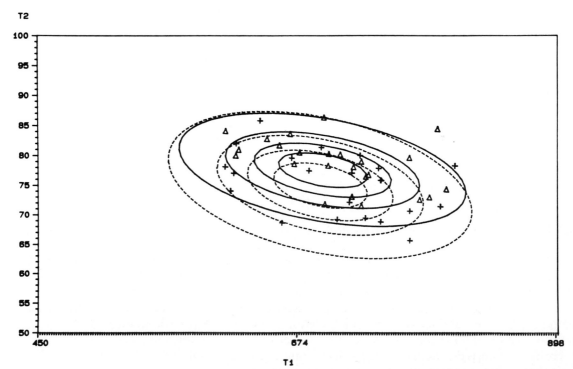

Figure 106–2. Overplot of data and bivariate normal probability contours for *T1* and *T2* of cortical white matter: left (Δ and solid line) and right (+ and dashed line).

A similar assessment for thalamus, internal capsule, caudate, and putamen yields the results that for all tissues in this study, (*T1, T2*) has the same distribution within tissue regardless of side of the brain studied.

TUMOR DETECTION VIA RIGHT/LEFT ANALYSIS

In the preceding section, we established that (*T1, T2*) values within a tissue are the same in probability distribution. This raises the anticipated possibility that tumors in a tissue on one side of the brain might be detected by failure of the pair of values (*T1, T2*) from one of the brain sides scanned in that tissue to fall within the contours given in the preceding section for that tissue.

Since readings are correlated within a subject, it is of interest to take the *differences of right and left side values in each subject* (within a tissue) and fit a bivariate normal distribution (see the preceding section on Summary Statistics for the initial discussion of these variables and the parameters). Then contours (as described in the preceding section) can be fitted and overplotted with the data points. For example, in the plot of Figure 106–3 we have, for cortical white matter, the variable (*T1* right)–(*T1* left) on the *x* axis, and (*T2* right)–(*T2* left) on the *y* axis. In a tumor detection screening, a patient with an (*x, y*) pair outside the outer contour would be flagged for further study for a possible cortical white matter abnormality.

Similar plots for thalamus, internal capsule, caudate, and putamen have been obtained and can be used similarly.

To approach the natural question, Are the zones that flag a patient for abnormality different for different tissue types? we overplot the graphs. This leads to the very

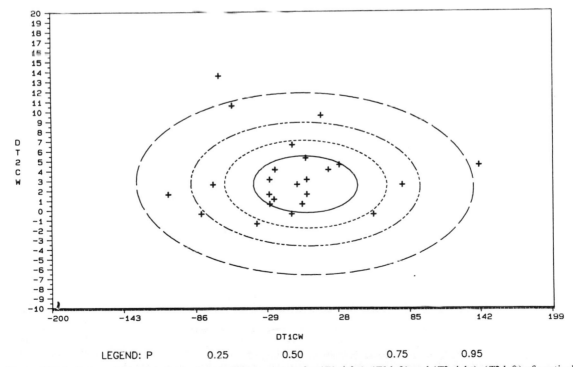

Figure 106–3. Data and bivariate normal probability contours for (*T1* right)–(*T1* left) and (*T2* right)–(*T2* left) of cortical white matter.

preliminary conclusion based on available data that all the zones are centered at the same point (0, 0) but that measurement differences are more variable in some tissues (those with larger contours) than in others. Thus, abnormalities will be harder to detect in some tissues than in others (due to the higher right/left variabilities in those tissues).

TISSUE DISCRIMINATION

The question, To what extent can tissue be discriminated via use of magnetic scan parameters? has already received a partial answer in earlier sections.

To assess the possibility of discriminating among tissue types of cortical white, caudate, thalamus, putamen, internal capsule, and corpus callosum, we will concentrate at this point on ($T1$, $T2$) parameters. (This analysis will be expanded to use of ^{1}H density parameters in upcoming work.) As these parameters have been shown earlier in this section to be bivariate normal within each of the tissue types under study, we can assess discrimination possibilities via examination of the degree of overlap/separation of these distributions.

In Figure 106–4, we overplot the 75 percent probability content contours for each of the six brain regions noted above. From this we can make the following preliminary conclusions (to be supplemented later by linear statistical discriminant analysis and quadratic statistical discriminant analysis, among others):

1. Thalamus and putamen are nearly identical in distribution of ($T1$, $T2$), with

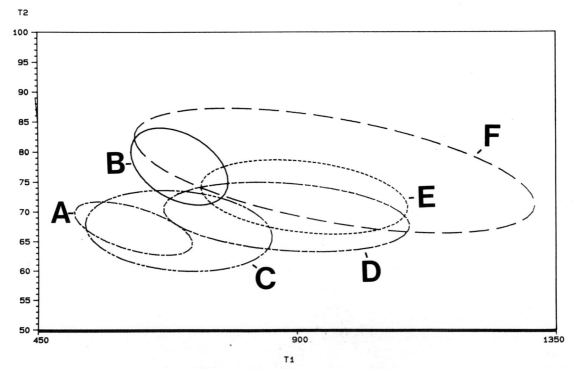

Figure 106–4. Overplot of 75 percent normal probability contours for $T1$ and $T2$ in six brain regions. Corpus callosum (A); cortical white matter (B); internal capsule (C); putamen (D); thalamus (E); and caudate (F).

putamen having slightly lower $T2$'s and lower and more variable $T1$'s. Hence in most cases it would not be possible to discriminate putamen from thalamus based on the values of $T1$ and $T2$ alone.

2. Corpus callosum covers a subregion of internal capsule's $(T1, T2)$ region. Hence, aside from anatomical considerations, corpus callosum would often be misclassified as internal capsule, while over half of internal capsule scans could be differentiated from corpus callosum.

3. Cortical white matter covers a subregion of the caudate region of $(T1, T2)$. This will have effects as just noted for corpus callosum and internal capsule.

4. The thalamus/putamen region is a subregion of the caudate region. This will have effects as just noted for corpus callosum and internal capsule.

5. Other overlaps are seen from the plot, e.g., the cortical white matter and thalamus/putamen regions of $(T1, T2)$ concentration have substantial overlap.

Thus, it has been shown from our first studies that distinct, i.e., nonidentical, regions of the $(T1, T2)$ magnetic scan parameter space contain the concentrations of values from different tissues in the brain. Since these different regions are not disjoint, 100 percent discrimination of healthy brain tissue types cannot be expected based on $T1$, $T2$ parameters alone at 1.5 tesla, though this will be attained in some cases; e.g., nearly 100 percent successful discrimination of corpus callosum and thalamus is expected. In practice, however, the MRI scan offers much additional information, in particular anatomical features. The important item to note is that different tissues have different characteristic regions of their $(T1, T2)$, and therefore it is reasonable to expect that other tissue types not involved in the present study will also differ from these and be able to be differentiated from them (e.g., for types such as abnormal versions of the tissues in the present study). This discrimination percentage will depend on the differentiation of regions between, for example, normal corpus callosum and abnormal corpus callosum, which will be the subject of later studies.

ADVANCED METHODS

Utilizing a far more extensive and homogeneous data set (the initial data set discussed above involved only 40 magnetic resonance imaging scans) incorporating an internal phantom for each of $T1$, $T2$, and ^{1}H density, we will both corroborate and refine the inferences already made on the basis of the preliminary data set. In addition, additional advanced statistical methods will be brought into play, including (1) multivariate analysis, which will allow us to supplement the qualitative graphical approaches displayed above with quantitative measures of multivariate normality, which is desirable since the graphical approach is limited to two or (at most) three dimensions and hence can be used to good advantage for $(T1, T2)$ analysis but approaches its limits as we move to analysis of $(T1, T2, {}^1H$ density);[31] (2) ridge regression analysis and ill-conditioning studies, which allow us to account for near-collinearity in the data set while obtaining estimates with lower mean squared error than are obtained by the usual least squares techniques; (3) logistic regression analysis, which allows discriminant models to be constructed for tissue discrimination using both quantitative and qualitative (zero-one) variables, i.e., variables such as $T1$, $T2$, ^{1}H density and also variables such as sex; and (4) sequential analysis (including two-stage analysis), which allows a rational decision as to "how many data" are needed to reach properly supported conclusions in the study. It is also possible (and indeed we are currently advancing this approach) to couple statistical and heuristic methods in a framework that may greatly improve tissue characterization from MRI data.

STATISTICAL-EXPERT-SYSTEMS AND EXPERT-STATISTICAL-SYSTEMS

In our preliminary studies, we are constructing an approach to a Statistical Expert System (with a PROLOG "Expert System" for logical control), or SES. An SES is a program package that incorporates advanced statistical techniques for analysis of the data sets in question, but needs supervision by practitioners in statistics in its running (to make choices of how to proceed at each decision node). An SES is the proper mode at the initial stages, where knowledge of the subject matter domain (of NMR and MRI) is being extracted from the data in sequential fashion.

Once the principles of the knowledge domain have been extracted from the data (e.g., for the brain) in preliminary studies, it is reasonable to proceed to the next stage, an Expert Statistical System (ESP). An ESP is a program package that not only incorporates advanced statistical techniques for analysis of the data sets in question but also does not need supervision by human statisticians in its running. Thus, an ESP is capable of "running itself," analyzing data in similar studies across a number of organs, or in other similar contexts, with only general directions from laboratory workers. Currently there are *no* ESPs available in *any* area (NMR/MRI or any other), though some are being worked on, besides ours. We expect our ESP to be one of the earliest available; further, we believe that ESPs in general will be, for most practitioners, one of the most exciting advances in statistics of the last quarter of the twentieth century.

Analysis of a small initial data set has yielded insights as to both needs of future studies (e.g., for an internal phantom for each $T1$, $T2$, and ^1H density), and as to variation in MRI parameters in the brain regions and sides, and their possible roles in tumor detection. These insights will be utilized in advanced analysis of larger data sets now in progress. The preliminary studies are leading to development of a Statistical Expert System, which our group intends to extend into enhance into an Expert Statistical System (ESP) environment.

ACKNOWLEDGMENTS

The authors gratefully acknowledge pilot project support from NIH and the General Electric Company. Various aspects of the project were facilitated by Dr. Robert Breger, Dr. James R. MacFall, and Teresa Harner.

References

1. Allen J: Anatomy of LISP. McGraw-Hill Computer Science Series, New York, McGraw-Hill Inc., 1978.
2. Berk KN: Validating regression procedures with new data. Technometrics *26*:331–338, 1984.
3. Bradley WJ, Waluch V, Yadley RA, Wykof RR: Comparison of CT and MR in 400 patients with suspected disease of the brain and cervical spinal cord. Radiology *152*:695, 1984.
4. Brant-Zawadzki M, Badami JP, Mills CM, Norman D, Newton TH: Primary intracranial tumor imaging: A comparison of magnetic resonance and CT. Radiology *150*:435, 1984.
5. Buchanan BA, Shortliffe EH: Rule-Based Expert Programs: The MYCIN Experiments of the Stanford Heuristic Programming Project. Reading, Massachusetts, Addison-Wesley, 1984.
6. Budinger TF, Lauterbur PC: Nuclear magnetic resonance technology for medical studies. Science *226*:288–298, 1984.
7. Bottomly PA, Foster TH, Argersinger RE, Pfeifer LM: General Electric Corporate R & D Technical Information Series, Report 84CRD072, 1984.
8. Cameron IL, Ord VA, Fullerton GD: Magn Reson Imaging *2*:97–106, 1984.
9. Clancey WJ, Shortliffe EH: Readings in Medical Artificial Intelligence. Reading, Massachusetts, Addison-Wesley, 1984.
10. Dixon WT: Simple proton spectroscopic imaging. Radiology *153*:189–194, 1984.
11. Dudewicz EJ: Basic statistical methods. *In* Juran JM (ed): Quality Control Handbook. 4th ed. New York, McGraw-Hill Book Company, 1988.

12. Edelstein WA, Bottomley PA, Hart HR, Smith LS: Signal, noise, and contrast in nuclear magnetic resonance (NMR) imaging. J Comput Assist Tomogr 7:391–401, 1983.
13. Fisher RA: The use of multiple measurements in taxonomic problems. Ann Eugenics 7:179–188, 1936.
14. Gomori JM, Grossman RI, Zimmerman RA, Goldberg HI, Bilanik LT: Intracranial hematosis: Imaging by high field MR. Radiology 157:87, 1985.
15. Kaufman L, Crooks L: Annual Postgraduate Course in MRI, CT, and Interventional Radiology, University of California at San Francisco, Jan., 1985.
16. Kowalski R: Logic For Problem Solving. Computer Science Series. New York, North-Holland Publishing Co., 1979.
17. Levy GC, Dudewicz EJ, Harner TJ, Wehrli FW, Breger R: A logic programming and expert statistical systems approach for tissue characterization in magnetic resonance imaging. Biometrical J. In press.
18. Lukes SA, Crooks LE, Aminoff MJ, Kaufman L, Panitch HS, Mills C, Norman B: Nuclear magnetic resonance in multiple sclerosis. Ann Neurol 13:592–601, 1983.
19. McFall JR, Wehrli FW, Breger RK, Johnson GA: Methodology for measurement and analysis of relaxation times in proton imaging. Physiological Chemistry and Physics. Symposium Issue on Magnetic Resonance, in press.
20. Nelson W: How to analyze data with simple plots. *In* Dudewicz EJ (ed): The ASQC Basic References in Quality Control: Statistical Techniques. Volume 1. Milwaukee, Wisconsin, American Society for Quality Control, 1979.
21. Newton TH, Potts DG: Advanced imaging techniques. Modern Neuroradiology, Vol. 2. San Anselmo, Clavadel Press, 1983.
22. Osbakken M: Nuclear magnetic resonance: Theory and review of cardiac applications. Am Heart J 108:574–590, 1984.
23. Partain CL, James AE, Rollo FD, Price RR (eds): Nuclear Magnetic Resonance (NMR) Imaging. Philadelphia, W. B. Saunders Co., 1983.
24. Randles RH, Broffitt J, Hogg RV: Discriminant analysis based on ranks. J Am Stat Assoc 73:379–384, 1978.
25. Randles RH, Broffitt J, Hogg RV: Generalized linear and quadratic discriminant functions using robust estimates. J Am Stat Assoc 73:564–568, 1978.
26. Royston JP: An extension of Shapiro and Wilk's W test for normality to large samples. Appl Stat 31:115–124, 1982.
27. Royston JP: Algorithm AS 181: The W test for normality. Appl Stat 31:176–180, 1982.
28. Royston JP: Some techniques for assessing multivariate normality based on the Shapiro-Wilk W. Appl Stat 32:121–133, 1983.
29. Royston JP: Algorithm AS 181 Correction: The W test for normality. Appl Stat 32:224, 1983.
30. Shapiro SS: How to test normality and other distributional assumptions. *In* Dudewicz EJ (ed): The ASQC Basic References in Quality Control: Statistical Techniques. Volume 3. Milwaukee, Wisconsin, American Society for Quality Control, 1980.
31. Siotani M, Hayakawa T, Fujikishi Y: Modern Multivariate Statistical Analysis. A Graduate Course and Handbook. Columbus, Ohio, American Sciences Press Inc., 1985.
32. Vale CD, Maurelli VA: Simulating multivariate nonnormal distributions. Psychometrika 48:465–471, 1983.
33. Webb WR, Gamsu G: Clinical NMR imaging of the chest and mediastinum. Diagn Imag Clin Med 53:22–28, 1984.
34. Wehrli FW et al: Fourth Annual Meeting of the Society for Magnetic Resonance in Medicine, Strategies for measurement and analysis of the intrinsic parameters in MR imaging. Abstracts, 1985, pp 195–196.
35. Weiss SM, Kulikowski CA: A model-based method for computer-aided medical decision-making. Artif Intell 11:145–172, 1978.
36. Weiss SM, Kulikowski CA: A Practical Guide to Designing Expert Systems. Totwik, New Jersey, Rowman & Allanheld, 1984.
37. Williams RD, Hricak H: Magnetic resonance imaging in urology. J Urol 132:641–649, 1984.
38. Wilson JR: Modelling multi-attribute populations with Johnson's translation system. University of Texas, Austin, 1983.

107

Current and Future Frontiers in Medical Imaging

C. LEON PARTAIN
GORDON L. BROWNELL
MASAHIRO IIO
RONALD R. PRICE

The frontiers of medical imaging are in a constant state of redefinition. New developments extend our boundaries, extend our outlook, and provide new direction for research. Frontiers emerge from past research, and those of the future are being established as this text is written. Research and development in medical imaging has been extremely active and phenomenally successful in many areas. In order to identify those frontiers likely to engage the most attention before the end of the century, it is necessary to examine the significant developments of the last three decades.

Initially, the field of medical imaging was defined almost totally by the principles of differential x-ray transmission utilizing elements in film-screen combinations, collimation, filtering, and patient positioning.[1] Nuclear medicine was born in the early and mid-1960s and has made significant contributions to medical imaging and to radioisotope therapy. Of primary importance are the added capabilities of functional dynamic imaging and specificity, especially with regard to the use of radioactive iodine and the evaluation of the thyroid gland.[2] This decade also saw the dramatic advance of ultrasound imaging with its associated portability, economy, and lack of risk. Ultrasound is integral to the acceleration of new physical interactions as a basis for the evolution of imaging modalities.[3]

In the early 1970s, x-ray techniques were extended to include improvements in angiography and interventional radiology.[4] The exceedingly rapid deployment of x-ray computed tomography into the field of medical imaging in the mid-1970s revolutionized diagnostic medicine, resulted in Nobel Prizes for the developers, and has remained one of the key frontiers in the 1980s.[5] The adoption of positron emission tomography (PET) as a diagnostic technique, although recognized within the same decade as an imaging breakthrough, has proceeded more slowly. However, the late 1970s brought rapid improvements in positron emission tomography. Today PET as a relatively recent addition is acknowledged as the second key frontier in medical imaging.[6]

The decade of the 1980s has witnessed the impressive clinical applications of magnetic resonance imaging. MRI, based upon the principle of nuclear magnetic resonance and primarily utilizing proton magnetic resonance imaging, is the third frontier of those medical imaging technologies involving active, rapidly developing research. This text has been dedicated to the description of medical applications, physical principles, instrumentation, and research involving this particular modality.

Major developments along these three frontiers can assist our glimpse into the future. Where do we go from here? Certainly questions remain as the potential of new and existing technologies continues to be examined. Will new external sources of energy continue to provide new data at less risk than any existing modalities? On the other hand, will new technologies allow the detection of inherent, natural, unperturbed energy processes to be observed and measured as the next revolution in diagnostic medicine? There are several possibilities to consider.

Current medical imaging modalities are of two basic types. They may be characterized or utilized as (1) external sources of energy or (2) internal, injectable or ingestable sources of energy. New frontiers in medical imaging may extend these two approaches and add a third—natural, internal energy emission. Consider now each category as a potentially fertile area for future development.

EXTERNAL SOURCES OF ENERGY

X-ray Fluorescence Tomography

X-ray fluorescence tomography (XFT) scanners typically utilize an external scan of low energy gamma rays such as Am-241 (E = 60 KeV). The gamma ray causes the removal of an inner shell electron from the isotope of interest. This empty shell is filled with a lower energy electron, resulting in the emission of a K-edge characteristic x-ray. For the assay of iodine concentration in the thyroid gland, the K-edge energy is 29 KeV, which is detected by a scintillation counter and scanner.[7] Future XFT scanners may be able to quantitatively assay the concentration in vivo of multiple isotopes of biomedical significance, including iron, lead, and gadolinium.

Electron-Paramagnetic Resonance

While the overwhelming majority of magnetic resonance imaging studies have utilized principles of nuclear magnetic resonance, the related electron-paramagnetic resonance (EPR) technology has the potential to provide different data related to substrate metabolism or an additional biochemical basis for anatomical distribution and imaging of pathophysiological processes.[8] Technical hurdles to be overcome include detector sensitivity and spatial registration of EPR data.

Free Radical Electron Spin Resonance Imaging

Free radicals are found in low concentration in the normal human body. In certain disease processes, for example, in cancer treated with radiation therapy, the concentration of free radicals is known to increase. This phenomenon has recently been proposed as a possible basis for medical imaging.[9] Problems with this approach, however, are the high frequency wave radiation (Giga-Hz range) required and the relatively low sensitivity of detectors.

Microwave Imaging

Several different portions of the electromagnetic spectrum have been utilized as a source of external energy. Any one of these has the potential to form the basis for a medical imaging modality. The source of energy in the wave band is hypothesized to result from the vibration of cell membranes and their oscillatory dipole movement.[10]

Limitations for medical imaging include short wave length penetration limitations and the need for a coupling medium.

Impedance Mapping

The spatial distribution of electrical impedance in the body is a measurable parameter that is a function of the resistance, inductance, and capacitance of body fluids and tissues.[11] Impedance is also a function of the frequency of the inherent or applied voltage. These maps should be unique for each chosen frequency and may be specific for particular pathologies. Patient safety and signal detection are two significant problem areas.

Free-Electron-Laser

Imaging by means of a free-electron-laser (FEL) is unique in three dimensions. First, light intensity is 10^6 to 10^8 times greater than conventional lasers. Moreover, coherent light (one frequency and in-phase) and tunable light (selectable wavelength) are additional valuable capabilities. Biomedical applications in imaging and in therapy result from these physical characteristics. Thus FEL imaging has the ability to (1) deposit energy nonthermally in such a way as to break chemical bonds, and (2) provide a tunable (variable frequency) energy source, which may be used as the basis for the spatial orientation mapping of spectral data.[12,13] Significant challenges for physicists and engineers do remain, including high cost and low availability of FEL technology, which requires a synchroton as an energy source. Limitations to penetrability also exist due to the frequency of light available and the corresponding deposition of energy.

INTERNAL, INJECTABLE OR INGESTABLE SOURCES OF ENERGY

Positron Emission Tomography

Positron emission tomography (PET) and MRI are described by some as the only existing truly functional imaging modalities.[14] This is due to the capability of PET to map, quantitate, and model the spatial and temporal distribution of metabolites, labeled with appropriate positron emitting radioisotopes, including C-11, N-13, O-15, F-18, Ga-68, and Rb-82. The data from PET are undeniably unique and the potential clinical application areas are numerous. PET facilities require a cyclotron, radiochemical laboratory, and scanner.[15] This combination of equipment, even with recent price reductions, is very expensive. The capital investment and operating costs exceed both x-ray CT and MRI. It follows, therefore, that the progressive evolution of PET centers in today's controlled environment (see Chapters 55 and 56) will be accompanied by careful evaluation of PET versus alternative and "equivalent" data sources. Thus, MRI and NMR-S enthusiasts sometimes claim that essentially the same spatial and temporal data are available from MRI and NMR spectroscopy.[16]

Single Photon Emission Computed Tomography

In addition to the competition of "equivalent data" available from MRI and NMR-S, the recent development of new single photon radiopharmaceuticals labeled with Tc-

99m and I-123 is challenging the practical implications of the claims of PET laboratories for unique data.[17] Single photon emission computed tomography (SPECT) investigations that generate equivalent data related to brain and myocardial perfusion may be available without the expense of PET. Further, I-123 labeled neurotransmitters also are challenging the presumed premier role of PET in evaluating basic brain functions in vivo. How many unique data do society need and how much can it afford are valid questions, which serious investigators are continuing to evaluate.

NATURAL INTERNAL ENERGY EMISSION

The living body is a perpetual source of continuing energy cycles. New technologies may be able to measure and observe directly those processes in a manner that yields spatial and temporal data adequate for functional medical imaging.

Infra-red and Ultra-violet Emission

The detection of thermal energy by means of a process known as thermography has received serious attention, but there has been limited clinical impact to date.[18] However, the noninvasive nature of this approach is most attractive if the technical problems of accurate detection and spatial display may be improved and related in a meaningful way to pathophysiology.

Electromagnetometer

The concept of external detection of electric and magnetic fields is sometimes referred to as electromagnetometry.[19] Owing to the tremendous impact of MRI, the idea of more sensitive detection and mapping of electric and magnetic fields is an intriguing possibility. The technical problems associated with detection and localization are yet to be solved.

Magnetic Mapping

The spatial and temporal in-vivo relationships of magnetic field distribution have been proposed as a noninvasive method to observe and measure normal and pathophysiological conditions.[20] Major challenges include signal/noise reduction and/or management as well as signal localization. Opportunities for improvement in signal/noise are focused on improved signal detection using SQID (superconducting quantum-interference-device) devices.[21] The clinical potential lies in the ability to detect small changes in magnetic fields as evidence of an early disease state.

Micro-wave Emission Imaging

The inherent emission of waves from the body has served as the basis for medical imaging[22] of peripheral structures such as the breast. Problems to be overcome before this technique can be considered practical are the penetrability limitation of short wave length (of the order of mm) microwave emission and the need for a transmission medium such as a water tank.

It is the hope of the editors of the second edition that this text has met its objective as a useful comprehensive text in magnetic resonance imaging. The difficulties of capturing the status of a rapidly developing technology need no elaboration. The intent of our concluding chapter has been to open a window on the possibilities that exist for even more dramatic and capable developments in the future. In a sense, we remain limited by our lack of foresight and creativity. It is, however, this human limitation that reminds us all that initial and ultimate sources of energy remain beyond human comprehension. This reality provides a continuing incentive in the attempt to bring under control those forces that are only partially understood. The urge to answer the question, What if . . . ? is strong indeed. Medicine and the people it serves stand to benefit from this continuing quest in diagnostic medical imaging.

References

1. Donizetti P: Shadow and Substance: The Story of Medical Radiography. Oxford, Pergamon Press, 1967.
2. Hendee W: Radioactive Isotopes in Biological Research. New York, John Wiley & Sons, Inc., 1973.
3. McDicken W: Diagnostic Ultrasonics. New York, John Wiley & Sons, Inc., 1976.
4. England I: Angiography: Choice of equipment. X-ray Focus 6:4, 1965.
5. Hounsfield G: Computerized transverse axial scanning (tomography). Part I. Description of system. Br J Radiol 46:1016, 1973.
6. Frackowiak RSJ, Lenzi GL, Jones T and Heather JD: Quantitative measurement of regional cerebral blood flow and oxygen metabolism in man using 15-O and positron emission tomography: Theory, procedure and normal values. J Comput Assist Tomogr 4:727–736, 1980.
7. Patton JA: Emission Tomography. *In* Coulam C, Erickson J, Rollo F, James A (eds): The Physical Basis of Medical Imaging. New York, Appleton-Century-Crofts, 1981.
8. Berliner LJ, Fujii H: Magnetic resonance imaging of biological specimens by electron paramagnetic resonance of multiple spin labels. Science 227:517–519, 1985.
9. Butler KW, Deslauriers R, Smith ICP: Effects of antimalarial drugs on oxygen consumption by erythrocytes infected with plasmodium berghei: An ESR study. Magn Reson Med 3:312–316, 1986.
10. Frohlich H: Long-range coherence and energy storage in biological systems. Int J Quantum Chem 11:641, 1968.
11. Barber DC, Brown BH: Construction of electrical resistivity images for medical diagnosis. SPIE Med Imag 767:23–27, 1987.
12. Robinson AL: Free electron laser sources explained. Science 235:27–29, 1987.
13. Proswitz D, Szoke A, Neil UK: High gain, free-electron-laser amplifiers: Design considerations and simulation. Phys Rev A 24:1436, 1981.
14. Raichle ME, Herocovitch P, Martin W, Markham J: Quantitative dynamic imaging of brain with positron-emitting radionuclides. *In* Magistretti PL (ed): Functional Radionuclide Imaging of the Brain. New York, Raven Press, 1983, p. 253.
15. Kessler RM, Partain CL, Price RR and James AE: Positron emission tomography: Prospects for clinical utility. Invest Radiol 22:529–537, 1987.
16. Scott K, Brooke HR, Fitzsimmons JR: Phosphorus NMR: potential application to diagnosis. *In* Partain CL, James AE, Rollo FD, Price RR (eds): Nuclear Magnetic Resonance (NMR) Imaging. Philadelphia, W.B. Saunders, 1983.
17. Drayer BP, Jaszczak R, King HF, Friedman A, et al: In vivo quantitation of regional cerebral blood flow: The SPECT-HIPD method. *In* Magistretti PL (ed): Functional Radionuclide Imaging of the Brain. New York, Raven Press, 1983, p 193.
18. Isard HJ, Ostrum BJ: Breast thermography: The mammatherm. Radiol Clin North Am 12:167–188, 1974.
19. Williamson SJ, Ramani GL, Kaufman L, Modena I: Biomagnetism: An Interdisciplinary Approach. New York, Plenum Press, 1982.
20. Singh M, Daria D, Henderson VW, Huth GC, Beaty J: Reconstruction of images from neuromagnetic fields. IEEE Trans Nucl Sci NS-31:585–589, 1984.
21. Leahy R, Jeffs B, Singh M, Brechner R: Evaluation of algorithm for a SQUID detector neuromagnetic imaging system. SPIE Med Imag 767:11–16, 1987.
22. Larsen LE, Jacobi JH: Microwaves offer promise as imaging modality. Diag Imag 11:44–47, November, 1982.

GLOSSARY OF
MRI TERMS

ABSORPTION LINE: Peak in NMR spectrum indicating absorption of radio frequency (rf) power by a spin system at a particular frequency.

ADIABATIC FAST PASSAGE: A technique that produces reorientation of the magnetization by sweeping either the external magnetic field or the applied frequency of an rf field through resonance (the Larmor frequency) in a time that is short compared with the relaxation times. Often used for the inversion of spins.

ALIASING: Also called wrap-around artifact, a phenomenon resulting from digitizing fewer than two samples per period in a periodic function. Can occur in MRI when object extends beyond field of view. Portions of object extending beyond field of view boundaries are aliased back to appear at artifactual locations. *See also* Nyquist limit.

ANALOG TO DIGITAL CONVERTER (ADC): Part of the electronic interface that produces a number, in digital, computer-readable form, that is proportional to a (analog) voltage, such as the detected MR signals.

ANGULAR FREQUENCY (ω): Frequency of oscillation or rotation expressed in radians, rather than revolutions or cycles, per second. There are 2π radians in a circle; therefore, $\omega = 2\pi f$, where f is the frequency in terms of cycles or revolutions per second, usually called Hertz (Hz).

ANGULAR MOMENTUM: A measure of rotational or spinning motion. Individual atomic nuclei possess an intrinsic angular momentum, i.e., they rotate about their axes. This intrinsic angular momentum is referred to as spin, or spin moment, and is measured in multiples of Planck's constant divided by 2π. In the absence of external torques, angular momentum remains constant. Generally, a nuclear magnetic dipole moment is associated with a nuclear spin. The ratio of the magnetic to spin moments is called the gyromagnetic ratio, or g-value, and may be positive or negative. A torque applied to a gyromagnetic body, such as that produced by a magnetic field acting on a spinning magnetic moment, induces a steady precession of the spin, at constant angle, about the magnetic field direction. This is known as Larmor precession or frequency.

ARTIFACTS: False features in the image produced either by the imaging processor or by the experimental methodology.

> *Aliasing artifact:* In MRI, this artifact occurs when the diameter of the imaged object exceeds the field of view. It is due to low sampling rates in the frequency-encoded direction. It has a more complex cause in the phase-encoded direction. The

* Compiled in part with the aid of the ACR Glossary of MRI Terms, 2nd ed., by S. Koenig, R. Brown, R. Price, and R. Tarr with permission of the American College of Radiology and Dr. Leon Axel, Chairman of the Subcommittee on MR nomenclature.

artifact appears as a series of ghost images along the frequency-encoded axis of the imaged object.

Asymmetric brightness: Uniform decrease in signal intensity along the frequency-encoded axis as a result of filters that are too narrow compared with the signal bandwidth. A similar artifact may be caused by nonuniformity in slice thickness, or by nonuniform receiver-coil sensitivity.

Chemical-shift artifact: Chemical shifts in tissue result from the difference in the Larmor frequency of hydrogen molecules in fat and in water. The chemical-shift artifact occurs only along the frequency-encoded axis as a low- or high-intensity band at one side of a structure with high fat content.

Bounce-point artifact: This artifact may occur when magnitude reconstruction is used with an inversion-recovery pulse sequence. The artifact occurs when $TI = 0.693 \times T1$ for any tissue, and $TR \gg T1$, and results in an absent signal.

Metallic artifacts: These artifacts are due to distortions of the main magnetic field caused by ferromagnetic materials. The spectrum of appearances includes spatial distortions, a region of signal void, a region of signal void surrounded by a zone of high intensity, or multiple high-intensity rings.

Motion artifact: Ghost images are due to the failure of compensatory gradients to completely eliminate the phase contribution of either the slice-select or the frequency-encoding gradient, when motion occurs in these planes. They may appear along the encoded axis or as blurring in the direction of motion. Temporal lag between phase encoding and signal read-out may cause ghost images along the phase-encoded axis.

Power gradient drop-off: This artifact is seen as a compression of the image along the faulty gradient axis and is due to power drop-off in the frequency- or phase-encoding gradient amplifiers causing the gradient to be less than that assumed by the computer software.

RF tip angle inhomogeneity: Produced by variation in rf energy required to tip protons 90 or 180 degrees within the selected slice volume. Presents as patchy areas of increased or decreased signal intensity.

Truncation artifact: Due to the inability of a truncated Fourier series or finite number of sine waves to perfectly describe abrupt changes in signal intensity. The artifact consists of multiple high- and low-intensity bands that parallel zones of such abrupt changes. This artifact may cause difficulty in the evaluation of complex anatomic areas, such as the larynx, and in the evaluation of small structures, such as the menisci of the knee. Also called Gibbs phenomenon.

Zeroline or star artifacts: Due to system noise or radio frequency interference; appear as a bright linear signal in a dashed pattern that decreases in intensity across the screen, either as a line or as a star pattern.

ATTENUATION: Reduction of power. Attenuation in electrical systems is commonly expressed in dB. (*See also* Decibel.)

ATTENUATOR: A device that reduces signal power by a specific fraction or ratio, commonly given in dB.

BANDWIDTH: In the case of pulsed radio frequency (rf) radiation, it is the range of frequencies present that combine to create a pulse. Also, it is the range of frequencies over which an amplifier or filter is effective.

BLOCH EQUATIONS: Phenomenological equations, proposed by the late Felix Bloch of Stanford University, that describe the motion of the macroscopic magnetization vector. The equations include the effects of external magnetic fields, both static and rf, and of longitudinal ($T1$) and transverse ($T2$) relaxation. They have been generalized by Torrey to include particle diffusion.

BOLTZMAN DISTRIBUTION: Energy distribution of a system of particles at thermal equilibrium. The relative number of particles N_1 and N_2 in two particular energy states with energies E_1 and E_2 is given by

$$\frac{N_1}{N_2} = \exp\left[-(E_1 - E_2)/kT\right]$$

where k is Boltzman's constant and T is the absolute temperature. In the case of a large ensemble of nuclear spins with moment μ in field B, the number of magnetic moments N_p (parallel) and N_a (antiparallel) alignment will be such that there will be a small majority of nuclear moments in the lower energy (parallel alignment) state.

CARR-PURCELL (CP) SEQUENCE: A sequence consisting of an initial 90 degree, followed by a series of equally spaced 180 degree, radio frequency (rf) pulses, often used to measure transverse relaxation (*T2*). This approach can minimize effects of molecular diffusion in a gradient, which often predominates in simpler spin-echo experiments.

CARR-PURCELL-MEIBOOM-GILL (CPMG) sequence: A modification of the Carr-Purcell rf pulse sequence, which uses a 90 degree phase shift between the initial 90 degree pulse and the subsequent series of 180 degree pulses. This reduces the cumulative effects of variations in the 180 degree pulses over the sample volume. (Alternatively, suppression of the effects of pulse error accumulation can be achieved by switching phases of the 180 degree pulses by 180 degrees.)

CHEMICAL SHIFT (σ): The difference in the Larmor frequency of a given nucleus when bound in different sites of a molecule, due to diamagnetic screening effects of the electron orbitals. Chemical shifts provide information about chemical structure and are usually expressed in parts per million (ppm) shift relative to some reference standard.

CHEMICAL-SHIFT IMAGING: A magnetic resonance imaging technique that provides mapping of the spatial distribution of a restricted range of chemical shifts corresponding to individual spectral lines or groups of lines.

CHEMICAL-SHIFT REFERENCE: A compound with which the chemical shifts of other compounds are compared. The reference standard can be used internally (i.e., dissolved in the sample) or can be external, either in a separate sample compartment or set by the software. Because of the need for possible corrections due to differential magnetic susceptibility between an external standard and the sample being measured, and which depend on the shape of the sample, the use of internal standards is generally preferred.

COHERENCE: A constant phase relationship between components of a rotating or oscillating system, or between the system and a reference signal.

COIL: Single or multiple loops of wire designed either to produce a magnetic field from a current flowing through the wire, or to detect a changing magnetic flux by the voltage it induces in the wire.

CONTINUOUS WAVE (Cw): A NMR spectroscopic technique that utilizes continuous rather than pulsed radio frequency irradiation, more common before the development of present-day Fourier technique.

CONTRAST: The relative difference of signal intensities in two adjacent regions of an image.

CONTRAST AGENT: A substance administered to a subject that selectively alters the image intensity of a particular anatomic or functional region. In MRI, this is usually accomplished by altering the relaxation times. *See also* Paramagnetic.

CONTRAST-TO-NOISE RATIO: The ratio of the absolute difference in intensities between two regions of an image to the level of random fluctuations in intensity due to noise.

CORRELATION FREQUENCY; CORRELATION TIME: The correlation frequency characterizes the high frequency limit of fluctuations in the local magnetic field experienced by a spin, often due to motion of that spin relative to others nearby. The correlation time is the reciprocal of the correlation frequency. Transverse and longitudinal relaxation times at a given field are functions of the correlation time and vary significantly with field whenever the Larmor frequency becomes comparable with the correlation frequency.

CPMG: Carr-Purcell-Meiboom-Gill sequence.

CROSSED COIL: Pair of rf coils arranged such that their magnetic fields are at right angles, to minimize their mutual magnetic interaction.

CRYOSTAT: Apparatus for maintaining a constant low temperature (often by means of liquid helium).

CT: X-ray computed tomography.

dB/dt: The rate of change of the magnetic flux density with time. Its magnitude is a potential concern for safety limits, since changing magnetic fields induce electrical voltages.

DECIBEL (dB): A measure of relative power. It is defined as $20 \log_{10}$ of the amplitude of the voltage in an electrical circuit relative to some standard, or $10 \log_{10}$ of the relative power.

DECOUPLING: Specific rf irradiation technique designed to remove multiple structure in a particular resonance due to spin-spin coupling with other nuclei. Also, a technique used to avoid interactions between coils, such as occur with separate rf transmitting and receiving coils.

DETECTOR: Portion of the rf receiver that demodulates an rf signal to recover the information contained in the frequency signal. Coherent detection involves a comparison with a reference oscillator.

DIAMAGNETIC: Property of a substance that tends to reduce the penetration of the substance by an external magnetic field. Diamagnetic effects are typically minute (ppm) unless the substance is superconducting, in which case the exclusion of field can be total.

DIFFUSION: The process by which molecules and other particles mix and migrate owing to thermal motion.

DIPOLE-DIPOLE INTERACTION: The interaction of two magnetic dipole moments due to the magnetic field that one generates at the location of the other. Fluctuation in this interaction due to random thermal motion is responsible for magnetic relaxation of both nuclear and atomic moments. In liquids and tissues, protons are generally relaxed by fluctuations in the dipole-dipole interaction with neighboring protons or paramagnetic ions.

DISPERSION: Variation of a quantity with energy in frequency. In NMR, variation of relaxation rates *R1* and *R2* with Larmor frequency (or magnetic field).

DRESS: Depth Resolved Surface Coil Spectroscopy. A method in which spectroscopic data are depth resolved by special applications of shaped rf pulses and gradients.

ECHO: *See* Spin echo.

ECHO PLANAR IMAGING: A technique of planar imaging in which a complete planar image is obtained from one selective excitation pulse. The FID is observed while periodically switching the *y*-magnetic field gradient in the presence of a static *x*-magnetic field gradient. The Fourier transform of the resulting spin-echo train can be used to produce an image of the excited plane.

ECHO TIME: See *TE*.

EDDY CURRENTS: Electrical currents induced in a conductor by a changing magnetic flux, produced either by motion of the conductor through a magnetic field or by a time dependence of the field. Eddy currents are a potential hazard to subjects in very high magnetic fields or rapidly varying gradients. They can also be a practical problem for superconducting magnets, or when induced in shim coils during gradient switching.

EXCITATION: Increasing the energy of a spin system above its Boltzman equilibrium value. If a net transverse magnetization is produced, an MR signal can be observed.

FARADAY SHIELD: Electrical conductor interposed between transmitter and/or receiver coil and patient to block out external electrical fields.

FAST FOURIER TRANSFORM (FFT): An efficient algorithm for calculating Fourier transforms of a given set of data.

FID: Free induction decay.

FIELD GRADIENT: In MRI, a spatial variation of the external magnetic field along a specific direction, e.g., a linear gradient has a constant variation with distance (*see* Gradient).

FIELD-FREQUENCY LOCK: A feedback control used to maintain resonance conditions in the presence of drift of the external field, usually done by monitoring the resonance frequency of a reference sample or line in a spectrum and adjusting the rf transmitter frequency accordingly.

FILLING FACTOR: A measure of the geometrical relationship of the rf coil and the object being studied. It affects the efficiency of irradiating the object and detecting MR signals, thereby affecting the signal-to-noise ratio and, ultimately, image quality.

FILTERING; FILTER: Filtering is a process that alters the relative frequency composition of a signal. A filter is a hardware or software implementation of filtering.

FILTERED BACK PROJECTION: An algorithm used in many technologies to reconstruct an image from a set of projection data (used in CT, MRI, PET, and SPECT).

FISP: Fast Imaging With Steady State Free Precession. Similar to FLASH, which uses small flip angles and gradient echoes, but in which the phase encoding is reversed after data collection. Image intensities are dependent on the ratio $T1/T2$.

FLASH: Fast Low Angle Shot. A fast scanning technique utilizing small flip angles and gradient echoes. Image intensities can be made to have $T1$ and $T2$ dependence.

FLIP ANGLE: The amount of rotation of the macroscopic magnetization vector produced by an rf pulse, measured with respect to the direction of the static magnetic field.

FLOW-RELATED ENHANCEMENT: The increase in image intensity that may be seen for flowing blood or other liquids using appropriate MR imaging techniques; due to the flux of equilibrium spins into the imaging region.

FOURIER-ACQUIRED STEADY-STATE (FAST): MR technique that utilizes variable tip angles in combination with short repetition times in order to allow decreased acquisition times with preserved image contrast.

FOURIER TRANSFORMATION: In MRI, a technique for resolving a complex waveform into the sum of its many frequency components. Fourier transformation of the FID signal gives the NMR spectrum of the sample. In the case of a single spin component resonant system, the spectrum full width at half height is inversely proportional to the time constant of the exponentially decaying FID signal, which by definition, is $1/T2$.

FREE INDUCTION DECAY (FID): The MR signal that follows a radio frequency (rf) pulse, usually 90 degrees. In practice, the initial part of the FID is not observable, owing to the electronics of the receiver (the receiver dead time) by the rf excitation.

FREQUENCY ENCODING: Encoding the distribution of sources of MR signals along a direction in space by generating the signal in the presence of a magnetic field gradient along that direction so that there is a corresponding gradient of resonance frequencies along that direction.

GAUSS (G): Unit of magnetic induction or flux, no longer standard. 1 tesla $= 10^4$ gauss. (Earth's magnetic field is 0.6 G.)

GIBBS PHENOMENON: A truncation artifact consisting of multiple bands of high and low-intensity bands that parallel zones of abrupt changes in signal intensity. *See also* Truncation artifact.

GOLAY COIL: Term for a particular kind of gradient coil commonly used to create magnetic field gradients perpendicular to the main magnetic field.

GRADIENT: The change in the value of a quantity with location in space; specifically, its first derivative. For example, a magnetic field that is not uniform, but is continuously changing in the *x* direction, has a magnetic field gradient in the *x* direction.

GRADIENT COILS: Current-carrying coils designed to produce a desired magnetic field gradient.

GRADIENT ECHO: A spin echo produced by reversing the direction of a magnetic field gradient or by applying balanced pulses of magnetic field gradient before and after a refocusing rf pulse so as to cancel out the position-dependent phase shifts that have accumulated because of the gradient.

GRASS: Gradient Recalled Acquisition in Steady State. A fast scan technique, similar to FLASH, that uses small flip angles and gradient echoes.

GYROMAGNETIC RATIO (γ): Ratio of the magnetic moment of a particle to its spin moment, usually expressed in dimensionless units. (*See* Angular momentum.)

HELMHOLTZ COIL: A pair of current-carrying coils, with well-defined geometries, designed to optimize the uniformity of the magnetic field near the center of Helmholtz pair. The distance between the two single wire loops is set equal to their radius.

HERTZ (Hz): The standard (SI) unit of frequency; the same as cycles per second.

HOMOGENEITY: Uniformity in space. In MR, the homogeneity of the magnetic field is an important criterion of the quality of the magnet.

HYBRID TECHNIQUE: MR fast scanning technique in which the phase-encoding gradient oscillates, allowing multiple views to be obtained with a single repetition, thereby smoothing motion-induced noise while retaining a relatively high signal-to-noise ratio.

INVERSION: A nonequilibrium state in which the macroscopic magnetization vector is oriented opposite to its equilibrium direction; produced either by adiabatic fast passage or by a 180 degree rf pulse. The rate of recovery of the magnetization to its equilibrium value is governed by the longitudinal relaxation time (*T1*).

INVERSION-RECOVERY PULSE SEQUENCE (IR): A pulse sequence that inverts the nuclear magnetization at a time of the order of *T1*; applied before the regular imaging pulse-gradient sequences. The subsequent partial relaxation of the magnetizations being imaged can be used to produce an image that is strongly weighted by *T1*.

INVERSION SPIN-ECHO PULSE SEQUENCE (ISE): A form of inversion recovery in which an initial 180 degree (inverting) pulse is followed in time *T1s* by a 90 degree measuring pulse. A subsequent 180 degree refocusing pulse creates a spin echo for read-out. The sequence can provide images with either *T2* weighting or almost pure *T1* weighting.

INVERSION TIME (*T1S*): In inversion recovery, the time between the middle of the 180 degree inverting rf pulse and the middle of the subsequent 90 degree measuring pulse; the latter is used to detect the amount of residual longitudinal relaxation.

ISOTOPE: Any of one or more species of atoms (elements) with the same atomic number but different atomic mass. Isotopes have different physical properties but nearly identical chemical properties.

LARMOR EQUATION: Relation between the Larmor precession frequency, the gyromagnetic ratio, and the magnetic field H_0.

$$\omega = H \text{ (radians/second)}$$

or

$$f_0 = \gamma H_0 / 2\pi \text{ (Hertz)}$$

where ω_0 or f_0 is the frequency, γ is the gyromagnetic ratio, and H_0 is the magnetic field strength. *See also* Angular momentum.

LARMOR FREQUENCY: The frequency of precession given by the Larmor equation. *See also* Angular momentum.

LATTICE: The thermal environment with which nuclei exchange magnetic energy.

LINE SCANNING: Class of MR imaging methods in which spin density distribution is determined along one line in space at a time. The line is scanned sequentially through a sample to obtain the total image.

LONGITUDINAL MAGNETIZATION (Mz): Component of the macroscopic magnetization vector along the static magnetic field. Following excitation by an rf pulse, Mz will return to its thermal equilibrium value Mo with a characteristic time constant $T1$, the longitudinal relaxation time. In solids, this time is often called the spin-lattice relaxation time.

LONGITUDINAL RELAXATION: Return of nonequilibrium longitudinal magnetization to its equilibrium value. Longitudinal relaxation involves exchange of energy between the magnetized nuclear spin system and the lattice.

LONGITUDINAL RELAXATION TIME $T1$ (SPIN-LATTICE RELAXATION TIME): *See* Longitudinal magnetization.

MACROSCOPIC MAGNETIZATION VECTOR M: The net magnetic moment per unit volume of a sample, the vector sum of all the nuclear magnetic moments.

MAGNETIC DIPOLAR MOMENT: The equivalent of a small bar magnet or current loop, characterized by the geometry of the magnetic field it produces.

MAGNETIC FIELD STRENGTH (H): Magnetic field is a vector quantity that produces torques on magnetic moments. It also induces the macroscopic magnetization M. Its SI unit is amperes/meter; an older unit is Oersted.

MAGNETIC INDUCTION OR FLUX DENSITY (B): A vector quantity related to H that exerts forces on wires carrying current. Often not distinguishable from H, the fundamental difference becomes important in strongly magnetized materials. There are no sources of B other than H. The SI unit is tesla.

MAGNETIC MOMENT, NUCLEAR: The magnetic moment associated a given nucleus. Nuclei with zero spin have zero magnetic moment, but not conversely. The relationship between nuclear spin and magnetic moments is complex.

MAGNETIC MOMENT, PARAMAGNETIC: The magnetic moment associated with a given electronic distribution of an ion or atom; also called "electronic moment." Electron spin resonance (ESR), also electron paramagnetic resonance (EPR), is the analog for the electronic moment of NMR for nuclear moments.

MAGNETIC RESONANCE (MR): The resonant absorption of electromagnetic energy by an ensemble of atomic nuclei or electrons situated in a magnetic field. The frequency of the magnetic resonance coincides with the frequency of the Larmor precession of the magnetic moments in the magnetic field.

MAGNETIC RESONANCE IMAGING (MRI): The use of magnetic resonance phenomena to create images of objects. Currently, this primarily involves imaging the distribution of water and aliphatic protons in the body. The signal intensity of a pixel, and the contrast between pixels, depends on the spin density [$N(H)$] and the relaxation times $T1$ and $T2$, their relative importance depending on the pulse sequence used. The relaxation times, and therefore the appearance of the image, can be altered by paramagnetic contrast-enhancing agents.

MAGNETIC SHIELDING: A method of restricting the range of the strong magnetic field that surrounds a magnet. This is most commonly done with the use of material with high permeability.

MAGNETIC SUSCEPTIBILITY χ: Measure of the extent to which a substance becomes magnetized in the presence of H. The magnetization is given by $M = 4\pi\chi H$. For diamagnetic materials, $\chi \leq 1$; for paramagnetic materials, $\chi \geq 1$.

MAST: Motion artifact suppression technique. A software technique to correct for motion occuring during data collection.

MAXWELL COIL: A particular type of gradient coil commonly used to create magnetic field gradients along the direction of the main magnetic field.

MEIBOOM-GILL SEQUENCE: A modification of the Carr-Purcell sequence intended to minimize effects resulting from inaccuracies in the 180 degree pulse lengths. (*See* CPMG.)

MULTIECHO IMAGING (ME): Spin-echo imaging using spin echoes acquired in series. A separate image is produced from each echo of the series.

MULTIPLE LINE-SCAN IMAGING (MLSI): Variation of sequential line-scan imaging techniques that can be used if selective excitation methods that do not affect adjacent lines are employed. Adjacent lines are imaged while waiting for relaxation of the first line toward equilibrium. This process can result in decreased image-acquisition time.

MULTIPLE SENSITIVE POINT: Sequential line-imaging technique utilizing two orthogonal oscillating magnetic field gradients, a steady-state free precession pulse sequence, and signal averaging to restrict the NMR spectrometer sensitivity to a desired line in the body.

MULTIPLE-SLICE IMAGING: Adjacent slices are imaged while waiting for relaxation of the first slice toward equilibrium, resulting in a decreased image-acquisition time for the set of slices.

NMR SIGNAL: Electromagnetic signal in the radio frequency range produced by Larmor precession of the transverse magnetization of the sample. Rotation of the transverse magnetization induces a signal voltage in a coil, which is amplified and demodulated by the receiver.

NOISE: That component of the reconstructed image due to random and unpredictable processes.

NUCLEAR MAGNETIC RELAXATION DISPERSION (NMRD): The magnetic field dependence (dispersion) of nuclear relaxation rates, also referred to as NMRD profiles.

NUCLEAR MAGNETIC RESONANCE (NMR): *See* MR.

NUCLEAR OVERHAUSER EFFECT (NOE): A change in the steady-state magnetization of a particular nucleus due to irradiation of a neighboring nucleus of a different isotope or element with which it is magnetically coupled. Such an effect can occur during decoupling and must be taken into account for accurate intensity determinations during such procedures.

NUCLEAR SPIN QUANTUM NUMBER (I): The angular momentum of a nucleus in units of $h/2\pi$. The number of possible quantitized orientations, and thus energy levels, for a given nucleus in a fixed magnetic field is equal to $2I + 1$.

NUCLEON: A proton or a neutron.

NUCLEUS: The positively charged central core of an atom composing nearly all its mass and consisting of protons and neutrons.

NUTATION: A slow, periodic variation of the angle of Larmor precession, generally produced by a resonant rf field.

NYQUIST LIMIT: Frequency of a signal beyond which aliasing will occur in the sampling process. This frequency is equal to one half of the sampling rate.

OERSTED: An old unit for H. It has the convenience that B in gauss, and H in Oersteds, have essentially the same numerical value in air.

PARAMAGNETIC: A substance with the property of becoming magnetized in the direction of an applied field, but not retaining this directional magnetization when the field is removed. The addition of a small amount of paramagnetic substance may greatly reduce the relaxation time of water. Most common paramagnetic substances contain transition metal ions or lanthanides: Gd^{+3}, Dy^{+3}, Ho^{+3}, Fe^{+3}, Fe^{+2}, Ni^{+2},

Cr^{+3}, and Mn^{+2}. O_2 is an exception. Substances with complexes of these ions with paramagnetic properties are being investigated for use as MRI contrast agents. *See* Magnetic susceptibility.

PARTIAL SATURATION (PS): Pulse sequence technique of applying repeated rf pulses in times on the order of or shorter than *T1*. Although this pulse sequence technique results in decreased signal amplitude, there is a possibility of generating images of increased contrast between regions with different relaxation times.

PARTIAL SATURATION SPIN ECHO (PSSE): Pulse sequence technique that utilizes partial saturation, but for which the signal is detected as a spin echo. Even though a spin echo is used, there will not necessarily be significant *T2* weighting unless the echo time (*TE*) is on the order of or longer than *T2*.

PASSIVE SHIMMING: Shimming by adjusting the position of suitable pieces of ferromagnetic metal within or around the main magnet of an MR system. This is in contrast to active shimming, which is achieved by adding extra gradient coils.

PERMANENT MAGNET: A magnet whose magnetic field originates from permanently magnetized material.

PERMEABILITY: Permeability equals $1 + 4\pi\chi$ for diamagnetic and paramagnetic substances, and more generally is given by the ratio B/H, an expression that holds for ferromagnetic substances.

PET: Positron emission tomography.

PHASE CYCLING: Techniques of excitation in which the phases of the exciting or refocusing rf pulses are systematically varied, and the resulting signals are then suitably combined in order to reduce or eliminate certain artifacts.

PHASE ENCODING: Process of encoding the distribution of sources of MR signals along a direction in space with different phases by applying a pulsed magnetic field gradient along that direction prior to detection of the signal.

PLANAR IMAGING: A type of MR imaging in which the information is gathered from an entire plane simultaneously.

POINT SCANNING: A type of MR imaging in which information is integrated one point at a time. A complete image is obtained by sequentially scanning throughout the sample. (Also called "sensitive point" imaging.)

PRECESSION: Rotation of the spin axis produced by a torque applied about an axis mutually perpendicular to the spin and the axis of the resulting rotation.

PROBE: The part of an NMR spectrometer that contains the sample and radio frequency (rf) coils.

PROJECTION PROFILE: A one-dimensional projection of nuclear spin density on the frequency axis.

PROJECTION-RECONSTRUCTION IMAGING: MR imaging technique in which a set of projection profiles of the body is obtained by observing MR signals in the presence of a suitable corresponding set of magnetic field gradients.

PULSE–90 DEGREES: RF pulse that rotates (nutates) the macroscopic magnetization vector 90 degrees in space about an axis at right angles to the main magnetic field and the applied rf field. This pulse will produce transverse magnetization from an initial longitudinal component, and conversely.

PULSE–180 DEGREES: RF pulse designed to rotate the macroscopic magnetization vector 180 degrees in space about an axis at right angles to the main magnetic field and RF field. Inversion of longitudinal magnetization is produced by these pulses.

PULSE LENGTH (WIDTH): Time duration of an rf pulse.

Q FACTOR: Most often, the coil quality factor. A measure of energy loss described as a ratio of energy in the system to energy that is lost in one oscillating radian. The Q factor affects the signal-to-noise ratio, since the detected signal increases proportionally to Q while the noise is proportional to the square root of Q.

QUENCHING: The sudden loss of superconductivity of a current-carrying coil.

RADIO FREQUENCY (**rf**): The part of the electromagnetic energy spectrum associated with radio waves. The approximate wavelengths involved range from 10^1 to 10^3 meters, with corresponding frequencies being 10^5 to 10^9 Hz.

RADIO FREQUENCY (**rf**) PULSE: A shaped burst of radio frequency radiation.

RARE: Rapid Acquisition with Relaxation Enhancement. A rapid scan technique that uses multiple spin echoes to produce separate phase-encoding projections.

RECEIVER COIL: Portion of the MR apparatus that picks up the NMR signal, for subsequent amplification and detection.

RELAXATION RATES: Inverse of the relaxation times. Longitudinal relaxation rate $R_1 = 1/T1$. Transverse relaxation rate $R_2 = 1/T2$.

RELAXATION TIMES: Characteristic NMR parameters of magnetized materials, particularly *T1* and *T2*. *T1* (longitudinal) is a measure of the time required for the longitudinal magnetization to return to thermal equilibrium with its surroundings. *T2* (transverse) is a measure of the decay time of the transverse (x,y) component of magnetization, when it is not due to loss of phase due to gradients of the magnetic field. In liquids and in tissue, both R_1 and R_2 of water protons and aliphatic protons arise from spin-spin interactions of a given proton with either its neighboring protons or a nearby paramagnetic ion.

RELAXOMETER, RELAXOMETRY: The measurement of relaxation rates, with length precision, over a range of magnetic field values and temperature requires a specialized instrument called a relaxometer. Relaxometry is the name for the discipline that involves all aspects of relaxation rate measurements and their interpretation. Relaxometry and relaxometer are analogs to, but quite distinct from, spectroscopy and spectrometer.

RESOLUTION: The limit set by noise, hardware, or software to the ability to perceive differences in neighboring parts of a spectrum in spectroscopy or regions of an image in MRI.

RESONANCE: A specific and large response of a physical system to excitation at a specific frequency near an absorption peak. In NMR experiments and MR imaging, the excitation is generated by rf energy.

ROPE: Respiratory Ordered Phase Encoding. A motion suppression technique that reorders the phase-encoding steps of the acquired image data according to the respiratory cycle.

ROTATING FRAME OF REFERENCE: A frame of reference that rotates at the Larmor frequency with respect to the laboratory frame. In this reference frame, the motion of the net magnetization describes a much simpler path than in the laboratory frame.

SADDLE COIL: Coil design that is commonly used when the static magnetic field is coaxial with the axis of the coil along the long axis of the body.

SAMPLING: The process of converting an analog signal into a series of digital values by measurement at a set of particular times. Aliasing will occur if the rate of sampling is less than twice the highest frequency.

SATURATION; PARTIAL SATURATION: After exposure to a single 90 degree rf pulse, if *T2* is much shorter than *T1*, the net transverse magnetization will disappear before significant repolarization of the spin occurs. The sample is said to be saturated during this time. If the pulse is less than 90 degrees, so that only a part of the signal disappears, the sample is said to be partially saturated.

SATURATION RECOVERY: A type of partial saturation in which the preceding pulses leave the spins in a state of saturation. In this condition, recovery at the time of the next pulse will have taken place from the initial condition of no magnetization.

SELECTIVE EXCITATION: Modulated rf exciting radiation designed to excite only a limited spatial region of the sample, defined by the field gradient.

SHIFT REAGENTS: Paramagnetic compounds designed to induce a shift in the resonance Larmor frequency of nuclei with which they interact.

SHIM COILS: Shaped coils used to produce small field gradients of an NMR magnet to reduce field inhomogeneities needed for NMR spectroscopic analysis.

SHIMMING: Correction of magnetic field inhomogeneity either by changing the configuration of coils or adding shim coils (active shimming) or by adding small pieces of metal (passive shimming).

SIGNAL AVERAGING: A process of averaging repeated signals acquired under similar conditions in a manner that suppresses the effects of noise.

SIGNAL-TO-NOISE RATIO: Term used to describe the relative contributions to a signal of the true signal and random superimposed noise signals.

SPECT: Single photon emission computer tomography.

SPECTRUM: The display of absorption peaks in the frequency domain of the MR signal.

SPIN: The intrinsic angular momentum of an electron or nucleus, usually given in units of $h/2\pi$, and called I. For electrons and protons, $I = 1/2$.

SPIN DENSITY (N): The number of resonating nuclei per unit volume of sample. The true spin density is generally not imaged directly, but can be calculated from signals derived using different interpulse times.

SPIN ECHO (SE): A phenomenon discovered by Erwin Hahn. The reappearance of an NMR signal arising from refocusing or rephasing of the various components of magnetization in the x,y plane. This usually results from the application of a 180 degree pulse (90 degree in the first experiments) after an initial 90 degree pulse and the decay of the initial FID. Measurement of $T2$ values by the Hahn method is complicated by effects of the magnetic field inhomogeneities. The Carr-Purcell and CPMG sequences, which apply a series of 180 degree pulses, can be used for more accurate measurements of $T2$.

SPIN-ECHO PULSE SEQUENCE: In MRI, a pulse sequence utilizing a 90 degree rf pulse followed in time ($TE/2$) by a 180 degree rf pulse that produces a spin echo at time TE. This can be used to produce images with strong $T2$ weighting if TE is approximately equal to the $T2$ of the tissues of interest. Some $T1$ weighting can be gained if the repetition time (TR) is approximately equal to the $T1$ value of the tissues of interest and if TE is much less than the $T2$ value of the tissues of interest.

SPIN TAGGING: Since nuclear magnetization retains its orientation for a time approximately equal to $T1$, this property can be used to trace spatial motion, such as flow, in a region for a time of the order of $T1$, by ''tagging'' the spins at the start and following the magnetization in space by imaging.

SPIN-WARP IMAGING: Fourier transform imaging in which the phase-encoding gradient pulses are applied for a constant duration but with varying amplitude. This method, as with other Fourier imaging techniques, is relatively tolerant of inhomogeneities in the magnetic field. Also called two-dimensional Fourier transformation (2-DFT) imaging.

STEADY-STATE FREE PRECESSION (SSFP): An MR pulse sequence technique in which a series of rf pulses are used with interpulse spacings that are short compared with $T1$ and $T2$.

STIR (SHORT $T1$ INVERSION RECOVERY): Variation of the inversion spin-echo (ISE) pulse sequence using short inversion times (TI). This pulse sequence allows increased image contrast, owing to synergism of $T1$ and $T2$ effects.

STEAM: Stimulated Echo Acquisition Mode. A fast scan technique that produces multiple $T1$ weighted images in the same scan.

SUPERCONDUCTING MAGNET: A magnet whose magnetic field originates from current flowing through a superconductor. Such a magnet must be enclosed in a cryostat.

SUPERCONDUCTOR: A substance whose electrical resistance disappears at temperatures near absolute zero, and below some critical maximum magnetic field. A commonly used superconductor is a niobium-titanium alloy embedded in a copper matrix.

SURFACE COIL: An rf sample coil that does not surround the body, but is placed close to the body surface to limit the region of the body contributing to the detected signal.

T1: See Longitudinal relaxation time.

T2: See Transverse relaxation time.

TE (ECHO TIME): Time between the center of an initial 90 degree pulse and the center of a subsequent spin echo.

TESLA (T): A unit of magnetic induction: 1 tesla $= 10^4$ gauss.

THERMAL EQUILIBRIUM: A state in which all parts of a system are at the same time-independent state, characterized by a temperature.

TI (INVERSION TIME): The time between the middle of the inverting (180 degree) rf pulse and the middle of the subsequent exciting (90 degree) pulse, used to measure the longitudinal magnetization in inversion recovery or inversion spin-echo pulse sequences.

TORQUE: A twisting moment, which produces or tends to produce rotation.

TR (REPETITION TIME): The time between the beginning of a pulse sequence and the beginning of the succeeding (essentially identical) pulse sequence.

TRANSVERSE MAGNETIZATION (M_{XY}): Component of the macroscopic magnetization at right angles to the static magnetic field. Precession of the transverse magnetization at the Larmor frequency gives rise to the detectable NMR signal. In liquids, the transverse magnetization will relax toward zero, its equilibrium value, with the characteristic time constant *T2*.

TRANSVERSE RELAXATION TIME ($T2$; SPIN-SPIN RELAXATION TIME): A measure of the decay time to lose transverse magnetization. *See* Relaxation times.

ZEUGMATOGRAPHY: The name given by Lauterbur to what has now become MRI. Taken from the Greek *zeugma* (to join together); referring to the combining of the static *B* field and its gradient with the NMR signal from tissue nuclei to produce a graphic image.

Appendix Tables

PROPERTIES OF BIOLOGICALLY SIGNIFICANT MAGNETIC NUCLEI

Isotope	Atomic Number	Atomic Weight	NMR Frequency MHz (at 1 tesla)	Spin	Natural Abundance (%)	Relative Sensitivity (Constant field)
H	1	1	42.5759	$\frac{1}{2}$	99.985	1.00
C	6	13	10.7054	$\frac{1}{2}$	1.108	1.59×10^{-2}
N	7	14	3.0756	1	99.63	1.01×10^{-3}
N	7	15	4.3142	$\frac{1}{2}$	0.37	1.04×10^{-3}
O	8	17	5.772	$\frac{5}{2}$	3.7×10^{-2}	2.91×10^{-2}
F	9	19	40.0541	$\frac{1}{2}$	100.0	0.833
Na	11	23	11.262	$\frac{3}{2}$	100.0	9.25×10^{-2}
P	15	31	17.235	$\frac{1}{2}$	100.0	6.63×10^{-2}
K	19	39	1.9868	$\frac{3}{2}$	93.1	5.08×10^{-4}
Ca	20	43	2.8646	$\frac{7}{2}$	0.145	6.40×10^{-3}
Fe	26	57	1.3758	$\frac{1}{2}$	2.19	3.37×10^{-5}

From CRC Handbook of Chemistry and Physics, 49th ed., Cleveland, The Chemical Rubber Co., 1968–69. Used by permission.

PHYSICAL CONSTANTS

Physical Quantity	Symbol	Value
Avogadro constant	N_A	6.0225×10^{26}/kmol
Boltzmann constant	k	1.38042×10^{-16}erg/degree
Bohr magneton	M_B	9.2732×10^{-21}erg/gauss
Electron rest mass	m_e	9.1085×10^{-28}gm
Electronic charge	e	1.602×10^{-19}coulomb
Permeability of free space	μ_0	$4\pi \times 10^{-7}$henry/meter
Planck's constant	h	6.625×10^{-27}erg sec
Speed of light	c	2.998×10^{10}cm/sec

SELECTED ELECTRICAL AND MAGNETIC QUANTITIES

Physical Quantity	Defined Units	Fundamental Units
Force	newton (N)	kg m/s^2
Energy	joule (J)	N m = kg m^2/s^2
Power	watt (W)	J/S = kg m^2/s^3
Electric charge	coulomb (C)	C
Electric current	ampere (A)	C/s
Magnetic inductance (L)	henry (H)	J/A^2 = kg m^2/s^2 A^2
Magnetic flux (ϕ)	weber (W)	J/A = kg m^2/s^2 A
Magnetic intensity (B)	tesla (T)	Wb/m^2 – kg/s^2 A
Magnetizing force (H)	oersted (O)	A/m
	(B = μH where μ is permeability)	
Magnetization (M)	oersted (O)	A/m
	(M = χH where χ is susceptibility)	

Permeability: (μ) of a material is the ratio of the magnetic intensities from a current-carrying coil of wire with and without the material present.
Susceptibility: (χ) of a material is related to the ability of a material to become magnetized when subjected to a magnetizing force, H.

APPROXIMATE RELAXATION TIMES OF SELECTED TISSUES

	T2* msec	T1 (0.5 T) msec	T1 (1.5 T) msec
Adipose	80	210	260
Liver	42	350	500
Muscle	45	550	870
White matter	90	500	780
Gray matter	100	650	920
CSF	160	1800	2400

* *T2* values are approximately field-strength independent.
From Sprawls P Jr: Physical Principles of Medical Imaging. Rockville, MD, Aspen Publishers, 1987. Used by permission.

Numbers in *italics* refer to illustrations; numbers followed by t refer to tables.